Supplements and New Media

for INSTRUCTORS

Instructor's Resource Manual
ISBN: 0-13-094150-6

This manual contains a wealth of material to help faculty plan and manage the fundamental nursing course. It includes detailed lecture outlines, learning outcomes, teaching suggestions, and more for each chapter. The IRM also guides faculty how to assign and use the text-specific Companion Website, www.prenhall.com/ramont and the CD-ROM that accompany the textbook. This supplement is available to faculty **free** upon adoption of the textbook.

Instructor's Resource CD-ROM
ISBN: 0-13-112452-8

This cross-platform CD-ROM provides Lecture Note PowerPoints, Animations, and illustrations in PowerPoint for use in classroom lectures. It also contains an electronic test bank. This supplement is available to faculty **free** upon adoption of the textbook.

Companion Website Syllabus Manager
www.prenhall.com/ramont

Faculty adopting this textbook have **free** access to the online Syllabus Manager feature of the Companion Website, www.prenhall.com/ramont. Syllabus Manager offers a whole host of features that facilitate the students' use of the Companion Website, and allows faculty to post syllabi and course information online for their students. For more information or a demonstration of Syllabus Manager, please contact a Prentice Hall Sales Representative.

also AVAILABLE

Wilson, Prentice Hall Nurse's Drug Guide
ISBN: 0-13-112968-6
This annual reference is the most complete source for drug administration information and the only source to identify prototype drugs.

Burke/LeMone/Mohn-Brown, Medical Surgical Nursing Care
ISBN: 0-13-028162-X
A care-oriented book, concretely focused on what LPNs and LVNs need to know and do in the medical-surgical setting.

Smith, Sandra Smith's Review for the NCLEX-PN 7E
ISBN: 0-13-028673-7
Nursing content review including thousands of questions to help students prepare for the NCLEX-PN.

Brown/Boyd/Twiname, LPN/LVN Student Nurse Handbook
ISBN: 0-13-094182-4
Free CD-ROM featuring an audio glossary of 800 terms and a flash-card maker accompany this "must-have" resource for practical/vocational nursing students.

Brief Table of Contents

UNIT I	The Nature of Nursing *1*
Chapter 1	Understanding Nursing 2
Chapter 2	Legal and Ethical Issues of Nursing 19
Chapter 3	Critical Thinking and Nursing Theory/Models 37
Chapter 4	The LVN/LPN and the Nursing Process 50

UNIT II	Introduction to Clinical Practice *71*
Chapter 5	Health Care Delivery Systems 72
Chapter 6	Safety 86
Chapter 7	Infection Control and Asepsis 111
Chapter 8	Admission, Transfer, and Discharge 137
Chapter 9	Documenting and Reporting 154

UNIT III	Promoting Physiological Health *179*
Chapter 10	Introduction to the Body 180
Chapter 11	Health Assessment 197
Chapter 12	Skin Integrity and Wound Care 222
Chapter 13	Hygiene 252
Chapter 14	Vital Signs 291
Chapter 15	Pain, The Fifth Vital Sign 324
Chapter 16	Oxygenation 344
Chapter 17	Nutrition, Fluids and Electrolytes, and Acid–Base Balance 375
Chapter 18	Urinary Elimination 404
Chapter 19	Gastrointestinal Elimination 436
Chapter 20	Activity, Rest, and Sleep 459

Chapter 21	Medications 499
Chapter 22	Perioperative Nursing 542
Chapter 23	Client Teaching 566

UNIT IV	Promoting Psychosocial Health *585*
Chapter 24	Life Span Development 586
Chapter 25	Client Communication 613
Chapter 26	Delivering Culturally Competent Care 629
Chapter 27	Sensory Perception 642
Chapter 28	Self-Concept 656
Chapter 29	Sexuality 667
Chapter 30	Stress and Coping 685
Chapter 31	Loss, Grieving, and Death 700

UNIT V	Becoming a Licensed Nurse *717*
Chapter 32	Introduction to Leadership 718
Chapter 33	Preparing to Take the Licensure Exam 731
Chapter 34	Finding That First Job 741

Appendices

I. 2003–2004 NANDA-Approved Nursing Diagnoses 757

II. Sample Critical Pathway for Client Following Total Mastectomy 759

III. Glossary 763

IV. NCLEX-PN Answers; Hints for Critical Thinking 779

Bibliography *807*

Index *817*

Fundamental
NURSING CARE

Fundamental
NURSING CARE

Roberta Pavy Ramont, RN, MS, Ed.Dc
Faculty
North Orange County Regional Occupational Program
Anaheim, California

Dolores Maldonado Niedringhaus, RN, BSN
Instructional Administrator of Medical Programs
North Orange County Regional Occupational Program
Anaheim, California

PEARSON
Prentice
Hall

Upper Saddle River, New Jersey 07458

Library of Congress Cataloging-in-Publication Data
Fundamental nursing care / [edited by] Roberta Pavy Ramont, Dolores Maldonado
  Niedringhaus.—1st ed.
    p. ; cm.
  Includes bibliographical references and index.
  ISBN 0-13-094156-5
  1. Nursing. I. Ramont, Roberta Pavy. II. Niedringhaus, Dolores Maldonado.
  [DNLM: 1. Nursing Care. 2. Nursing Process. 3 Nursing, Practical. WY 100 F9779 2004]
RT41.F873 2004
610.73—dc21   2003054865

Publisher: Julie Levin Alexander
Executive Assistant & Supervisor: Regina Bruno
Editor-in-Chief: Maura Connor
Executive Editor: Barbara Krawiec
Managing Development Editor: Marilyn Meserve
Development Editor: Rachel Bedard
Assistant Editor: Yesenia Kopperman
Editorial Assistants: Jennifer Dwyer & Sheba Jalaluddin
Director of Manufacturing and Production: Bruce Johnson
Managing Production Editor: Patrick Walsh
Production Liason: Mary C. Treacy
Production Editor: Linda Begley, Rainbow Graphics
Manufacturing Manager: Ilene Sanford
Manufacturing Buyer: Pat Brown
Design Director: Cheryl Asherman
Senior Design Coordinator: Maria Guglielmo Walsh
Cover Designer: Mary Siener
Manager of Media Production: Amy Peltier
Media Development Editor: John J. Jordan
New Media Project Manager: Lisa Rinaldi
New Media Production: Eclectic Multimedia
Senior Marketing Manager: Nicole Benson
Marketing Assistant: Janet Ryerson
Channel Marketing Manager: Rachele Triano
Composition: Rainbow Graphics
Cover Printer: LeHigh Press
Printer/binder: RR Donnelley/Ohio

Pearson Education LTD.
Pearson Education Australia PTY, Limited
Pearson Education Singapore, Pte. Ltd
Pearson Education North Asia Ltd
Pearson Education, Canada, Ltd
Pearson Educación de Mexico, S.A. de C.V.
Pearson Education—Japan
Pearson Education Malaysia, Pte. Ltd
Pearson Education, Upper Saddle River, New Jersey

Notice: Care has been taken to confirm the accuracy of the
information presented in this book. The authors, editors, and
the publisher, however, cannot accept any responsibility for
errors or omissions or for consequences from application of
the information in this book and make no warranty, express or
implied, with respect to its contents.

The authors and the publisher have exerted every effort to
ensure that drug selections and dosages set forth in this text
are in accord with current recommendations and practice at
time of publication. However, in view of ongoing research,
changes in government regulations, and the constant flow of
information relating to drug therapy and drug reactions, the
reader is urged to check the package inserts of all drugs for
any change in indications of dosage and for added warnings
and precautions. This is particularly important when the recommended agent is a new and/or infrequently employed drug.

The authors and publisher disclaim all responsibility for
any liability, loss, injury, or damage incurred as a consequence, directly or indirectly, of the use and application of
any of the contents of this volume.

All photographs/illustrations not credited on page, under
or adjacent to the piece, were photographed/rendered on
assignment and are the property of Pearson
Education/Prentice Hall Health.

10 9 8 7 6 5 4 3 2 1
ISBN 0-13-094156-5

Guide to Key Features

The end is just the beginning...

Student practical and vocational nurses from around the country told us that they start their chapter reading from the end of the chapter. So, to ensure students' success in the classroom, on the NCLEX-PN exam and in the workplace, we put dynamite preview/review materials in a three-page Chapter Review at the end of each chapter, right where students will benefit the most from them!

Key Terms by Topics provides an overview for organizing study

Key Points provide a quick highlight of lifelong need-to-know items

EXPLORE MediaLink provides multi-modal reinforcement for all learners

For Further Study provides references to related chapters to connect related content

Critical Thinking Care Map prepares students step-by-step for much needed on-the-job critical thinking leading to clinical success, including:
- ◆ NCLEX-PN Focus Area
- ◆ Case Study
- ◆ Nursing Diagnosis
- ◆ Data Collection
- ◆ Reporting
- ◆ Nursing Care
- ◆ Documentation

NCLEX-PN Preparation includes:
- ◆ Test-Taking Tip that provides a focused study hint to help promote NCLEX-PN success
- ◆ NCLEX-PN style questions that provide content preview/review, as well as invaluable practice for taking the test

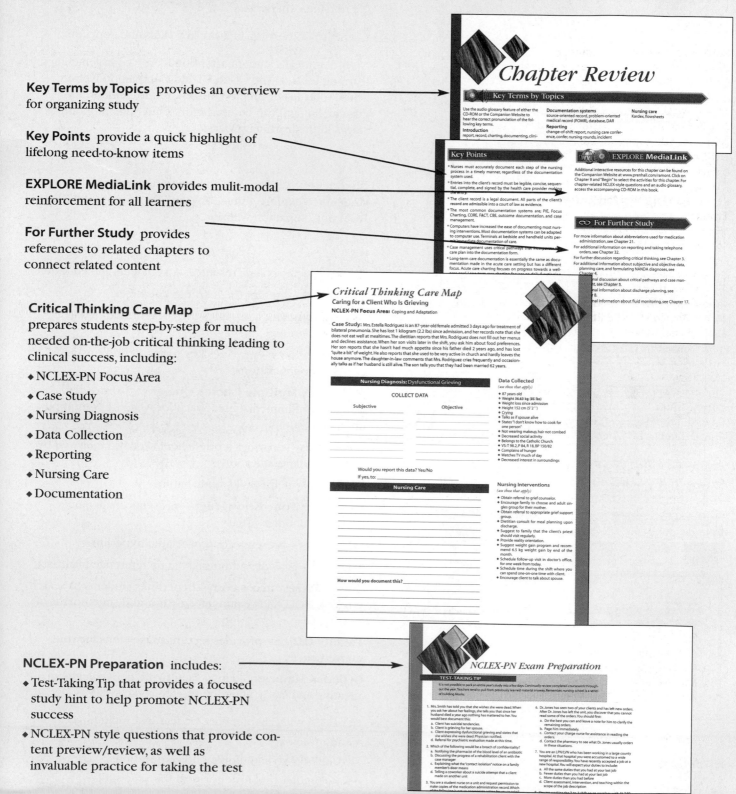

Student success is built-in from the start...

Sharing Experiences from student and practicing LPNs and LVNs throughout the country give insights about real-life nursing experiences

Learning Outcomes identify key skills and concepts

MediaLink calls student attention to key complementary learning tools on the CD-ROM and Companion Website. These tools foster preview, review, reinforcement, and enrichment and can be used more than once, at multiple stages in the learning process

MediaLink Tab icons located along page margins prompt students to explore animations and activities on the CD-ROM or Companion Website

www.prenhall.com/ramont, a free website provides chapter-specific on-line resources for students and educators!

Objectives—present the learning outcomes

Chapter Outline—provides the content outline for student reference

Audio Glossary—provides key terms, definitions, and correct pronunciations

NCLEX-PN Multiple Choice Questions—provides practice and immediate feedback for NCLEX-PN multiple choice questions

Case Study—provides a brief client scenario followed by critical thinking questions

Study Tip—helps build study habits

Challenge Your Knowledge—presents challenging questions about a visual

Web Links—presents content-related hyperlinks

Toolbox—provides additional handy reference materials

www.LPNresources.com—hyperlinks students to search engines, NCLEX-PN exam information, and state boards of nursing

Faculty Office—provides lecture suggestions for your convenience

Syllabus Manager—allows faculty the convenience of creating and easily updating an electronic syllabus

CD-ROM with chapter-specific features, including:

- Audio Glossary
- NCLEX-PN style multiple choice questions
- Case Studies that foster critical thinking skills
- Animations

Need-to-know concepts and skills are readily accessible and easily memorable...

Client Teaching, Population Focus, and Nutrition boxes (identifiable in green) provide information on age-specific and other special needs of groups of clients, and help students prepare for client instruction

---

BOX 6-9

CLIENT TEACHING

HOW TO PREVENT BACK INJURIES

* Become consciously aware of your posture and body mechanics.
* When standing for a period of time, periodically flex one hip and knee and rest your foot on an object if possible.
* When sitting, keep your knees slightly higher than your hips.
* Use a firm mattress that provides good body support at natural body curvatures.
* Exercise regularly to maintain overall physical condition; include exercises that strengthen the pelvic, abdominal, and lumbar muscles.
* Avoid exercises that cause pain or require spinal flexion with straight legs (e.g., toe-touching and sit-ups) or spinal rotation (twisting).
* When moving an object, spread your feet apart to provide a wide base of support.
* When lifting an object, distribute the weight between large muscles of the legs and arms.
* Wear clothing that allows you to use good body mechanics and comfortable low-heeled shoes that provide good foot support and will not cause you to slip, stumble, or turn your ankle.

Nursing Care Checklist boxes (identifiable in blue) provide students with a ready-reference summary of important nursing interventions

---

BOX 6-2

NURSING CARE CHECKLIST

PREVENTING FALLS IN HEALTH CARE AGENCIES

☑ Orient clients on admission to their surroundings, and explain the call system.
☑ Carefully assess the client's risk for falling.
☑ Alert all personnel to the client's risk for falling.
☑ Assign clients at risk for falls to rooms near the nursing station where they can be more closely supervised.
☑ Encourage the client and family to use the call bell to request assistance; ensure that the bell is within easy reach.
☑ Answer call bells promptly.
☑ Place bedside tables and overbed tables near the bed or chair so that clients do not overreach and consequently lose their balance.
☑ Always keep hospital beds in the low position when not providing care so that clients can move in or out of bed easily.
☑ Keep side rails up and the bed in the low position for sedated and unconscious clients when they are unattended.
☑ Lock wheels on beds, wheelchairs, and stretchers.
☑ Ensure that the client wears nonskid footwear.
☑ Use bed or chair safety monitoring devices prn.

BOX 12-3 ASSESSING COMMON PRESSURE SITES

* Be sure there is good lighting, preferably natural or fluorescent.
* Regulate the environment before beginning the assessment so that the room is neither too hot nor too cold. Heat can cause the skin to flush; cold can cause the skin to blanch or become cyanotic.
* Inspect pressure areas for any whitish or reddened spots; discoloration can be caused by impaired blood circulation to the area. It should disappear in a few minutes when rubbing restores circulation.
* Inspect pressure areas for abrasions and excoriations. An abrasion (wearing away of the skin) can occur when skin rubs against a sheet (e.g., when the client is pulled). Excoriations (loss of superficial layers of the skin) can occur when the skin has prolonged contact with body secretions or excretions or with dampness in skinfolds.
* Palpate the surface temperature of the skin over the pressure areas. Normally, the temperature is the same as that of the surrounding skin. Increased temperature is abnormal and may be due to inflammation or blood trapped in the area.
* Palpate over bony prominences and dependent body areas for the presence of edema, which feels spongy.

Assessment boxes (identifiable in orange) summarize what data to collect during assessment and identify common manifestations or risk factors the nurse may observe

---

BOX 2-1 BASIC NURSING CARE ERRORS RESULTING IN NEGLIGENCE

Assessment Errors
Failing to
* Gather and chart client information adequately.
* Recognize the significance of certain information (e.g., laboratory values, vital signs).

Planning Errors
Failing to
* Chart each identified problem.
* Use language in the care plan that other caregivers understand.
* Ensure continuity of care by ignoring the care plan.
* Give discharge instructions that the client understands.

Intervention Errors
Failing to
* Administer and document medications correctly.
* Interpret and carry out a doctor's orders.
* Perform nursing tasks correctly.
* Pursue the physician if the doctor doesn't respond to calls or notify the nurse-manager if the physician is unavailable.

Miscellaneous boxes (identifiable in aqua) highlight content on law, health care systems, and other diverse content

---

B
Figure 1-12. **A.** The Knights of Saint Lazarus (established circa 1200) dedicated themselves to the care of people with leprosy, syphilis, and chronic skin conditions. In the mid-thirteenth century, leprosy was viewed as an incurable and terminal disease. **B.** Modern male nurses work side by side with their female colleagues to provide care to hospitalized clients. Source: (1–12A) © Bettmann/CORBIS. Reprinted with permission.

Full-color Visuals enable students to visualize key skills and concepts

---

Tables help students categorize and visualize information

TABLE 4-2	USE OF THE SENSES IN COLLECTING DATA
SENSES	EXAMPLE OF CLIENT DATA
Vision	Overall appearance (body size, general weight, posture, grooming); signs of distress or discomfort; facial and body gestures; skin color and lesions; abnormalities of movement; nonverbal demeanor (e.g., signs of anger or anxiety); religious or cultural artifacts (e.g., books, icons, candles, beads)
Smell	Body or breath odors
Hearing	Breath and heart sounds; bowel sounds; ability to communicate; language spoken; ability to initiate conversation; ability to respond when spoken to; orientation to time, person, and place; thoughts and feelings about self, others, and health status
Touch	Skin temperature and moisture; muscle strength (e.g., hand grip); pulse rate, rhythm, and volume; palpatory lesions (e.g., lumps, masses, nodules)

Students learn to deliver safe, effective nursing care as team members in different care environments...

Nursing Care is presented in the five-step nursing process format, applicable to the practical/vocational nurse's scope of practice.

Discharge Considerations focus student attention on their role in preparing clients and families to achieve or maintain health after discharge

Case Studies that bring specific disorders into "real life" emphasize the holistic aspects of nursing care

Critical Thinking Questions that conclude each case study allow students to apply their new-found learning

Clinical Alerts call attention to clinical roles and responsibilities for heightened awareness, monitoring and/or reporting

Procedures give step-by-step instructions and rationales for fundamental nursing actions. "Short-cut" icons (described in Chapter 4) reinforce essential preliminary steps in client care. "Live" documentation samples illustrate good record-keeping

Units come together with critical thinking...

After each unit, **Thinking Strategically** pages give students an opportunity to reflect on unit topics in terms of important nursing curriculum themes. Short scenarios and project ideas call for **critical thinking** about unit content from a variety of angles and enable students to move forward from a more integrated perspective.

◆ **Collaborative Care Strategies** challenge students to think concretely about health care settings and to envision the many health care workers who may participate in a client's care

◆ **Conflict Resolution** issues help students think ahead about potentially difficult situations

◆ **Critical Thinking questions** highlight specific challenges new nurses will face as they strive to provide the best possible care

◆ **Culturally Competent Care** strengthens the student's confidence by providing information and scenarios to familiarize them with cultural patterns and differences

◆ **Time Management** items offer hints for efficiency and organization

◆ **Communication and Team Building** presents ideas and activities for becoming a stronger communicator and a more effective professional

◆ **Community Care Strategies** discuss the nurse's role and responsibility in and beyond the workplace

◆ **Compassionate Caring** focuses on the caring and empathy that are at the core of the nursing profession

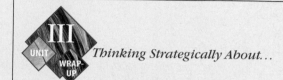

UNIT III WRAP-UP   *Thinking Strategically About...*

You are a newly graduated LPN assigned to a medical–surgical unit. You have been assigned to three clients.

Mr. Ramos is a 58-year-old male who was admitted for a prostatectomy (TURP) this morning. He is predominantly Spanish speaking, though he knows a few words of English and understands a little if he is spoken to slowly. He has returned from surgery. Initially, he was sedated but begins to be more alert. He appears agitated and is yelling loudly at his roommate, who puts on his call light to summon the nurse. The roommate states, "Mr. Ramos is trying to climb out of bed and he is frightening me."

Mr. Drew is a 53-year-old male who was admitted directly from his physician's office with chest pain. His BP is 168/90 with tachycardia (heart rate 102). He is diaphoretic and is complaining of nausea.

Mr. Melezack is a 64-year-old male who had a colon resection 3 days ago. His NG tube has been clamped and he has been started on clear liquids. It was reported that he tolerated them well. The doctor has ordered that the tube can be removed if there is no nausea or vomiting.

TIME MANAGEMENT

You have received report. Using your knowledge of the three clients' diagnoses and present needs, prioritize your care for the shift.

CRITICAL THINKING

Mr. Drew's lab work has come back. You observe that his CPK values are within normal limits and that his chest pain is relieved with sublingual nitroglycerin spray. He will be discharged in the morning, and you are to begin his discharge planning. In your teaching plan, state what activities would decrease the chance of recurrent angina and the risk factors that need to be controlled to decrease effects of heart disease.

COMPASSIONATE CARING

Mr. Ramos is frightening his roommate and trying to climb out of bed. He has an IV line and a three-way catheter, which is draining dark red urine with clots. Outline the steps you would take to protect Mr. Ramos from himself and to relieve the concerns of the roommate.

COMMUNICATION AND TEAM BUILDING

The client care assistant reports to you that Mr. Melezack is complaining of abdominal pain. He has vomited and asks to see you right away. After you go to his room to assess his present status, you will need to document and report your findings to the appropriate individuals. Write a medical record entry, using the focus charting method. State what information needs to be reported and to whom.

Roberta: *To the memory of my mentor and nursing instructor Mary Anne Aldinger, who taught me how to relate to students. To Russell and Doris Pavy, my parents, who always believed that I could do whatever I set my mind to.*

Dee: *To my husband Lee, my children Jamie and Josh, and my mother Dora, whose love and patience have always made the difference in my life.*

Preface

Fundamental Nursing Care arose from a desire to provide the best possible fundamentals book for LPNs and LVNs. For years, LPNs and LVNs in training have had to use RN-level textbooks, sifting out material and "translating" it from the RN point of view. This text, however, begins and ends with what LPNs and LVNs need to know and do. It identifies their scope of practice and affirms their importance in the larger health care system.

Increasingly, LPNs and LVNs are the nurses who come in direct contact with the health care consumer. They will be bedside nurses, team members, supervisors of unlicensed health care workers, and client educators. They will function in settings as diverse as acute care hospitals, long-term care facilities, and clients' homes. They must be competent, professional, articulate, and compassionate to win the confidence of their clients. We undertook this project to meet their growing needs.

To make this text "user friendly," we incorporated student feedback and our own wish lists from using other textbooks. The result is a practical book with ideas for many types of learners. By presenting solid information about studying, test taking, and time management, we help create more successful students and, in time, more successful nurses. By highlighting the role of men, we reflect the fact that nursing is becoming increasingly gender equal. By providing technology assistance with the text and support materials, we aid students in long-distance or computer-assisted programs.

Fundamental Nursing Care is a print and electronic product with a wealth of resources for students and instructors. It consists of textbook (with enclosed CD-ROM), instructor's resource manual, and student workbook. Electronic media are also available, including a test bank, links to valuable LPN/LVN Web sites, PowerPoints, a "toolbox" of teaching adjuncts, and a variety of visuals and critical thinking exercises.

This text is in alignment with the NCLEX-PN test plan. It does not "teach to the test," but it demonstrates how information relates to the broad categories of the test plan. It incorporates focus area information into all clinical chapters, and provides NCLEX-PN–style testing in every review section.

Organization

This book is organized to be accessible to students. Most LPN/LVN programs are designed from simple to complex,

building on knowledge and skills already obtained. The chapters of *Fundamental Nursing Care* are organized in the same manner and with a consistent format.

Unit I describes the history, laws, ethics, and basic theories of nursing. It provides a sketch of the health care system and a full discussion of the nursing process, with specifics about the role of vocational/practical nurses. **Units II, III, and IV** cover clinical aspects of care. Only skills and competencies that are within the scope of practice are included, making this text a truly LPN/LVN-level book. **Unit V** discusses teamwork and leadership, the NCLEX-PN licensure exam, and strategies for entering the workforce.

◆ Features

CHAPTER OPENING PAGE

- ◆ **Learning Outcomes**—Identify key skills and concepts.
- ◆ **Sharing Experiences**—Words of wisdom from practical/vocational nurse educators, students, and practicing LPNs/LVNs around the country support students to be competent, caring nurses.
- ◆ **MediaLink**—Provides reference to the **Audio Glossary** and multimedia supplements on the CD-ROM or Companion Website.
- ◆ **MediaLink Tabs**—Icons on page margins that prompt students to explore animations and activities.

END-OF-CHAPTER REVIEW

- ◆ **Key Terms by Topic**—Provides an overview for organizing study.
- ◆ **Key Points**—Highlights lifelong need-to-know items.
- ◆ **EXPLORE MediaLink**—Provides multimodal reinforcement for all learners, with references to the **free** student CD-ROM and the **free** Companion Website.
- ◆ **For Further Study**—Supplies references to related chapters to broaden understanding.
- ◆ **Critical Thinking Care Map**—Prepares students step by step for on-the-job critical thinking that leads to clinical success. It includes NCLEX-PN exam focus area, Case Study, Nursing Diagnosis, Data Collection, Reporting, and more!
- ◆ **NCLEX-PN Exam Preparation**—Test-Taking Tips focus study and help promote NCLEX success. NCLEX-PN–style questions contain content preview/review, as well as invaluable practice for taking the test.

WRAP-UP ITEMS

◆ **Thinking Strategically About. . .**—Challenges students to respond to unit-based scenarios from the viewpoint of curriculum themes.
◆ **Bibliography and Appendices**—Compile readings, full Glossary, answers with rationales, and more, to aid study and research.

VISUALS, INCLUDING TABLES AND COLOR-CODED BOXES

◆ **Nursing Care Checklist Boxes (identifiable in blue)**—Provide students with a ready-reference summary of important nursing interventions.
◆ **Population Focus Boxes and Client Teaching Boxes (identifiable in green)**—Help students meet age-specific and other special needs of different groups of clients.
◆ **Assessment Boxes (identifiable in orange)**—Identify signs and symptoms related to particular conditions.
◆ **Miscellaneous Boxes (identifiable in aqua)**—Highlight information for easy retrieval and review.
◆ **Full-Color Visuals**—Enable students to visualize key skills and concepts.
◆ **Tables**—Help students categorize and visualize data.

NURSING PROCESS

◆ **Nursing Care**—Specially formatted sections highlight traditional steps of the nursing process within the LPN/LVN scope of practice.
◆ **Case Studies**—Bring disorders in clinical chapters into "real life."
◆ **Critical Thinking in the Nursing Process**—Questions conclude each case study and allow students to apply their new-found learning.
◆ **Procedures with Sample Documentation**—Present key steps, rationales, and models for charting.
◆ **Clinical Alerts**—Emphasize clinical situations that require heightened awareness, monitoring, or reporting.

◆ Acknowledgments

Each author owes much gratitude to a special LVN/LPN who helped her achieve her career path. With this text, we hope to repay some of our debt, assisting today's LVN/LPN students to become the outstanding nurses of the twenty-first century.

ROBERTA RAMONT

When I was 19, nursing was the farthest thing from my mind. I was working at a job I disliked immensely, when I ended up in a hospital bed. An LPN student cared for me. She saw I was lost and looking for direction in my life, and she took time to talk. She suggested I consider a career in nursing. At first, it seemed like an outrageous idea, but after a month, I signed up for a nurse's aide training class at the very same hospital. Things went well until one winter morning I bathed a client

with the window open slightly. The instructor suggested I resign, saying this lack of attention would prevent me from being a good care provider. I was devastated. While I was crying in the back of the cafeteria, my LPN "guardian angel" appeared once again. She didn't coddle me or allow me to make excuses. Instead, she said that if I really wanted to be a nurse, I shouldn't let anything or anyone stand in my way. "Go to the instructor," she told me. "Tell her that you want to learn, you want to correct your mistakes, and tell her that you are not going to quit." This occurred almost 40 years ago. Since then, I have learned much about caring for clients, about dealing with students, and, most of all, much about myself. I have learned that we as nurses must encourage people to consider health care as a life's work, and we must always try to excel, even in the midst of discouragement.

DEE NIEDRINGHAUS

In contrast to Roberta, I wanted to be a nurse ever since I could remember. I signed up to be a Candy Striper as soon as they would take me. When I started out, I was very timid; I was afraid to go into a room to make a bed! Luckily for me, I met an LVN who was kind, caring, and enjoyed being a nurse. I loved working with her. As a senior in high school, I took a nursing assistant class there, and the LVN who had had such an influence on me was still working at the hospital. When I completed my nursing assistant class, she wrote me a letter of recommendation for the Los Angeles County School of Nursing. I had no doubts; I wanted to be a nurse, and this kind of support certainly helped.

A project such as this could never have been accomplished without the contributions of many people. We first thank our students. In our quest to teach you nursing, we have learned much from you about persistence, motivation, culture, and life. You are our future and we are confident that you will be a credit to the profession.

We want to thank the many nursing colleagues who have provided us with their encouragement and insight and helped to shape the book. Their experience as practitioners and as instructors helped to inform the content. Our contributors provided knowledge, skill, and time to write selected chapters in the text. Reviewers provided quality assurance for the book as well as a nationwide perspective. They validated the content and provided broader perspective as this book came into being. We thank the Prentice Hall author team of Kozier, Erb, Berman, and Burke for the vast wealth of material that laid the foundation for this book.

This project required the support, skills, and expertise of many people. Barbara Krawiec, our editor, adopted our proposal as a concept and made it happen. Her knowledge, calm demeanor, and endless attention to detail have been our inspiration. Rachel Bedard, our developmental editor, is the best. She skillfully turned our manuscript into a book. Our weekly conversations kept this project on track. We worked and laughed and accomplished a dream. Thank you, Rachel, for keeping us focused on the goal even when the day-to-day details clouded the view. Tia Himpsl, Rachel's right hand, rose to dozens of organizational challenges and worked through many weekends to keep the book on schedule. Sheba Jalaluddin and Jennifer Dwyer, editorial assistants, attended to many critical details. Mary Treacy, production editor, tracked and recorded all the pieces of the project, problem-solved, and monitored quality.

Our special thanks are also due to many others. Marilyn Meserve, managing editor, guided important editorial aspects from behind the scenes. Yesenia Kopperman, assistant editor, coordinated the test bank. Patrick Walsh (managing production editor), Ilene Sanford, and Pat Brown (manufacturing managers) guided scheduling, production, and manufacturing. Linda Begley and her capable staff at Rainbow Graphics copy-edited and produced the book. Cheryl Asherman, art director, and Maria Guglielmo created a visually clear and inviting format. Bridget Straton, research analyst, brought the voices of educators and students to life. John Jordan, Amy Peltier, Lisa Rinaldi, and Steve Hartner made all the media components happen. Nicole Benson, marketing manager, Rachele Strober, and Janet Ryerson enthusiastically worked to convey the features and benefits of these materials. Our thanks to all of you!

Roberta Pavy Ramont, RN, MS, Ed.Dc

Roberta Pavy Ramont has been an instructor of Vocational Nursing at North Orange County Regional Occupational Program (NOCROP) in Anaheim for 12 years. She received her initial nursing education at Cooper Hospital School of Nursing in Camden, New Jersey; her baccalaureate degree from the University of Redlands; and a masters in Psychology–School Counseling from the University of LaVerne. She is presently a doctoral candidate in Educational Leadership at Alliant International University.

Roberta credits her entrance into nursing to an LPN student who cared for her during an illness and who recognized her potential. She also credits the continued support and encouragement of her parents, who always demonstrated that anything worth achieving is worth 100% effort.

Roberta began her nursing career working in intensive care, but quickly realized that she wanted to focus on keeping people healthy. She worked for an agency visiting well-child clinics, schools, and homes, and later worked in maternal and infant care, childbirth preparation, and physicians' offices. When she moved to California, she found a job working with the developmentally disabled in a state hospital, and was quickly promoted to unit supervisor. The LVNs she hired to care for residents with physical and cognitive deficits were an inspiration; they brought joy and self-respect to the residents' lives by focusing on residents' accomplishments, not their disabilities. When state regulations changed, Roberta continued to work with students with special needs.

In 1985, a diagnosis of cancer led to six years with numerous treatments and surgeries. As a hospital client, Roberta was able to observe nurses at work. She became concerned that many of them seemed just to be doing a job. When she had a chance to teach, and found she enjoyed sharing knowledge and insights with students, she was eager to pass on some of the "lost art" of nursing. A job as instructor of a nursing assistant class quickly

developed into an opportunity to teach LVNs. Over the years she has been able to share with hundreds of students what it means to be a nurse. She feels that nursing students need two things: roots (to understand the rich heritage of nursing they will carry into the future) and wings (to develop skills that make them competent, safe nurses who can think and function with confidence).

Roberta served as curriculum chair for health careers education at NOCROP. She has worked on projects to identify academic standards taught in the career technical classes and to develop rubrics for alternate assessment of student work. She has served as advisor for Health Occupation Students of America, and recently was installed as Cal-HOSA Inc. Board of Directors Chair. She was President of the California Association of Health Careers Educators (CAHCE) in 2000–2001, and was awarded their Lillian Runge Memorial Scholarship for Continuing Education in 2002. She is a member of Society of Pediatric Nurses and Pi Lambda Theta, International Honor Society in Education.

Roberta has served on the NCLEX-PN writing panel. She developed seminars on the adult learner and technology in the classroom. She has taught teacher credentialing classes for San Diego University and is on a task force with the California Department of Education of Teacher Credentialing for Health Occupations teachers.

Roberta and Fred, her husband of 32 years, have three children: twin daughters Amy (an RN) and Alicia (mom to Haley and T.J. and an early childhood teacher), and son Tom (who recently completed grad school). When time permits Roberta enjoys reading and traveling.

Dolores Maldonado Niedringhaus

Dee's nursing career began right after graduation from Nursing School at USC/LACMC (Los Angeles County Medical Center), when she moved to Orange County and applied for a graduate nursing position. She was hired on the spot at what used to be Orange County Hospital. Although it was much smaller than LACMC (the rooms had only had five beds instead of eight to ten), it was a challenge. As the county hospital, it was always busy. The first year she worked PM shift on an orthopedic floor, where once there were prisoners in four rooms with guards. Sometimes conditions were so crowded that clients had spaces in the halls. This was a growthful time. The doctors were interns

and residents; all the staff worked together and learned how to be creative, innovative, and inventive.

After her marriage Dee transferred to a day shift position on the surgical floor, dealing with all types of surgical specialties (EENT, Plastic Surgery, Thoracic Surgery, and General Surgery). In team nursing there, Dee was fortunate to have as colleagues two excellent LVNs, who did most of the dressings and wound care and helped with medications. Dee's nursing techniques developed as she learned from these nurses. After working at this hospital for 12 years in various areas, she was chosen to work a new unit as the surgical specialist. It was the first outpatient unit developed at what was now UCIMC (University of California at Irvine Medical Center).

A chance request brought her to teaching. One summer a colleague needed a substitute instructor for a nursing assistant program run by North Orange County Regional Occupational Program. Those two months changed her nursing career. She was hooked on and loved teaching. When she was offered a full-time position teaching a day nursing assistant program, she taught this for a year. She then took a position teaching vocational nurses, and for 15 years taught Fundamentals I & II, Integumentary, Gastrointestinal, Endocrine, and Leadership modules. She began the first HOSA (Health Occupations Students of America) chapters, which became very successful and continue today. She also instructed classes for Health Career Instructors and was the chairman for Cal-HOSA Inc. Currently Dee is an Instructional Administrator of Medical Programs at North Orange County ROP.

Contributor Team

Chapters

Charlene Adams, BS
Case Manager
Central Coast Community Health Clinic
Paso Robles, CA

Susan Balke, RN, MSN, GNP
Director, Education Services
St. Joseph Regional Health Center
Bryan, TX

Peggy Bohannon, RN, MS
Director, School of Vocational Nursing
Lee College
Baytown, TX

Donna Breed, RN, BSN
Instructor
North Orange County Regional Occupational
    Program
Anaheim, CA

Rosemary Brown, BSN, RN-c
Nursing Instructor
Idaho State University Practical Nursing Program
Pocatello, ID

Paige Fletcher, RN, MSN
Associate Professor
Austin Community College
Austin, TX

Amy J. Fukushima, RN
O.B./Acute Care Nursery
French Hospital Medical Center
San Luis Obispo, CA

Janis Grimland, RN, BSN
Program Director
Hill College
Clifton, TX

David Oswandel, BS
Instructor
Pikes Peak Community College
Colorado Springs, CO

Stephanie Randall, RN
Vocational Nursing Coordinator
Concorde Career Institute
Arlington, TX

Betty Richardson, PhD, APRN, BC, CNAA,
    LPC, LMFT
Professor Emeritus
Austin Community College
Austin, TX

Mickle Ward-Ellison, RN, MS
Director of Nursing Related Programs
Kennedy-King College/Dawson Technical Institute
Chicago, IL

M. Angela Webster, MSN, RN, PHN
Associate Dean of Nursing, West Haven University
Cypress, California
Faculty, Casa Loma College
Van Nuys, California

Ron Zack, RN, MA
Hospice Preferred Choice
Orange, CA

Sharing Experiences Quotes

Tina M. Banzhof, LPN
Community Hospital
Lancaster, PA

Bonnie L. Boroski, RN, MSN
LPN Program Director
Greater Johnstown Area Vocational Technical
    School
Johnstown, PA

Alexis Chavarria, LPN student
Idaho State University
Pocatello, ID

Denise Foster, LVN
North Orange County Regional Occupational
    Program
Anaheim, CA

Kelly C. Goetz, LVN
Fullerton, CA

Valarie Gray, LPN student
Idaho State University
Pocatello, ID

Sandy Groff, LPN, DON
Colonial Hall Assisted Living
Willow Street, PA

LaReta Gugelman, LPN student
Idaho State University
Pocatello, ID

Christine Haggard, LVN
Clinical Research
Austin, TX

Maria Hughes, LVN
Concorde Career Institute
Arlington, TX

Renay Jones, LVN student
North Orange County Regional Occupational
    Program
Anaheim, CA

Margaret Kamara, LPN student
Idaho State University
Pocatello, ID

Lana Knapp, LPN student
Idaho State University
Pocatello, ID

Michelle Marshall, LVN
North Orange County Regional Occupational
    Program
Anaheim, CA

Mohammad Naz, LVN student
North Orange County Regional Occupational
    Program
Anaheim, CA

Susan Palmer, RN, ADN
Parkmoor View Medical Center
Colorado Springs, CO

Jane Pond, LPN
Lewis Memorial Christian Home
President, LPN Association of Indiana
Springfield, IL

Briseida Ramirez, LVN student
North Orange County Regional Occupational
    Program
Anaheim, CA

Stephanie Randall, RN
Vocational Nursing Coordinator
Concorde Career Institute
Arlington, TX

Eric Reed, LPN student
Idaho State University
Pocatello, ID

Mark S. Reef, LPN, BSN, RN
Howard Community Hospital
Kokomo, IN

Melinda Barrowcliff-Reyes, LVN student
Cal-HOSA State Officer
North Orange County Regional Occupational
    Program
Anaheim, CA

Darrin Rodriguez, LPN student
Idaho State University
Pocatello, ID

Marilyn Runnells, LVN
North Orange County Regional Occupational
    Program
Anaheim, CA

Martha Solis, LVN
North Orange County Regional Occupational
    Program
Anaheim, CA

Rose Syass, LPN
The Manor Retirement Center
Las Vegas, NV

Ginger L. Taft, LPN student
Idaho State University
Pocatello, ID

Valerie A. Gordon-Tate, LVN, LPN
Pediatric Home Care Nurse
Newport News, VA

Jessica Thielmann, LVN student
North Orange County Regional Occupational
    Program
Anaheim, CA

Shawna Thurman, LVN student
Austin Community College
Austin, TX

Deborah Tovar, LVN
High Desert Medical Group
Lancaster, CA

Holly Zamora, LPN student
Idaho State University
Pocatello, ID

Student CD-ROM and Companion Website: www. prenhall.com/ramont

Susan Balke, RN, MSN, GNP
Director, Education Services
St. Joseph Regional Health Center
Bryan, TX

Marti Burton, RN, BS
Former Practical Nursing Instructor
Author of Practical Nursing Curriculum
Oklahoma Department of Career and Technology
 Education
Stillwater, OK

Terri Quillen, RN
Parish Nurse
Greenwood, IN

Stephanie Randall, RN
Vocational Nursing Coordinator
Concorde Career Institute
Arlington, TX

**Betty Richardson, PhD, APRN, BC, CNAA,
 LPC, LMFT**
Professor Emeritus
Austin Community College
Austin, TX

Frances M. Warrick, MS, RN
Program Coordinator Vocational Nursing
El Centro College
Dallas, TX

 ## Student Workbook

Helen Barnes, MSN, RN
Instructor
Long Beach City College
Long Beach, CA

Rita Callahan, RN, BSN
Instructor
Southwestern College
San Diego, CA

Lora Lee Crawford, RN, BSN
Instructor
Emanuel Turlock Vocational School
Turlock, CA

Pamela Darensburg-Jude, LVN (Teach Cred)
LVN Instructor
College of Marin and Glendale Career College
Los Angeles, CA

Beverly Drake, RN, BSN, PHN
Assistant Professor
Porterville College
Porterville, CA

Joyce Moody Flores, MSN, RN
Professor, Porterville College
Porterville, CA

Anita Garman, RN, MSN
Assistant Director
Emanuel Turlock Vocational School
Turlock, CA

Olma Guerra-Weaver, LVN
Lab Skills/Clinical Instructor
Coastal Bend College
Beeville, TX

Anita Holt, RN, BSN, MSN
Professor Vocational Nursing Program
Southwest College
Vista, CA

Yazmin Mojica, RN, BSN, MA
Founder/ President, National NCLEX® Solutions
Educator/Consultant
Walnut, CA

Myrtle Jo Neely, RN, BSN
Vocational Nursing Instructor
St. Philips College
San Antonio, TX

Stephanie Randall, RN
Vocational Nursing Coordinator
Concorde Career Institute
Arlington, TX

Carolyn Reese, RN, BSN
Vocational Nursing Instructor
Critical Care Nurse at St. Joseph Regional Health
 Center
Blinn College
Bryan, TX

**Betty Richardson, PhD, APRN, BC, CNAA,
 LPC, LMPT**
Professor Emeritus
Austin Community College
Austin, TX

Sharron Rust, RN
VN Program Director
Clarendon College
Clarendon, TX

Rox Ann Sparks, RN, MICN, ASSN
Vocational Nursing Instructor
Merced College
Merced, CA

Gloria Spencer, RN, BSN, MSN
Director, Vocational Nursing Program–Brownsville
University of Texas at Brownsville and Texas
 Southmost College
Brownsville, TX

Rose Sprull, RN, BSN
Vocational Nursing Instructor
St. Philips College
San Antonio, TX

Angela Stephens, RN
LVN Instructor
Hanford Adult School
Hanford, CA

Jean C. Stevenson, RN, BS, MHA
Director of Nursing Education
Four-D Success Academy, Inc.
Colton, CA

Linda Stewart, LVN
Instructor
Blinn College
Bryan, TX

Doreen Story, RN, BSN
Retired LVN Instructor
Glendale Career College
Glendale, CA.

Eva Talastas, RN, MSN
Nursing Department Head
Long Beach City College
Long Beach, CA

Peggy Wells, RN, BS, MS
Instructor
Long Beach College
Long Beach, CA

Rebecca Zielinski, RN
Program Director
Concorde Career Institute
Arlington, TX

Instructor's Resource Manual and IRM CD-ROM

Susan Balke, RN, MSN, GNP
Director, Education Services
St. Joseph Regional Health Center
Bryan, TX

Marti Burton, RN, BS
Former Practical Nursing Instructor
Author of Practical Nursing Curriculum
Oklahoma Department of Career and Technology
 Education
Stillwater, OK

Terri Quillen, RN
Parish Nurse
Greenwood, IN

Stephanie Randall, RN
Vocational Nursing Coordinator
Concorde Career
Arlington, TX

**Betty Richardson, PhD, APRN, BC, CNAA,
 LPC, LMFT**
Professor Emeritus
Austin Community College
Austin, TX

Frances M. Warrick, MS, RN
Program Coordinator Vocational Nursing
El Centro College
Dallas, TX

Test Manager

Author

Vivian Bingman, R.N., M.Ed.
Former Director, Practical Nursing Program
Mid-Del Technology Center
Midwest City, Oklahoma

Contributors

Marti Burton, RN, BS
Former Practical Nursing Instructor
Author of Practical Nursing Curriculum
Oklahoma Department of Career and Technology
 Education
Stillwater, OK

Frances M. Warrick, MS, RN
Program Coordinator Vocational Nursing
El Centro College
Dallas, TX

Reviewer Panel

Cheryll Alt, RN, BSN
Program Director, Practical Nurse Program
MSU Great Falls College of Technology
Great Falls, MT

Cynthia Amerson, RN, BSN, MS
Director of Nursing
Northeast Texas Community College
Mt. Pleasant, TX

LaVon Barrett, RN, BSN
Instructor of Vocational Nursing
Amarillo College
Amarillo, TX

Julia Barton, RN, BSN, MEd
Instructor
Ohio Hi Point Career Center
Bellefontaine,OH

Thelma Blouch, RN, BSN
Instructor
Lebanon County Career and Tech Center
Lebanon, PA

Carole Bomba, RN, MSN
Assistant Professor of Nursing
William Rainey Harper College
Palatine, IL

Adrienne Bowlus, RN, MSN
Instructor
Apollo School of Practical Nursing
Lima, OH

Denise Brehmer, RN, MSN
Assistant Professor of Nursing
Ivy Tech State College
Kokomo, IN

Rebecca A. Cappo, RN, MSN
Coordinator
Lenape LPN Program
Ford City, PA

Patricia Collins, RN, MSN, MSEd, EdD
Director of Nurse Education
Westshore Community College
Scottville, MI

Barbara Daniel, MEd, MS, CRNP
Professor of Nursing
Cecil Community College
North East, MD

Karen D. Danielson, RN, MSN
Associate Professor
Practical Nursing Program
North Central State College
Mansfield, OH

Sally Flesch, PhD, RN
Professor of Allied Health
Black Hawk College
Moline, IL

Brad Foley, BSN, CNN
Instructor
Minneapolis Community Technical College
Minneapolis, MN

Connie L. Geiser, BSN, RN
Nurse Educator
Southeastern Community College
West Burlington, IA

Candace Gioia, RN, BSN, CNOR
Health Care Coordinator and Instructor
Pinellas Technical Education Center
Clearwater, FL

Teresa Grooms, RN, BSN
Nursing Instructor
Southern State Community College
Hillsboro, OH

Pamela Gwin, RN-c
Director Vocational Nursing Program
Brazosport College
Lake Jackson, TX

Joan M. Lang, RN, BSN, MA
Nursing Professor
Hawkeye Community College
Waterloo, IA

Eloise Lewis-Kiilu, RN, BSN
Assistant Professor
Ivy Tech State College
Columbus, OH

Christine Martin, RN
Faculty, ADN Program
Berkshire Community College
Pittsfield, MA

Marina Martinez-Kratz, RN-c, MS
Assistant Professor of Nursing
Jackson Community College
Jackson, MI

Sharon E. Moran, RN, MPH, CS
Associate Professor of Nursing
Hawaii Community College
Hilo, HI

Mary Nielsen, RN, MSN
Instructor
University of Montana College of Technology
Missoula, MT

Diane Okeson, EdD, ARNP/CNS
Assistant Professor
Emporia State University
Emporia, KS

Judith Pelletier
Massachusetts Bay Community College
Framingham, MA

Lynne Peterson, RN, MEd, MSN
Coordinator of Nursing Program
Hocking College
Nelsonville, OH

Jennifer Ponto, RN, BSN
Instructor
South Plains College
Levelland, TX

LuAnn J. Reicks, RN-c, MSN
Instructor
Iowa Central Community College
Fort Dodge, IA

Mickey Ryan, RN, BSN
Former Instructor
Apollo School of Practical Nursing
Lema, OH

Margi Schultz, RN, MSN
Assistant Director of Nursing
GateWay Community College
Phoenix, AZ

Nettie Seale, RN, MEd
Instructor of Practical Nursing
Kiamichi Technology Center
Stiger, OK

Lyndi C. Shadbolt, MS, BSN, RN
Assistant Professor of Nursing
Amarillo College
Amarillo, TX

Beverly Smith, RN, BSN
Director
San Jacinto College District North Campus
Houston, TX

Juanita J. Smith, RN, BSN
Instructor
Lorain County Community College
Elyria, OH

Sue E. Smith, MSN, MEd
Assistant Professor
Iowa Western Community College
Harlan, IA

Rox Ann Sparks, MICN, AASN
Instructor Vocational Nursing
Merced College
Merced, CA

Deborah L. Stevenson, RN
Nursing Instructor
Midlands Technical College
Columbia, SC

Nancy Vrabec, PhD, RN-c
Associate Dean, Nursing
Milwaukee Area Technical College
Milwaukee, WI

Ellen F. Wirtz, RN-c, MN
Chair, Practical Nursing
Helena Career Tech of UM
Helena, MT

Cindy W. Yount, RN, MSN
Nursing Program Director
Rockingham Community College
Wentworth, NC

Contents

UNIT I   The Nature of Nursing   1

Chapter 1   Understanding Nursing 2

Understanding Nursing Through History 3

  Influences on the Development of Nursing 3

  Leading Nurses of History 5

  Male Nurses in History 7

  Licensed Practical and Vocational Nurses
  in History 8

Understanding Contemporary Nursing Practice 8

  Definitions of Nursing 8

  Factors Influencing Contemporary Nursing 10

  Opportunities for LPNs/LVNs in Contemporary
  Nursing 11

Understanding Nursing Education 13

  Academic Success Skills 13

Chapter 2   Legal and Ethical Issues of Nursing 19

Understanding Legal Issues 20

Kinds of Legal Actions 20

  Civil Law 20

  Criminal Law 22

Regulation of Nursing Practice 23

  Credentialing 23

  Nurse Practice Acts 23

  Standards of Practice 23

Legal Roles of Nurses 23

  Provider of Service 23

  Employee or Contractor for Service 24

  Citizen 24

Nursing Responsibilities and Protections 24

  Good Samaritan Acts 24

  Professional Liability Insurance 25

  Nurses as Witnesses 25

  Student Nurses 25

Selected Legal Aspects of Nursing Practice 25

  Privileged Communication 25

  Informed Consent 25

  Carrying Out Physician's Orders 26

  Providing Competent Nursing Care 27

  Record Keeping 27

  The Incident Report 27

  Reporting Crimes, Torts, and Unsafe Practices 27

  Americans with Disabilities Act 27

  Controlled Substances 29

  Sexual Harassment 29

Understanding Ethical Issues 29

Ethical Concepts 29

Moral Concepts 30

Nursing Ethics 31

  Origins of Ethical Problems in Nursing 31

  Making Ethical Decisions 31

  Specific Ethical Issues 32

  Allocation of Health Resources 33

  Management of Computerized Information 33

  Advocacy 33

**Chapter 3   Critical Thinking and Nursing
                        Theory/Models 37**

Critical Thinking 38

  Methods of Problem Solving 38

  Applying Critical Thinking to Nursing 38

  Using Critical Thinking to Make Nursing
  Decisions 39

  Practicing Critical Thinking 40

Theories and Models 42

  Introduction to Nursing Theories 42

  Non-nursing Models 42

  Significance of Models and Theories 43

**Chapter 4   The LVN/LPN and the Nursing
                        Process 50**

Components of the Nursing Process 51

  Role of the LPN/LVN in the Nursing Process 51

Assessment 52

  Collecting Data 52

  Types of Data 52

  Sources of Data 53

  Data Collection Methods 53

  Documenting Data 54

Diagnosis 54

  Components of a NANDA Nursing Diagnosis 55

  Two-Part and Three-Part Nursing Diagnosis
  Statements 55

Planning 56

  Types of Planning 56

  Nursing Care Plans 56

  The Planning Process 58

  LVNs/LPNs and Long-Term Care Planning 63

  Nursing Process Case Studies 63

Implementation 63

  Types of Nursing Interventions 63

Implementing Skills **64**

Basic Procedures for Nursing Interventions **64**

Process of Implementing **64**

Evaluation 65

Procedure 4-1 Basic Procedure Steps and Admission
Information **66**

**UNIT II   Introduction to Clinical
Practice 71**

Chapter 5   Health Care Delivery Systems 72

Types of Health Care 73

Health Promotion and Illness Prevention **73**

Diagnosis and Treatment **73**

Rehabilitation and Health Restoration **73**

Levels of Health Care 73

Types of Health Care Settings 73

Outpatient Settings **74**

Inpatient Settings **75**

Mixed Settings **77**

Rights and Health Care 77

Patient's Bill of Rights **77**

Providers of Health Care 77

Nurse **78**

Physician **78**

Physician's Assistant **78**

Unlicensed Assistive Personnel **78**

Dentist **78**

Pharmacist **78**

Dietitian or Nutritionist **78**

Physiotherapist **78**

Respiratory Therapist **78**

Occupational Therapist **78**

Paramedical Technologists **78**

Social Worker **78**

Spiritual Support Person **79**

Case Managers **79**

Alternative Care Providers **79**

Factors Affecting Health Care Delivery 79

Increasing Number of Elderly **79**

Advances in Technology **79**

Women's Health **79**

Uneven Distribution of Services **79**

Access to Health Care **80**

Homeless Populations **80**

Demographic Changes **80**

Contemporary Frameworks for Care 80

Managed Care **80**

Case Management **80**

Models of Care 80

Client-Focused Care **80**

Case Method **81**

Functional Method **81**

Team Nursing **81**

Primary Nursing **82**

Health Care Economics 82

Payment Sources **82**

Prospective Payment System **82**

Insurance Plans **82**

Chapter 6   Safety 86

Factors That Affect Safety 87

Age and Development **87**

Lifestyle **87**

Mobility and Health Status **87**

Sensory–Perceptual Alterations **87**

Cognitive Awareness **87**

Emotional State **87**

Ability to Communicate **87**

Safety Awareness **87**

Preventing Specific Hazards 87

Scalds and Burns **89**

Fires **89**

Falls **89**

Suffocation or Choking **90**

Excessive Noise **91**

Electrical Hazards **92**

Radiation **92**

Preventing Equipment-Related Accidents 92

Hospital and Institutional Safety 92

Infectious Waste **92**

Hazardous Waste **93**

Disaster Plan **93**

Emergency Codes **94**

Emergency Nursing and First Aid **94**

Cardiopulmonary Resuscitation **94**

Restraining Clients 95

Legal Implications of Restraints **95**

Selecting a Restraint **97**

Kinds of Restraints **97**

NURSING CARE 98

Assessing 98

Diagnosing, Planning, and Implementing 99

Evaluating 100

Discharge Considerations 100

**Nursing Process Case Study: Client
with a Fractured Hip 101**

Personal Safety for Nurses **101**
Body Mechanics **101**
Procedure 6-1 Using a Bed or Chair Exit Safety
Monitoring Device **106**
Critical Thinking Care Map: Caring for a Client with Risk
for Injury **109**

Chapter 7   Infection Control and Asepsis **111**
Microorganisms **112**
Types of Microorganisms **112**
Controlling Microorganisms **113**
Controlling Communicable Diseases **113**
Infection **113**
Types of Infections **113**
Chain of Infection **114**
Factors That Increase Susceptibility to Infection **115**
Nonspecific Defenses **116**
Specific or Immune Defenses **116**
Controlling Microorganisms in the
Environment **116**
Using Asepsis **117**
Protective Precautions **118**
Collaborative Care **119**
NURSING CARE **120**
Assessing **120**
Diagnosing, Planning, and Implementing **121**
Evaluating **121**
Discharge Considerations **122**
Nursing Process Case Study: Client with Respiratory
Infection **122**
Procedure 7-1 Hand Washing **124**
Procedure 7-2 Donning and Removing Sterile Gloves (Open
Method) **126**
Procedure 7-3 Donning Personal Protective Equipment **127**
Procedure 7-4 Establishing and Maintaining a Sterile Field **129**
Critical Thinking Care Map: Caring for a Client
with a Stasis Ulcer **135**

Chapter 8   Admission, Transfer, and Discharge **137**
Admitting a Client **138**
Common Responses to Hospital Admission **138**
Cultural Considerations **138**
Admission Procedure Guidelines **138**
NURSING CARE **141**
Assessing **141**
Diagnosing, Planning, and Implementing **141**
Evaluating **143**
Nursing Process Case Study: Admission of a Client
from Emergency Unit **143**
Transferring a Client **144**

Common Responses to Transfer **144**
Transfer Guidelines **144**
NURSING CARE **144**
Assessing **144**
Diagnosing, Planning, and Implementing **144**
Evaluating **146**
Discharging a Client **146**
Discharge Guidelines **146**
Common Responses to Discharge **146**
NURSING CARE **146**
Assessing **146**
Diagnosing, Planning, and Implementing **149**
Evaluating **149**
Critical Thinking Care Map: Caring for a Client Prior
to Discharge **152**

Chapter 9   Documenting and Reporting **154**
Purposes of Client Records **155**
Communication **155**
Planning Client Care **155**
Legal Documentation **155**
Education, Research, and Health Care Analysis **155**
Auditing **155**
Reimbursement **155**
Guidelines for Recording **155**
Date and Time **155**
Timing **155**
Legibility **156**
Permanence **156**
Accepted Terminology **156**
Correct Spelling **156**
Signature **156**
Accuracy **156**
Sequence **158**
Continued Notes **159**
Appropriateness and Completeness **159**
Conciseness **159**
Legal Prudence **159**
Additional Tips for Documentation **159**
Confidentiality of Client Records **159**
Ensuring Confidentiality of Computer Records **159**
Documentation Systems **160**
Source-Oriented Record **160**
Problem-Oriented Medical Record **160**
Types of Documentation Methods **161**
SOAP **161**
PIE/APIE Charting **162**
Focus Charting **163**
CORE **164**
Charting by Exception **164**

FACT **164**

Outcome Documentation **164**

Computerized Documentation **164**

Case Management **165**

Reporting **167**

Change-of-Shift Reports **167**

Telephone Reports **167**

Telephone Orders **168**

Fax and E-mail Communication **168**

Nursing Care Conference **168**

Nursing Rounds **168**

Interdisciplinary Care Plan Meetings **168**

Incident Reports **168**

NURSING CARE 169

Assessing 169

Diagnosing, Planning, and Implementing 169

Evaluating 173

Nursing Process Case Study: Client with Altered Protection 173

Critical Thinking Care Map: Caring for a Client Who Is Grieving 175

UNIT III   Promoting Physiological Health **179**

Chapter 10   Introduction to the Body **180**

Cells **181**

Cell Structure **181**

Cell Division **182**

Tissues **183**

Epithelial Tissue **183**

Connective Tissue **184**

Muscle Tissue **185**

Nervous Tissue **185**

Body Systems **185**

Integumentary System **185**

Nervous System **185**

Endocrine System **187**

Skeletal System **187**

Muscular System **188**

Circulatory System **189**

Lymphatic System **189**

Respiratory System **189**

Digestive System **189**

Urinary System **191**

Reproductive System **191**

Anatomic Positions **192**

Body Planes **193**

Body Cavities **193**

Chapter 11   Health Assessment **197**

Physical Health Assessment **198**

Complete Assessment **198**

Focused Assessment **198**

Preparing the Client **198**

Methods of Examination **201**

Inspection **201**

Auscultation **201**

Palpation **201**

Percussion **204**

NURSING CARE 204

Assessing 204

Diagnosing, Planning, and Implementing 209

Evaluating 210

Nursing Process Case Study: Client with Postpartum Bleeding 210

Procedure 11-1 Focused Physical Assessment by Body Systems **211**

Critical Thinking Care Map: Caring for a Client with Activity Intolerance 220

Chapter 12   Skin Integrity and Wound Care **222**

Skin Integrity **223**

Types of Wounds **223**

Wound Healing **223**

Phases of Wound Healing **224**

Kinds of Wound Drainage **224**

Complications of Wound Healing **225**

Factors Affecting Wound Healing **225**

Collaborative Care **226**

NURSING CARE 231

Assessing 231

Diagnosing, Planning, and Implementing 232

Evaluating 236

Discharge Considerations 236

Pressure Ulcers **236**

Risk Factors **236**

Stages of Pressure Ulcer Formation **237**

Collaborative Care **237**

NURSING CARE 240

Assessing 240

Diagnosing, Planning, and Implementing 241

Evaluating 242

Discharge Considerations 242

Nursing Process Case Study: Client with Pressure Ulcer 242

Procedure 12-1 Wound Dressings **244**

Procedure 12-2 Obtaining a Specimen of Wound Drainage **246**

Procedure 12-3 Irrigating a Wound 247
Critical Thinking Care Map: Caring for a Debilitated Client 250

Chapter 13   Hygiene 252

Skin, Foot, and Nail Care 253
   Types of Baths 253
   Feet 254
   Nails 254
NURSING CARE 254
   Assessing 254
   Diagnosing, Planning, and Implementing 256
   Evaluating 258
   Discharge Considerations 258
   Nursing Process Case Study: Client with Diabetes 258
Hair Care 259
NURSING CARE 259
   Assessing 259
   Diagnosing, Planning, and Implementing 260
   Evaluating 261
Mouth Care 261
NURSING CARE 262
   Assessing 262
   Diagnosing, Planning, and Implementing 263
   Evaluating 265
Eye Care 265
NURSING CARE 265
   Assessing 265
   Diagnosing, Planning, and Implementing 265
   Evaluating 267
   Discharge Considerations 267
Ear Care 268
   Cleaning the Ears 268
   Care of Hearing Aids 268
Nose Care 268
Supporting a Hygienic Environment 268
   Hospital Beds 269
   Intravenous Rods 270
   Making Beds 270
Procedure 13-1 Bathing Clients 272
Procedure 13-2 Providing Hair Care 276
Procedure 13-3 Providing Oral Care 279
Procedure 13-4 Removing, Cleaning, and Inserting a Hearing Aid 282
Procedure 13-5 Changing a Bed 284
Critical Thinking Care Map: Caring for a Client with Oral Cavity Problems 289

Chapter 14   Vital Signs 291

Body Temperature 292
   Regulation of Body Temperature 293
   Alterations in Body Temperature 293
   Temperature Assessment Methods 295
NURSING CARE 297
   Assessing 297
   Diagnosing, Planning, and Implementing 297
   Evaluating 297
   Discharge Considerations 298
Pulse 298
   Factors Affecting Pulse Rate 298
   Pulse Sites 298
NURSING CARE 300
   Assessing 300
   Diagnosing, Planning, and Implementing 301
   Evaluating 301
   Discharge Considerations 301
   Nursing Process Case Study: Client with Left-Sided Heart Failure 301
Respirations 302
   Mechanics and Regulation 302
NURSING CARE 302
   Assessing 302
   Diagnosing, Planning, and Implementing 303
   Evaluating 303
Blood Pressure 304
   Determinants of Blood Pressure 304
   Factors Affecting Blood Pressure 305
   Hypertension 305
   Hypotension 305
   Blood Pressure Equipment 306
   Blood Pressure Assessment Sites 308
   Methods 308
NURSING CARE 309
   Assessing 309
   Diagnosing, Planning, and Implementing 309
   Evaluating 309
Procedure 14-1 Assessing Body Temperature 311
Procedure 14-2 Assessing Pulse 313
Procedure 14-3 Assessing Respirations 317
Procedure 14-4 Assessing Blood Pressure 318
Critical Thinking Care Map: Caring for a Client after a Heart Attack 322

Chapter 15   Pain, The Fifth Vital Sign 324

Types of Pain 325
Concepts Associated with Pain 326
Physiology of Pain 326

Transmission and Perception 326
Gate Control Theory 327
Responses to Pain 328
Factors Affecting the Pain Experience 328
Collaborative Care 328
Key Factors in Pain Management 331
Acknowledging and Accepting 331
Assisting Support Persons 331
Reducing Misconceptions about Pain 331
Reducing Fear and Anxiety 331
Preventing Pain 331
Barriers to Pain Management 332
Routes for Opiate Delivery 333
NURSING CARE 333
Assessing 333
Diagnosing, Planning, and Implementing 338
Evaluating 339
Nursing Process Case Study: Client
with Pain 340
Critical Thinking Care Map: Caring for a Client
with Postoperative Pain 342

Chapter 16   Oxygenation 344
Structure and Function of the Respiratory System 345
Structure of the Respiratory System 345
Pulmonary Ventilation 345
Alveolar Gas Exchange 346
Transport of Oxygen and Carbon Dioxide 346
Respiratory Regulation 347
Alterations in Respiratory Function 347
Structure and Function of the Cardiovascular System 348
The Heart 348
Blood Vessels 349
Blood 350
Alterations in Cardiovascular Function 350
Treatment of Oxygenation Problems 351
Collaborative Care 351
Oxygen Therapy 353
NURSING CARE 355
Assessing 355
Diagnosing, Planning, and Implementing 355
Evaluating 359
Discharge Considerations 359
Nursing Process Case Study: Client
with Hemothorax 359
Procedure 16-1 Measuring Pulse Oximetry 361
Procedure 16-2 Administering Oxygen by Nasal Cannula
or Face Mask 362
Procedure 16-3 Providing Tracheostomy Care 364
Procedure 16-4 Suctioning 367

Procedure 16-5 Applying a Sequential Compression
Device 370
Critical Thinking Care Map: Caring for a Client with
Pneumonia 373

Chapter 17   Nutrition, Fluids and Electrolytes,
and Acid–Base Balance 375
Nutrition 376
Nutrients 376
Water 376
Macronutrients 376
Micronutrients 377
Standards for a Healthy Diet 378
NURSING CARE 379
Assessing 379
Diagnosing, Planning, and Implementing 380
Evaluating 383
Discharge Considerations 383
Nursing Process Case Study: Client with Altered
Nutrition 383
Fluid and Electrolytes, and Acid–Base Balance 384
Body Fluids and Electrolyte Balance 384
Composition of Body Fluids 384
Regulating Body Fluids 385
Acid–Base Balance 386
Acid–Base Regulators 386
Acid–Base Imbalances 387
Respiratory Acidosis 387
Respiratory Alkalosis 387
Metabolic Acidosis 387
Metabolic Alkalosis 388
NURSING CARE 388
Assessing 388
Diagnosing, Planning, and Implementing 388
Assisting with IV Therapy 390
Evaluating 391
Discharge Considerations 391
Procedure 17-1 Monitoring Blood Glucose 392
Procedure 17-2 Inserting and Removing
Nasogastric Tubes 392
Procedure 17-3 Administering a Tube Feeding 396
Procedure 17-4 Discontinuing an Intravenous Infusion 399
Critical Thinking Care Map: Caring for a Client with Risk
for Deficient Fluid Volume 402

Chapter 18   Urinary Elimination 404
Structure and Function of the Urinary System 405
Kidneys 405
Ureters 405
Bladder 405
Urethra 406
Urination 406

Factors Affecting Urinary Function **406**
    Psychosocial Factors **406**
    Fluid and Food Intake **407**
    Medications **407**
    Muscle Tone and Activity **407**
Pathologic Conditions **407**
    Altered Urine Production **408**
    Altered Urinary Elimination **408**
    Collaborative Care **408**
NURSING CARE **408**
    Assessing **408**
    Diagnosing, Planning, and Implementing **408**
    Evaluating **420**
    Discharge Considerations **420**
    Nursing Process Case Study: Client with Abdominal Injury **420**
Procedure 18-1 Collecting a Urine Specimen for Culture and Sensitivity by Clean Catch **422**
Procedure 18-2 Applying a Condom Catheter **423**
Procedure 18-3 Female Urinary Catheterization Using a Straight Catheter **425**
Procedure 18-4 Male Urinary Catheterization Using a Straight Catheter **427**
Procedure 18-5 Inserting a Retention (Indwelling) Catheter **428**
Procedure 18-6 Irrigating a Catheter or Bladder (Closed System) **431**
Critical Thinking Care Map: Caring for a Client with Altered Urinary Elimination **434**

Chapter 19   Gastrointestinal Elimination **436**
Physiology of Defecation **437**
    Large Intestine **437**
    Rectum and Anal Canal **437**
Factors That Affect Defecation **438**
    Age and Development **438**
    Diet **439**
    Fluids **439**
    Activity **439**
    Psychological Factors **439**
    Defecation Habits **439**
    Medications **439**
    Diagnostic Procedures **439**
    Anesthesia and Surgery **439**
    Pathologic Conditions **439**
    Pain **439**
Common Fecal Elimination Problems **439**
    Constipation **439**
    Fecal Impaction **440**
    Diarrhea **440**

    Bowel Incontinence **441**
    Flatulence **441**
Fecal Diversion Ostomies **441**
    Permanence **441**
    Anatomic Location **441**
    Ostomy Management **441**
    Collaborative Care **442**
NURSING CARE **443**
    Assessing **443**
    Diagnosing, Planning, and Implementing **443**
    Evaluating **448**
    Discharge Considerations **448**
    Nursing Process Case Study: Client with Constipation **448**
Procedure 19-1 Changing a One-Piece, Drainable Bowel Diversion Ostomy Appliance **450**
Procedure 19-2 Administering an Enema **452**
Critical Thinking Care Map: Caring for a Client with Ulcerative Colitis **456**

Chapter 20   Activity, Rest, and Sleep **458**
Activity **459**
Normal Movement **459**
    Alignment and Posture **459**
    Joint Mobility **459**
Factors Affecting Body Alignment and Activity **460**
    Growth and Development **460**
    Physical Health **460**
    Mental Health **460**
    Nutrition **460**
Effects of Immobility **460**
    Musculoskeletal System **461**
    Cardiovascular System **461**
    Respiratory System **462**
    Metabolic System **462**
    Urinary System **462**
    Gastrointestinal System **463**
    Integumentary System **463**
    Psychoneurologic System **463**
    Collaborative Care **463**
NURSING CARE **464**
    Assessing **464**
    Diagnosing, Planning, and Implementing **466**
    Evaluating **472**
    Nursing Process Case Study: Client in Traction **473**
Rest and Sleep **473**
Physiology of Sleep **473**
    NREM Sleep **474**
    REM Sleep **474**

Functions of Sleep 474
Factors Affecting Sleep 474
    Illness 474
    Environment 475
    Lifestyle 475
    Emotional Stress 475
    Alchohol and Stimulants 475
    Smoking 475
    Diet 475
    Motivation 475
    Medications 475
Common Sleep Disorders 475
    Insomnia 475
    Hypersomnia 475
    Narcolepsy 475
    Sleep Apnea 476
    Parasomnias 476
    Sleep Deprivation 476
    Collaborative Care 476
NURSING CARE 477
    Assessing 477
    Diagnosing, Planning, and Implementing 477
    Evaluating 479
    Discharge Considerations 479
Procedure 20-1 Providing Passive Range-of-Motion Exercises 480
Procedure 20-2 Moving a Client in Bed 484
Procedure 20-3 Transferring a Client 488
Procedure 20-4 Assisting a Client to Walk 492
Procedure 20-5 Providing a Back Massage 494
Critical Thinking Care Map: Caring for a Client with Sleep Problems 497

Chapter 21 Medications 499
Drug Standards 500
    Legal Aspects of Drug Administration 501
Effects of Drugs 501
    Actions of Drugs on the Body 502
    Factors Affecting Medication Action 503
Medication Orders 503
    Essential Parts of a Medication Order 503
    Communicating a Medication Order 503
Systems of Measurement 507
    Metric System 507
    Apothecaries' System 508
    Household System 508
    Converting Units of Weight and Measure 508
    Calculating Dosages 509
Equipment 510
    Syringes 510
    Needles 510

Routes of Administration 511
    Oral Medications 511
    Nasogastric and Gastrostomy Medications 512
    Parenteral Medications 512
    Topical Medications 513
NURSING CARE 513
    Assessing 513
    Diagnosing, Planning, and Implementing 513
    Evaluating 520
    Nursing Process Case Study: Client with an Emergency Appendectomy 521
Procedure 21-1 Administering Oral Medications 524
Procedure 21-2 Preparing Medications 527
Procedure 21-3 Administering Injections 530
Procedure 21-4 Administering Ophthalmic Instillations 534
Procedure 21-5 Administering Otic Instillations 536
Procedure 21-6 Administering Vaginal Instillations 537
Critical Thinking Care Map: Caring for a Client with IDDM (Insulin-Dependent Diabetes Mellitus) 540

Chapter 22 Perioperative Nursing 542
Preoperative Phase 543
    Preoperative Consent 543
    Screening Tests 543
NURSING CARE 544
    Assessing 544
    Diagnosing, Planning, and Implementing 544
    Evaluating 546
Intraoperative Phase 546
    Types of Anesthesia 546
Postoperative Phase 546
    Immediate Postanesthetic Phase 546
    Preparing for Ongoing Care of the Postoperative Client 547
NURSING CARE 547
    Assessing 547
    Diagnosing, Planning, and Implementing 550
    Evaluating 553
    Discharge Considerations 553
    Nursing Process Case Study: A Postsurgical Client 553
Procedure 22-1 Teaching Moving, Leg Exercises, Deep Breathing, and Coughing 555
Procedure 22-2 Applying Antiemboli Stockings 557
Procedure 22-3 Managing Gastrointestinal Suction 558
Procedure 22-4 Cleaning a Sutured Wound and Applying a Sterile Dressing 561
Critical Thinking Care Map: Caring for a Client with an Amputated Arm 564

Chapter 23   Client Teaching **566**

Learning **567**

    Learning Theories **567**

    Applying Learning Theories **568**

    Factors That Facilitate Learning **568**

    Factors That Inhibit Learning **570**

Teaching **571**

    Teaching Clients and Their Families **571**

    Teaching in the Community **571**

    Teaching Health Personnel **572**

NURSING CARE 572

    Assessing 572

    Motivation 573

    Diagnosing, Planning, and Implementing 573

    Evaluating 577

    Nursing Process Case Study: Client with Laceration 579

Critical Care Thinking Map: Caring for a Client with Deficient Knowledge 582

UNIT IV   Promoting Psychosocial Health **585**

Chapter 24   Life Span Development **586**

Processes of Growth and Development **587**

    Relationship between Growth and Development **587**

Conception and Prenatal Development **588**

Neonates and Infants (Birth to 1 Year) **589**

    Physical Development **589**

    Psychosocial Development **591**

    Cognitive Development **591**

    Moral Development **591**

    Health Assessment and Promotion **591**

Toddlers (1 to 3 Years) **592**

    Physical Development **592**

    Psychosocial Development **594**

    Cognitive Development **594**

    Moral Development **594**

    Spiritual Development **594**

    Health Assessment and Promotion **594**

Preschoolers (4 and 5 Years) **594**

    Physical Development **594**

    Psychosocial Development **597**

    Cognitive, Moral, and Spiritual Development **597**

    Health Assessment and Promotion **597**

School-Age Children (6 to 12 Years) **597**

    Physical Development **598**

    Psychosocial Development **598**

    Cognitive, Moral, and Spiritual Development **598**

    Health Assessment and Promotion **599**

Adolescents (12 to 18 Years) **599**

    Physical Development **599**

    Psychosocial Development **600**

    Cognitive Development **600**

    Moral Development **600**

    Spiritual Development **600**

    Health Assessment and Promotion **601**

Young Adults (20 to 40 Years) **601**

    Physical Development **601**

    Psychosocial Development **601**

    Cognitive, Moral, and Spiritual Development **601**

    Health Assessment and Promotion **601**

Middle-Aged Adults (40 to 65 Years) **601**

    Physical Development **602**

    Psychosocial Development **602**

    Cognitive, Moral, and Spiritual Development **602**

    Health Assessment and Promotion **602**

Older Adults (Over 65 Years) **603**

    Physical Changes **603**

    Psychosocial Development **603**

    Cognitive Development **607**

    Moral Development **608**

    Spiritual Development **608**

    Health Assessment and Promotion **608**

NURSING CARE 608

    Assessing 608

    Diagnosing, Planning, and Implementing 608

    Evaluating 608

    Nursing Process Case Study: Client with Involutional Depression 608

Critical Thinking Care Map: Caring for a Client with Risk for Injury 611

Chapter 25   Client Communication **613**

Factors Influencing Communication **614**

    Development **614**

    Personal Space **614**

    Roles and Relationships **614**

    Environment **614**

    Group Communication **614**

Modes of Communication **616**

    Verbal Communication **618**

    Nonverbal Communication **618**

Therapeutic Communication **619**

    Therapeutic Techniques **619**

    Barriers to Communication **619**

Principles of Communication
for the Clinical Setting **619**

Attentive Listening **620**

Interviewing **620**

Kinds of Interview Questions **620**

Planning the Interview and Setting **620**

Stages of an Interview **622**

NURSING CARE 623

Assessing 623

Diagnosing, Planning, and Implementing 624

Evaluating 624

**Nursing Process Case Study: Client Affected
by Nurse Communication Barriers 624**

**Critical Thinking Care Map: Caring for a Client
with Anorexia 627**

Chapter 26 Delivering Culturally Competent
Care **629**

Concepts Related to Culture **630**

Culture and Health Care **631**

Health Beliefs and Practices **631**

Cultural Patterns **632**

Culturally Sensitive Care **635**

Barriers to Cultural Sensitivity **636**

NURSING CARE 636

Assessing 636

Diagnosing, Planning, and Implementing 637

Evaluating 637

Discharge Considerations 637

**Nursing Process Case Study: Providing Culturally
Sensitive Care 638**

**Critical Thinking Care Map: Caring for a Child Receiving
Home Remedies 640**

Chapter 27 Sensory Perception **642**

Components of the Sensory Process **643**

Sensory Reception and Perception **643**

Sensory Alterations **643**

Sensory Deprivation **643**

Sensory Overload **644**

Sensory Deficits **644**

Sensory Aids **644**

Factors Affecting Sensory Function **644**

Developmental Stage **644**

Culture **644**

Stress **645**

Medications and Illness **645**

Lifestyle and Personality **645**

The Confused Client **645**

NURSING CARE 645

Assessing 645

Diagnosing, Planning, and Implementing 647

Evaluating 651

Discharge Considerations 651

Nursing Process Case Study: Client in ICU 651

**Critical Thinking Care Map: Caring for the Client
with Sensory–Perceptual Alteration 654**

Chapter 28 Self-Concept **656**

Formation of Self-Concept **657**

Components of Self-Concept **657**

Body Image **657**

Role Performance **659**

Personal Identity **659**

Self-Esteem **659**

Factors Affecting Self-Concept **659**

NURSING CARE 659

Assessing 659

Diagnosing, Planning, and Implementing 661

Evaluating 663

**Nursing Process Case Study: Client
with Self-Concept Issues 663**

**Critical Thinking Care Map: Caring for a Client
with an Amputation 665**

Chapter 29 Sexuality **667**

Sex Versus Sexuality **668**

Pediatric and Adolescent Considerations **668**

Puberty **668**

Sexual Abuse **668**

Culture and Sexuality **671**

STD Prevention **671**

Prevention of Unwanted Pregnancies **671**

Screening for Cancer **672**

Maternal and Infant Considerations **673**

Pregnancy and Postpartum **673**

Infertility **674**

Adult Health Considerations **674**

Sexual Orientation **675**

Normal Sexual Response **675**

Geriatric Health Considerations **678**

Factors Affecting Sexual Response **678**

NURSING CARE 679

Assessing 679

Diagnosing, Planning, and Implementing 679

Evaluating 680

**Nursing Process Case Study: Client with Ineffective
Sexuality Patterns 680**

**Critical Thinking Care Map: Caring for a Client
with Altered Sexuality 683**

Chapter 30   Stress and Coping 685

Concepts of Stress **686**
  Sources of Stress **687**
  Models of Stress **687**
  Indicators of Stress **688**
Coping **690**
  Defense Mechanisms **690**
NURSING CARE 691
  Assessing 691
  Diagnosing, Planning, and Implementing 691
  Evaluating 694
  Discharge Considerations 695
  Nursing Process Case Study: Client with Stress 695
Stress Management for Nurses 696
**Critical Thinking Care Map: Caring for a Client
with Myocardial Infarction 698**

Chapter 31   Loss, Grieving, and Death 700

Loss and Grief **701**
Grief, Bereavement, and Mourning **701**
  Stages of Grieving **701**
  Manifestations of Grief **701**
  Factors Influencing Loss and Grief Responses **701**
NURSING CARE 703
  Assessing 703
  Diagnosing, Planning, and Implementing 704
  Evaluating 704
  **Nursing Process Case Study: Client with Metastatic
  Carcinoma of the Bowel 705**
Dying and Death **705**
  Responses to Dying and Death **705**
  Definitions and Signs of Death **706**
  Legalities Related to Death **706**
  Death-Related Religious and Cultural Practices **708**
  Hospice and Home Care **708**
NURSING CARE 709
  Assessing 709
  Diagnosing, Planning, and Implementing 709
  Evaluating 711
**Critical Thinking Care Map: Caring for a Client
with Anticipatory Grieving 713**

**UNIT V   Becoming a Licensed
              Nurse 717**

Chapter 32   Introduction to Leadership 718
Licensure **719**
  Suspension or Revocation **719**
  Standards of Care **719**
  Nurse Practice Acts **719**
  Health Insurance Portability and Accountability
  Act (HIPPA) **720**

Leadership **721**
  Types of Leaders **721**
  Team Leading **722**
  Delegation **722**
Reporting Techniques **722**
  Shift Report **722**
  Written Report **723**
Paperwork Responsibilities **724**
  Physician's Orders **724**
  Incident Reports **725**
Conflict Resolution **725**
  Stages of Conflict **725**
Nursing Trends **727**
  Nursing Care Delivery Methods **727**
  Men in Nursing **728**
Community Service **728**

**Chapter 33   Preparing to Take the Licensure
              Exam 731**

Development of the NCLEX-PN **732**
  Availability of the NCLEX-PN **732**
Understanding the NCLEX-PN Plan **732**
  Cognitive Levels of Questions **732**
  Test Plan Framework **732**
  Computerized Adaptive Testing (CAT) **733**
Preparing and Reviewing for the Exam **735**
  Preparing for the Exam **735**
  Reviewing for the Exam **735**
Evaluating Your Readiness to Take the Examination **736**
Applying to Take the NCLEX-PN **736**
Coping with Test Anxiety **736**
  Ways to Overcome Test Anxiety **737**
Taking the Examination **737**
Waiting for Your Results **738**

Chapter 34   Finding That First Job 741
Portfolio **742**
  Work Samples **742**
  Writing Samples **742**
  Community Service **742**
  Clinical Evaluation **742**
  Sample Thank You Letter **742**
  Sample Letter of Resignation **743**
Job Search **743**
  The Cover Letter **743**
  Résumé **744**
  References **748**
  Application **748**

Interviews **748**

Awaiting a Response **750**

The Hiring Process 750

Orientation **750**

Profession/Professionalism **751**

Probationary Period and Performance Evaluation **751**

Pursuing Your Career 752

Continuing Education **752**

Career Ladder **752**

Professional Organizations **752**

Networking and Collaboration **752**

Appendices

2003–2004 NANDA-Approved Nursing Diagnoses 757

Sample Critical Pathway for Client Following Total Mastectomy 759

Glossary 763

NCLEX-PN Answers; Hints for Critical Thinking 779

Bibliography 807

Index 817

Fundamental
NURSING CARE

UNIT I

The Nature of Nursing

Chapter 1 ▶ Understanding Nursing

Chapter 2 ▶ Legal and Ethical Issues of Nursing

Chapter 3 ▶ Critical Thinking and Nursing Theory/Models

Chapter 4 ▶ The LVN/LPN and the Nursing Process

Chapter 1

Understanding Nursing

SHARING experiences

Taking the time to plan a schedule and incorporate study time into my day has served me *well in developing organizational and time management skills.*

Shawna Thurman, VN student, Austin Community College, Austin, TX.

LEARNING outcomes

After completing this chapter, you will be able to:

- Discuss historical and contemporary factors influencing the development of nursing.
- Discuss the history of practical/vocational nursing.
- Identify the essential aspects of nursing.
- Describe the contribution made by men to nursing.
- Identify four major areas within the scope of LVN/LPN practice.
- Identify the purposes of nurse practice acts and standards for nursing practice.
- Relate essential nursing values to attitudes, personal qualities, and professional behaviors.
- Describe three important aspects of academic survival in nursing education.

"To look backward for a while is to refresh the eye, to restore it and to render it more fit for its prime function of looking forward," say the authors of *The Power to Heal*. Margaret Fairless Barber's statement sums up why the study of nursing history is important to every nurse beginning his or her career. The rich heritage that has gone before has shaped the nursing profession of the twenty-first century. **Nursing** has been defined by the American Nurses Association (ANA) in their Social Policy Statement in 1980 as "the diagnosis and treatment of human responses to actual and potential health problems" (ANA, 1980). While this is now considered to be the official definition of nursing, nursing has been described through the ages by many different actions and activities. Nurses have always been providers of health care, but they haven't always been the "Lady with the Lamp" or the "Angel of Mercy" or even the caring helper in starched white uniform and crisp cap (Figure 1-1 ◆).

Nursing today is far different from nursing as it was practiced 50 years ago. Standing at the beginning of the twenty-first century, we can only imagine how things will be at the end. The nursing profession must prepare for the future, but it must not forget past events while it considers today's issues and the effect they have on society.

Understanding Nursing Through History

INFLUENCES ON THE DEVELOPMENT OF NURSING

Nursing has undergone dramatic change in response to societal needs and influences. A look at nursing's beginnings reveals its continuing struggle for autonomy and professionalization. In recent decades, a renewed interest in nursing history has produced a growing amount of related literature. This section highlights only selected aspects of events that have influenced nursing practice.

Religion

Although many of the world's religions encourage benevolence, Western nursing was strongly influenced by the Christian value of "love thy neighbor as thyself" and Christ's parable of the Good Samaritan. During the third and fourth centuries, several wealthy matrons of the Roman Empire, including Marcella, Fabiola (Figure 1-2 ◆), and Paula, converted to Christianity and used their wealth to provide houses of care and healing (the forerunner of hospitals) for the poor, the sick, and the homeless.

These "deaconess groups" were suppressed during the Middle Ages by Western churches. However, groups of nursing providers resurfaced occasionally throughout the centuries. In 1836, Theodore Fliedner reinstituted the Order of Deaconesses and opened a small hospital and training school in

Figure 1-1. ◆ Although the modern-day nurse rarely wears a cap, it continues to be the symbol of the profession. Mother & daughter carry on the tradition. *Source:* Thom Palmer, Thom Palmer Photography, Yorba Linda, CA.

Figure 1-2. ◆ Wealthy Roman matrons like Fabiola (circa A.D. 400)—viewed by some as the patron saint of early nursing—used position and wealth to establish hospitals for the sick. Fabiola by Jean Jaques Henner (1829–1905 French). *Source:* SuperStock.

Figure 1-3. ◆ Considered to be the founder of modern nursing, Florence Nightingale (1820–1910) was influential in developing nursing education, practice, and administration. Her 1859 publication, *Notes on Nursing: What it Is and What It Is Not,* was intended for all women. *Source:* © Bettmann/CORBIS. Reprinted with permission.

Figure 1-4. ◆ Sojourner Truth (1797–1863), abolitionist, underground railroad agent, preacher, and women's rights advocate was a nurse for 4 years during the Civil War and worked as a nurse and counselor for the Freedom Relief Association after the war. *Source:* Courtesy of the National Portrait Gallery, Smithsonian Institution.

Kaiserswerth, Germany. Florence Nightingale (Figure 1-3 ◆) received her "training" in nursing at the Kaiserswerth School.

Early religious values, such as self-denial, spiritual calling, and devotion to duty and hard work, have dominated nursing throughout its history. Nurses' commitment to these values often resulted in exploitation and few monetary rewards. For some time, nurses themselves believed it was inappropriate to expect economic gain from their "calling."

War

Throughout history the need for nurses always increased during times of war. During the Crimean War (1854–1856), the inadequacy of care given to soldiers led to a public outcry in Great Britain. The role Florence Nightingale played in addressing this problem is well known. She was asked by Sir Sidney Herbert of the British War Department to recruit a group of female nurses to provide care to the sick and injured in the Crimea. Nightingale and her nurses transformed the military hospitals by setting up kitchens, a laundry, recreation centers, and reading rooms and by organizing classes for orderlies. Nightingale is credited with performing miracles. The mortality rate in the Barrack Hospital in Turkey, for example, was reduced to 1 percent.

During the American Civil War (1861–1865), several nurses contributed greatly to a country torn by internal strife. Harriet Tubman and Sojourner Truth (Figure 1-4 ◆) provided care and safety to slaves fleeing to the North on the "Underground Railroad." Mother Biekerdyke and Clara Barton searched the battlefields and gave care to injured and dying soldiers. Noted authors Walt Whitman and Louisa May Alcott volunteered as nurses to give care to injured soldiers in military hospitals.

Nurses continued to provide care and assistance through the turn of the twentieth century and the first World War. However, World War II casualties created an acute shortage of care. It was at this time that auxiliary health care workers became prominent. Practical nurses, aides, and technicians provided much of the actual nursing care under the instruction and supervision of registered nurses. At the same time, medical specialties arose to meet the needs of hospitalized clients. Nurse Ruby Bradley was the most decorated woman ever to serve in the U.S. military. As a POW for 37 months in a Japanese prison camp, she slowly starved so that children could eat. She dropped to 86 pounds and was able to smuggle surgical supplies into the POW camp under her ill-fitting uniform. Miss Bradley earned 34 medals and citations for bravery, including two Bronze Stars. Dr. Elizabeth Norman, in her book *We Band of Angels,* wrote about the sacrifice, terror, and contribution of nurses involved in the Bataan March. Military nurses experienced life, death, joy, and sorrow all within the time span of a duty shift.

It is estimated that between 4,000 and 15,000 nurses served during the Vietnam War. Very little has been written to document nurses' contributions during that time, but their work is commemorated near the Vietnam Memorial in Washington, D.C. (Figure 1-5 ◆).

Nurses continue to provide care to military personnel as well as civilians. Nurses served with distinction during Desert Storm and more recently treated victims of terrorist attacks at home and in Afghanistan. The combat nurse through the years has been on the cutting edge. Risk and ingenuity in the war zone have been responsible for many accepted nursing practices used today.

Societal Attitudes

Society's attitudes about nurses and nursing have significantly influenced professional nursing. Before the mid-1800s, nursing was without organization, education, or social status. The

Figure 1-5. ◆ Nurses served with distinction during the Vietnam War, but little has been written about them.

Figure 1-6. ◆ Sairy Gamp, a character in Dickens's book *Martin Chuzzlewit*, epitomizes nurses in the early 1800s. *Source:* © Bettmann/CORBIS. Reprinted with permission.

prevailing attitude was that a woman's place was in the home and that no respectable woman should have a career. Society's attitudes about nursing during much of the 1800s are reflected in the writings of Charles Dickens. The character of Sairy Gamp (in his 1896 novel *Martin Chuzzlewit*—Figure 1-6 ◆) epitomizes the nurse of the day, who lived and worked in appalling environments. Dickens characterized nurses' work as a repugnant form of domestic service, for which little or no special training was required. This portrayal greatly influenced attitudes toward nurses and training.

The "Guardian Angel" or "Angel of Mercy" image arose in the latter part of the nineteenth century, largely because of the work of Florence Nightingale. After Nightingale brought respectability to the nursing profession, nurses were viewed as noble, compassionate, moral, religious, dedicated, and self-sacrificing. Another image that arose in the early nineteenth century was the nurse as doctor's handmaiden. This image evolved when women did not yet have the right to vote, when family structures were largely paternalistic, and when the use of scientific knowledge was viewed as a male domain.

LEADING NURSES OF HISTORY

Nightingale (1820–1910)

Florence Nightingale's contributions to nursing are well documented. Her achievements in improving the standards for the

care of war casualties in Crimea earned her the title "Lady with the Lamp" (see Figure 1-3). Her efforts in reforming hospitals and in producing and implementing public health policies also made her an accomplished political nurse. She was the first nurse to exert political pressure on government. She is also recognized as nursing's first scientist–theorist for her work *Notes on Nursing: What It Is, and What It Is Not.*

When she returned from Crimea, a grateful English public gave Nightingale an honorarium of £4500. She used this money to establish the Nightingale Training School for Nurses in 1860. At St. Thomas Hospital in London, England, she taught her straightforward requirements.

Nightingale believed that nursing education should develop both the intellect and character of the nurse. Accordingly, she gave students a solid background in sciences to understand the theory behind their care. To develop character, she assigned readings in the humanities to increase their understanding of human ethics and morals. She believed that nurses should never stop learning. To her nurses she wrote, "To nurse is a field of which one may safely say: there is no end in what we may be learning everyday" (Schuyler, 1992). The school served as a model for other training schools. Its graduates traveled to other countries to manage hospitals and to institute nurse-training programs.

Nightingale's vision of nursing, which included public health and health promotion roles for nurses, was only partially addressed in the early days. The focus first was on developing the profession within hospitals. Although Miss Nightingale died in 1910, her influence continues in nursing today.

Barton (1812–1912)

Clara Barton (Figure 1-7 ◆) was a schoolteacher who volunteered as a nurse during the American Civil War. Her respon-

Figure 1-7. ◆ Clara Barton (1812–1912) organized the American National Red Cross, which linked with the International Red Cross when the U.S. Congress ratified the Geneva Convention in 1992. *Source:* © Bettmann/CORBIS. Reprinted with permission.

sibility was to organize the nursing services. Barton is noted for her role in establishing the American Red Cross, which linked with the International Red Cross when the United States Congress ratified the Treaty of Geneva (Geneva Convention). In 1882, Barton persuaded Congress to ratify this treaty, so that the Red Cross could perform humanitarian efforts in times of peace.

Wald (1867–1940)
Lillian Wald (Figure 1-8 ◆) is considered the founder of public health nursing. Wald and Mary Brewster were the first to offer trained nursing services to the poor in the New York slums. Their home among the poor on the upper floor of a tenement, called the Henry Street Settlement and Visiting Nurse

Figure 1-8. ◆ Lillian Wald (1867–1940) founded the Henry Street Settlement and Visiting Nurse Service (circa 1893), which provided nursing and social services and organized educational and cultural activities. She is considered to be founder of public health nursing. *Source:* University of Iowa, College of Nursing, Iowa City, IA.

Service, provided nursing and social services, and also organized educational and cultural activities. Soon after the founding of the Henry Street Settlement, school nursing was established as an adjunct to visiting nursing.

Dock (1858–1956)
Lavinia Dock (Figure 1-9 ◆) was a feminist, as well as a prolific writer, political activist, suffragette, and friend of Wald. She participated in protest movements for women's rights that resulted in the 1920 passage of the 19th Amendment to the U.S. Constitution, granting women the right to vote. In addition, Dock campaigned for legislation to allow nurses rather than physicians to control their profession. In 1893, Dock, Mary Adelaide Nutting, and Isabel Hampton Robb founded the American Society of Superintendents of Training Schools for Nurses of the United States and Canada. This was a precursor to the current National League for Nursing.

Sanger (1879–1966)
Margaret Higgins Sanger (Figure 1-10 ◆) a public health nurse from New York, has had a lasting impact on women's health care. Imprisoned for opening the first birth control information clinic in America, she is considered the founder of Planned Parenthood.

Breckinridge (1881–1965)
After World War I, the Frontier Nursing Service (FNS) was established by a notable pioneer nurse, Mary Breckinridge (Figure 1-11 ◆). In 1918, she worked with the American Committee for Devastated France, distributing food, clothing, and supplies to rural villages and taking care of sick children. In 1921, Breckinridge returned to the United States with plans to provide health care to the people of rural America.

In 1925 Breckinridge and two other nurses began the Frontier Nursing Service in Leslie County, Kentucky. Within

Figure 1-9. ◆ Nursing leader and suffragist Lavinia L. Dock (1885–1956) was active in the protest movement for women's rights that resulted in the United States constitutional amendment allowing women to vote in 1920. *Source:* Courtesy of Millbank Memorial Library, Teachers' College, Columbia University. Reprinted with permission.

Figure 1-10. ◆ Nurse activist Margaret Sanger, considered to be the founder of Planned Parenthood, was imprisoned for opening the first birth control information clinic in Baltimore in 1916. *Source:* © Bettmann/CORBIS. Reprinted with permission.

this organization, Breckinridge started one of the first midwifery training schools in the United States.

Kenney (1886–1952)

Sister Elizabeth Kenney, an Austrian nurse, is remembered for her efforts to fight poliomyelitis. She devised a method for treatment of poliomyelitis by stimulating and reeducating affected muscles. In the early 1940s she came to the United States. She gained the support of the American Medical Association and in 1943 established the Elizabeth Kenney Institute in Minneapolis, Minnesota, to train nurses and physiotherapists in her methods. Sister Kenney's death in 1952

Figure 1-11. ◆ Mary Breckinridge, a nurse who practiced midwifery in England, Australia, and New Zealand, founded the Frontier Nursing Service in Kentucky in 1925 to provide family-centered health care to rural populations. *Source:* Reprinted with permission of Frontier Nursing Service.

prevented her from seeing the introduction of the Salk vaccine program, which has virtually put an end to the disease she dedicated her life to treating.

MALE NURSES IN HISTORY

Women were not the sole providers of nursing services. The first nursing school in the world was started in India in about 250 B.C. Only men were considered to be "pure" enough to fulfill the role of nurse at that time. In Jesus's parable in the New Testament, the good Samaritan paid an innkeeper to provide care for the injured man. Paying a man to provide nursing care was fairly common. During the Crusades, several orders of knights provided nursing care to their sick and injured comrades and also built hospitals (Figure 1-12A ◆). The organization and management of their hospitals set a

A

B

Figure 1-12. ◆ **A.** The Knights of Saint Lazarus (established circa 1200) dedicated themselves to the care of people with leprosy, syphilis, and chronic skin conditions. In the mid-thirteenth century, leprosy was viewed as an incurable and terminal disease. **B.** Modern male nurses work side by side with their female colleagues to provide care to hospitalized clients. *Source:* (1-12A) © Bettmann/CORBIS. Reprinted with permission.

standard for the administration of hospitals throughout Europe at that time. St. Camillus de Lellis started out as a soldier and later turned to nursing. He started the sign of the Red Cross and developed the first ambulance service. Friar Juan de Mena was shipwrecked off the south Texas coast in 1554. He is the first identified nurse in what would become the United States. James Derham, a black slave who worked as a nurse in New Orleans in the late 1700s, saved the money he earned to purchase his freedom. Later, he studied medicine and became a well-respected physician in Philadelphia. During the Civil War, both sides had military men who cared for the sick and wounded.

In 1876, only three years after the first U.S. nurse received her diploma from New England Hospital for Women and Children, the Alexian brothers opened their first hospital in the United States and a school to educate men in nursing.

During the years from the Civil War to the Korean War, men were not permitted to serve as nurses in the military. Today, men have resumed their historical place in the profession. As the history of nursing continues to be written, men and women will work side by side (Figure 1-12B). In the years to come the profession will be without gender distinction.

LICENSED PRACTICAL AND VOCATIONAL NURSES IN HISTORY

The site for the first training for practical nurses was at the Young Women's Christian Association (YWCA) in New York City in 1892. The following year this became the Ballard School. The program of study was 3 months long, and the participants studied special techniques for caring for the sick as well as a variety of homemaking techniques.

Much of the care during this time was done in the client's home, making the LPN a home health or visiting nurse. Eleven years later, a second school, the Thompson Practical Nursing School, was established.

In 1914, the state legislature in Mississippi passed the first laws governing the practice of Practical Nurses. Other states were slow to follow. By 1940, only six states had passed such laws. In 1955, the state board test pool of the NLN Education Committee established the procedures for testing graduates of approved practical/vocational education programs in all states. Graduates who passed the examination became licensed practical nurses (LPNs) or, in California and Texas, licensed vocational nurses (LVNs). Each state set its own passing score.

Today, a graduate of an approved LPN/LVN training program is eligible to take the National Council Licensing Examination for Practical Nursing (**NCLEX-PN**). The examination is computerized, with a "pass" score that is standardized throughout the United States. All states have licensing laws. *Interstate endorsement* (reciprocity between states) exists. This means that an LPN/LVN from one state can apply for licensure in another state without retesting. It is the responsibility of the individual nurse to contact the board of nursing in the jurisdiction where he or she wishes to work. The nurse must apply for licensure and for information regarding the scope of practice within that state. See Table 1-1 ◆ for important events in the history of practical/vocational nursing.

 Understanding Contemporary Nursing Practice

An understanding of contemporary nursing practice includes a look at definitions of nursing, recipients of nursing, scope of nursing, factors influencing contemporary nursing practice, and opportunities for LPNs/LVNs in contemporary nursing practice.

DEFINITIONS OF NURSING

Many definitions of nursing exist, but some misrepresent the complex knowledge and skill of professional nursing. Common dictionary definitions, for example, still refer to the nurse as "a person, usually a woman, trained to care for the sick." Today, however, many men are choosing to become nurses. Nurses also provide preventive and health-promoting care to well clients, not just care to the sick.

Florence Nightingale defined nursing as "the act of utilizing the environment of the patient to assist him in his recovery" (Nightingale, 1860). Nightingale considered a clean, well-ventilated, and quiet environment essential for recovery. In 1966, Virginia Henderson wrote, "The unique function of the nurse is to assist the individual, sick or well, in the performance of those activities contributing to health or its recovery (or to peaceful death) that he would perform unaided if he had the necessary strength, will, or knowledge, and to do this in such a way as to help him gain independence as rapidly as possible" (Henderson, 1966, p. 3).

A number of nurse theorists have developed theoretical definitions of nursing (see Chapter 3). 🔗 These are important because they describe the interrelationship among nurses, nursing, the client, and the intended client outcome—health.

Certain themes are common to many of these definitions:

◆ Nursing is caring.
◆ Nursing is an art.
◆ Nursing is a science.
◆ Nursing is client centered.
◆ Nursing is holistic.
◆ Nursing is adaptive.
◆ Nursing is concerned with health promotion, health maintenance, and health restoration.
◆ Nursing is a helping profession.

Recipients of Nursing Care

The recipients of nursing are sometimes called consumers, sometimes patients, and sometimes clients. A **consumer** is

TABLE 1-1	IMPORTANT HISTORICAL EVENTS FOR LPN/LVNs	
DATE	EVENT	IMPORTANCE
1893	Ballard School at YMCA Brooklyn, NY	First formal training for practical nurses
1914	Mississippi Legislature passed license laws for practical nurses	First laws passed to govern the practice of practical nurses
1917	Smith-Hughes Act	Provided federal funding for vocationally oriented schools of practical nursing
1918	Third school established	Even with new schools and federal assistance, the need for nurses could not be met because of the demand created by the war and epidemics.
1941	The association of Practical Nurse Schools was founded. The name was changed to National Association of Practical Nurse Education (NAPNE) in 1942.	Standards for practical nurse education were established.
1944	U.S. Department of Education commissioned an intensive study differentiating tasks of the practical nurse.	The outcome of the study differentiated tasks performed by the practical nurse from those performed by the registered nurse. State boards of nursing established tasks which could be performed by both groups.
1945	New York established mandatory licensure for practical nurses.	The first state to require licensure; by 1955 all other states had followed suit.
1949	The National Federation of Licensed Practical Nurses (NFLPN) was founded by Lillian Kuster. The name was changed to the National Association of Licensed Practical Nurse Education and Services in 1959.	The discipline now had an official organization with membership limited to LPN/LVNs.
1955	All states passed licensing laws for practical/vocational nurses.	Practice of nursing by licensed practical nursing was regulated in all states.
1961	The National League of Nursing established a Department of Practical Nursing.	Through this department schools of practical nursing could be accredited by the NLN.
1965	American Nurses Association published a position paper that influenced the attitude about practical/vocational nursing.	The paper clearly defined the two levels of nursing: registered nursing and technical nursing. The exclusion of the term practical/vocational nurse necessitated that the LPN/LVN prove his/her worth to provide valuable nursing interventions under the direction of a registered nurse.
1994	Computerized NCLEX-PN examination available to graduates of practical/vocational nursing programs in all states.	Allowed for more availability of test dates and interstate endorsement of licensure.

an individual, a group of people, or a community that uses a service or commodity. People who use health care products or services are consumers of health care. **A patient** is a person who is waiting for or undergoing medical treatment and care. The word *patient* comes from a Latin word meaning "to suffer" or "to bear." Traditionally, the person receiving health care has been called a patient, and people become patients when they seek assistance because of illness. Some nurses believe that the word patient implies passive acceptance of the decisions and care of health professionals. Because nurses interact with family, friends, and healthy people as well as those who are ill, nurses increasingly refer to recipients of health care as *clients*.

A **client** is a person who engages the advice or services of someone who is qualified to provide this service. Therefore, a client is a collaborator, a person who is also responsible for his or her own health. The health status of a client is the responsibility of the individual in collaboration with health professionals. In this book, *client* is the preferred term, although consumer and patient may be used in some instances.

Scope of Nursing

Nurses provide care for individuals, families, and communities. Nursing practice involves four areas: promoting health and wellness, preventing illness, restoring health, and caring for the dying.

PROMOTING HEALTH AND WELLNESS. Wellness is a state of well-being. It means engaging in attitudes and behavior that enhance the quality of life and maximize personal potential. Nurses promote wellness in individuals and groups who are healthy or ill. This may involve activities to enhance healthy lifestyles, to prevent drug and alcohol misuse, to restrict smoking, and to prevent accidents and injury in the home and workplace.

PREVENTING ILLNESS. Illness may be defined as the highly individualized response a person has to a disease. The goal of illness prevention programs is to maintain optimal health by preventing disease. Nursing activities that prevent illness include immunizations, prenatal and infant care, and prevention of sexually transmitted disease.

RESTORING HEALTH. Restoring health focuses on the ill client. This help extends from early detection through the recovery period. Nursing activities include the following:

◆ Providing direct care to the ill person, such as administering medications, assisting with activities of daily living, and specific procedures and treatments
◆ Performing diagnostic and assessment procedures, such as measuring blood pressure and examining feces for occult blood
◆ Consulting with other health care professionals about client problems
◆ Teaching clients about recovery activities, such as exercises that will hasten recovery after a stroke
◆ Rehabilitating clients to their optimal functional level following physical or mental illness, injury, or chemical addiction

CARE OF THE DYING. This area of nursing practice involves comforting and caring for people of all ages who are dying. It includes helping clients live as comfortably as possible until death and helping support persons cope with death. Nurses carry out these activities in homes, hospitals, and extended care facilities. Some agencies, called hospices, are specifically designed for this purpose (see Chapter 31). 🔗

FACTORS INFLUENCING CONTEMPORARY NURSING

Social forces strongly influence the nursing profession. These forces usually affect the entire health care system. Nursing, as a major component of that system, cannot avoid the effects.

Economics

Greater financial support provided through public and private health insurance programs has increased the demand for nursing care. Health services such as emergency room care, mental health counseling, and preventive physical examinations have become more accessible to many people. Costs of health care have also increased during the past two decades.

REIMBURSEMENT. In 1982, Medicare revised its payment system to hospitals and physicians. Reimbursement fees were established that related to the client's medical diagnosis. This classification system is known as **diagnostic-related groups (DRGs).** The system has categories that establish pretreatment diagnosis billing categories.

Since the implementation of this legislation, clients in hospitals are more acutely ill than before. Clients once considered ill enough to be hospitalized are now treated at home. However, health care costs continue to rise.

CONSUMER DEMANDS. Consumers of nursing services (the public) have become an increasingly effective force in changing nursing practice. On the whole, people are better educated and have more knowledge about health and illness than in the past. Consumers also have become more aware of others' needs for care. The ethical and moral issues raised by poverty and neglect have made people more vocal about the needs of minority groups and the poor.

The public's concepts of health and nursing have also changed. Most now believe that health is a right of all people, not just a privilege of the rich. Furthermore, many people now want more than freedom from disease. They want energy, vitality, and a feeling of wellness. The consumer has become an increasingly active participant in making decisions about health and nursing care.

FAMILY STRUCTURE. New family structures influence the need for and provision of nursing services. People may live far from their extended families. Children may be raised by single parents, or both parents may work to support an extended family. These family units need support services, such as day care or elder care centers.

Adolescent mothers also need specialized nursing services, both while they are pregnant and after their babies are born. These young mothers usually have the normal needs of teenagers as well as those of new mothers. Many teenage mothers are raising their children alone with little, if any, assistance from the child's father. This type of single-parent family is especially vulnerable, because motherhood compounds the difficulties of adolescence. Since many of these families live in poverty, the children often do not receive preventive immunizations and are at increased risk for nutritional and other health problems.

Science and Technology

Advances in science and technology affect nursing practice. For example, people with acquired immune deficiency syndrome (AIDS) can receive new drug therapies to prolong life and delay the onset of AIDS-associated diseases. Nurses must be knowledgeable about the action of such drugs and the needs of clients receiving them. As physicians expand their knowledge base and technical skills, nurses acquire complementary knowledge and skills and adapt to meet the new needs of clients.

In some settings, technologic advances have required that nurses become highly specialized. Nurses frequently use sophisticated computerized equipment to monitor or treat clients. As technologies change, nursing education changes, and nurses need more education to practice effective, safe nursing care.

The Women's Movement

The women's movement has empowered nurses to identify "the commonality and interconnectedness of nurses' experience as women and men and as health care workers." This enables nurses to develop a clearer group identity, which can lead to greater empowerment and involvement in effective political action (Mason, Backer, & Georges, 1993, p. 107). Recently, the federal government has been challenged in its funding of research about women's health problems. As a result, a new concern for women's issues has emerged.

Nurse Practice Acts

Nurse practice acts, or legal acts for professional nursing practice, regulate the practice of nursing in the United States and Canada. Each state in the United States and each province in Canada has its own act.

Although practice acts may differ in various jurisdictions, they all have a common purpose: to protect the public. The title of nurse can legally be used *only* by an individual who is licensed as a registered nurse or a licensed practical or vocational nurse. For additional information, see Chapter 32. ⊂⊃

Nursing Standards

Within the nursing education program, the nurse develops, clarifies, and internalizes professional values. The National Federation of Licensed Practical Nurses Inc. has identified specific standards (Box 1-1 ◆). These should be adhered to by LPN/LVNs in all areas of practice.

OPPORTUNITIES FOR LPN/LVNS IN CONTEMPORARY NURSING

Practice Settings

In the past, the acute care hospital was the major practice setting open to most nurses. Today the LPN/LVN works in hospitals, in clients' homes, community agencies, ambulatory clinics, health maintenance organizations (HMOs), and skilled nursing facilities (see Chapter 5). ⊂⊃ See also Chapter 34 for a description of opportunities available to the LPN/LVN. ⊂⊃

LPN/LVNs work under their own license under direct supervision of a physician or a registered nurse. LPN/LVNs may be involved in clinical planning meetings because of their expertise, but they are required to do this less than other licensed health care providers. Their primary duty is the delivery of care to the client.

Professional Organizations

Operation under the umbrella of a professional organization differentiates a profession from an occupation.

NATIONAL ASSOCIATION FOR PRACTICAL NURSE EDUCATION AND SERVICE.
The National Association for Practical Nurse Education and Service (NAPNES) was established in 1941. This was the first national organization for the practical/vocational level of nursing. NAPNES was responsible for the accreditation of LPN/LVN education programs from 1945 until 1984.

NATIONAL FEDERATION OF LICENSED PRACTICAL NURSES.
In 1949, Lillian Custer founded the National Federation of Licensed Practical Nurses (NFLPN). This organization is considered to be the official membership organization for LPNs and LVNs. Only individuals with those licenses may join the organization. The National League for Nursing, formed in 1952, is an organization of both individuals and agencies. In 1961 the NLN established the Council for Practical Nursing Programs. This arm of the organization assumed responsibility for promoting the interests of LPN/LVNs in the NLN. All of these organizations provide continuing education opportunities and publish literature of interest to the LPN/LVN.

Student Organizations

NFLPN welcomes LVN/LPN students as members. NFLPN provides leadership for nearly one million licensed practical and vocational nurses employed in the United States. It also fosters high standards of practical/vocational nursing education and practice so that the best nursing care will be available to every client. The NFLPN serves as the central source of information on what is new and changing in practical/vocational nursing education and practice on the local, state, and national level. The organization is a three-tiered concept of local, state, and national enrollment. By participating in local, state, and national meetings and conferences, the VN/PN student can learn firsthand how a professional organization works to maintain the professional status of the membership. NFLPN also encourages continuing education and publishes a quarterly magazine, *Practical Nursing Today*. Through relationships with the National Council of State Boards of Nursing and the U.S. Congress, the NFLPN enables policy makers to better understand the role of practical/vocational nursing in the nation's health care delivery system (NFLPN, 10/31/2000).

Health Occupation Students of America (HOSA)

HOSA is a nationally recognized career technical student organization, which was founded in 1976. HOSA provides a unique program of leadership and team-building development, motivation, and recognition experience. HOSA is an instructional tool integrated into the health careers classroom by the instructor. It is an intracurricular activity, which reinforces technical skills and supports service to the community. HOSA helps to develop the "total person." The national organization is made up of health occupation students from 37 affiliated states and Puerto Rico. HOSA's membership is made

MediaLink ● Responsibilities of an Employee

Education

The licensed practical/vocational nurse:

1. Shall complete a formal education program in practical nursing approved by the appropriate nursing authority in a state.
2. Shall successfully pass the National Council Licensure Examination for Practical Nurses.
3. Shall participate in initial orientation within the employing institution.

Legal/Ethical Status

The licensed practical/vocational nurse:

1. Shall hold a current license to practice nursing as an LP/VN in accordance with the law of the state wherein employed.
2. Shall know the scope of nursing practice authorized by the Nursing Practice Act in the state wherein employed.
3. Shall have a personal commitment to fulfill the legal responsibilities inherent in good nursing practice.
4. Shall take responsible actions in situations wherein there is unprofessional conduct by a peer or other health care provider.
5. Shall recognize and commit to meet the ethical and moral obligations of the practice of nursing.
6. Shall not accept or perform professional responsibilities that the individual knows (s)he is not competent to perform.

Practice

The licensed practical/vocational nurse:

1. Shall accept assigned responsibilities as an accountable member of the health care team.
2. Shall function within the limits of educational preparation and experience, as related to the assigned duties.
3. Shall function with other members of the health care team in promoting and maintaining health, preventing disease and disability, caring for and rehabilitating individuals who are experiencing an altered health state, and contributing to the ultimate quality of life until death.
4. Shall know and utilize the nursing process in planning, implementing, and evaluating health services and nursing care for the individual patient or group.
   a. Planning: The planning of nursing includes:
      1. Assessment of health status of the individual patient, the family, and community groups
      2. Analysis of the information gained from assessment
      3. Identification of health goals
   b. Implementation: The plan for nursing care is put into practice to achieve the stated goals and includes:
      1. Observing, recording, and reporting significant changes that require intervention or different goals
      2. Applying nursing knowledge and skills to promote and maintain health, to prevent disease and disability, and to optimize functional capabilities of an individual patient

      3. Assisting the patient and family with activities of daily living and encouraging self-care as appropriate
      4. Carrying out therapeutic regimens and protocols prescribed by an RN, physician, or other persons authorized by state law
   c. Evaluation: The plan for nursing care and its implementations are evaluated to measure the progress toward the stated goals and will include appropriate persons and/or groups to determine:
      1. The relevancy of current goals in relation to the progress of the individual patient
      2. The involvement of the recipients of care in the evaluation process
      3. The quality of the nursing action in the implementation of the plan
      4. A reordering of priorities or new goal setting in the care plan
5. Shall participate in peer review and other evaluation processes.
6. Shall participate in the development of policies concerning the health and nursing needs of society and in the roles and functions of the LP/VN.

Continuing Education

The licensed practical/vocational nurse:

1. Shall be responsible for maintaining the highest possible level of professional competence at all times.
2. Shall periodically reassess career goals and select continuing education activities that will help to achieve these goals.
3. Shall take advantage of continuing education opportunities that will lead to personal growth and professional development.
4. Shall seek and participate in continuing education activities that are approved for credit by appropriate organizations, such as the NFLPN.

Specialized Nursing Practice

The licensed practical/vocational nurse:

1. Shall have had at least one year's experience in nursing at the staff level.
2. Shall present personal qualifications that are indicative of potential abilities for practice in the chosen specialized nursing area.
3. Shall present evidence of completion of a program or course that is approved by an appropriate agency to provide the knowledge and skills necessary for effective nursing services in the specialized field.
4. Shall meet all of the standards of practice as set forth in this document.

Source: National Federation of Licensed Practical Nurses, Inc. Copyright 1991.

up of secondary, postsecondary, and collegiate students. Health care professionals, alumni, and business and industry members are welcome. There is also an associate membership category for students who are interested in health careers but who are not enrolled in a program. Through participation, the LVN/LPN student can network with other health career students. Involvement in a student organization demonstrates to students the benefits of participating in professional organizations once they have graduated.

 # Understanding Nursing Education

LPN/LVN training programs can be found in many different types of schools. In some states they are part of high schools. In others, they are in community college settings, vocational training centers, or private schools.

The length of the programs is dictated by the governing nursing board of each state. Some programs can be completed in about 9 months. Others take up to 2 years. Some are full time day-school programs. Others are part time, with classes and clinical experience held in the evenings and on weekends.

ACADEMIC SUCCESS SKILLS

When students enroll in a program of study, they bring with them varying degrees of life experience, educational backgrounds, and ethnic/cultural influences. The age of LPN/LVN students within a class may range from young adult to near retirement. Students may be realizing a lifelong dream to be a nurse. They may be making a career change. They may be preparing for their first job. No matter what the circumstance or their previous experience, they all will need to dedicate themselves to study for a period of 9 months or more.

How to Read the Textbook

Reading is one of the most basic academic skills. Reading enhances learning and reinforces lecture material. Many methods can be used to extract information from the assigned reading material. Once one or more of these techniques have been mastered, the student will be able to decrease reading time while improving comprehension. See Table 1-2 ◆ for textbook reading guidelines.

Textbook reading should begin the day you purchase the book. Begin by reading the preface and other material in the front of the book. Become familiar with how the book is organized and any special features that will make your reading and studying easier. Review the table of contents and look over the appendices. By spending a few minutes becoming familiar with the book, you will be ready to use your book when the first reading assignment is given. The textbook is a great reference as well a source for clarifying lecture material.

Read textbook assignments before the class in which the material will be covered. Reading beforehand will help you organize your thoughts, and help you spell and define words

TABLE 1-2	TEXTBOOK MASTERY STRATEGIES
SP2CSD (Supermarket Theme)	
S – Shop	What's available/overview main idea
P – Purchase	Selectivity—picking out what you want
C – Consume	Read
C – Chew	Cluster ideas/record
S – Swallow	Recitation
D – Digest	Review/relationship
S2RQ2R	
S – Survey	Bold, main idea, headings
R – Read	Read, general overview
R – Record	Write down concepts
QR – Question and Recite	Use key concepts question and recite information
R – Review	Review what you wrote down
SQ3R (Most famous system, most applicable to technical manuals) Overview, look over headings, of entire chapter, italicized information, summary—define study unit	
S – Survey	Look for heads and turn headings into questions
Q – Question	Read to answer questions
3R – Read Recite Review	Recite answers to questions Review to check your memory (reflect—create ties to the big picture)

that may be used in lecture. Although many students use highlighter pens while reading, it is much better to save the highlighter for reviewing lectures notes or marking the location of answers to the chapter's study questions (Porter).

How to Take Tests

ANSWERING MULTIPLE-CHOICE QUESTIONS. Most tests given in nursing programs will be objective, multiple-choice tests. These are the same types of questions used on the NCLEX-PN exam. Multiple-choice questions can evaluate your knowledge of facts as well as your ability to apply that knowledge within a client care scenario. Each question will consist of a stem and four answer choices. Read each question completely in order to understand what is being asked. Then read each of the choices. Try to eliminate one or more of the choices. Examine each choice to see if anything is incorrect within the answer itself. Watch out for choices that are correct and accurate on their own, but that do not answer the question as it is written. See Box 1-2 ◆ for an example.

Multiple-choice questions can test knowledge, comprehension, and application and ability to analyze. Table 1-3 ◆ provides examples and comparison of each type.

Questions that include choices such as "all of the above" or "none of the above" have been eliminated from the NCLEX-PN examination. However, some textbooks have them as study questions, and some instructors may test with them. A choice of this type can be confirmed or eliminated easily. If you have identified one choice as being correct, then

TABLE 1-3	TEST QUESTIONS AND LEVELS OF LEARNING		
LEVELS	**INFORMATION REQUIRED**	**EXAMPLE**	**RATIONALE**
Knowledge question	Requires recall of information. To answer a knowledge question, you need to commit facts to memory. Knowledge questions expect you to know terminology, specific facts, trends, sequences, classifications, categories, criteria, structures, principles, generalizations, or theories.	When administering medications, qid means: a. Once a day b. Twice a day c. Three times a day d. Fours times a day	To answer this questions correctly you have to know the meaning of the abbreviation qid (fours times a day).
Comprehension question	Requires you to understand information. To answer a comprehension question, not only must you commit facts to memory but it is essential that you can translate, interpret, and determine the implications of the information. You demonstrate understanding when you translate or paraphrase information, interpret or summarize information, or determine the implications, consequences, corollaries, or effects of information. Comprehension questions expect you not only to know but also to understand the information being tested. You do not necessarily have to relate it to other material or see its fullest implications.	To evaluate the therapeutic effect of a cathartic, the nurse should assess the client for: a. Increased urinary output b. A decrease in anxiety c. A bowel movement d. Pain relief	To answer this question, you not only have to know that a cathartic is a potent laxative that stimulates the bowel, but that the increase in peristalsis will result in a bowel movement (answer c).
Application question	Require you to utilize knowledge. To answer an application question, you must take remembered and comprehended concepts and apply them to concrete situations. The abstractions may be theories, technical principles, rules of procedures, generalizations, or ideas that have to be applied in a scenario. Application questions test your ability to use information in a new situation.	An elderly client's skin looks, dry, thin, and fragile. When providing back care, the nurse should: a. Apply a moisturizing body lotion b. Wash back with soap and water c. Massage back using short kneading strokes d. Leave excess lubricant on the client's skin	To answer this question, you must know that dry, thin, fragile skin is common in the elderly and that moisturizing lotion helps the skin to retain water and become more supple. When presented with this scenario, you have to apply your knowledge concerning developmental changes in the elderly and the benefits of using moisturizing lotion.
Analysis question	Requires you to interpret a variety of data and recognize the commonalities, differences, and interrelationships among present ideas. Analysis questions make assumptions that you know, understand, and can apply information. Now you must identify, examine, dissect, evaluate, or investigate the organization, systematic arrangement, or structure of the information presented in the question. This type of question tests your analytical ability.	A client who is undergoing cancer chemotherapy says to the nurse, "This is no way to live." Which of the following responses uses reflective technique? a. "Tell me more about what you are thinking." b. "You sound discouraged today." c. "Life is not worth living?" d. "What are you saying?"	To answer this question, you must understand the communication techniques of reflection, clarification, and paraphrasing. You must also analyze the statements and identify which techniques are represented. This question requires you to understand, interpret, and differentiate information to know that the correct answer would be c.

BOX 1-2 EXAMPLE OF MULTIPLE-CHOICE QUESTION

Which of the following men was responsible for the reduction of maternal death related to infection transmitted by way of unwashed hands?

1. Joseph Lister
2. Louis Pasteur
3. Ignaz Semmelweis
4. Karl Crede

Although all four people were involved in prevention of infection and/or disease, the correct answer is 3. Ignaz Semmelweis was the person who discovered that puerperal fever was related to examination of mothers in the intra– and postpartum period by doctors who had not washed their hands after performing autopsies.

TABLE 1-4 KEY WORDS IN ESSAY EXAMS

KEY WORD	EXPLANATION
Compare	To point out similarities and differences
Contrast	To point out differences only
Define	Several connotations: (1) to give the meaning of, (2) to explain or describe essential qualities, (3) to place it in the class to which it belongs and set it off from other items in the same class.
Describe	Enumerate (list) the special features of the topic. Shows how the topic is different from similar or related items. Give an account of, tell about, and give a word picture of.
Discuss	Present various sides or points, talk over, consider the different sides. A discussion is usually longer than an explanation of the same subject.
Explain	Make plain or clear, interpret, tell "how" to do.
Identify	Show recognition
Illustrate	Describe in narrative form using "word pictures" to provide examples
Justify	Provide supporting data for opinions or actions
List or Name	Present a group of names or items in a category
Outline	Give information systematically in headings and subheadings
Summarize	Present in condensed form; give main points briefly

you can eliminate "none of the above." If you can identify one choice that is incorrect, then "all of the above" can also be eliminated. If you can identify at least two answers as correct, then the question qualifies as an "all of the above" answer.

If you are able to narrow your choice to two options, don't spend too much time deciding between them. More likely than not, your first impression is correct. Once you have identified your choice, don't go back and change it unless you later figure out the correct response with absolute certainty. (The NCLEX-PN exam is discussed again in detail in Chapter 33. ↺)

Using visualization, you may be able to picture something the instructor wrote on the board during a lecture. You may be able to "see" in your mind a poster or handout that was used during a class presentation. With some practice, you may be able to visualize a word or a passage that you read in the textbook.

Answering the study questions at the end of each chapter and in the student workbook will help you improve your ability to select correct answers in objective tests.

ANSWERING ESSAY, SHORT-ANSWER, OR CALCULATION QUESTIONS. Answers to these types of questions will need to be extracted from your memory. Read the question carefully to determine what is being asked. Some students find it helpful to develop a brief outline before beginning an essay question. Check with the instructor to see if this can be written on the test paper or if you are permitted to use an additional sheet. The outline can help organize thought and can serve as a checkpoint that all the important information was included. Usually, a number of key introductory words appear in essay questions (Table 1-4 ◆). Look for these words, and do only what is required of you. Many low grades are caused by ignoring these key words.

Calculation questions are particularly troubling for many students who have convinced themselves that they can-

not do math. Although math may be difficult, it is a necessary skill for a nurse. With extra practice, calculations are possible to learn. There are several methods for calculations (see Chapter 21). ↺

It is important to show your work on calculations. If you are unable to calculate the correct answer, your instructor can review your work, and will be able to tell you where you went wrong. Memorizing formulas and frequently used conversions will make calculations on tests and in the clinical area much easier.

How to Manage Your Time

The "average" vocational/practical nursing student is far from average, so proposing a management template that would work for everyone is impossible. Still, being organized and having a plan will help you work within your time constraints. Learning to manage your time is a skill that will benefit you during the nursing program and also in jobs and in life.

Learning how to be a good student may be the most important lesson during the first few weeks of your nursing program. Study skills will support you throughout your student days and as you prepare for exams. The time taken to perfect these skills will be hours well spent. See Figure 1-13 ◆ for a sample time management schedule.

The following suggestions for time management may be useful:

◆ Obtain a blank calendar or planner for the entire year.
◆ Fill in holidays, vacations, and class and clinical days as soon as you know them.
◆ Add due dates, tests, homework, and projects as they are assigned.
◆ Schedule study time by writing it on your calendar or planner.
◆ Schedule personal time for relaxation and being with other people.

Group study time can also be very useful when you participate regularly. Learn to plan your group study time, just as you would plan other parts of your day. To prepare for group sessions, review your lecture notes. Think of four or five questions that can be discussed with the group. Make sure you have read the textbook assignment.

It is a good idea to break a study session down into segments. For example, a 2-hour session might include 30 minutes of lecture note review, 20 minutes of shared questions and answers, a 10-minute break, 30 minutes of quizzing, and 30 minutes of review of class objectives. This plan gives focus to the study time. The change in activities also helps to sustain people's interest and energy level.

Note: The bibliography listings for this and all chapters have been compiled at the back of the book.

	Monday	Tuesday	Wednesday	Thursday	Friday	Saturday	Sunday
0600	Sleep	Sleep	Sleep	Shower/dress	Shower/dress	Shower/dress	Sleep
0700	Shower/dress	Shower/dress	Shower/dress	Clinical	Clinical	Work	Sleep
0800	Class	Class	Class				Shower/dress
0900							Breakfast
1000							Church
1100							
1200	Lunch	Lunch	Lunch	Lunch	Lunch	Lunch	
1300	Class	Class					
1400		Library	Group project				Dinner with family
1500							
1600							
1700	Dinner	Dinner	Dinner	Dinner	Dinner	Dinner	
1800						Movie	
1900	Study group	Study	Study	Study			Laundry
2000							Study
2100			Personal time	Personal time			
2200	Personal time	Personal time	Sleep	Sleep	Personal time		Personal time
2300	Sleep	Sleep	Sleep	Sleep	Sleep		Sleep

Figure 1-13. ◆ Sample Time Management Schedule.

Chapter Review

Key Terms by Topics

Use the audio glossary feature of either the CD-ROM or the Companion Website to hear the correct pronunciation of the following key terms.

Introduction
nursing

Understanding nursing through history
NCLEX-PN

Understanding contemporary nursing practice
consumer, patient, client, wellness, illness

Factors influencing contemporary nursing
diagnostic-related groups (DRGs), nurse practice acts

Understanding nursing education
knowledge, comprehension, application, analysis

Key Points

◆ Historical perspectives of nursing practice reveal recurring themes. For example, women have traditionally cared for others, but often in subservient roles. Nursing values include compassion, devotion to duty, and hard work. Wars increase the need for nurses and medical specialists. Visionary leaders have made notable contributions to improving the status of nursing.

◆ The essence of nursing is caring for and caring about people as holistic beings.

◆ The scope of nursing practice includes promoting wellness, preventing illness, restoring health, and caring for the dying.

◆ Traditionally, the majority of nurses were employed in hospital settings. Today, more nurses are working in home health care, ambulatory care, and community health settings.

◆ Nurse practice acts vary among states and provinces, and nurses are responsible for knowing the act that governs their practice.

◆ Standards of clinical nursing practice provide measurement criteria for the effectiveness of nursing care and for professional performance behaviors.

◆ Professional and student organizations help the nursing profession and individual nurses. Participation in nursing associations encourages individual growth and helps nurses influence policies that affect nursing practice.

EXPLORE MediaLink

Additional interactive resources for this chapter can be found on the Companion Website at www.prenhall.com/ramont. Click on Chapter 1 and "Begin" to select the activities for this chapter.

For chapter-related NCLEX-style questions and an audio glossary, access the accompanying CD-ROM in this book.

∞ For Further Study

For more information about theories of nursing, see Chapter 3.

To find out more about care of the dying, see Chapter 31.

For further information concerning health care settings and job opportunities for LPN/LVNs, see Chapter 5 and Chapter 34.

To learn more about nurse practice acts and licensure, see Chapter 2 and Chapter 32.

For more information about the NCLEX-PN exam, see Chapter 33.

For additional information regarding calculations and calculation questions, see Chapter 21.

NCLEX-PN Exam Preparation

TEST-TAKING TIP

Wrong choices tend to be very brief or very long. In general, look for the average, safe, acceptable, common "garden variety" answers.

1. Florence Nightingale, considered to be the founder of modern nursing, received her training at:
   a. Crimea
   b. Kaiserwerth, Germany
   c. London, England
   d. Italy

2. What famous American author also served as a nurse during the Civil War?
   a. Charles Dickens
   b. Robert Frost
   c. Walt Whitman
   d. Gore Vidal

3. Who was the founder of the American Red Cross?
   a. Lavinia Dock
   b. Clara Barton
   c. Lillian Wald
   d. Mary Breckinridge

4. A question that requires you to use knowledge, as well as take remembered and comprehended abstractions and apply them to concrete situations, is what type of question?
   a. Knowledge
   b. Comprehension
   c. Application
   d. Analysis

5. The Ballard School of practical nursing was established in Brooklyn, New York, in what year?
   a. 1876
   b. 1893
   c. 1907
   d. 1918

6. What is the significance of the Smith-Hughes Act for LPN/LVNs?
   a. Required licensure for practical nurses
   b. Differentiated practice of LPN/LVNs from RNs
   c. Provided federal funds to support practical nurse education
   d. Established computerized testing centers for licensure exams

7. What differentiates a profession from an occupation?
   a. Required licensure
   b. Educational programs
   c. Professional organizations
   d. Nationally recognized testing

8. In 1949, Lillian Kuster founded which of the following organizations?
   a. Health Occupation Students of America (HOSA)
   b. National Council for State Boards of Nursing
   c. National Federation of Licensed Practical Nurses (NFLPN)
   d. Henry Street Settlement House

9. The NCLEX-PN examination consists of
   a. Essay questions and math calculations
   b. A practical demonstration to evaluate skills
   c. Multiple-choice questions that test knowledge, comprehension, application, and analysis
   d. A different test for each licensure jurisdiction

10. The nurse practice act provides
    a. The NCLEX-PN test plan
    b. The scope of practice for LPN/LVNs in individual states
    c. Guidelines for the ethical practice of nursing
    d. Questions to prepare for the licensing exam

Answers for Review Questions appear in Appendix IV.

Legal and Ethical Issues of Nursing

SHARING experiences

Being a nurse is more than a profession, it is a way of life. To be a nurse, certain attributes must be present in our professional life as well as our daily life. Whether it is helping someone live or helping someone die, we must be able to act upon attributes. What could be a nobler thing than to be a part of making a difference for the sake of humanity?

Ginger Taft, PN student, Idaho State University, Pocatello, ID.

LEARNING outcomes

After completing this chapter you will be able to:

- Differentiate crimes from torts, and give examples in nursing.
- Define unprofessional conduct: negligence, assault/battery, false imprisonment, invasion of privacy, and defamation.
- Describe standards of care, agency policies, and nurse practice acts that affect the scope of nursing practice.
- Describe the purpose of the Good Samaritan Act and Americans with Disabilities Act.
- Identify ways nurses and nursing students can minimize their chances of liability and the purpose of professional liability insurance.
- Discuss how privileged communication applies to the nurse–client relationship.
- Describe the purpose and essential elements of informed consent.
- List information that needs to be included in an incident report.
- Discuss the problem of the chemically impaired nurse.
- Discuss the problem of sexual harassment in nursing.
- Explain the uses and limitations of professional codes of ethics.
- Discuss common ethical issues currently facing health care professionals.
- Discuss the advocacy role of the nurse.

MediaLink

www.prenhall.com/ramont

Use the address above to access the free, interactive Companion Website created for this textbook. Get hints, instant feedback, and textbook references to chapter-related NCLEX-style questions. Link to other interesting sites.

Audio Glossary:
Use the Companion Website, or the CD-ROM disk enclosed with your textbook to hear the pronunciation of key terms in the chapter.

Checking the medication administration record (MAR) against the armband at the bedside everytime can prevent cases of mistaken identity, which are costly to the client and render the nurse liable for malpractice.

Intentional Torts

In the United States, the terms *assault* and *battery* are often heard together, but each has its own meaning. **Assault** can be described as an attempt or threat to touch another person unjustifiably. Assault precedes battery; it is the act that causes the person to believe a battery is about to occur. For example, the person who threatens someone by making a menacing gesture with a club or a closed fist is guilty of assault. In nursing, a nurse who threatens a client with an injection after the client refuses to take the medication orally would be committing assault.

Battery is the willful touching of a person (or the person's clothes, or even something the person is carrying) that may or may not cause harm. To be illegal, however, the touching must be wrong in some way. For example, it must be done without permission, be embarrassing, or cause injury. In the previous example, if the nurse followed through on the threat and gave the injection without the client's consent, the nurse would be committing battery. Even though the physician ordered the medication and even if the client benefits from the administration of the medication, the nurse is still liable.

In Canada, the term *battery* is not used. Instead, there are three categories of assault: assault with intent to injure (like threatening someone with a knife), assault causing bodily injury, and sexual assault.

To perform procedures without consent is considered battery. (See discussion on Informed Consent later in this chapter.)

False imprisonment is the "unlawful restraint or detention of another person against his or her wishes." False imprisonment does not require force; the fear of force to restrain or detain the individual is sufficient (Bernzweig, 1996). False imprisonment accompanied by forceful restraint or threat of restraint is battery.

Nurses may suggest under certain circumstances that a client remain in the hospital room or in bed, but the client must not be detained against the client's will. The client has a right to insist on leaving, even though it may be detrimental to health. The client can leave by signing an absence without authority (AWA) or against medical advice (AMA) form. As with assault or battery, client competency is a factor in determining whether there is a case of false imprisonment or a situation of protecting a client from injury. Agencies usually have clear policies about the application of restraints to guide nurses in such dilemmas. See Chapter 6 for information about restraints. ⌘

Invasion of privacy is a direct wrong of a personal nature that injures the feelings of the person and does not take into account the effect of revealed information on the standing of the person in the community. Privacy is the right of individuals to withhold themselves and their lives from public scrutiny, or the right to be left alone. Liability can result if the nurse breaches confidentiality by passing along confidential client information to others or intrudes into the client's private domain.

Necessary discussion about a client's medical condition is usually considered appropriate, but unnecessary discussions and gossip are considered a breach of confidentiality. Necessary discussion involves only those people engaged in the client's care. Four major categories of confidential client information must be reported: (1) vital statistics, such as births and deaths; (2) infections and communicable diseases, such as syphilis; (3) child or elder abuse; and (4) violent incidents, such as knife wounds. As of 4/14/2003, health care agencies and providers must adhere to the Health Insurance Portability and Accountability Act of 1996 (HIPPA). See Chapter 32 for Act guidelines. ⌘

False Communication

Defamation is communication that is false, or made with a careless disregard for the truth, and that results in injury to the reputation of a person. Both libel and slander are wrongful actions that come under the heading of defamation. **Libel** is defamation by means of print, writing, or pictures. Writing in the nurse's notes that a physician is incompetent because he didn't respond immediately to a call is an example of libel. **Slander** is defamation by the spoken word, stating information or false words, which can cause damage to a person's reputation. An example of slander would be for the nurse to tell a client that another nurse is incompetent.

If a comment is made in private criticizing that person's competence, it is not defamation since a third party did not hear it. It is slander only if it is communicated to a third party.

Nurses are allowed to make statements that could be considered defamatory, but only as a part of nursing practice and only to a physician or another health care team member caring directly for the client.

Loss of Client Property

Client property, such as jewelry, money, eyeglasses, and dentures, is a constant concern to hospital personnel. Today, agencies are taking less responsibility for property and are generally requesting clients to sign a waiver on admission relieving the hospital and its employees of any responsibility for property. Situations arise, however, in which the client cannot sign a waiver and the nursing staff must follow prescribed policies for safeguarding the client's property (see Chapter 8). ⌘ Nurses are expected to take reasonable precautions to safeguard a client's property, and they can be held liable for its loss or damage if they do not exercise reasonable care.

CRIMINAL LAW

A **crime** is an act committed in violation of public (criminal) law and punishable by a fine or imprisonment. A crime does not have to be intended in order to be a crime. For example, a nurse may commit a crime by accidentally giving a client an additional and lethal dose of a narcotic to relieve discomfort.

Crimes are classified as either felonies (or in Canada, indictable offenses) or misdemeanors (or in Canada, summary conviction offenses). A *felony* is a crime of a serious nature, such as murder, punishable by a term in prison. In some areas, second-degree murder is called manslaughter. A nurse who accidentally gives an additional and lethal dose of a narcotic can be accused of manslaughter.

Crimes are punished through criminal action by the state or province against an individual. A *misdemeanor* is an offense of a less serious nature and is usually punishable by a fine, a short-term jail sentence, or both. A nurse who slaps a client's face could be charged with a misdemeanor.

Regulation of Nursing Practice

CREDENTIALING
Credentialing is the process of determining and maintaining competence in nursing practice. The credentialing process is one way in which the nursing profession maintains standards of practice and accountability for the educational preparation of its members. Credentialing includes licensure, registration, certification, and accreditation.

Licensure and Registration
There are two types of licensure and registration: mandatory and permissive. In the United States, nursing licensure is mandatory in all states. However, in Canada, those who are not licensed or registered can perform nursing duties. Permissive licensure and registration exists in some situations in Canada, although registration and licensure is mandatory in most provinces of Canada.

A nurse in any state or province can have his or her license revoked for just cause. These causes are defined in the nurse practice acts. They include: incompetent nursing practice, professional misconduct, and conviction of a crime such as using illegal drugs or selling drugs illegally. In each situation, all the facts are generally reviewed by a committee at a hearing. Nurses are entitled to be represented by legal counsel at such a hearing. If the nurse's license is revoked as a result of the hearing, either the nurse can appeal the decision to a court of law or, in some states, an agency is designated to review the decision before any court action is initiated.

Certification
Most certifications are awarded to advanced practice nurses. However, an LPN/LVN can be certified in long-term care through NFLPN.

Accreditation/Approval of Basic Nursing Education Programs
Accreditation is a process by which a private organization, such as the National League for Nursing (NLN), or governmental agency, such as the state board of nursing, appraises and grants accredited status to institutions, programs, or services that meet predetermined standards. Minimum standards for basic nursing education programs are established in each state of the United States and in each province in Canada. State accreditation or provincial approval is granted to schools of nursing that meet the minimum criteria.

NURSE PRACTICE ACTS
Each state in the United States has a nurse practice act, and each province in Canada has a nurse practice act or an act for professional nursing practice. Nurse practice acts legally define and describe the scope of nursing practice, which the law seeks to regulate, thereby protecting the public as well. See http://www.ncsbn.org/public/regulation/boards_of_nursing_board.htm or www.ncsbn.org for National Council State Boards of Nursing.

State boards of nursing have Internet Web sites which provide valuable information on the nurse practice acts and scope of practice for the LPN/LVN.

STANDARDS OF PRACTICE
Another way the nursing profession attempts to ensure that its practitioners are competent and safe to practice is through the establishment of standards of practice. These standards are often used to evaluate the quality of care nurses provide. Standards of practice for the LPN/LVN are outlined in the **scope of practice,** a document developed by the board of nursing that governs practice within each state.

 # Legal Roles of Nurses

Nurses have three separate, interdependent legal roles, each with rights and associated responsibilities: provider of service, employee or contractor for service, and citizen. As the nurse carries out these roles, the issue of liability must be considered. **Liability** means being legally responsible for one's acts and omissions. When a nurse carries out treatments ordered by the physician, the responsibility for the nursing activity is the nurse's. When a nurse is asked to carry out an activity that the nurse believes could injure the client, the nurse's legal responsibility is to refuse to carry out the order and report this to the nurse's supervisor.

PROVIDER OF SERVICE
The nurse is expected to provide safe and competent care so that harm (physical, psychological, or material) to the recipient of the service is prevented.

EMPLOYEE OR CONTRACTOR FOR SERVICE

A nurse who is employed by an agency works as a representative of the agency. A nurse who is employed directly by a client, for example, a private nurse, may have a written contract with that client to provide professional services for a certain fee. If the nurse becomes ill or dies and cannot fufill the contract, that is understood. But if a nurse does not fulfill the contract because his or her car broke down or because of personal problems, the nurse broke the contract.

A nurse employed by a hospital functions within an employer–employee relationship, in which the nurse represents and acts for the hospital and therefore must function within the policies of the employing agency. The employer assumes responsibility for the conduct of the employee and can also be held responsible for malpractice by the employee. The nurse's conduct, therefore, is the hospital's responsibility.

This does not mean that the nurse cannot be held liable as an individual. If the employee's actions are extraordinarily inappropriate, the employer might not be held liable. For example, if a nurse hits a client in the face, the employer would not be responsible because this behavior is inappropriate. Criminal acts, such as assisting with criminal abortions or taking drugs from a client's supply for personal use, would also be considered extraordinarily inappropriate behavior. Nurses can be held liable for failure to act as well. For example, a nurse who sees another nurse hitting a client and fails to do anything to protect the client may also be considered negligent.

The nurse has obligations to the employer, the client, and other personnel. Nurses must give appropriate care and perform only those responsibilities that they are competent to perform.

The nurse is expected to respect the rights and responsibilities of other health care team members. For example, the nurse explains nursing activities to a client, but does not have the right to comment on the client's medical care in a way that disturbs the client or criticizes the physician. The nurse also has the right to expect reasonable and prudent conduct from other health professionals.

Collective Bargaining

Collective bargaining is the formalized decision-making process between representatives of management and representatives of labor to negotiate wages and conditions of employment, including work hours, working environment, and fringe benefits of employment (e.g., vacation time, sick leave, and personal leave). Through a written agreement, both employer and employees legally commit themselves to observe the terms and conditions of employment.

When collective bargaining breaks down because an agreement cannot be reached, the employees usually call a strike. A *strike* is an organized work stoppage by a group of employees to express a grievance, enforce a demand for changes in conditions of employment, or solve a dispute with management.

Because nursing practice is a service to people (often ill people), striking presents a moral dilemma to many nurses. Actions taken by nurses can affect the safety of people. When faced with a strike, each nurse must make an individual decision to cross or not to cross a picket line.

Arbitration (an agreement negotiated by a designated impartial person) may be required to prevent a strike or may be used to settle a strike.

CITIZEN

The rights and responsibilities of the nurse in the role of citizen are the same as those of any individual under the legal system. Nurses move in and out of these roles when carrying out professional and personal responsibilities.

 # Nursing Responsibilities and Protections

GOOD SAMARITAN ACTS

Good Samaritan acts are laws designed to protect health care providers who provide assistance at the scene of an emergency against claims of malpractice unless it can be shown that there was a gross departure from the normal standard of care or willful wrongdoing on their part. Gross negligence usually involves further injury or harm to the person. For example, an injured child left on the side of the road may be struck by an automobile when the nurse leaves to obtain help.

In the United States, most state statutes do not require citizens to render aid to people in distress. Such assistance is considered more of an ethical than a legal duty. A few states and provinces, however, have enacted legislation that requires people to stop and aid persons in danger (Hall, 1996, p. 139). In Canada, some provinces specify that it is the responsibility of people to give aid at the scene of an accident.

To encourage citizens to be "Good Samaritans," most states have now enacted legislation releasing a Good Samaritan from legal liability for injuries caused under such circumstances, even if the injuries resulted from negligence of the person offering emergency aid.

It is generally believed that a person who renders help in an emergency, at a level that would be provided by any reasonably prudent person under similar circumstances, cannot be held liable. The same reasoning applies to nurses, who are among the people best prepared to help at the scene of an accident. If the level of care a nurse provides is of the caliber that would have been provided by any other nurse, then the nurse will not be held liable. Guidelines for nurses who choose to render emergency care are:

◆ Limit actions to those normally considered first aid if possible.
◆ Do not perform actions that you do not know how to do.

- Offer assistance, but do not insist.
- Do not leave the scene until the injured person leaves or another qualified person takes over.

PROFESSIONAL LIABILITY INSURANCE

Because of the increase in the number of malpractice lawsuits against health professionals, nurses are advised in many areas to carry their own liability insurance. Most hospitals have liability insurance that covers all employees, including all nurses. However, some smaller facilities, such as "walk-in" clinics, may not. Thus the nurse should always check with the employer at the time of hiring to see what coverage the facility provides. A physician or a hospital can be sued because of the negligent conduct of a nurse, and the nurse can also be sued and held liable for negligence or malpractice. Because hospitals have been known to countersue nurses when they have been found negligent and the hospital was required to pay, nurses are advised to provide their own insurance coverage and not rely on hospital-provided insurance.

Additionally, nurses often provide nursing services outside of employment-related activities, such as being available for first aid at children's sport or social activities or providing health screening and education at health fairs. Neighbors or friends may seek advice about illnesses or treatment for themselves or family members. In such situations, the nurse may be tempted to give advice, but it is always advisable for the nurse to refer the friend or neighbor to the family physician. The nurse may be protected from liability under Good Samaritan acts when nursing service is volunteered. However, if the nurse receives any compensation or if there is a written or verbal agreement outlining the nurse's responsibility to the group, the nurse needs liability coverage to cover legal expenses in the event that the nurse is sued.

Students and teachers of nursing are unlikely to be covered by the insurance carried by hospitals and health agencies. It is advisable for them to check with their school about the coverage that applies to them. In some states, hospitals do not allow nursing students to provide nursing care without liability insurance.

NURSES AS WITNESSES

A nurse may be called to testify in a legal action for a variety of reasons. The nurse may be a defendant in a malpractice or negligence action or may have been a member of the health care team that provided care to the plaintiff. If a nurse is going to testify, he or she should consult an attorney first. If the action is against the nurse's employer, the same attorney will assist the nurse. If the action is against the nurse, he or she should retain a separate attorney.

A nurse may also be asked to provide testimony as an expert witness. An *expert witness* has special training, experience, or skill and offers an opinion on some issue within the nurse's area of expertise. Nurses usually are called to help a judge or jury understand evidence pertaining to the extent of damage or the standard of care.

STUDENT NURSES

Nursing students are responsible for their own actions and liable for their own acts of negligence committed during the course of clinical experiences. When they perform duties that are within the scope of professional nursing, such as administering an injection, they are legally held to the same standard of skill and competence as a licensed nurse. Lower standards are not applied to the actions of nursing students.

Students in clinical situations must be assigned activity within their capabilities and be given reasonable guidance and supervision. Nursing instructors are responsible for assigning students to the care of clients and for providing reasonable supervision.

To fulfill responsibilities to clients and to minimize chances for liability, nursing students need to

- Make sure they are prepared to carry out the necessary care for assigned clients.
- Ask for additional help or supervision in situations for which they feel inadequately prepared.
- Comply with the policies of the agency in which they obtain their clinical experience.
- Comply with the policies and definitions of responsibility supplied by the school of nursing.

Students who work as part-time or temporary nursing assistants or aides must also remember that legally they can perform only those tasks that appear in the job description of a nurse's aide or assistant. Even though a student may have received instruction and acquired competence in administering injections or suctioning a tracheostomy tube, the student cannot legally perform these tasks while employed as an aide or assistant. While acting as a paid worker, the student is covered for negligent acts by the employer, not the school of nursing.

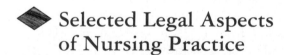

Selected Legal Aspects of Nursing Practice

PRIVILEGED COMMUNICATION

A *privileged communication* is information given to a professional person who is forbidden by law from disclosing the information in a court without the consent of the person who provided it. See the discussion of invasion of privacy.

Legislation regarding privileged communications is highly complicated. Many states with statutes granting privileged communications between the client and various health care providers do not extend the privilege to nurse–client communication.

INFORMED CONSENT

Informed consent is an agreement by a client to accept a course of treatment or a procedure after complete information has been provided by a health care provider. Information includes the risks of the treatment and facts relating to it. Usually, the client signs a form provided by the agency. The form is a record of the informed consent, not the informed consent itself.

Obtaining informed consent for specific medical and surgical treatments is the responsibility of a physician. This responsibility is delegated to nurses in some agencies, and no laws prohibit the nurse from being part of the information-giving process. However, it is not appropriate for the nurse to obtain informed consent.

Witnessing Informed Consent

Often, the nurse's responsibility is to witness the giving of informed consent for medical procedures. This involves the following:

◆ Witnessing the exchange between the client and the physician
◆ Establishing that the client really did understand, that is, was really informed
◆ Witnessing the client's signature

If a nurse witnesses only the client's signature and not the exchange between the client and the physician, the nurse should write "witnessing signature only" on the form. If the nurse finds that the client really does not understand the physician's explanation, then the physician must be notified.

Obtaining informed consent for nursing procedures is the responsibility of nurses when they perform direct care such as insertion of nasogastric tubes or medication administration.

It can be a challenge to determine the amount and type of information required for the client to make an informed decision. General guidelines include:

◆ The purposes of the treatment
◆ What the client can expect to feel or experience
◆ The intended benefits of the treatment
◆ Possible risks or negative outcomes of the treatment
◆ Advantages and disadvantages of possible alternatives to the treatment (including no treatment)

There are three major elements of informed consent:

1. The consent must be given voluntarily.
2. The client must have the capacity and competence to understand.
3. The client must be given enough information to be the ultimate decision maker.

To give informed consent voluntarily, the client must not feel coerced. Sometimes fear of disapproval by a health professional can be the reason the client gives consent. Such consent is not voluntarily given.

Technical words and language barriers can keep clients from understanding information about the procedure. If a client cannot read, the consent form must be read to the client before it is signed. If the client does not speak the same language as the health professional who is giving the information, an interpreter must be provided.

A client who is confused, disoriented, or sedated is not considered functionally competent (able to understand and give informed consent).

Ensuring informed consent is also important when providing nursing care in the home. Because home care often occurs over an extended period of time, the nurse has many opportunities to ensure that the plan of treatment is accepted.

Exceptions

Three groups of people cannot provide consent. The first is a dependent child, under the age of 18 (minor). In most areas, a parent or guardian must give consent before minors can obtain treatment. Adults who have the mental capacity of a child and who have an appointed guardian also fall into this category. There are some exceptions. Some states allow minors to give consent for such procedures as blood donations, treatment for drug dependence and sexually transmitted disease, and procedures for obstetric care. Minors who are married, pregnant, parents, members of the military, or emancipated (living on their own) may be legally allowed to give their own consent. These statutes may vary by state or province.

The second group includes persons who are unconscious or injured so that they are unable to give consent. In these situations, consent is usually obtained from the closest adult relative if existing statutes permit. In a life-threatening emergency, if consent cannot be obtained from the client or a relative, the law generally agrees that consent is implied (agreed to).

The third group consists of mentally ill persons who have been judged by professionals to be incompetent. State and provincial mental health acts or similar statutes generally provide definitions of mental illness and specify the rights of the mentally ill under the law as well as the rights of the staff caring for such clients.

CARRYING OUT PHYSICIAN'S ORDERS

Nurses are expected to analyze procedures and medications ordered by the physician. It is the nurse's responsibility to seek clarification of ambiguous or seemingly erroneous orders from the prescribing physician. Clarification from any other source is unacceptable and regarded as a departure from competent nursing practice.

There are several categories of orders that nurses must question to protect themselves legally:

◆ Question any order a client questions. For example, if a client who has been receiving an intramuscular injection tells the nurse that the doctor changed the order from an injectable to an oral medication, the nurse should recheck the order before giving the medication.
◆ Question any order if the client's condition has changed. The nurse is considered responsible for notifying the physician of any significant changes in the client's condition, whether the physician requests notification or not. For

example, if a client who is receiving an intravenous infusion suddenly develops a rapid pulse, chest pain, and a cough, the nurse must notify the physician immediately and question continuance of the ordered rate of infusion.

◆ Question and record verbal orders to avoid miscommunications. In addition to recording the time, the date, the physician's name, and the orders, the nurse documents the circumstances that occasioned the call to the physician, reads the orders back to the physician, and documents that the physician confirmed the orders as the nurse read them back.

◆ Question any order that is illegible, unclear, or incomplete. Misinterpretations in the name of a drug or in dose, for example, can easily occur with handwritten orders. The nurse is responsible for ensuring that the order is interpreted the way it was intended and that it is a safe and appropriate order.

PROVIDING COMPETENT NURSING CARE

Competent practice is a major legal safeguard for nurses. Nurses need to provide care that is within the legal boundaries of their practice and within the boundaries of agency policies and procedures. Nurses therefore must be familiar with their various job descriptions, which may be different from agency to agency. All nurses are responsible for ensuring that their various education and experience is adequate to meet the responsibilities delineated in their job descriptions.

Competency also involves care that protects clients from harm. Nurses need to anticipate sources of client injury, educate clients about hazards, and implement measures to prevent injury.

Application of the nursing process is another essential aspect of providing safe and effective client care. Clients need to be assessed and monitored appropriately and involved in care decisions. All assessments and care must be documented accurately. Effective communication can also protect the nurse from negligence claims. Nurses need to approach every client with sincere concern and include the client in conversations. In addition, nurses should always acknowledge when they don't know the answer to a client's questions, tell the client they will find out the answer, and then follow through.

Methods of legal protection for nurses are summarized in Box 2-2 ◆.

RECORD KEEPING

The client's medical record is a legal document and can be produced in court as evidence. Often, the record is used to remind a witness of events surrounding a lawsuit, because several months or years usually elapse before the suit goes to trial. The effectiveness of a witness's testimony can depend on the accuracy of such records. Nurses, therefore, need to keep accurate and complete records of nursing care provided to clients. Failure to keep proper records can constitute negligence and be the basis for tort liability. Insufficient or inaccurate assessments and documentation can hinder proper diagnosis and

treatment and result in injury to the client. See Chapter 9 for types of records and facts about recording. ⌘

THE INCIDENT REPORT

An incident report is an agency record of an accident or unusual occurrence. Incident reports are used to make all the facts available to agency personnel, to contribute to statistical data about accidents or incidents, and to help health personnel prevent future incidents or accidents. All accidents are usually reported on incident forms. Some agencies also report other incidents, such as the occurrence of client infection or the loss of personal effects. Box 2-3 ◆ lists the information to be included in an incident report. The report should be completed as soon as possible, and filed according to agency policy. As incident reports are not part of the client's medical record, the facts of the incident should also be noted in the medical record. Do not record in the client record that an incident report has been completed.

The incident report should be completed by the person who identifies that the incident occurred. This may not be the same person actually involved with the incident. For example, the nurse who discovers that an incorrect medication has been administered completes the form even if it was another nurse who administered the medication. In addition, all witnesses to an incident, such as a client fall, are listed on the incident form even if they were not directly involved.

Incident reports are often reviewed by an agency risk management committee, which decides whether to investigate the incident further. Nurses may be required to answer such questions as what they believe precipitated the accident, how it could have been prevented, and whether any equipment should be adjusted. Incident reports are discussed further in Chapter 32. ⌘

REPORTING CRIMES, TORTS, AND UNSAFE PRACTICES

Nurses may need to report nursing colleagues or other health professionals for practices that endanger the health and safety of clients. For instance, alcohol and drug use, theft from a client or agency, and unsafe nursing practice should be reported. Reporting a colleague is not easy. The person reporting may feel disloyal, incur the disapproval of others, or perceive that chances for promotion are endangered. When reporting an incident or series of incidents, the nurse must be careful to describe observed behavior only and not make inferences as to what might be happening. Reporting these events is referred to as "whistle-blowing." Many states have laws that prevent wrongful termination of whistle-blowers by employers. Reporting illegal, unethical, or incompetent performance is an expectation found in the code of ethics of the National Federation of Licensed Practical Nurses.

AMERICANS WITH DISABILITIES ACT

The Americans with Disabilities Act (ADA), passed by the United States Congress in 1990 and fully implemented in

BOX 2-2
NURSING CARE CHECKLIST

LEGAL PRECAUTIONS FOR NURSES

☑ Function within the scope of your education, job description, and area nurse practice act. This enables you to function within the scope of the description and know what is and what is not expected.

☑ Follow the procedures and policies of the employing agency.

☑ Build and maintain good rapport with clients. Keeping clients informed about diagnostic and treatment plans, giving feedback on their progress, and showing concern for the outcome of their care prevent a sense of powerlessness and a buildup of hostility in the client.

☑ Always identify clients, particularly before initiating major interventions (e.g., surgical or other invasive procedures or when administering medications or blood transfusions).

☑ Observe and monitor the client accurately. Communicate and record significant changes in the client's condition to the physician.

☑ Promptly and accurately document all assessments and care given. Records must show that the nurse provided and supervised the client's care daily.

☑ Be alert when implementing nursing interventions and give each task your full attention and skill.

☑ Perform procedures appropriately. Negligent incidents during procedures generally relate to equipment failure, improper technique, and improper performance of the procedure. For instance, the nurse must know how to safeguard the client in the event that a respirator or other equipment fails.

☑ Make sure the correct medications are given in the correct dose, by the right route, at the scheduled time, and to the right client. See Chapter 21 for more detailed information about the administration of medications. ⊙⊃

☑ When delegating nursing responsibilities, make sure that the person who is delegated a task understands what to do and that the person has the required knowledge and skill. As the delegating nurse, you can be held liable for harm caused by the person to whom the care was delegated.

☑ Protect clients from injury. Inform clients of hazards and use appropriate safety devices and measures to prevent falls, burns, or other injuries.

☑ Report all incidents involving clients. Prompt reports enable those responsible to attend to the client's well-being, to analyze why the incident occurred, and to prevent recurrences.

☑ Always check any order that a client questions and ensure that verbal orders are accurate and documented appropriately. Question and confirm standing orders if you are inexperienced in a particular area.

☑ Know your own strengths and weaknesses. Ask for assistance and supervision in situations for which you feel inadequately prepared.

☑ Maintain your clinical competence. For students, this demands study and practice before caring for clients. For graduate nurses, it means continued study, including maintaining and updating clinical knowledge and skills.

BOX 2-3 INFORMATION TO INCLUDE IN AN INCIDENT REPORT

◆ Identify the client by name, initials, and hospital or identification number.

◆ Give the date, time, and place of the incident.

◆ Describe the facts of the incident. Avoid any conclusions or blame. Describe the incident as you saw it even if your impressions differ from those of others.

◆ Identify all witnesses to the incident.

◆ Identify any equipment by number and any medication by name and number.

◆ Document any circumstance surrounding the incident, for example, that another client was experiencing cardiac arrest.

1994, prohibits discrimination on the basis of disability in employment, public services, and public accommodations. The purposes of the act are:

◆ To provide a clear and comprehensive national mandate for eliminating discrimination against individuals with disabilities

◆ To provide clear, strong, consistent, enforceable standards addressing discrimination against individuals with disabilities

◆ To ensure that the federal government plays a central role in enforcing standards established under the act

An employer may not refuse to hire a nurse with disabilities if the nurse is able to fulfill the duties of the work role. The ADA also enables individuals of normal intelligence who have a physical or learning disability to pursue a nursing curriculum through alternative learning methods.

CONTROLLED SUBSTANCES

United States and Canadian laws regulate the distribution and use of controlled substances such as narcotics, depressants, stimulants, and hallucinogens. Misuse of controlled substances leads to criminal penalties. See Chapter 21 for the legal aspects of drug administration.

The Impaired Nurse

The term **impaired nurse** refers to a nurse whose practice has been negatively affected because of chemical abuse, specifically the use of alcohol and drugs. Chemical dependence in health care workers has become a problem because of the high levels of stress involved in many health care settings and the easy access to addictive drugs. Substance abuse is the most common reason for actions against nurses' licenses. Between 10 and 15 percent of nurses are estimated to be chemically impaired. This is about the same percentage as in the general population. Employers must have sound policies and procedures for identifying situations that involve a possibly impaired nurse. Intervention in such situations is important to protect clients and to get treatment for the impaired nurse quickly.

A variety of programs have been developed to assist impaired nurses to recover. In many states, impaired nurses who enter an intervention program for treatment (diversion program) are closely supervised and restricted in practice, but do not have to surrender their nursing license.

SEXUAL HARASSMENT

Sexual harassment is a violation of the individual's rights and a form of discrimination. In 1987, the law prohibiting sexual discrimination was clarified to apply to all educational and employing institutions receiving federal funding. The Equal Employment Opportunity Commission (EEOC) defines **sexual harassment** as "unwelcome sexual advances, requests for sexual favors, and other verbal or physical conduct

of a sexual nature" occurring in the following circumstances (EEOC, 1980, sections 3950.10–3950.11):

◆ When submission to such conduct is considered, either explicitly or implicitly, a condition of an individual's employment
◆ When submission to or rejection of such conduct is used as the basis for employment decisions affecting the individual
◆ When such conduct interferes with an individual's work performance or creates an "intimidating, hostile, or offensive working environment"

In health care, both clients and health care professionals may experience sexual harassment. Because sexual harassment is generally related to a power imbalance, female nurses are more likely to experience sexual harassment from male physicians or administrators. Nurses may be "sexually propositioned," "suggestively touched," or "sexually insulted" during their career. Such behavior is considered sexual harassment and can negatively affect client care. For example, to avoid uncomfortable situations, a nurse may refuse to care for the clients of a particular offensive physician or work on a unit with an offensive administrator, or a nurse may avoid calling a physician to report changes in client status or to suggest changes to improve client care.

The victim or the harasser may be male or female. The victim does not have to be of the opposite sex. Furthermore, the victim does not have to be the person harassed. Anyone who is affected by the offensive conduct may be considered a victim. Nurses must develop skills of assertiveness to deter sexual harassment in the workplace. (See also Box 29-7, Nursing Strategies for Inappropriate Sexual Behavior.)

Nurses must be familiar with the sexual harassment policy and procedures that are in place in every institution. These will include information regarding the grievance policy, the person to whom incidents should be reported, and the resolution process.

Understanding Ethical Issues

In the course of their daily work, nurses deal with such fundamental events as birth, suffering, and death. They must decide the morality of their own actions when they face these ethical issues. The present cost-driven environment of managed care tends to give highest priority to business values. This creates new moral problems and exaggerates old ones. It is more critical than ever for nurses to make sound moral decisions. Therefore, nurses need to develop understanding of the ethical dimensions of nursing practice by examining their values. Early on in their practice, nurses must look ahead to the kinds of moral problems they are likely to face and begin to understand how values influence their decisions.

Ethical Concepts

Values are freely chosen, enduring beliefs or attitudes about the worth of a person, object, idea, or action. Values are important because they influence decisions and actions. Values are often taken for granted. In the same way that people are not aware of their breathing, they usually do not think about their values; they simply accept them and act on them. The word *values* usually brings to mind such things as honesty, fairness, friendship, safety, or family unity. Of course, not all values are moral values. For example, some people hold money, work, power, and politics as values in their lives.

Although values consist of freely chosen and enduring beliefs and attitudes, beliefs and attitudes are related, but not identical, to values.

Values are learned through observation and experience. They are transmitted to others through the influence of environment—that is, by family and peer groups, by cultural, ethnic, and religious groups: For example, if a parent consistently demonstrates honesty in dealing with others, the child will probably begin to value honesty. Nurses should keep in mind the influence of values on health. In some cultures, folk healers are valued over treatment by a physician.

Beliefs or opinions are interpretations or conclusions that people accept as being true; they do not necessarily involve values. For example, the statement, "I believe if I study hard I will get a good grade" expresses a belief that does not involve a value. By contrast, the following statement, "Good grades are really important to me. I believe I must study hard to obtain good grades" involves both a belief and a value.

Attitudes are mental positions or feelings toward a person, object, or idea (e.g., acceptance, compassion, openness). Attitudes are often judged as bad or good, positive or negative; whereas beliefs are judged as correct or incorrect.

The term **ethics** has several meanings in common use. It refers to (a) a method of inquiry that helps people to understand the morality of human behavior (i.e., it is the study of morality), (b) the practices or beliefs of a certain group (e.g., medical ethics, nursing ethics), and (c) the expected standards of moral behavior of a particular group as described in the group's formal code of professional ethics. **Bioethics** is ethics as applied to life (e.g., decisions about abortion or euthanasia). Nursing ethics refers to ethical issues that occur in nursing practice. The National Federation of Licensed Practical Nurses (NFLPN) holds nurses accountable for their legal and ethical conduct in the Nursing Practice Standards for the Licensed Practical/Vocational Nurse (1998).

◆ Moral Concepts

Morality (or morals) is similar to ethics, and many use the terms interchangeably. *Morality* usually refers to private, personal standards of what is right and wrong in conduct, character, and attitude. Sometimes the first clue to the moral nature of a situation is an aroused conscience or an awareness of feelings such as guilt, hope, or shame. Another indicator is the tendency to respond to the situation with words such as *ought, should, right, wrong, good*, and *bad*. Moral issues are concerned with important social values and norms; they are not about trivial things.

Nurses should distinguish between morality and law. An action can be legal but not moral. For example, an order for full resuscitation of a dying client is legal, but one could still question whether the act is moral. On the other hand, an action can be moral but illegal. For example, if a child at home

stops breathing, it is moral but not legal to exceed the speed limit when driving to the hospital.

Moral principles are statements about broad, general, philosophic concepts such as autonomy and justice. They provide the foundation for moral rules, which are specific prescriptions for actions. Principles are useful in ethical discussions because even if people disagree about which action is right in a situation, they may be able to agree on the principles that apply. Such an agreement can serve as the basis for a solution that is acceptable to all parties.

Autonomy refers to the right to make one's own decisions. Nurses who follow this principle recognize that each client is unique, has the right to be what that person is, and has the right to choose personal goals.

Honoring the principle of autonomy means that the nurse respects a client's right to make decisions even when those choices seem not to be in the client's best interest. It also means treating others with consideration. In a health care setting, this principle is violated, for example, when a nurse disregards a client's report of the severity of his or her pain.

Nonmaleficence is duty to do no harm. Although this would seem to be a simple principle to follow, in reality it is complex. Harm can mean intentional harm, risk of harm, and unintentional harm. In nursing, intentional harm is never acceptable. However, the risk of harm is not always clear. A client may be at risk of harm during a nursing intervention that is intended to be helpful. For example, a client may react adversely to a medication, and caregivers may or may not always agree on the degree to which a risk is morally permissible.

Beneficence means "doing good." Nurses are obligated to do good, that is, to implement actions that benefit clients and their support persons. However, doing good can also pose a risk of doing harm. For example, a nurse may advise a client about a strenuous exercise program to improve general health, but should not do so if the client is at risk of a heart attack.

Justice is often referred to as fairness. Nurses often face decisions in which a sense of justice should prevail. For example, a nurse making home visits finds one client tearful and depressed, and knows she could help by staying for 30 more minutes to talk. However, that would take time from her next client, who is a diabetic who needs a great deal of teaching and observation. The nurse will need to weigh the facts carefully in order to divide her time justly among her clients.

Fidelity means to be faithful to agreements and promises. By virtue of their standing as professional caregivers, nurses have responsibilities to clients, employers, government, and society, as well as to themselves. Nurses often make promises such as: "I'll be right back with your pain medication," "You'll be all right," "I'll find out for you." Clients take such promises seriously, and so should nurses.

Veracity refers to telling the truth. Although this seems straightforward, in practice, choices are not always clear. Should a nurse tell the truth when it is known that it will cause harm? Does a nurse tell a lie when it is known that the lie will relieve anxiety and fear? The loss of trust in the nurse and the anxiety caused by not knowing the truth, for example, usually outweigh any benefits derived from lying. Lying to sick or dying people is rarely justified.

Nursing Ethics

In the past, nurses looked on ethical decision making as the physician's responsibility. However, no one profession is responsible for ethical decisions, nor does expertise in one discipline such as medicine or nursing necessarily make a person an expert in ethics. As situations become more complex, input from all caregivers becomes increasingly important.

Most health care institutions have ethics committees. Ethical standards of the Joint Commission on Accreditation of Healthcare Organizations (JCAHO) support nurses' involvement on these committees.

Ethics committees typically review cases, write guidelines and policies, and provide education and counseling. They ensure that relevant facts of a case are brought out, provide a forum in which diverse views can be expressed, provide support for caregivers, and can reduce legal risks.

A **code of ethics** is a formal statement of a group's ideals and values. It is a set of ethical principles that (a) is shared by members of the group, (b) reflects their moral judgments over time, and (c) serves as a standard for their professional actions. Codes of ethics usually have higher requirements than legal standards, and they are never lower than the legal standards of the profession. Nurses are responsible for being familiar with the code that governs their practice.

International, national, state, and provincial nursing associations have established codes of ethics.

Nursing codes of ethics have the following purposes:

1. Inform the public about the minimum standards of the profession and help them understand professional nursing conduct.
2. Provide a sign of the profession's commitment to the public it serves.
3. Outline the major ethical considerations of the profession.
4. Provide general guidelines for professional behavior.
5. Guide the profession in self-regulation.
6. Remind nurses of the special responsibility they assume when caring for the sick.

ORIGINS OF ETHICAL PROBLEMS IN NURSING

Nurses' growing awareness of ethical problems has occurred largely because of (a) social and technologic changes, and (b) nurses' conflicting loyalties and obligations.

Social and Technologic Changes

Social changes, such as the women's movement and a growing consumerism, also expose problems. Presently, the large num-

ber of people without health insurance, the high cost of health care, and workplace redesign under managed care are all raising issues of fairness and allocation of resources.

Technology creates new issues that did not exist in earlier, simpler times. Before monitors, respirators, and parenteral feedings, there was no question about whether to "allow" an 800-gram premature infant to die. Today, with treatments that can prolong biologic life almost indefinitely, the questions are: Should we do what we know we can? Who should be treated—everyone, only those who can pay, only those who have a chance to improve?

Conflicting Loyalties and Obligations

Because of their unique position in the health care system, nurses experience conflicts among their loyalties and obligations to clients, families, physicians, employing institutions, and licensing bodies. Client needs may conflict with institutional policies, physician preferences, needs of the client's family, or even laws of the state. According to the nursing code of ethics, the nurse's first loyalty is to the client. However, it is not always easy to determine which action best serves the client's needs. For instance, a nurse may think that a client needs to be told a truth that others have been withholding. But this might damage the client–physician relationship, in the long run causing harm to the client rather than the intended good.

MAKING ETHICAL DECISIONS

Responsible ethical reasoning is rational and systematic. It should be based on ethical principles and codes rather than on emotions, intuition, fixed policies, or precedent. (A precedent is an earlier similar occurrence.)

A good decision is one that is in the client's best interest and at the same time preserves the integrity of all involved. Nurses have ethical obligations to their clients, to the agency that employs them, and to physicians. Therefore, nurses must weigh competing factors when making ethical decisions (Box 2-4 ◆). See also Chapter 3, the section on critical thinking. ∞

Although the nurse's input is important, in reality several people are usually involved in making an ethical decision.

MediaLink ◆ Nursing Code of Ethics

BOX 2-4 EXAMPLES OF NURSES' OBLIGATIONS IN ETHICAL DECISIONS

◆ Maximize the client's well-being.
◆ Balance the client's need for autonomy with family members' responsibilities for the client's well-being.
◆ Support each family member and enhance the family support system.
◆ Carry out hospital policies.
◆ Protect other clients' well-being.
◆ Protect the nurse's own standards of care.

Therefore collaboration, communication, and compromise are important skills for health professionals. When nurses do not have the autonomy to act on their moral or ethical choices, compromise becomes essential.

Integrity-preserving compromises are most likely to be produced by collaborative decision making. See Box 2-5 ◆ for strategies to enhance ethical decisions and practice.

SPECIFIC ETHICAL ISSUES

The ANA Center for Ethics and Human Rights conducted a survey at the 1994 ANA convention that indicated the following as some of the ethical problems nurses encounter most frequently: cost-containment issues that jeopardize client welfare and access to health care (resource allocation); end-of-life decisions; breaches of client confidentiality (e.g., computerized information management); use of advance directives; informed consent and procedures; and issues in the care of HIV/AIDS clients (Scanlon, 1995). These and other issues are discussed in this section.

Acquired Immune Deficiency Syndrome (AIDS)

Because of its association with sexual behavior, prostitution, illicit drug use, and inevitable physical decline and death, AIDS bears a social stigma. Nurses caring for AIDS clients frequently have conflicting feelings of anger, fear, sympathy, fatigue, helplessness, and self-enhancement.

According to an ANA position statement on HIV Infections and Nursing Students, "Nursing Curriculum including current HIV information should be provided by faculty with expertise in HIV disease at the onset of the academic program and as applicable throughout their course . . . Each school of nursing should demonstrate the availability of a post-exposure management program for students who sustain exposure to blood and certain body fluids in the clinical prac-

tice setting . . . Nursing students should be assured workplace/clinical setting protections consistent with those of employees according to OSHA Standards . . . Nursing students and applicants to nursing programs should not be deprived of access to schools of nursing nor dismissed based solely on HIV positive status . . . There must be confidentiality of all HIV-related information to safeguard nursing students' right to privacy" (ANA, 2001).

Other ethical issues center on testing for HIV status and for the presence of AIDS in health professionals and clients. Questions arise as to whether testing should be mandatory or voluntary and to whom test results should be given. The U.S. Public Health Service, Centers for Disease Control and Prevention (CDC) provides recommendations as to which persons should be considered for HIV antibody counseling and testing. It also recommends that voluntary testing be made available to anyone, including all health care professionals. In addition, the CDC recommends that HIV-positive health care professionals avoid performing "exposure prone procedures" (CDC, 2001).

Abortion

Abortion is a highly publicized issue about which many people, including nurses, feel very strongly. Debate continues, pitting the principle of sanctity of life against the principle of autonomy and the woman's right to control her own body. This is an especially volatile issue because no public consensus has yet been reached.

Most state and provincial laws have provisions known as conscience clauses that permit individual physicians and nurses, as well as institutions, to refuse to assist with an abortion if doing so violates their religious or moral principles. However, nurses have no right to impose their values on a client. Abortion laws provide specific guidelines for nurses about what is legally permissible, although the Supreme Court and state legislatures continue to struggle with the issue of abortion.

Organ Transplantation

Organs for transplantation may come from living donors or from donors who have just died. Many living people choose to become donors by giving consent under the Uniform Anatomical Gift Act. Ethical issues related to organ transplantation include allocation of organs, selling of body parts, involvement of children as potential donors, consent, clear definition of death, and conflicts of interest between potential donors and recipients. In some situations, a person's religious belief may also present conflict. For example, certain religions forbid the mutilation of the body, even for the benefit of another person.

End-of-Life Issues

Some of the most frequent disturbing ethical problems for nurses involve issues that arise around death and dying. These

> ### BOX 2-5 STRATEGIES TO ENHANCE ETHICAL NURSING PRACTICE
>
> - Become aware of your own values and the ethical aspects of nursing.
> - Be familiar with nursing codes of ethics.
> - Respect the values, opinions, and reponsibilities of other health care professionals that may be different from your own.
> - Participate in or establish ethics rounds. Ethics rounds using hypothetical real cases incorporate the traditional teaching approach for clinical rounds, but focus on the ethical dimensions of client care rather than the client's clinical diagnosis and treatment.
> - Serve on institutional ethics committees.
> - Strive for collaborative practice in which nurses function effectively in cooperation with other health care professionals.

include euthanasia, assisted suicide, termination of life-sustaining treatment, and withdrawing or withholding of food and fluids.

Many moral problems surrounding the end of life can be resolved if clients complete advance directives. Presently, all 50 of the United States have enacted advance directive legislation (Scanlon, 1996, p. 94). Advance directives direct caregivers as to the client's wishes about treatments, providing an ongoing voice for clients when they have lost the capacity to make or communicate their decisions. See Chapter 31 for a full discussion of advance directives. ∞

EUTHANASIA AND ASSISTED SUICIDE. *Euthanasia,* a Greek word meaning "good death," is popularly known as "mercy killing." Active euthanasia involves actions to directly bring about the client's death, with or without client consent. An example of this would be the administration of a lethal medication to end the client's suffering. Regardless of the caregiver's intent, active euthanasia is forbidden by law and can result in criminal charges of murder.

Active euthanasia includes assisted suicide, or giving clients the means to kill themselves if they request it (e.g., providing pills or a weapon). Nurses should recall that legality and morality are not one and the same. Determining whether an action is legal is only one aspect of deciding whether it is ethical. The questions of suicide and assisted suicide are still controversial in our society. The American Nurses Association's position statement on assisted suicide (1995) states that active euthanasia and assisted suicide are in violation of the Code for Nurses.

Passive euthanasia involves the withdrawal of extraordinary means of life support, such as removing a ventilator or making a client a "no code."

TERMINATION OF LIFE-SUSTAINING TREATMENT. Antibiotics, organ transplants, and technologic advances (e.g., ventilators) help to prolong life, but not necessarily to restore health. Clients may specify that they wish to have life-sustaining measures withdrawn, they may have advance directives on this matter, or they may appoint a surrogate decision maker. There is no ethical or legal distinction between the withholding or withdrawing of treatments. However, it is usually more troubling for health care professionals to withdraw a treatment than to decide initially not to begin it. Nurses must understand that a decision to withdraw treatment is not a decision to withdraw care. As the primary caregivers, nurses must ensure that sensitive care and comfort measures are given as the client's illness progresses.

WITHDRAWING OR WITHHOLDING FOOD AND FLUIDS. It is generally accepted that providing food and fluids is part of ordinary nursing practice and, therefore, a moral duty. However, when food and fluids are administered by tube to a dying client, or are given over a long period of time to an unconscious client who is not expected to improve, then some consider it to be an extraordinary, or heroic, measure. A nurse is morally obligated to withhold food and fluids when it is more harmful to administer them than to withhold them. In addition, "It is morally as well as legally permissible for nurses to honor the refusal of food and fluids by competent patients in their care" (ANA, 1988, p. 3). The ANA Code for Nurses supports this position through the nurse's role as a client advocate and through the moral principle of autonomy.

ALLOCATION OF HEALTH RESOURCES

Allocation of health care goods and services, including organ transplants, artificial joints, and the services of specialists, has become an especially urgent issue as medical costs continue to rise and more stringent cost-containment measures are implemented.

Nursing care is also a health resource. Most institutions have been implementing "workplace redesign" in order to cut costs. As a result, nursing units are staffed with fewer nurses and more unlicensed caregivers. Nurses must continue to look for ways to balance economics and caring in the allocation of health resources.

MANAGEMENT OF COMPUTERIZED INFORMATION

In keeping with the principle of autonomy, nurses are obligated to respect clients' privacy and confidentiality. Clients must be able to trust that nurses will reveal details of their situations only as appropriate and will communicate only the information necessary to provide for their health care. Computerized client records make sensitive data accessible to more people and accent issues of confidentiality. Nurses should help develop and follow security measures and policies to ensure appropriate use of client data. For example, nurses should not give their system security codes to allow unauthorized persons access to computer files.

ADVOCACY

An **advocate** is one who expresses and defends the cause of another. A client advocate is an advocate for clients' rights. The health care system is complex and many clients are too ill to deal with it. If they are to keep from "falling through the cracks," clients need an advocate to cut through the layers of bureaucracy and help them get what they require. Values basic to client advocacy are shown in Box 2-6 ◆.

The overall goal of the client advocate is to protect clients' rights. Being an effective client advocate involves

◆ Being assertive
◆ Recognizing that the rights and values of clients and families must take precedence when they conflict with those of health care providers
◆ Being aware that conflicts may arise over issues that require consultation, confrontation, or negotiation between the nurse and administrative personnel or between the nurse and physician

- Working with unfamiliar community agencies and lay practitioners
- Knowing that advocacy may require political action—communicating a client's health care needs to government and other officials who have the authority to do something about these needs

Note: The bibliography listings for this and all chapters have been compiled at the back of the book.

BOX 2-6
VALUES BASIC TO CLIENT ADVOCACY

- The client is a holistic, autonomous being who has the right to make choices and decisions.
- Clients have the right to expect a nurse–client relationship that is based on shared respect, trust, and collaboration in solving problems related to health and health care needs, and consideration of their thoughts and feelings.
- Clients are responsible for their own health.
- It is the nurse's responsibility to ensure the client has access to health care services that meet health needs.

Chapter Review

Key Terms by Topics

Use the audio glossary feature of either the CD-ROM or the Companion Website to hear the correct pronunciation of the following key terms.

Kinds of legal actions
law, tort, negligence, malpractice, statute of limitations, assault, battery, false imprisonment, invasion of privacy, defamation, libel, slander, crime

Regulation of nursing practice
scope of practice

Legal roles of nurses
liability

Selected legal aspects of nursing practice
impaired nurse, sexual harassment

Ethical concepts
values, beliefs, attitudes, ethics, bioethics

Moral concepts
autonomy

Nursing ethics
code of ethics, advocate

Key Points

◆ Accountability is an essential concept of professional nursing practice under the law.

◆ Nurses need to understand laws that regulate and affect nursing practice to ensure that the nurses' actions are consistent with current legal principles and to protect the nurse from liability.

◆ Nurse practice acts legally define and describe the scope of nursing practice that the law seeks to regulate.

◆ Nurses can be held liable for intentional torts, such as invasion of privacy, defamation, assault and battery, and false imprisonment; and for unintentional torts, such as negligence and malpractice.

◆ Negligence or malpractice of nurses can be established when (a) the nurse (defendant) owed a duty to the client, (b) the nurse failed to carry out that duty according to standards, (c) the client (plaintiff) was injured, and (d) the client's injury was caused by the nurse's failure to follow the standard.

◆ Good Samaritan acts protect health professionals from claims of malpractice when they offer assistance at the scene of an emergency, provided that there is no willful wrongdoing or gross departure from normal standards of care.

◆ Chemical dependence in health care workers has become a problem because of the high levels of stress involved in many health care settings and the easy access to addictive drugs. The nurse needs to know the proper reporting of nursing colleagues who are chemically impaired.

◆ Sexual harassment is a violation of the Individual's right and a form of discrimination. Sexual harassment can happen to both nurses and clients. The nurse needs to be aware of strategies to deter harassing behavior.

◆ Nursing students need to make certain that they are prepared to provide the necessary care to assigned clients and to ask for help or supervision in situations for which they feel inadequately prepared.

◆ Moral issues and ethical problems are created as a result of advances in technology and nurses' conflicting loyalties and obligations.

◆ Client advocacy involves concern for an action on behalf of another person or organization in order to bring about change.

EXPLORE MediaLink

Additional interactive resources for this chapter can be found on the Companion Website at www.prenhall.com/ramont. Click on Chapter 2 and "Begin" to select the activities for this chapter.

For chapter-related NCLEX-style questions and an audio glossary, access the accompanying CD-ROM in this book.

For Further Study

See Chapter 6 for more information about providing a safe client environment and the correct use of restraints.

See Chapter 8 for policies for safeguarding client's property.

See Chapter 9 for information about types of records and how to document care.

See Chapter 21 for information about administering medications and documenting their administration.

See Chapter 29 for ways to deal with sexual harassment.

See Chapter 31 for more information about advance directives.

For more information on HIPPA and on incident (or occurrence) reports, see Chapter 32.

NLCEX-PN Exam Preparation

1. A client has signed the consent for surgery, which is scheduled for the morning. You enter the room and find the client crying. The client tells you, "I don't want to have surgery, but the doctor and my family tell me I must." You are faced with which of the following ethical dilemmas?

   a. Has the client been given informed consent?

   b. Do the client and family disagree on treatment?

   c. Is the client anxious about surgery?

   d. Has the treatment team followed the principle of beneficence?

2. You are assigned a client who has been placed in restraints. You fail to follow the hospital policy on frequency of assessment and periodic release of restraints. Your behavior could be considered which of the following?

   a. Negligence

   b. False imprisonment

   c. Ethical misconduct

   d. Defamation

3. In the course of administering medications, your client states, "I don't take that yellow pill every day and I took it at home yesterday." Without verifying the physician's orders, you say to the client, "Your doctor wants you to have this, so you must take it now!" Later, you check the order and find that it is an every-other-day order (q.o.d.) You are guilty of which of the following?

   a. A crime

   b. Assault

   c. Negligence

   d. Misdemeanor

4. When you are performing your morning assessment on a client you notice there is a bruise in the area where the last injection was given. When you ask the client to turn onto that side, she complains that it is sore. You state, "The night nurse is incompetent; no one gets a bruise like that from an injection." You have used which type of false communication?

   a. Libel

   b. Slander

   c. Breach of confidence

   d. Invasion of privacy

5. If a nurse fails to report a client's complaint, resulting in client suffering, the nurse can be liable for which type of malpractice?

   a. Mistaken identity

   b. Failure to observe and take appropriate action

   c. Intentional tort

   d. Performing a procedure without consent

6. Which of the following is a responsibility of the National League of Nursing?

   a. Enforcing nurse practice acts

   b. Issuing nursing licenses once the exam has been passed

   c. Providing approval and accreditation of basic nursing programs

   d. Assessing credentials of foreign-trained nurses

7. An incident report should be completed by which of the following individuals?

   a. The nurse involved in the incident

   b. The immediate supervisor of the nurse involved in the incident

   c. The nurse who discovers the incident

   d. The risk management department of the facility

8. The Americans with Disabilities Act:

   a. Can be interpreted by the employer

   b. Enables a person with a learning disability, who is physically able, to pursue a nursing curriculum through alternate methods

   c. Provides retraining for nurses who have been injured on the job

   d. Prohibits setting lifting requirements for nursing jobs

9. The right of the person to make his or her own decisions is related to which principle?

   a. Respect for the person

   b. Autonomy

   c. Justice

   d. Nonmaleficence

10. Your supervisor has asked you to serve on the committee to develop guidelines for the new computerized client record system. Co-workers are concerned about confidentiality. The best response to their concerns would be:

    a. Medical records on the Internet are guaranteed to be secure.

    b. The best ways we can protect the client's information is by following security policies and keeping our security codes private.

    c. There is no way to protect confidentiality, but the benefits of the system outweigh the risks.

    d. As long as we save after each entry, the records are secure.

Answers for Review Questions appear in Appendix IV.

Critical Thinking and Nursing Theory/Models

SHARING experiences

Give clients time to respond. Make sure they understand. Teaching is not over just because you've finished your speech.

Valerie A. Gordon-Tate, LPN, Newport News, VA.

LEARNING outcomes

After completing the chapter you will be able to:

- Discuss characteristics, skills, and attitudes of critical thinking.
- Explain the importance of critical thinking to the nursing process.
- Define *nursing theory*.
- Compare selected nursing theories in terms of nursing, client/person, health, and environment.
- Identify areas in which the LPN/LVN can incorporate nursing theory into nursing practice.

MediaLink

www.prenhall.com/ramont

Use the address above to access the free, interactive Companion Website created for this textbook. Get hints, instant feedback, and textbook references to chapter-related NCLEX-style questions. Link to other interesting sites.

Audio Glossary:
Use the Companion Website, or the CD-ROM disk inclosed with your textbook, to hear the pronunciations of key terms in the chapter.

Nursing instructors as well as staff nurses in the clinical setting continually challenge nursing students to become critical thinkers. Beginning PN/VN students certainly may be puzzled by these instructions. From the very beginning of the training program, the PN/VN student needs to begin to think like a nurse. Thinking like a nurse is different from thinking like a doctor or a teacher or a lawyer. How the nurse views the client, and the types of problems we deal with in practice when providing care, are what defines thinking for the nurse.

A nurse's thinking is not limited to problem solving or decision making. Nurses must also make reliable observations, draw sound conclusions, create new information and ideas, evaluate other people's way of reasoning, and improve their own self-knowledge. Critical thinking goes hand-in-hand with the nursing process. As you work your way through this chapter and Chapter 4, you will begin to see how the pieces fit together.

You will develop many critical skills and abilities, such as information gathering, focusing, remembering, organizing, analyzing, generating, integrating and evaluating. As you progress through your program, you will encounter increasingly more complex situations. This is the challenge of nursing: *critical reflective practice based on sound reasoning of intelligent minds committed to safe, effective client care.* To accomplish this goal you will be required to reason about nursing by reading, writing, listening, and speaking critically. By thinking critically about nursing, you will gain in-depth knowledge about practicing nursing as a professional.

◆ Critical Thinking

The thinking process that guides nursing practice must be organized, logical, purposeful, and disciplined rather than random or undirected. Paul and Elder (2001) describe **critical thinking** as "the art of thinking about thinking." *Critical,* in this context, does not mean "eager to find fault" but instead "capable of judging carefully and accurately."

METHODS OF PROBLEM SOLVING

LPN/LVNs must problem-solve and make decisions that require the use of cognitive critical-thinking skills. When solving problems the nurse makes inferences, sorts out facts from opinions, evaluates the credibility of information sources, and uses a variety of other cognitive skills. The LPN/LVN employs questioning skills when listening to an end-of-shift report, reviewing a history or progress notes, planning care, or discussing a client's care with colleagues.

Types of Reasoning

The nurse learns to approach problems from several angles in order to apply reasoning skills. Figure 3-1 ◆ highlights the different factors that go into the process of reasoning.

Two other skills used in critical thinking are inductive and deductive reasoning.

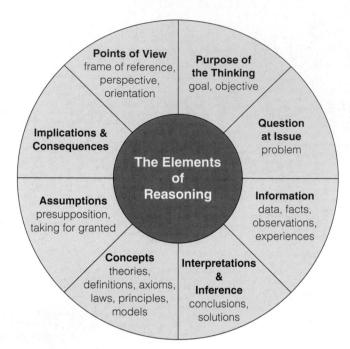

Figure 3-1 ◆ The elements of reasoning. *Source:* Adapted from "Critical Thinking" by R. Paul, 1993, Dillion Beach, CA. Foundation for Critical Thinking, www.criticalthinking.org. Reprinted with permission.

• **Inductive reasoning** forms generalizations from a set of facts or observations. Inductive reasoning is like looking at the pieces of a jigsaw puzzle and attempting to describe the whole (without seeing a picture of the completed puzzle). As the person puts more and more pieces together, the whole picture becomes clearer. For example, the nurse who observes that a client has dry skin, poor turgor, sunken eyes, and dark amber urine may make the generalization that the client appears dehydrated.

• **Deductive reasoning** is reasoning from the general to the specific. In deductive reasoning, the thinker sees the whole picture (from the box cover) and puts the puzzle together by organizing the pieces into border pieces, colors, or specific shapes. For example, nurses know that people who have experienced several days of vomiting and diarrhea are likely to be dehydrated. In a client who has had vomiting and diarrhea for two days, the nurse would confirm this generalization deductively by checking skin turgor, appearance of the client's eyes, and color and quantity of the client's urine.

By using critical thinking, the nurse also separates facts, inferences, judgments, and opinions (Table 3-1 ◆). See Box 3-1 ◆ for characteristics of a critical thinker.

APPLYING CRITICAL THINKING TO NURSING

LVN/LPNs use their critical-thinking skills in a variety of ways:

• Nursing students must take knowledge from the classroom and apply it to real-life client situations. LPN/LVN stu-

TABLE 3-1 DIFFERENTIATING TYPES OF STATEMENTS

STATEMENT	DESCRIPTION	EXAMPLE
Facts	Can be verified through investigation	Birth control pills do not protect against sexually transmitted diseases (STDs).
Inferences	Conclusions drawn from the facts, going beyond facts to make a statement about something not currently known	A person in a sexual relationship with a client with an STD should not rely on birth control pills alone but should consider using a method that provides a physical barrier.
Judgments	Evaluation of facts or information that reflect values or other criteria; a type of opinion	Having multiple sexual partners can lead to serious health consequences.
Opinions	Beliefs formed over time that include judgments and may fit facts or be in error	It is wrong not to wait until marriage to have sex.

dents will study life span development, nutrition, communication, and psychosocial issues. They will also take nursing courses where they can acquire a strong foundation in nursing knowledge and skill.

- Nurses deal with change in stressful environments. Treatments, medications, and technology change constantly, and a client's condition may change from minute to minute. When unexpected situations arise, critical thinking enables the nurse to recognize important cues, respond quickly, and adapt interventions to meet specific client needs.
- During the course of a workday, nurses make vital decisions of many kinds. These decisions may be made independently by the LPN/LVN or in collaboration with an RN or other team member. It is important that the decisions be sound. LPN/LVNs use critical-thinking skills when collecting information. For example, during routine visits with the client, nurses must decide which observations to report to the physician immediately and which to note in the client record for the physician to address later.

Nurses function effectively some part of every day without thinking critically. Small decisions like selecting clothes or deciding what to eat for lunch are based primarily on habit and require minimal thinking. Psychomotor skills in nursing, like operating a familiar piece of equipment, often involve minimal thinking. But the higher-order skills of critical thinking are put into play as soon as a new idea is encountered or a less-than-routine decision must be made. When setting priorities for the day, a nurse employs critical thinking.

USING CRITICAL THINKING TO MAKE NURSING DECISIONS

The Nursing Process
One model for making decisions is the nursing process. It is the systematic method of assessing, planning, providing, and evaluating nursing care (see Chapter 4). Critical thinking is used throughout the nursing process (Table 3-2 ◆).

Nurses use critical thinking to resolve problems related to direct client care. The nurse obtains information that clarifies the nature of the problem and suggests possible solutions. The nurse then carefully evaluates the possible solutions and chooses the best one to implement. The nurse monitors the situation carefully over time to ensure its initial and continued effectiveness. The nurse does not discard the other solutions but keeps them in mind. They may be useful if the first solution is not effective, or if a different client with a similar problem prefers an alternative solution. Therefore, problem solving for one situation contributes to the nurse's body of knowledge for problem solving in similar situations.

NURSING DECISIONS. Nurses make many types of decisions throughout the day. They make value decisions (e.g., to keep

BOX 3-1 CHARACTERISTICS OF CRITICAL THINKERS

As Critical Thinkers:
- We analyze our thinking.
- We expose the egocentric (self-centered) roots of our thinking to close scrutiny.
- We expose inappropriate standards and replace them with sound ones.
- We learn how to raise our thinking to conscious examination, to free ourselves from traps of undisciplined, instinctive thought.
- We develop tools for analyzing and assessing our participation in the logical systems in which we live.
- We take explicit intellectual and emotional command of who we are, what we are, and the ends to which our lives are tending.
- We learn how to govern the thoughts that govern us.

TABLE 3-2 QUESTIONS ABOUT CRITICAL THINKING THROUGHOUT THE NURSING PROCESS

NURSING PROCESS	QUESTIONS TO ASK
Collecting data for the assessment	Are the data complete? What other data do I need? What are the possible sources of the data? What assumptions and biases do I have about the situation? What is the client's point of view?
IMPLEMENTING AND PLANNING FOR THE NURSING DIAGNOSIS	
Diagnosing	What do these data mean? What else could be happening? Are there any gaps in the data? How are these data similar and how are they different? What assumptions or biases do I have in this situation? Have my assumptions affected my interpretation of the data?
Planning	What are the goals for the client? What do I want to accomplish? How are my goals related to what the client wants to accomplish? What are the expected outcomes for this client? What interventions are to be used? How much involvement can the client and family have at this time?
Implementing	What is the client's current status? What are the most critical steps in this intervention? How must I alter the interventions to best meet this client's needs and maintain the principles of safety? What is the client's response during and after the intervention? Is there a need to alter the intervention in any way? If so, how?
Evaluating	Were the interventions successful in helping the client to meet the desired goals? How could things have been done differently? What data do I need to make new decisions? Where will I get the data? Were there assumptions, biases, or points of view that I missed that affected the outcomes?

client information confidential) and time management decisions (e.g., taking clean linens to the client's room at the same time as the medication in order to save steps). They make scheduling decisions (e.g., to bathe the client before visiting hours) and priority decisions (e.g., which interventions are most urgent and which can be postponed or delegated).

Decision making is a critical-thinking process for choosing the best actions to meet a desired goal. Nurses must make decisions and assist clients to make decisions. When faced with several client needs at the same time, the nurse must decide which client to assist first. When a client is trying to make a decision about what course of treatment to follow, the nurse may need to provide information or resources the client can use in making a decision. See Table 3-3 ◆ for description of a seven-step decision making process.

PRACTICING CRITICAL THINKING

A nurse cannot develop or maintain critical thinking without practice. As you examine all sides of issues and learn to respect opposing viewpoints, you will become more aware of thinking errors and of ways you can broaden your own thinking. Every chapter in this text provides review questions to strengthen your thinking. Chapters 6 through 31 also provide Critical Thinking Case Studies and Care Maps to encourage you to apply your thinking skills to nursing situations. ∞

Critical Thinking Care Map

As LPN/LVNs collect assessment data about a client, they use critical thinking skills to organize data into subjective and objective information. These data contribute to the development of Nursing Diagnoses (see Chapter 4). ∞ LPN/LVNs also use critical thinking to determine whether data should be reported (and to whom), and which interventions would be appropriate for specific Nursing Diagnoses. They think critically when they frame their narrative notes for the client's chart.

A Sample Critical Thinking Care Map is shown on page 41. The Case Study supplied will focus on one of the NCLEX-PN Focus Areas, to help you think in terms of the

This line provides an appropriate nursing diagnosis.

This line provides the appropriate NCLEX-PN focus area.

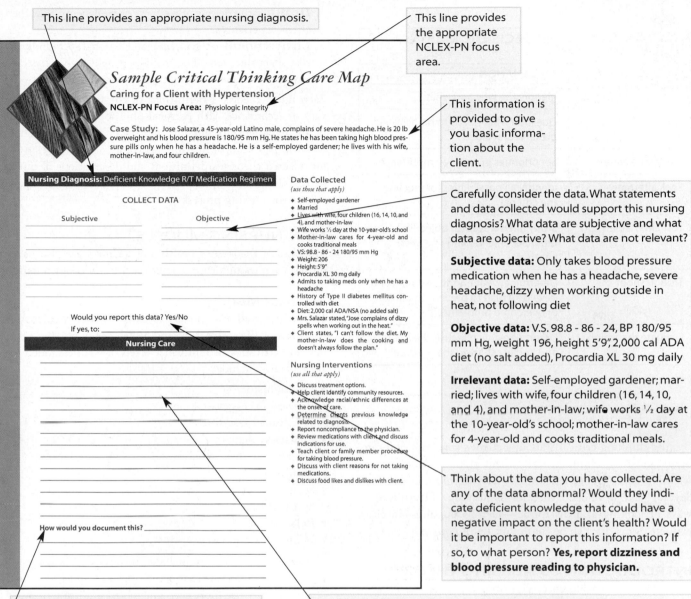

Sample Critical Thinking Care Map

Caring for a Client with Hypertension

NCLEX-PN Focus Area: Physiologic Integrity

Case Study: Jose Salazar, a 45-year-old Latino male, complains of severe headache. He is 20 lb overweight and his blood pressure is 180/95 mm Hg. He states he has been taking high blood pressure pills only when he has a headache. He is a self-employed gardener; he lives with his wife, mother-in-law, and four children.

Nursing Diagnosis: Deficient Knowledge R/T Medication Regimen

COLLECT DATA

Subjective

Objective

Would you report this data? Yes/No

If yes, to: _____

Nursing Care

How would you document this? _____

Data Collected
(use those that apply)

◆ Self-employed gardener
◆ Married
◆ Lives with wife, four children (16, 14, 10, and 4), and mother-in-law
◆ Wife works ⅟₂ day at the 10-year-old's school
◆ Mother-in-law cares for 4-year-old and cooks traditional meals
◆ VS: 98.8 - 86 - 24 180/95 mm Hg
◆ Weight: 206
◆ Height: 5'9"
◆ Procardia XL 30 mg daily
◆ Admits to taking meds only when he has a headache
◆ History of Type II diabetes mellitus controlled with diet
◆ Diet: 2,000 cal ADA/NSA (no added salt)
◆ Mrs. Salazar stated, "Jose complains of dizzy spells when working out in the heat."
◆ Client states, "I can't follow the diet. My mother-in-law does the cooking and doesn't always follow the plan."

Nursing Interventions
(use all that apply)

◆ Discuss treatment options.
◆ Help client identify community resources.
◆ Acknowledge racial/ethnic differences at the onset of care.
◆ Determine clients previous knowledge related to diagnosis.
◆ Report noncompliance to the physician.
◆ Review medications with client and discuss indications for use.
◆ Teach client or family member procedure for taking blood pressure.
◆ Discuss with client reasons for not taking medications.
◆ Discuss food likes and dislikes with client.

This information is provided to give you basic information about the client.

Carefully consider the data. What statements and data collected would support this nursing diagnosis? What data are subjective and what data are objective? What data are not relevant?

Subjective data: Only takes blood pressure medication when he has a headache, severe headache, dizzy when working outside in heat, not following diet

Objective data: V.S. 98.8 - 86 - 24, BP 180/95 mm Hg, weight 196, height 5'9", 2,000 cal ADA diet (no salt added), Procardia XL 30 mg daily

Irrelevant data: Self-employed gardener; married; lives with wife, four children (16, 14, 10, and 4), and mother-in-law; wife works ⅟₂ day at the 10-year-old's school; mother-in-law cares for 4-year-old and cooks traditional meals.

Think about the data you have collected. Are any of the data abnormal? Would they indicate deficient knowledge that could have a negative impact on the client's health? Would it be important to report this information? If so, to what person? **Yes, report dizziness and blood pressure reading to physician.**

This question allows you to practice your documentation. It is not necessary to document all the data or interventions for this exercise. For example, the assessment documentation might be:

1/5/05 Client admitted through ER following dizzy spell at work. BP 180/95, complaining of severe headache. Hx of hypertension, treated with Procardia XL 30 mg. q.d. Client admits to taking meds only when he has a headache.

Marge Smith, LPN

Consider the client's deficient knowledge about the medication regimen. Make a decision about which interventions are relevant and which are not relevant.

Relevant interventions: Acknowledge racial/ethnic differences at the onset of care. Determine clients previous knowledge related to diagnosis. Review medications with client and discuss indications for use. Teach client or family member procedure for taking blood pressure. Discuss with client reasons for not taking medications. Report noncompliance to the physician.

Irrelevant interventions: Discuss treatment options. Help client identify community resources. Discuss food likes and dislikes with client.

broad categories of nursing you will master in order to achieve this level of nursing. An appropriate nursing diagnosis will be supplied, and you will select and sort the **subjective data** (apparent only to the person being affected) and **objective data** (detectable by an observer)

that apply to *this nursing diagnosis.* You will decide whether the data require you to report immediately to a supervisor or physician. You will select appropriate interventions from the list provided. And, you will practice documenting the important information.

TABLE 3-3	SEVEN-STEP DECISION-MAKING PROCESS	
STEPS	**EXPLANATION**	
Identify the purpose	Identify the why and what.	
Set the criteria	Question what needs to be: achieved, preserved, avoided	
Weigh the criteria	Set priorities in order of importance.	
Seek alternatives	Identify all possibilities for meeting the criteria.	
Test alternatives	Study alternatives for objective rationale for choosing one over another.	
Troubleshoot	Determine what might go wrong and develop a plan to prevent, minimize, or overcome problems.	
Evaluate the action	Determine how effective they were and if they achieved the purpose.	

 ## Theories and Models

Besides thinking critically about a client's condition and care, nurses must also think critically about nursing itself. Starting with Florence Nightingale, nurses have been doing just that. Several have developed theories of nursing. **Theories** are ways of looking at a discipline—such as nursing—in clear, explicit terms that can be communicated to others.

INTRODUCTION TO NURSING THEORIES

Until 1859, when Florence Nightingale penned her *Notes on Nursing—What Nursing Is and Is Not,* nursing practice was based on theory borrowed from medicine. Nursing continues to draw upon the medical community for knowledge, but since the middle of the last century nursing has begun to develop its own unique theory. Theory development gained momentum in the 1960s and has progressed since then through the work of several nurse theorists and nurses. Each theory bears the name of the person or group who developed it and reflects the beliefs of the developer.

Essential Elements in Nursing Theory

Nursing theories address and specify relationships about four major ideas. These four concepts are central to nursing.

1. Nursing—the attributes, characteristics, and actions of the nurse providing care on behalf of, or in conjunction with the client.
2. Person or client—the recipient of nursing care (includes individuals, families, and communities).

3. **Health**—the degree of wellness or well-being that the client experiences.
4. **Environment**—the internal and external surroundings that affect the client. This includes people in the physical environment, such as families, friends, and significant others.

Each nurse theorist's definitions of the four major concepts vary in accordance with personal philosophy, scientific orientation, experience in nursing, and the effects of experience on the theorist's view of nursing. See Table 3-4 ◆ (pages 44–47) for selected theorist's definitions and descriptions of nursing, person/client, health, and environment as well as the application to the nursing process.

NON-NURSING MODELS

Models and theories of health and wellness are also used by nurses, even though they are not specifically about nursing.

Wellness Model

Nurses use wellness models to assist clients in identifying health risks, lifestyle habits, and health behaviors. Beliefs, values, and attitudes also influence levels of wellness. Such models generally include:

◆ Health history
◆ Physical fitness evaluation
◆ Nutritional assessment
◆ Life-stress analysis
◆ Lifestyle and health habits
◆ Health beliefs
◆ Sexual health
◆ Spiritual health
◆ Relationships
◆ Health risk appraisal

Non-nursing models are included in LPN/LVN training programs to assist the nurse in gathering data and processing it. Nurses usually use more than one model at a time in order to obtain a complete client history.

Body Systems Model

One common non-nursing model is the Body Systems Model. This is closely related to the medical model. The client is assessed and treated according to the body system affected by the primary or presenting medical diagnosis. When a client has a disease process with multisystem effects, however, this model has significant limitations.

Body systems reviewed in this model are:

◆ Integumentary system
◆ Respiratory system
◆ Cardiovascular system
◆ Nervous system
◆ Musculoskeletal system
◆ Gastrointestinal system
◆ Genitourinary system
◆ Reproductive system

Maslow's Hierarchy of Needs

Another non-nursing model is Maslow's Hierarchy of Needs, which the nurse uses to identify needs and to set priorities of care.

Maslow's hierarchy of needs clusters data in order of importance. Survival needs form the base of the pyramid; once met, other needs take priority, as follows:

◆ Physiologic needs (survival needs)
◆ Safety and security needs
◆ Love and belonging needs
◆ Self-esteem needs
◆ Self-actualization needs

See Chapter 24 and Figure 4-4 for more information.

Developmental Theories

Developmental theories are used by the nurse to treat the client holistically. The concept of **holistic** treatment takes into account that the client is a physical, mental, emotional, and spiritual being. No single aspect of the client can be isolated if holistic treatment is to be provided.

Several physical, psychosocial, cognitive, and moral developmental theories may be used by the nurse. The theories and theorists are discussed in Chapter 24 as they relate to life-span development. At some point in your curriculum, you will study them in depth.

SIGNIFICANCE OF MODELS AND THEORIES

Why is it important for an LPN/LVN to have an understanding of nursing theories? A theoretical understanding of nursing helps you view your clients as more than a medical diagnosis for which you will perform nursing tasks. This understanding will help you develop a personal nursing philosophy. It will help you to understand and participate in the nursing process and collaborate with registered nurses and other staff. It also will help you to discern the differences in scope between levels of nursing practice. Most schools of nursing and health care agencies have developed their own structured assessment tools. Many of these are based on selected nursing theories.

Today, the LPN/LVN has a great deal of responsibility and must think critically to make sound decisions. Understanding the four concepts that are central to nursing will help the LPN/LVN process information and make appropriate judgments. As nurses progress in formal education or lifelong learning, they will learn to develop a personal theory of nursing. Understanding the basic principles prepares LVN/LPNs for the future.

TABLE
3-4

SELECTED NURSING THEORIES AND THE NURSING PROCESS

THEORY	NURSING	PERSON/CLIENT	HEALTH
Nightingale's Environmental Theory	Provision of optimal conditions to enhance the person's reparative processes and prevent the reparative process from being interrupted.	An individual with vital reparative processes to deal with disease and desirous of health but passive in terms of influencing the environment or nurse.	Health: Being well and using one's powers to the fullest extent. Health is maintained through prevention of disease via environmental health factors. Disease is a reparative process nature institutes because of some want of attention.
Orem's General Theory of Nursing	A helping or assisting service to persons who are wholly or partly dependent—infants, children, and adults—when they, their parents, guardians, or other adults responsible for their care are no longer able to give or supervise their care. A creative effort of one human being to help another human being. Nursing is deliberate action, a function of the practical intelligence of nurses, and action to bring about humanely desirable conditions in persons and their environments. It is distinguished from other human services and other forms of care by its focus on human beings.	A unity who can be viewed as functioning biologically, symbolically, and socially and who initiates and performs self-care activities on own behalf in maintaining life, health, and well-being; self-care activities deal with air, water, food, elimination, activity and rest, solitude and social interaction, prevention of hazards to life and well-being, and promotion of human functioning.	Health is a state that is characterized by soundness or wholeness of developed human structures and of bodily and mental functioning. It includes physical, psychologic, interpersonal, and social aspects. Well-being is used in the sense of individuals' perceived condition of existence. Well-being is a state characterized by experiences of contentment, pleasure, and certain kinds of happiness; by spiritual experiences; by movement toward fulfillment of one's self-ideal; and by continuing personalization. Well-being is associated with health, with success in personal endeavors, and with sufficiency of resources.
Neuman's System Model	A unique profession in that it is concerned with all of the variables affecting an individual's response to stressors, which are intra-, inter-, and extrapersonal in nature. The concern of nursing is to prevent stress invasion, or, following stress invasion, to protect the client's basic structure and obtain or maintain a maximum level of wellness. The nurse helps the client, through primary, secondary, and tertiary prevention modes, to adjust to environmental stressors and maintain client system stability.	Open system consisting of a basic structure or central core of survival factors surrounded by concentric rings that are bounded by lines of resistance, a normal line of defense, and a flexible line of defense. The total person is a composite of physiologic, psychologic, sociocultural, and developmental variables.	Wellness is the condition in which all parts and subparts of an individual are in harmony with the whole system. Wholeness is based on interrelation-ships of variables that determine the resistance of an individual to any stressor. Illness indicates lack of harmony among the parts and subparts of the system of the individual. Health is viewed as a point along a continuum from wellness to illness; health is dynamic (i.e., constantly subject to change). Optimal wellness or stability indicates that all a person's needs are being met. A reduced state of wellness is the result of unmet systemic needs. The individual is in a dynamic state of wellness–illness, in varying degrees, at any given time.

ENVIRONMENT	COLLECTING DATA FOR ASSESSMENT	PLANNING AND IMPLEMENTING THE DIAGNOSIS	EVALUATING
Environment: The major concepts for health are ventilation, warmth, light, diet, cleanliness, and absence of noise. Although the environment has social, emotional, and physical aspects, Nightingale emphasized the physical aspects.	"The most important practical lesson that can be given to nurses is to teach them what to observe, how to observe, what symptoms indicate improvement, what the reverse indicates, which are of importance, which are not, which are the evidence of neglect, and what kind of neglect." In this statement Nightingale was teaching the first step.	**Diagnose/Plan:** The concept of nursing diagnoses came much later, but she did identify particular needs and problems presented by the patient. Through observation she was able to title problems such as lack of appetite or difficulty breathing so that they could be addressed immediately. Nurses were able to plan care, basing it on the prioritizing of patients needs. **Implementing:** The plan of care was directly related to Nightingale's theory of environment. Nurses were not only responsible for personal care of the patient but were also responsible for washing the floors and walls and maintenance of the stove to provide warmth in the environment.	The patient's progress was evaluated and reassessed by observation. She determined that the evaluation of client's status was critical to the process of providing adequate care, and to determine if care should be continued or altered.
The environment is linked to the individual, forming an integrated and interactive system.	Involves collecting data about the client's capacities (knowledge, skills, and motivation) to perform universal, developmental, and health-deviation self-care requisites. Determines self-care deficits.	**Diagnosing:** Stated in terms of the client's limitations for maintaining self-care (a deficit in self-care agency). **Planning:** Involves considering and designing, with the client's participation, an appropriate nursing system (wholly compensatory, partially compensatory, supportive-educative, or a mix) that will help the client achieve an optimal level of self-care (i.e., enhance the client's self-care agency). **Implementing:** Assisting the client by acting for or doing for, guiding, supporting, providing a developmental environment, and teaching.	Determining the client's level of achievement in resolving self-care deficits and in performing self-care.
Both internal and external environments exist and a person maintains varying degrees of harmony and balance between them. It is all factors affecting and affected by the system.	Proper assessment requires consideration of both the client's and the care giver's perceptions of the basic structure, the lines of resistance and defense, and the internal and external environment.	**Diagnosing:** The nursing diagnosis must be a comprehensive statement that emcompasses the client's general condition and circumstances, including actual and potential variances from wellness. **Planning:** The diagnostic statements are used to formulate and prioritize the client's needs and to identify interactions. **Implementing:** Nursing interventions focus on retaining or maintaining system stability. Interventions are carried out on three preventative levels: primary, secondary, and tertiary.	The final stage of nursing process according to Neuman occurs when the client's outcomes are evaluated to confirm their attainment or guide reformulation of the goals.

(continued)

TABLE 3-4 SELECTED NURSING THEORIES AND THE NURSING PROCESS (*continued*)

THEORY	NURSING	PERSON/CLIENT	HEALTH
Roy's Adaptation Model	Nursing involves the care and well-being of human persons; the value-based stance of the discipline is rooted in beliefs about the human person. As a science, nursing is a developing system of knowledge about persons used to observe, classify, and relate the processes by which persons positively affect their health status. As a practice discipline, nursing's scientific body of knowledge is used to provide an essential service to people, that is, to promote the ability to affect health positively.	A biopsychosocial being who is in constant interaction with the environment and who has four modes of adaptation, based on physiologic needs, self-concept (physical self, moral-ethical self, self-consistency, self-ideal and expectancy, and self-esteem), role function, and interdependence relations. Persons are coextensive with their physical and social environments. Persons and the earth are one; they are in God and of God.	A state and a process of being and becoming an integrated and whole person. Lack of integration represents lack of health.
Leininger's Culture Care, Diversity, and Universality Theory	A learned humanistic art and science that focuses on personalized behaviors, functions, and processes to promote and maintain health or recovery from illness. It has physical, psychosocial, and cultural significance for those being assisted. It uses a problem-solving approach, as depicted in the Sunrise Model, and uses three models of action: culture care preservation, culture care accommodation, and culture care repatterning.	Human beings are caring and capable of feeling concern for others; caring about human beings is universal, but ways of caring vary across cultures.	A state of well-being that is culturally defined, valued, and practiced. Is universal across cultures but is defined differently by each culture. It includes health systems, health care practices, health patterns, and health maintenance and promotion.

ENVIRONMENT	COLLECTING DATA FOR ASSESSMENT	PLANNING AND IMPLEMENTING THE DIAGNOSIS	EVALUATING
All the conditions, circumstances, and influences surrounding and affecting the development and behavior of persons or groups; the input into the person as an adaptive system involving both internal and external factors.	Involves two levels. First-level assessment includes collecting data about output behaviors related to the four adaptive modes (physiologic, self-concept, role function, and interdependence modes). Second-level assessment includes collecting data about internal and external stimuli (focal, contextual, or residual) that are influencing the identified behaviors.	**Diagnosing:** Focuses on adaptation problems and uses one of three alternative methods: 1. Stating behaviors within one mode with their most relevant influencing stimuli. 2. Clustering behavioral information and labeling it according to indicators of positive adaptation and a typology of common adaptation problems related to each mode. Roy provides a typology of indicators of positive adaptation and a typology of commonly recurring adaptation problems according to each of the four modes. 3. Labeling a behavioral pattern when more than one mode is being affected by the same stimuli. **Planning:** Setting goals in terms of behaviors the client is to achieve and planning nursing interventions to promote the effectiveness of the client's coping mechanisms and adaptive behaviors. **Implementing:** Altering and manipulating the focal, contextual, and residual stimuli by increasing, decreasing, or maintaining them.	Determining the client's output behaviors with those identified in the goals.
Not specifically defined, but concepts of world view, social structure, and environmental context are closely related to the concept of culture.	Must take into account biocultural variations in health and illness, (e.g. assessing cyanosis, jaundice, anemia, and related clinical manifestations of disease in darkly pimented clients).	**Diagnosing:** Focuses on meeting health care needs in the context of clients patterns. **Planning:** The nurse plans, negotiates, and accommodates the client's specific cultural wants and needs (e.g., food preferences, religious practices, and treatment practices). **Implementing:** Health care personel should work toward an understanding of care and the values, health beliefs, and lifestyles of different cultures, which will form the basis for providing culture-specific care.	When the client chooses to follow only folk medicine/treatment and refuses all prescribed medical or nursing interventions, nursing goals for the client need to be adjusted.

Note: The bibliography listings for this and all chapters have been compiled at the back of the book.

Chapter Review

Key Terms by Topics

Use the audio glossary feature of either the CD-ROM or the Companion Website to hear the correct pronunciation of the following key terms.

Critical thinking
critical thinking, inductive reasoning, deductive reasoning

Practicing critical thinking
objective data, subjective data

Theories and models
theories

Introduction to nursing theories
health, environment

Non-nursing models
holistic

Key Points

- Critical thinking is a purposeful mental activity in which ideas are produced and evaluated and judgments made.

- Critical thinking is reasonable, rational, reflective, autonomous, creative, and fair and inspires an attitude of inquiry that focuses on deciding what to believe or do. When nurses incorporate creativity into their thinking, they are able to find unique solutions to unique problems.

- Critical thinkers have certain attitudes: independence of thought, humility, courage, integrity, perseverance, empathy, and fair-mindedness.

- Everyone has at least some level of critical-thinking skill, and that skill can be developed with practice.

- Nursing theories help us view the client more completely or understand the goals of nursing better.

- Nursing theories explore the meaning of "client, environment, health, and nursing" and add perspective to our own individual ways of approaching our profession.

- Non-nursing theories help nurses as they gather and process data, particularly when completing a client history.

EXPLORE MediaLink

Additional interactive resources for this chapter can be found on the Companion Website at www.prenhall.com/ramont. Click on Chapter 3 and "Begin" to select the activities for this chapter.

For chapter-related NCLEX-style questions and an audio glossary, access the accompanying CD-ROM in this book.

For Further Study

For more information about the development of Nursing Diagnoses, see Chapter 4.

For additional information about development theories, see Chapter 24.

For Maslow's Hierarchy of Needs, see Figure 4-4.

NCLEX-PN Exam Preparation

1. There are four concepts that are central to nursing theory: nursing, client, environment, and health. Which of the following interventions is aimed at addressing the environment?
   a. Teaching a community class on proper nutrition.
   b. Actively listening to a client who expresses concerns about an upcoming surgery.
   c. Limiting external stimulation for a client who has increased intracranial pressure (ICP).
   d. Instructing a client to do active range of motion (AROM) exercises in preparation for walking following a CVA (cerebral vascular accident).

2. The Neuman Systems Model's unique focus is on:
   a. Responses to the constantly changing environment
   b. Clients' reactions to stress
   c. Nurses' actions related to therapeutic self-care
   d. Culturally competent care

3. Critical thinking can be described as:
   a. Finding fault with statements or facts
   b. The art of thinking about thinking
   c. Making decisions considering only one point of view
   d. Random and undirected

4. Critical thinking and the nursing process go hand-in-hand. The nurse should consider personal assumptions or biases about the situation during what phase of the nursing process?
   a. Assessment/data collection
   b. Diagnosing
   c. Planning
   d. Evaluation

5. The environmental theory is attributed to which of the following nursing theorists?
   a. Florence Nightingale
   b. Sister Callista Roy
   c. Betty Neuman
   d. Madeleine Leininger

6. An application of critical thinking to the client teaching process requires that the nurse be aware of potential pitfalls and limitations in thinking. Which of the following actions takes this into account?
   a. Evaluate cognitive ability of the client.
   b. Give the client written instructions and allow them time to read them.
   c. Instruct the client to call the home health nurse if problems develop.
   d. Arrange for family member to be present during teaching.

7. The client is recovering from a myocardial infarction. Using your critical thinking skills, which of the following observations would need to be reported immediately?
   a. Blood pressure 118/74; pulse, 72; capillary refill, 1 second; SaO_2 98%.
   b. Blood pressure 138/88; pulse, 86; capillary refill, 3 seconds; SaO_2 95%.
   c. Blood pressure 100/50; pulse, 90; capillary refill, 4 seconds; SaO_2 97%.
   d. Blood pressure 120/88; pulse, 78; capillary refill, 2 seconds; SaO_2 97%.

8. Your neighbor is a nurse at the community hospital. She is a member of the union. The union has called for a strike. All the nurses at the hospital will go on strike. This sequence of thinking is called:
   a. Inductive reasoning
   b. Deductive reasoning
   c. Opinion
   d. Belief

9. The dominant, distinctive, and unifying feature of nursing was identified as human caring by which of the following theorists?
   a. Dorothea Orem
   b. Sister Callista Roy
   c. Betty Neuman
   d. Madeleine Leininger

10. Research has shown that children under 18 years who are given aspirin products during a viral infection are at risk for developing Reye's syndrome. Of the following statements, which is an example of deductive reasoning about this subject?
    a. The American Academy of Pediatrics recommends that children under the age of 18 not be given aspirin products.
    b. All children are at risk for developing Reye's syndrome.
    c. Parents who give children aspirin during a viral infection are negligent.
    d. Parents should treat fever with cooling measures rather than medication.

The LVN/LPN and the Nursing Process

SHARING experiences

The nursing process has been extremely helpful to me throughout my entire VN program. It has given me a foundation on which to base my nursing care, and has led me to make impor- *tant health care decisions regarding the type of care given to each individual. It has also given me a more organized approach to client care and lets me focus on my love of helping others.*

Melinda Barrowcliff-Reyes, Cal-HOSA State Officer, Region 4 Vice-President, VN Student, NOCROP, Anaheim, CA.

LEARNING outcomes

After completing this chapter, you will be able to:
- Identify essential characteristics of the nursing process.
- Describe the components of the nursing process.
- Identify the purpose of assessing.
- Differentiate objective and subjective data and primary and secondary data.
- Identify three methods of data collection, and give examples of how each is useful.
- Describe the importance and the elements of nursing diagnoses.
- Identify basic steps in the diagnostic process.
- Discuss the planning step of the nursing process.
- Discuss the activities of the implementing phase.
- Explain the value of evaluating and how evaluating relates to other phases of the nursing process.

MediaLink

 www.prenhall.com/ramont

Use the address above to access the free, interactive Companion Website created for this textbook. Get hints, instant feedback, and textbook references to chapter-related NCLEX-style questions. Link to other interesting sites.

Audio Glossary:
Use the Companion Website, or the CD-ROM disk enclosed with your textbook, to hear the pronunciation of key terms in the chapter.

The **nursing process** is a systematic, logical method of providing individualized nursing care. Box 4-1 ◆ provides characteristics of the nursing process. The purposes of the nursing process are:

◆ To identify a client's health status and actual or potential health care problems or needs
◆ To establish plans to meet the identified needs
◆ To deliver specific nursing interventions to meet those needs

The components of the nursing process follow a logical sequence, but more than one component may be involved at any one time (Figure 4-1 ◆).

In 1961, the nursing process was defined at the Catholic University of America. It was developed as a template for thinking that was exclusively for nursing. Although the process was designed with registered nurses in mind, use of the nursing process provides a common way of thinking for all licensed nurses. All licensed nurses collect data for assessment. They plan, implement, and evaluate. LPNs and LVNs, through the data they collect and through their ongoing evaluation of the client, contribute to the nursing diagnoses that RNs are responsible for making.

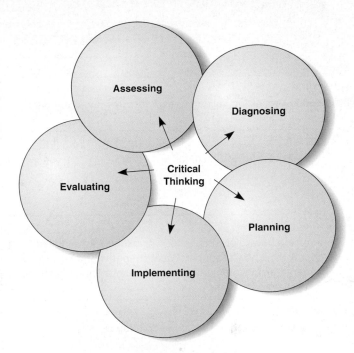

Figure 4-1. ◆ The nursing process in action

 ## Components of the Nursing Process

The nursing process consists of five steps: assessing, diagnosing, planning, implementing, and evaluating. Nursing theorists may use different terms to describe these steps. For exam-

ple, nursing diagnosis may sometimes be called analysis. Implementation (implementing) may be called intervention or intervening. However, the activities of the nurse using the process are similar. An overview of the five-phase nursing process is shown in Table 4-1 ◆.

The nursing process "provides the framework in which nurses use their knowledge and skills to express human caring" and to help clients meet their actual and potential health problems. The nursing process has unique properties that enable it to respond to the changing health status of the client.

ROLE OF THE LPN/LVN IN THE NURSING PROCESS

LPN/LVNs, as important members of the health care team, should be familiar with all aspects of the nursing process. They should be specially educated in those aspects that fall within their scope of practice. Within each step of the nursing process, there will be functions performed by the LPN/LVN, functions carried out in collaboration with or under the direction of the RN, and functions implemented by the RN. The importance of understanding the entire process cannot be overemphasized.

The nursing process:

1. Helps students transfer classroom knowledge to the clinical setting
2. Provides structure and guidance for LPN/LVNs as they provide client care

This chapter will define specific duties that can be carried out by the LPN/LVN.

BOX 4-1 CHARACTERISTICS OF THE NURSING PROCESS

◆ The system is open and flexible to meet the unique needs of client, family, group, or community.
◆ It is cyclic and dynamic. Because all phases are interrelated, there is no absolute beginning or end.
◆ It is client centered; it individualizes the approach to each client's particular needs.
◆ It is interpersonal and collaborative. It requires the nurse to communicate directly and consistently with clients to meet their needs.
◆ It is planned.
◆ It is goal directed.
◆ It permits creativity for the nurse and client in devising ways to solve the stated health problem.
◆ It emphasizes feedback, which leads either to reassessment of the problem or to revision of the care plan.
◆ It is universally applicable. The nursing process is used as a framework for nursing care in all types of health care settings, with clients of all age groups.

TABLE 4-1 OVERVIEW OF THE NURSING PROCESS	
COMPONENT AND DESCRIPTION	**PURPOSE**
Assessing Collecting, organizing, validating, and documenting client data	To establish a database about the client's response to health concerns or illness and the ability to manage health care needs
Diagnosing Analyzing and synthesizing data	To identify client strengths and health problems that can be prevented or resolved by collaborative and independent nursing interventions To develop a list of nursing diagnoses and collaborative problems
Planning Determining how to prevent, reduce, or resolve the identified client problems; how to support client strengths; and how to implement nursing interventions in an organized, individualized, and goal-directed manner	To develop an individualized care plan that specifies client goals/desired outcomes and related nursing interventions
Implementing Carrying out the planned nursing interventions	To assist the client to meet desired goals/outcomes; promote wellness; prevent illness and disease; restore health; and facilitate coping with altered functioning
Evaluating Measuring the degree to which goals/outcomes have been achieved and identifying factors that positively or negatively influence goal achievement	To determine whether to continue, modify, or terminate the plan of care

 Assessment

Assessment is the systematic collection, organization, *validation* (proving or supporting), and documentation of *data* (information). All phases of the nursing process depend on accurate and complete data collection. Nursing assessments focus on a client's responses to a health problem. The Joint Commission on Accreditation of Healthcare Organizations (JCAHO, 2001) recommended that each client receive a documented assessment on admission to an agency. The initial assessment is usually done by the RN.

In some situations, ongoing assessments are also done only by RNs. This may be stated in the nurse practice act of the state or may be a management decision of a particular facility. The LPN/LVN is responsible for contributing by collecting data. The LPN/LVN is also responsible for reading the assessment prior to beginning care of assigned clients.

The assessment process involves four closely related activities: collecting data, organizing data, validating data, and documenting data.

COLLECTING DATA

Data collection is the process of gathering information about a client. It must be both systematic and continuous, and it must reflect a client's changing health status.

A client's **database** (baseline data) includes information from many sources: (1) the nursing health history, (2) nurse's

physical assessment, (3) the physician's history and physical examination, (4) results of laboratory and diagnostic tests, and (5) information contributed by other health personnel. (See Components of a Nursing Health History in Box 4-2. ◆)

Client data should include past history as well as current problems. For example, a history of an allergic reaction to penicillin is a vital piece of historical data. Current data relate to present circumstances, such as pain, nausea, or sleep patterns. To collect data accurately, both the client and nurse must participate actively.

TYPES OF DATA

Data can be subjective or objective. **Subjective data,** also referred to as **symptoms,** are apparent only to the person affected. Itching, pain, and feelings of worry are examples of subjective data. Subjective data include the client's sensations, feelings, values, beliefs, attitudes, and perception of personal health status and life situation. Information supplied by family members and significant others is also considered subjective.

Objective data, also referred to as **signs,** are detectable by an observer or can be tested against an accepted standard. They can be seen, heard, felt, or smelled. For example, a discoloration of the skin or a blood pressure reading are objective data. During the head-to-toe assessment, the nurse obtains the objective data needed to validate subjective data. A complete database of both subjective and objective data provides a baseline for

BOX 4-2 COMPONENTS OF A NURSING HEALTH HISTORY

Biographic Data
Client's name, address, age, sex, marital status, occupation, religious preference, health care financing, and usual source of medical care

Chief Complaint or Reason for Visit
The answer given to the question "Why did you come here today?"

History of Present Illness
◆ Provocation or palliation: what causes it, what relieves it
◆ Quality and quantity: type of pain and intensity
◆ Region or radiation: where it is, where it goes
◆ Scale of pain: 1 to 10
◆ Timing: when it began, how long it lasts, and how often it occurs

Past History
◆ Childhood illnesses
◆ Childhood immunizations
◆ Allergies
◆ Accidents and injuries
◆ Hospitalization for serious illnesses
◆ Medication: all currently used prescription and over-the-counter medication, such as aspirin, nasal spray, vitamins, or laxatives

Family History of Illness
◆ Heart disease, cancer, genetic abnormality

Lifestyle
◆ Personal habits: tobacco, alcohol, coffee, etc.
◆ Diet
◆ Sleep/rest patterns
◆ Activities of daily living (ADLs): any difficulties in performing the basic activities
◆ Recreation/hobbies

Social Data
◆ Client's support system: family, friends, professional counseling
◆ Ethnic affiliation
◆ Highest level of education
◆ Occupation and employment: Has illness affected ability to work?
◆ Health insurance
◆ Home and neighborhood conditions (if applicable)

Psychological Data
◆ Major stressors
◆ Usual coping pattern
◆ Communication style

comparing the client's responses to nursing and medical interventions. Examples of objective and subjective data (also called **manifestations**) are shown in Box 4-3 ◆.

SOURCES OF DATA
The client is the *primary source* of data. All sources other than the client are considered *secondary sources*. The nurse should indicate on the nursing history when the data are obtained from a secondary source (a parent, a cousin, a friend).

Client Records
The nurse must always consider the information in client records in light of the present situation. For example, if the most recent medical record is 10 years old, it is likely that the client's health practices and coping behaviors have changed.

DATA COLLECTION METHODS
The primary methods used to collect data are observing, interviewing, and examining. Observation occurs whenever the nurse is in contact with the client or support persons. Interviewing is used mainly while taking the nursing health history.

Observing
Observation is gathering data by using the senses. Although nurses observe mainly through sight, most of the senses are engaged during careful observations. Examples of client data observed through four of the five senses are shown in Table 4-2 ◆.

BOX 4-3 EXAMPLES OF SUBJECTIVE AND OBJECTIVE DATA

Subjective
◆ "I feel weak all over when I exert myself."
◆ Client states he has a cramping pain in his abdomen. States, "I feel sick to my stomach."
◆ "I'm short of breath."
◆ "He doesn't seem so sad today," wife states.
◆ "I would like to see the chaplain before surgery."

Objective
◆ Blood pressure 90/50
◆ Apical pulse 104
◆ Skin pale and diaphoretic
◆ Vomited 100 mL green-tinged fluid
◆ Abdomen firm and slightly distended
◆ Active bowel sounds auscultated in all four quadrants
◆ Lung sounds clear bilaterally; diminished in right lower lobe
◆ Cried during interview
◆ Holding open Bible
◆ Has small silver cross on bedside table

TABLE 4-2	USE OF THE SENSES IN COLLECTING DATA	
SENSES	**EXAMPLE OF CLIENT DATA**	
Vision	Overall appearance (body size, general weight, posture, grooming); signs of distress or discomfort; facial and body gestures; skin color and lesions; abnormalities of movement; nonverbal demeanor (e.g., signs of anger or anxiety); religious or cultural artifacts (e.g., books, icons, candles, beads)	
Smell	Body or breath odors	
Hearing	Breath and heart sounds; bowel sounds; ability to communicate; language spoken; ability to initiate conversation; ability to respond when spoken to; orientation to time, person, and place; thoughts and feelings about self, others, and health status	
Touch	Skin temperature and moisture; muscle strength (e.g., hand grip); pulse rate, rhythm, and volume; palpatory lesions (e.g., lumps, masses, nodules)	

Observation involves interpretation of data. The LPN/LVN and the RN work together (**collaborate**) to determine the meaning of the observation.

Interviewing

An **interview** is a planned communication or a conversation with a purpose. In interviews, the nurse gets or gives information; identifies problems of mutual concern; evaluates change; teaches; and provides support, counseling, or therapy. (See Chapter 25 for interviewing and communication techniques. ∞) Interviewing is a process the nurse applies in most phases of the nursing process. During the assessment phase, however, the primary purpose of the interview is to gather data. One example of the interview is the admission questionnaire. (See Chapter 8 for more about admitting a client. ∞)

Examining

The physical **examination** or physical assessment is a systematic data-collection method that uses the senses of sight, hearing, smell, and touch to detect health problems. To conduct the examination, the nurse uses techniques of inspection, auscultation, palpation, and percussion. Inspection, auscultation, and palpation are described in Chapter 11. ∞ Additional training is needed in order to practice percussion.

DOCUMENTING DATA

To complete the assessment phase, the nurse records client data. Accurate documentation is essential and should include all data collected about the client's health status. Data are recorded in a factual manner and not interpreted by the nurse. For example, the nurse records the client's breakfast intake (objective data) as "coffee 240 mL, juice 120 mL, 1 egg, and 1 slice of toast," not as "appetite good" (a judgment). A judgment or conclusion such as "appetite good" or "normal appetite" may have different meanings for different people.

To increase accuracy, the nurse records subjective data in the client's own words. Restating what someone says increases

the chance of changing the original meaning. Details of recording are discussed in Chapter 9. ∞

Diagnosis

Diagnosis is the second phase of the nursing process. In this phase, nurses use critical-thinking skills to interpret assessment data and identify client strengths and problems. As mentioned, this phase is the responsibility of the RN. The LPN/LVN discusses the collected data with the RN. The RN identifies appropriate nursing diagnoses for the client and initiates the nursing care plan.

A **nursing diagnosis** is a statement about an alteration in the client's health status. It refers to a condition that nurses are licensed to treat. A *medical diagnosis* is made by a physician and refers to a condition that only a physician can treat. Table 4-3 ◆ compares medical and nursing diagnoses, and collaborative problems.

The identification and development of nursing diagnoses began formally in 1973, and the First Canadian Conference took place in 1977. In 1982, the conference group accepted the name North American Nursing Diagnosis Association (NANDA), recognizing the participation and contributions of nurses in the United States and Canada. NANDA updates its list of nursing diagnoses every two years (see Appendix I). ∞

Definitions

In 1990, NANDA adopted an official working definition of *nursing diagnosis:* "Nursing diagnosis is a clinical judgment about individual, family, or community responses to actual and potential health problems/life processes. Nursing diagnoses provide the basis for selection of nursing interventions to achieve outcomes for which the nurse is accountable."

Linda Carpenito provided a definition of nursing diagnosis which is perhaps easier to understand. According to her, nursing diagnoses are " . . . actual or potential health problems

	TABLE 4-3 COMPARISON OF MEDICAL AND NURSING DIAGNOSES AND COLLABORATIVE PROBLEMS		
CATEGORY	MEDICAL DIAGNOSES	NURSING DIAGNOSES	COLLABORATIVE PROBLEMS
Description of the Term	Describe disease and pathology; do not consider other human response; usually consist of not more than three words	Describe human responses to disease process or health problems; consist of a one-, two-, or three-part statement, usually including problem and etiology	Involve human responses—mainly physiologic complications of disease, test, or treatments; consist of a two-part statement of situation/ pathophysiology and the potential complication
Example	Myocardial infarction	Activity Intolerance related to decreased cardiac output	Potential complication of myocardial infarction: congestive heart failure (CHF)
Duration	Remains the same while disease is present	Can change frequently	Present when disease or situation is present
Treatment Orders	Physician orders primary interventions to prevent and treat	Nurse plans interventions to prevent and treat the nursing diagnosis	Nurse collaborates with physician and other health care professionals to prevent and treat
Nursing Focus	Implement medical orders for treatment and monitor status of condition	Provide interventions for the nursing diagnosis	Prevent and monitor for onset or status of condition

which nurses, by virtue of their education and experience, are capable and licensed to treat" (Carpenito, 2002).

These definitions imply the following:

◆ Registered nurses are responsible for making nursing diagnoses. LPN/LVNs and other nursing personnel contribute data to the process of diagnosing, and implement specified nursing care.
◆ Nursing diagnoses describe a continuum of health states: deviations from health, presence of risk factors, and areas of improved health.
◆ The domain of nursing diagnosis includes only those health states that nurses are educated and licensed to treat. For example, nurses are not educated to diagnose or treat diseases like diabetes mellitus. This task is legally within the practice of medicine. Yet nurses can diagnose and treat Deficient Knowledge, Ineffective Individual Coping, or Imbalanced Nutrition, all of which may accompany diabetes mellitus.
◆ A nursing diagnosis is a statement made only after thorough, systematic data collection.

COMPONENTS OF A NANDA NURSING DIAGNOSIS

A nursing diagnosis has three components: the problem, qualifier(s), and etiology.

Problem (Diagnostic Label)

The problem statement, or *diagnostic label,* describes the client's health problem or response for which nursing theory is given in clear, concise terms. (See Appendix I. ⊶) The purpose of the

nursing diagnosis is to direct the formation of client goals and desired outcomes. It may also suggest some nursing interventions.

Defining characteristics are the cluster of manifestations (signs and symptoms) that indicate the presence of a particular diagnostic statement.

Qualifiers

When a NANDA label is followed by the word "(specify)", the nurse states the area in which the problem occurs. For example, Deficient Knowledge (medications) or Deficient Knowledge (dietary adjustments) specify the particular area in which teaching is needed.

Qualifiers are added to some NANDA statements to give additional meaning to the diagnostic statement. For example:

◆ *Impaired* (made worse, weakened, damaged, reduced, deteriorated)
◆ *Decreased* (smaller in size, amount, or degree)
◆ *Ineffective* (not producing the desired effect)

Etiology (Related Factors and Risk Factors)

The **etiology** piece of the nursing diagnosis identifies factors contributing to, or probable causes of, the health problem. It gives direction to the required nursing therapy and enables the nurse to individualize the client's care.

TWO-PART AND THREE-PART NURSING DIAGNOSIS STATEMENTS

Most nursing diagnoses are written as two-part or three-part statements. Basic two-part statements are used for potential

BOX 4-4 BASIC THREE-PART DIAGNOSTIC STATEMENT

Problem
Situational Low Self-Esteem related to (r/t)

Etiology
Rejection by husband as manifested by (a.m.b.)

Signs and Symptoms
Hypersensitivity to criticism; states, "I don't know if I can manage by myself" and rejects positive feedback

problems or "at risk for" statements. They include the problem (NANDA label) and the etiology. The two parts are joined by the words *related to* to imply a relationship. Some NANDA labels contain the word *specify*. For these, the RN adds words to indicate the problem more specifically. For example, "Noncompliance (specify)" might become "Noncompliance (diabetic diet)" related to denial of having disease.

Basic three-part statements are used for actual problems. The basic three-part nursing diagnosis statement is called the PES format and includes:

1. Problem (P): Statement of the client's response (NANDA label).
2. Etiology (E): Factors contributing to or probable causes of the response.
3. Signs and symptoms (S): Defining characteristics manifested by the client. An example of a three-part nursing diagnosis statement is given in Box 4-4 ◆.

◆ Planning

Planning is the third step in the nursing process. Planning is a systematic phase of the nursing process that involves decision making and problem solving. In planning, the nurse refers to the client's assessment data and diagnostic statements for direction in formulating client goals. All planning is aimed at preventing, reducing, or eliminating the client's health problems. The product of the planning phase is a client care plan.

The input of the LPN/LVN and support persons is essential if a plan is to be effective. Nurses do not plan for the client, but encourage the client to participate as actively as possible in shaping a plan. In a home setting, the client's support people and caregivers are the ones who implement the plan of care. Its effectiveness depends largely on them.

According to the NCLEX-PN test plan, the LPN/LVN's role in the planning phase is to do the following:

1. Assist in the formation of the goals of care:
   ◆ Participate in identifying nursing interventions required to achieve goals
   ◆ Communicate client needs that may require alteration of the goals of care
2. Assist in developing the plan of care:
   ◆ Involve the client and healthcare team members in the selection of nursing interventions.
   ◆ Plan for the client's safety, comfort, and maintenance of optimum functioning.
   ◆ Select nursing interventions for delivery of client's care (Anderson 2000, 233.)

TYPES OF PLANNING
Planning begins with the first client contact and continues until the nurse–client relationship ends, usually when the client is discharged from the health care agency.

Initial Planning
The RN who performs the admission assessment usually develops the initial comprehensive plan of care. Planning should be initiated as soon as possible after the initial assessment, especially because of the trend toward shorter hospital stays. The LPN/LVN can assist with data collection.

Ongoing Planning
Ongoing planning is done by all nurses who work with the client. As nurses obtain new information and evaluate the client's responses to care, they can individualize the initial care plan further.

Discharge Planning
Discharge planning involves anticipating and planning for needs after discharge. It is a crucial part of comprehensive health care and should be addressed in each client's care plan. Although many clients are discharged to other agencies (e.g., nursing homes), follow-up care is increasingly being delivered in the home. Effective discharge planning begins at first client contact and involves comprehensive and ongoing assessment to obtain information about the client's ongoing needs. For more about discharge planning, see Chapter 8. 🔗

NURSING CARE PLANS
The end product of the planning phase of the nursing process is a formal or informal plan of care. An informal plan is a plan of action that exists in the nurse's mind. For example, the nurse may think, "Mrs. Phan is very tired. I will need to reinforce her teaching after she is rested." A formal nursing **care plan** is a written guide that organizes information about the client's care. LPN/LVN students will practice writing care plans as part of their study of the nursing process. This process is discussed below.

Standardized Care Plan for Nursing Diagnosis of DEFICIENT FLUID VOLUME		
Etiology	**Desired Outcomes**	**Nursing Order** (Identify Frequency)
√Decreased oral intake	√Urinary output > 30 mL/hr	√Monitor intake and output q _1_ h
√Nausea	√Urine specific gravity 1.005±1.025	√Weigh daily
__Depression	√Serum Na⁺ normal	√Monitor serum electrolyte levels X 1 or until normal
√Fatigue, weakness	√Mucous membranes moist	√Check skin turgor and mucous membranes q _8_ h
__Difficulty swallowing	√Skin turgor good	√Monitor temperature q _4_ h
__Other:_____	√No weight loss	√Administer prescribed IV therapy (Monitor according to protocol for ™Intravenous Therapy) 1000 mL D₅ LR at 100 mL/hr
√Excess fluid loss	√8-hour intake = _400 mL oral_	√Offer oral liquids q _1_ h
√Fever or increased metabolic rate	Other:	Type _clear, cold_____
√Diaphoresis		√Instruct client regarding amount, type, and schedule of fluid intake.
√Vomiting		√Assess understanding of type of fluid loss; teach accordingly
__Diarrhea		√Mouth care prn with _mouthwash_
__Burns		√Institute measures to reduce fever (eg, lower room temperature, remove bed covers, offer cold liquids.)
__Other_____		Other Nursing Orders:_____
		Monitor urine specific gravity
Defining Characteristics		_q shift_____
√Insufficient intake		_____
√Negative balance of intake and output		_____
√Dry mucous membranes		_____
√Poor skin turgor		_____
__Concentrated urine		_____
__Hypernatremia		
√Rapid, weak pulse		
__Falling B/P		
__Weight loss		

Plan Initiated by: _M. Medina RN_____ **Date** _4-15-05_____

Plan/outcomes evaluated_____ **Date**_____

Plan/outcomes evaluated_____ **Date**_____

Client: _Amanda Aquilini_____

Figure 4-2. ◆ A standardized care plan for nursing diagnosis of Deficient Fluid Volume.

The most obvious benefit of a formal written care plan is that it provides continuity of care. When nurses use the client's nursing diagnoses to develop goals and nursing interventions, the result is a holistic, individualized plan of care that will best meet the client's unique needs.

Standardized care plans specify the nursing care for groups of clients with common needs (e.g., all clients with myocardial infarction). See Figure 4-2 ◆ for a standardized care plan. Individualized care plans are tailored to meet the unique needs of a specific client—needs that are not addressed by the standardized plans.

Care plans include the actions nurses must take to address the client's nursing diagnoses and produce the desired outcomes and a timeline for accomplishing the goal. The complete plan of care for a client is made up of several different documents (see Chapters 9 and 11). ∞

Kardex Care Plans

Kardex is a trade name for a system in which client information and instructions for some of the client's care are kept on a large card in a central file, making information quickly accessible. The Kardex (Figure 4-3 ◆) usually contains information about diet, activity levels, self-care/hygiene needs, treatments, and procedures. Kardex information may change frequently. It is usually recorded in pencil so that the Kardex can be changed and kept up to date. It is a temporary record for ongoing care, and it does not become part of the client's medical record.

Computerized Care Plans

Computers are increasingly being used to create and store nursing care plans. The computer can also generate both standardized and individualized care plans. Nurses access the client's stored care plan from a centrally located terminal at the nurses' station or from terminals in client rooms. Examples of a computerized student care plan can be found on the companion website.

Regardless of whether care plans are handwritten, computerized, or standardized, nursing care must be individualized to fit the unique needs of each client. The nurse uses standardized care plans for predictable, commonly occurring problems and an individual plan for unusual problems or problems that need special attention.

Student Care Plans

Because student care plans are a learning activity as well as a plan of care, they may be more lengthy and detailed than care plans used by working nurses. To help students learn to write a care plan, educators generally require that it be individualized. They may also require a column be included for "Rationale" after the nursing intervention column. A **rationale** is the scientific principle given as the reason for selecting a particular nursing intervention. Table 4-4 ◆ shows how such a care plan would be made.

Guidelines for Writing Nursing Care Plans

The student may find it helpful to follow these guidelines when writing nursing care plans:

1. Date and sign the plan. The date the plan is written is essential for evaluation, review, and future planning. The nurse's signature demonstrates accountability to the client and to the nursing profession, since the effectiveness of nursing actions can be evaluated.
2. Use these category headings: "Nursing Diagnoses," "Goals/Desired Outcomes," "Nursing Orders/Interventions," "Rationales," and "Evaluation." Include a date for the evaluation of each goal.
3. Use standardized medical or English abbreviations and key words, not complete sentences, to communicate your ideas. For example, write "Turn and reposition q2h" rather than "Turn and reposition the client every two hours." (See Table 9-1 for a list of standard medical abbreviations. ∞)
4. Refer to procedure books or other sources of information rather than including all the steps on a written plan.
5. Tailor the plan to the unique characteristics of the client by ensuring that the client's choices, such as preferences about the times of care and the methods used, are included. This reinforces the client's individuality and sense of control. For example, the written nursing order "Provide prune juice at breakfast rather than regular juice" indicates that the client was given a choice of beverages.
6. Ensure that the nursing plan incorporates preventive and health maintenance aspects as well as restorative ones. For example, carrying out the order "Provide active-assistance ROM (range-of-motion) exercises to affected limbs q2h" prevents joint contractures and maintains muscle strength and joint mobility.
7. Ensure that the plan contains orders for ongoing assessment of the client (e.g., "Inspect incision q8h").
8. Include collaborative and coordination activities in the plan. For example, the nurse might ask a nutritionist or physical therapist about specific aspects of the client's care.
9. Include plans for the client's discharge and home care needs. It is often necessary to consult and make arrangements with the community health nurse, social worker, and specific agencies that supply client information and needed equipment.

THE PLANNING PROCESS

Setting Priorities

Priority setting is the process of identifying nursing diagnoses and interventions in order from most important or critical to least important. Life-threatening problems, such as loss of respiratory or cardiac function, are given highest priority. Health-threatening problems, such as pain and decreased coping ability, are assigned medium priority because they may result in delayed development or cause destructive physical or emotional changes. A low-priority problem is one that arises

MediaLink Computerized Student Care Plan and Template

CLIENT KARDEX WITHOUT MED

ACTIVITIES	HYGIENE	ALLERGIES	VITAL SIGNS
_____ Bedrest_____	_____ Bed Bath	_____ _____	_____ TPR q _____
_____ BRP_____	_____ Self Bath		_____ BP q _____
_____ Dangle_____	_____ Shower	**Diet**	_____ Oral_____ Rectal_____ Axill.
_____ Chair_____	_____ Tub	_____ NPO	_____ _____
_____ Ambulate_____	_____ Assist/Partial	_____ Clear Liquids	
_____ Turn_____	_____ Skin Care	_____ Full Liquids	**IV THERAPY**
_____ Wheelchair_____	_____ Sitz Bath	_____ Soft	_____ Peripheral
_____ Walker_____	_____ Dentures	_____ Regular	_____ Subclavian / Jugular
_____ Up Ad Lib_____	_____ Oral Care	_____ Isolation, Compromised Host	_____ Heparin Lock
_____ High Risk For Fall	_____ Trach Care	_____ Bland	_____ TPN
		_____ Force Fluids	_____ Blood
BLADDER/BOWEL	**TRAITS**	_____ Other (Specify)	_____ _____
_____ Foley Catheter	_____ Paraplegic	_____ _____	_____ _____
Insert Date_____	_____ Hemiplegic R/L		_____ IV (Type)
Ostomy (Type) _____	_____ Blind	**FEEDING**	
_____ Incontinent	_____ Deaf		**ADDITIONAL INFO.**
_____ Ostomy Care	_____ Speech Impediment	_____ Feed	_____
_____ Catheter Care	_____ Glasses	_____ Prepare Food	_____
_____ Peri Care	_____ Diabetic	_____ Feed Self	_____
_____ Diaper/Pads	_____ Literacy Level	_____ Tube Feedings	_____
_____ Other	_____ Foreign Lang.	Amt. _____	_____
_____ _____	_____ Other (Specify)	_____	**ISOLATION**
_____ _____	_____ _____	_____ Gastrostomy Tube	

DATE	TREATMENTS	DATE	IV FLDS / ADDITIVES / RATE
_____	Neuro Checks_____	_____	_____
_____	Activity_____	_____	_____
_____	Bath Complete_____ Assist_____ Self_____	_____	_____
_____	I & O_____	_____	_____
_____	Foley_____	_____	_____
_____	NG Tube_____	DATE	RESPIRATORY THER.	DATE	PHYSICAL THERAPY
_____	Drains_____	_____	_____	_____	_____
_____	Telemetry_____				
_____	Dressing Change_____				
_____	Decubitus Care_____				
_____	Limit Fluids_____				
_____	Other_____				

DAILY WT.	RESUSCITATION	NOTIFY IN EMERGENCY	DIET
Time_____	Yes _____ No _____	_____	Type_____
Bedscales Standing	Date Ordered _____	_____	_____
SAFETY	**PRECAUTIONS**	_____	Snacks_____

Bedrails Posey Restrain	Type	**CONSULTS**	Feed Yes_____ No_____

Adm. Date	To ICU	To Floor	Age	Sex	Height	Weight	1.	DATE	SURGERY
							2.		

ROOM #	CLIENT NAME	DIAGNOSIS	PHYSICIAN

HMA NU0006A (REV. 7/91)

Figure 4-3. ◆ Kardex. *Source:* Courtesy of Community Hospital of Lancaster, PA.

TABLE 4-4	PARTIAL CARE PLAN WITH RATIONALES FOR CLIENT WITH PNEUMONIA		

Nursing Diagnosis: Ineffective Airway Clearance related to viscous secretions and shallow chest expansion secondary to fluid volume deficit, pain, and fatigue.

DESIRED OUTCOMES	EVALUATION STATEMENTS	NURSING ORDERS	RATIONALE
Demonstrates adequate air exchange, as evidenced by			
1. Absence of pallor and cyanosis (skin and mucous membranes)	1. Goal partially met. Skin and mucous membranes not cyanotic, but still pale.	a. Monitor respiratory status q4h; rate, depth, effort, skin color, mucous membranes, amount and color of sputum. b. Monitor results of blood gases, chest x-ray studies, and incentive spirometer volume as available. c. Monitor level of consciousness. d. Auscultate lungs q4h.	a, b, c, d. To identify progress toward or deviations from goal. Ineffective Airway Clearance leads to poor oxygenation, evidenced by pallor, cyanosis, lethargy, drowsiness. *Retain nursing orders to continue to identify progress. Goal status indicates problem not resolved.*
2. Using correct breathing/coughing technique after instruction	2. Goal partially met. Uses correct technique when pain well controlled by narcotic analgesics.	e. Vital signs q4h (TPR, BP).	e. Inadequate oxygenation causes increased pulse rate. Respiratory rate may be decreased by narcotic analgesics or increased by dyspnea and anxiety.
3. Productive cough	3. Goal met. Cough productive of moderate amounts of thick, yellow, pink-tinged sputum.	f. Instruct in breathing and coughing techniques. Remind to perform and assist q3h. Support and encourage. (4/17/01, JW) g. Administer prescribed expectorant; schedule for maximum effectiveness.	f. Does not need to be reinstructed as client demonstrates correct techniques. May still need support and encouragement because of fatigue and pain. g. Helps loosen secretions so they can be coughed up and expelled.
4. Demonstrating symmetric chest excursion of at least 4 cm	4. Goal not met. Chest excursion = 3 cm.	h. Maintain Fowler's or semi-Fowler's position.	h. Gravity allows for fuller lung expansion by decreasing pressure of abdomen on diaphragm.

from normal developmental needs or that requires only minimal nursing support. Table 4-5 ◆ gives examples of setting priorities for client care.

Nurses frequently use Maslow's hierarchy of needs when setting priorities. (See Figure 4-4 ◆, page 62.) In Maslow's hierarchy, physiologic needs that are basic to life (like air, food, and water) are listed at the base of the pyramid. They receive higher priority than the need for security or activity. Growth needs, such as self-esteem, are not perceived as "basic" in this framework. So, nursing diagnoses such as Ineffective Airway Clearance and Impaired Gas Exchange would take priority over nursing diagnoses like Anxiety or Ineffective Coping.

Establishing Client Goals/Desired Outcomes

After establishing priorities, the nurse and client set goals for each nursing diagnosis. On a care plan the goals/desired out-

comes describe, in terms of observable client responses, what the nurse hopes the client will achieve by implementing the nursing orders. (*Note:* The terms **goal** and **desired outcome** are used interchangeably in this text.)

LONG-TERM AND SHORT-TERM GOALS. Goals may be short term or long term. A short-term goal might be, "Client will raise right arm to shoulder height by Friday." In the same context, a long-term goal might be, "Client will regain full use of right arm in 6 weeks." Long-term goals are often used for clients who live at home and have chronic health problems and for clients in nursing homes, extended-care facilities, and rehabilitation centers.

DEVELOPING DESIRED OUTCOMES FROM NURSING DIAGNOSES. Goals are drawn from and relate to the client's nursing diagnoses. The problem clause contains the unhealthy

TABLE 4-5	PRIORITIZING NURSING DIAGNOSES FOR A CLIENT WITH PNEUMONIA	
NURSING DIAGNOSIS	**PRIORITY**	**RATIONALE**
Ineffective Airway Clearance related to (1) viscous secretions secondary to fluid volume deficit and (2) shallow chest expansion secondary to pain and fatigue	High priority	Loss of respiratory functioning is a life-threatening problem. The nurse's primary concern must be to promote the client's oxygenation by addressing the etiologies of this problem.
Deficient Fluid Volume: intake insufficient to replace fluid loss related to fever and diaphoresis	High priority	Severe fluid volume deficit is life threatening. Although not that severe for this client, it is a high-priority problem because it is also a contributing factor for Ineffective Airway Clearance. Collaborative efforts to improve hydration have already begun (intravenous fluids). The nurse must immediately and continuously assess and promote hydration.
Anxiety related to (1) difficulty breathing and (2) concerns over work and parenting roles	Medium priority	Although the client is concerned about work and parenting roles, these are not a threat to life. Also, treatment of her high-priority problem, Ineffective Airway Clearance, will relieve one of the etiologies of this problem (dyspnea). Meanwhile, the nurse must provide symptomatic relief of the client's anxiety during periods of dyspnea because extreme anxiety could further compromise oxygenation by causing her to breathe ineffectively and increasing the rate at which she uses oxygen.
Imbalanced Nutrition: Less than Body Requirements related to decreased appetite, nausea, and increased metabolism secondary to disease process	Low priority	This problem is not currently health threatening, but it could be if it were to persist. It will almost certainly resolve in a day or two as the medical problem is treated. If the medical problem does not resolve quickly, this will change to a medium priority.
Risk for Altered Family Processes related to mother's illness and temporary unavailability of father to provide child care	Low priority	Client's child is currently being cared for. If the husband returns as planned, this potential problem will not develop into an actual problem. No interventions are needed at present, except for continued assessment and reassurance.

response; it states what should change. For example, if the nursing diagnosis is "Risk for Deficient Fluid Volume related to diarrhea and inadequate intake secondary to nausea," the related goal statement might be: "Maintain fluid balance, as evidenced by urinary output in balance with fluid intake, normal skin turgor, and moist mucous membranes."

In this example, a general goal (fluid balance) is stated as the opposite of the problem (Deficient Fluid Volume) and then followed by a list of observable desired outcomes. If achieved, the outcomes would be evidence that the problem, Deficient Fluid Volume, has been prevented.

For every nursing diagnosis, there must be at least one desired outcome that, when achieved, directly demonstrates resolution of the problem clause.

COMPONENTS OF GOAL/DESIRED OUTCOME STATEMENTS. Goal/desired outcome statements should usually have the following four components:

◆ *Subject.* The subject, a noun, is the client, any part of the client, or some attribute of the client, such as the client's pulse or urinary output. The subject may be omitted in goals; it is assumed that the subject is the client unless indicated otherwise.

◆ *Action verb.* The verb specifies an action the client is to perform, for example, what the client is to do, learn, or experience. Some examples of action verbs are listed in Box 4-5 ◆.

◆ *Measurable outcome modifiers.* Conditions or modifiers may be added to the verb to explain the circumstances under which the behavior is to be performed. They explain:

   ◆ *How*—Walks with the help of a walker
   ◆ *When*—After attending two group diabetes classes, lists signs and symptoms of diabetes
   ◆ *Where*—When at home, maintains weight at existing level
   ◆ *What*—Discusses Food Pyramid and recommended daily servings

◆ *Criteria of desired performance.* The criteria indicate the standard by which a performance is evaluated, or the level at which the client will perform the behavior. These criteria may specify time or speed, accuracy, distance, and quality. Examples include:

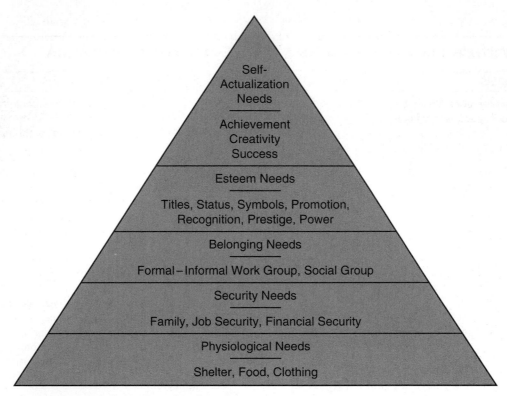

Figure 4-4. ◆ Maslow's Hierarchy of Needs

◆ To establish a time-achievement criterion, the nurse asks, *"How long?"*—"Weighs 75 kg by April"

◆ To establish an accuracy criterion, the nurse asks, *"How well?"*—"Lists five out of six signs of diabetes in 2 weeks"

◆ To establish distance, the nurse asks, *"How far?"*—"Walks one block per day"

◆ To establish quality, the nurse asks, *"What is the expected standard?"* —"Administers insulin using aseptic technique in 3 days"

WRITING GOALS/DESIRED OUTCOMES. Students should follow these guidelines when writing desired outcomes:

BOX 4-5
EXAMPLES OF ACTION VERBS

Apply	Explain	Share
Assemble	Help	Sit
Breathe	Identify	Sleep
Choose	Inject	State
Compare	List	Talk
Define	Move	Transfer
Demonstrate	Name	Turn
Describe	Prepare	Verbalize
Differentiate	Report	
Discuss	Select	

---

1. Write goals/outcomes in terms of client responses, not nurse activities. Begin each goal statement with "the client will" to focus on client behaviors and responses. Avoid statements that start with *enable, facilitate, allow, let,* or *permit,* which indicate what the nurse hopes to accomplish, not what the client will do.
   Correct: Client will drink 100 cc of water per hour (client behavior).
   Incorrect: Maintain client hydration (nursing action).

2. Be sure that desired outcomes are realistic for the client's capabilities, limitations, and designated time span, if it is indicated. Limitations include finances, equipment, family support, social services, physical and mental condition, and time. For example, the outcome "Measures insulin accurately" may be unrealistic for a client who has poor vision due to cataracts.

3. Ensure that the goals/desired outcomes are compatible with the therapies of other professionals. For example, the outcome "Will increase the time spent out of bed by 15 minutes each day" is not compatible with a physician's prescribed therapy of bed rest.

4. Make sure that each goal is derived from only one nursing diagnosis. For example, the goal "The client will increase the amount of nutrients ingested and show progress in the ability to feed self" is derived from two nursing diagnoses: Feeding Self-Care Deficit and Imbalanced Nutrition: Less than Body Requirements.

5. Use observable, measurable terms for outcomes. Avoid words that are vague and require interpretation or judg-

ment by the observer. Phrases like "increase daily exercise" and "improve knowledge of nutrition" can mean different things to different people. They are not clear and specific enough to guide the nurse when evaluating client responses.

6. Make sure the client considers the goals important and values them. The nurse must actively listen to the client to determine personal values, goals, and desired outcomes in relation to current health concerns. Clients are usually motivated to reach goals they consider important. They may resist goals they feel they are told they "should do."

Table 4-6 ◆ shows how outcomes are derived from nursing diagnoses.

LVNS/LPNS AND LONG-TERM CARE PLANNING

The LVN/LPN working in long-term or home care may be assigned greater responsibilities related to care planning. Once the initial assessment has been completed by the RN, the care plan will be developed as a collaborative process. The LPN/LVN will be responsible for implementing, evaluating, and reporting back to the RN on the achievement of the client's goals. Most long-term facilities and home care agencies have regularly scheduled client care conferences so that the health care team can interact and plan for the client's future needs.

NURSING PROCESS CASE STUDIES

In Chapters 6 through 31, the clinical chapters, you will be presented with a Nursing Process Case Study. ⊘ Each study provides an opportunity for you to review the use of care plans and to test your critical thinking skills. Discussion of the critical thinking questions is provided in Appendix IV. ⊘

 Implementation

Implementation is the fourth step of the nursing process, in which selected nursing interventions and activities occur. **Nursing interventions** are the actions that are initiated

by the nurse to achieve client goals. The specific strategies should focus on eliminating or reducing the cause of the nursing diagnosis.

TYPES OF NURSING INTERVENTIONS

Nursing interventions are identified and written during the planning step of the nursing process. However, they are actually performed during the implementing step. McCloskey and Bulechek (2000) define a *nursing intervention* as "any treatment, based upon clinical judgment and knowledge, that a nurse performs to enhance patient/client outcomes." Nursing interventions include:

◆ *Direct care.* An intervention performed through interaction with the client such as giving a back massage

◆ *Indirect care.* An intervention performed away from but on behalf of the client, such as obtaining a referral for physical therapy.

◆ *Nurse-initiated.* **Independent interventions** are those activities that nurses are licensed to initiate on the basis of their knowledge and skills. An example of an independent action is planning and providing special mouth care for a client based on a diagnosis of Impaired Oral Mucous Membranes.

◆ *Physician-initiated.* **Dependent interventions** are activities carried out under the physician's orders or supervision, or according to specified routines.

◆ **Collaborative actions.** Collaborative nursing activities reflect the overlapping responsibilities between health personnel. A collaborative problem is a type of potential problem that nurses manage using both independent and physician-prescribed interventions. Independent nursing interventions for a collaborative problem focus mainly on monitoring the client's condition and preventing development of the potential complication. For example, the physician might order physical therapy to teach the client crutch-walking. The nurse would be responsible for informing the physical therapy department and for coordinating the client's care to include the physical therapy sessions. When the client returns to the nursing unit, the

TABLE 4-6	**DERIVING DESIRED OUTCOMES FROM NURSING DIAGNOSES**	
NURSING DIAGNOSIS	**OPPOSITE HEALTHY RESPONSE (GOALS)**	**DESIRED OUTCOMES**
Impaired Physical Mobility: inability to bear weight on left leg, related to inflammation of knee joint	Improved mobility Ability to bear weight on left leg	Ambulate with crutches by end of the week. Be able to stand without assistance by end of the month.
Ineffective Airway Clearance related to poor cough effort, secondary to incision pain and fear of damaging sutures	Effective airway clearance	Lungs will be clear to auscultation during entire postoperative period. No skin pallor or cyanosis by 12 hours postoperation. Within 24 hours after surgery, will demonstrate good cough effort.

nurse would assist with crutch-walking and collaborate with the physical therapist to evaluate the client's progress.

The nurse is responsible for explaining, assessing the need for, and administering the medical orders. The RN writes nursing orders to individualize the medical order based on the client's status. For example, for a medical order of "Progressive ambulation, as tolerated," the nursing orders might be:

1. Dangle for 5 min, 12 h postop.
2. Stand at bedside 24 h postop; observe for pallor, dizziness, and weakness.
3. Check pulse before and after ambulating. Do not progress if pulse 110.

Usually, several possible interventions can be identified for each nursing diagnosis. The nurse's task is to choose those that are most likely to achieve the desired client outcomes.

IMPLEMENTING SKILLS

Nurses employ a wide variety of skills in providing client care.

Cognitive (intellectual) skills include problem solving, decision making, critical thinking, and creative thinking. They are crucial to safe, intelligent nursing care.

Interpersonal skills are all the verbal and nonverbal activities people use when communicating directly with one another. The effectiveness of a nursing action often depends largely on the nurse's ability to communicate with others. Even when giving medication to a client, the nurse needs to understand the client and in turn be understood. A nurse who is delegating a nursing action also needs to be understood. Communication skills are discussed in detail in Chapter 25. ⌾

Interpersonal skills are necessary for all nursing activities. Caring, comforting, referring, counseling, and supporting are just a few. They include conveying knowledge, attitudes, feelings, interest, and appreciation of the client's cultural values and lifestyle.

Technical skills are "hands-on" skills such as manipulating equipment, giving injections, doing dressing changes, moving, lifting, and repositioning clients. These tasks, called **procedures** or psychomotor skills, always require communicating with the client. However, they also require knowledge and, frequently, manual dexterity. The number of technical skills expected of a nurse has greatly increased in recent years because of the increased use of technology, especially in acute care hospitals.

BASIC PROCEDURES FOR NURSING INTERVENTIONS

All procedures follow a basic format. You need to perform several steps whenever you begin a procedure. These steps provide safeguards for the client and aid in your organization. Procedure 4-1, Basic Procedure Steps and Admission Information, demonstrates the use of the procedure template.

The LPN/LVN should develop an understanding of the rationale (scientific reasoning) for each intervention. You will find rationales in italics for many steps of the procedures.

PROCESS OF IMPLEMENTING

The process of implementing normally includes: reassessing the client, determining the nurse's need for assistance, implementing nursing orders, delegating and supervising, and documenting nursing actions.

Reassessing the Client

Just before implementing an order, the nurse must reassess the client to make sure the intervention is still needed, because the client's condition may have changed. For example, Gayle Fischer has a nursing diagnosis of Disturbed Sleep Pattern related to anxiety and unfamiliar surroundings. During rounds, the nurse discovers that Gayle is sleeping and therefore defers the back rub that had been planned as a relaxation strategy.

New data may indicate a need to change the priorities of care or the nursing strategies. For example, a nurse begins to teach Ms. Eves, who has diabetes, how to give herself insulin injections. Shortly after beginning the teaching, the nurse realizes that Ms. Eves is not concentrating on the lesson. Subsequent discussion reveals that she is worried about her eyesight and fears she is going blind. Realizing that the client's level of stress is interfering with her learning, the nurse ends the lesson and documents the clients concern on the teaching plan. The physician should be informed so that arrangements can be made for a consultation if needed. The nurse also should validate the client's concerns and communicate actions that have been taken.

Determining the Nurse's Need for Assistance

When implementing some nursing strategies, the nurse may require assistance for one of the following reasons:

◆ The nurse is unable to implement the nursing strategies safely alone (e.g., turning an obese client in bed).
◆ Assistance would reduce stress on the client (e.g., turning a person who experiences acute pain when moved).
◆ The nurse lacks the knowledge or skills to implement a particular nursing activity (e.g., a nurse who is not familiar with a particular model of oxygen mask needs assistance the first time it is applied).

Implementing Nursing Orders (Strategies)

It is important to explain to the client what will be done, what sensations to expect, and what the client is expected to do. For many nursing actions, it is also important to ensure the client's privacy, for example, by closing doors, pulling curtains, or draping the client.

Delegating and Supervising

The LPN/LVN may have the opportunity to delegate to nursing assistants or other unlicensed staff.

It is the responsibility of the delegator to assess the capabilities of the staff member being assigned the task. Delegating does not relieve the nurse of the ultimate responsibility for the task. When in doubt, the nurse and the unlicensed person should work together until the unlicensed person's understanding of the assigned task and ability to perform it are confirmed.

Documenting Nursing Actions

After carrying out the nursing orders, the nurse completes the implementing phase by recording the interventions and client responses in the nursing progress notes. These are a part of the agency's permanent record for the client. Nursing actions must not be recorded in advance because, on reassessment, the nurse may find that the action should not or cannot be implemented. For example, a nurse is authorized to inject 10 mg of morphine sulfate subcutaneously to a client, but the nurse finds that the client's respiratory rate is 4 breaths per minute. This finding contraindicates the administration of morphine (a respiratory depressant). The nurse withholds the morphine and reports the client's respiratory rate to the nurse in charge and/or physician.

The nurse may record routine or recurring activities (e.g., mouth care) at the end of a shift. In the meantime, the nurse maintains a personal record of these interventions. Many agencies have special forms for this type of recording.

In some instances, it is important to record a nursing action immediately after it is implemented. Recorded data about a client must be up to date, accurate, and available to other nurses and health care professionals. This is particularly true of the administration of medications and treatments. Immediate recording helps safeguard the client, for example, from receiving a second dose of medication.

Nursing actions are communicated verbally as well as in writing. When a client's health is changing rapidly, the charge nurse and/or the physician may want to be kept up to date with verbal reports.

Interdisciplinary documentation forms require the nurse to chart in a timely manner. When others are using the same form, delayed charting may find the nurse without a place to document, making it necessary to document a late entry.

Nurses also give verbal reports at a change of shift and on a client's discharge to another unit or health agency. For information on documenting and reporting, see Chapter 9.

◆ Evaluation

Evaluation is the fifth and last phase of the nursing process, but many times the evaluation phase is overlooked. **Evaluation** is review of interventions to determine their effectiveness. An intervention may be discarded as ineffective without taking time to discover why it did not work. One thing that sets the LPN/LVN apart from a CNA is the knowledge and ability to evaluate.

Clients need to be evaluated all day long. The best way to evaluate an intervention is to determine if the objective from the written care plan has been met, and if not, why not. Through evaluating, nurses accept responsibility for their actions, indicate interest in the results of the nursing actions, and demonstrate a desire to replace ineffective actions with more effective ones. After determining whether a goal has been met, the nurse writes an evaluative statement (either on the care plan or in the nurse's notes). These notes help the RN to review and modify the nursing care plan, so that individualized nursing care can continue. Once the care plan is modified, the nursing process cycle begins again.

Note: The bibliography listings for this and all chapters have been compiled at the back of the book.

PROCEDURE 4-1

Basic Procedure Steps and Admission Information

EQUIPMENT

- ◆ Admission kit
- ◆ Thermometer
- ◆ Blood pressure cuff and stethoscope

- ◆ Appropriate scale of client's need
- ◆ Urine container (if UA needed)
- ◆ Kardex, care plan
- ◆ Client's medical record

1. Check physician's orders (Figure 4-5A ◆). *All dependent nursing interventions require a physician's order.*

2. Gather all equipment (Figure 4-5B). *Collecting all necessary equipment prior to beginning procedure will save steps, time, and assure that you will have what you need to complete procedure correctly.*

3. Introduce self (Figure 4-5C). *Giving your full name and title will help the client feel more comfortable and will help gain his or her cooperation.*

4. Identify the client (Figure 4-5D). *Address the client by Mr., Mrs., Ms., followed by first and last name. Compare the armband to the name and medical record number on the client's chart, in order to make sure procedure is being done on the correct client.*

5. Provide privacy (Figure 4-5E). *By closing the door or pulling the bed curtain you can assure the client that their confidentiality will be maintained.*

6. Explain the procedure (Figure 4-5F). *This will help relieve client anxiety and help establish rapport between you and the client.*

7. Wash hands (Figure 4-5G). *Hand washing is the most important thing that the nurse can do to stop the spread of infectious disease. This should be done prior to any client contact.*

8. Put on gloves if necessary. Some facilities say, "If it's wet and you are not, put on gloves." Other facilities may require gloves for all client contact. (Figure 4-5H). (*Note: Throughout the text, steps 1–8 will be identified with icons only to remind you to complete the steps before starting the procedure.*) Rationales follow the procedure steps in italics.

9. Place a hospital gown on the client and assist him or her into bed. *Wearing a hospital gown will be necessary during*

the physical assessment, the client will be more comfortable in the bed during the assessment.

10. Explain equipment and hospital routine. *To assist the client to adjust to hospital environment with minimal distress.*

11. Open and place admission kit on the bedside table. Fill and place water pitcher and cup on the overbed-table

Figure 4-5. ◆ Icons of initial nursing actions: **(A)** Check the physician's order; **(B)** Gather the necessary equipment; **(C)** Introduce yourself to the client; **(D)** Identify the client (check the client's wristband against the chart); **(E)** Provide privacy as needed (close the curtain); **(F)** Explain the procedure; **(G)** Wash your hands. Hand washing is the single most effective way to prevent disease transmission. **(H)** Don gloves as needed. (If the client is wet and you're not, wear gloves.)

unless the client is NPO (nothing by mouth). *Supplies and water will be easily accessible to the client.*

12. Record personal belongings on the admission form and encourage family to take valuables home. (Valuables can be placed in hospital safe if no family is available). *This will serve as a checklist on discharge to be sure all belongings are sent home with client. Valuables should not be kept at the bedside to prevent loss.*

13. Obtain client's height and weight using a bed or floor scale. *Height and weight needs to be available for physician and pharmacy for proper dosage of medication, and as a baseline of client's nutritional status.*

14. Take vital signs. *This is a baseline to determine the client's status.*

15. Collect data for the client's health history. *A complete history provides a total picture of client's condition and present health problems.*

16. Complete the bedside assessment (if this is within the LPN/LVN's scope in your area of practice). *To obtain as much data as possible about the client's chief complaint.*

17. Document the procedure. *"If it is not documented, it is not done." (Each procedure in the clinical chapters will provide a sample documentation.)*

18. Obtain a urine specimen, and notify laboratory, x-ray, and EKG of client's admission. *Client may need to have admission laboratory studies, EKG, and chest x-ray done as a baseline.*

19. Document all findings in the client's medical record on the admission form. *Complete, accurate, timely documentation is necessary to provide continuity of care.*

20. Collaborate with the RN to write and initiate the care plan. *Initiation of care plan will be the first step on client's road to recovery.*

21. Notify the physician that the client has been admitted and obtain orders if they are not on the floor. *It is important that the physician be notified in a timely manner so that treatment can begin as soon as possible.*

◆ SAMPLE CHARTING (DOCUMENTATION)

9/9/05	Admission procedure completed on a 28-year-old female, admitted with pneumonia. See admission form for vital signs and assessment. U.A. obtained and sent to lab. Blood sample drawn by lab for CBC and blood culture. Bedside portable chest obtained. Hospital routine and equipment explained. Client resting in bed. Dr. Katz's exchange notified. M. Smith LPN

Chapter Review

Key Terms by Topics

Use the audio glossary feature of either the CD-ROM or the Companion Website to hear the correct pronunciation of the following key terms.

Introduction
nursing process

Assessment
assessment, data collection, database, subjective data (symptoms), objective data

(signs), manifestations, observation, collaborate, interview, examination

Diagnosis
diagnosis, nursing diagnosis, etiology

Planning
planning, care plan, rationale, priority setting, goal/desired outcome

Implementation
implementation, nursing interventions, interventions (dependent, independent), collaborative actions, procedures

Evaluation
evaluation

Key Points

♦ The nursing process is a systematic, rational method of planning and providing individualized nursing care.

♦ The goals of the nursing process are to identify a client's actual or potential health care needs, to establish plans to meet the identified needs, and to deliver and evaluate specific nursing interventions to meet those needs.

♦ The nursing process provides a framework for nurses' accountability and responsibility.

♦ The nursing process is organized into five interrelated, interdependent phases: assessing, diagnosing, planning, implementing, and evaluating.

♦ The client is the primary source of data. Secondary sources are family, friends, health team members, the health record, and pertinent literature.

♦ The client care plan provides a guideline for delivery care and critiquing each phase of the nursing process.

EXPLORE MediaLink

Additional interactive resources for this chapter can be found on the Companion Website at www.prenhall.com/ramont. Click on Chapter 4 and "Begin" to select the activities for this chapter.

For chapter-related NCLEX-style questions and an audio glossary, access the accompanying CD-ROM in this book.

For Further Study

See chapter 8 for more about admitting a client.

Inspection, auscultation, and palpation are described in Chapter 11.

For details about discharge planning, see "Continuity of Care" in Chapter 8.

Communication skills and interviewing techniques are discussed in detail in Chapter 25.

For information on documenting recording and reporting, see Chapter 9.

NCLEX-PN Exam Preparation

1. Assessment can be distinguished from evaluation in which of the following ways?
   a. Assessment is done throughout the nursing process; evaluation is done only when the client is ready for discharge.
   b. Assessment is done by the LPN/LVN; evaluation is always done by the RN.
   c. Assessment identifies the client's current status, while evaluation determines the client's progress toward a desired outcome.
   d. Assessment is based on subjective data while evaluation is based on objective data.

2. The second phase of the nursing process involves analyzing data and identifying health problems, risks, and strengths. This phase is known as:
   a. Planning
   b. Evaluating
   c. Diagnosing
   d. Implementing

3. In your collaboration with the RN it is determined that the client has a nursing diagnosis of impaired mobility. Which of the following statements is an appropriately written client goal for this problem?
   a. Encourage ambulation 3×/day.
   b. Client will walk the length of the hall 2×/per day, with the assistance of two staff members, in 2 days.
   c. Client's ability to ambulate will improve by the second day of hospitalization.
   d. Assist client to sit in chair for meals.

4. Rationales can be described as:
   a. Scientific reasons that support the choice of a particular nursing intervention
   b. Subjective data for identifying client problems
   c. Methods used to evaluate client outcomes
   d. Steps of nursing procedures

5. The final nursing task of the planning phase is:
   a. Choosing the appropriate interventions
   b. Evaluating the effectiveness of the interventions
   c. Delegating interventions to unlicensed personnel
   d. Writing the care plan

6. Of the following statements from a care plan, identify which one is a rationale.
   a. Vital signs q4h (T and BP)
   b. Cough productive of moderate amount of pink-tinged sputum
   c. Inadequate oxygenation causes increase in pulse rate.
   d. Demonstrates adequate air exchange as evidenced by (AEB) absence of cyanosis.

7. The nursing care plan is put into action during what phase of the nursing process?
   a. Planning
   b. Implementing
   c. Assessing
   d. Evaluating

8. Delegating and supervision occur in which stage of the nursing process?
   a. Assessing
   b. Diagnosis
   c. Planning
   d. Implementing

9. Evaluation statements consist of two parts:
   a. Conclusion and supporting data
   b. Desired outcome and rationale
   c. Problem status and client's response
   d. Reassessment and data comparison

10. The nursing process can be described as a(n):
    a. Strategy for implementing evidence based nursing practice
    b. Holistic nursing assessment
    c. Organized framework for professional nursing practice
    d. Contributing factor for nursing diagnosis

Answers for Review Questions appear in Appendix IV.

Thinking Strategically About...

Carlos, a licensed vocational nurse with several years' experience, begins working in a long-term care facility. Within a few weeks, it becomes apparent that the night nurse is treating elderly clients unkindly, and there seems to be an increase in reported skin tears on the nights when she works. He speaks to this nurse about his concerns, but he sees no change in the situation. One morning, arriving at work early for a staff meeting, he overhears her verbally abusing a confused resident who will not take his medications. Carlos reports his observation to the Director of Nursing. When there is still no improvement, Carlos returns to the manager and says that he is considering speaking to the administrator or making a formal complaint to the state nursing board.

The alleged abuser is a long-time employee at the facility and popular with the nursing assistants and other staff. When the supervisor finally speaks to her about the complaint, the identity of the reporter becomes clear. Carlos is ostracized by most of the staff. He is criticized in front of residents and family members, and the night nurse continuously makes racial slurs when referring to him with other staff members. After several months, Carlos feels he can no longer tolerate the working conditions and accepts a job at another facility.

COMMUNITY

Why could this nurse's action or inaction be considered a community issue?

CRITICAL THINKING

- Would you consider Carlos to be a "whistle-blower"?
- Was Carlos's decision to report what he observed a legal or an ethical issue?
- Does Carlos have any legal recourse for his treatment?

COMMUNICATION

Consider the instances of communication that occurred in this case study: between the abusive nurse and the client, between the two nurses, between Carlos and the Director of Nursing, and between the staff and Carlos. In pairs or small groups, role-play these interactions as you think they probably occurred.

CONFLICT RESOLUTION

As a class or in an essay, review Carlos's decisions using Table 3-3 (page 42) as a guide. What other alternatives might Carlos have had? How could the DON have handled the situation differently?

UNIT

II

Introduction to Clinical Practice

Chapter 5 Health Care Delivery Systems

Chapter 6 Safety

Chapter 7 Infection Control and Asepsis

Chapter 8 Admission, Transfer, and Discharge

Chapter 9 Documenting and Reporting

Chapter 5

Health Care Delivery Systems

SHARING experiences

"I have always enjoyed helping people. As I have aged, I have noticed that the health care industry has become more of a money-making enterprise than a service available to whoever needs it. So, as I am on my way to becoming a nurse, I really want to do my part in reforming health care to be what it should be and not what it is."

Alexis Chavarria, PN student, Idaho State University, Pocatello, ID.

LEARNING outcomes

After completing this chapter, you will be able to:
- Differentiate primary, secondary, and tertiary health care delivery services.
- Compare the characteristics of nursing in the outpatient setting to those of institutionalized nursing care.
- Describe the functions and purposes of the health care agencies outlined in this chapter.
- Discuss health care as a right and the essentials of the Patient's Bill of Rights.
- Identify the roles of various health care professionals.
- Differentiate between the various models of care.
- Compare various systems of payment for health care services.

A **health care system** is the totality of services offered by all health disciplines. Health care services are commonly categorized according to type and level.

 ## Types of Health Care

Three types of services are often described: (1) health promotion and illness prevention, (2) diagnosis and treatment, and (3) rehabilitation and health restoration.

HEALTH PROMOTION AND ILLNESS PREVENTION

Based on the notion of maintaining an optimum level of wellness, the U.S. Department of Health and Human Services has developed a systematic approach to health improvement. The report, *Healthy People 2010* (2000), "focuses on improving health—the health of each individual, the health of the communities, and the health of the nation." However, the *Healthy People 2010* goals and objectives cannot by themselves improve the health status of the nation; instead, they need to be recognized as a part of a larger systemic approach to health improvement.

Since the 1980s more and more people are recognizing the advantages of staying healthy and avoiding illness. Health-promotion programs address areas such as adequate and proper nutrition, weight control and exercise, and stress reduction. Health-promotion activities emphasize the important role clients play in maintaining their own health and encourage them to maintain the highest level of wellness they can achieve. Recent transitions in health care also reflect a growing support for community-based nursing and health care that capitalizes on health-promotion activities.

The health care delivery system also offers illness prevention programs. They may be directed at the client or the community and involve such practices as providing immunizations, identifying risk factors for illnesses (e.g., cardiovascular disease), and helping people take measures to prevent these illnesses from occurring.

DIAGNOSIS AND TREATMENT

Traditionally, the largest segment of the health care delivery system has been dedicated to the diagnosis and treatment of illness. Hospitals and physicians' offices were the major agencies offering these services. More recently, however, community-based agencies have been instrumental in providing these services. For example, clinics in some communities provide mammograms and education regarding the early detection of cancer of the breast. Voluntary HIV testing and counseling is another example of the shift in services from traditional health care settings to community-based agencies. Some shopping malls and shopping centers have walk-in clinics that provide diagnostic screening tests, such as screening for cholesterol and high blood pressure.

REHABILITATION AND HEALTH RESTORATION

Rehabilitation is a process of restoring ill or injured people to optimum and functional levels of wellness. Rehabilitative care emphasizes the importance of assisting clients to function adequately in the physical, mental, social, economic, and vocational areas of their lives. The goal of rehabilitation is to help people move to their previous level of health (i.e., to their previous capabilities) or to the highest level they are capable of given their current health status. Rehabilitation may begin in the hospital but will eventually lead clients back out into the community for further treatment and follow-up once health has been restored.

 ## Levels of Health Care

Health care delivery services can also be categorized according to the complexity or level of the services provided: primary, secondary, or tertiary. See Table 5-1 ◆ for the levels of care and the kinds of services provided at each level. Nurses play a key role in health-promotion activities and in providing primary health care, whether in the hospital or in the community.

 ## Types of Health Care Settings

Health care agencies and settings are both varied and numerous. Some agencies provide a number of services; for example, a hospital may provide acute inpatient services, outpatient or ambulatory care services, and emergency services. In addition, the same services may be found in other community-based agencies. For example, hospice services may be provided in the hospital, in the home, or in another agency within the community.

A client may be categorized as an inpatient or an outpatient. An *inpatient* is a person who enters a setting such as a

TABLE 5-1	TYPES OF HEALTH CARE SERVICES BY INCREASING COMPLEXITY	
LEVEL	**NURSING SERVICES**
Primary	Health promotion Preventive care (e.g., immunization) Health education Environmental protection Early detection and treatment
Secondary	Emergency care Diagnosis and treatment (complex) Acute care
Tertiary	Long-term care Care of the dying Rehabilitation

hospital and remains for at least 24 hours. An *outpatient* is a person who requires health care but does not need to stay in an institution such as a hospital.

Because the array of health care services and agencies is so great, nurses often need to help clients choose the service that best suits their needs. Clients may be seen in any number of these agencies, depending on their care and ability to pay for the services. Traditional nursing roles and responsibilities are also changing in response to the movement of client care from the hospital into the community. The LPN/LVN are currently being employed in almost every type of health care setting.

OUTPATIENT SETTINGS

Public Health
Health agencies at the state, county, or city level vary according to the need of the area. Their funds, generally from taxes, are administered by elected or appointed officials. Local health departments (county, bicounty, or tricounty) traditionally have responsibility for developing programs to meet the health needs of the people, providing the necessary staff and facilities to carry out these programs, continually evaluating the effectiveness of the programs, and monitoring changing needs. State health organizations are responsible for assisting the local health departments. In some remote areas, state departments also provide direct services to people.

The Centers for Disease Control and Prevention (CDC) in Atlanta, Georgia, administers a broad program related to surveillance of diseases. By means of laboratory and epidemiologic investigations, data are made available to the appropriate authorities. The CDC also publishes recommendations about the prevention and control of infections and administers a national health program. The federal government also administers a number of Veterans Administration (VA) services in the United States.

Physicians' Offices
In North America, the physician's office is a traditional primary care setting. The majority of physicians either have their own offices or work with several other physicians in a group practice. Clients usually go to a physician's office for routine health screening, illness diagnosis, and treatment. People often seek consultation from physicians when they are experiencing symptoms of illness or when a significant other considers the person to be ill.

Nurses employed in physician's offices have a variety of roles and responsibilities. Some nurses carry out traditional functions including client registration, preparing the client for an examination, obtaining health information, and providing information. Other functions may include obtaining specimens, assisting with procedures, and providing some treatments.

Ambulatory Care Centers
Ambulatory care centers are being used more frequently in many communities. Most ambulatory care centers have diag-

nostic and treatment facilities providing medical, nursing, laboratory, and radiological services, and they may or may not be attached to or associated with an acute care hospital. Some ambulatory care centers provide services to people who require minor surgical procedures that can be performed outside the hospital. Nurses in ambulatory care centers may have specialized knowledge and skills to enable them to assist physicians with procedures. The term *ambulatory care center* has replaced the term *clinic* in many places.

General Clinics
The term *clinic* can refer to a department inside or outside the hospital, managed by a group of physicians or by nurses. Some may provide a specialized type of health service such as infant immunizations. Nurses in clinics perform many of the same functions as nurses employed in a physician's office.

Industrial Clinics
The industrial clinics are gaining importance as a setting for employee health care. Employee health has long been recognized as important to productivity. Nursing functions in industrial health care include work safety and health education, annual employee health screening for tuberculosis, and maintaining immunization information. Other functions may include screening for such health problems as hypertension and obesity, caring for employees following injury, and counseling.

Home Health Care Agencies
The implementation of prospective payment (discussed later in this chapter) and the resulting earlier discharge of clients from hospitals have made home care an essential aspect of the health care delivery system. As concerns about the cost of health care have escalated, the use of the home as a care delivery site has increased. In addition, the scope of services offered in the home has broadened. Home health care agencies offer education to clients and families, as well as provide comprehensive care to acute, chronic, and terminally ill clients. Once the RN has opened the home care case, the LPN/LVN may be assigned to provide care and to supervise the home health aide or the individual providing homemaker services.

There are several different types of home health agencies. These include:

◆ Official or public agencies are operated by state or local governments and financed primarily by tax funds.
◆ Voluntary or private not-for-profit agencies are supported by donations, endowments, charities such as the United Way, and third-party reimbursement. Because these agencies are not-for-profit, they are exempt from federal income tax.
◆ Private, proprietary agencies are for-profit organizations and are governed by either individual owners or national corporations. Some of these agencies participate in third-party reimbursement; others rely on "private-pay" sources.

◆ Institution-based agencies operate under a parent organization, such as a hospital.

Regardless of the type of agency, all home health agencies must meet specific standards for licensing, certification, and accreditation. See Box 5-1 ◆ for the unique aspects of home-care nursing.

Day Care Centers

Day care centers serve many functions and many age groups. A relatively new concept is centers that provide care for adults who cannot be left at home alone but do not need to be in an institution. Elder care centers often provide care involving socializing, exercise programs, and stimulation. Some centers provide counseling and physical therapy. Nurses who are employed in adult day care centers may provide medications, treatments, and counseling, thereby facilitating continuity between day care and home care. Adult day care is another work opportunity for the LPN/LVN.

INPATIENT SETTINGS

Hospitals

Hospitals traditionally have provided restorative care to the ill and injured. Although hospitals are chiefly viewed as institutions that provide care, they have other functions, such as providing sources for health-related research and teaching.

BOX 5-1 UNIQUE ASPECTS OF HOME HEALTH NURSING

The nurse:

◆ Functions independently
◆ Must establish rapport with client and family
◆ Provides care while family is present

The family:

◆ May feel more free to question advice
◆ Will set their own schedule and priorities
◆ Has more responsibility for care of client

Positive Aspects

◆ Setting is more intimate and relaxed.
◆ Behaviors are more natural.
◆ Cultural beliefs and practices are more visible.
◆ Multigenerational interaction can take place.

Negative Aspects

◆ Caregiver demands may continue for months or years.
◆ Living conditions and support systems may be inadequate.
◆ There is risk of psychological or physical problems for caregiver.

Hospitals are classified by the services they provide. General hospitals admit clients requiring a variety of services, such as medical, surgical, obstetric, pediatric, and psychiatric services. Other hospitals offer only specialty services, such as psychiatric or pediatric care. Hospitals can be further described as acute care or chronic (long-term) care. An acute care hospital provides assistance to clients who are acutely ill or whose illness and need for hospitalization are relatively short term. Long-term care hospitals provide services for longer periods, sometimes for years or the remainder of the client's life.

The variety of health care services hospitals provide usually depends on their size and location. The large urban hospitals usually have inpatient beds, emergency services, diagnostic facilities, ambulatory surgery centers, pharmacy services, intensive and coronary care services, and multiple outpatient services provided by clinics. Some large hospitals have other specialized services such as spinal cord injury and burn units, oncology services, and infusion and dialysis units. In addition, some hospitals have substance abuse treatment units and health promotion units. Small rural hospitals often are limited to inpatient beds, radiology and laboratory services, and basic emergency services. The number of services a rural hospital provides is usually directly related to its size and its distance from an urban center.

Hospitals in the United States have undergone massive changes. Many hospitals have merged with other hospitals or have been sold to large multihospital for-profit corporations.

Another change relates to the client population. Most clients in hospitals are seriously ill and require complex nursing care. With the increasing acuity (severity) of illness among clients, general hospitals have virtually become complex care centers. Because so many of the seriously ill are elderly, some general hospitals are becoming acute care hospitals solely for the elderly.

Nurses in hospitals have multiple responsibilities including the coordination of client care, assessing and monitoring client health, and providing direct care. The LPN/LVN works closely with the RN and provides much of the direct client care. Acute hospital nursing care gives the LPN/LVN an excellent opportunity to observe RN level of practice, and to consider his/her current position as a career ladder. Many LPNs/LVNs decide to continue their education while employed in the acute hospital.

Extended-Care (Long-Term Care) Facilities

Traditionally, all extended-care facilities were called nursing homes. Extended-care facilities now include skilled nursing facilities (intermediate care) and extended-care facilities (long-term care) that provide personal care for those who are chronically ill or are unable to care for themselves without assistance. Traditionally, extended-care facilities provided care only for elderly clients, but now they provide care to clients of all ages who require rehabilitation or custodial care. As clients are being discharged earlier from acute care hospitals, some clients may still require supplemental care in an extended-care facility before they return home.

Because long-term illness occurs most often in the elderly, long-term care facilities have programs that are oriented to the needs of this age group. These facilities are intended for people who require not only personal services (bathing, hygiene, assistance with daily activities, etc.), but also some regular nursing care and occasional medical attention. However, the type of care provided varies considerably. Some facilities admit and retain only residents who are able to dress themselves and are ambulatory. Other extended-care facilities provide bed care for clients who are more incapacitated. These facilities can, in effect, become the client's home, and consequently the people who live there are frequently referred to as residents rather than patients or clients.

In 1987, as part of the **Omnibus Budget Reconciliation Act (OBRA),** the Congress of the United States passed legislation to bring a measure of quality improvement to the nursing home and extended-care facility industry. In response to a growing concern about whether minimal essential standards were being met in many facilities, OBRA instituted requirements for nurse's aide training. Specific requirements include a 75-hour training program for nurse's aides and competence evaluations of the aides.

Specific guidelines govern the admission procedures for clients admitted to an extended-care facility. Insurance criteria, treatment needs, and nursing care requirements must all be assessed beforehand. Many skilled nursing facilities exist as units within a hospital but are regulated by federal, state, and local governmental bodies to make sure they are meeting the requirements for a long-term care facility. If a client in a hospital needs to be transferred to such a unit, the client is discharged from the hospital and then admitted to the long-term care unit. Extended-care and skilled nursing facilities are becoming increasingly popular means for managing the health care needs of clients who require additional care but do not meet the criteria for remaining in the hospital. Often, these extended-care facilities have client waiting lists for admission. Nurses in extended-care facilities assist clients with their daily activities, provide care when necessary, and coordinate rehabilitation activities (Figure 5-1 ◆).

Licensed practical/vocational nurses have an increased level of responsibility in the long-term care setting. They may function in a charge nurse position, being responsible for coordination of client care, working with physicians and supervision of unlicensed nursing assistants. They will administer medications and treatments and serve as a liaison between families and needed services.

Retirement and Assisted-Living Centers

Retirement or assisted-living centers consist of separate houses, condominiums, or apartments for residents. Residents live relatively independently. However, many of these facili-

Figure 5-1. ◆ The LPN/LVN charge nurse in the long-term setting serves as a liaison between resident, family, and physician.

ties offer meals, laundry services, nursing care, transportation, and social activities. Some centers have a separate hospital to care for residents with short-term or long-term illness. Often, these centers also work collaboratively with other community services including case managers, social services, and a hospice to meet the needs of the residents who live there. The retirement or assisted-living center is intended to meet the needs of people who are unable to remain at home but do not require hospital or nursing home care. Nurses in retirement and assisted-living centers provide limited care to residents, usually related to the administration of medications and minor treatments. An LPN/LVN may be the only licensed nurse in an assisted living facility.

Rehabilitation Centers

Rehabilitation centers usually are independent community centers or special units. However, because rehabilitation ideally starts the moment the client enters the health care system, nurses who are employed on pediatric, psychiatric, or surgical units of hospitals also help to rehabilitate clients. Rehabilitation centers play an important role in assisting clients to restore their health and recuperate. Drug and alcohol rehabilitation centers, for example, help free clients of drug and alcohol dependence, and assist them to reenter the community. Physical rehabilitation centers help clients to regain purpose, function, and dignity. The focus is to assist them to function at the maximum level and return to their community. Today, the concept of rehabilitation is applied to all illness (physical and mental), to injury, and to chemical addiction. Nurses in the rehabilitation setting coordinate client activities and ensure that clients are complying with their treatments. This type of nursing often requires specialized skills and knowledge.

MIXED SETTINGS

Hospice Services

The hospice movement provides a variety of services to the terminally ill, their families, and support persons. In the 1970s, the movement gained momentum, through the work of such people as Elisabeth Kübler-Ross, whose books challenged prevailing attitudes, and Cicely Saunders, founder of St. Christopher's Hospice in London, England. Saunders believed that the physical and social environments of dying people are as important as medical interventions on their behalf. The central concept of the hospice movement, as distinct from the acute care model, is not saving life but improving or maintaining the quality of life until death. The LPN/LVN works under the direction of an RN case manager to provide care for terminally ill clients in their home, long-term care facilities or in inpatient hospice centers. For additional information, see Chapter 31.

Crisis Centers

Crisis centers provide emergency services to clients experiencing life crises. These centers may operate out of a hospital or in the community, and most provide 24-hour telephone service. Some also provide direct counseling to people at the center or in their homes. The primary purpose of a crisis center is to help people cope with an immediate crisis and then provide guidance and support for long-term therapy. The LPN/LVN with specialized training may be employed and work with RNs, counselors, and psychologists in these settings.

Mutual Support and Self-Help Groups

There are mutual support or self-help groups that focus on nearly every major health problem or life crisis people experience. Alcoholics Anonymous, which formed in 1935, served as the model for many of these groups. The National Self-Help Clearinghouse provides information on current support groups and guidelines about how to start a self-help group. Many of these groups are facilitated by lay volunteers, although social workers or other health care professionals carry out responsibilities for self-help groups.

◆ Rights and Health Care

The movement for clients' rights in health care arose in the late 1960s. Today, clients are also seeking more self-determination and control over their own bodies when they are ill. Informed consent, confidentiality, and the right of the client to refuse treatment are all aspects of this self-determination. Today, the goals of health include the return of autonomy and independence to the client and the acceptance of good health as a responsibility of the client, the care providers, and society. These goals cannot be met unless clients accept active responsibility for their health and health care, and unless clients and care providers have mutual respect.

When people are ill, they are frequently unable to assert their rights as they would if they were healthy. Asserting rights requires energy and an underlying awareness of one's rights in the situation.

PATIENT'S BILL OF RIGHTS

In 1973, the American Hospital Association (AHA) published *A Patient's Bill of Rights* to promote the rights of hospitalized clients. These were revised in 1992. Included in this bill of rights are the right of clients to considerate and respectful care; consideration of privacy for clients, including confidentiality of all records and communications regarding their care; and the right to make decisions about their care, including the right to refuse a treatment or plan of care. In addition, clients have a right to make a statement such as a living will, which should be followed by the agency as permitted by law.

The AHA bill of rights states that clients have the right to review all their medical records and have them explained; to receive requested care and services, provided these are reasonable; and to be informed of any business arrangements among institutions or people involved in their care. In addition, clients have the right to be informed of resources that can be used to resolve a dispute or grievance and of hospital policies and practices that relate to client care, treatment, and responsibilities, and to be informed of hospital charges and available payment methods. Furthermore, the AHA bill states that clients have the right to refuse to participate in any research study, to expect a reasonable continuity of care, and to have options explained when hospital care is no longer appropriate.

The Patient Bill of Rights, by federal law, must be explained verbally and signed by the client before care can be provided. Verification of compliance is an important nursing function at the time of admission. The client should be asked about any advance directive (e.g., not to be resuscitated in the event of a cardiac arrest), and this information must be on the client's record. If the hospital's policy limits its ability to implement any advance directive, the client has a right to be informed of this before any problem arises. See details about advance directives in Chapter 31.

If a client lacks decision-making capacity, is legally incompetent, or is a minor, these rights can be exercised on the client's behalf by a designated surrogate or proxy decision maker.

◆ Providers of Health Care

The providers of health care, also referred to as the health care team or health professionals, are health personnel from different disciplines who coordinate their skills to assist clients and perhaps their support persons. Their mutual goal is to restore a client's health and promote wellness. The choice of personnel for a particular client depends on the needs of the client. In the present system of health care in North America, health teams commonly include the personnel that follow.

NURSE

The role of the nurse varies with the needs of the client. As nursing roles have expanded, new dimensions for nursing practice have been established. See Chapter 1 for the roles of the nurse. ⊕ Nurses can pursue a variety of practice specialties (e.g., critical care, mental health, oncology). A registered nurse (RN) assesses a client's health status, identifies health problems, and develops and coordinates care. A licensed vocational nurse (LVN), also referred to as a licensed practical nurse (LPN), provides direct client care under the direction of a registered nurse.

PHYSICIAN

The physician is responsible for medical diagnosis and for determining the therapy required by a person who has a disease or injury. The physician's traditional role is the treatment of disease and trauma (injury); however, many physicians are now including health promotion and disease prevention in their practice. Some physicians specialize in specific areas such as surgery or oncology.

PHYSICIAN'S ASSISTANT

Physician's assistants (PAs) perform certain tasks under the direction of a physician. They diagnose and treat certain diseases and injuries.

UNLICENSED ASSISTIVE PERSONNEL

Unlicensed assistive personnel (UAPs) are health care staff such as certified nurse assistants, hospital attendants, nurse technicians, and orderlies who assume aspects of client care that do not require nursing judgment. These tasks include bathing, assisting with feeding, exercise, and range of motion. Individual facilities may provide training for unlicensed personnel to perform additional tasks.

DENTIST

Dentists diagnose and treat dental problems. Dentists are also actively involved in preventive measures to maintain healthy oral structures (e.g., teeth and gums). Many hospitals, especially long-term care facilities, have dentists on staff.

PHARMACIST

A pharmacist prepares and dispenses pharmaceuticals in hospital and community settings. The role of the pharmacist in monitoring and evaluating the actions and effects of medications on clients is becoming increasingly prominent. A clinical pharmacist is a specialist who guides physicians in prescribing medications. A pharmacy technician/assistant is also recognized in some states. This person administers medications to clients or works in the pharmacy under the direction of the pharmacist.

DIETITIAN OR NUTRITIONIST

When dietary and nutritional services are required, the dietitian or nutritionist may be a member of a health team. A dietitian, often a registered dietitian (RD), has special knowledge about the diets required to maintain health and to treat disease. Dietitians in hospitals generally are concerned with therapeutic diets, may design special diets to meet the nutritional needs of individual clients, and supervise the preparation of the meals to ensure that clients receive the proper diet.

A nutritionist is a person who has special knowledge about nutrition and food. The nutritionist in a community setting recommends healthy diets and gives broad advisory services about the purchase and preparation of foods. Community nutritionists often function at the preventive level. They promote health and prevent disease, for example, by advising families about balanced diets for growing children and pregnant women.

PHYSIOTHERAPIST

The physiotherapist (PT), or physical therapist, assists clients with musculoskeletal problems. They provide physical therapy in response to a physician's order. The physiotherapist's functions include assessing clients' mobility and strength, providing therapeutic measures (e.g., exercises and heat applications to improve mobility and strength), and teaching new skills (e.g., how to walk with an artificial leg). Some physiotherapists provide their services in hospitals; however, independent practitioners establish offices in communities and serve clients either at the office or in the home.

RESPIRATORY THERAPIST

A respiratory therapist (RT) is skilled in therapeutic measures used in the care of clients with respiratory problems. These therapists are knowledgeable about oxygen therapy devices, intermittent positive pressure breathing respirators, artificial mechanical ventilators, and accessory devices used in inhalation therapy.

OCCUPATIONAL THERAPIST

An occupational therapist (OT) assists clients with an impaired function to gain the skills to perform activities of daily living. The therapist also teaches skills that are therapeutic and at the same time provide some satisfaction.

PARAMEDICAL TECHNOLOGISTS

Paramedical means having some connection with medicine. Laboratory technologists examine specimens such as urine, feces, blood, and discharges from wounds to provide exact information that facilitates the medical diagnosis and the prescription of a therapeutic regimen. The radiologic technologist assists with a wide variety of x-ray film procedures, from simple chest radiography to more complex fluoroscopy. The nuclear medicine technologist uses radioactive substances to provide diagnostic information.

SOCIAL WORKER

A social worker counsels clients and support persons about social problems, such as finances, marital difficulties, and adoption of children. It is not unusual for health problems to produce problems in living and vice versa. The current trend toward shorter acute care hospitalizations has led to an increased need for rehabilitative services in skilled nursing facilities or in the home. Thus, social workers, who usually make the placement arrangements, are playing an increasingly important role on the health care team.

SPIRITUAL SUPPORT PERSON

Chaplains, pastors, rabbis, priests, and so on serve as part of the health care team by attending to the spiritual needs of clients. In most facilities, local clergy volunteer their services on a regular or on-call basis. Hospitals affiliated with specific religions, as well as many large medical centers, have full-time chaplains on staff. They usually offer regularly scheduled religious services. The nurse is often instrumental in identifying the client's desire for spiritual support and notifying the appropriate person.

CASE MANAGERS

The case manager's role is to ensure fiscally sound, appropriate care in the best setting. This role is often filled by the member of the health care team who is most involved in the client's care. Depending on the nature of the client's concerns, the case manager may be a nurse, a social worker, an occupational therapist, a physical therapist, or any member of the health care team.

ALTERNATIVE CARE PROVIDERS

Chiropractors, herbalists, acupuncturists, and other nontraditional health care providers are playing increasing roles in the contemporary health care system. These providers may practice alongside traditional health care providers, or clients may use their services in conjunction with, or in lieu of, traditional therapies.

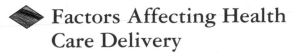 # Factors Affecting Health Care Delivery

Today's health care consumers have greater knowledge about their health than in previous years and they are increasingly influencing health care delivery. Formerly, people expected a physician to make decisions about their care; today, however, consumers expect to be involved in making any decisions. Consumers have also become aware of how lifestyle affects health. As a result, they desire more information and services related to health promotion and illness prevention. A number of other factors affect the health care delivery system.

INCREASING NUMBER OF ELDERLY

By the year 2020 it is estimated that the number of adults over the age of 65 years will be nearly 50 million in the United States (Abrams, Beers, & Berkow, 1995). Long-term illnesses are prevalent among this group and frequently require special housing, treatment services, financial support, and social networks.

The frail elderly, considered to be people over age 85, are projected to be the fastest-growing population in North America and will constitute 14 percent of the elderly population by 2030 (Lee & Estes, 1990, p. 77).

Because only 5 percent of older people are institutionalized with health problems, substantial home management and nursing support services are required to assist those in their homes and communities.

ADVANCES IN TECHNOLOGY

Scientific knowledge and technology related to health care are rapidly increasing. Improved diagnostic procedures and sophisticated equipment permit early recognition of diseases that might otherwise have remained undetected. New antibiotics and medications are continually being manufactured to treat infections and multiple drug-resistant organisms. Surgical procedures that were nonexistent 20 years ago are common today. Laser and microscopic procedures streamline the treatment of diseases that required surgery in the past. Computers, bedside charting, and the ability to store and retrieve large volumes of information in databases are commonplace in health care organizations. All the technologic advances and specialized treatments and procedures come, unfortunately, with a high price tag.

WOMEN'S HEALTH

The women's movement has been instrumental in changing health care practices. Examples are the provision of childbirth services in more relaxed settings such as birthing centers, and the provision of overnight facilities for parents in children's hospitals. Traditionally, women's health issues have focused on the reproductive aspects of health, disregarding many health care concerns that are unique to women. Today, research and treatment focuses on many areas of women's health care such as breast cancer, osteoporosis, abuse, treatment of sexually transmitted diseases (STDs), and issues on aging. An expert panel on women's health of the American Academy of Nursing (AAN) recommends that "understanding women's health requires more than a biomedical view; it requires awareness of the context of women's lives" (AAN Panel on Women's Health, 1997, p. 7).

UNEVEN DISTRIBUTION OF SERVICES

Serious problems in the distribution of health services exist in the United States. In many remote and rural area locations, there are insufficient health care professionals and services available to meet the health care needs of individuals. Uneven distribution is evidenced by the relatively higher number of physicians and nurses per capita in the New England states and the lowest number in the South.

Because of the highly specialized techniques and new knowledge that have emerged during the past 30 years, an increasing number of health care personnel provide specialized services. This specialization leads to fragmentation of care and, often, increased cost of care. To clients, it may mean receiving care from 5 to 30 people during their hospital experience. This seemingly endless stream of personnel is often confusing and frightening.

ACCESS TO HEALTH CARE

Another problem plaguing individuals is access to health care. Low income has been associated with relatively higher rates of infectious diseases, problems with substance abuse, rape, violence, and chronic diseases. The use of health care services is also affected by unemployment and poverty. Even though some government assistance is available, eligibility for and benefits varies considerably from state to state.

HOMELESS POPULATIONS

The growing number of homeless individuals in towns and cities is a major health problem. The homeless differ from those who are poor. They are alone, lack some type of permanent residence, and are disaffiliated from family and friends. Limited access to health care services and compliance from the client contributes to their general poor health of the homeless in the United States. See Box 5-2 ◆ for factors contributing to health problems of the homeless.

DEMOGRAPHIC CHANGES

The characteristics of the North American family have changed considerably in the last few decades. The numbers of single-parent families and alternative family structures have increased markedly. Most of the single-parent families are headed by women, many of whom work and require assistance with child care or when a child is sick at home.

Recognition of cultural and ethnic diversity is also increasing. Health care professionals and agencies are aware of this diversity and are employing means to meet the challenges it presents.

BOX 5-2

POPULATION FOCUS

Risk Factors for Health Problems in the Homeless

◆ Poor physical environment resulting in increased susceptibility to infections
◆ Inadequate rest and privacy
◆ Improper nutrition
◆ Poor access to facilities for personal hygiene
◆ Exposure to the elements
◆ Lack of social support
◆ Few personal resources
◆ Questionable personal safety (physical assault is a constant threat)
◆ Inadequate health care
◆ Poor compliance with treatment plans

 ## Contemporary Frameworks for Care

A number of approaches to client care support continuity of care and cost-effectiveness. They include managed care, case management, and client-focused care.

MANAGED CARE

Managed care describes a health care system whose goals are to provide cost-effective, quality care that focuses on improved outcomes for groups of clients. The care of a client is carefully planned from initial contact to the conclusion of the specific health problem. In managed care, health care providers and agencies collaborate so as to render the most appropriate, fiscally responsible care possible. Managed care emphasizes cost controls, customer satisfaction, health promotion, and preventive services. Health maintenance organizations (HMOs) and preferred provider organizations (PPOs) are examples of provider systems committed to managed care.

CASE MANAGEMENT

Case management describes a range of models for integrating health care services for individuals or groups. Various case management models strive to provide cost-effective care and ensure quality outcomes. Generally, case management involves nurse–physician teams that assume collaborative responsibility for planning, assessing needs, and coordinating, implementing, and evaluating care for groups of clients from preadmission to discharge or transfer and recuperation. A case manager, however, may be a social worker or other appropriate professional.

Case management may be used as a cost-containment strategy in managed care. Case management is usually the responsibility of the RN. Occasionally in a long-term care setting, an LPN/LVN may be specially trained to carry out these duties. Both case management and managed care systems often use **clinical pathways** to track the client's progress (Figure 5-2 ◆). These are very valuable for planning care and providing client teaching and discharge planning.

 ## Models of Care

CLIENT-FOCUSED CARE

Client-focused care is a delivery model that brings all services and care providers to the clients. The supposition is that if activities normally provided by auxiliary personnel (e.g., physical therapy, respiratory therapy, electrocardiographic [ECG] testing, and phlebotomy) are moved closer to the client, the number of personnel involved and the number of steps involved to get the work done are decreased. Proponents of this type of system believe that clients will perceive improved care and service and the agency will achieve cost savings.

Cross-training, development of multiskilled workers who can perform tasks or functions in more than one discipline, is

	OUTCOME INTERVENTION	T	I	T	EXCEPTIONS/*	OUTCOME STATUS:
Pain Mgmt.	**Patient will verbalize/indicate comfort or tolerance of pain.** *Location & pain rating (0-10 pain scale) q 4 hrs w/a. **PCA/CEA/IM analgesics.** Comfort measures_Back rub_	1700	LJ	1600 1800	C/O pain of "10" in R knee cea at 6 cc/hr. ↑ to 8cc/hr c̄ no relief. Dr. Green notified. Percocet tablet given p.o. Still c/o pain at "8" on scale.	1800_LJ_ M/Ⓝ 0600____M/N
Endocrine	**Patient will have no s/s of hypo/ hyperglycemia.**					1800_LJ_ Ⓜ/N 0600____M/N

Signature	Initials	Signature	Initials	Signature	Initials
Laura Jiminez RN	LJ				

Date @ 0700:   2/1/04   To Date @ 0700:   2/2/04

Figure 5-2. ◆ Example of Critical Pathway. *Source:* Critical Pathways for Collaborative Care by Beyea, S. C. Reprinted by permission of Pearson Education, Inc. Upper Saddle River, NJ.

an essential element of client-focused care. For example, a health care worker may be taught to obtain a 12-lead ECG and perform phlebotomy. Individuals who are already certified in one profession can take on a second certification such as medical laboratory and x-ray technology, nursing and respiratory therapy, physical therapy, and occupational therapy. Cross-training will be integral to the managed care system in the future. Contemporary configurations for the delivery of nursing include collaborative arrangements such as managed care, case management, and client-focused care discussed earlier. Other models specifically designed for the provision of nursing are the case method, the functional method, team nursing, primary nursing, differentiated practice, shared governance, and partners in practice.

CASE METHOD

The **case method,** also referred to as total care, is one of the earliest nursing models developed. In this client-centered method, one nurse is assigned to and is responsible for the comprehensive care of a group of clients during an 8- or 12-hour shift. Facilities that function under the case method employee RNs only for bedside care. With the shortage of nursing personnel during World War II, the case method

could no longer be the chief mode of care for clients. Many hospitals reinstituted a form of total care, called primary care, beginning in the mid-1970s and continuing for many years.

FUNCTIONAL METHOD

The **functional method** focuses on the jobs to be completed (e.g., bedmaking, temperature measurement). In this task-oriented approach, personnel with less preparation than the professional nurse perform less complex care requirements. It is based on a production and efficiency model that gives authority and responsibility to the person assigning the work, for example, the head nurse. Clearly defined job descriptions, procedures, policies, and lines of communication are required. The functional approach to nursing is economical and efficient and permits centralized direction and control. Its disadvantages are fragmentation of care and the possibility that nonquantifiable aspects of care, such as meeting the client's emotional needs, may be overlooked.

TEAM NURSING

In the early 1950s, Eleanor Lambertson and her colleagues proposed a system of team nursing to overcome the fragmentation of care resulting from the task-oriented functional approach and to meet increasing demands for professional nurses created by advances in technologic aspects of care. **Team nursing** is the delivery of individualized nursing care to clients by a nursing team led by a professional nurse. A nursing team consists of RNs, LPNs, and often nurse's aides. This team is responsible for providing coordinated nursing care to a group of clients during an 8- or 12-hour shift.

With the advent of managed care, team nursing is experiencing a resurgence. In this revisited form of team nursing, licensed nursing personnel (RNs and LPNs) are frequently paired with an unlicensed assistive person (UAP). The licensed nurse retains responsibility and authority for client care but delegates appropriate tasks to the UAP. Contemporary proponents of this model believe the team approach increases the efficiency of the licensed nurse. Opponents state that inpatients' high acuity of illness leaves little to be delegated. Team nursing is providing increased opportunity for the LPN/LVN in the acute care setting.

PRIMARY NURSING

Primary nursing, a system in which one nurse is responsible for total care of a number of clients 24 hours a day, 7 days a week, was introduced at the Loeb Center for Nursing and Rehabilitation, the Bronx, New York, in the early 1960s. It is a method of providing comprehensive, individualized, and consistent care.

Primary nursing uses the nurse's technical knowledge and management skills. The primary nurse assesses and prioritizes each client's needs, identifies nursing diagnoses, develops a plan of care with the client, and evaluates the effectiveness of care. Associates provide some care, but the primary nurse coordinates it and communicates information about the client's health to other nurses and other health professionals. Primary nursing encompasses all aspects of the professional role, including teaching, advocacy, decision making, and continuity of care. The primary nurse is the first-line manager of the client's care with all its inherent accountabilities and responsibilities. With today's nursing shortage and high cost of healthcare, this model of nursing care is being replaced.

 # Health Care Economics

Although efforts have been made to control the costs of health care, these costs continue to increase. Employers, legislators, insurers, and health care providers continue to collaborate in efforts to resolve the issues surrounding how to best finance health care costs.

PAYMENT SOURCES

Medicare and Medicaid

In the United States, the 1965 **Medicare** amendments (Title 18) to the Social Security Act provided a national and state health insurance program for older adults. Medicare is divided into two parts: Part A is available to the disabled and people 65 years and over. It provides insurance toward hospitalization, home care, and hospice care. Part B is voluntary and provides partial coverage of physician services to people eligible for Part A. Clients pay a monthly premium for this coverage.

Medicare does not cover dental care, dentures, eyeglasses, hearing aids, or examinations to prescribe and fit hearing aids. Most preventive care, including routine physical examinations and associated diagnostic tests, is also not included.

Medicaid was also established in 1965 under Title 19 of the Social Security Act. Medicaid is a federal public assistance program paid out of general taxes to people who require financial assistance. Medicaid is paid by federal and state governments. Each state program is distinct. Some states provide very limited coverage, whereas others pay for dental care, eyeglasses, and prescription drugs.

Supplemental Security Income

In addition, disabled or blind persons may be eligible for special payments called **Supplemental Security Income (SSI)** benefits. These benefits are also available to people not eligible for Social Security, and payments are not restricted to health care costs. Clients often use this money to purchase medicines or to cover costs of extended health care.

PROSPECTIVE PAYMENT SYSTEM

In 1983 the United States, Congress passed legislation putting the **prospective payment system (PPS)** into effect. This legislation limits the amount paid to hospitals that are reimbursed by Medicare. Reimbursement is made according to a classification system known as **diagnostic-related groups (DRGs).** Prospective payment or billing is formulated before the client is even admitted to the hospital; thus, the record of admission, rather than the record of treatment, now governs payment. DRG rates are set in advance of the prospective year during which they apply and are considered fixed except for major, uncontrollable occurrences.

INSURANCE PLANS

A variety of plans have come into existence to finance health care in the United States. These include private insurance and group insurance. Each individual and group plan offers different options for consumers to consider when choosing a prepaid health care program.

Private Insurance

Commercial health insurance carriers offer a wide range of coverage plans. There are two types of private insurance: not-for-profit (e.g., Blue Shield) and for-profit (e.g., commercial companies such as Metropolitan Life, Travelers, and Aetna). Private health insurance is known as third-party reimbursement because the insurance company pays either the entire bill or, more often, 80 percent of the costs of health care services. With private insurance health plans, the insurance company reimburses the health care provider a fee for each service provided (fee-for-service).

These insurance plans may be purchased either as an individual plan or as part of a group plan through a person's employer, union, student association, or similar organization.

Group Plans

Health care group plans provide blanket medical service in exchange for a predetermined monthly payment. Each group plan offers different options for consumers to consider when choosing a prepaid health care program.

HEALTH MAINTENANCE ORGANIZATIONS. A **health maintenance organization (HMO)** is a group health care agency that provides basic and supplemental health maintenance and treatment services to voluntary enrollees. A fee is set without regard to the amount or kind of services provided.

The HMO plan emphasizes client wellness; the better the health of the person, the fewer HMO services are needed and the greater the agency's profit. Members of HMOs choose a primary care provider (PCP), who evaluates their health status and coordinates their care. The PCP has two options: treat the condition or refer the client to a specialist. To reduce costs, HMOs will pay for a specialty physician's services only if the PCP has made the referral. It is an expectation between the HMO and physicians being reimbursed under their plans that PCPs will treat clients and reduce costs whenever possible. Thus, under HMO plans, clients are limited in their ability to select health care providers and services. Because health promotion and illness prevention are highly emphasized in HMOs, nurses in HMOs focus on these aspects of care.

PREFERRED PROVIDER ORGANIZATIONS. The **preferred provider organization (PPO)** has emerged as another alternative in the health care delivery system. PPOs consist of a group of physicians and perhaps a health care agency (often a hospital) that provide an insurance company or employer with health services at a discounted rate. One advantage of the PPO is that it provides clients with a choice of health care providers and services. Physicians can belong to one or several PPOs, and the client can choose among the physicians belonging to the PPO. A disadvantage of PPOs is that they tend to be slightly more expensive than HMO plans and if individuals wish to join a PPO, they might have to pay more for the additional choices. PPOs were first established in 1980 in the United States.

PREFERRED PROVIDER ARRANGEMENTS. **Preferred provider arrangements (PPAs)** are similar to PPOs. The main difference is that the PPAs can be contracted with individual health care providers, whereas PPOs involve an organization of health care providers.

INDEPENDENT PRACTICE ASSOCIATIONS. **Independent practice associations (IPAs)** are somewhat like HMOs and PPOs. The difference is that clients pay a fixed prospective payment to the IPA, and the IPA pays the provider. The provider receives a fixed fee for services given. At the end of the fiscal year, any surplus money is divided among the providers; any loss is assumed by the IPA.

PHYSICIAN/HOSPITAL ORGANIZATIONS. Physician/hospital organizations (PHOs) are joint ventures between a group of private practice physicians and a hospital. PHOs combine both resources and personnel to provide managed care alternatives and medical services. PHOs work with a variety of insurers to provide services. A typical PHO will include primary care providers and specialists.

A PHO may be part of an **integrated delivery system (IDS).** Such a system incorporates acute care services, home health care, extended and skilled care facilities, and outpatient services. Most integrated delivery systems provide care throughout the life span. An IDS enhances continuity of care and communication between professionals and various agencies providing managed care.

Note: The bibliography listings for this and all chapters have been compiled at the back of the book.

Chapter Review

Key Terms by Topics

Use the audio glossary feature of either the CD-ROM or the Companion Website to hear the correct pronunciation of the following key terms.

Introduction
health care system

Types of health care settings
Omnibus Budget Reconciliation Act (OBRA)

Factors affecting health care delivery
managed care, case management, clinical pathways

Models of care
client-focused care, case method, functional method, team nursing, primary nursing

Health care economics
Medicare, Medicaid, Supplemental Security Income (SSI), prospective payment system (PPS), diagnostic-related groups (DRGs), health maintenance organization (HMO), preferred provider organization (PPO), preferred provider arrangements (PPAs), independent practice associations (IPAs), integrated delivery system (IDS)

Key Points

- Health care delivery services can be categorized as primary, secondary, or tertiary, and generally, they can also be grouped by the type of service: (1) health promotion and illness prevention, (2) diagnosis and treatment, and (3) rehabilitation.

- Health care can be considered a right of all people.

- Hospitals provide a wide variety of services on an inpatient and outpatient basis. Hospitals can be categorized as for-profit or not-for-profit, public or private, acute care or long-term care. Many other settings, such as clinics, offices, and day care centers, also provide care.

- Various providers of health care coordinate their skills to assist a client. Their mutual goal is to restore a client's health and promote wellness.

- The many factors affecting health care delivery include health care consumers, women's health, the increasing number of elderly people, advances in knowledge and technology, economic factors, fragmentation of care, increased costs, health care of the homeless, uneven distribution of health services, demographic changes, and access to health care.

- There are a number of frameworks for client health care, including managed care, case management, client-focused care, and partners in practice.

- In the United States, health care is financed largely through government agencies and private organizations that provide health care insurance, prepaid plans, and federally funded programs.

EXPLORE MediaLink

Additional interactive resources for this chapter can be found on the Companion Website at www.prenhall.com/ramont. Click on Chapter 5 and "Begin" to select the activities for this chapter.

For chapter-related NCLEX-style questions and an audio glossary, access the accompanying CD-ROM in this book.

For Further Study

For more information about hospice services, see Chapter 31.

For additional information about advance directives, see Chapter 31.

To find out more about the roles of nurses, see Chapter 1.

NCLEX-PN Exam Preparation

1. The Patient Bill of Rights was published in 1973 for the purpose of:
   a. Protecting the hospital from frivolous law suits.
   b. Insuring respectful care, privacy, and the client's right to refuse care.
   c. Providing the staff with "Do not resuscitate" orders.
   d. Authorizing third party payment for outpatient services.

2. The Omnibus Budget Reconciliation Act (OBRA)
   a. Instituted specific training requirements for nurse's aides working long-term care.
   b. Outlined guidelines for death with dignity.
   c. Governs Medicare payments for individuals receiving social security.
   d. Set the nurse–client ratio in acute care hospitals.

3. A homeless client is brought by a police officer to the emergency room for treatment. Which of the following would you recognize as a major contributing factor for his/her health problems?
   a. Mistrust of the system and health care providers
   b. Transportation for follow-up visits
   c. Poor physical environment exacerbating chronic health problems.
   d. Lack of motivation to work and provide for self

4. Team nursing is defined as:
   a. A system in which a nurse is responsible for the total care of a number of clients for 24 hours a day 7 days per week
   b. A client-centered method in which a client has consistent contact with one nurse during a shift
   c. A delivery model that brings all services and care providers to the client
   d. The delivery of individualized nursing care by a professional nurse (LPN/LVN) and an unlicensed assistive person (UAP)

5. National health insurance for individuals over the age of 65 is called:
   a. Medicaid
   b. Medi-cal
   c. Medi-soft
   d. Medicare

6. Diagnostic-related groups (DRGs) are:
   a. Physician groups that specialize in diagnostic procedures
   b. A part of integrated delivery systems
   c. A prospective payment system
   d. Part of the Canadian Health Care system

7. Which of the following is not considered to be a paramedical technologist?
   a. Occupational therapist
   b. Physiotherapist
   c. Laboratory technician
   d. Spiritual support person

8. One of the benefits of managed care can be to:
   a. Ensure consumer access to the most effective treatment
   b. Reduce the number of days a client is hospitalized
   c. Eliminate the nursing shortage
   d. Be effective only in a primary nursing model

9. The physician's office where you work is paid monthly by the insurance company by the number of enrollees, not the service provided. You understand that the office is part of a(n):
   a. IPA—independent practice association
   b. HMO—health maintenance organization
   c. PPO—preferred provider organization
   d. PHO—physician/hospital organization

10. Preventive care such as immunizations are classified as what type of health care service?
    a. Primary
    b. Secondary
    c. Tertiary
    d. Prospective

Answers for Review Questions appear in Appendix M

Chapter 6

Safety

SHARING experiences

"As an LPN, you will see some hard things to deal with—injuries, disabilities, illness—and there will be days you ask yourself "Why do I do this?" But then you will see the faces of people whose family member you just helped and see the happiness that you have created, and you will remember why. This is the reason you are an LPN."

Eric Reed, PN student, Idaho State University, Pocatello, ID.

LEARNING outcomes

After completing this chapter, you will be able to:

- Discuss factors that affect people's ability to protect themselves from injury.
- Carry out a focused safety assessment interview.
- Identify common potential hazards in the home.
- Plan strategies to maintain safety in the health care setting, home, and community.
- Describe the use and legal implications of restraints.
- List desired outcomes to use in evaluating the selected strategies for injury prevention.
- Describe proper techniques for lifting and transferring patients.
- Describe ways to prevent back injuries while delivering client care.

A fundamental concern of nurses, which extends from the bedside to the home and to the community, is prevention of accidents and injury, as well as assisting the injured. Motor vehicle accidents, falls, drowning, fire and burns, poisoning, inhalation and ingestion of foreign objects, and firearm use are major causes of accidental injury and death.

Nurses need to be aware of what constitutes a safe environment for a particular person, or for a group of people, in home and community settings. Accidents are often caused by human conduct and can be prevented.

Factors That Affect Safety

The ability of people to protect themselves from injury is affected by such factors as age and development, lifestyle, mobility and health status, sensory–perceptual alterations, cognitive awareness, emotional state, ability to communicate, safety awareness, and environment. Nurses need to assess each of these factors when they plan care or teach clients to protect themselves.

AGE AND DEVELOPMENT

Through knowledge and accurate assessment of the environment, people learn to protect themselves from many injuries. Young children's curiosity often exceeds their judgment. However, through knowledge and experience, children do learn what is safe and what is potentially harmful. Elderly people can have difficulty with movement and diminished senses, which contribute to the likelihood of injury.

Measures to ensure the safety of people of all ages focus on two things:

1. Observation or prediction of potentially harmful situations so that harm can be avoided
2. Client education that empowers clients to safeguard themselves and their families from injury

Specific age-related potential hazards and preventive measures are discussed later in this chapter. See Box 6-1 ◆ for safety measures for each age group.

LIFESTYLE

Lifestyle factors that place people at risk include unsafe work environments; residence in neighborhoods with high crime rates; access to guns and ammunition; insufficient income to buy safety equipment or make necessary repairs; and access to illicit drugs, which may also be contaminated by harmful additives. Risk-taking behavior is a factor in some accidents.

MOBILITY AND HEALTH STATUS

People who have impaired mobility due to paralysis, muscle weakness, and poor balance or coordination are obviously prone to injury. Clients with spinal cord injury and paralysis of both legs may be unable to move even when they perceive discomfort. Hemiplegic clients or clients with leg casts often have poor balance and fall easily. Clients weakened by illness or surgery are not always fully aware of their condition.

SENSORY–PERCEPTUAL ALTERATIONS

Accurate sensory perception of environmental stimuli is vital to safety. People with impaired touch perception, hearing, taste, smell, and vision are highly susceptible to injury. A person who does not see well may trip over a toy or not see an electric cord. Deaf people do not hear a siren in traffic, and people with impaired olfactory sense may not smell burning food or escaping gas.

COGNITIVE AWARENESS

Awareness is the ability to perceive environmental stimuli and body reactions and to respond appropriately through thought and action. Clients with impaired awareness include people lacking in sleep, unconscious or semiconscious persons, disoriented people (i.e., those who may not understand where they are or what to do to help themselves), people who perceive stimuli that do not exist, and people whose judgment is altered by disease or medications (such as narcotics, tranquilizers, hypnotics, and sedatives). Mildly confused clients may momentarily forget where they are, wander from their rooms, or misplace personal belongings.

EMOTIONAL STATE

Extreme emotional states can alter the ability to perceive environmental hazards. Stressful situations can reduce a person's level of concentration, cause errors of judgment, and decrease awareness of external stimuli. Depressed people may think and react to environmental stimuli more slowly than usual.

ABILITY TO COMMUNICATE

People with diminished ability to receive and convey information are also at risk for injury. Aphasic clients, people with language barriers, and those unable to read are among them. For example, a person who cannot interpret the sign "No smoking—Oxygen in use" may cause a fire.

SAFETY AWARENESS

Information is crucial to safety. Clients in unfamiliar environments frequently need specific safety information. Lack of knowledge about unfamiliar equipment, such as oxygen tanks, intravenous tubing, and hot packs, is a potential hazard. Healthy clients need knowledge about water safety, car safety, fire prevention, ways to prevent the ingestion of harmful substances, and preventive measures for age-related hazards.

Preventing Specific Hazards

Measures to prevent specific hazards or accidents (such as burns, fire, falls, poisoning, suffocation, and electrocution) are critical aspects of nursing care. Teaching clients about safety is another important aspect. Nurses usually have opportunities to teach while providing care.

BOX 6-1

POPULATION FOCUS

SAFETY MEASURES THROUGHOUT THE LIFESPAN

Newborns and Infants

◆ Use a federally approved car seat at all times (including coming home from hospital). Place children in back seat when traveling in a car.
◆ Never leave the infant unattended on a raised surface.
◆ Check the temperature of the infant's bath water and formula prior to using.
◆ Hold the infant upright during feeding. Do not prop the bottle. Cut food in small pieces, and do not feed the infant peanuts or popcorn.
◆ Investigate the infant's crib for compliance with federal safety regulations: slats no more than 2⅜ inches apart, lead-free paint, height of crib sides, tight fit of mattress to crib.
◆ Use a playpen with sides made of small-sized netting. Never leave playpen sides down.
◆ Provide large, soft toys with no small detachable or sharp-edged parts.
◆ Use guard-gates on stairs and screens on windows. Supervise the infant in the walker, swing, and highchair.
◆ Cover electric outlets. Coil cords out of reach.
◆ Place plants, household cleaners, and wastebaskets out of reach. Lock away potential poisons, such as medicines, paint, and gasoline.

Toddlers

◆ Continue to use federally approved car seat or seat belts at all times.
◆ Teach children not to put objects in the mouth, including pills (unless given by parent).
◆ Keep objects with sharp edges (such as furniture and knives) out of children's reach.
◆ Place hot pots on back burners with handles turned inward.
◆ Keep cleaning solutions, insecticides, and medicines in locked cupboards.
◆ Keep windows and balconies screened.
◆ Teach children to swim. Fence in pools, and supervise at all times. Do not overfill bathtub. Do not let toddlers play near ditches or wells.
◆ Teach children not to run or ride a tricycle into the street.
◆ Obtain a low bed when the child begins to climb.
◆ Cover outlets with safety covers or plugs.

Preschoolers

◆ Do not allow children to run with candy or other objects in the mouth.
◆ Teach children not to put small objects in the mouth, nose, and ears.
◆ Remove doors from unused equipment, such as refrigerators.

◆ Teach preschoolers to cross streets safely and obey traffic signals.
◆ Check Halloween treats before allowing children to eat them. Discard loose or open candy.
◆ Teach children to play in safe areas, not on streets and railroad tracks.
◆ Teach preschoolers the dangers of playing with matches and playing near charcoal grill, fire, and heating appliances.
◆ Teach children to keep parents informed of their whereabouts and to avoid strangers.
◆ Teach preschoolers not to walk in front of swings and not to push others off playground equipment.

School-Age Children

◆ Teach children safety rules for recreational and sports activities: Never swim alone; always wear a life jacket when in a boat; and wear a protective helmet and knee and elbow pads when needed.
◆ Supervise contact sports and activities in which children aim at a target (e.g., archery or darts).
◆ Teach children to obey all traffic and safety rules for bicycling, skateboarding, and roller skating.
◆ Teach children to use light or reflective clothing when walking or cycling at night.
◆ Teach children safe ways to use the stove, garden tools, and other equipment.
◆ Supervise children when they use saws, electric appliances, tools, and other potentially dangerous equipment.
◆ Teach children not to play with fireworks, gunpowder, or firearms. Keep firearms unloaded, locked up, and out of reach.
◆ Teach children to avoid excavations, quarries, vacant buildings, and playing around heavy machinery.
◆ Teach children the effects of drugs and alcohol on judgment and coordination.

Adolescents

◆ Have adolescents complete a driver's education course, and take practice drives with them in various kinds of weather.
◆ Set firm limits on automobile use, namely, never to drive after drinking or using drugs, and never to ride with a driver who has done so. Encourage adolescents to call home for a ride if they have been drinking, assuring them they can do so without a reprimand.
◆ Teach adolescents to wear a safety helmet when riding motorcycles, scooters, and other sports vehicles. Teach safety rules for water sports.
◆ Encourage adolescents to use proper equipment when participating in sports. Schedule a physical examination

before participation, and be certain there is medical supervision for all athletic activities.

- Encourage adolescents to swim, jog, and go boating in groups so they can obtain help in case of an accident.
- Teach rules for hunting and the proper care and use of firearms.
- Inform the adolescent of the dangers of drugs, alcohol, and unprotected sex. Be alert to changes in the adolescent's mood and behavior. Listen to and maintain open communication with the adolescent. Open communication is a powerful preventive measure.
- Set a good example of behavior that the adolescent can follow.

Young Adults

- Reinforce motor vehicle safety: Drive defensively, use "designated drivers" if alcohol is consumed, routinely check brakes and tires, and use seat and shoulder belts or car seats for all passengers.
- Remind the young adult to repair potential fire hazards, such as electric wiring.
- Reinforce water safety: Know the depth of a pool before diving; supervise backyard pools and other water activities.
- Discuss evaluating the potential for workplace injuries or death when making decisions about a career or occupa-

tion. Encourage the young adult to participate actively in programs that reduce occupational hazards.

- Discuss avoiding excessive sun radiation by limiting exposure, using sun-blocking agents, and wearing protective clothing. Explain the skin changes that may indicate a cancerous condition.
- Encourage young adults who are unable to cope with the pressures, responsibilities, and expectations of adulthood to seek counseling.

Middle-Aged Adults

- Reinforce motor vehicle safety: Use seat belts and drive within the speed limit. Test visual acuity periodically.
- Make certain stairways are well lighted and uncluttered.
- Equip bathrooms with hand grasps and nonskid bath mats.
- Test smoke detectors and fire alarms regularly.
- Keep all machines and tools in good working condition at work and at home. Follow safety precautions when using machinery.

Older Adults

- Encourage the client to have regular vision and hearing tests.
- Assist the client to have a home hazard appraisal.
- Encourage the client to keep as active as possible.

SCALDS AND BURNS

A *scald* is a burn from a hot liquid or vapor, such as steam. A burn results from excessive exposure to thermal, chemical, electric, or radioactive agents.

In health care agencies, the risk of scalds and burns is greater for clients whose skin sensitivity to temperature is impaired. Scalds can occur from overly hot bath water, and burns from therapeutic applications of heat (see Chapter 20). ⊕ It is important for the nurse to assess how well clients can protect themselves and what special precautions, if any, need to be taken.

FIRES

Fires continue to be a constant risk in both health care settings and homes. Agency fires usually result from malfunctioning electric equipment or combustion of anesthetic gas.

Agency Fires

In health care agencies, fire is particularly hazardous when people are incapacitated and unable to leave the building without assistance. This makes it extremely important for nurses to be aware of the fire safety regulations and fire prevention practices of the agency in which they work. When a fire occurs, the nurse follows four sequential priorities. Using the acronym RACE can help you remember the procedure (Figure 6-1 ◆):

Rescue clients in immediate danger
Alarm (Pull alarm or call to report)
Contain the fire
Extinguish the fire

Extinguishing the fire requires knowledge of three categories of fire, classified according to the type of material that is burning:

Class A: Paper, wood, upholstery, rags, ordinary rubbish
Class B: Flammable liquids and gases
Class C: Electrical

The right type of extinguisher must be used to fight the fire. Each extinguisher has picture symbols showing the type of fire for which it is to be used. Directions for use are also attached. When using an extinguisher, remember PASS:

Point
Aim
Squeeze
Sweep

FALLS

People of any age can fall, but infants and older adults are particularly prone to falling and serious injury. Falls are the leading cause of accidents among older adults. They are also a major cause of hospital and nursing home admissions. Most falls occur in the home and are a major threat to the indepen-

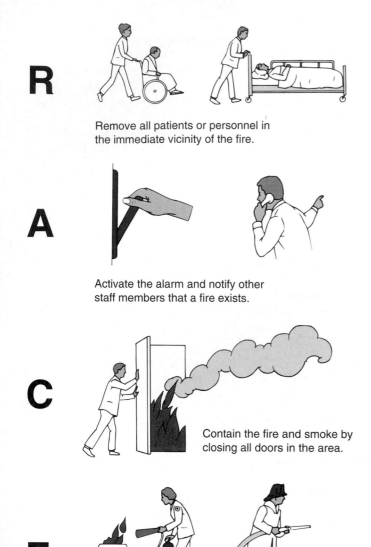

R Remove all patients or personnel in the immediate vicinity of the fire.

A Activate the alarm and notify other staff members that a fire exists.

C Contain the fire and smoke by closing all doors in the area.

E Extinguish the fire, if it is a very small fire, or allow the fire department to extinguish it.

Figure 6-1. ◆ The RACE system for protecting clients in case of fire.

dence of older adults. Fear of falling is common in older adults, even in those who have not experienced a fall. This fear is of particular concern for those who live alone and who anticipate being helpless and unable to summon help after a fall. For these individuals the nurse can make the following recommendations:

- Encourage daily or more frequent contact with a friend or family member.
- Install a personal emergency response system.
- Maintain a physical environment that prevents falls.

Risk factors and associated preventive measures are shown in Table 6-1 ◆.

Prevention of falls in health care agencies is an ongoing concern. Health care environments are designed with many safety features. These include railings along corridors; call bells at each bedside; safety bars in toilet areas; locks on beds, wheelchairs, and stretchers; side rails on beds; and nightlights. In addition, nurses can implement measures to decrease the incidence of falls, as described in Box 6-2 ◆.

Safety monitoring devices are also available to prevent falls. Some monitoring systems use a chair or bed sensor (Figure 6-2 ◆); others use a leg band. These devices trigger an alarm when the client attempts to get out of bed or a chair unassisted. Procedure 6-1 describes how to use these devices.

SUFFOCATION OR CHOKING

Suffocation, or *asphyxiation,* is lack of oxygen due to interrupted breathing. Suffocation occurs when the air source is cut off for any reason. One common reason for choking is food or a foreign object becoming lodged in the throat. The universal sign of distress in this case is observation of the victim grasping and pointing to the neck and throat area without speaking. The emergency response is the Heimlich maneuver, or abdominal thrust, which can dislodge the foreign object and reestablish an airway (see Figure 6-3 ◆).

BOX 6-2
NURSING CARE CHECKLIST

PREVENTING FALLS IN HEALTH CARE AGENCIES

☑ Orient clients on admission to their surroundings, and explain the call system.

☑ Carefully assess the client's risk for falling.

☑ Alert all personnel to the client's risk for falling.

☑ Assign clients at risk for falls to rooms near the nursing station where they can be more closely supervised.

☑ Encourage the client and family to use the call bell to request assistance; ensure that the bell is within easy reach.

☑ Answer call bells promptly.

☑ Place bedside tables and overbed tables near the bed or chair so that clients do not overreach and consequently lose their balance.

☑ Always keep hospital beds in the low position when not providing care so that clients can move in or out of bed easily.

☑ Keep side rails up and the bed in the low position for sedated and unconscious clients when they are unattended.

☑ Lock wheels on beds, wheelchairs, and stretchers.

☑ Ensure that the client wears nonskid footwear.

☑ Use bed or chair safety monitoring devices prn.

TABLE 6-1	RISK FACTORS FOR FALLS AND PREVENTIVE MEASURES
RISK FACTOR	**PREVENTIVE MEASURES**
Poor vision	Ensure eyeglasses are functional. Ensure appropriate lighting. Mark doorways and edges of steps as needed. Keep the environment tidy.
Cognitive dysfunction (confusion, disorientation, impaired memory, or judgment)	Set safe limits to activities. Remove unsafe objects.
Impaired gait or balance and difficulty walking because of lower extremity dysfunction (e.g., arthritis)	Wear shoes or well-fitted slippers with nonskid soles. Use ambulatory devices as necessary (cane, crutches, walker, braces, and wheelchair). Provide assistance with ambulation as needed. Monitor gait and balance. Adapt living arrangements to one floor if necessary. Encourage exercise and activity as tolerated to maintain muscle strength, joint flexibility, and balance. Ensure uncluttered environment with securely fastened rugs.
Difficulty getting in and out of chair or in and out of bed	Encourage client to request assistance. Keep the bed in the low position. Install grab bars in bathroom. Provide raised toilet seat.
Orthostatic hypotension	Instruct client to rise slowly from a lying to sitting to standing position, and to stand in place for several seconds before walking.
Urinary frequency or receiving diuretics	Provide a bedside commode. Assist with voiding on a frequent and scheduled basis.
Weakness from disease process or therapy	Encourage client to summon help. Monitor activity tolerance.
Current medication regimen that includes sedatives, hypnotics, tranquilizers, narcotic analgesics, diuretics	Attach side rails to the bed. Keep the rails in place when the bed is in the lowest position. Monitor orientation and alertness status. Encourage annual or more frequent review of all medications prescribed.

Figure 6-2. ◆ Bed exit monitoring device; the sensor is usually placed under the client's buttocks in bed. *Source:* Courtesy of J.T. Posey Company. Reprinted with permission.

EXCESSIVE NOISE

Excessive noise is a health hazard that can cause hearing loss, depending on the overall level of noise, the frequency range of the noise, the duration of exposure, and individual susceptibility. When ill or injured, people are frequently sensitive to noises that normally would not disturb them. Loud voices, the clatter of dishes, and even a nearby television can disturb clients, some of whom react angrily. Physiologic effects of noise include (a) increased heart and respiratory rates, (b) increased muscular activity, (c) nausea, and (d) hearing loss, if the noise is sufficiently loud.

Noise can be minimized in several ways. Acoustic tile on ceilings, walls, and floors as well as drapes and carpeting absorb sound. Background music can mask noise and have a calming effect on some people. It is important for nurses to minimize noise in the hospital setting and to encourage clients to protect their hearing as much as possible.

Figure 6-3. ◆ Performing the Heimlich maneuver. *Source:* © Elena Dorfman.

ELECTRICAL HAZARDS

All electric equipment must be properly grounded. The electric plug of grounded equipment has three prongs. The two short prongs transmit the power to the equipment. The third, longer prong is the grounding device, which carries short circuits or stray electric current to the ground. (See Figure 6-4 ◆.) Grounding prongs offer a path of least resistance to stray electric currents.

Faulty equipment (e.g., equipment with a frayed cord) presents a danger of electric shock or may start a fire. For example, an electric spark near certain anesthetic gases or a high concentration of oxygen can cause a serious fire. Electric shock occurs when a current travels through the body to the ground rather than through electric wiring, or from static electricity that builds up on the body. Using machines in good repair, wearing shoes with rubber soles, standing on a nonconductive floor, and using nonconductive gloves are all ways to prevent shock.

RADIATION

Radiation injury can occur from overexposure to radioactive materials used in diagnostic and therapeutic procedures.

Figure 6-4. ◆ Three-pronged grounded plug. *Source:* Ambularm Co.

Clients being examined using radiography or fluoroscopy generally receive minimal exposure, and few precautions are necessary. Nurses need to protect themselves, however, from radiation when some clients are receiving radiation therapy. Exposure to radiation can be minimized by (a) limiting the time near the source; (b) providing as much distance as possible from the source; and (c) using shielding devices such as lead aprons when near the source. Nurses need to become familiar with agency protocols related to radiation therapy.

Preventing Equipment-Related Accidents

Risk assessment in the health care setting must include risks related to procedures and equipment. Whether giving a medication or assisting a client out of bed, nurses need to follow safeguards to prevent errors or accidents. Most health care agencies establish protocols that are designed to prevent accidents. When in doubt about a course of action, the nurse should consult the appropriate written guidelines before proceeding.

When an accident or error does occur, most agencies require that the incident be reported. The nurse completes the report immediately after taking whatever action is required to safeguard the client, and notifying the charge nurse. For additional information about incident reports, see Chapters 2 and 32. ⊕

Hospital and Institutional Safety

The Occupational Safety and Health Administration (OSHA) is under the Department of Labor of the federal government. Its purpose is to make sure that every worker in the United States is employed in a safe environment. Employees are required to follow OSHA regulations. Fines are imposed for violations. Student nurses are not specifically addressed in the regulations. However, they are expected to comply with health care facility policies and procedures.

INFECTIOUS WASTE

OSHA has developed two standards dealing with infection control activities in the health care setting: The Bloodborne Pathogens Standards and the Occupational Exposure to Tuberculosis Standard. Health care facilities are required to develop exposure control plans. It is important that students and nurses be familiar with the requirements.

Disposal of Used or Soiled Equipment from an Isolation Room

Most facilities have policies and procedures in place that state specifically how to dispose of equipment and supplies that have been contaminated. Be familiar with these policies! Materials may be disposed of, cleaned, disinfected, or sterilized. Some equipment and supplies are for single use only. Other materials are meant to be used many times.

Bagging is a technique recommended by the Centers for Disease Control and Prevention (CDC) for removal of materials from a client's room. The purpose is to prevent exposure from items contaminated with body secretions. The bag must be impervious to microorganisms. The bags may come in colors (e.g., red) and have labels that indicate they contain infectious materials.

The CDC recommends placing contaminated disposable items in the plastic bags that line the waste containers. Nondisposable or reusable items should be put into a labeled bag before being removed from the client's room and sent to a central processing area for decontamination. Rubber, plastic, metal, and glass items should be bagged separately. (Metal and glass can be autoclaved, but rubber and plastic needed to be exposed to gas sterilization.)

Special procedure trays should be disassembled and bagged as indicated above. Soiled linens or clothing should be bagged and sent to the facility laundry or home. Linens should be handled as little as possible. They should be rolled into a bundle before being placed in the bag (do not shake the linens). Laboratory specimens should be put into a leak proof container. If the container is contaminated on the outside, it should be put in a plastic bag before sending it to the laboratory. Dishes are often made of paper and are disposed of in the refuse container. Blood pressure equipment, if kept in the room, needs no special precautions. If it becomes contaminated, follow the agency's cleaning procedures. Nondisposable thermometers should be disinfected after use according to agency protocols. Needles, syringes, and "sharps" should be placed in a puncture-resistant container kept in the room. Clients' personal objects (such as toys) that are contaminated should be bagged and sent home for cleaning. For additional information on infection control see Chapter 7. ⚭

HAZARDOUS WASTE

Every work area is responsible for having Material Safety Data Sheets (MSDS) available for all chemicals used in that work area. Common substances considered to be hazardous include bleach and other disinfectants. Chemotherapeutic or antineoplastic agents are among the most hazardous substances for nurses. As an LPN/LVN you will not be administering these drugs without special training.

Each person is responsible for knowing the chemical used. The containers must be labeled with the chemical name as well as the function. The labels must also tell any danger or hazard that may exist with that chemical or ingredients and the name, address, and phone number of the manufacturer. Always read the label before using. If labels become illegible, do not use the bottle and report it so bottle or label can be replaced. Know where the MSDS are kept and how to access them. Even more information about the chemical can be found on the sheets. See Box 6-3 ◆ for required information.

BOX 6-3
MSDS REQUIRED INFORMATION

- ◆ The name of the substance, the manufacturer, and the date the MSDS was prepared.
- ◆ Other names the chemical(s) may be called or listed and exposure limits.
- ◆ Physical characteristics are described. This may include how a chemical looks and smells, melting and boiling points, how easily it dissolves or if it does not, and whether it floats or sinks in water.
- ◆ Fire and explosion data tell you if a substance is flammable or combustible and lowest temperature at which it could catch fire. It also tells you the safest way to put out a fire with this chemical.
- ◆ Reactivity tells you what happens when the chemical comes in contact with air, water, or other chemicals. This part tells you when it might burn, explode, or release dangerous vapors.
- ◆ Health Hazards lists how a chemical might enter your body (e.g., inhalation, ingestion, absorption through skin, or injection).
- ◆ Use, handling, and storage describes how to clear up a spill or leak in addition to handling, storage, and disposal of the chemical.
- ◆ Special protective precautions explain any need for personal protective equipment (PPE) (such as goggles or a respirator) or signs or other equipment (such as ventilation hood over a lab or pharmacy area) when using the chemical.

DISASTER PLAN

Disaster can be external or internal or a combination for a health care facility. **External disasters** include events outside the hospital which produce a large number of victims (e.g., fires, plane or train accidents, earthquakes, or violent civil disturbances). **Internal disasters** are events within the hospital that interrupt services and produce victims (e.g., utility interruption or chemical spill). Disasters such as earthquakes with building damage, tornadoes, and floods are both internal and external.

Teamwork and cooperation are essential to any disaster plan. Many communities hold annual disaster drills in cooperation with hospitals, police and fire departments, and public works offices. Mock disasters can provide much valuable information for all involved agencies.

Triage is an important consideration during a disaster. Clients in the hospital will be assessed for possible discharge if necessary. Victims are prioritized according to their care needs, from most severe to least. Victims are identified by universal EMS (Emergency Medical Services) disaster triage codes:

- ◆ Red: The most severely injured—likely need surgery or hospitalization in intensive care unit (ICU)

◆ Yellow: Significant injuries—require quick attention to prevent worsening of condition; may require hospitalization after treatment

◆ Green: Persons who are "walking wounded" and have non–life-threatening injuries that must eventually be treated to restore client to normal functioning; may not require hospitalization

◆ Black: Deceased, DOA, code blue; transported to morgue.

Not all victims arrive at the hospital with an EMS Triage tag. The "walking wounded" may arrive by private car and will need to be assessed in the emergency room.

Health care workers during a disaster must be willing to perform tasks as assigned by the supervisor. During this time personal communication should be put on hold in order not to tie up communication systems. It is important to observe client confidentiality and not perpetuate rumors. Each person should stay in his or her assigned area until directed to do otherwise. The facility will usually have a public information officer who will make statements to the media; it is imperative that all questions be referred to that person or office. Don't fall into the trap of giving unauthorized information.

EMERGENCY CODES

All health care facilities have emergency codes. Eleven codes have been identified. There is a real push to have all hospitals use a universal code system. Code Red and Code Blue are widely accepted, but much work is needed to bring other codes into line in all facilities. See Box 6-4 ◆ for commonly used emergency codes. It is important that both students and nurses know the specific codes used in each facility where they work or are affiliated.

EMERGENCY NURSING AND FIRST AID

You may be called on to deal with health care emergencies inside and outside of the health care facility. Nurses who give emergency care in the community should seek first aid training. Such training provides the individual with specific skills that can be used to serve and protect the community. It is important to administer first aid treatment and/or cardiopulmonary resuscitation (CPR) in the manner in which you have been trained (Figure 6-5 ◆).

Any nurse who volunteers his or her time at community activities to provide first aid should contact the local Red Cross to obtain a first aid certification.

CARDIOPULMONARY RESUSCITATION

CPR certification is required for health care professionals by most health care facilities (Box 6-5 ◆). Both the American Heart Association and the Red Cross provide certification programs that meet these requirements. Many facilities and schools provide the classes for employees and students. It is important to maintain current certification as a nurse as well

---

BOX 6-4
EMERGENCY CODES

◆ Code Red: Fire
◆ Code Blue: Medical emergency adult
◆ Code White: Medical emergency pediatric
◆ Code Pink: Infant Abduction
◆ Code Purple: Child Abduction
◆ Code Yellow: Bomb Threat
◆ Code Grey: Combative Person
◆ Code Silver: Person with a weapon and/or hostage situation
◆ Code Orange: Hazardous material spill/release
◆ Code Triage Internal: An internal disaster
◆ Code Triage External: An external disaster

Note: Codes may vary by facility. Be sure to know the color coding of the facility in which you work!

BOX 6-5
CPR OVERVIEW

CPR for Adult by Health Care Provider

If you find an unresponsive adult, place flat on back on a firm surface. Move an injured adult only if necessary, and turn head, neck, and body as a unit.

1. Shout for help. If alone, phone the emergency response number or 911 and retrieve the automated external defibrillator (AED) and emergency equipment.
2. **A** Open the Airway.
   Perform a head tilt–chin lift.
   If neck injury is suspected, use jaw thrust.
3. **B** Check for Breathing (look, listen, and feel).
   If breathing is not adequate, provide 2 slow breaths.
   Use bag–mask with oxygen or barrier device.
   Be sure chest rises with each breath.
   If chest does not rise, reopen the airway and try again.
4. **C** Check for signs of Circulation (pulse, breathing, coughing, or movement).
   Signs of circulation but no breathing:
   Provide rescue breathing (1 breath every 4 to 5 seconds).
   No pulse, no signs of circulation present:
   If AED is available: Power on, attach electrodes, follow prompts.
   If no AED, perform chest compressions:
   —Compress lower half of sternum.
   —Rate approximately 100 times per minute.
   —15 compressions, then 2 breaths (repeat).
5. CPR: Provide 15 compressions and 2 breaths (repeat) until client is intubated, then 5 compressions to 1 ventilation (repeat).

Source: Adapted from Guidelines of American Heart Association, 2000.

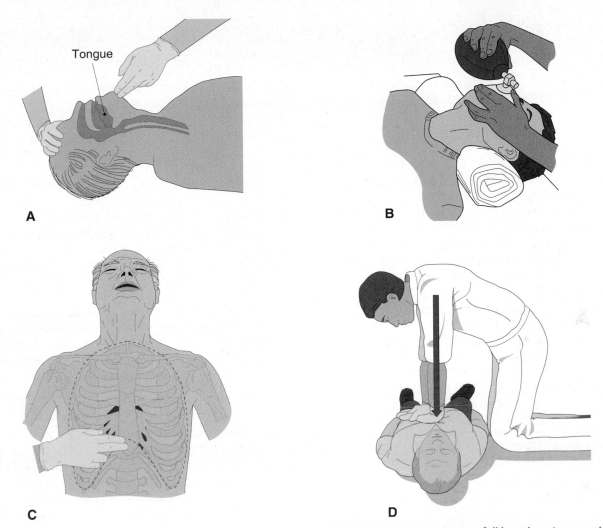

Figure 6-5. ◆ CPR. **A.** Use the head tilt/chin lift method to open the airway. **B.** If not breathing, give two full breaths using a pocket mask, mouth shield, or bag–valve mask. Observe the chest rise and fall during ventilation. **C.** Locate the compression site by following the edge of the rib cage to the notch where the ribs join the sternum. **D.** Position your hands and begin chest compressions with your arms vertical over the victim.

as a responsible citizen. Guidelines change periodically. Those holding a CPR card should refer to the guidelines frequently and practice the skills on a regular basis. For more information, contact the local provider of CPR certification classes.

◆ Restraining Clients

Restraints are protective devices used to limit the physical activity of the client or a part of the body. They can be classified as physical or chemical. Physical restraints are any manual method or physical or mechanical device, material, or equipment attached to the client's body. They cannot be removed easily, and they restrict the client's movement. Chemical restraints are psychotropic agents used to control disruptive behavior.

The purpose of restraints is to ensure the physical safety of the person who is being restrained, or of other persons whom the restrained person may otherwise harm. Nurses are encouraged to reduce the use of restraints and use safe alternatives whenever possible. Alternatives to restraints are shown in Box 6-6 ◆.

To safeguard clients in long-term care facilities, the United States government regulated the use of mechanical restraints. The Omnibus Budget Reconciliation Act (OBRA) clearly states that restraints should be applied only as a last resort. Regulations also require that (a) restraints be applied only under a physician's written order, one that specifies why the restraint is used and for how long it will be used; (b) the client agree to be restrained; and (c) the client be free of physical restraints not required to treat the client's medical symptoms.

LEGAL IMPLICATIONS OF RESTRAINTS

Because restraints restrict a person's ability to move freely, their use has legal implications. See Box 6-7 ◆ for the legal implications of using restraints.

BOX 6-6
NURSING CARE CHECKLIST

ALTERNATIVES TO RESTRAINTS

☑ Assign nurses in pairs to act as "buddies" so that one nurse can observe the client when the other leaves the unit.

☑ Place unstable clients in an area that is constantly or closely supervised.

☑ Prepare clients before a move, in order to limit relocation shock and resultant confusion.

☑ Stay with a client using a bedside commode or bathroom if the client is confused or sedated or has a gait disturbance or a high risk score for falling.

☑ Monitor all the client's medications and, if possible, attempt to lower or eliminate dosages of sedatives or psychotropic drugs.

☑ Position beds at their lowest level from the floor to facilitate getting in and out of bed.

☑ Replace full-length side rails with half- or three-quarter-length rails to prevent confused clients from climbing over rails or falling from the end of the bed.

☑ Use rocking chairs to help confused clients expend some of their energy so that they will be less inclined to wander.

☑ Wedge pillows or pads against the sides of wheelchairs to keep clients well positioned.

☑ Place a removable lap tray on a wheelchair to provide support and help keep the client in place.

☑ To quiet agitated clients, try a warm beverage, soft lights, a back rub, or a walk.

☑ Use "environmental restraints," such as pieces of furniture or large plants as barriers, to keep clients from wandering beyond appropriate areas.

☑ Place a picture or other personal item on the door to clients' rooms to help them identify their room.

☑ Try to determine the causes of the client's *"sundown syndrome"* (nocturnal wandering and disorientation as darkness falls, associated with dementia). Possible causes include poor hearing, poor eyesight, or pain.

☑ Establish ongoing assessment to monitor changes in physical and cognitive functional abilities and risk factors.

BOX 6-7 LEGAL IMPLICATIONS FOR USE OF RESTRAINTS

To protect clients and to avoid legal problems, the nurse should follow these guidelines:

◆ Know the agency's restraint policies. Policies should cover all types of physical and chemical restraints and specify how and when to apply them and what procedures to follow.

◆ When determining the need for a restraint, always assess the underlying reason for a client's restlessness, agitation, or confusion.

◆ Apply restraints only when necessary for the client's health and safety, not for convenience or to cope with understaffing.

◆ Avoid being influenced by a family member's advice not to restrain the client, even when the person offers to sit with the client. Nurses cannot legally delegate responsibility to a family member.

◆ Try to obtain a physician's order before applying a restraint. If the client needs to be restrained immediately, apply the restraint and then notify the physician as soon as possible. In many agencies, standing orders allow the use of restraints under certain circumstances, provided that a written order is obtained from the physician within 24 hours.

◆ Recognize the competent adult's right to make decisions regarding personal care and treatment, and obtain appro-

priate consent. Check agency policies if necessary restraint is refused. An agency may require the client to sign a release of liability should injury result; otherwise, the agency has the option of refusing to continue care. For clients who are declared legally incompetent, obtain consent from an appointed guardian or surrogate as permitted under law.

◆ Keep in mind the principle of least restriction; that is, restrain the client only to the extent necessary to accomplish the restraint's purpose.

◆ Make sure that a physical restraint fits properly.

◆ When a restraint is applied, document:
a. The specific behavior that made it necessary
b. The type of restraint used
c. The substance of explanations given to the client and support persons
d. The client's consent
e. The exact times the restraint was applied and removed
f. The client's behavior while the restraint was applied
g. The frequency of care given while the restraint was applied and removed (e.g., assessment of circulation and range-of-motion exercises)
h. Notification of the physician

◆ Periodically reevaluate the need for the restraint.

SELECTING A RESTRAINT

Before selecting a restraint, nurses need to understand its purpose clearly and measure it against the following five criteria:

1. It restricts the client's movement as little as possible. If a client needs to have one arm restrained, do not restrain the entire body.

2. It does not interfere with the client's treatment or health problem. If a client has poor blood circulation to the hands, apply a restraint that will not aggravate that circulatory problem.

3. It is readily changeable. Restraints need to be changed frequently, especially if they become soiled. Keeping other guidelines in mind, choose a restraint that can be changed with minimal disturbance to the client.

4. It is safe for the particular client. Choose a restraint with which the client cannot self-inflict injury. For example, a physically active child could incur injury trying to climb out of a crib if one wrist is tied to the side of the crib. A jacket restraint would restrain the child more safely.

5. It is the least obvious to others. Both clients and visitors are often embarrassed by a restraint, even though they understand why it is being used. The less obvious the restraint, the more comfortable people feel.

KINDS OF RESTRAINTS

There are several kinds of restraints (Figures 6-6 ◆ through 6-8). Among the most common are the jacket restraint, the belt restraint, the mitt or hand restraint, limb restraints, elbow restraints, mummy restraints, and crib nets. Geri chairs and wheelchairs used to confine client activity can also be considered restraints. There are several types of vest restraints, but all are essentially sleeveless jackets (vests) with straps (tails) that can be tied to the bed frame under the mattress or to the legs of a chair (see Figure 6-7 ◆). These body restraints are used to ensure the safety of confused or sedated clients in beds or wheelchairs. The Food and Drug Administration (FDA) advises that manufacturers place "front" and "back" labels on vest restraints.

Belt or safety strap body restraints (see Figure 6-6B) are used to ensure the safety of all clients who are being moved on stretchers or in wheelchairs. Some wheelchairs have a soft padded safety bar that attaches to side brackets that are installed under the arm rests. To prevent the person from slumping forward, the nurse then attaches a shoulder "Y" strap to the bar and over the client's shoulders to the rear handles. Other safety belt models have a three-loop design. One loop surrounds the person's waist and attaches to the rear handles. If such restraints are unavailable, the nurse can place a

A

B

C

Figure 6-6. ◆ **A.** Poncho-type vest restraint. Put vest on client, with front/back opening placed according to manufacturer's recommendations. Pull the tie on the end of the vest flap across the chest, and place it through the slit on the opposite side of the chest. Repeat for the other tie. Use a half-bow knot to secure each tie. Do not tie the vest to the head of the bed. Fasten the ties together behind the chair using a square knot. Ensure that the client is positioned appropriately to enable maximum chest expansion for breathing. **B.** Belt restraint (safety belt). Attach the belt around the client's waist and fasten it at the back of the chair. If the client is bedridden or on a stretcher, one portion of the belt (the longer portion) is placed beneath the client, and the shorter portion is over the client's gown, with a finger width between the belt and the client. Belt restraints need to be applied to all clients on stretchers even when the side rails are up. **C.** Mitt restraint. Make sure the fingers can be slightly flexed and are not caught under the hand. Follow the manufacturer's directions for securing the mitt. Remove the mitt at least every 2 to 4 hours for washing and exercising the client's hand. Assess the client's hand circulation shortly after the mitt is applied and at regular intervals. Monitor for feelings of numbness or discomfort or inability to move the fingers. *Source:* Jenny Thomas Photography, photos A and B.

A

B

C

Figure 6-7. ◆ **A, B.** Wrist or ankle restraint. Pad bony prominences to prevent skin breakdown. Pull the tie of the commercially made restraint through the slit or through the buckle, and secure the tie to the bed frame. **C.** Elbow restraint. Place the child's elbow in the center of the restraint. Make sure that the ends of the tongue depressors are covered by padded material to prevent irritation. Wrap the restraint smoothly around the arm and secure it with safety pins, ties, or tape. Pinning it to the child's shirt prevents it from sliding down the arm. Monitor for tightness and obstructed blood circulation. *Source:* Jenny Thomas Photography, photo A.

folded towel or small sheet around the client's waist and fasten it at the back of the wheelchair. Belt restraints may also be used for certain clients confined to bed or to chairs.

A mitt or hand restraint (Figure 6-6C) is used to prevent confused clients from using their hands or fingers to scratch and injure themselves. For example, a confused client may need to be prevented from pulling at intravenous tubing or a bandage following surgery. Hand or mitt restraints allow the client to be ambulatory and/or to move the arm freely rather than be confined to a bed or a chair. (See legend for Figure 6-6C.)

Limb restraints (Figure 6-7A and B ◆) are generally made of cloth. They may be used to immobilize a limb, primarily for therapeutic reasons (e.g., to maintain an intravenous infusion).

Elbow restraints (Figure 6-7C) are used to prevent infants or small children from flexing their elbows to touch or scratch a skin lesion or to reach the head when a scalp vein infusion is in place. This restraint consists of a piece of material with pockets into which plastic or wooden tongue depressors are inserted to provide rigidity.

The mummy restraint is a special folding of a blanket or sheet around a child to prevent movement during a procedure such as gastric washing, eye irrigation, or collection of a blood specimen. See Figure 6-8 ◆ for application instructions.

General guidelines for applying and monitoring restraints are presented in Box 6-8 ◆ (See page 100.).

Attaching restraints to bed or chair requires the use of knots, which must be secure but easily untied by staff in an emergency situation. See Figure 6-9 ◆ for instructions on tying a half-bow knot and Figure 6-10 ◆ for a square knot.

A   **B**

Figure 6-8. ◆ Making a mummy restraint. **A.** Use a blanket about twice the length of the infant's body. Fold down one corner, and place the baby's shoulders on it in the supine position. Fold the right side of the blanket over the infant's body, leaving the left arm free (1). The right arm is in a natural position at the side. **B.** Fold the excess blanket at the bottom up under the infant (2). With the infant's left arm in a natural position beside the body, fold the left side of the blanket over the infant, including the arm, and tuck the blanket under the body (3).

NURSING CARE

◆ ASSESSING

Assessing clients at risk for accidents and injury involves (a) noting risk indicators in the nursing history and physical examination; (b) using specifically developed risk assessment tools; and (c) evaluating the client's home environment.

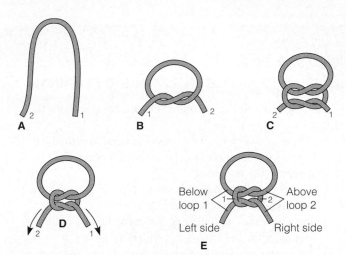

Figure 6-9. ◆ To make a half-bow (quick-release) knot, first place the restraint tie under the side frame of the bed (or around a chair leg). **A.** Bring the free end up, around, under, and over the attached end of the tie and pull it tight. **B.** Again take the free end over and under the attached end of the tie, but this time make a half-bow loop. **C.** Tighten the free end of the tie and the bow until the knot is secure. To untie the knot, pull the end of the tie and then loosen the first cross over the tie.

Figure 6-10. ◆ To make a square (reef) knot: **A.** Form a "U" loop. **B.** Pass one end (1) over and under the other. **C.** Take the same end (1), and pass it over, under, and over the other. **D.** Pull knot tight. **E.** When the knot is tied correctly, the ties on each side are both either above or below the loop. Attach the other end of the commercial restraint to the movable portion of the bed frame, never to the side rails or to the nonmoving bed frame. If the ties are attached to the movable portion, the wrist or ankle will not be pulled when the bed position is changed.

The nursing history and physical examination can reveal considerable data about the client's safety practices and risks for injury. Data include age and developmental level; general health status; mobility status; presence or absence of physiologic or perceptual deficits such as olfactory, visual, tactile, taste, or other sensory impairments; altered thought processes or other impaired cognitive or emotional capabilities; substance abuse; any indications of abuse or neglect; and an accident and injury history. A safety history also needs to include the client's awareness of hazards, knowledge of safety precautions both at home and work, and any perceived threats to safety.

Risk Assessment Tools

Risk assessment tools are available to determine clients at risk both for specific kinds of injury, such as falls, or skin impairment. In general, these tools direct the nurse to appraise the factors affecting safety as they have been outlined earlier. See Figure 12–4 for one skin impairment assessment tool.

◆ DIAGNOSING, PLANNING, and IMPLEMENTING

A primary NANDA diagnostic label related to safety issues is Risk for Injury: A state in which the individual is at risk for injury as a result of environmental conditions interacting with the individual's adaptive and defense resources. One of the subcategories of this diagnosis may be preferred when the nurse wants to isolate suitable interventions. These subcategories are:

◆ Risk for Poisoning
◆ Risk for Suffocation
◆ Risk for Trauma

(Refer to Appendix I for a complete list of nursing diagnoses related to safety. ⊙)

When planning care to prevent accidents and injury, the nurse considers all factors affecting the client's safety, specifies desired outcomes, and selects nursing activities to meet these outcomes. The major goal for clients with safety risks is to prevent accidents and injury. To meet this goal clients often need to change their health behavior and may need to modify the environment.

Desired outcomes associated with preventing injury depend on the individual client. Examples of desired outcomes follow. The nurse needs to individualize these for clients. The client:

◆ Describes methods to prevent specific hazards (e.g., falls, suffocation, choking, fires, drowning, electric shock).
◆ Reports use of home safety measures (e.g., fire safety measures, smoke detector maintenance, fall prevention strategies, burn prevention measures, poison prevention measures, safe storage of hazardous materials, firearm safety precautions, electrocution prevention, water safety precautions, bicycle safety, motor vehicle safety).
◆ Alters home physical environment to reduce the risk of injury.

BOX 6-8
NURSING CARE CHECKLIST

APPLYING AND MONITORING RESTRAINTS

☑ Apply the selected restraint. Obtain consent from the client or guardian.

☑ Ensure that a physician's order has been provided, or in an emergency, obtain one within 24 hours after applying the restraint.

☑ Assure the client and the client's support people that the restraint is temporary and protective. A restraint must never be applied as punishment for any behavior or merely for the nurse's convenience.

☑ Apply the restraint in such a way that the client can move as freely as possible without defeating the purpose of the restraint.

☑ Ensure that limb restraints are applied securely but not so tightly that they impede blood circulation to any body area or extremity.

☑ Assess the restraint every 30 minutes. Some facilities have specific forms to be used to record ongoing assessment.

☑ Release all restraints at least every 2 to 4 hours, and provide range-of-motion (ROM) exercises (see Chapter 20) and skin care (see Chapter 12).

☑ If more than one limb is restrained, remove one restraint at a time. When a restraint is temporarily removed, do not leave the client unattended.

☑ Reassess the continued need for the restraint at least every 8 hours. Include an assessment of the underlying cause of the behavior necessitating use of the restraints.

☑ Immediately report to the nurse in charge and record on the client's chart any persistent reddened or broken skin areas under the restraint.

☑ At the first indication of cyanosis or pallor, coldness of a skin area, or a client's complaint of a tingling sensation, pain, or numbness, loosen the restraint and exercise the limb.

☑ Apply a restraint so that it can be released quickly in case of an emergency and with the body part in a normal anatomic position.

☑ Provide emotional support verbally and through touch.

☑ Determine that restraint is in good condition and is the appropriate size for the client.

☑ Explain to client and support people the purpose and procedure for using the restraint.

☑ Document relevant information for all types of restraints.

☑ Record on the client's chart the time the physician was notified, the type of restraint applied, the time it was applied, the reason for its application, the client's response to the restraint, and the times that the restraints are removed and skin care given.

☑ Record any other interventions, assessments, and explanations to client and significant others.

☑ Adjust the nursing care plan as required, for example, to include releasing the restraint q2h, assessing circulation, sensation, and motion of restrained extremities; providing skin care, and providing range-of-motion exercises.

- Describes emergency procedures for poisoning and fire.
- Describes age-specific risks or work safety risks or community safety risks.
- Demonstrates correct use of child safety seats.
- Demonstrates correct administration of cardiopulmonary resuscitation.

Nursing interventions to meet desired outcomes are largely directed toward helping the client and family to:

- Identify environmental hazards in home and community.
- Demonstrate safety practices appropriate to the home health care agency, community, and workplace.
- Demonstrate safe childrearing practices or lifestyle practices.

◆ EVALUATING

In preventing client injury, the nurse's role is largely one of education. The nurse evaluates whether the client has learned about safety hazards, incorporated safety practice into behavior, and acquired skills to perform in the event of certain emergencies.

◆ DISCHARGE CONSIDERATIONS

If clients require an alarm system when they return home, caregivers would need instruction in its setup and use. Instruct them to test the monitoring device every 12 to 24 hours to ensure that it is working. Also, have them check the volume of the alarm to be sure they can hear it.

If a client is in danger of falling, remind caregivers to:

- Clear the floor of wires or loose rugs.
- Provide lighting at night between bedroom and bathroom.
- Encourage clients to rise in stages from lying to sitting to standing, and to get their balance before starting to walk.
- Provide assistive devices (cane, walker) as needed.

Nursing Process Case Study:
CLIENT WITH FRACTURED HIP

Mr. Moore is a 72-year-old widower who is recovering from a fall in which he fractured his hip and underwent surgical repair 1 week ago. He will be staying with his son for 2 weeks after he is discharged from the hospital, but he is eager to return to his own home. Once he is home, his son will visit nightly after work. He will receive Meals on Wheels once a day, and a home health care attendant will visit weekly to assist him with hygienic care until he is more independent. Mr. Moore's wife died 3 years ago, but he has remained independent and continued his social functions. He lives in a small three-bedroom house with his dog and cat, and he enjoys gardening. Prior to fracturing his hip, he walked his dog daily. After the initial visit from the RN, you will be his home health care nurse.

Assessment Home care nurse (LVN) visit on second day in own home. HHA assisted with shower and dressing. Doing well, physically no complaints of pain. VS stable T98.2, P74, R18, and BP 132/84. Surgical incision well healed, no redness or drainage, open to air. AAO × 4. Throw rugs and furniture in pathway from bed to bathroom. Safety devices installed in bathroom. Grab-bar, raised toilet seat. Family members' phone numbers programmed on speed-dial on phone. Client states, "It is so good to be home, I had the best night's sleep last night." Walked 20 feet from front door to car. Looking forward to being able to walk dog.

Diagnosis

- Ineffective Health Maintenance
- Chronic Confusion
- Impaired Physical Mobility

Expected Outcomes

Mr. Moore will:

- Follow mutually agreed upon health care maintenance plan
- Participate in activities of daily living at the maximum of functional ability
- Demonstrate use of adaptive equipment (e.g., walker) to increase mobility

Planning and Implementation

- Assess client's awareness of deficits that may result from normal aging.
- Give client information about community resources for the elderly (Meals on Wheels, home visitors, transportation to appointments).
- Use reminiscence and life review therapeutic interventions. Ask questions such as "What was really important to you as you look back?"
- Monitor client for physiological causes, including pain, medication effects.
- Obtain any assistive devices needed for activity.

- Initiate a walking program in which the client walks with or without help every day as part of daily routine.

Evaluation Two weeks after discharge Mr. Moore is in his own home. You make your first home visit.

- Client and family have established regular schedule of caretakers and family members' visits to allow independence.
- Meals on Wheels scheduled 6 days per week.
- Client spending one weekend day with family.
- Mr. Moore is able to shower and dress with assistance of home health aide. Home safety evaluation reveals that night-lights have been installed and furniture has been rearranged for easy access from bedroom to bath.
- PT home visits 2× per week. Able to get in and out of bed. Using walker in house and outside when accompanied.

Critical Thinking in the Nursing Process

1. While hospitalized, Mr. Moore experienced some mild confusion during the night, but his nurses decided not to restrain him. What are the best reasons for avoiding the use of restraints for clients such as Mr. Moore?
2. What are some of the more obvious factors that may affect Mr. Moore's safety as he returns home?
3. What strengths do you note about Mr. Moore that may protect him from injury when he returns home?

See discussion of Critical Thinking in Appendix IV.

 Personal Safety for Nurses

Nurses routinely protect the safety of the client for whom they care. However, little thought is given to the nurse's personal safety until the nurse sustains an injury. A nurse cannot provide for clients effectively unless he or she is free from injury.

BODY MECHANICS

Body mechanics is the term used to describe safe, efficient use of the body to move objects and carry out activities of daily living. The purpose of body mechanics is to ensure safe and efficient use of appropriate muscle groups to maintain balance, reduce fatigue and energy expended, and prevent injury.

Body mechanics involves the concepts of alignment and posture discussed earlier. When a person moves, the center of gravity shifts continuously in the direction of moving body parts. The closer the line of gravity is to the center of the base of support, the greater the person's stability (Figure 6-11A ◆). Conversely, the closer the line of gravity is to the edge of the base of support, the more precarious the balance (Figure 6-11B). If the line of gravity falls outside the base of support, the person falls (Figure 6-11C).

Body balance can be greatly enhanced by (a) widening the base of support and (b) lowering the center of gravity, bringing it closer to the base of support. The base of support

Figure 6-11. ◆ **A.** Balance is maintained when the line of gravity falls close to the base of support. **B.** Balance is precarious when the line of gravity falls at the edge of the base of support. **C.** Balance cannot be maintained when the line of gravity falls outside the base of support.

may be easily widened by spreading the feet farther apart. The center of gravity is readily lowered by flexing the hips and knees until a squatting position is achieved. Use of these two techniques is vital to nurses to prevent work-related back injuries.

Preventing Back Injuries
Many factors increase the potential for lower back injury. Low back pain can be caused by a number of factors, from injuries to the effects of aging.

Undesirable twisting can be prevented by facing the direction of movement squarely, whether pushing, pulling, or sliding, and by moving the object directly toward or away from one's center of gravity (Figure 6-12 ◆).

clinical ALERT

Twisting (rotation) of the thoracolumbar spine and **stooping** (acute flexion of the back with hips and knees straight) must always be avoided because of their potential for causing back injury.

LOW BACK SPRAIN AND STRAIN. The muscles of the low back provide power and strength for activities such as standing, walking, and lifting. A strain of the muscle can occur when the muscle is poorly conditioned or overworked. The ligaments of the low back interconnect the five vertebral bones and provide support or stability for the low back. A sprain of the low back can occur when a sudden, forceful movement injures a liga-

Hold object close to body

Turn whole body; don't twist

Push or pull rather than twist

Figure 6-12. ◆ Correct body mechanics for the proper method of caring or moving an object.

ment that has become stiff or weak through poor conditioning or overuse. These injuries, or sprain and strain, are the most common causes of low back pain. Although you cannot totally halt the progress of these effects, they can be slowed by regular exercise, knowing the proper way to lift and move objects, proper nutrition, and good posture. See Box 6-9 ◆ for guidelines for preventing back injury in nurses or in clients.

Lifting

When a person lifts or carries an object, the object's weight becomes part of body weight. This weight change affects the center of gravity, which becomes displaced in the direction of the added weight. To counteract this potential imbalance, body parts (e.g., arm, trunk) move away from the weight, so the center of gravity is maintained at the same point in the base of support. By holding an object as close to the body as possible, the lifter avoids displacing the center of gravity and achieves greater stability.

People can lift more weight when using a lever. Human bones function as levers—the joint is the **fulcrum** (fixed point about which a lever moves) and the muscles exert the force (Figure 6-13 ◆). Lifting involves movement against gravity, so the nurse must use major muscle groups of the thighs, knees, upper and lower arms, abdomen, and pelvis to prevent back strain.

Figure 6-13. ◆ Using the arm as a lever.

Another technique based on the principle of leverage may be used when lifting objects from floor to waist level. In this technique, the back and knees are flexed until the load is at thigh level. Then the back straightens slowly while the knees remain flexed to provide thrust (Figure 6-14 ◆). This maneuver provides for better balance and leverage. The muscles work together (in *synchronization*), which helps prevent injury. When an object is lifted to knee level, the abdominal and lumbar muscles contract for leverage and pull. The thigh and leg muscles exert the upward thrust to bring the object off the floor. When an object is lifted from mid-thigh to waist level, force is primarily exerted by leg and thigh muscles, while back and lumbar muscles remain contracted.

For all lifting positions, it is necessary to maintain a distance of 30 cm (12 inches) or more between the feet and to keep the load close to the body, especially when it is at knee

---

BOX 6-9

CLIENT TEACHING

HOW TO PREVENT BACK INJURIES
- Become consciously aware of your posture and body mechanics.
- When standing for a period of time, periodically flex one hip and knee and rest your foot on an object if possible.
- When sitting, keep your knees slightly higher than your hips.
- Use a firm mattress that provides good body support at natural body curvatures.
- Exercise regularly to maintain overall physical condition; include exercises that strengthen the pelvic, abdominal, and lumbar muscles.
- Avoid exercises that cause pain or require spinal flexion with straight legs (e.g., toe-touching and sit-ups) or spinal rotation (twisting).
- When moving an object, spread your feet apart to provide a wide base of support.
- When lifting an object, distribute the weight between large muscles of the legs and arms.
- Wear clothing that allows you to use good body mechanics and comfortable low-heeled shoes that provide good foot support and will not cause you to slip, stumble, or turn your ankle.

A   **B**   **C**

Figure 6-14. ◆ Stages in lifting an object from the floor to the waist: **A.** Move close to the object, and begin with the back and knees flexed to grasp the object. **B.** Start the lift by keeping the back flexed while the knees begin to straighten so that the leg muscles can exert an upward thrust. **C.** Keep the back and knees in a less flexed, but not straight, position.

TABLE 6-2 SUMMARY OF GUIDELINES AND PRINCIPLES RELATED TO BODY MECHANICS

GUIDELINES	PRINCIPLES
Plan the move or transfer carefully. Free the surrounding area of obstacles and move required equipment near the head or foot of the bed.	Appropriate preparation prevents potential falls and injury and safeguards the client and equipment.
Obtain the assistance of other people or use mechanical devices to move objects that are too heavy. Encourage clients to assist as much as possible by pushing or pulling themselves to reduce your muscular effort. Use arms as levers whenever possible to increase lifting power.	The heavier an object, the greater the force needed to move the object.
Adjust the working area to waist level, and keep the body close to the area. Elevate adjustable beds and overbed tables or lower the side rails of beds to prevent stretching and reaching.	Objects that are close to the center of gravity are moved with the least effort.
Provide a firm, smooth, dry bed foundation before moving a client in bed or use a pull sheet.	Less energy is required when you reduce the friction between the object moved and the surface on which it is moved.
Always face the direction of the movement.	Ineffective use of major muscle groups occurs when the spine is rotated or twisted.
Start any body movement with proper alignment. Stand as close as possible to the object to be moved. Avoid stretching, reaching, and twisting, which may place the line of gravity outside the base of support.	Balance is maintained and muscle strain is avoided as long as the line of gravity passes through the base of support.
Before moving an object, increase your stability by widening your stance and flexing your knees, hips, and ankles.	The wider the base of support and the lower the center of gravity, the greater the stability.
Before moving an object, contract your gluteal, abdominal, leg, and arm muscles to prepare them for action.	The greater the preparatory isometric tensing, or contraction of muscles, before moving an object, the less the energy required to move it, and the less likelihood of musculoskeletal strain and injury.
Avoid working against gravity. Pull, push, roll, or turn objects instead of lifting them. Lower the head of the client's bed before moving the client up in bed.	Moving an object along a level surface requires less energy than moving an object up an inclined surface or lifting it against the force of gravity. Pulling creates less friction than pushing.
Use your gluteal and leg muscles rather than the sacrospinal muscles of your back to exert an upward thrust when lifting. Distribute the work load between both arms and legs to prevent back strain.	The synchronized use of as many large muscle groups as possible during an activity increases overall strength and prevents muscle fatigue and injury.
When pushing an object, enlarge the base of support by moving the front foot forward. When pulling an object, enlarge the base of support by either moving the rear leg back if facing the object or moving the front foot forward if facing away from the object.	Balance is maintained with minimal effort when the base of support is enlarged in the direction in which the movement will occur.
When moving or carrying objects, hold them as close as possible to your center of gravity.	The closer the line of gravity to the center of the base of support, the greater the stability.
Use the weight of the body as a force for pulling or pushing, by rocking on the feet or leaning forward or backward.	Body weight adds force to counteract the weight of the object and reduces the amount of strain on the arms and back.
Alternate rest periods with periods of muscle use to help prevent fatigue.	Continuous muscle exertion can result in muscle strain and injury.

level. Before attempting to lift, the nurse must ensure that there are no hazards on the floor, there is a clear path for moving the object, and the nurse's base of support is secure.

Pushing and Pulling

When pushing or pulling an object, a person maintains balance with the least effort when the base of the support is enlarged in the direction in which the movement is to be produced or opposed. It is easier and safer to pull an object toward one's own center of gravity than to push it away, because the person can exert more control of the object's movement when pulling it.

Pivoting

Pivoting is a technique in which the body is turned in a way to avoid twisting of the spine. To pivot, place one foot ahead of the other, raise the heels very slightly, and put the weight on the balls of the feet. When the weight is off the heels, the frictional surface is decreased and the knees are not twisted when turning. Keeping the body aligned, turn (pivot) about 90 degrees in the desired direction. The foot that was forward will now be behind. A summary of principles and guidelines related to body mechanics is shown in Table 6-2 ◆.

Note: The bibliography listings for this and all chapters have been compiled at the back of the book.

PROCEDURE 6-1

Using a Bed or Chair Exit Safety Monitoring Device

A bed or chair safety monitor (Figure 6-15 ◆) is an electronic device with a position-sensitive switch that triggers an audio alarm when the client attempts to get out of the bed or chair unassisted. When activated, the alarm alerts the nurse and provides an opportunity for the nurse to intervene.

PURPOSES

◆ To alert the nurse that the client is attempting to get out of bed
◆ To help decrease the risk of client falls

EQUIPMENT

◆ Alarm and control device
◆ Connection to nurse call system (optional)
◆ Sensor device

Figure 6-15. ◆ Bed exit monitoring device; the sensor is usually placed under the client's buttocks. *Source:* Courtesy of J. T. Posey Company. Reprinted with permission.

INTERVENTIONS

1. Explain to the client and support people the purpose and procedure for using safety monitoring.
   ◆ Explain that the device does not limit mobility in any manner; rather, it alerts the staff when the client is about to get out of bed or a chair.
   ◆ Explain that the nurse must be called when the client needs to get out of bed. *These measures reduce anxiety and protect the client from injury.*

2. Obtain the appropriate sensor device and control unit.

3. Test the battery device and alarm sound. *This ensures that the device is functioning properly prior to use.*

4. Apply the sensor pad or leg band.
   ◆ Place the leg band according to the manufacturer's recommendations. The usual position for a bed or chair sensor is under the mattress (see Figure 6-15) or chair cushion directly beneath the client's buttocks. For clients at high risk of falling, the sensor may be placed under the shoulders. *Placement must be individualized to the client's needs.*
   ◆ For a bed or chair device set the time delay for determining the client's movement patterns from 1 to 12 seconds.
   ◆ Connect the sensor pad to the control unit and the nurse call system. *The alarm device is position sensitive. For example, when a leg band approaches a near-vertical position (such as in*

walking, crawling, or kneeling as the client attempts to get out of bed), the audio alarm is triggered, causing a sharp, shrill sound.

5. Instruct the client to call the nurse when the client wants or needs to get up, and assist as required. *This reassures the client that he or she will not be confined indefinitely.*
   ◆ Before assisting the client to rise, deactivate the alarm by unsnapping the alarm device from the elastic band. *This prevents the alarm from being triggered.*
   ◆ Assist the client back to bed, and reattach the alarm device to the sensor. *The alarm provides a safeguard against client injury.*

6. Ensure client safety with additional safety precautions.
   ◆ Place call light within client reach, lift all side rails, and lower the bed to its lowest position. *The alarm device is not a substitute for other precautionary measures.*
   ◆ Place monitoring device stickers on the client's door, chart, and Kardex. *This communicates use of the alarm to other personnel.*

7. Document relevant data. *An action that is not documented is not legally considered to be done.*
   ◆ Record that monitoring device is intact when applied.
   ◆ Record all assessments.
   ◆ Record all safety precautions and interventions discussed and employed. *Documentation is crucial for client safety and to ensure quality of care.*

◆ SAMPLE DOCUMENTATION

Date	Focus		
Time 0930	Safety	D	Attempting to climb out of bed over side rail. Confused. Stated "I need to go home, and feed my dogs."
		A	Reoriented, placed call light within reach. Instructed to call before attempting to get o.o.b. Wander-guard® attached to left ankle. Relocated to room close to nurses' station. Explained that the alarm will sound if he leaves the bed. Contacted family members to reassure client that the dogs are being cared for. Instruct nursing assistant to check q 15 min and respond immediately to alarm.
1030		R	Alarm activated 3 times within one hour. Asked that alarm be removed. Resting quietly after reorientation. K. Adams LPN

Chapter Review

Key Terms by Topics

Use the audio glossary feature of either the CD-ROM or the Companion Website to hear the correct pronunciation of the following key terms

Preventing specific hazards
suffocation

Hospital and institutional safety
bagging, external disasters, internal disasters, triage

Personal safety for nurses
body mechanics, stooping, twisting, fulcrum

Key Points

- Education is a major health protection strategy in preventing accidents.
- When planning to meet safety needs of clients, nurses need to consider physical factors in the environment and the psychological and physiologic state of the individual.
- Accidents are a major cause of death among individuals of all ages in the United States and Canada.
- Hazards to safety occur at all ages and vary according to the age and development of the individual.
- To ensure safety, focus on (a) observing or predicting situations that are potentially harmful and (b) educating clients to safeguard themselves and their families. It is often necessary to modify the environment to make it safe.
- Nurses must be familiar with the fire procedures in the health care agency where they practice. In the event of a fire, the nurse must (1) protect clients from injury, (2) report, (3) contain, and (4) put out the fire.
- To prevent falls, the nurse must provide constant surveillance for infants and young children and assess older clients' safety needs carefully.
- Prolonged exposure to excessive noise can produce hearing loss. Ill or injured people may be especially sensitive to noises.
- Accidents can be prevented by using grounded outlets and plugs, putting protective covers over outlets, and making sure that electric wiring and circuits meet safety standards.
- In hospitals, radioactive substances are used for both diagnostic and treatment purposes. Follow agency policy to safeguard clients and staff from unsafe exposure.
- Side rails and handrails protect hospitalized clients from falls. Restraints keep clients from falling and from inflicting injuries on themselves and others.
- Because restraints restrict a client's basic freedom to move, they should be used as a last resort. Careful assessment and accurate, complete documentation are important when restraints are used.

EXPLORE MediaLink

Additional interactive resources for this chapter can be found on the Companion Website at www.prenhall.com/ramont. Click on Chapter 6 and "Begin" to select the activities for this chapter. For chapter-related NCLEX-style questions and an audio glossary, access the accompanying CD-ROM in this book.

Animation:
- Naproxen
- Penicillin

∞ For Further Study

For additional information on infection control, see Chapter 7.

See Figure 12–4 for an example of a skin assessment tool.

For more about bathing a client, see Chapter 13.

For therapeutic applications of heat and cold, see Chapter 20.

For directions on passive range-of-motion (PROM) exercises, see Chapter 20.

For additional information about incident reports, see Chapter 2 and Chapter 32.

Critical Thinking Care Map

Caring for a Client with Risk for Injury

NCLEX-PN Focus Area: Safety

Case Study: George Whitman is a 75-year-old man with a history of Parkinson's disease. He was admitted to the hospital following a fall, which resulted in an intertrochanteric fracture of his right hip. The fracture was treated with an open reduction internal fixation (ORIF). For the past 7 days he has been in the transitional care unit receiving physical therapy and mobility training. He is presently able to ambulate with a walker.

Nursing Diagnosis: Ineffective Protection

COLLECT DATA

Subjective	Objective
_____	_____
_____	_____
_____	_____
_____	_____
_____	_____

Would you report this data? Yes/No

If yes, to: _____

Nursing Care

_____

_____

_____

_____

_____

_____

_____

_____

_____

_____

_____

_____

How would you document this? _____

_____

_____

_____

_____

Data Collected
(use those that apply)

- Client's wife expressed concerns about his upcoming discharge.
- Lives with wife in a two-story house
- Does yard work
- Socializes with the neighbors
- Daughter and three grandchildren live 75 miles away
- Mrs. Whitman and the daughter feels the couple should move to a retirement apartment.
- Mr. Whitman expressed, "Selling the house would be a sign that I am just giving up."
- Rigidity due to the Parkinson's
- Soft diet—difficulty in swallowing
- Large bruise on his left leg and right forearm
- Routine medications: Sinemet 25/100 tid, Tasmar 100 tid, DSS capsule 100 mg daily, ferrous sulfate 325 mg qd, Heparin 5,000 U sq bid
- VS: BP 140/88, P 76, R 20, T 98.2° F
- Lab results: H&H 13.2 40.4, PT 13.5 sec, PTT 90 sec

Nursing Interventions
(use those that apply)

- Monitor risk for bleeding.
- Assess pain severity on 1–10 scale.
- Help client perform prescribed exercises q 8 hrs.
- Refer family to appropriate community resources.
- Observe client for cause of impaired mobility.
- Evaluate client for signs of depression.
- Observe for causes of inability to feed self independently.
- Take temperature, pulse, and blood pressure q 4 hrs.
- Observe nutritional status.
- Teach client and family signs of bleeding, precautions to take to prevent bleeding.
- Work with dietitian to improve nutritional status.
- Teach caregiver feeding techniques that prevent choking.

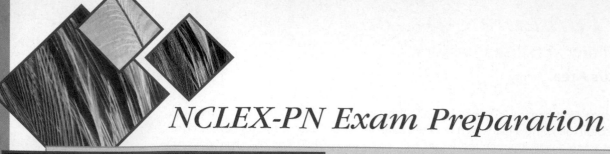

NCLEX-PN Exam Preparation

1. You are asked to teach a parenting class on safety at a community center. One of the parents asks why young children are so prone to accidents. Of the following, which is the best answer?
   a. Young children are uncoordinated, so they are more likely to fall.
   b. Misbehavior results in many injuries to children.
   c. Young children's curiosity exceeds their judgment.
   d. Parental neglect results in many accidents.

2. Restraining a client without a physician's order stating type of restraint and how long it will be used is considered to be:
   a. False imprisonment
   b. Allowed for short time periods
   c. Allowed if family members agree
   d. Allowed by facility policy

3. A young child is restrained following surgery to the face. The child is in a crib and is attempting to climb out. Which of the following would be the most appropriate type of restraint?
   a. Wrist restraint
   b. Belt restraint
   c. Mitten restraints
   d. Vest restraint

4. Your client is being discharged following a total hip replacement. You provide discharge instructions involving home safety in the presence of the son. Which of the following statements would demonstrate the need for more teaching?
   a. "Dad will be staying with us until he is completely recovered."
   b. "We have removed the throw rugs from the bedroom and bathroom."
   c. "Dad will need to use the walker only when leaving the house."
   d. "When Dad gets out of bed, we will have him get up slowly and gain his balance before walking."

5. The safe and efficient use of the body to move objects and carry out activities of daily living is:
   a. Physical therapy
   b. Body mechanics
   c. A nursing intervention
   d. Occupational therapy

6. The government agency responsible for a safe work environment is the:
   a. CDC
   b. OSHA
   c. JCAHO
   d. Department of Labor

7. You are assigned to care for a client in isolation. After you have changed the bed, you need to remove the soiled linen from the room. What is the procedure for dealing with soiled linen?
   a. Linen remains in the room until the client is discharged.
   b. Carry the rolled-up linen to the soiled linen without touching your uniform.
   c. Place the soiled linen in a bag, which is held by another person outside the isolation room.
   d. Dispose of the linen in the refuse container.

8. During a community disaster drill you are assigned to triage. Which of the following describes your understanding of triage duties? You will:
   a. Assign duties to disaster workers
   b. Serve as the public information officer for the media
   c. Prioritize victims according to their care needs
   d. Greet the "walking wounded" at the ER

9. Clients with paralysis of both legs are at risk for injury because of:
   a. Inevitable muscle atrophy
   b. The use of pain or other medication
   c. Inability to move even when they perceive discomfort
   d. The likelihood of incontinence

10. Extreme emotional stress can alter the ability to perceive environmental hazards. Which of the following is the reason for this?
    a. Stressful situations can reduce a person's level of concentration.
    b. Stress can diminish the person's ability to receive and convey information.
    c. Stress can diminish one's ability to respond appropriately through thought and action.
    d. Stressful situations can suppress the ability to perceive environmental stimuli.

Answers for Review Questions, as well as discussion of Case Study and Critical Thinking Care Map questions, appear in Appendix IV.

Infection Control and Asepsis

SHARING experiences

I entered nursing as a career because I wanted to make a difference. [The people I care for] appreciate a smile and a caring heart when they are away from home and not feeling well. I often try to see myself through the [other person's] eyes, and approach my profession as a person who is there to assist someone who is not able to help themselves.

I feel most inspired by a sincere thank you. Even an unspoken one can be just as gratifying, as long as I can be a part of easing [their] discomfort, helping them cope with their fears, or ridding them of the pain.

Deborah Tovar, LVN, High Desert Medical Group, Lancaster, CA.

LEARNING outcomes

After completing this chapter, you will be able to:

- Discuss helpful and harmful actions of micoorganisms.
- Name six links in the chain of infection.
- State some risks of nosocomial infections.
- Explain the difference between nonspecific and specific defense systems of the body.
- State who is most at risk for developing an infection.
- List relevant nursing diagnoses for people who have an infection or are at risk of developing an infection.
- List measures that break links in the chain of infection.
- Explain the meaning of medical and surgical asepsis.
- Describe standard precautions and precautions for blood-borne pathogens.
- List different types of isolation precaution systems and demonstrate aseptic techniques including: hand washing, establishing and maintaining a sterile field, donning personal protective equipment, and donning and removing sterile gloves.

Infection control is a primary concern in nursing care. Nurses play an important role in establishing a biologically safe environment for their clients.

Microorganisms

Microorganisms are tiny living bodies that are visible only with a microscope. They are classified as bacteria, viruses, fungi, and parasites. Microorganisms are present in the environment and on body surfaces (such as the skin), in the intestinal tract, and any area open to the outside environment (e.g., mouth, upper respiratory tract, lower urinary tract, and vagina). Although we frequently refer to microorganisms as "germs," most are harmless and some are even helpful because they perform essential functions for the body.

TYPES OF MICROORGANISMS

Bacteria are the most common type of disease-causing microorganisms. They can live in and be transported through the air, water, food, soil, inanimate objects, and body tissues or fluids. **Viruses** are the smallest known disease-causing agent. They must enter living cells in order to reproduce. Viral infections are generally self-limiting (e.g., rhinovirus which causes the common cold). Others can result in serious illness or death (hepatitis, herpes, and human immunodeficiency virus [HIV]). **Fungi** are either yeasts or molds. Examples are the fungi that cause athlete's foot and yeast infections. **Parasites** live on other living organisms. Examples are protozoa (which cause malaria), helminths (worms), and arthropods (mites, ticks, and fleas).

Helpful Actions of Microorganisms

Resident flora (normal flora) are harmless microorganisms. They can be found in and on the body. Many of them perform useful protective functions. For example, intestinal flora help to synthesize vitamin K, which is important to the body's blood clotting mechanism. Various other microorganisms make antibiotic-like substances and toxic substances that slow or stop the growth of other organisms. The process of *colonization* occurs when strains of microorganisms become resident flora. Resident flora can grow in or on the body and not cause disease. However, if a person's defenses are weak, flora may invade a part of the body they normally would not, and cause illness. *Escherichia coli (E. coli)*, a normal resident flora of the intestinal tract, causes illness if transmitted elsewhere. (See Table 7-1 ◆ for some common resident organisms.)

Harmful Actions of Microorganisms

An **infection** is defined as an invasion of the body by a disease-causing organism called the *infectious agent*. Microorganisms that cause disease are called **pathogens**. A "true" pathogen causes disease or infection in a healthy person. An *opportunistic pathogen* causes a disease only in a susceptible person, that is, someone who has a poor defense system.

TABLE 7-1	EXAMPLES OF COMMON RESIDENT ORGANISMS
BODY AREA	**ORGANISMS**
Skin	*Staphylococcus epidermidis* *Propionibacterium acnes* *Staphylococcus aureus* *Corynebacterium xerosis* *Pityrosporum oxale* (yeast)
Nasal passages	*Staphylococcus aureus* *Staphylococcus epidermidis*
Oropharynx	*Streptococcus pneumoniae*
Bronchi, lungs	None
Mouth	*Streptococcus mutans* *Lactobacillus* *Bacteroides* *Actinomyces*
Stomach	None
Esophagus	None
Intestine	*Bacteroides* *Fusobacterium* *Eubacterium* *Lactobacillus* *Streptococcus* *Enterobacteriaceae* *Shigella* *Escherichia coli*
Urethral orifice	*Staphylococcus epidermidis*
Urethra (lower)	*Proteus*
Bladder, ureters, kidneys	None
Vagina	*Lactobacillus* *Bacteroides* *Clostridium* *Candida albicans*
Blood, lymph system	None

A **disease** occurs when the signs and symptoms of the infection are distinctive and the person's health is recognized as being different from the normal. Disease causes a detectable change in the way the body functions. In some cases, the microorganism will not cause any signs or symptoms of disease, and the infection is called *asymptomatic* or *subclinical*.

Various microorganisms are stronger than others and are called more *virulent*. **Virulence** refers to the organism's ability to produce disease. Microorganisms also differ in their strength and their communicability (how easily they can be spread). A **communicable disease** is one that is spread or transmitted by direct or indirect contact. The transmission of an organism can be caused by a **vector** or vehicle (an insect, or a used drinking glass, for instance). Microorganisms can also be airborne and carried by air currents.

 ## Controlling Microorganisms

CONTROLLING COMMUNICABLE DISEASES

Infectious diseases are the major cause of death throughout the world. They account for a significant threat to public health and for many deaths annually in the United States. The World Health Organization (WHO) works on the international level to protect people from communicable forms of disease. In the United States, the Centers for Disease Control and Prevention (CDC) is the main agency concerned with protecting the public from disease and controlling its spread on a national level. Health departments in states, counties, and cities follow epidemics and illnesses when hospitals, physicians, and other health care givers make reports.

 ## Infection

TYPES OF INFECTIONS

There are two types of infections: local and systemic. A **local infection** occurs when the microorganisms are in only a specific part of the body. A **systemic infection** exists when the microorganisms spread and begin to damage other body areas. The person has *bacteremia* if the microorganisms enter the blood stream. When bacteremia spreads through all of the body's systems, the condition is called **septicemia.**

Acute infections occur suddenly or last a short time. *Chronic infections* happen slowly over a long period of time and may last months or years.

Infections that occur as a result of health care delivery in a health care setting (such as a clinic or hospital) are called **nosocomial infections.**

A microorganism that comes from the client's own body and causes a nosocomial infection is referred to as being from an *endogenous* source. If the organism causing the infection comes from the health care environment or personnel, it is from an *exogenous* source. The three most common microorganisms causing exogenous infections are *E. coli, Staphylococcus aureus,* and *Enterococcus* species. (See Table 7-2 ◆.)

Many factors contribute to nosocomial infections. An infection directly caused by any diagnostic or therapeutic source is called an **iatrogenic infection.** An example of this would be bacteremia caused by an infected or contaminated intravenous (IV) site. Failure to perform appropriate hand hygiene is considered to be the leading cause of health-care-associated infections and spread of multi-resistant organ-

TABLE 7-2	NOSOCOMIAL INFECTIONS	
MOST COMMON ORGANISMS	**CAUSES**	
Urinary Tract *Escherichia coli* *Enterococcus* species *Pseudomonas aeruginosa*	Catheterization technique Contamination of closed drainage system Inadequate hand washing	
Surgical Sites *Staphylococcus aureus* *Enterococcus* species *Pseudomonas aeruginosa*	Inadequate hand washing Improper dressing change technique	
Bloodstream Coagulase-negative staphylococci *Staphylococcus aureus* *Enterococcus* species	Inadequate hand washing Improper intravenous fluid, tubing, and site care technique	
Pneumonia *Staphylococcus aureus* *Pseudomonas aeruginosa* *Enterobacter* species	Inadequate hand washing Improper suctionIng technique	

isms and has been recognized as a substantial contributor to outbreaks (CDC, 2002).

Clinical GuIdelines

Recommendations by the CDC for hand washing and hand antisepsis follow:

◆ When hands are visibly dirty or contaminated with proteinaceous material or are visibly soiled with blood or body fluids, wash hands with either a non-antimicrobial soap and water or an antimicrobial soap and water.

◆ If hands are not visibly soiled, use alcohol-based hand rub for routinely decontaminating hands in all other clinical situations.

◆ When decontaminating hands with an alcohol-based hand rub, apply product to palm of one hand and rub together, covering all surfaces of hands and fingers, until hands are dry (CDC, 2002).

See Procedure 7-1 for handwashing instructions.

Drug-Resistant Pathogens

In recent years a major concern with nosocomial infections has been resistant organisms. Three classifications of these are methicillin-resistant *Staphylococcus aureus* (MRSA), vancomycin-resistant *Enterococci* (VRE), and multi-drug-resistant tuberculosis (MDR TB). The overuse of anibiotics, as well as the tendency of clients not to complete a prescribed course of treatment, have produced resistant organisms. Hospitalized clients whose immune systems are already compromised are at the greatest risk. MRSA also can cause illness in persons outside the hospital and health care facilities. Cases in the community have been associated with recent antibiotic use and sharing of contaminated items and living in crowded areas.

The practice of good hygiene and the responsible use of antibiotic therapy are the best ways to prevent public health problems and life-threatening infections.

CHAIN OF INFECTION

The chain of infection is made up of six links (Figure 7-1 ◆): microorganism, reservoir, portal of exit, mode of transmission, portal of entry, and susceptibility of the host.

Agent

The first link in the chain of infection is the infectious *(etiologic) agent*. Several factors affect whether or not a microorganism invades the body and causes an infection. These factors include the number of organisms present, how virulent or potent they are, and whether the organisms can live in the host's body. Some organisms, such as smallpox, infect almost all of the people who are exposed to it. Others, like the tuberculosis bacillus, infect only a small percentage of people who are exposed and susceptible. Some organisms live in a **carrier,** which is a person or animal that has the microorganism living inside of them. The carrier doesn't have any signs or symptoms but is a potential source of infection for others. In some diseases the individual is a temporary carrier during the incubation period, the convalescence or recovery time, or the

postconvalescent period. These carriers are called *incubatory* or *convalescent carriers*. In contrast, *chronic carriers* are in the carrier state for long periods of time.

Reservoir

The second link in the chain of infection is the place where the microorganism naturally lives, its **reservoir.** The source, or reservoir, of the microorganism can be many different places: the person him- or herself, other humans, animals, plants, insects, birds, or the environment. Food, water, milk, or anything that can be ingested could also be considered a reservoir (see Table 7-3 ◆). The more a person's resistance is lowered, the more susceptible the person becomes and the more easily he or she will be infected from the reservoir of microorganisms.

Portal of Exit from the Reservoir

The third link in the chain is the *portal of exit,* a way of leaving the reservoir. The microorganism must leave the reservoir in order to spread the infection. Any body fluid can provide an exit from the source. Wound drainage, blood, urine, feces, mucus, or any break in the skin or mucus membrane can all provide a portal of exit.

Methods or Modes of Transmission

The fourth link in the chain of infection is a **method, or mode, of transmission.** It is the manner in which the microorganism gets to the host. There are three modes of transmission. The first is direct transmission. This occurs immediately when the infected person touches, bites, kisses, or has sexual intercourse with another. Direct transmission (as in sneezing, coughing, or spitting) also occurs through droplet spread if the source and the host are within three feet of each other. Droplet sprays can enter through the conjunctiva and the mucus membranes of the eye, or through the nose or mouth of a susceptible person.

The second method is indirect transmission. This form of transmission requires a vector or vehicle to carry the microorganism to the host. *Vector-borne transmission* could occur when an animal or insect bites or injects the microorganism through saliva into the host, or leaves feces or other material on the host's traumatized skin. *Vehicle-borne transmission* occurs when infectious material is introduced into the host though a portal of entry by way of a substance. Water, food, blood products, or contact with a *fomite* (an inanimate object such as a toy, cooking or eating utensil, or contaminated instrument) are all examples of vehicle-borne transmission. When a person eats poorly cooked chicken contaminated with the *Salmonella* species and becomes ill, the microorganism was transmitted by a vehicle.

The third method of transmission is airborne transmission. This usually involves droplet nuclei, the remains of droplets coming from an infected person. An example is when someone infected with tuberculosis coughs. The organism goes into the air, and another individual then inhales it into his or her lungs. Dust particles can also carry infectious spores,

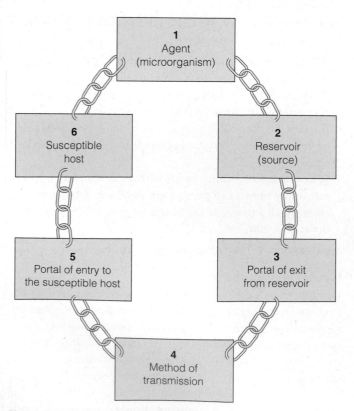

Figure 7-1. ◆ The chain of infection.

TABLE 7-3	HUMAN RESERVOIRS, COMMON INFECTIOUS MICROORGANISMS, AND PORTALS OF EXIT	
BODY AREA (SOURCE)	**COMMON INFECTIOUS ORGANISMS**	**PORTALS OF EXIT**
Respiratory tract	Parainfluenza virus *Mycobacterium tuberculosis* *Staphylococcus aureus*	Nose or mouth through sneezing, coughing, breathing, or talking; endotracheal tubes or tracheostomies
Gastrointestinal tract	Hepatitis A virus *Salmonella* species	Mouth: saliva, vomitus; anus: feces; ostomies: drainage tubes (e.g., nasogastric or T-tubes)
Urinary tract	*Escherichia coli* enterococci *Pseudomonas aeruginosa*	Urethral meatus and urinary diversion ostomies
Reproductive tract (including genitals)	*Neisseria gonorrhoeae* *Treponema pallidum* Herpes simplex virus type 2 Hepatitis B virus	Vagina: vaginal discharge; urinary meatus: semen, urine
Blood	Hepatitis B virus (HBV) Human immunodeficiency virus (HIV) *Staphylococcus aureus* *Staphylococcus epidermidis*	Open wound, needle puncture site, any disruption of intact skin or mucous membrane surfaces
Tissue	*Staphylococcus aureus* *Escherichia coli* *Proteus* species *Streptococcus* beta-hemolytic A or B	Drainage from cut or wound

viruses, and bacteria. Microorganisms can be inhaled into the lungs when dust is disturbed and becomes airborne.

Portal of Entry

The fifth link in the chain of infection is a *portal of entry* into the host. Intact skin can be a barrier to any infectious microorganism. However, broken skin provides an easy portal of entry for a pathogen. Most microorganisms enter the body through the same routes they use to leave it. For example, an organism that was inhaled into the lungs can be then coughed out to infect someone else.

Susceptible Host

The sixth link in the chain of infection is the *susceptibility of the host*. The body provides natural defenses to fight off infection. Any individual who has difficulty combating microorganisms and is at risk for developing an infection is called a **susceptible host**. A *compromised host* is someone who has a higher risk for getting an infection, for one or more reasons. An example would be a geriatric client with emphysema; this person is at a higher risk for developing pneumonia than someone of the same age without emphysema.

FACTORS THAT INCREASE SUSCEPTIBILITY TO INFECTION

Age is a factor influencing the risk of infection. Both the very young and the elderly have reduced defenses. Newborns have immature immune systems and are protected for only the first

2 or 3 months by immunities they received from their mother. Immunizations against communicable diseases are started at about 2 months of age, when the infant's immune system can respond.

The immune system becomes weak in the elderly, and as they age they develop infections more easily. The CDC recommends annual immunizations for them against influenza and pneumonia, particularly if they have histories of cardiac, renal, respiratory, or metabolic diseases.

Heredity may also influence the development of infections. People may have a genetic susceptibility to them.

Stressors in life can influence susceptibility to infection. Stressors can be physical, emotional, or both. The nature, number, and duration of the stressors may all influence whether or not the individual develops an infection. Stressors elevate blood cortisol, and prolonged elevation decreases anti-inflammatory responses; drains energy stores, causing exhaustion; and decreases resistance to infection.

Nutrition plays a role in resistance to infection. Good nutrition provides ample proteins, which allow the body to manufacture antibodies. Medical therapies may contribute to the development of infection. Radiation treatments for cancer and diagnostic procedures that penetrate the skin or sterile body cavities are examples of procedures that increase infection risk.

Medications can increase the chance of infection if they depress bone marrow production of white blood cells (leukocytes). Also, corticosteroids (steroids) slow down the inflammatory response needed to fight infection. Antibiotics may kill not only infectious organisms but also the resident flora. This would allow other strains, which would not normally grow, to multiply. Some microorganisms may become resistant to certain medications, making them more difficult to overcome.

Other diseases (*pathologies*) that lessen the body's defense system increase the risk for infection. Some examples are pulmonary diseases (emphysema, asthma), burns, peripheral vascular diseases, diseases of the blood, and diabetes mellitus.

NONSPECIFIC DEFENSES

The body has normal defenses to protect it against infection. **Nonspecific defenses** include anatomic and physiologic barriers and the inflammatory response.

◆ Intact skin protects against bacteria. Fungi can live on the skin but cannot penetrate it. Resident flora (bacteria) on the skin stop other bacteria from growing. The skin's slight acidity also inhibits bacterial growth.
◆ Moist mucous membranes and cilia in the nose trap microorganisms, dust, and foreign materials.
◆ Special cells in the lungs (called macrophages or phagocytes) ingest microorganisms and foreign particles.
◆ Saliva in the mouth helps to prevent infection by its washing action.
◆ Tears (which have an enzyme in them) wash away organisms and protect the eyes.
◆ Stomach acids protect the stomach from infection. Resident flora in the large intestine stop the growth of other microorganisms.
◆ Vaginal secretions have a pH that stops the growth of many disease-producing bacteria.
◆ The flow of urine flushes the urethra and keeps bacteria from entering the bladder.

Inflammatory Response

The **inflammatory response** is a local nonspecific defense reaction of tissues when they are exposed to infection or injury. The inflammatory response destroys or dilutes microorganisms and prevents their spread. There are five primary signs of inflammation: pain, swelling, redness, heat, and (if there is severe injury) weakened function of a body part. Inflammation of a part is indicated by the suffix *-itis*. For example, appendicitis is inflammation of the appendix.

There are three stages to the inflammatory response:

◆ *First stage: Vascular and cellular response.* During the cellular and vascular response, blood vessels first constrict at the site of injury. This is quickly followed by dilation of small vessels in the area, which causes increased blood flow and redness (*hyperemia*) with increased warmth. Fluid enters the interstitial space, causing edema and irritation to the nerve endings and producing pain. Blood flow eventually slows down in the capillaries, and *leukocytes* (white blood cells) move out of them into the tissues to work against the microorganisms.

◆ *Second stage: Exudate production.* The exudate consists of dead phagocytic cells (cells that attacked the microorganism). During this stage the microorganisms are killed. The exudate is removed when it drains into the lymphatic system channels or leaves the body as drainage. The major types of exudates are: serous, purulent, and hemorrhagic (sanguineous). (See types of cultures in Chapters 16, 18, 19, and 22. ⬗)
◆ *Third stage: reparative phase.* In the reparative phase, the tissues regenerate cells that are similar or identical in structure and function to the dead cells. Some tissues (like skin) regenerate well; others (like nerve tissue) regenerate little if at all. The sequence of repair of damaged tissue is discussed in detail in Chapter 12. ⬗

SPECIFIC OR IMMUNE DEFENSES

Specific defenses are also known as *immune* defenses. They work against identified foreign proteins such as bacteria, fungi, viruses, and other infectious agents, which are considered to be invading agents and are called **antigens.**

The resistance of the body to infection is known as **immunity** (see Table 7-4 ◆). In *active immunity* the body produces its own antibodies to natural antigens (e.g., infection), or artificial antigens (e.g., vaccines). During *passive immunity* the person receives natural antibodies (e.g., from a nursing mother) or artificial antibodies (e.g., from an injection of immune serum) produced from another source. Two systems are working and overlapping during the immune response.

Antibody-Mediated Defense

The *antibody-mediated defense* (also called circulating or *humoral* immunity) defense depends primarily on the B lymphocytes. They are mediated by antibodies produced from B cells, which flow through the blood stream. These antibodies are also called *immunoglobulins (Ig)* and are part of the body's plasma proteins. The B cells are activated and attack when they recognize a foreign invader. Their response makes five different classes of antibody molecules: IgM, IgG, IgA, IgD, and IgE. If IgM is found, it means there is a current infection. If IgG antibodies are present, it means there was a past infection with the development of immunity.

Cell-Mediated Defense

The *cell-mediated defense* acts through the T-cell system. When there is exposure to an antigen, the lymphoid tissue produces and releases large numbers of T cells into the lymphatic fluid and system. If T-cell immunity is lost, people cannot defend themselves against most viral, bacterial, and fungal infections. An example of depressed T-cell function is human immunodeficiency virus (HIV) infection.

CONTROLLING MICROORGANISMS IN THE ENVIRONMENT

Maintaining a clean environment helps to inhibit the growth and multiplication of organisms. The very process of cleaning

TABLE 7-4

TYPES OF ACQUIRED IMMUNITY

TYPE	ANTIGEN OR ANTIBODY SOURCE	DURATION
Active	Antibodies are produced by the body in response to an antigen.	Long
Natural	Antibodies are formed in the presence of active infection in the body.	Lifelong
Artificial	Antigens (vaccines or toxoids) are administered to stimulate antibody production.	Many years: the immunity must be reinforced by booster inoculations
Passive	Antibodies are produced by another source, animal or human.	Short
Natural	Antibodies are transferred naturally from an immune mother to her baby through the placenta or in colostrum.	6 months to 1 year
Artificial	Immune serum (antibody) from an animal or another human is injected.	2 to 3 weeks

slows down the growth of microorganisms. **Antiseptics** (agents that inhibit the growth of some microorganisms) and **disinfectants** (agents that destroy pathogens other than spores) help to keep control of the environment.

Disinfecting requires the use of a disinfectant solution or spray that contains a chemical preparation, such as phenol or iodine compounds. These substances should not be used on tissue since they are often caustic or toxic. Both antiseptics (which can be used on tissue) and disinfectants have bactericidal and/or bacteriostatic properties. A **bactericidal agent** destroys bacteria, while a **bacteriostatic agent** prevents growth and reproduction of only some bacteria. Ultraviolet light is a type of nonionizing radiation that can be used to disinfect. However, its rays do not penetrate deeply. Important points to remember when disinfecting are listed in Box 7-1 ◆. Using boiling water for a minimum of 15 minutes is a good method for the home setting, although many spores and viruses are not destroyed by this method.

Sterilizing destroys all microorganisms, viruses, and spores. Moist heat (steam) can be used under pressure or as a free agent to sterilize. Autoclaves provide steam under pressure, with temperatures ranging from 121 to 123°C (250 to 254°F) and 15 to 17 lbs of pressure. Free steam at 100°C (212°F) must be used for at least 30 minutes for 3 consecutive days. Gas sterilization is effective for heat-sensitive items. An example is ethylene oxide gas. However, it may be toxic to humans and should be used with caution. Radiation can also be employed in sterilization. Ionizing radiation is often used for foods and drugs that are sensitive to heat, although it is a very costly process.

USING ASEPSIS

Asepsis is the absence of disease-causing microorganisms. **Sepsis** is the opposite, the presence of infection. It can take many forms in the human body. **Aseptic technique** is used to prevent the possibility of transferring microorganisms from one place or person to another.

Medical Asepsis

Medical asepsis includes all practices that are used to confine a specific microorganism to a specific area, or to limit the number of microorganisms, their growth, and their transmission. Objects are referred to as clean or dirty in medical asepsis. *Clean* means the absence of almost all microorganisms. *Dirty* (soiled or contaminated) means there are microorganisms present that may cause an infection.

Surgical Asepsis

Surgical asepsis is also called *sterile technique,* and it means every practice that keeps an object or an area completely free of microorganisms and spores. When dealing with sterile areas of the body, only surgical asepsis should be used.

BOX 7-1
NURSING CARE CHECKLIST

USING BACTERICIDAL AND BACTERIOSTATIC AGENTS

When disinfecting, remember to:

☑ Use the recommended concentration of the solution and keep it on the area for the required amount of time.

☑ Know the type and number of infectious organisms. Make certain no soap is present on the item since some disinfectants will not work when soap is present.

☑ Keep the room temperature within a normal range since some disinfectants will not work otherwise.

☑ Be certain there is no organic material (e.g., blood, pus, excretions) present because the disinfectants may be inactivated.

☑ Treat all exposed surface areas and crevices.

PROTECTIVE PRECAUTIONS

Many infection control measures are used in institutions to prevent the spread of microorganisms. Standard Precautions (Figure 7-2 ◆) are practiced in all health care facilities. They are precautions referring to all body fluids, especially those associated with bloodborne pathogens (e.g., hepatitis B and C, and HIV infections). In 1996, the CDC presented new guidelines for isolation precautions that included two levels: Tier 1 or Standard Precautions, and Tier 2 or Transmission-Based Precautions.

Figure 7-2. ◆ Standard Precautions for infection control. *Source:* Courtesy of BREVIS Corporation.

Standard Precautions

Standard Precautions are used in the care of all clients. They are applied to all body fluids, blood, secretions, excretions (except sweat), mucous membranes, and nonintact skin.

Transmission-Based Precautions

Transmission-Based Precautions are used in addition to Standard Precautions for any client with known or suspected infections that are spread by airborne or droplet transmission or by physical contact. Airborne nuclei are those agents smaller than 5 microns (e.g., tuberculosis, measles, varicella). Droplets are particles larger than 5 microns (e.g., diphtheria, streptococcal pharyngitis, mumps, pneumonia). Contact transmission occurs by touching items in the client's environment that are contaminated.

ISOLATION PRACTICES. Isolation practices are initiated after assessing the client's condition. Institutional policies, nursing assessment, and laboratory study results are used to make the decision to place an individual in an isolated environment. Other factors that must be considered are the status of the client's defense mechanisms, the source of the infection, and its mode of transmission.

TRANSPORTING CLIENTS WITH INFECTIONS. Clients with infections are not transported outside of their own rooms unless absolutely necessary. If they need to be moved to another area, the environment must be protected to avoid contamination of it and others. The client should wear a mask if the infection is airborne, and all draining wounds should be covered with dressings that will not leak. The area the client is going to should be advised of the infectious condition so that they can take precautions and maintain the environment. The client should wear clean clothing, so as not to contaminate wheelchairs or transportation carts.

COLLABORATIVE CARE

Laboratory Tests

Some laboratory work with abnormal values indicates infection. Elevated white blood cell counts with changes in specific types of cells are seen on the differential count. Neutrophils increase with bacterial infections. Lymphocytes are elevated with viral infections. The erythrocyte sedimentation rate (ESR) increases with the inflammatory response. Cultures of body fluids and any drainage can identify specific infectious organisms.

Equipment

PERSONAL PROTECTIVE EQUIPMENT. Particular items are used to protect the personnel and the client when administering care. They include gloves, gowns, and masks.

Gloves are used to protect the nurse's hands from coming in contact with body fluids and contaminated items. They also protect the client from the nurse's microorganisms.

Gloves reduce the transmission of microorganisms from one client to another, or to any object (*fomite*) where they might grow. Hands are washed before and after wearing gloves.

For many activities, only clean gloves are worn, and no special technique is used to put them on. Sterile gloves are worn if the nurse works with a wound or when the nurse's hands enter a body orifice. A specific technique is used to apply and to remove sterile gloves (Procedure 7-2). If a gown is worn, the cuff of the glove is pulled over the gown's sleeve (Figure 7-3 ◆).

Gowns are used only once before being either discarded or laundered. Gowns should be water resistant and clean. Sterile gowns are used in surgery and in cases of reverse isolation (wherein the client is protected from organisms carried by the staff) or when the nurse is changing dressings on extensive wounds (e.g., burns). No special technique is used to put on a clean gown or to take it off if it is not visibly soiled. If there is a large amount of contamination, the nurse should avoid touching the area and roll the gown up with the soiled area inside. The gown is then disposed of in the proper container. Sterile gowns are grasped at the crease near the neck and held away from the body. They are allowed to unfold without touching anything. If the gown's outer surface does touch something, it is contaminated. The nurse's hands are put into the shoulders and sleeves without touching the outside of the gown. The hands can be put through the cuff if using the open method of sterile gloving. A coworker will tie the gown at the

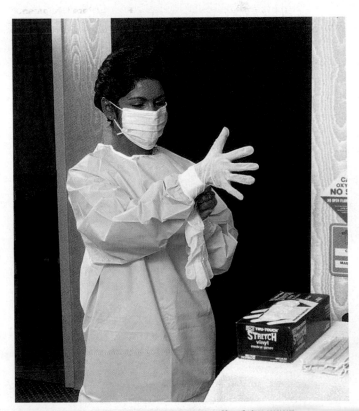

Figure 7-3. ◆ Pull gloves up over the cuffs of the gown.

neck and at the back without touching the outside surface (Procedure 7-3).

Face masks are worn to stop the spread of microorganism and airborne droplets from either the nurse to the client, or the client to the nurse. They also protect against splatters from body fluids. Many face masks now have transparent protective eye coverings for protection. Otherwise, protective glasses or goggles should be worn if there is a possibility of body fluid splatters. The CDC recommends those close to the client should wear masks if the infection is transmitted by large particle droplets, or by all persons entering the room if the infection is transmitted by small particle or droplet nuclei. Masks should be disposable and worn only once. They should be replaced if they become wet or soiled. They are to be disposed of in the appropriate waste container.

Particulate respirators are also used to protect against droplet transmission. Some are disposable. There are many different types on the market. The CDC recommends those with a rating of N95, which means a category N respirator that has 95% efficiency and meets the tuberculosis control criteria.

When removing soiled protective equipment, remove the gloves first (if the gown is tied in the front, undo the ties before removing the gloves). After removing the gloves, remove the mask, holding it by the strings. Remove the gown next. Finally, remove any eyewear. Wash the hands and wrists thoroughly.

CLEANING REUSABLE EQUIPMENT. Washing items to remove any organic material is important. Cold water rinses should be done first, because hot water coagulates the protein of organic material and causes it to stick to items. Then wash items in hot water with soap to emulsify and dislodge dirt. Abrasive action with stiff-bristled brushes will help to remove material from crevices in equipment. Rinse articles with warm to hot water and dry thoroughly. Items are now considered clean. However, the process is not complete until the basin or sink and any brushes or tools used for cleaning the items are also cleaned with a disinfectant.

DISPOSAL OF USED OR SOILED EQUIPMENT FROM AN ISOLATION ROOM. Most facilities have policies and procedures in place that state specifically how to dispose of equipment and supplies that have been contaminated. Be familiar with these policies! Materials may be disposed of, cleaned, disinfected, or sterilized. Some equipment and supplies are for single use only. Other materials are meant to be used multiple times.

Bagging is a technique recommended by the CDC for removal of materials from a client's room. The purpose is to prevent exposure from items contaminated with body secretions. The bag must be impervious to microorganisms. The bags may come in colors (e.g., red) and have labels that indicate they contain infectious materials.

The CDC recommends placing contaminated disposable items in the plastic bags that line the waste containers. Nondisposable or reusable items should be put into a labeled bag before being removed from the client's room and sent to a central processing area for decontamination. Rubber, plastic, metal, and glass items may be bagged separately. (Metal and glass can be autoclaved, but rubber and plastic need to be exposed to gas sterilization.)

Special procedure trays should be disassembled and bagged as indicated above. Soiled linens or clothing should be bagged and sent to the facility laundry or home. Linens should be handled as little as possible. They should be rolled into a bundle before being placed in the bag (do not shake the linens). Laboratory specimens should be put into a leakproof container. If the container is contaminated on the outside, it should be put in a plastic bag before it is sent to the laboratory. Dishes are often made of paper and are disposed of in the refuse container. Blood pressure equipment, if kept in the room, needs no special precautions. If it becomes contaminated, follow the agency's cleaning procedures. Nondisposable thermometers should be disinfected after use according to agency protocols. Needles, syringes, and "sharps" should be placed in a puncture-resistant container kept in the room (see Chapter 21). Clients' personal objects (such as toys) that are contaminated should be bagged and sent home for cleaning.

NURSING CARE

◆ ASSESSING

The client history is one of the most important parts of the assessment. Among the many facts it presents, it tells you the background of all the symptoms and what the client has done to cope with the problem. The nursing history allows the nurse to assess the client's degree of risk for developing an infection and symptoms that suggest the presence of an infection. Along with reviewing the chart, the nurse will interview the client in order to collect objective data that are significant. Such data would include anything that might influence the development of an infection, history of recurring infections, immunization history, nutritional status, emotional stressors, and current medications and/or therapeutic measures.

Subjective data can be obtained from clients when they are asked about any symptoms they have experienced that may indicate infection. These include headache, lethargy, nausea or vomiting, and pain.

Along with data already collected, the nurse looks for signs and symptoms of infection associated with specific body systems. Sneezing or watery, discolored discharge from the nose suggests sinus infection. Cloudy urine may indicate bladder infection. Vital signs also show changes, such as increased temperature, pulse, and respirations. Other observations may include anorexia and lymph node enlargement.

DIAGNOSING, PLANNING, and IMPLEMENTING

The primary nursing diagnosis for the transmission of pathologic microorganisms is *Risk for Infection*. Some of the specific risk factors include: traumatized or broken skin, stasis of body fluids, altered peristalsis, change in pH of secretions, decreased ciliary action, and wound contamination. Contributing factors to the nursing diagnosis include immunosuppression, anemia, and suppressed inflammatory response.

Other contributing nursing diagnoses that may result from the infection are: impaired physical mobility, altered nutrition, pain due to tissue damage, fever related to infection, fluid and electrolyte imbalances, anxiety, low self-esteem, and impaired social interaction.

Nursing goals in the planning stage of the nursing process include:

- Restoring and maintaining body defenses against infection
- Preventing the spread of infection and its complications
- Maintaining hydration to prevent fluid and electrolyte imbalances

To achieve these goals, nursing care must include thorough aseptic technique, supporting the host's defenses, client teaching that emphasizes protective measures to prevent infections and their spread, and appropriate hydration measures. Some common nursing interventions for the client at risk for infection include:

- Help the client as necessary with routine hygiene (including oral hygiene) and skin care. *Practicing consistent and good hygiene reduces the numbers of microorganisms. Maintaining intact skin prevents the possibility of infection.*
- Appropriately dispose of, or change, any clothing or linens, bandages, or dressing whenever they become soiled or wet. *Microorganisms grow easily and live in soiled or wet cloth.*
- Dispose of feces and urine appropriately. *Human waste contains many microorganisms that can cause infection or transfer bacteria and viruses to others.*
- Cover all containers of fluid (e.g., water bottles) at the client's bedside. *Uncapped containers holding liquids increase the risk of contamination and microbial growth.*
- Empty all drainage containers (e.g., suction bottles, catheter bags) before they become full, and at the end of each nursing shift, or according to agency policy. Hold containers steady and level to prevent spillage. *Body fluids and drainage contain microorganisms that grow and increase in numbers and can potentially be transmitted to others.*
- When giving care, avoid reaching over, talking, sneezing, or coughing across open wounds. Also, cover the mouth and nose when coughing or sneezing. *This limits the number of microorganisms falling from the caregiver's skin or escaping from the respiratory tract and prevents contamination of the wound.*
- Start all client care using aseptic precautions. *Anyone may have infectious microorganisms that can potentially be transmitted to others.*
- Wash hands before and after any client contact. *Correct hand washing controls and prevents the spread and transmission of microorganisms.*
- Wear masks and eye protection when caring for clients who have infections transmitted by droplets from the respiratory tract, or when sprays of body fluid may occur (e.g., during wound irrigations). *Masks and eye protection reduce the spread of microorganisms from droplet and body substance contamination.*
- Wear gloves (and gowns if there is a possibility of soiling clothing) when handling any secretions or excretions from the client. *Gloves and gowns prevent contamination with microorganisms by contact.*
- Provide every client with his or her own individual hygiene and personal care items. *This prevents cross contamination of microorganisms from others.*
- Use sterile technique for all invasive procedures (e.g., injections, catheterizations, suctioning) and for open wounds. *When the body's natural defense mechanisms (e.g., skin, body cavities) are penetrated, the barriers to microorganisms are broken.*
- Only use appropriate puncture-proof containers for all used needles, knife blades, and syringes. *Infectious diseases can be transmitted to health care workers and others by puncture injuries from contaminated needles, blades, and syringes.*
- Provide a balanced diet for the client. *A well-balanced diet provides all the nutrients needed to maintain and build body tissues.*(See Chapter 17.)

Practicing Sterile Technique

Many client care procedures require the use of sterile technique. Objects are only sterile when free of all microorganisms. When practicing sterile technique, the basic principles of surgical asepsis are used.

A **sterile field** is a microorganism-free area. Nurses use sterile drapes and the inside of sterile wrappers to create the sterile field (Procedure 7-4). Some general concepts to keep in mind when creating and working with a sterile field are listed in Box 7-2 ◆.

◆ EVALUATING

During the evaluation process, the nurse reviews both positive and negative outcomes of the care and instructions given to the client. Revisions in care are made as needed until the desired result is achieved. Examples of positive outcomes and obtaining stated goals in client care are:

BOX 7-2
NURSING CARE CHECKLIST

CREATING AND MAINTAINING A STERILE FIELD

☑ Wear sterile gloves to work with the equipment on the field, or use sterile forceps to move items around on it.

☑ Never reach across a sterile field once it is established. (Microorganisms can be dropped on it and cause contamination.)

☑ If the field becomes wet, it is considered contaminated.

☑ If an unsterile object touches a sterile object, it is then contaminated.

☑ The edges of the sterile field are considered unsterile.

☑ If an object is below the nurse's waist level or is out of sight, it is considered unsterile.

☑ If objects must be left open to the air for a prolonged period of time, cover the sterile field with sterile drapes to prevent contamination by airborne microorganisms.

☑ Nursing qualities that are essential in maintaining a sterile field are alertness, honesty, and conscientiousness.

☑ Follow the old adage: "If there is any doubt about sterility, the object or field is unsterile."

- All dressings are kept dry and are changed when they are soiled or become wet.
- The client eats a well-balanced diet and has adequate fluid intake in order to maintain nutrition and hydration.
- Clients participate in self-care to the degree possible, and good hygiene is maintained.
- All contaminated equipment and linens are disposed of appropriately and according to agency standards.
- All containers holding human waste or drainage are disposed of appropriately.
- All materials used for invasive procedures (e.g., needles, syringes, catheters) are disposed of safely.

◆ DISCHARGE CONSIDERATIONS

Education is an important aspect of the nurse's role in treating a client with an infection or potential for infection. Some appropriate points follow:

- Teach clients and their significant others why articles must be clean, disinfected, or sterilized.
- Teach clients and significant others to wash their hands before eating or handling food, after toileting, or after handling any infectious materials.

- Educate or remind clients and significant others about the importance of immunizations and booster shots.

Clients and support people must often provide home care of a person with an infectious disease or partially healed wound. The following instructions can be useful:

- Wash hands carefully before and after any hands-on care.
- Keep fingernails clean, short, and well-trimmed.
- If there is no running water, use commercially available hand-washing agents that require no water.
- Use bactericidal soap and paper towels when washing hands.
- Teach young children hand washing as soon as they can participate.
- Keep pets out of the area when setting up for and performing sterile procedures.
- Clean and wipe dry a flat surface for the sterile field.
- Dispose of all soiled materials in a waterproof bag. Check with the home care nurse as to how to dispose of medical refuse.

Nursing Process Case Study:
CLIENT WITH RESPIRATORY INFECTION

Mrs. Chase is a 76-year-old woman who has a 10-year history of emphysema. She has a history of smoking a pack a day for 25 years, and continues to do so. Recently, she began coughing much more frequently and expectorating larger volumes of colored mucus. She was admitted to the hospital with complaints of fatigue, coughing, a poor appetite, and a fever with chills. She is sitting on the edge of the bed, coughing, with her hand pressing against her chest. There are used tissues scattered all over the bed.

Assessment Vital signs: BP 146/88, P 90, R 22 and shallow, T 101.4° F, pain 4/10 in the chest while coughing and less between episodes. Weight is 108 lbs. Height 5′6″. The client's skin is hot, flushed, and dry. Skin turgor is fair. She is alert and oriented, but restless and anxious. She coughs frequently and expectorates moderate amounts of thick, yellow–green–tinged mucus. She has a barrel chest, and on auscultation slight wheezes are heard in both lungs. Nail beds show slight cyanosis. Specimens of blood and sputum had already been collected. The white blood cell count (WBC) is elevated. The sputum specimen shows a streptococcal upper respiratory tract infection. The chest x-ray shows bilateral pneumonia. Mrs. Chase states she had been caring for her young grandchild who had a "strep throat."

Diagnosis The following priority nursing diagnoses are established for Mrs. Chase:

- Risk for Infection due to decreased ciliary action in lungs.

- Deficient Fluid Volume related to high fever and poor appetite.
- Impaired Gas Exchange related to rapid respirations, copious secretions, alveolar destruction, and air trapping.
- Ineffective Airway Clearance related to increased secretions and a weak cough.
- Deficient Knowledge related to infectious process and status of compromised host.

Expected Outcomes The expected outcomes for the plan of care are that Mrs. Chase will:

- Regain prior lung function.
- Maintain adequate hydration and circulating blood volume.
- Improve gas exchange as demonstrated by respirations within normal limits, normal pulse, and blood gases.
- Maintain a patent airway with decreased volume of secretions.
- Understand and be able to verbalize the process of contamination, susceptibility to infection, and how to prevent spread of organisms.

Planning and Implementation The following nursing interventions are implemented for Mrs. Chase. Ongoing assessments are done to monitor her condition.

- Monitor character of respirations including rate and rhythm, blood gases, and skin color every 2 to 4 hours.
- Auscultate breath sounds. Encourage deep breathing and coughing.
- Monitor vital signs q4h and intake and output q shift.
- Encourage fluids. Find out what liquids she likes and offer her 8 ounces of preferred fluid every hour.
- Have client deep breathe and cough q2h while awake. Position in semi-Fowler's or Fowler's position. Change client's position from back to sides often.

- Document volume of secretions as well as color and character. Request order for chest physiotherapy. Suction as necessary. See also Chapter 16.
- Administer medications (antibiotics, analgesics, expectorants, antitussives) on time.
- Teach Mrs. Chase to limit her exposure to others who are ill, because her history of emphysema and advanced age make her more susceptible to infection.
- Discuss hand-washing techniques, and emphasize that she should wash her hands after coughing or sneezing into them, and after handling objects used by other ill persons.
- Remind her to throw contaminated tissues into a waste container, to maintain a clean environment.

Evaluation At the end of the shift, Mrs. Chase's lung sounds were improved with less wheezing. Mucus was clear in color, thin, and "easier to cough out." The rate, rhythm, and character of her respirations were adequate. Her blood gases were within normal limits, and she showed no signs of cyanosis. Her temperature was 99.9°F and her pulse was 82. She was resting easily with her oxygen on. She was eating and taking fluids well with good urinary output.

Critical Thinking in the Nursing Process

1. Why was caring for her ill grandchild endangering Mrs. Chase's health?
2. What is the connection between the used tissues and the spread of infection?
3. Which of Mrs. Chase's assessment findings are consistent with a bacterial infection?

Note: The bibliography listings for this and all chapters have been compiled at the back of the book.

PROCEDURE 7-1

Hand Washing

PURPOSES

◆ To reduce the number of microorganisms on the hands
◆ To reduce the risk of transmission of microorganisms to clients
◆ To reduce the risk of cross-contamination among clients
◆ To reduce the risk of transmission of infectious organisms to oneself

EQUIPMENT

◆ Soap
◆ Warm running water
◆ Towels

INTERVENTIONS

1. Prepare and assess the hands.
   ◆ File the nails short. *Short nails are less likely to harbor microorganisms, scratch a client, or puncture gloves.*
   ◆ Remove all jewelry. Some nurses prefer to slide their watches up above their elbows. Others pin the watch to the uniform. *Microorganisms can lodge in the settings of jewelry and under rings. Removal facilitates proper cleaning.*
   ◆ Check hands for breaks in the skin, such as hangnails or cuts. Use lotions to prevent hangnails and cracked, dry skin. *A nurse who has broken skin areas may have to change work assignments or wear gloves for protection.*

2. Turn on the water and adjust the flow.
   ◆ There are five common types of faucet controls:
   a. Hand-operated handles.
   b. Knee levers. Move these with the knee to regulate flow and temperature (Figure 7-4 ◆).

c. Foot pedals. Press these with the foot to regulate flow and temperature (Figure 7-5 ◆).
d. Elbow controls. Move these with the elbows instead of the hands.
e. Infrared controls. The water runs when motion is detected at a preset distance.
   ◆ Adjust the flow so that the water is warm. Warm water removes less of the protective oil of the skin than hot water.

3. Wet the hands thoroughly by holding them under the running water, and apply soap to the hands.
   ◆ Hold the hands lower than the elbows so that the water flows from the arms to the fingertips. *The water should flow from the least contaminated to the most contaminated area; the hands are generally considered more contaminated than the lower arms.*
   ◆ Apply 2 to 4 mL (1 tsp) of liquid soap; rub it firmly between the hands.

Figure 7-4. ◆ A knee-lever faucet control. *Source: © Elena Dorfman.*

Figure 7-5. ◆ A foot-pedal faucet control. *Source: © Elena Dorfman.*

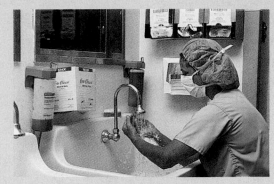

Figure 7-8. ◆ The hands are held higher than the elbows during a hand wash before sterile technique.

Figure 7-6. ◆ Interlacing the fingers during hand washing. *Source:* © Elena Dorfman.

4. Thoroughly wash and rinse the hands.
- ◆ Wash hands for a minimum of 10 seconds. For a more thorough washing, extend the time for wetting, washing, and rinsing.
- ◆ Use firm rubbing and circular movements to wash the palm, back, and wrist of each hand. Interlace the fingers and thumbs and move the hands back and forth (Figure 7-6 ◆), continuing the motion for 10 seconds. *The circular action helps remove microorganisms mechanically. Interlacing the fingers and thumbs cleans between the fingers.*
- ◆ Rinse the hands.

5. Thoroughly dry the hands and arms.
- ◆ Dry hands and arms thoroughly with a paper towel. *Moist skin becomes chapped readily; chapping produces lesions.*
- ◆ Discard the paper towel in the appropriate container.

6. Turn off the water.
- ◆ Use a dry paper towel to grasp a hand-operated control (Figure 7-7 ◆). *This prevents the nurse from picking up microorganisms from the faucet handles.*

VARIATION: HAND WASHING BEFORE STERILE TECHNIQUES

- ◆ Apply the soap and wash as described in step 4, but hold the hands higher than the elbows during this hand wash. Wet the hands and forearms under the running water, letting it run from the fingertips to the elbows so that the hands become cleaner than the elbows. (Figure 7-8 ◆). *In this way, the water runs from the area with the fewest microorganisms to areas with a relatively greater number.*
- ◆ Apply the soap and wash as described earlier in step 3, maintaining the hands uppermost.
- ◆ After washing and rinsing, use a towel to dry one hand thoroughly in a rotating motion from the fingers to the elbow. Use a clean towel to dry the other hand and arm. *A clean towel prevents the transfer of microorganisms from one elbow (least clean area) to the other hand (cleanest area).*

◆ SAMPLE DOCUMENTATION

10-30-2005	
0930	Handwashing done for 3 minutes per hospital protocol prior to clean dressing change. A Parsons, LVN

Figure 7-7. ◆ Using a paper towel to grasp the hand-operated faucet. *Source:* © Elena Dorfman.

PROCEDURE 7-2

Donning and Removing Sterile Gloves (Open Method)

PURPOSES

◆ To enable the nurse to handle sterile objects freely
◆ To prevent clients at risk (e.g., those with open wounds) from becoming infected by microorganisms on the nurse's hands

EQUIPMENT

◆ Package of sterile gloves

INTERVENTIONS

1. Open the package of sterile gloves.
  ◆ Place the package of gloves on a clean dry surface. *Any moisture on the surface could contaminate the gloves.*
  ◆ Some gloves are packed in an inner as well as an outer package. Open the outer package without contaminating the gloves or the inner package (see Procedure 7-3).
  ◆ Remove the inner package from the outer package.
  ◆ Open the inner package as in step 2 of Procedure 7-3 or according to the manufacturer's directions. *Some manufacturers provide a numbered sequence for opening the flaps and folded tabs to grasp for opening the flaps.* If no tabs are provided, pluck the flap so that the fingers do not touch the inner surfaces. *The inner surfaces, which are next to the sterile gloves, will remain sterile.*

2. Put the first glove on the dominant hand.
  ◆ If the gloves are packaged so that they lie side by side, grasp the glove for the dominant hand by its cuff (on the palmar side) with the thumb and first finger of the nondominant hand. Touch only the inside of the cuff (Figure 7-9 ◆). *The hands are not sterile. By touching only the inside of the glove, the nurse avoids contaminating the outside.*

Figure 7-9. ◆ Picking up the first sterile glove.

Figure 7-10. ◆ Putting on the first sterile glove.

or
If the gloves are packaged one on top of the other, grasp the cuff of the top glove as above, using the opposite hand.
  ◆ Insert the dominant hand into the glove and pull the glove on. Keep the thumb of the inserted hand against the palm of the hand during insertion (Figure 7-10 ◆). *If the thumb is kept against the palm, it is less likely to contaminate the outside of the glove.*
  ◆ Leave the cuff turned down.

3. Put the second glove on the nondominant hand.
  ◆ Pick up the other glove with the sterile gloved hand, inserting the gloved fingers under the cuff and holding the gloved thumb close to the gloved palm (Figure 7-11 ◆). *This helps prevent accidental contamination of the glove by the bare hand.*

Figure 7-11. ◆ Picking up the second sterile glove.

◆ Pull on the second glove carefully. Hold the thumb of the gloved first hand as far as possible from the palm (Figure 7-12 ◆). *In this position, the thumb is less likely to touch the arm and become contaminated.*

◆ Adjust each glove so that it fits smoothly, and carefully pull the cuffs up by sliding the fingers under the cuffs.

4. Remove and dispose of used gloves.

Figure 7-12. ◆ Putting on the second sterile glove.

◆ To remove sterile gloves that are soiled with secretions, hold the palmar surface below the cuff and turn it inside out. Insert fingers into the second glove, and turn it inside out while removing it (Figure 7-13 ◆).

◆ **SAMPLE DOCUMENTATION**

10-3-2004	
0700	Donned sterile gloves according to institutional protocol. Changed dressing. Wound pink, granulation tissue visible. P. Morgan, LVN

A

B

C

Figure 7-13. ◆ **A.** Plucking the palmar surface below the cuff of a contaminated glove **B.** Inserting fingers to remove the second contaminated glove. **C.** Holding contaminated gloves, which are inside out.

PROCEDURE 7-3
Donning Personal Protective Equipment

PURPOSES

◆ To enable the nurse to work close to a sterile field and handle sterile objects freely

◆ To protect clients from becoming contaminated with microorganisms on the nurse's hands, arms, and clothing

EQUIPMENT

◆ A sterile pack containing a sterile gown

◆ A package of sterile gloves

INTERVENTIONS

DONNING A STERILE GOWN

1. Open the package of sterile gloves.
   - ◆ Remove the outer wrap from the sterile gloves and leave the gloves in their inner sterile wrap on the sterile field. *If the inner wrapper is not touched, it will remain sterile.*
2. Unwrap the sterile gown pack.
3. Wash and dry hands carefully.
   See "Variation" at the end of Procedure 7-1 and review agency practice.
4. Put on the sterile gown.
   - ◆ Grasp the sterile gown at the crease near the neck, hold it away from you, and permit it to unfold freely without touching anything, including the uniform. *The gown will be unsterile if its outer surface touches any unsterile objects.*
   - ◆ Put the hands inside the shoulders of the gown, and work the arms partway into the sleeves without touching the outside of the gown (Figure 7-14 ◆).
   - ◆ If donning sterile gloves by using the closed method (*see below*), work the hands down the sleeves only to the proximal edge of the cuffs.
     or
     If donning sterile gloves by using the open method, work the hands down the sleeves and through the cuffs.
   - ◆ Have a co-worker wearing a hair cover and mask grasp the neck ties without touching the outside of the gown and pull the gown upward to cover the neckline of your uniform in front and back. The co-worker ties the neck ties. Gowning continues at step 4.

DONNING STERILE GLOVES (CLOSED METHOD)

1. Open the sterile wrapper containing the sterile gloves.
   - ◆ Open the sterile glove wrapper while the hands are still covered by the sleeves (Figure 7-15 ◆).
2. Put the glove on the nondominant hand. Figures 7-16 ◆ through 7-18 show a right-handed person.

Figure 7-15. ◆ Opening the sterile glove wrapper. *Source:* © Jenny Thomas.

   - ◆ With the dominant hand, pick up the opposite glove with the thumb and index finger, handling it through the sleeve.
   - ◆ Lay the glove on the opposite gown cuff, thumb side down, with the glove opening pointed toward the fingers (Figure 7-16 ◆). Position the dominant hand palm upward inside the sleeve.
   - ◆ Use the nondominant hand to grasp the cuff of the glove through the gown cuff, and firmly anchor it.
   - ◆ With the dominant hand working through its sleeve, grasp the upper side of the glove's cuff, and stretch it over the cuff of the gown. *This covers the nonsterile skin of the wrist and creates a solid sterile area from gloves to gown.*
   - ◆ Pull the sleeve up to draw the cuff over the wrist as you extend the fingers of the nondominant hand into the glove's fingers (Figure 7-17 ◆).
3. Put the glove on the dominant hand.
   - ◆ Place the fingers of the gloved hand under the cuff of the remaining glove.
   - ◆ Place the glove over the cuff of the second sleeve.
   - ◆ Extend the fingers into the glove as you pull the glove up over the cuff (Figure 7-18 ◆).
   Completion of Gowning
4. Complete gowning as follows:
   - ◆ Have a co-worker wearing a hair cover and mask hold the waist tie of your gown, using sterile gloves or a sterile forcep or drape. *This approach keeps the ties sterile.*

Figure 7-14. ◆ Putting on a sterile gown. *Source:* © Jenny Thomas.

Figure 7-16. ◆ Positioning the first sterile glove for the nondominant hand. *Source:* © Jenny Thomas.

◆ Make a three-quarter turn, then take the tie and secure it in front of the gown.
or
Have a co-worker wearing sterile gloves take the two ties at each side of the gown and tie them at the back of the gown, making sure that your uniform is completely covered. *Both methods ensure that the back of the gown remains sterile.*

◆ When worn, sterile gowns should be considered sterile in front from the waist to the shoulder. The sleeves should be considered sterile from 2 inches above the elbow to the cuff, since the arms of a scrubbed person must move across a sterile field. Moisture collection and friction areas such as the neckline, shoulders,

Figure 7-18. ◆ Extending the fingers into the second glove of the dominant hand. *Source:* © Jenny Thomas.

underarms, back, and sleeve cuffs should be considered unsterile.

Figure 7-17. ◆ Pulling on the first sterile glove. *Source:* © Jenny Thomas.

◆ **SAMPLE DOCUMENTATION**

10-31-2005	
0700	Prior to entering reverse isolation, sterile gown, gloves, and mask applied utilizing proper procedure, and according to institutional protocol. P. Morgan, LVN

PROCEDURE 7-4

Establishing and Maintaining a Sterile Field

PURPOSE

To maintain the sterility of supplies and equipment

EQUIPMENT

◆ Package containing a sterile drape
◆ Sterile equipment as needed (e.g., wrapped sterile gauze, wrapped sterile bowl, antiseptic solution, sterile forceps)

INTERVENTIONS

1. Confirm the sterility of the package.
   ◆ Ensure that the package is clean and dry. *If moist, it is considered contaminated and must be discarded.*
   ◆ Check the sterilization expiration dates on the package, and look for any indications that it has been previously opened

2. Open the package.

TO OPEN A WRAPPED PACKAGE ON A SURFACE
   ◆ Place the package in the center of the work area so that the top flap of the wrapper opens away from you. *This position prevents the nurse from subsequently reaching directly over the exposed sterile contents, which could contaminate them.*

Figure 7-19. ◆ Opening the first flap of a sterile wrapped package.

◆ Reaching around the package (not over it), pinch the first flap on the outside of the wrapper between the thumb and index finger (Figure 7-19 ◆). *Touching only the outside of the wrapper maintains the sterility of the inside of the wrapper.* Pull the flap open, laying it flat on the far surface.

◆ Repeat for the side flaps, opening the top one first. Use the right hand for the right flap, and the left hand for the left flap (Figure 7-20 ◆). *By using both hands, the nurse avoids reaching over the sterile contents.*

◆ Pull the fourth flap toward you by grasping the corner that is turned down (Figure 7-21 ◆). Make sure that the flap does not touch any object. *If the inner surface touches any unsterile article, it is contaminated.*

TO OPEN A WRAPPED PACKAGE WHILE HOLDING IT

◆ Hold the package in one hand with the top flap opening away from you.

Figure 7-20. ◆ Opening the second flap to the side.

Figure 7-21. ◆ Pulling the last flap toward oneself by grasping the corner.

◆ Using the other hand, open the package as described above, pulling the corners of the flaps well back and not reaching across the contents of the package (Figure 7-22 ◆). *The hands are considered contaminated, and at no time should they touch the contents of the package.*

TO OPEN COMMERCIALLY PREPARED PACKAGES

Commercially prepared sterile packages and containers usually have manufacturer's directions for opening.

◆ If the flap of the package has an unsealed corner, hold the container in one hand and pull back on the flap with the other hand (Figure 7-23 ◆).

◆ If the package has a partially sealed edge, grasp both sides of the edge, one with each hand, and pull apart gently.

3. Establish a sterile field by using a drape.

◆ Open the package containing the drape as described in step 2.

◆ With one hand, pluck the corner of the drape that is folded back on the top.

◆ Lift the drape out of the cover and allow it to open freely without touching any objects (Figure 7-24 ◆). *If the drape touches the outside of the package or any unsterile surface or object, it is considered contaminated.*

◆ Discard the cover.

Figure 7-22. ◆ Opening a wrapped package while holding it.

Figure 7-23. ◆ Opening a sterile package that has an unsealed corner. *Source:* © Elena Dorfman.

◆ With the other hand, carefully pick up another corner of the drape, holding it well away from yourself.
◆ Lay the drape on a clean and dry surface, placing the bottom (ie, the freely hanging side) farthest from you (Figure 7-25 ◆). *By placing the lowermost side farthest away, the nurse avoids leaning over the sterile field and contaminating it.*

4. Add necessary sterile supplies.

TO ADD WRAPPED SUPPLIES TO A STERILE FIELD
◆ Open each wrapped package as described in the preceding steps.
◆ With the free hand, grasp the corners of the wrapper and hold them against the wrist of the other hand (Figure 7-26 ◆). *The unsterile hand is now covered by the sterile wrapper.*
◆ Place the sterile bowl, drape, or other supply on the sterile field by approaching from an angle rather than holding the arm over the field.
◆ Discard the wrapper.

TO ADD COMMERCIALLY PACKAGED SUPPLIES TO A STERILE FIELD
◆ Open each package as previously described.
◆ Hold the package 15 cm (6 in) above the field and allow the contents to drop on the field (Figure 7-27 ◆). *Keep in*

Figure 7-25. ◆ Placing a drape on a surface.

Figure 7-26. ◆ Adding wrapped sterile supplies to a sterile field.

Figure 7-24. ◆ Allowing a drape to open freely without touching any objects.

Figure 7-27. ◆ Adding commercially packaged gauze to a sterile field.

mind that 2.5 cm (1 in.) around the edge of the field is considered contaminated. At a height of 15 cm (6 in), the outside of the package is not likely to touch and contaminate the sterile field.

TO ADD STERILE SOLUTION TO A STERILE BOWL

Sterile liquids (e.g., normal saline) frequently need to be poured into metal or nonabsorbent containers within a sterile field. *Unwrapped bottles or flasks that contain sterile solution are considered sterile on the inside and contaminated on the outside because the bottle may have been handled. Bottles used in an operating room may be sterilized on the outside as well as the inside, however, and these are handled with sterile gloves.*

◆ Before pouring any liquid, read the label three times to make sure you have the correct solution and concentration (strength).

◆ Obtain the exact amount of solution, if possible. *Once a sterile container has been opened, its sterility cannot be ensured for future use unless it is used again immediately.*

◆ Remove the lid or cap from the bottle and turn the lid upside down before placing it on a surface that is not sterile. *Inverting the lid keeps the inside surface sterile, because it is not allowed to touch an unsterile surface.*

◆ Hold the bottle at a slight angle so that the label is uppermost. *Any solution that flows down the outside of the bottle during pouring will not damage the label or make it unreadable.*

◆ Hold the bottle of fluid at a height of 10 to 15 cm (4 to 6 in) over the bowl and to the side of the sterile field so that as little of the bottle as possible is over the field. *At this height, there is less likelihood of contaminating the sterile field by touching the field or by reaching an arm over it.*

◆ Pour the solution gently to avoid splashing the liquid. *If the sterile drape is on an unsterile surface, moisture will contaminate the field by allowing the movement of microorganisms through the sterile drape.*

◆ Replace the lid securely on the bottle if you plan to use it again, and provide the date and time of opening according to agency policy. *Replacing the lid immediately maintains the sterility of the inner aspect of the lid and the solution. In many agencies a sterile container of solution that is opened is used only once and then discarded.*

5. Use sterile forceps to handle certain sterile supplies. Forceps are commonly used for such techniques as changing a sterile dressing and shortening a drain. Transfer forceps are usually used to move a sterile article from one place to another, for example, transferring sterile gauze from its package to a sterile dressing tray. Forceps may be discarded or resterilized after use. Commonly used forceps include hemostats, or artery forceps (Figure 7-28 ◆), and tissue forceps (Figure 7-29 ◆).

◆ Keep the tips of wet forceps lower than the wrist at all times, unless you are wearing sterile gloves (Figure 7-30 ◆). *Gravity prevents liquids on the tips of the forceps from flowing to the handles*

Figure 7-28. ◆ Hemostats. **A.** Curved. **B.** Straight.

Figure 7-29. ◆ Tissue forceps. **A.** Plain. **B.** Toothed.

Figure 7-30. ◆ Holding forceps with an ungloved hand, keeping the tips lower than the wrist.

and later back to the tips, thus making the forceps unsterile. The handles are unsterile once they are held by the bare hand.

◆ Hold sterile forceps above waist level. *Items held below waist level are considered contaminated.*

◆ Hold sterile forceps within sight. *While out of sight, forceps may, unknown to the user, become unsterile. Any forceps that go out of sight should be considered unsterile.*

◆ When using forceps to lift sterile supplies out of a commercially prepared package, be sure that the forceps do not touch the edges or outside of the wrapper. *The edges and outside of the package are exposed to the air and handled and are thus unsterile.*

◆ When placing forceps whose handles were in contact with the bare hand, position the handles outside the sterile area. *The handles of these forceps harbor microorganisms from the bare hand.*

◆ Deposit a sterile item on a sterile field without permitting moist forceps to touch the sterile field when the surface under the absorbent sterile field is unsterile and a barrier drape is not used. *A barrier drape is resistant to moisture (e.g., blood and antiseptics) and should be used whenever a procedure involves the use of liquids. Made of chemically treated cotton or synthetic materials, barrier drapes prevent a sterile field from becoming unsterile when the drape becomes wet. If the underlying surface is sterile (e.g., a plastic container), the field will not become unsterile when moist.*

◆ SAMPLE DOCUMENTATION

10-26-2004	
1400	A sterile field was set up according to hospital protocol using aseptic technique for abdominal wound irrigation and dressing change. ———— M. Stuart, LVN

Chapter Review

Use the audio glossary feature of either the CD-ROM or the Companion Website to hear the correct pronunciation of the following key terms.

Microorganisms
bacteria, viruses, fungi, parasites, resident flora, infection, pathogen, disease, virulence, communicable disease, vector

Types of infection
local infection, systemic infection, septicemia, nosocomial infections, iatrogenic infection

Chain of infection
carrier, reservoir, transmission, susceptible host

Factors that increase susceptibility to infection
nonspecific defenses, inflammatory response, specific defenses, antigens, immunity

Controlling microorganisms
antiseptics, disinfectants, bactericidal agent, bacteriostatic agent, asepsis, sepsis, aseptic technique, medical asepsis, surgical asepsis

Protective precautions
Standard Precautions, Transmission-Based Precautions

Nursing Care
sterile field

Key Points

- Microorganisms are everywhere in our environment and in or on our body. Most of them are harmless and perform essential functions.
- Infections are invasions and growth of microorganisms in a body tissue.
- Microorganisms are different in their strength and communicability.
- The medical and nursing communities use aseptic technique to prevent the transfer of microorganisms from one place or person to another.
- Nosocomial infections occur as a result of health care delivery in a health care setting.
- The chain of infection is composed of six links, all of which must be present to cause the infectious process.
- Specific defenses are immune defenses and work against identified foreign proteins and other infectious agents.
- Age is a factor that affects the risk of infection. Both the very young and the elderly have reduced defenses.
- Cleaning, disinfecting, and sterilizing are proven ways of inhibiting the growth and multiplication of microorganisms and of maintaining the environment.
  Isolation practices that protect the client, the health care provider, and others are initiated after assessing the client's condition. They are practiced according to institutional policies and the recommendations of the CDC.
- If there is any doubt about sterility, the object or field is unsterile.

EXPLORE MediaLink

Additional interactive resources for this chapter can be found on the Companion Website at www.prenhall.com/ramont. Click on Chapter 7 and "Begin" to select the activities for this chapter.

For chapter-related NCLEX-style questions and an audio glossary, access the accompanying CD-ROM in this book.

Animations:
- HIV cells
- Naproxen
- Zidovudine
- HIV
- Penicillin

For Further Study

For more information on obtaining different types of cultures, see Chapters 12, 16, 18, and 19.

For more information on wound healing, see Chapter 12.

For further information about nutrition in healing, see Chapter 17.

For more about using sterile technique, see Chapter 22.

Critical Thinking Care Map

Caring for a Client with a Stasis Ulcer

NCLEX-PN Focus Area: Physiological Integrity

Case Study: George Gower has been admitted to the hospital with an open wound from an arterial stasis ulcer on his inner right lower leg. The wound has increased in size and is now draining small amounts of yellow–green secretions. There is a foul odor. The WBC count is elevated and he has an oral temperature of 101°F.

Nursing Diagnosis: Risk for Infection

COLLECT DATA

Subjective	Objective
_____	_____
_____	_____
_____	_____
_____	_____
_____	_____
_____	_____

Would you report this data? Yes/No

If yes, to: _____

Nursing Care

_____
_____
_____
_____
_____
_____
_____
_____
_____
_____
_____
_____
_____
_____

How would you document this? _____
_____
_____
_____
_____

Data Collected
(use those that apply)

- Complains of burning pain in area of wound
- Yellow–green secretions
- Foul odor from wound and secretions
- Poor pedal pulses
- Says his foot is cold
- States elevating his foot hurts his hip
- Edema around wound and feet are swollen
- Feet appear slightly cyanotic
- Says he hasn't washed right leg in several days
- States he left wound open because "air is good for it"

Nursing Interventions
(use those that apply)

- Administer analgesics as ordered by physician.
- Report poor pedal pulses and edema.
- Look for hazards in the environment.
- Consult with physical therapist about positioning.
- Cleanse wound and apply wound dressings as ordered.
- Keep feet warm.
- Elevate feet.
- Keep the leg uncovered.
- Put feet in a dependent position.
- Teach client about airborne contamination.
- Consult with dietitian regarding diet.
- Keep the leg immobilized.

NCLEX-PN Exam Preparation

1. A man has a history of a draining wound infection in his lower right leg. He was admitted with a wet, soiled dressing and the following vital signs: BP 136/70, P 90, R 20, T 100.6°F. A nursing priority would be:
   a. Elevation of the right leg
   b. Placing the person in isolation
   c. Medicating the client for an elevated temperature
   d. Changing the wound dressing

2. A client was admitted with active tuberculosis and was coughing up moderate amounts of pink-tinged sputum. She was placed in isolation. The nurse was aware the type of isolation initiated would:
   a. Be Tier 1 or Standard Precautions
   b. Be Tier 2 or Transmission-Based Precautions
   c. Include only the use of clean gowns
   d. Require the use of masks by the client while in the room

3. After administering care to the client, the nurse needed to remove a tray of soiled instruments from the room. The nurse knew it was necessary to "bag" the materials. Some of the items were metal, while others were made of plastic. The nurse knew:
   a. Everything could be placed into one bag as long as it was labeled properly
   b. The metal items must be bagged and sent for autoclaving, and the plastic items could be disposed
   c. The items must be separated into plastic in one bag for gas sterilization, and metal into another in order to be autoclaved
   d. The type of bag didn't matter as long as it was labeled "isolation"

4. A child was admitted with an infectious pneumonia and placed in isolation. The exact organism had not yet been identified. The family was instructed to take all clothing and extra toys home. Client education for the parents would include:
   a. Instructing them to wash all the clothing and toys in very hot water before putting them away
   b. Throwing all the clothes and toys away
   c. Telling them nothing special needed to be done to the clothing and toys
   d. "Airing" the clothes and toys to destroy the organisms

5. A client with infectious tuberculosis needed to go to the radiology department for a chest x-ray. The nurse was aware that appropriate nursing care included:
   a. Calling the radiology department and telling them the client was still in isolation
   b. Covering the client with a blanket and providing tissues
   c. Telling the transport person to wear a mask for protection
   d. Putting a mask and gloves on the client to prevent the spread of organisms

6. The nurse is assisting the physician with an irrigation of a draining abdominal wound by preparing the sterile tray. She knew sterility of the tray must be maintained at all times. During the process the nurse:
   a. Used sterile forceps while reaching across it to move the contents around
   b. Wore clean gloves to handle the contents of the tray
   c. Allowed the open tray to stand unattended for a period of 20 minutes and then covered it with a towel
   d. Put on sterile gloves to handle the contents of the tray

7. A client who was admitted with pneumonia and placed in isolation has a history of HIV+ (AIDS). Before leaving the room, the nurse will remove all soiled personal protective equipment. The nurse knew the order of removal was:
   a. Remove the gown, then mask, then gloves
   b. Take off the mask, the gloves, and then the gown
   c. Remove the gloves, then the mask, and finally the gown
   d. Take off the gown first, then either the mask or gloves

8. An 82-year-old client with a history of emphysema was being seen for a possible upper respiratory tract infection (URI). Several family members had been ill with colds during the previous week. The nurse is aware that the client may be considered:
   a. A susceptible host
   b. A compromised host
   c. In no special danger of the infection since the family was ill last week
   d. Having a chronic URI

9. You have been assigned to represent your unit on the infectious control committee. The committee is discussing the CDC hand hygiene recommendations. Of the following guidelines suggested for implementation in your hospital, which one demonstrates an understanding of the CDC's recommendations?
   a. Health care providers will wear gloves at all times when providing client care.
   b. Disinfecting hands following glove removal is not necessary.
   c. Waterless hand cleaner is effective on hands that are not visibly soiled with blood and body fluids.
   d. Waterless alcohol-based hand cleaner must be removed with paper towels in order to remove pathogens from hands.

10. When seen in the clinic, a client had already developed an inflammatory response in the area of a wound on the left hand. The nurse knew this was an appropriate observation when he noted:
    a. The client complaining of itching around the area of the wound
    b. A moderate amount of drainage weeping from the wound
    c. Swelling, redness, and heat around the wound
    d. Bruising around the wound

Answers for Review Questions, as well as discussion of Case Study and Critical Thinking Care Map questions, appear in Appendix IV.

Admission, Transfer, and Discharge

Chapter

8

SHARING experiences

"*Set your expectations for yourself high and then strive daily to meet them. Learn to be flexible and adaptable to be employable in today's changing health care environment.*"

Bonnie Boroski, Coordinator of Practical Nursing, Greater Johnstown Area Vocational Technical School, Johnstown, PA.

LEARNING outcomes

After completing the chapter, you will be able to:
- Discuss the common reactions that a client might have to the admission, transfer, and discharge processes.
- Describe the environment in which the client may experience dehumanization.
- Describe the procedural steps for admission, transfer, and discharge.
- Discuss how nursing process applies to admission, transfer, and discharge.
- Discuss the importance of discharge planning.
- Explain the nurse's responsibility related to discharge instructions.

MediaLink

www.prenhall.com/ramont

Use the address above to access the free, interactive Companion Website created for this textbook. Get hints, instant feedback, and textbook references to chapter-related NCLEX-style questions. Link to other interesting sites.

Audio Glossary:
Use the Companion Website, or the CD-ROM disk enclosed with your textbook, to hear the pronunciation of key terms in the chapter.

Everyone, during the course of a lifetime, experiences changes in health status. At times, these changes will require medical treatment in a hospital or other health care facility. The person in need of such medical care, the client, will be admitted, possibly transferred, and eventually discharged from the hospital or other health care setting.

This chapter addresses the processes of admission, transfer, and discharge of clients in these settings. It also includes the responsibilities of the nurse in helping clients through these processes successfully, with caring attention to the client's needs and concerns. Many research studies conducted in health care settings demonstrate that nursing care, and specifically the quality of the client–nurse interaction, is a part of medical treatment that affects the client's health status.

The goal of nursing care is to ensure the continuity of individualized client care during admission, transfer, and discharge. The nursing process is used (see Chapter 4) as a framework for achieving these objectives. ⊙⊃ In this chapter, the nursing process is applied in the discussion of each section: admission, transfer, and discharge.

◆ Admitting a Client

COMMON RESPONSES TO HOSPITAL ADMISSION

Hospital **admission** is entry into the hospital. It is usually a very stressful time for a client and his or her family or significant others. The nurses who initially provide assistance with admission and orientation will influence the client's reaction to hospitalization and treatment. Therefore, it is important to make a positive first impression. Each individual client deserves to be greeted in a caring manner that demonstrates concern and respect.

The admission process elicits many different responses from clients. Clients' responses, while unique, are influenced by their particular gender, age, culture, religion, and **coping behaviors** (behaviors such as crying, acting angry, overeating, or smoking, which people perform in times of crisis or stress in an attempt to deal with their feelings). The client's responses are also related to needs identified by Maslow (see Figure 4-4 and discussion in Chapter 24). ⊙⊃

Two of the most common responses to hospital admission are anxiety and fear of the unknown. Clients already are vulnerable to these responses because of the medical need for which they are entering the hospital. Anxiety causes emotional discomfort. It may have physical effects as well (increase vital signs). Fear of the unknown causes a sense of insecurity. Clients can be helped to feel more secure by reassuring them that their needs will be met promptly and their questions answered thoroughly.

Unfortunately, the health care environment promotes **dehumanization** (removal of unique human qualities) by asking clients to surrender their belongings, privacy, and independence. A loss of self-identity occurs when individuals are referred to as a number, a diagnosis, a nickname, or when they are called by their first name without having given permission. Children have other anxieties and fears that may be expressed during the admission process. For example, they are likely to experience separation anxiety if their parents are not allowed to stay with them throughout the admission procedures.

It is the nurse's responsibility to help protect the client from feeling dehumanized by anticipating and avoiding situations that are likely to provoke these feelings. In addition, the nurse must strive to help reduce the specific fears and anxieties of each client. The client's integrity and personal dignity must always be maintained (see Chapter 23). ⊙⊃

CULTURAL CONSIDERATIONS

Culture is a set of learned attitudes and behaviors associated with particular values, ethnic traditions, and religious beliefs. Clients come from many different cultures, and so have a variety of attitudes and beliefs related to illness and medical treatment. Clients' views about health care and their behavior during hospitalization may be expressions of their cultural beliefs. Often, the client's views are different from the nurse's view. Regardless of the cultural differences between the nurse and the client, it is the nurse's obligation to provide culturally sensitive care (see Chapter 26). ⊙⊃

Suggestions for communicating with culturally diverse clients during the admission, transfer, and discharge procedures include the following:

1. Address clients by their last name. In some cultures, the informal use of first names is offensive. It is best to ask clients how they wish to be addressed.
2. Respect the clients' values and beliefs about health care and illness.
3. Use culturally sensitive language (this may include African-American instead of black, gay or lesbian instead of homosexual, etc.). Take your cues from the client.
4. Use clear, common English. The use of slang is usually not appropriate.
5. If a language barrier exists, find an interpreter. Unless specifically requested, this should not be a member of the client's family.

Further steps to improve cultural sensitivity are discussed in detail in Chapter 26. ⊙⊃

ADMISSION PROCEDURE GUIDELINES

Each health care facility has its own policies concerning admission procedures. Immediately upon entering the hospital, the client usually goes to the admitting office, where clerical personnel start the admission process. However, clients may also be admitted directly from the emergency department or physician's office.

The client's medical record is initiated in the admitting department (Figure 8-1 ◆). It usually includes demographic data, such as age, gender, birthday, Social Security number, next of kin, and insurance information. At this time clients are usually informed about their legal rights. Forms for durable power

ADMISSION DATA

Date _4-16-05_ Time _3:15 p.m._ Primary Language _English_
Arrived Via: ☐ Wheelchair ☐ Stretcher ☑ Ambulatory
From: ☐ Admitting ☐ ER ☑ Home ☐ Nursing Home ☐ Other
Admitting M.D. _R. Katz_ Time Notified _5 p.m._

ORIENTATION TO UNIT

	YES	NO		YES	NO
Arm Band Correct	☑	☐	Visiting Hours	☑	☐
Allergy Band	☑	☐	Smoking Policy	☑	☐
Telephone	☑	☐	TV, Lights, Bed Controls,		
Electrical Policy	☑	☐	Call Lights, Side Rails	☑	☐
Educational Mat©	☑	☐	Nurses Station	☑	☐
(TV Brochure)	☑	☐			

Family M.D. _R. Katz_
Weight _125 lb._ Height _5ft. 2in._ BP:R — L _122 / 80_
Temp. _103F_ Pulse _92, weak_ Resp. _28, shallow_
Source Providing Information ☑ Patient ☐ Other_____
Unable to Obtain History ☐ _____
Reason for Admission (Onset, Duration, Pt. ⓒ Perception) _"Chest cold" X2 weeks S.O.B. on exertion. "Lung pain, fever." "Dr. says I have pneumonia."_

ALLERGIES & REACTIONS

Drugs _Penicillin_
Food/Other_____
Signs & symptoms _Rash, nausea_
Blood Reaction ☐ Yes ☑ No Dyes/Shellfish ☐ Yes ☑ No

MEDICATIONS

Current Meds	Dose/Freq.	Last Dose
Synthroid	0.1 mg, daily	4-16, 8 a.m.

Disposition of Meds: ☑ Home ☐ Pharmacy ☐ Safe *At Bedside

MEDICAL HISTORY

☑ No Major Problems   ☐ Gastro_____
☐ Cardiac_____   ☐ Arthritis_____
☐ Hyper/Hypotension_____   ☐ Stroke_____
☐ Diabetes_____   ☐ Seizures_____
☐ Cancer_____   ☐ Glaucoma_____
☐ Respiratory_____   ☑ Other _Childbirth - 1998_

Surgery/Procedures	Date
Appendectomy	1988
Partial thyroidectomy	2001

SPECIAL ASSISTIVE DEVICES

☐ Wheelchair ☐ Contacts ☐ Venous ☐ Dentures
☐ Braces ☐ Hearing Aid Access ☐ Partial
☐ Cane/Crutches ☐ Prosthesis Device ☐ Upper
☐ Walker ☐ Glasses ☐ Epidural Catheter ☐ Lower
☐ Other _None_

VALUABLES

Client informed Hospital not responsible for personal belongings.
Valuables Disposition: ☐ Client ☐ Safe ☐ Given to_____
Client/SO Signature _None_

PSYCHOSOCIAL HISTORY

Recent Stress _None_
Coping Mechanism _Not assessed because of fatigue_
Support System _Husband, coworkers, friends_
Calm: ☑ Yes ☐ No_____
Anxious: _Facial muscles tense; trembling_
Religion _Catholic, would want Last Rites_
Tobacco Use: ☐ Yes ☑ No_____
Alcohol Use: ☐ Yes ☑ No_____
Drug Use: ☐ Yes ☑ No_____

NEUROLOGICAL

Oriented: ☑ Person ☑ Place ☑ Time ☐ Confused ☐ Sedated
☐ Alert ☐ Restless ☑ Lethargic ☐ Comatose
Pupils: ☑ Equal ☐ Unequal ☑ Reactive ☐ Sluggish
☐ Other _3mm._
Extremity Strength: ☑ Equal ☐ Unequal
Speech: ☑ Clear ☐ Slurred ☐ Other_____

MUSCULO-SKELETAL

Normal ROM of Extremities ☑ Yes ☐ No
☑ Weakness ☐ Paralysis ☐ Contractures ☐ Joint swelling ☑ Pain
☐ Other ↘ _related to fatigue_ _when coughing_ ↙

RESPIRATORY

Pattern: ☐ Even ☐ Uneven ☑ Shallow ☑ Dyspnea
☑ Other _diminished breath sounds_
Breathing Sounds: ☐ Clear ☑ Other _inspiratory crackles_
Secretions: ☐ None ☑ Other _pink, thick sputum_
Cough: ☐ None ☑ Productive ☐ Nonproductive

CARDIOVASCULAR

Pulses: Apical Rate _92-W_ ☑ Reg. ☐ Irregular ☐ Pacemaker
S = Strong W = Weak A = Absent D = Doppler
Radial R _92_ L — Pedal R — L —
Edema: ☑ Absent ☐ Present Site_____
Perfusion: ☐ Warm ☐ Dry ☑ Diaphoretic ☐ Cool (Hot)

GASTROINTESTINAL

Oral Mucosa ☐ Normal ☑ Other _pale and dry_
Bowel Sounds: ☑ Normal ☐ Other _Abd. soft_
Wt. Change ☐ ☑ N/V Stool Frequency/Character _1/day soft_
Last B/M _4-15-05_ ☐ Ostomy (type)_____
Equip._____

GENITOURINARY

Urine: Last Voided _This morning_
☐ Normal ☐ Anuria ☐ Hematuria ☐ Dysuri ☐ Incontinent
☑ Other ↓ _amount & frequency since ill_
☐ Catheter (type)_____ Other_____
LMP _4-1-05_ ☐ Vaginal/Penile Discharge
Other_____

SELF CARE

Need Assist with: ☐ Ambulating ☐ Elimination
☐ Meals ☑ Hygiene ☐ Dressing
while fatigued

Amanda Aquilini [F. age 28]
_#4637651_

✿ **NORTH BROWARD HOSPITAL DISTRICT**
NURSING ADMINISTRATION ASSESSMENT

Figure 8-1. ◆ Adult Admission Assessment *Source:* Courtesy of North Broward Hospital District.

NUTRITION

General Appearance: ☑ Well Nourished ☐ Emaciated ☐ Other _____

Appetite: ☐ Good ☐ Fair ☑ Poor - X2 days

Diet _Liquid_ Meal Pattern _3/day_

☐ Feeds Self ☐ Assist ☐ Total Feed

SKIN ASSESSMENT

Color: ☐ Normal ☐ Flushed ☑ Pale ☐ Dusky ☐ Cyanotic ☐ Jaundiced ☑ Other _Cheeks flushed, hot_

General Description _Surgical scars; RLQ abdomen; anterior neck_

_____

_____

_____

_____

Note Cultures Obtained _____

_____

_____

PRESSURE SORE ™AT RISK[SCREENING CRITERIA

OVERALL SKIN CONDITION

Grade

☐ 0	Turgor (elasticity adequate, skin warm and moist)
☑ 1	Poor turgor, skin cold & dry
☐ 2	Areas mottled, red or denuded
☐ 3	Existing skin ulcer/lesions

BOWEL AND BLADDER CONTROL

Grade

☑ 0	Always able to ask for bedpan
☐ 1	Incontinence of urine
☐ 2	Incontinence of feces
☐ 3	Totally incontinent Confined to bed

REHABILITATIVE STATE

Grade

☐ 0	Fully ambulatory
☑ 1	Ambulated with assistance
☐ 2	Chair to bed ambulation only
☐ 3	Confined to bed
☐ 4	Immobile in bed

NUTRITIONAL STATE

Grade

☐ 0	Eats all
☑ 1	Eats very little
☐ 2	Refuses food often
☐ 2	Tube feeding
☐ 4	Intravenous feeding

MENTAL STATE

Grade

☑ 0	Alert and clear
☐ 1	Confused
☐ 2	Disoriented/senile
☐ 3	Stuporous
☐ 4	Unconscious

CHRONIC DISEASE STATUS (i.e. COPD, ASCVD, Peripheral Vascular Disease, Diabetes, or Renal Disease, Cancer, Motor or Sensory Deficits, Elderly, Other)

Grade

☑ 0	Absent
☐ 1	One Present
☐ 2	Two Present
☐ 3	Three or more Present

TOTAL _____ Refer to Skin Care Protocol

FALLS SCREENING

If one or more of the following are checked institute fall precautions/plan of care

☐ History of Falls ☐ Unsteady Gait ☐ Confusion/Disorientation ☐ Dizziness

If two or more of the following are checked institute fall precautions/plan of care

☐ Age over 80 ☐ Utilizes cane, walker, w/c ☐ Sleeplessness

☐ Impaired vision ☐ Impaired hearing ☐ Urgency/frequency in elimination

☐ Multiple Diagnoses ☐ Medication/Sedative /Diuretic etc.

☐ Inability to understand or follow directions

NURSE SIGNATURE/TITLE	DATE	TIME
Mary Medina, RN	4-16-05	3:30p.m.
NURSE SIGNATURE/TITLE	**DATE**	**TIME**

EDUCATION/DISCHARGE PLANNING

1. What do you know about your present illness? _"Dr. says I have pneumonia." "I will have an I.V."_
2. What information do you want or need about your illness? _____
3. Would you like family/SO involved in your care? _Husband, Michael_
4. How long do you expect to be in the hospital? _"1-2 days_
5. What concerns do you have about leaving the hospital?—

CHECK APPROPRIATE BOX

Will client need post discharge assistance with ADLs/physical functioning? ☐ Yes ☑ No ☐ Unknown

Does client have family capable of and willing to provide assistance post dishcarge? ☑ Yes ☐ No ☐ Unknown ☐ No family

Is assistance needed beyond that which family can provide? ☐ Yes ☑ No ☐ Unknown

Previous admission in the last six months? ☐ Yes ☑ No ☐ Unknown

Client lives with _Husband and child_

Planned discharge to _Home_

Comments _Fatigue and anxiety may have interfered with learning. Re-teach anything covered at admission, later._

_____

Social Services Notified ☐ Yes ☑ No

ADVANCE DIRECTIVES:

Does client have a Living Will? ☑ Yes ☐ No If Yes, please obtain a copy for the medical record. If unable to obtain a copy, document intent of Advace Directive in the medical record. Please refer to Interdisciplinary Patient/Family Education Record for documentation of Education regarding Advance Directives/Living Will.

Is the client an Organ Donor? ☑ Yes ☐ No If no, explain in progress notes.

If "No", provided information on organ donation ☐ Yes ☐ No

NARRATIVE NOTES

S–c/O sharp chest pain when coughing and dyspnea on exertion. States unable to carry out regular daily exercise for past week. Coughing relieved "if I sit up and sit still." Nausea associated with coughing. Having occasional "chills." Occasionally becomes frightened stating, "I can't breathe." Well groomed but "too tired to put on make-up."

O--Chest expansion < 3cm, no nasal flaring or use of accessory muscles. Breath sounds and insp. crackles in ℞ upper and lower chest.

Assesses own supports as "good" (eg, relationship c–husband). Is "worried" about daughter. States husband will be out of town until tomorrow. Left 3-year-old daughter with neighbor. Concerned too about her work (is attorney). "I'll never get caught up." Had water at noon—no food today. Informed of need to save urine for 24 hr. specimen. IV D5W LR 1000 mL started in ℞ arm, 100 mL/hr. Slow capillary refill. Keeping head of bed ↑ to facilitate breathing.

✿✿ **NORTH BROWARD HOSPITAL DISTRICT**
NURSING ADMINISTRATION ASSESSMENT

Figure 8-1. ◆ (continued)

of attorney and do not resuscitate (DNR) orders are presented. The client may sign or waive them, but most facilities require that these forms be in the client's file. If the person does not sign the forms, a notation is made to document that the client waived the signature (see more about legal issues in Chapter 2). 🔗

The admitting clerk places an identification bracelet on the client's arm. The bracelet is worn throughout the client's stay in the facility. When all the appropriate information is collected and the client is ready to be transferred to the room, the admitting personnel notifies the nurse or unit clerk. The client is usually transported to the nursing unit by wheelchair.

The nurse should prepare the room before the client arrives on the unit. A room that is neat and clean, with good lighting, appropriate temperature, and equipped with basic supplies, makes a client feel welcome and safe. When the client arrives on the unit, he or she should be greeted warmly and with a smile. The greeting is a way to begin the client–nurse relationship on a positive note.

Orientation

All new clients are oriented to the hospital unit. **Orientation** is the introduction of clients to the people and the facility in which they are admitted. It starts with the nurse introducing him- or herself and explaining roles of the staff who care for the client. If the client is in a semiprivate room, the roommate is also introduced. Important elements to include in the orientation are listed in Box 8-1 ◆.

Client's Valuables and Clothing

Clients may bring jewelry, money, credit cards, prescription medications, and other valuables with them to the hospital. During the admission process they should be instructed to give those items to a family member to take home. If this is not possible, the valuables can usually be stored in the hospital safe. The hospital's policy for storing personal items should be explained carefully to the client and family. An inventory with a general description of each item (such as a gold colored ring with a clear stone, instead of gold diamond ring) should be documented on the proper forms required by the hospital (Figure 8-2 ◆). The client and a designated member of the hospital staff must sign these forms.

The client may keep personal items such as clothing, glasses, contact lenses, dentures, and hearing aid in the room. These items must also be listed on the inventory sheet. When forms are completed and signed, a copy is given to the client and a copy is placed on the client's medical record.

NURSING CARE

◆ ASSESSING

The initial assessment should be started once the client is settled into the room. The Joint Commission on Accreditation of

---

BOX 8-1
NURSING CARE CHECKLIST

ORIENTING A CLIENT ON ADMISSION

When admitting a person to a facility, the nurse should provide the following information and instructions:

☑ The location of the room in relation to the nurse's desk.
☑ How to use the intercom system.
☑ How to call the nurse's station from the bed and bathroom.
☑ How to use the phone.
☑ How to adjust the bed. (The bed should always be in the low position when the client enters.)
☑ How to operate the television.
☑ Location of the bathroom.
☑ How to adjust the lights.
☑ Time meals are served.
☑ Location of personal care items.
☑ Hospital policies that apply to the clients, such as visiting times.
☑ A gown and instructions on how to wear it (if the client doesn't have a gown or pajamas). Assist them to change if necessary.
☑ Explanation of why an identification band is necessary.
☑ Information about when laboratory or other diagnostic tests will be performed.
☑ Information about when the physician usually visits.

Healthcare Organizations (JCAHO) requires that a registered nurse perform the admission assessment. Subjective and objective data are collected throughout the interview, medical history, and physical assessment. However, the RN may delegate parts of the assessment to the practical/vocational nurse. This may include baseline information such as level of consciousness, vital signs, skin condition, height and weight, bowel sounds, lung sounds, specimen collection, and clarification of the client's questions and concerns. The collected data are then organized, prioritized, and reviewed. They are used to construct nursing diagnoses and to identify areas in which the client may need teaching before discharge. (See Chapter 11 for more on focused head-to-toe assessment; Chapter 14, for vital signs assessment; and Chapter 18, for obtaining urine specimens.) 🔗

When the client is admitted, the physician is notified, and orders are requested if they were not sent with the client from the admitting office.

◆ DIAGNOSING, PLANNING, and IMPLEMENTING

As mentioned, some common nursing diagnoses of clients at admission are Anxiety, Fear, Powerlessness, Social Isolation,

Valuables		
Cash		
Currency	Coins	
Watch and Jewelry		
Wallet		
Keys		
Driver's License		
Insurance Cards		
Credit Cards		
Documents		
Admitting Date Time Received by Dept Use		
Disposition of Valuables	Client/Designate Signature Date	
	Witness Signature Date	
Envelope No.		
This facility assumes **NO RESPONSIBILITY** for the loss or damage of personal property not enclosed within the envelope		
Client Identification		
Client Valuables Record		
Adapted from form courtesy of Community Hospital of Lancaster, PA		

Figure 8-2. ◆ Excerpt from client's valuables record. *Source:* Courtesy of Community Hospital of Lancaster.

and Disturbed Personal Identity. For example, the RN might write "Anxiety related to unfamiliar hospital environment" as an admission nursing diagnosis.

As part of the planning process, the client's short- and long-term goals are set by the nurse and client. The client's choices and decisions about his or her health care are discussed and noted at this time. Nursing interventions are then planned to help the client reach these goals. Common interventions follow:

◆ Orient the client to the hospital staff and environment (see Box 8-1). It is important for the client to know who should receive what information and to become acquainted with various caregiver roles. For example: "You will be visited by a laboratory technician who will draw some blood for examination." It is equally important for the client to know where the nurse's station and lounge are in relation to the room. Familiarity increases comfort.

* Monitor client's level of understanding. Becoming familiar with the client's educational, cultural, and familial background makes communication easier. It also will make your choice of words more appropriate.

* Provide the opportunity for clients to place belongings in the room as they wish, and assist as needed. This simple courtesy helps the client avoid feeling a loss of control and encourages a sense of ownership of the environment.

* Provide the opportunity for the client to ask questions. Answer only what you know and obtain the answer quickly to what you do not know. Do not appear hurried during the admission process. Appearing hurried will prevent the client from asking questions and will increase stress.

EVALUATING

The evaluation step is measured by assessing whether or not the goals have been met. For example, for a client with anxiety, an evaluation statement might be: Client states "less anxious" after orientation. The plan of care is consistently reevaluated to determine if the client's changing needs are being met as treatment progresses.

Nursing Process Case Study:
ADMISSION OF A CLIENT
FROM EMERGENCY UNIT

David Reynolds is a 42-year-old accounting executive with chest pain admitted from the emergency unit. Janet, the admitting nurse, introduces herself and welcomes him to the cardiovascular unit. As Janet begins to obtain Mr. Reynolds's vital signs, he says: "I got this really sharp pain at work. Someone called the ambulance and also called my wife. She should have been here by now." He adds: "My father died of a heart attack at 47." While Mr. Reynolds was in the ER, he was examined by the cardiologist, who admitted him for observation and diagnostic tests. Mr. Reynolds is not receiving intravenous fluids. His right hand is on the left side of his neck. He says he is feeling his pulse.

Assessment Mr. Reynolds's temperature is 100°F. Radial pulse is 120 and regular. Apical pulse is 118 and regular. Respirations are 28, audible and shallow. BP is 160/94.

Mr. Reynolds rates his pain as a 4 on a scale of 1 to 10. He says he is just a "little nauseated." His color is pink, and his skin is cool and dry. He is frowning, his face appears taut, and his hands are shaking. Janet is asking Mr. Reynolds about his pain—when it started, its character, and the location. She

also asks him if this pain has ever been present before. He says he has never had pain this sharp or in his chest before but has had some pain in his stomach on occasion after eating a lot late at night. Mr. Reynolds interrupts Janet's questioning: "Where the heck is my wife? I could be buying the big one here! I wonder if she went to the wrong hospital."

Diagnosis The current nursing diagnoses for Mr. Reynolds are:

* Pain (midline chest)
* Nausea
* Fear
* Anxiety

Expected Outcomes The current expected outcomes specify that Mr. Reynolds will:

* Obtain relief from pain
* Obtain relief from nausea
* State his fears
* Become less anxious
* Regain and maintain vital signs within normal limits

Planning and Implementation The interventions indicated for Mr. Reynolds are:

* Orient to the unit.
* Explain the purpose of admission (observation and diagnosis).
* Position for greater comfort in breathing.
* Respond to need for information regarding wife.
* Encourage to talk about fears.
* Listen attentively to concerns.
* Welcome questions.
* Arrange room (client belongings) according to preferences.
* Monitor vital signs frequently as specified by physician's orders.
* Assess rate, rhythm, and character of pulse and respiration.
* Assess pain occurrence, including intensity, duration, and location.
* Assess skin color.
* Assess presence of nausea.
* Explain diagnostic procedures ordered (procedure and purpose).

Evaluation By the third day of hospitalization, Mr. Reynolds has learned that he did not have a heart attack (myocardial infarction) but instead has a peptic ulcer. Treatment for the ulcer is continuing. Discharge planning has begun. Stress management will be one of the teaching initiatives.

Critical Thinking in the Nursing Process

1. What nursing care problems did Mr. Reynolds present at the time of admission that would be reported to the nurse team leader?
2. What aspects of Mr. Reynolds's verbal and nonverbal communication were significant indicators of fear and anxiety?

3. What effect would arranging Mr. Reynolds's room according to his preferences have in reducing his anxiety?

 ## Transferring a Client

COMMON RESPONSES TO TRANSFER

The client may require **transfer** (a move) to another unit in the hospital or to a different health care facility as a result of a client or physician request. The usual reasons for transfer are:

- The client may request another room (e.g., the client may need a quieter environment).
- The client's health condition may change and require more specialized nursing care (e.g., a severely elevated heart rate may require that the client be moved into intensive care).
- The client's condition may improve, permitting transfer from ICU to a medical/surgical or a transitional care unit (TCU).
- The client's condition may require a transfer to another facility (e.g., from an acute care setting to a rehab unit).
- The client may be disturbing others.

Transferring from one room, department, or facility to another is always somewhat stressful for the client and significant others. Clients may be concerned about people not being informed or about staff losing their belongings during the transfer. Anxieties tend to be lessened when the client is being transferred to a step-down or rehabilitation unit. However, when the physician orders the transfer for the purpose of having the client receive more specialized care (such as intensive care), the client's initial response is fear. Concerned that his or her condition has worsened, the client's fears may escalate into fear of death. Obviously, whatever the client's response, individualized nursing care is required.

TRANSFER GUIDELINES

Each hospital has written policies for transferring a client. The procedure usually requires the following:

1. A physician's order
2. Informing the client and family about the reason for the transfer
3. Assisting the client to gather all belongings
4. Completion of the required documentation

Figure 8-3 ◆ illustrates one type of transfer form.

NURSING CARE

 ### ASSESSING

While it is not the practical/vocational nurse's responsibility to determine if, where, or when a client is transferred, he or she may participate in the process. The nurse may be involved in assessing and reporting client problems related to transfer. The LPN or LVN may also assist in implementing transfer procedures as directed by the registered nurse.

The following are common assessment issues related to transfer:

1. Client's health status. Physical and emotional support may be necessary throughout the process of transfer.
2. The client's and significant others' level of understanding about the reason for the transfer.
3. Safety precautions. Special equipment (such as wheelchair, stretcher, and portable IV apparatus) may be required to ensure client safety.

 ### DIAGNOSING, PLANNING, and IMPLEMENTING

Nursing diagnoses for clients who are being transferred are identified upon reviewing assessment issues. The following are examples:

- Deficient Knowledge related to need for transfer
- Potential for Injury related to the transfer procedure
- Anxiety related to a new environment

Implementation of the care plan or nursing actions address client issues directly related to the nursing diagnoses. All nursing actions related to transfer should be directed toward managing the transfer process in an efficient and calm manner. These nursing actions include:

- Explanation of the transfer process. Sharing information with the client and significant others decreases anxiety. It also generally increases compliance.
- Safety precautions. There is risk for injury in transfer situations. Also, if the transfer is delayed, there is potential for client discomfort. (For example, the client may have to wait a long time on a transfer bed or in a wheelchair. Clients in hospital gowns may become chilled.)
- Checking and recording vital signs. It is important to document client status before transfer. This documentation can be used as a reference point should the client's condition change.

clinical ALERT

Report

It is important to report all aspects of the transfer process immediately upon completion. Reporting completion of a transfer will allow several steps to occur:

1. Details about room number and client status at the time of transfer will be communicated.
2. The physician will be notified, usually by the unit clerk, that the client has been transferred.
3. The empty room will be cleaned and prepared for the next client.

The nurse may be directed to accompany the client to the new environment. If so, it is the nurse's responsibility to ensure that

SKILLED NURSING FACILITY (SNF)
Transfer Record

Client's Name ———————————————— DOB ——————— Insurance No. ————————

SNF Name ——

Hosp. Admission Date ———————— Discharge Date ———————— SNF Admission Date ————————

Principal Diagnosis (es):

Surgical Procedures and Dates:

Client Allergies:

Diet:

Physician Transfer Orders: (Medicines, Therapy, Lab Work, etc.)

Physician's Signature ————————————————————————

Nursing Evaluation:

Date of Foley Insertion ———————————— Date of Late BM ————————

Decubitus size / condition ————————————

Nursing Assessment:

Nurse's Signature ————————————————————————

Community Hospital
of Lancaster
LANCASTER, PENNSYLVANIA

Figure 8-3. ◆ Skilled nursing facility transfer record. Source: Courtesy of Community Hospital of Lancaster.

the client is greeted by the staff member of the new unit or facility who will be caring for the client. When accompanying a client to a new environment, it is also necessary to inform the registered nurse manager that transfer has occurred. Any change in the client's health status during transfer, or any problem encountered during the process, is also reported to the registered nurse who will oversee the client's care.

EVALUATING

After transfer, the nurse evaluates whether the client's vital signs and general health status have remained stable, and determines whether the transfer was completed safely. The time of transfer and the client's reaction to transfer are also noted.

Discharging a Client

Discharge is the official procedure by which the client leaves the health care facility and returns home or to another setting. Written permission from the physician is required for discharge. The situation of a client leaving the hospital or health care facility without the written permission of a physician and **against medical advice (AMA)** is reported to the registered nurse manager immediately. If the client is rational and a court order does not exist to detain the client, he or she cannot be forcibly detained. The nurse or designated supervisor is responsible for notifying the physician. The client and supervisor sign and complete the proper forms. If the client refuses to sign the forms, this is documented in the client's medical record.

Clients are generally discharged from the hospital and return home because their condition has improved or has become stable. Client discharge to another health care facility may occur for various reasons. For example, the discharged client may be a resident of a nursing home or may require the type of care received in a rehabilitation center. Clients may be discharged by wheelchair to their personal vehicle or by wheelchair or stretcher to some other form of transport such as an ambulance. Depending on the condition of the client at the time of discharge and the type of facility receiving the client, a nurse may accompany the client. In many health care facilities, there is a particular time for discharge of clients (for example, 11 A.M.), which precedes a designated admission time. Regardless of the policies and procedures in a health care setting, it is the nurse's responsibility to manage discharge efficiently and in a manner that ensures the client's physical and emotional comfort.

DISCHARGE GUIDELINES

Each hospital has written guidelines about the discharge procedure. They generally consist of the following:

♦ Written physician's order for discharge.
♦ Completion of discharge documentation (Figure 8-4 ♦).
♦ Notification of discharge sent to the business office.
♦ Assisting the client to prepare for discharge.
♦ Ensuring that all client belongings are assembled for discharge.
♦ Explanation of referral agencies and information about people or groups to contact (if this is not required prior to discharge).
♦ Completion of the teaching process. This includes all discharge instructions related to medication, nutrition and diet, self-care, allowable activity, and future appointments. Figure 8-5 ♦ provides a sample of discharge instructions.
♦ Transporting the client to the discharge location.

Appointments such as those to physical therapy and referral to agencies such as home health are usually arranged by the social worker assigned to the client. Appointments and referrals are also sometimes scheduled by the nurse manager, discharge planner, or the unit clerk. The client or significant others may be instructed by the nurse or social worker in making the referral.

Referrals and appointments are ordered by the physician. An exception to a physician-ordered referral may occur when the client requests information regarding a particular problem or disease. The nurse may then refer the client to an organization by providing the name and number and perhaps some printed material. For example, a newly diagnosed diabetic client may ask where he or she can learn more about the disease and perhaps join a support group. In instances such as this, referral to community services is part of the nursing responsibility of promoting health education.

COMMON RESPONSES TO DISCHARGE

Most clients are excited and happy to be returning home. Others may be anxious about the support they will receive at home or about the consequences and nature of continued convalescence. Those who are going to an unfamiliar destination may feel uncomfortable. Clients generally feel concerned about how to care for themselves and how to follow the discharge instructions precisely.

NURSING CARE

ASSESSING

The LPN/LVN may collect data about the following issues prior to discharge:

♦ Client's physical and emotional readiness for discharge. The nurse should provide the opportunity to listen to the client's feelings related to discharge. These concerns could be related to wondering how well the client will continue

Discharge Charting

Content Items marked with (✓) required on all Clients	Identified Client/Family Educational Needs		Date	Instruction Educator's Initials	Learner's Resonse	Date	Instruction Educator's Initials	Learner's Response
	Pre-op	Other						
Teaching/Miscellaneous:								
OR / PACU Routine								
Report Time to Hospital								
Waiting Area/visitors								
SCD's								
IV Therapy								
Incision / Wound Care								
NPO status								
Drain Tubes								
Other:								
Rehabilitation Needs:								
Cane/Crutch/Walker Training/Transfer Training								
Hip/Knees/Back/Ankle/Upper Extremity Exercise								
Sling/Splint/Corset/Braces								
TENS								
CPM								
Total Hip Precautions								
ADL Adaptive Equipment								
Energy Conservation / Joint Protection								
Body Mechanics								
Safety								
Other:								
Lifestyle Changes / Interventions								
Activity Level								
Other:								
Community Resources								
Specify								
Grief Counseling / Training								

 COMMUNITY HOSPITAL OF LANCASTER LANCASTER, PENNSYLVANIA

Figure 8-4. ◆ Discharge teaching from interdisciplinary client/family education record. *Source: Courtesy of Community Hospital of Lancaster.*

ADDRESSOGRAPH

MEMORIAL CARE®
ANAHEIM MEMORIAL MEDICAL CENTER

DISCHARGE INSTRUCTIONS

For medical questions, call your physician.
For medical emergencies, dial 9-1-1 immediately.

CLIENT NAME: _____

REASON FOR YOUR HOSPITAL STAY: _____

DATE ADMITTED:_____ DATE DISCHARGED: _____

DIET: REGULAR   SPECIAL (see "special instructions" below)

BATHING: AS DESIRED   LIMITS (see "special instructions" below)

PAIN MANAGEMENT: MEDICATION TREATMENT OUTPATIENT FOLLOW-UP

ACTIVITY: NORMAL   LIMITS (see "special instructions" below)

YOU CAN RESUME NORMAL ACTIVITIES WHEN: _____

_____

_____

PRE-PRINTED INSTRUCTIONS PROVIDED & REVIEWED INCLUDING FOOD/DRUG AND

OTHER INTERACTIONS (LIST TITLE): _____

Home Health Services Ordered: _____

_____

_____

Co. _____ # _____

Medical Equipment Ordered: _____

_____

_____

Co. _____ # _____

Assisted Daily Living Needs: _____

_____

List of Homemaker Agencies Given? _____

Other Services Ordered/Resources Contacted?

_____

Co. _____ # _____

SPECIAL INSTRUCTIONS: _____

_____

_____

THINGS TO LET YOUR DOCTOR KNOW ABOUT: _____

_____

PHYSICIAN APPOINTMENTS / REFERRALS:

1. _____
   DATE   PHYSICIAN/SPECIALTY   PHONE

2. _____
   DATE   PHYSICIAN/SPECIALTY   PHONE

3. _____
   DATE   PHYSICIAN/SPECIALTY   PHONE

4. _____
   DATE   PHYSICIAN/SPECIALTY   PHONE

MEDICATION INSTRUCTIONS

NO.	DRUG / DOSE	ROUTE	TIME(S)	PURPOSE	DATE/TIME LAST GIVEN
1					/
2					/
3					/
4					/
5					/
6					/
7					/
8					/
9					/
10					/

11 Pain Medication: _____ CALL YOUR DOCTOR WITH QUESTIONS REGARDING PAIN.

Prescription Given? ____ Yes ____ No   Medication Information Discussed? ____ Yes ____ No   Medication Side Effects Discussed? ____ Yes ____ No

Client requests additional information about medication ____ Yes ____ No   Pharmacy contacted ____ Yes ____ No   By whom: _____

Client verbalizes an understanding of above discharge instructions and states where to obtain medications.

Figure 8-5. ◆ Discharge instruction sheet for client. *Source:* Courtesy of Anaheim Memorial Medical Center.

to progress at home or whether medical supplies or equipment will be accessible in the home.

◆ Support system for client. Significant others must become part of the discharge process. The nurse listens to their concerns about the client's return home or to a designated facility.

◆ Understanding discharge instructions. Assessing how the client interprets the instructions is essential. Confusion about diet, medication, special procedures, or exercise and activity may be present.

◆ Progress expectations. The client may not understand what to expect regarding convalescence. Clients may wonder how long they will need certain types of treatment or how long they will have certain symptoms.

◆ Home environment and safety. Clients may feel insecure about home safety. They may feel that their living space will not accommodate the medical supplies and equipment they need.

 clinical **ALERT**

Report

LPNs/LVNs should inform the registered nurse of all concerns stated by the client that could potentially affect the client's continued progress toward wellness. Questions and concerns specifically related to discharge instructions and progress expectations should always be discussed with the registered nurse. In some instances, the registered nurse will refer questions to or obtain answers from the physician.

◆ DIAGNOSING, PLANNING, and IMPLEMENTING

Two of the most common nursing diagnoses that are identified when discharging clients are Insecurity Regarding Self-Care and Deficient Knowledge. The planning and implementation of the nursing process related to discharge occur in response to these diagnoses.

Discharge planning actually begins with hospital admission. Teaching that was identified at admission and introduced during a client's stay is reinforced on the day of discharge. Written guidelines often are provided (see Figure 8-4). Underlying all care and treatment the client receives is the goal to restore the client, if possible, to the level of wellness that preceded hospitalization.

In collaboration with the RN, the LVN/LPN helps the client to clarify goals for discharge by assisting the client in anticipating and solving problems. For example, the client who lives alone may realize that he or she will need help to carry out activities of daily living (ADLs) and to follow discharge instructions. A goal would be set to obtain help and support from significant others, home health care, or other available agencies. The social worker may be notified and may provide special assistance in obtaining help and support.

Client outcomes and timelines are also developed to help the client and family in the transition. For example, for a very weak client, an initial goal might be to work gradually toward full participation in ADLs over a period of two weeks (if this is in keeping with physician orders). The plan may include slowly increasing the time spent on each activity, or selecting one or two activities to complete and gradually increasing the number as strength permits.

The example of problem solving given above relates to planning (goal setting), but it is also an example of the implementation process associated with discharge. Perhaps the most important nursing actions at discharge are those directed toward giving the client the appropriate oral presentation and written resources related to discharge instructions. For example, if a particular diet is recommended, then the nutritionist can be contacted to discuss the diet with the client and provide helpful materials and menu ideas. Printed instructions are available on many topics and in almost every language (examples: insulin self-administration, dressing changes, and mobility devices). Large-print materials are also available.

However, the nurse must not simply give the client a pack of printed brochures or information sheets and consider the discharge process complete. Printed materials are intended as an information supplement and as a reference. Every discharge instruction should be explained verbally to the client. During oral instruction, the client should be encouraged to ask questions. The client should paraphrase the instructions, and the nurse should listen carefully to determine whether the client interprets the instructions accurately. Whenever possible, the nurse should ask the client to demonstrate procedures listed in the discharge instructions.

In addition to discharge instructions related to medical care, the client should also be informed about what to expect in convalescence, what symptoms to report and to whom, and what to regard as an emergency. Often, a number of physicians in different specialties have attended the client. The client may be confused about which one to call. Review physician names and phone numbers and scheduled appointments, or give directions for scheduling appointments.

The most important fact about discharge is not a set of discharge instructions but the client's departure. Saying goodbye and wishing the client well are aspects of nursing care that, in themselves, promote client well-being. An acknowledged departure provides closure for the client and for the nursing staff and can be personally satisfying to both.

EVALUATING

Evaluation of the discharge process involves reporting to the nurse manager that discharge is completed. There is usually a release form (obtained from the business office at the time of discharge) that is returned to the nurse manager. Details about the discharge (time, who accompanied client, type of transportation) and the client's reaction are recorded on the medical record.

Either at the time of discharge or shortly after (through the mail), the client is given the opportunity to evaluate the nursing care and other aspects of hospitalization. Each facility has its own procedure for reviewing and disseminating the information. Generally, though, evaluations are shared with the nursing staff in the form of reports.

Note: The bibliography listings for this and all chapters have been compiled at the back of the book.

Chapter Review

Key Terms by Topics

Use the audio glossary feature of either the CD-ROM or the Companion Website to hear the correct pronunciation of the following key terms.

Admitting a client
admission, coping behaviors, dehumanization, orientation

Transferring a client
transfer

Discharging a Client
discharge, against medical advice (AMA)

Key Points

* Nurses can significantly affect how the client views and experiences the admission, transfer, and discharge processes.
* The client's feelings about admission help to determine the success of the hospital stay.
* The LPN/LVN participates in the baseline assessment of the new client.
* Common reactions of newly admitted client include anxiety, loss of independence, loss of identity and, in children, separation anxiety.
* Nurses are responsible for giving culturally sensitive care.
* The client's belongings and valuables must be properly identified and safely stored.
* Client transfer requires adherence to certain procedures designed to keep the client safe and comfortable during the process.
* Discharge planning and teaching actually begin during the admission process.
* The emphasis of nursing care during the discharge process is to assist the client in understanding the discharge instructions accurately and planning for any problems that may arise.

EXPLORE MediaLink

Additional Interactive resources for this chapter can be found on the Companion Website at www.prenhall.com/ramont. Click on Chapter 8 and "Begin" to select the activities for this chapter.

For chapter-related NCLEX-style questions and an audio glossary, access the accompanying CD-ROM in this book.

For Further Study

For further information about needs as identified by Maslow, see Figure 4-4 and discussion in Chapter 24.

For more about maintaining the client's integrity and personal dignity, see Chapter 23.

For more details on the nursing process, see Chapter 4.

Further steps to improve cultural sensitivity are discussed in detail in Chapter 26.

For additional information about legal issues, see Chapter 2.

For further study on head-to-toe assessment, see Chapter 11; for vital signs assessment, Chapter 14; and for obtaining urine specimens, Chapter 18.

Critical Thinking Care Map

Caring for a Client Prior to Discharge

NCLEX-PN Focus Area: Coping and Adaptation

Case Study: Amanda Carr is an 86-year-old client being discharged from the Rehabilitation Unit to an assisted living center. Two months ago, after a fall, she had a hip replacement. She has been in the medical center's rehab unit since that time. Before surgery, she lived with her two cats in a second-floor apartment with an outdoor metal staircase. Mrs. Carr is scheduled to leave the hospital in 1 week. She is resisting discharge planning and insists she is returning home. "My cats need me, and I can make do."

Nursing Diagnosis: Ineffective Individual Coping

COLLECT DATA

Subjective

_____
_____
_____
_____
_____
_____
_____

Objective

_____
_____
_____
_____
_____
_____

Would you report this data? Yes/No

If yes, to: _____

Nursing Care

_____
_____
_____
_____
_____
_____
_____
_____
_____
_____
_____
_____
_____

How would you document this? _____
_____
_____
_____
_____

Data Collected

(*use those that apply*)

- "My cats need me, and I can make do."
- Daughter says client very independent
- Unsafe environment at home (outdoor entry and metal stairs)
- Chart indicates noncompliance with discharge plan to assisted living facility.
- Height 5'9"
- Weight 100 lbs
- Reports "Nurses all mumble."

Nursing Interventions

(*use those that apply*)

- Maintain a calm, quiet manner.
- Demonstrate firmness in seeking cooperation.
- Assess level of understanding regarding discharge and transfer.
- Explain purpose of transfer to assisted living.
- Encourage statement of concerns.
- Isolate from other clients.
- Allow time to answer questions about the assisted living facility.
- Inquire about family members who live in the area.

NCLEX-PN Exam Preparation

1. Which statement is least dehumanizing to a client?
   a. "The new total abdominal hysterectomy client has been oriented to room."
   b. "Billy, the 24-year-old with the femur fracture, will need crutches ordered."
   c. "The client in 256 needs a pair of slippers."
   d. "Miss Smith, who just came back from surgery, is requesting a private room."

2. The nurse's understanding of culturally sensitive communication is best illustrated by:
   a. Referring to a Native American as Indian
   b. Addressing clients by first name to reduce anxiety
   c. Speaking in a loud but clear voice using simple words
   d. Arranging an interpreter for the Hispanic client who speaks no English

3. What is the priority goal for a client during admission, transfer, and discharge?
   a. Ensuring the continuity of individualized care
   b. Beginning discharge planning after the physician writes discharge orders
   c. Assisting the adult client to use the proper coping skills throughout his or her stay
   d. Assessing the adult client's knowledge regarding the disease process

4. All the following tasks need to be completed prior to transfer of a client in respiratory distress. Which is the **priority** task?
   a. Answer the client's and significant others' questions related to visiting hours in the intensive care unit (ICU).
   b. Call the registered nurse (RN) to answer the significant others' questions related to the transfer process.
   c. Give report to the RN.
   d. Arrange for and place the adult client on portable oxygen prior to transfer.

5. The RN delegates the admission of a new client. In what aspects of the admission process should the LPN/LVN participate?
   a. Formulation of the nursing diagnosis related to anxiety caused by the admission process
   b. Collection of data regarding the confused client's mental status and placing him or her in restraints
   c. Collection of baseline subjective and objective data delegated by the RN
   d. Development of the treatment plan to ensure the client progresses to the optimal level of independence

6. A newly admitted adult client in an acute care facility says to the nurse, "Please put my wallet, watch, and rings in the drawer for me." Which of the following best expresses facility policy about valuables?

   a. "Don't worry, I'll leave your things in the drawer here next to your bed."
   b. "Is there a family member here who could take these things home for you?"
   c. "Valuables all need to be stored in the safe."
   d. "I need to inventory and document your personal belongings."

7. In caring for all of the following persons, which one is most in need of discharge planning?
   a. A 70-year-old male, who is being discharged to the skilled unit for rehabilitation
   b. A 24-year-old female, who broke her left tibia while skiing and who lives with her husband
   c. A 38-year-old female, who is a newly diagnosed diabetic beginning insulin therapy
   d. A 64 year old, African-American male with a 20-year history of hypertension, controlled by medication

8. A female client is new to the unit, and diagnostic tests are ordered. The client does not have a readable identification band in place. What should the LPN/LVN do?
   a. Call registration to replace the identification band before sending her for the test.
   b. Report this to the charge RN, then send her for the test.
   c. Replace the identification band after sending the client for the test.
   d. Ask the client for her name, send her for the test so there is no delay in treatment, and replace the identification band when she returns.

9. A client is admitted to the pediatric unit. When caring for pediatric clients, which principle is most important to remember?
   a. Encourage the parents to stay with the child throughout the admission process.
   b. Hold the pediatric client to build trust during the admission process.
   c. Speak in a normal tone and clearly.
   d. Reassure the child that the shot will not hurt.

10. The LPN/LVN is preparing to transfer an adult client to the Intensive Care Unit from the Surgical Unit. The nurse can improve the client's comfort by which intervention?
    a. Prior to transfer, position the client on his side to allow visualization of the hall as he is transferred.
    b. Call the client by her first name when you introduce her to the intensive care staff.
    c. Reinforce the need for transfer to intensive care and answer any questions the client or significant others may have.
    d. Give a bedside report to the ICU nurse so the client can hear their condition is stable and they will be less anxious.

Answers for Review Questions, as well as Case Study and Critical Thinking Care Map questions, appear in Appendix IV.

Chapter 9

Documenting and Reporting

SHARING experiences

"The hardest thing to get used to in computerized documentation was not having something in our hand to look at. At first, documentation and information retrieval took a lot longer because we forgot how to navigate to certain areas, but it got faster as we went along. Not having typed before made it very challenging for some of us [who had to use] the hunt-and-peck method of typing. Having terminals in the client's rooms was the best, though. That's where we needed information a lot of the time and it's so easy to look it up right there, especially when your instructor or family is asking questions."

Comments by Vocational Nursing Class II, Fall 2002, Extended Health Education, Arlington, TX.

LEARNING outcomes

After completing this chapter, you will be able to:

- Identify and discuss guidelines for effective recording that meet legal and ethical standards.
- List the measures used to maintain the confidentiality of records, including computer records.
- Discuss reasons for keeping client records.
- Identify essential guidelines for reporting client data.
- Identify abbreviations and symbols commonly used for charting.
- Describe the nurse's role in reporting, conferring, and making referrals.
- Compare and contrast different documentation systems.
- Explain how various forms in the client record are used to document steps of the nursing process.
- Compare and contrast the documentation needed for clients in acute care, home health care, and long-term care settings.

MediaLink

 www.prenhall.com/ramont

Use the address above to access the free, interactive Companion Website created for this textbook. Get hints, instant feedback, and textbook references to chapter-related NCLEX-style questions. Link to other interesting sites.

Audio Glossary:
Use the Companion Website, or the CD-ROM disk enclosed with your textbook, to hear the pronunciation of key terms in the chapter.

Effective communication among health professionals is vital to the quality of client care. Generally, health personnel communicate through discussion, reports, and records. A *discussion* is an informal conversation between two or more health care personnel to identify a problem or establish strategies to resolve a problem. A **report** is an oral, written, or computer-based communication intended to convey information to others. For example, nurses always report on clients at the end of a work shift. A **record** is a written or computer-based collection of data. The process of making an entry on a client record is called *recording*, **charting**, or **documenting.** A **clinical record,** also called a *chart* or *client record*, is the formal, legal document that provides evidence of a client's care. Although health care organizations use different systems and forms for documentation, all client records have similar information.

Each health care organization has policies about recording and reporting client data, and each nurse is accountable for practicing according to these standards. Agencies also indicate which nursing assessments and interventions must be recorded by a nurse and those items that may be delegated to unlicensed personnel. In addition, the Joint Commission on Accreditation of Healthcare Organizations (JCAHO) has policies on information management which specify that record keeping should be timely, accurate, confidential, and client specific (JCAHO, 2000).

 ## Purposes of Client Records

COMMUNICATION
The client record serves as the vehicle by which different health professionals who interact with a client communicate with each other. This prevents fragmentation, repetition, and delays in client care. The record also provides a central location for notifying health professionals of the client's needs, progress, and current health status.

PLANNING CLIENT CARE
Each health professional uses data from the client's record to plan care for that client. A physician, for example, may determine that laboratory tests reveal the presence of a certain microorganism and then orders an antibiotic. Nurses then use baseline and ongoing assessments to determine effectiveness of interventions and the nursing care plan. The record also provides a base from which all disciplines may coordinate the client's care.

LEGAL DOCUMENTATION
The client's record is a legal document and is admissible in court as evidence. In some jurisdictions, however, the record is considered inadmissible as evidence when the client objects, because information the client gives to the physician is confidential. A record is usually considered the property of the agency. The client generally has a right to a copy of the information, though the client will need to make a written request for the information and may need to pay a copying fee.

EDUCATION, RESEARCH, AND HEALTH CARE ANALYSIS
Students use client records as an essential educational tool. A record can frequently provide a comprehensive view of the client, the illness, treatment strategies, and factors that affect the outcome of the illness. The information contained in a record can be a valuable source of data for research. Review of treatment plans for clients with the same health problems can yield helpful information for treating new clients.

Likewise, information from records may assist health care planners to identify agency needs. It can highlight overused and underused hospital services. It can identify services that cost the agency money and those that generate revenue.

AUDITING
An audit is a review of records. Client records are audited for quality assurance. Accrediting agencies such as JCAHO may review client records to determine if a particular health agency is meeting its stated standards.

REIMBURSEMENT
Documentation also helps a facility receive reimbursement from the federal government. For a facility to obtain payment through Medicare, the client's clinical record must contain the correct diagnosis-related group (DRG) codes and reveal that the appropriate care has been given.

 ## Guidelines for Recording

Because the client's record is a legal document and may be used to provide evidence in court, many factors are considered in recording. Health care personnel must not only maintain the confidentiality of the client's record but also meet legal standards in the process of recording.

DATE AND TIME
- Document the date and time with each entry.
- Make entries as soon as possible after performing an assessment or intervention.
- Record the time either using conventional time, denoting A.M. or P.M., or using the 24-hour clock (military time). Follow agency policy (Figure 9-1 ◆).
- Avoid block-style charting in which an entire shift is documented under one date and time.

TIMING
- Follow agency policy regarding the frequency of documenting.
- Adjust frequency of documentation as a client's condition indicates. An unstable client requires more frequent assessment and documentation than a stable client.
- Never record nursing care before it is provided.

Figure 9-1. ◆ 24-hour clock.

LEGIBILITY

♦ Make all entries legible and easy to read to prevent inter-pretation errors.
♦ Print your entries if your cursive writing is difficult to read.
♦ Follow agency policy regarding handwritten recording of nurse's notes.

PERMANENCE

♦ Make all entries on the client's record in blue or black ink according to agency policy. This ensures that the record is permanent and that changes can be identified.

ACCEPTED TERMINOLOGY

♦ Use only commonly accepted abbreviations, symbols, and terms specified by agency policy. See Table 9-1 ◆ for com-mon abbreviations and Table 9-2 ◆ for common symbols. See Chapter 21 for abbreviations related to medication administration. ⊘
♦ Write a term out in full if in doubt about whether to use an abbreviation.

CORRECT SPELLING

♦ Use correct spelling to ensure accuracy in documentation.
♦ Look words up in a dictionary or other resource book if unsure of the correct spelling.
♦ Spell similar medication names correctly to avoid medica-tion errors. (For example, *Celebrex* and *Cerebyx* are two decidedly different medications.)

SIGNATURE

♦ Sign entries made in the nurses' notes at the time you make the entry.

♦ Use the name and title in the signature. For example, the signatures "Susan J. Green, LPN" or "S. Green, LPN" would be correct, depending on facility policy.
♦ Use correct title abbreviations: RN for registered nurse, LPN for licensed practical nurse, LVN for licensed voca-tional nurse, SN for student nurse in an RN program, and SVN/SPN for student vocational/practical nurse. (Some schools use VNS or PNS for Vocational/Practical Nursing student.)

ACCURACY

♦ Check that you have the correct chart by verifying the client's name and identification information stamped or written on each page before making any entry or filing a report.
♦ Make accurate notations—ones that consist of facts or observations rather than opinions or interpretations. Describe what you see and hear, not what what you think or interpret for client actions.
♦ Quote the client directly in the client's exact words when documenting client's concerns. For example, "Stated: 'I'm worried about my leg.'"
♦ Chart specific data rather than using general terms such as large, good, or normal that can be misinterpreted. For example, "2 cm by 3 cm bruise" is more accurate than "large bruise."
♦ Document a description of behavior you observed rather than using terms such as anxiety or agitation.

TABLE 9-2 COMMONLY USED SYMBOLS

SYMBOL	TERM	SYMBOL	NUMBER
>	greater than	$\bar{o}$	0
<	less than	$\overline{ss}$	1/2
=	equal to	ī	1
↑	increased	īi	2
↓	decreased	īii	3
♀	female	īv	4
♂	male	v̄	5
°	degree	v̄i	6
#	number; fracture	v̄ii	7
ʒ	dram	v̄iii	8
℥	ounce	īx	9
×	times	x̄	10
@	at		

TABLE 9-1 COMMONLY USED ABBREVIATIONS

ABBREVIATION	TERM	ABBREVIATION	TERM
abd	abdomen	nil (o⁻)	none
ABO	the main blood group system	no. (#)	number
ac	before meals (ante cibum)	NPO (NBM)	nothing by mouth (per os)
ADL	activities of daily living	NS (N/S)	normal saline
ad lib	as desired (ad libitum)	O_2	oxygen
adm	admitted or admission	od	daily (omni die)
am	morning (ante meridiem)	OD	right eye (oculus dexter); overdose
amb	ambulatory	OOB	out of bed
amt	amount	os	mouth or opening
approx	approximately (about)	OS	left eye (oculus sinister)
bid	twice daily (bis in die)	pc	after meals (post cibum)
BM (bm)	bowel movement	PE (PX)	physical examination
BP	blood pressure	per	by or through
BR	bed rest	pm	afternoon (post meridiem)
BRP	bathroom privileges	po	by mouth (per os)
C⁻ (C)	with	postop	postoperative (ly)
C	Celsius (centigrade)	preop	preoperative (ly)
CBC	complete blood count	prep	preparation
CBR	complete bed rest	prn	when necessary (pro re nata)
Cl	client	pt	patient
c/o	complains of	q	every (quaque)
DAT	diet as tolerated	qd	every day (quaque die)
dc (disc)	discontinue	qh (q1h)	every hour (quaque hora)
drsg	dressing	q2h, q3h, and so on	every 2 hours, 3 hours, and so on
Dx	diagnosis	qhs	every night at bedtime (quaque hora somni)
ECG (EKG)	electrocardiogram	qid	four times a day (quater in die)
F	Fahrenheit	req	requisition
fld	fluid	Rt (rt, R)	right
GI	gastrointestinal	S (s⁻)	without (sine)
GP	general practitioner	SI	seriously ill
gtt	drops (guttae)	spec	specimen
h (hr)	hour (hora)	stat	at once, immediately (statim)
H_2O	water	tid	three times a day (ter in die)
hs	at bedtime (hora somni)	TL	team leader
I&O	intake and output	TLC	tender loving care
IV	intravenous	TPR	temperature, pulse, respirations
Lab	laboratory	Tr	tincture
liq	liquid	VO	verbal order
LMP	last menstrual period	VS (vs)	vital signs
lt (L)	left	WNL	within normal limits
meds	medications	wt	weight
mL (ml)	milliliter		
mod	moderate		
neg	negative		

◆ Correct an error in documentation by drawing a single line through it and writing the word error above it, with your initials or name, depending on agency policy.

◆ Do not erase, overwrite, blot out, or use correction fluid. The original entry must remain visible.

◆ Write on every line but never between lines.

◆ Draw a line through any blank space and sign the notation. In this way, no additional information can be recorded at any other time or by any other person.

◆ Never leave blank lines above your entry or between your entries (Figure 9-2 ◆).

SEQUENCE

◆ Document events in the order in which they occur: assessments, interventions, and client responses.

◆ Make a late entry by clearly labeling your entry as late according to facility policy. For example, "Late entry 12/1/05 0400" or "1/1/06 0400 Late entry" could be correct.

◆ Do not make a late entry more than 24 hours after the event. This is not usually permitted (see Figure 9-2).

Date	Time	Nursing Note
1/1/04	0015	BP 150/82, P 92 irregular/irregular EKG leads in place, Resp 22
		unlabored O_2 2L/min via N/C. NG tube placement verified via
		auscultation and litmus strip testing, low intermittent suction
		continues. C/O nausea, phenergan 25mg suppository given rectally.
		Color normal for race, skin warm and dry to touch. --------S. Oradei LPN
----------	--------	--- ----
1/1/04	0200	Wakeful watching TV states relief of nausea. ----------------S. Oradei LPN
1/1/04	0600	~~BP 152/90~~ error S.O. -- BP 152/80, P 90 irregular/irregular EKG leads
		in place. Resp 24 unlabored O_2 2L/min via NC occasional dry
		non-productive cough, lung sounds clear to auscultation. Denies
		nausea at this time. ---S. Oradei LPN
1/1/04	0400	Late entry – Telemetry unit reports irregular signal. Leads checked,
		lead left low chest loose, pad replaced and lead reattached. Verified
		signal with telemetry.---S. Oradei LPN
1/1/04	0700	Vomited approximately 100cc of dark green liquid, black flecks noted
		in emesis. Denies nausea prior to emesis---(Continued) --S. Oradai LPN
Jones, Adam (male - 51y/o) / 410A / Dr. A. Amsterdamm / Partial Gastrectomy , A.Fib, HTN / NKDA

Date	Time	Nursing Notes
1/1/04	0700	(Continued) – and denies nausea at this time. BP 168/90, P 100
		irregular/irregular, Resp 26 O_2 2L/min via N/C, no cough noted at this
		time. Color pale, skin moist. .----------------------------------S. Oradai LPN
1/1/04	0715	Dr. Amsterdamm notified of client condition, no new orders noted.
		--S. Oradai LPN
01/01/04	0800	Dr. Amsterdamm to see client. New orders noted for IV Zantac BID, and labs to be
		drawn stat. Lab & Pharmacy notified.--------------------------- *K. Hamrick LPN*

Figure 9-2. ◆ Sample narrative notes with error correction, a skipped line, and a continued note.

CONTINUED NOTES

◆ Continue entries to another page by indicating that the note continues and signing the entry. On the next page, enter the date/time of the note and start it by indicating that it is a continuation (see Figure 9-2).

APPROPRIATENESS AND COMPLETENESS

◆ Record only information that pertains to the client's health problems and care.
◆ Record all assessments, dependent and independent nursing interventions, client problems, client comments and responses to interventions and tests, progress toward goals, and communication with other disciplines.
◆ Document any care that was omitted and include why it was omitted and who was notified.

CONCISENESS

◆ Do not use the client's name or the word *client* in documentation. This helps keep notes brief and saves time.
◆ End each thought or sentence with a period; it is not necessary to use complete sentences.
◆ Write notes so that data that follows a comma is associated with the data that preceded it.

LEGAL PRUDENCE

◆ Document accurately and completely to protect the health care staff, the facility, and the client. The clinical record is a legal document that provides proof of the quality of care given to a client.
◆ Follow the general principle, "If it isn't charted, it wasn't done."
◆ Follow agency policy and procedures for intervention and documentation in all situations, especially high-risk situations.
◆ Do not record the words "incident report completed" in the nursing notes when an unexpected event occurs. Incident reports are for the agency's use and are not generally a part of the client's record.

ADDITIONAL TIPS FOR DOCUMENTATION

Special care is needed when caring for clients with the same last name to prevent documentation mistakes. Many agencies have a policy about flagging charts when name confusion could occur. Do not identify charts by room number only.

When you are charting, be sure to use objective, factual information rather than opinions or interpretations. It is more accurate, for example, to write that a client "refused medication" (fact) than to write that the client "was uncooperative" (opinion). To write that a client "was crying" (observation) is preferable to noting that the client "was depressed" (interpretation).

Not all data about a client should be recorded. Any personal information the client shares that does not pertain to the client's health problems and care is inappropriate for the record.

Recording irrelevant information may be considered an invasion of the client's privacy and could be considered libelous.

For the best legal protection, the nurse should not only adhere to professional standards of nursing care but also follow agency policy and procedures for intervention and documentation in all situations, especially high-risk situations. Below is an example of such documentation:

1100 hours—Complained of feeling dizzy. Raised side rails and instructed to stay in bed and ring call bell if requiring assistance. 1130 hours—found beside bed on floor. Said, "I climbed over these rails all by myself." When asked about pain, replied, "I feel fine but a little dizzy." Helped into bed. BP 100/60 P 90 R 24. Dr. RJ Naden notified. _____ RS Woo LVN

Documentation is the determining factor in a great percentage of malpractice cases involving client care, so it is important that you document client care clearly, concisely, and accurately.

◆ Confidentiality of Client Records

The client's record is protected legally as a private record of the client's care. Access to the record is restricted to health professionals directly involved in giving care to the client. Insurance companies, for example, have no legal right to demand access to medical records, even though they may be determining compensation to the client. Therefore, a client who is making a claim for compensation may ask to have the medical history used as evidence. In order for an agency to provide the requested information, the client must sign an authorization for review, copying, or release of information from the record. This form must specifically indicate what information is to be released and to whom. A nurse should not allow access to a client's record by significant others or any person other than the health care providers who are directly involved in the care of the client.

For purposes of education and research, most agencies allow student and graduate health professionals access to client records. The records are used in client conferences, clinics, rounds, and written papers or client studies. The student is bound by a strict ethical code to hold all information in confidence. It is the responsibility of the student and health professionals to protect the client's privacy by not using a name or any statements in the notations that would identify the client. Additionally, it is very important for staff and students to maintain confidentiality with worksheets and assignment sheets. Caution must be used to ensure that papers are not left where visitors and clients may see them.

ENSURING CONFIDENTIALITY OF COMPUTER RECORDS

Because of the increased use of computerized client records, health care agencies have developed policies and procedures to ensure the privacy and confidentiality of client information stored in computers. The following are some suggestions for ensuring the confidentiality of computerized records:

1. Each health care worker needs a password to enter and sign off computer files. Do not share this password with anyone. Do not write down your password where others may find it.
2. After logging on, never leave a computer terminal unattended. If your agency provides hand-held computers, ensure that you do not leave it unattended.
3. Do not leave client information displayed on the monitor where others may see it.
4. Follow agency procedures for documenting sensitive material. The confidentiality of computerized documents is the same as with paper charts.

Documentation Systems

A number of documentation systems are in current use: source-oriented record, problem-oriented record, PIE, Focus Charting, charting by exception, FACT, CORE, outcome documentation, computerized documentation, and case management.

SOURCE-ORIENTED RECORD

The traditional client record is source oriented. Each person or department makes notations in a separate section or sections of the client's chart In the **source-oriented record,** information about a particular problem is distributed throughout the record. For example, if a client had *left hemiplegia* (paralysis of the left side of the body), data about this problem might be found in the physician's history sheet, on the physician's order sheet, in the nurses' notes, in the physical therapist's record, and in the social service record. See Table 9-3 ◆ for the components of a source-oriented record.

Narrative charting is a traditional part of the source-oriented record. It consists of written notes that include routine care, normal findings, and client problems. There is no right or wrong order to the information, although chronological order is most frequently used. Currently, narrative recording is being replaced by other systems, such as PIE and Focus. Narrative charting is expedient in emergency situations or when the space provided on a flow sheet is insufficient for the information which needs to be documented (see Figure 9-2 for an example of a narrative note).

Source-oriented records are convenient because care providers from each discipline can easily locate the forms on which to record data and it is easy to trace the information specific to one's discipline. The disadvantage is that information about a specific problem is scattered throughout the chart, so it can be difficult to find chronological information on a client's problems and progress.

PROBLEM-ORIENTED MEDICAL RECORD

In the **problem-oriented medical record (POMR),** or *problem-oriented record (POR),* established by Lawrence Weed in the 1960s, the data are arranged according to the individual problems the client has rather than the source of the information. All of the members of the health care team contribute to the same problem list, plan of care, and progress notes. Plans for each active or potential problem are drawn up, and progress notes are recorded for each problem.

The advantages of POMR are that it encourages collaboration, and that the problem list in the front of the chart alerts caregivers to the client's needs and makes it easier to track the status of each problem. Its disadvantages are that caregivers differ in their ability to use the required charting format, it takes constant vigilance to maintain an up-to-date problem list, and it is somewhat inefficient because assessments and interventions that apply to more than one problem must be repeated.

The POR has four basic components: database, problem list, plan of care, and progress notes. In addition, flowsheets and discharge notes are added to the record as needed.

Database

The **database** is all of the information known about the client gathered from a variety of sources: nursing assessment, physician's history, and family. Data are constantly updated as the client's health status changes.

Problem List

The problem list (Figure 9-3 ◆) is derived from the database. It is usually kept at the front of the chart and serves as an index to the numbered entries in the progress notes. Problems are listed in the order in which they are identified, and the list is continually updated as new problems are identified and others resolved. All caregivers may contribute to the problem list, which includes the client's physiologic, psychological, social, cultural, spiritual, developmental, and environmental needs. Physicians write problems as medical diagnoses, surgical procedures, or symptoms; nurses write problems as nursing diagnoses.

As the client's condition changes or more data are obtained, it may be necessary to "redefine" problems. Figure 9-3 illustrates how this has been done for Problems 1B, 1C, and 2.

Plan of Care

The initial list of orders or plan of care is made with reference to the active problems. The person who lists the problem generates problem specific care plans. Physicians write physician's orders or medical care plans; nurses write nursing orders or nursing care plans. The RN usually writes nursing orders. The written plan in the record is listed under each problem in the progress notes (discussed next) and is not isolated as a separate list of orders.

Progress Notes

All health professionals involved in a client's care make progress notes in the POR/POMR on the same type of sheet. Updated progress notes are numbered to correspond to the problems on the record.

TABLE 9-3	COMPONENTS OF THE SOURCE-ORIENTED RECORD
FORM	**INFORMATION**
Admission (face) sheet	Legal name, birth date, age Social Security number Address Marital status; closest relatives or person to notify in case of emergency Date, time, and admitting diagnosis Food or drug allergies Name of admitting (attending) physician Insurance information Any assigned diagnosis-related group (DRG)
Initial nursing assessment	Findings from the initial nursing history and physical health assessment
Graphic record	Body temperature, pulse rate, respiratory rate, blood pressure, daily weight, and special measurements, such as fluid intake and output
Daily care record	Activity, diet, bathing, and elimination records; may also include restraints, isolation precautions
Special flowsheets	Examples: 24-hour fluid balance record
Medication record (see Chapter 33)	Name, dosage, route, time, date, site of regularly administered medications Name or initials of person administering the medication
Narrative nurses' notes	Pertinent assessment of client Specific nursing care including teaching and client's responses Client's complaints and how client is coping
Medical history and physical examination	Past and family medical history, present medical problems, differential or current diagnoses, findings of physical examination by the physician
Physician's order sheet	Medical orders for medications, treatments, and so on
Physician's progress notes	Medical observations, treatments, client progress, and so on
Consultation records	Reports by medical and clinical specialists
Diagnostic reports	Examples: laboratory reports, x-ray reports, CT scan reports
Consultation reports	Physical therapy, respiratory therapy
Client discharge plan and referral summary	Started on admission and completed upon discharge; includes nursing problems, general information, and referral data

◆ Types of Documentation Methods

There are several methods for documenting data in the progress notes: SOAP, which has evolved into SOAPIE and SOAPIER in some facilities; PIE or APIE; Focus Charting; charting by exception; FACT, CORE, or DAE format; outcome documentation; and case management.

SOAP

SOAP is an acronym for subjective data, objective data, assessment, and planning.

S—Subjective data are information obtained from what the client says. They describe the client's perceptions and expe-

rience of the problem. When possible, the nurse quotes the client's words; otherwise, they are summarized. Subjective data are included only when they are important and relevant to the problem. Refer to the section on Accuracy for more information regarding quoting the client.

O—Objective data consist of information that is measured or observed by use of the senses (e.g., vital signs, laboratory and x-ray results). Examples of subjective and objective data are provided in Chapter 4. ⟨⟩

A—Assessment is the interpretation or conclusions drawn about the subjective and objective data. During the initial assessment, the problem list is created from the database, so the initial "A" entry should be a statement of the problem, such as in a nursing diagnosis. In all subsequent

No.	Date Entered	Date Inactive	Client Problem
#1	3/9/05		CVA resulting in Rt hemiplegia and left-sided weakness
#1A	3/9/05		Self-care deficit (hygiene, toileting, grooming, feeding)
#1B	3/9/05		Impaired physical mobility (unable to turn and position self) Redefined 2/7/03
#1C	3/9/05		Total urinary incontinence Redefined 1/17/02
#1D	3/9/05		Progressive dysphasia
#2	3/9/05		Constipation r/t immobility Redefined 6/10/01
#3	3/9/05		History of depression
#4	3/9/05		Essential hypertension
~~#5~~	~~6/6/05~~	~~7/11/05~~	~~Pruritus~~
#2	*6/10/05*		*Risk for constipation r/t insufficient fiber intake*
#1C	1/17/06		Nocturnal urinary incontinence
#1B	2/7/07		Impaired physical mobility (needs major assistance to transfer and walk)

Figure 9-3. ◆ Client problem list in the POR system.

SOAP notes for that problem, the "A" should describe the client's condition and level of progress rather than merely restating the diagnosis or problem.

P—The plan is the plan of care designed to resolve the stated problem. The person who entered the problem into the record writes the initial plan. All subsequent plans, including revisions, are entered into the progress notes.

Over the years, the SOAP format has been modified. The acronyms SOAPIE and SOAPIER refer to formats that add interventions, evaluation, and revision.

I—Intervention refers to the specific interventions that have actually been performed by the caregiver.

E—Evaluation includes client responses to nursing interventions and medical treatments. This is primarily reassessment data.

R—Revision reflects care plan modifications suggested by the evaluation. Changes may be made in desired outcomes, interventions, or target dates.

See Figure 9-4 ◆ for an example of progress notes using the SOAP, SOAPIER, and PIE formats.

PIE/APIE CHARTING

PIE charting, which is similar to SOAPIE charting, stands for problem, intervention, and evaluation and is based on the nursing process. PIE charting consists mainly of assessment flowsheets and progress notes. On admission, the nurse, generally an RN, completes a thorough assessment and identifies and documents specific problems on the progress notes using NANDA diagnoses. If there is no NANDA diagnosis for the client's particular problem, then a problem statement is formulated based

SOAP Format

2/13/05 #5 Generalized pruritus

1400 S—"My skin is itchy on my
         back and arms, and it's been
         like this for a week."

      O—Skin appears clear—no rash
         or irritations noted. Marks where
         client has scratched noted on
         left and right forearms. Allergic
         to elastoplast but has not been
         in contact.
         No previous history of pruritus.

      A—Altered comfort (pruritus): cause
         unknown.

      P—Instructed to not scratch skin.
         —Applied calamine lotion to back
         and arms at 1430 h.
         —Cut fingernails.
         —Assess further to determine
         whether recurrence associated
         with specific drugs or foods.
         —Refer to physician and
         pharmacist for assessment.
         S. Myers LVN

SOAPIER Format

2/13/05 #5 Generalized pruritus

1400 S—"My skin is itchy on my
         back and arms, and it's been
         like this for a week."

      O—Skin appears clear—no rash
         or irritation noted. Marks where
         client has scratched noted on
         left and right forearms. Allergic
         to elastoplast but has not been
         in contact.
         No previous history of pruritus.

      A—Altered comfort.

      P—Instruct to not scratch skin.
         —Apply calamine lotion
         as necessary.
         —Cut nails to avoid scratches.
         —Assess further to determine
         whether recurrence associated
         with specific drugs or foods.
         —Refer to physician and
         pharmacist for assessment.

      I —Instructed not to scratch skin.
         Applied calamine lotion to back
         and arms at 1430 h.
         Assisted to cut fingernails.
         Notified physician and
         pharmacist of problem.

1600 E—States, "I'm still itchy. That
         lotion didn't help."

      R—Remove calamine lotion and
         apply hydrocortisone ungt. as
         ordered.   S. Myers LVN

APIE Format

2/13/05 #5 Generalized pruritus r/t unknown cause

1400   States, "My skin is itchy on my
         back and arms, and it's been like
         this for a week." Skin appears clear.
         No rash or irritations noted. Marks
         where client has scratched noted
         on left and right forearms. Allergic
         to elastoplast but has not been in
         contact. No previous history of
         pruritus.
         Instructed not to scratch skin.
         Applied calamine lotion to back
         and arms at 1430 h.
         Assisted to cut fingernails.
         Notified physician and pharmacist
         of problem.
         States, "I'm still itchy. That
         lotion didn't help."
         S. Myers LVN

Figure 9-4. ◆ SOAPIER and PIE charting examples. Nurse's signature is required whenever charting is done.

on the NANDA format (see Chapter 4). 🔗 Each problem is numbered P1, P2, P3, and so on. As problems are revised, the numbers are changed to P1A, P1B, and so on. Interventions and evaluations are numbered similarly (see Figure 9-4).

After the initial assessment, 24-hour flowsheets are used, which include specific assessment criteria in a structured format. Some PIE systems use APIE wherein "A" stands for assessment. The assessment data are included in your problem list to support the PIE portion of the documentation.

The PIE or APIE system eliminates the traditional care plan by incorporating an ongoing care plan into the progress notes. The major disadvantage is that the nurse must review all of the progress notes before giving care, to determine which problems are current and which interventions were effective.

FOCUS CHARTING

Focus Charting is intended to make the client and client concerns and strengths the focus of care. Three columns for recording are usually used: date and time, focus, and progress notes (see the example at the end of this section). The focus may be a condition, a nursing diagnosis, a behavior, a sign or symptom, an acute change in the client's condition, or a client's strength. The progress notes are organized into data (**D**), action (**A**), and response (**R**), referred to as **DAR.** The data category consists of observations of client status and behaviors, including data from flowsheets (e.g., vital signs, pupil reactivity). The nurse records both subjective and objective data in this section.

The action category includes immediate and future nursing actions. It may also include any changes to the plan of care. The response category describes the client's response to any nursing and medical care.

The Focus Charting system provides a holistic perspective of the client and the client's needs. It also provides a framework for the progress notes (DAR). The three components do not need to be recorded in order and each note does not need to have all three categories. Flowsheets are frequently used on the client's chart to augment recording data.

Date/Hour	Focus	Progress Notes
2/11/04 0900	Neuro status	**D**: Unresponsive to verbal stimuli; responsive to painful stimuli. Pupils pinpoint and equal. Dr. Ward visited. **A**: Neuro assessment and V/S q2h. **R**: See flowsheets. S. Myers LVN

CORE

The CORE documentation system focuses on the nursing process. It consists of a database, plans of care, flowsheets, progress notes, and discharge summary. CORE documentation calls for assessing the client's functional and cognitive status within 8 hours of admission (Springhouse, 1995, p. 91).

The progress notes use a DAE format:

Data
Action
Evaluation

This system has been found to be most useful in acute care and long-term care facilities.

CHARTING BY EXCEPTION

Charting by exception (CBE) is a documentation system in which only significant findings or exceptions to norms are recorded. CBE involves three distinct components:

1. Unique flowsheets that highlight significant findings and define assessment parameters and findings. The flowsheets include a sheet for the nursing and physician orders to perform assessments or interventions, the graphic record (see Figure 9-5 ◆), the client teaching record, and the client discharge note.
2. Documentation by reference to the agency's printed standards of nursing practice. This eliminates much of the repetitive charting of routine care. An agency using CBE must develop its own specific standards or definitions of nursing practice that identify the minimum criteria for client care or status regardless of clinical area. Some units may also have unit-specific standards unique to their type of client; for example, "The nurse must ensure that the unconscious client has oral care at least q4h." Documentation of care according to these specified standards involves only a check mark in the routine standards box on the graphic record. If all the standards are not implemented an asterisk or other mark is made on the flowsheet with reference to the nurses' notes. All exceptions to the standards are fully described in narrative form on the nurses' notes.
3. Documentation forms at the bedside. Flowsheets are kept at the client's bedside for immediate recording. This eliminates the need to transcribe data from the nurse's worksheet to the permanent record.

FACT

The FACT system of documentation is named for its elements. It has many similarities to CBE and is designed to eliminate redundant and irrelevant data and inconsistencies in recording. The four main elements are:

Flowsheets that are individualized
Assessment sheet that is standardized with baseline parameters
Concise integrated progress notes and flowsheets that are used to document the client's condition and response
Timely entries that are recorded after care is given

To use FACT documentation, the nurse must start with a complete database on each client. Only significant information and exceptions to the normal are recorded. The comprehensive assessment is recorded on an assessment action flowsheet. Another flowsheet is used for frequent assessments, such as blood pressure or neurological assessments. Progress notes are written in narrative style to document a client's clinical progress and any significant changes in health status.

This system of documentation is computer ready, and it eliminates duplication and supports consistent language.

OUTCOME DOCUMENTATION

This system of documentation focuses on a client's behavior. It presents the client's condition in relation to predetermined outcomes, such as, "The client's blood pressure will be 120/80 while sitting by the time of discharge."

The standards that are used to evaluate outcomes are specific client behavior, a specific standard, the conditions under which the behaviors occur, and a target date or time by which the behaviors occur.

COMPUTERIZED DOCUMENTATION

Computerized clinical record systems are rapidly being developed as a way to manage the huge volume of information required in contemporary health care. Nurses use computers to store the client's database, add new data, create and revise care plans, and document client progress (Figure 9-6 ◆). Some institutions have a computer terminal at each client's bedside, or nurses carry a small handheld unit, enabling the nurse to document care immediately after it is given.

Multiple flowsheets are not needed in computerized record systems. Information can be easily retrieved in a variety of formats, because the data is cross-indexed within the computer's program. For example, the computer can provide results of a client's blood test, a schedule of all clients on the unit who are to have surgery during the day, a suggested list of interventions for a nursing diagnosis, a graphic chart of a client's vital signs, or a printout of all the progress notes for a client. Many systems can generate a work list for the shift, with a list of all the treatments, procedures, and medications needed by the client. It is also possible to run a computer query to find out whether documentation was missed or medication is due.

Figure 9-5. ◆ Graphic flow sheet. *Source:* Courtesy of Community Hospital of Lancaster.

Computers make care planning and documentation relatively easy. To record nursing actions and client responses, the nurse either chooses from standardized lists of terms or types narrative information into the computer. Automated speech-recognition technology may allow nurses to enter data by voice and have it converted to written documentation. Handwriting-recognition technology reduces the need for typing on the handheld units. Selected pros and cons of computer documentation are shown in Box 9-1 ◆.

CASE MANAGEMENT

The case management model emphasizes quality, cost-effective care delivered within an established length of stay (LOS). This model uses a multidisciplinary approach to planning and documenting client care, using critical pathways, and is most effective when there is a predictable outcome. These forms identify the outcomes that certain groups of clients are expected to achieve on each day of care, along with the interventions necessary for each day. See Chapter 5 for more infor-

Figure 9-6. ◆ The nurse using a bedside computer. *Source:* © Elena Dorfman.

mation about critical pathways and case management. ⊘⊘ See Appendix II for a sample critical pathway. ⊘⊘

Along with critical pathways, the case management model incorporates graphics and flowsheets. Progress notes typically use some type of charting by exception. For example, if goals are met, no further charting is required. Goals that are not met are called *variances*. Deviations or variances are unexpected occurrences that affect the planned care or the client's responses to care. When a variance occurs, the nurse writes a note documenting the unexpected event, the cause, and actions taken to correct it. Or, the note may justify the actions taken. See Table 9-4 ◆ for an example of how a variance might be documented.

The case management model promotes collaboration and teamwork among caregivers, helps to decrease length of stay, and makes efficient use of time. Because care is goal focused, the quality may improve. However, critical pathways work best for clients with one or two diagnoses and few individualized needs. Clients with multiple diagnoses (e.g., a

BOX 9-1 SELECTED PROS AND CONS OF COMPUTER DOCUMENTATION

Pros

- ◆ Nurses can use their time efficiently.
- ◆ The system links various sources of client information.
- ◆ Client information, requests, and results are sent and received quickly.
- ◆ Bedside terminals can synthesize information from monitoring equipment.
- ◆ Computer records can facilitate a focus on client outcomes.
- ◆ Information is legible.
- ◆ The system incorporates and reinforces standards of care.
- ◆ Standard terminology improves communication.
- ◆ Bedside terminals eliminate need to take notes on a worksheet before recording.
- ◆ Bedside terminals permit the nurse to check an order immediately before administering a treatment or medication.
- ◆ Links to monitors improve accuracy of documentation.

Cons

- ◆ Client's privacy may be infringed on if security measures are not used.
- ◆ Breakdowns make information temporarily unavailable.
- ◆ System is expensive.
- ◆ Extended training periods may be required when a new or updated system is installed.

client with a hip fracture, pneumonia, diabetes, and pressure sore) or those with an unpredictable course of symptoms (e.g., a neurological client with seizures) are difficult to document on a critical path.

TABLE 9-4	EXAMPLE OF VARIANCE DOCUMENTATION (PORTION OF A CRITICAL PATHWAY)

An elderly client has had a below-the-knee amputation. On the third postoperative day he has a temperature of (102°F) (38.8°C). Lung sounds are clear and he is not coughing. The nurse notices redness and skin breakdown over the client's sacrum. The critical pathway outcomes specified for Day 3 are "Oral temperature <100°F" (37.7°C) and "Skin intact over bony prominences." The nurse should chart the following variances:

DATE/TIME	VARIATION	CAUSE	ACTION TAKEN/PLANS
4/16/04 0900	Elevated temperature	Possible sepsis	4/16—Blood cultures ×3 per order. Monitor temp. q1h. Monitor I&O, hydration, and mental status.
4/16/04 1130	Impaired skin integrity: pressure sore on sacrum	Client does not move about in bed unless reminded	4/16—Positioned on L side. Turn side-to-side q2h while awake. On every client contact, remind client to move about in bed. Apply Duoderm daily after bath.

◆ Reporting

Reports can be either oral or written. The purpose of reporting is to communicate specific information to a person or group of people. A report should be concise, including pertinent information but no extraneous detail.

CHANGE-OF-SHIFT REPORTS

A **change-of-shift report** is a report given to all nurses on the next shift. Its purpose is to provide continuity of care for clients by providing the new caregivers a quick summary of client needs and details of care to be given.

Change-of-shift reports may be written or given orally, either in a face-to-face exchange or by audiotape recording. The face-to-face report permits the listener to ask questions during the report. Written and tape-recorded reports are often briefer and less time consuming. Reports are sometimes given at the bedside, and clients as well as nurses may participate in the exchange of information. See Box 9-2 ◆ for key elements of a change-of-shift report. Also see information on reporting in Chapter 32. ↩

TELEPHONE REPORTS

Health professionals frequently report about a client by telephone. Nurses inform physicians about a change in a client's condition; a radiologist reports the results of an x-ray study; a nurse may confer with a nurse on another unit about a transferred client.

The nurse receiving a telephone report should document the date and time, the name of the person giving the information, and what information was received, and should sign the notation. For example:

> June 8/05 10:35 A.M. GL Messina, laboratory technician, reported by telephone that Mrs. Sara Ames's hematocrit was 39/100 ml. _____ Barbara Ireland LPN

If there is any doubt about the information given over the telephone, the person receiving the information should repeat it back to the sender to ensure accuracy.

When giving a telephone report to a physician, it is important that the nurse be concise and accurate. Begin with name and relationship to the client (e.g., "This is Jana Gomez; I'm calling about your patient, Dorothy Mendes. I'm her nurse on the 7 P.M. to 7 A.M. shift.").

Telephone reports usually include the client's name and medical diagnosis, changes in nursing assessment, vital signs related to baseline vital signs, significant laboratory data, and related nursing interventions. The nurse should have the client's chart ready to give the physician any further information.

After reporting, the nurse should document the date, time, and content of the call. (See Table 32-2 for guidelines for calling physician ↩ .) For example:

BOX 9-2 KEY ELEMENTS OF A CHANGE-OF-SHIFT REPORT

◆ Follow a particular order (e.g., follow room numbers in a hospital).

◆ Provide basic identifying information for each client (e.g., name, room number, bed designation).

◆ For new clients, provide the reason for admission or medical diagnosis (or diagnoses), surgery (date), diagnostic tests, and therapies in past 24 hours.

◆ Include significant changes in client's condition and present information in order (i.e., assessment, nursing diagnoses, interventions, outcomes, and evaluation). For example, "Mr. Ronald Oakes said he had an aching pain in his left calf at 1400 hours. Inspection revealed no other signs. Calf pain is related to altered blood circulation. Rest and elevation of his legs on a footstool for 30 minutes provided relief."

◆ Provide exact information, such as "Ms. Jessie Jones received Demerol 100 mg intramuscularly at 2000 hours," not "Ms. Jessie Jones received some Demerol during the evening."

◆ Report clients' need for special emotional support. For example, a client who has just learned that his biopsy results revealed malignancy and who is now scheduled for a laryngectomy needs time to discuss his feelings before preoperative teaching is begun.

◆ Include current nurse-prescribed and physician-prescribed orders.

◆ Provide a summary of newly admitted clients, including diagnosis, age, general condition, plan of therapy, and significant information about the client's support people.

◆ Report clients who have been transferred or discharged from the unit.

◆ Clearly state priorities of care and care that is due after the shift begins. For example, in a 7:00 A.M. report the nurse might say, "Mr. Li's vital signs are due at 0730, and his IV bag will need to be replaced by 0800." Give this information at the end of that client's report, as memory is best for the first and last information given.

◆ Be concise. Don't elaborate on background data or routine care (e.g., do not report "Vital signs at 0800 and 1200" when that is the unit standard). Do not report coming and going of visitors unless there is a problem or concern, or visitors are involved in teaching and care. Social support and visits are the norm.

2/24/05 12 noon 24-year-old Asian female admitted from ER to room 301B with c/o burning and pain URQ. BP 120/80, P 100, R 22, T 99.8. Had received Demerol 100 mg IM in ER at 11:10. States pain "10" on a scale of 1 to 10. See Admission Sheet for admission assessment. _____K.Hamrick LVN 2/24/05 12:30 states pain unchanged. Color pale and perspiring profusely. BP 100/60, P 105, R 24, T 100.4. Dr. Burns notified via telephone new order noted for stat MRI of abd. _____K. Hamrick LVN

TELEPHONE ORDERS

Physicians often order a therapy (e.g., a medication) for a client by telephone. Most agencies have specific policies about telephone orders. Some agency policies require that only registered nurses take telephone orders. (See also Chapter 32. ⬛)

When the physician gives the order, write it down and repeat it back to the physician to ensure accuracy. Question the physician about any order that is ambiguous, unusual (e.g., an abnormally high dosage of a medication), or contraindicated by the client's condition. When preparing to receive verbal or telephone orders, you should have the client's chart with you so that you may verify allergies or review current medication orders while the physician is talking to you. These efforts will prevent you from having to contact the physician to clarify the order or provide omitted information. Then transcribe the order onto the physician's order sheet, indicating it as a verbal order (VO) or telephone order (TO). Refer to Box 9-3 ◆ for guidelines concerning telephone orders.

Once the order is transcribed on the physician's order sheet, the order must be countersigned by the physician within a time period described by agency policy. Many acute

---

BOX 9-3
NURSING CARE CHECKLIST

GUIDELINES FOR TELEPHONE ORDERS

☑ Do not accept an order from a prescriber you do not know.

☑ Ask the prescriber to speak slowly and clearly.

☑ Ask the prescriber to spell out the name of the medication.

☑ Question the drug, dosage, or changes if they seem inappropriate for this client.

☑ Read the order back to the prescriber at the end. Use words for abbreviations (i.e., three times a day for tid).

☑ When writing a dosage always put a zero "0" before a decimal (i.e., 0.3 mL) but never after a decimal (i.e., 6 mg, not 6.0 mg).

☑ Write out units (i.e., 20 units of insulin, not 20 u of insulin).

☑ Follow agency protocol about the prescriber's protocol for signing telephone orders (i.e., within 24 hours).

---

care hospitals require that this be done within 24 hours, while most long-term care facilities require physician signatures within 72 hours.

FAX AND E-MAIL COMMUNICATION

Faxing and e-mailing are convenient ways of sending large amounts of information, laboratory results, or copies of progress notes. These routes of communication should not be used in emergency situations as a primary method of communication. In the nurse's notes, document how the information was sent and the date and time of the fax or e-mail.

When faxing or e-mailing information, a follow-up phone call is needed to ensure that the information was received. You should also document the follow-up call. Include the person's name who verified receipt of the fax or e-mail, as well as the date and time of your call.

NURSING CARE CONFERENCE

A **nursing care conference** is a meeting of a group of nurses to discuss possible solutions to certain problems of a client, such as inability to cope with an event or lack of progress toward reaching goals.

To **confer** is to consult another person or persons for advice, information, ideas, or instructions. Nursing conferences are most effective when there is a climate of respect—that is, nonjudgmental acceptance of others even though their values, opinions, and beliefs may seem different. Nurses will gain the most information and insight about a client's situation by listening with an open mind to what others are saying, even when there is disagreement (see Chapter 3 ⬛).

NURSING ROUNDS

Nursing rounds are procedures in which a group of nurses visit selected clients at each client's bedside to:

◆ Obtain information that will help plan nursing care.
◆ Provide clients the opportunity to discuss their care.
◆ Evaluate the nursing care the client has received.

To help clients participate in nursing rounds, nurses need to use terms that clients can understand.

INTERDISCIPLINARY CARE PLAN MEETINGS

Skilled nursing units, rehabilitation facilities, and long-term care facilities have regularly scheduled meetings where care is coordinated for a common care plan. Often nursing services or social workers are the primary coordinators for these meetings.

INCIDENT REPORTS

An **incident** can be defined as any unexpected event. A medication error and a fall are examples of incidents. Each agency defines what it considers an incident, which forms need to be completed, and which protocols are to be implemented. An incident event needs to be documented in the nurse's notes. However, the words "incident report completed" should not be included in the nurse's notes. Incident reports are for the agency's use. They are not generally part of the client's medical record. Incident reports are discussed in Chapter 32.

NURSING CARE

The client record should describe the client's ongoing status and reflect the full range of the nursing process. Regardless of the records system used in an agency, nurses document the same types of evidence of the nursing process on a variety of forms throughout the clinical record (Table 9-5 ◆).

◆ ASSESSING

Admission Nursing Assessment

A comprehensive admission assessment, also referred to as an initial assessment, initial database, nursing history, or nursing assessment, is completed when the client is admitted to the nursing unit. The initial nursing assessment is a snapshot of the client's condition and needs upon admission. This comprehensive and accurate evaluation of the client guides care and interventions. See Figure 8-1 for an example of an admission assessment document.

◆ DIAGNOSING, PLANNING, and IMPLEMENTING

Nursing Care Plans

The JCAHO Accreditation Manual for Hospitals (2002) requires that the clinical record include evidence of client assessments, nursing diagnoses and/or client needs, nursing interventions, and client outcomes, but the standards no longer require a separate nursing care plan. Depending on the records system being used, the nursing care plan may be separate from the client's chart, recorded in progress notes and other forms in the client record, or incorporated into a multi-disciplinary plan of care.

There are two types of nursing care plans: traditional and standardized. The traditional care plan is written for each client. The form varies from agency to agency according to the needs of the client and the department. Most forms have three columns: one for nursing diagnoses, a second for expected outcomes, and a third for nursing interventions. See Chapter 4 for additional information.

Standardized care plans have been developed to save documentation time. These plans are based on an institution's standards of practice; they help maintain the quality of nursing care. However, the nurse must individualize standardized plans in order to address individual client needs well. To do this, the nurse selects from a list of interventions relating to a specific nursing diagnosis, then fills in data specific to the client.

Kardexes

The **Kardex** (see Figure 4-3) is a widely used, concise method of organizing and recording data about a client, making information quickly accessible to all health professionals. The system consists of a single card or a series of cards kept in a portable index file or on computer-generated forms. The cards for a particular client can be quickly turned up to reveal specific data. The Kardex may or may not become a part of the client's permanent record. In some organizations it is a temporary worksheet written in pencil for ease in recording when frequent changes in details of a client's care must be made. The information on Kardexes may be organized into sections, for example:

- ◆ Pertinent information about the client, such as name, room number, age, religion, marital status, admission date, physician's name, diagnosis, type of surgery and date, occupation, and next of kin
- ◆ List of intravenous fluids, with dates of infusions; medications may also be listed
- ◆ List of daily treatments and procedures, such as dressing changes, postural drainage, or measurement of vital signs
- ◆ List of diagnostic procedures ordered
- ◆ Allergies
- ◆ Specific data on how the client's physical needs are to be met, such as type of diet, assistance needed with feeding, elimination devices, activity, hygienic needs, and safety precautions (e.g., use of side rails)
- ◆ A problem list, stated goals, and a list of nursing approaches to meet the goals and relieve the problems

Although much of the information on the Kardex may be recorded by the nurse in charge or a delegate (e.g., the ward clerk), any nurse who cares for the client plays a key role in initiating the record and keeping the data current. Students must be cautious to not plan care solely based on information found on the Kardex, it is necessary to check orders with the physician's orders.

TABLE 9-5	DOCUMENTING THE NURSING PROCESS	
STEP[a]	**DOCUMENTATION FORMS**	
Assessment	Initial assessment form, various flowsheets	
Nursing diagnosis	Nursing care plan, Kardex, critical path, progress notes, problem list	
Planning	Nursing care plan, critical path	
Intervention	Progress notes, flowsheets	
Evaluation	Progress notes	

[a]All steps are recorded on discharge/referral summaries

Flowsheets

Flowsheets, also called abbreviated progress notes, enable nurses to record nursing data quickly and concisely and provide an easy-to-read record of the client's condition over time (see Figure 9-5).

The time parameters for flowsheets can vary from minutes to months. In a hospital intensive care unit a client's blood pressure may be monitored by the minute, whereas in an ambulatory clinic a client's blood glucose level may be recorded once a month.

Flowsheets commonly used are the graphic (clinical) record; the fluid intake and output record, the medication record, and daily nursing care records.

Graphic (Clinical) Record

This record (Figure 9-5) indicates body temperature, pulse, respiratory rate, blood pressure, weight, and, in some agencies, other significant clinical data such as admission or postoperative day, bowel movements, appetite, and activity.

24-Hour Fluid Balance Record

All routes of fluid intake and all routes of fluid loss or output are measured and recorded on this form. Information about ways to measure and record specific amounts of fluid intake and output are described in Chapter 17. ⊂⊃ This record is often called an I&O Sheet.

Medication Record

Medication flowsheets are also called medication administration records (MARs). They usually include designated areas for the date of the medication order, the expiration date, the medication name and dose, the frequency of administration and route, and the nurse's signature. Some records also include a place to document the client's allergies. A sample medication record is shown in Chapter 21. ⊂⊃ When changes are made to the MAR, the initials of the nurse making the changes and the date of the changes should be included. Frequently, facilities will use a colored highlighter to cross through medications which have been discontinued (dc), for easy identification.

Daily Nursing Care Record

Daily nursing care for activities of daily living (ADLs) are most frequently recorded on a flowsheet such as the one in Figure 9-7 ◆. These records may include categories related to diet, hygiene, activity, elimination, treatments, protective precautions, diagnostic studies, and so on. Depending on the agency, licensed nurses may delegate the completion of this flowsheet to unlicensed staff.

Progress Notes

Progress notes made by nurses provide information about the progress a client is making toward achieving the desired outcomes. Therefore, in addition to assessment and reassessment data, progress notes include information about client problems and nursing interventions. The format used depends on the documentation system in place in the institution. Various kinds of nursing progress notes were discussed earlier in this chapter.

Nursing Discharge/Referral Summaries

Discharge notes are completed when the client is being discharged. See Figure 8-4 in the discharge planning section of Chapter 8, and the assessment parameters suggested when preparing clients to go home. ⊂⊃ Many discharge forms combine the discharge plan, including instructions for care, and the final progress note. Many forms are designed with checklists to facilitate data recording.

If the client is being transferred to another institution or to a home setting where a visit by a home health nurse is required, the discharge note takes the form of a referral summary. Regardless of format, the nurse includes some or all of the elements noted in Box 9-4 ◆ in discharge and referral summaries.

Long-Term Care Documentation

Requirements for documentation in long-term care settings are based on professional standards, federal and state regulations, and the policies of the health care agency. The kind and frequency of documentation required are determined by the Health Care Financing Administration (HCFA) and the Omnibus Budget Reconciliation Act (OBRA) of 1987. The OBRA law, for example, requires that (a) a comprehensive assessment (the Minimum Data Set [MDS] for Resident Assessment and Care Screening) be performed within 14 days of a client's admission to a long-term care facility, (b) a formulated plan of care must be completed within 7 days of completion of the MDS, and (c) the comprehensive assessment and care screening process must be reviewed every 90 days.

> ### clinical ALERT
>
> The ability of the nurse to be aware of his/her clients' status is essential for identifying changes in condition. In long term care, a client's condition can change significantly in hours, and the nurse must be alert to these changes.
>
> **Report**
> The nurse must document and report changes in a client's condition within 24 hours to the physician and the client's family, and institute appropriate care measures.

Documentation also must comply with requirements set by Medicare and Medicaid. These requirements vary with the level of service provided and other factors. For example, Medicare provides little reimbursement for care provided in long-term care facilities except for services that require skilled care such as chemotherapy, tube feedings, ventilators, and so on. For such clients, the nurse must provide daily documentation to verify the need for service and reimbursement.

Nurses need to familiarize themselves with regulations that influence the kind and frequency of documentation

PeaceHealth

MED /SURG / TELE / ONC
DAILY CARE RECORD

Date: _____

12	13	14	15	16	17	18	19	20	21	22	23

Pain Intervention Key:
1. Medicated   4. Repositioned
2. Cold   5. Diversion
3. Heat   6. PCA/Epidural

Sedation Scale:
0 – None; alert
1 – Mild; occasionally drowsy, easy to arouse
2 – Moderate; frequently drowsy, easy to arouse
3 – Severe; somnolent, difficult to arouse

Diversion Therapies Key:
A - Audio   V - Visual   T - Tactile

Hygiene Key:
S–Self   A–Assist   D–Depend
CB – Complete bath
SH – Shower   PC – Peri Care
OC – Oral Care   HS – HS Care
FC – Foley Care

Toileting Key:
BRP – Bathroom Privileges
C – Commode   U – Urinal
BP – Bed Pan   I – Incontinent
FC – Foley Catheter

Activity Key:
S–Self   A–Assist   D–Depend
BR – Bed Rest   T – Turn
C – Chair   AMB – Ambulate

Positioning Key:
R – Right   L – Left   S – Supine

12	13	14	15	16	17	18	19	20	21	22	23

Pulmonary Toilet Key:
IS – Incentive Spirometer
C&DB – Cough & Deep Breathe
RT – Respiratory Therapy

Diet Function Key:
FS – Feeds Self
A – Setup Assist
CS – Constant Supervision
F – Total Feed
FF – Force Fluids
RF – Restrict Fluids

Dysphagia Eval Key:
CH – Choke   CO – Cough
V – Change in Voice   N – None

Oversight of Care: Initials Indicate RN Delegation and Oversight of Care:

Initials	Signature	Initials	Signature	Initials	Signature

Figure 9-7. ◆ Daily record of care. *Source:* Courtesy of PeaceHealth St. John Medical Center, Longview, WA. Used with permission.

> ## BOX 9-4
> ## NURSING CARE CHECKLIST
>
> ### DISCHARGE OR REFERRAL SUMMARY
>
> The nurse would include some or all of the following in the client summary for discharge or referral:
>
> ☑ Description of client's physical, mental, and emotional status at discharge or transfer
> ☑ Resolved health problems
> ☑ Unresolved continuing health problems and continuing care needs; may include a review-of-systems checklist (e.g., integumentary, respiratory, cardiovascular problems)
> ☑ Treatments that are to be continued (e.g., wound care, oxygen therapy)
> ☑ Current medications
> ☑ Restrictions that relate to
>   ◆ Activity such as lifting, stair climbing, walking, driving, work
>   ◆ Diet
>   ◆ Bathing such as sponge bath, tub, or shower
> ☑ Functional/self-care abilities in terms of vision, hearing, speech, mobility with or without aids, meal preparation and eating, preparing and administering medications, and so on
> ☑ Comfort level
> ☑ Support networks including family, significant others, religious adviser, community self-help groups, home care and other community agencies available, and so on
> ☑ Client education provided in relation to disease process, activities and exercise, special diet, medications, specialized care or treatments, follow-up appointments, and so on
> ☑ Discharge destination (e.g., home, nursing home) and mode of discharge (e.g., walking, wheelchair, ambulance)
> ☑ Referral services (e.g., social worker, home health nurse)

required in long-term care facilities. Usually, the nurse completes a nursing care summary at least once a week for clients requiring skilled care and every 2 to 4 weeks for those requiring intermediate care. Clients in a skilled nursing unit within a long-term care facility should be assessed daily or each shift, depending on the skilled services needed by the client. Summaries should address the following:

◆ Specific problems noted in the care plan
◆ Mental status
◆ Activities of daily living (ADLs)
◆ Rehabilitative or restorative interventions, with comments about progress made

◆ Hydration and nutrition status
◆ Safety measures needed (e.g., bed rails)
◆ Medications and treatments
◆ Skin condition and wound treatments if applicable
◆ Preventive measures

Nurses should also keep a record of visits and phone calls to the client from family, friends, and others.

Home Care Documentation

The Health Care Financing Administration (HCFA), a branch of the Department of Health and Human Services, mandated that home health care agencies standardize their documentation methods to meet requirements for Medicare and Medicaid and other third-party disbursements. Two records are required: (a) a home health certification and plan of treatment form and (b) a medical update and client information form. The nurse assigned to the home care client usually completes the forms, which must be signed by both the nurse and the attending physician. Box 9-5 ◆ provides guidelines for home health care documentation.

> ## BOX 9-5
> ## NURSING CARE CHECKLIST
>
> ### HOME CARE DOCUMENTATION
>
> ☑ Complete a comprehensive nursing assessment and develop a plan of care to meet Medicare and other third-party payer requirements. Some agencies use the certification and plan of treatment form as the client's official plan of care.
> ☑ Write a progress note at each client visit, noting any changes in the client condition; nursing interventions performed (including education and instructional brochures and materials provided to the client and home caregiver); client responses to nursing care; and vital signs as indicated.
> ☑ Provide a monthly progress nursing summary to the attending physician and to the reimburser to confirm the need to continue services.
> ☑ Keep a copy of the care plan in the client's home and update it as the client's condition changes.
> ☑ Report changes in the plan of care to the physician and document that these were reported. Medicare and Medicaid will reimburse only for the skilled services provided that are reported to the physician.
> ☑ Encourage the client or home caregiver to record data when appropriate.
> ☑ Write a discharge summary for the physician to approve the discharge and to notify the reimbursers that services have been discontinued. Include all services provided, the client's health status at discharge, outcomes achieved, and recommendations for further care.

Some home health agencies provide nurses with laptop or handheld computers to make records available in multiple locations. With the use of a modem, the nurse can add new client information to records at the agency without traveling to the office.

 ## EVALUATING

Evaluation of client status, goals, and outcomes is an ongoing part of the nursing process. Documentation of client changes are recorded on progress notes daily. Periodic evaluations are performed and documented at regular intervals, depending on client status and institutional policy.

Nursing Process Case Study: CLIENT WITH ALTERED PROTECTION

Amy is a 14-year-old girl who is popular in school. She has recently been diagnosed with Leukemia. Amy lives with her mother, father, and two brothers who are also active in school activities. The physician has ordered Amy be started on chemotherapeutics and corticosteroids.

Assessment VS: T 99.2, P 72, R 16, BP 124/68.

Client states:
"I have several of my friends coming to visit me tonight."
"I don't like to eat much. I have to keep my weight down."
"I have Leukemia. I'm not sure what that means."
"I get tired easily."

Diagnosis Altered Protection related to chemotherapy and cortisone therapy.

Expected Outcomes

Client will not have symptoms of infection.
Client will demonstrate knowledge and understanding of asepsis.
Client will demonstrate understanding of need for balanced diet.
Client will demonstrate understanding of need for energy conservation.

Planning and Implementation

- VS every 4 hours.
- Monitor white blood cell (WBC) levels.
- Administer medications per doctor's orders.
- Post signs regarding neutropenic precautions.
- Provide age-appropriate education (to client and family) regarding the following:

- Client teaching regarding hand washing and need for asepsis.
- Observe return demonstration of proper hand washing.
- Client will verbalize understanding of asepsis.
- Client teaching regarding neutropenic precautions.
- Client verbalizes understanding of precautions.
- Client verbalizes willingness to comply with precautions.
- Age-appropriate education for visiting friends.
- Client education regarding proper nutrition.
- Client verbalizes understanding of need for balanced diet (without raw/uncooked foods).
- Obtain dietitian consult regarding dietary needs.
- Client teaching regarding energy conservation.
- Client verbalizes understanding regarding grouping activities and resting between activities.
- Client teaching regarding signs and symptoms of infection
- Client is able to verbalize signs and symptoms of infection and verbalizes understanding of need to immediately report signs/symptoms if noted.

Evaluation Two days after admission Amy has met all of her educational needs. She verbalizes that she is unhappy about not being able to have plants in her room but is willing to comply. You note that she is washing her hands regularly and wears a mask when her friends come to visit. The dietitian reports that Amy is not eating a balanced diet and has scheduled further meetings with both Amy and her parents. She must be reminded to rest during the day, especially when friends are visiting. Amy's parents are supportive and cooperative with protocols. Amy is 48 hours into her chemotherapy and corticosteroids treatments, and is free of any signs of infection at this time.

Critical Thinking in the Nursing Process

1. What is Amy's priority need at this time?
2. Amy's friends do not understand why Amy wears a mask. They say that they thought you couldn't catch cancer.
3. Four days into her treatment Amy reports a sore throat. Her VS are T 101.4°F, P 92, R 18, and BP 136/74. What is your next action and why?
4. Ten days into her treatment Amy is upset about her "fat face" and wants to know what is causing it. When you tell her it is a side effect of the steroids, she wants to know why she's taking them. How would you explain the indications of steroids?

Note: The bibliography listings for this and all chapters have been compiled at the back of the book.

Chapter Review

Use the audio glossary feature of either the CD-ROM or the Companion Website to hear the correct pronunciation of the following key terms.

Introduction
report, record, charting, documenting, clinical record

Documentation systems
source-oriented record, problem-oriented medical record (POMR), database, DAR

Reporting
change-of-shift report, nursing care conference, confer, nursing rounds, incident

Nursing care
Kardex, flowsheets

Key Points

- Nurses must accurately document each step of the nursing process in a timely manner, regardless of the documentation system used.

- Entries into the client's record must be legible, concise, sequential, complete, and signed by the health care provider making the entry.

- The client record is a legal document. All parts of the client's record are admissible into a court of law as evidence.

- The most common documentation systems are; PIE, Focus Charting, CORE, FACT, CBE, outcome documentation, and case management.

- Computers have increased the ease of documenting most nursing interventions. Most documentation systems can be adapted to computer use. Terminals at bedside and handheld units permit immediate documentation of care.

- Case management uses critical pathways that incorporate the care plan into the documentation form.

- Long-term care documentation is essentially the same as documentation made in the acute care setting but has a different focus. Acute care charting focuses on progress towards a wellness goal. Long-term care charting focuses on daily functioning and maintenance of function with the use of restorative and preventive measures. Long-term care charting is also less frequent.

- Accuracy is important in the home care setting because there are fewer care givers. Documentation in the home care setting is used to obtain reimbursement from third-party payers and to justify continued home care.

- Confidentiality must be maintained at all times, regardless of location of care, documentation method, or whether computers are used or not.

EXPLORE MediaLink

Additional interactive resources for this chapter can be found on the Companion Website at www.prenhall.com/ramont. Click on Chapter 9 and "Begin" to select the activities for this chapter. For chapter-related NCLEX-style questions and an audio glossary, access the accompanying CD-ROM in this book.

For Further Study

For more information about abbreviations used for medication administration, see Chapter 21.

For additional information on reporting and taking telephone orders, see Chapter 32.

For further discussion regarding critical thinking, see Chapter 3.

For additional information about subjective and objective data, planning care, and formulating NANDA diagnoses, see Chapter 4.

For additional discussion about critical pathways and case management, see Chapter 5.

For additional information about discharge planning, see Chapter 8.

For additional information about fluid monitoring, see Chapter 17.

Critical Thinking Care Map

Caring for a Client Who Is Grieving

NCLEX-PN Focus Area: Coping and Adaptation

Case Study: Mrs. Estella Rodriguez is an 87-year-old female admitted 3 days ago for treatment of bilateral pneumonia. She has lost 1 kilogram (2.2 lbs) since admission, and her records note that she does not eat well at mealtimes. The dietitian reports that Mrs. Rodriguez does not fill out her menus and declines assistance. When her son visits later in the shift, you ask him about food preferences. Her son reports that she hasn't had much appetite since his father died 2 years ago, and has lost "quite a bit" of weight. He also reports that she used to be very active in church and hardly leaves the house anymore. The daughter-in-law comments that Mrs. Rodriguez cries frequently and occasionally talks as if her husband is still alive. The son tells you that they had been married 62 years.

Nursing Diagnosis: Dysfunctional Grieving

COLLECT DATA

Subjective	Objective

Would you report this data? Yes/No

If yes, to: _____

Nursing Care

_____
_____
_____
_____
_____
_____
_____
_____
_____
_____

How would you document this? _____
_____
_____
_____
_____

Data Collected
(use those that apply)

- 87 years old
- Weight 36.63 kg (85 lbs)
- Weight loss since admission
- Height 152 cm (5'2'')
- Crying
- Talks as if spouse alive
- States "I don't know how to cook for one person"
- Not wearing makeup, hair not combed
- Decreased social activity
- Belongs to the Catholic Church
- VS: T 98.2, P 84, R 18, BP 150/82
- Complains of hunger
- Watches TV much of day
- Decreased interest in surroundings

Nursing Interventions
(use those that apply)

- Obtain referral to grief counselor.
- Encourage family to choose and adult singles group for their mother.
- Obtain referral to appropriate grief support group.
- Dietitian consult for meal planning upon discharge.
- Suggest to family that the client's priest should visit regularly.
- Provide reality orientation.
- Suggest weight gain program and recommend 6.5 kg weight gain by end of the month.
- Schedule follow-up visit in doctor's office, for one week from today.
- Schedule time during the shift where you can spend one-on-one time with client.
- Encourage client to talk about spouse.

NCLEX-PN Exam Preparation

1. Mrs. Smith has told you that she wishes she were dead. When you ask her about her feelings, she tells you that since her husband died a year ago nothing has mattered to her. You would best document this:

   a. Client has suicidal tendencies.
   b. Client is grieving for her spouse.
   c. Client expressing dysfunctional grieving and states that she wishes she were dead. Physician notified.
   d. Referral for psychiatric evaluation made at this time.

2. Which of the following would be a breach of confidentiality?

   a. Notifying the pharmacist of the blood level of an antibiotic
   b. Discussing the progress of a rehabilitation client with the case manager
   c. Explaining what the "contact isolation" notice on a family member's door means
   d. Telling a coworker about a suicide attempt that a client made on another unit

3. You are a student nurse on a unit and request permission to make copies of the medication administration record. Which of the following is not an appropriate action for you to take?

   a. Mark through the identifying information with a thick marker.
   b. Remember to initial the copy as you give medications.
   c. Return the forms at the end of the day for shredding.
   d. Tell the unit manager how you plan to keep the copies secure during your shift.

4. Mr. Alexander tells you that he didn't like his care and is going to sue. He is demanding a copy of his records. You would tell him:

   a. He will need to contact medical records and complete necessary paperwork before he may receive a copy.
   b. Since he's going to sue, he cannot have a copy of his records for legal reasons.
   c. The chart belongs to the facility and he has no right to it.
   d. There is a $100 copy fee and it will take 6 to 8 weeks to receive it.

5. You are making an entry into the nurse's notes and discovered that you forgot to enter something that happened half an hour ago. You would best correct this omission by:

   a. Crossing through the entry you are now making, write error, initial it, and then make the entry you forgot to enter earlier.
   b. Make the entry now with the current time since that is when you are documenting it.
   c. Make the entry with the time the event happened, and label it a late entry.
   d. Do nothing—it's too late.

6. Dr. Jones has seen two of your clients and has left new orders. After Dr. Jones has left the unit, you discover that you cannot read some of the orders. You should first:

   a. Do the best you can and leave a note for him to clarify the remaining orders.
   b. Page him immediately.
   c. Contact your charge nurse for assistance in reading the orders.
   d. Contact the pharmacy to see what Dr. Jones usually orders in these situations.

7. You are an LPN/LVN who has been working in a large county hospital. At that hospital you were accustomed to a wide range of responsibility. You have recently accepted a job at a new hospital. You will expect your duties to include:

   a. All the same duties that you had at your last job
   b. Fewer duties than you had at your last job
   c. More duties than you had before
   d. Client assessment, intervention, and teaching within the scope of the job description

8. You are working the 7-to-3 shift on an oncology unit. At 7:30 this morning you changed a client's surgical dressing and assessed the site. You are documenting it at 8:00. What time would you enter into the nurse's notes?

   a. 0730
   b. 0800
   c. 7-to-3 shift
   d. No time is needed if you use the flowsheet.

9. You are working at a long-term care facility and lab reports have just come in. You plan to fax the lab results to the individual doctors. You should:

   a. Not fax lab reports, as this is unreliable.
   b. Follow up with a phone call to the physician's office to ensure receipt of the fax.
   c. Fax the lab results and include a request for the office staff to call you if they don't get the fax.
   d. Call the abnormal lab values in to the office.

10. You are doing walking rounds with the on-coming nurse. You come to room 402 and stand in the doorway to discuss the conditions and progress of the clients in bed A and bed B. You should be aware that:

    a. This is normal procedure.
    b. If you are not careful, you may create a breach of confidentiality.
    c. Walking rounds are only done on critical care units.
    d. Taped reports are a better form of shift-to-shift communication.

Answers for Review Questions, as well as discussion of Case Study and Critical Thinking Care Map questions, appear in Appendix IV.

Thinking Strategically About...

Deborah Mason, LPN, has been assigned to work with Laurene Carter, a triage nurse, in the emergency department of a large metropolitan hospital in the Southwest. Ms. Mason is responsible for conducting an "intake inquiry." This inquiry includes a brief history ("the chief complaint") and taking client vital signs. The information is charted and verbally communicated to Ms. Carter, who determines in which area of the ED the client is to be treated and escorts them there.

José Suarez, age 58, arrives at the ED, accompanied by his wife Mariela. Mr. Suarez is diaphoretic and visibly short of breath. Mr. Suarez reports that he feels like he has influenza, like he had a few years ago, except he doesn't have a sore throat. Petechiae are visible on his forearms. In broken English, he explains that he picks tomatoes at a small ranch and sells them to families living on the nearby military testing base, as well as to tourists. Mrs. Suarez interrupts him repeatedly in Spanish during the intake inquiry. He gestures impatiently and says, "She wants me to tell you I had to bury four dead sheep last week at the ranch." In recent weeks, there have been three reported cases of anthrax in the state.

CRITICAL THINKING

- What is the priority nursing concern for Mr. Suarez?
- Does Mr. Suarez's condition suggest any special safety concerns?

COLLABORATIVE CARE

Based on information gained from this scenario, what members of the health care team might need to be involved in assessment of Mr. Suarez?

CULTURAL COMPETENCY

- What must be done to ensure that Mr. and Mrs. Suarez have the best possible communication with hospital staff?
- What cultural influences are apparent in the case study above?

COMPASSIONATE CARE

What interventions might the nurse use to assist Mr. Suarez while he is in the ED?

UNIT III

Promoting Physiological Health

Chapter 10 ▸ Introduction to the Body

Chapter 11 ▸ Health Assessment

Chapter 12 ▸ Skin Integrity and Wound Care

Chapter 13 ▸ Hygiene

Chapter 14 ▸ Vital Signs

Chapter 15 ▸ Pain, The Fifth Vital Sign

Chapter 16 ▸ Oxygenation

Chapter 17 ▸ Nutrition, Fluids and Electrolytes, and Acid–Base Balance

Chapter 18 ▸ Urinary Elimination

Chapter 19 ▸ Gastrointestinal Elimination

Chapter 20 ▸ Activity, Rest, and Sleep

Chapter 21 ▸ Medications

Chapter 22 ▸ Perioperative Nursing

Chapter 23 ▸ Client Teaching

Chapter 10

Introduction to the Body

SHARING experiences

My greatest joy in nursing has been being able to share my experiences in the medical field to help educate others.

Denise Foster, LVN, North Orange County Regional Occupational Program, Anaheim, CA.

LEARNING outcomes

After completing this chapter, you will be able to:

- Define the terms *anatomy* and *physiology*.
- Describe the levels of organization of the human body from the very simple to the very complex.
- Describe the structure of a cell.
- Understand the functions of the cell organelles.
- Describe and understand the forms of cell division: mitosis and meiosis.
- Describe the four main tissue classifications.
- Explain the difference between exocrine and endocrine glands.
- List the major body systems and describe the general function of each.
- List and define the directional terms for the body.
- List and define the three planes used to divide the body.
- List the different body cavities and the organs found in each.

MediaLink

 www.prenhall.com/ramont

Use the address above to access the free, interactive Companion Website created for this textbook. Get hints, instant feedback, and textbook references to chapter-related NCLEX-style questions. Link to other interesting sites.

Audio Glossary:
Use the Companion Website, or the CD-ROM disk enclosed with your textbook, to hear the pronunciation of key terms in the chapter.

The study of the human body or, more specifically, anatomy and physiology, is absolutely essential for anyone considering a career in the health sciences. In fact, anyone can benefit from this knowledge. With rapid advances being made in the fields of biology and health care, people are being asked to make important decisions about their health and the health of their families. A basic understanding of anatomy and physiology can help people to make informed decisions.

So what exactly do the terms anatomy and physiology mean? **Anatomy** is the study of body structure, including size, shape, and composition. **Physiology** is the study of how the body functions. These two fields of study form the basis for the practice of medicine.

 Cells

CELL STRUCTURE
The body, like all living things, is organized from the very simple to the very complex. The most basic level begins with simple chemicals. Those chemicals come together to form a structure known as a *cell.* Cells with similar structure and functions form *tissues*. Tissues work together to form *organs,* which are a group of two or more tissue types that perform a specialized function. Organs with the same functional purpose are called *organ systems.* Organ systems work together to produce a living organism, in this case the human body. When all the components are working properly and are in balance, the body is said to be in **homeostasis.** Anything that upsets that balance is considered a disease. The study of anatomy and physiology begins at the level of the cell.

From the simplest microorganism to the complex human being, all living things share one common characteristic: they are made of cells. The cell is the basic unit of all life (Figure 10-1 ◆). It is the simplest structure that possesses all

the characteristics of life: organization, metabolism, responsiveness, homeostasis, growth, and reproduction.

There are many types of cells all with different functions and characteristics. Despite these differences, cells are very similar at the structural level.

The "skin" of a cell is known as the **cell membrane** or plasma membrane. This membrane is a double-layered structure composed of phospholipids, cholesterol, and proteins. *Phospholipids* are fats or fat-like substances that contain the element phosphorus. The lipid nature of the cell membrane allows fat-soluble materials to enter and exit the cells through a process known as diffusion. The presence of *cholesterol* strengthens the cell membrane and helps to maintain its flexibility.

There are several different *proteins* in the cell membrane; their functions generally fall into one of the five following categories:

1. **Receptors,** points of attachment for certain materials such as hormones on the surface of the cell membrane
2. **Enzymes,** proteins that catalyze the chemical reactions that occur at the cell membrane
3. **Channels,** openings that permit the passage of certain materials into or out of the cell
4. **Transporters,** proteins that actively move materials that are too big for the channels through the cell membrane in both directions
5. **Antigens,** markers that identify the type of cell and help the immune system determine whether the cell should be present within the organism or whether it is foreign to the organism

Cytoplasm
The main substance filling the inside of the cell is a *colloidal* (jellylike) suspension known as **cytoplasm.** This suspension consists of minerals, nutrients, and enzymes in water. Many of the cell's chemical reactions occur in the cytoplasm, and most of the organelles are found there.

Organelles
Within the cell are structures, often bound in their own membranes, known as *organelles* (meaning "little organs"). These are special subdivisions, similar to the human body's organs, which carry out many of the functions of the cell.

NUCLEUS. The most prominent organelle is the **nucleus.** All cells in the human body (except for mature red blood cells) possess a nucleus. Because it contains the genetic material or deoxyribonucleic acid (DNA) of the cell, the nucleus is often referred to as the control center. The nucleus is contained within a double-layered nuclear membrane. Inside the nucleus is a sphere known as the *nucleolus,* which is composed of DNA, ribonucleic acid (RNA), and protein. Ribosomal RNA (used in protein synthesis) is produced here.

RIBOSOMES. Ribosomes are made up of ribosomal RNA and protein. They are found on the surface of rough ER and float-

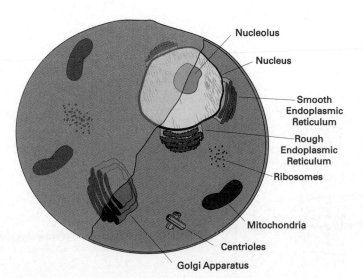

Figure 10-1. ◆ Human cell. *Source:* Drawing by Thomas Ramont

Labels in figure: Nucleolus, Nucleus, Smooth Endoplasmic Reticulum, Rough Endoplasmic Reticulum, Ribosomes, Mitochondria, Centrioles, Golgi Apparatus ing freely within the cytoplasm. Ribosomes are the site of protein synthesis by the cell.

ENDOPLASMIC RETICULUM (ER).

The **endoplasmic reticulum** is a network of membrane bound tubules that extend from the cell membrane to the nuclear membrane. The ER functions as a transport system for the lipids and proteins needed for cell function. The endoplasmic reticulum is often referred to as *rough* or *smooth,* depending on whether it has ribosomes on its surface or not. When ribosomes are not present, smooth ER synthesizes lipids. Rough ER contains ribosomes; the proteins synthesized by these ribosomes are transported by the ER.

MITOCHONDRIA.

Mitochondria are large organelles surrounded by a double membrane. Often referred to as "power plants," they are the site of the aerobic phase of cellular respiration where **adenosine triphosphate (ATP)** is produced. Since ATP is the energy compound of cells, large numbers of mitochondria are found in cells that require large amounts of energy, like muscle cells.

GOLGI APPARATUS.

The **Golgi apparatus** consists of layers of flat, membranous sacs. They are the site where carbohydrates are synthesized and sorted, along with other material, for secretion from the cell. Additionally, proteins are processed and modified within the Golgi apparatus.

LYSOSOMES.

Lysosomes are small membranous sacs that contain digestive enzymes. Their functions include breaking down waste and foreign materials, and helping to destroy bacteria engulfed by white blood cells known as phagocytes.

CENTRIOLES.

A pair of rod-shaped structures known as *centrioles* is located outside the nucleus. They provide attachment points for the spindle fibers that help separate the chromosomes during cell division.

CILIA AND FLAGELLA.

Some cells contain small projections known as cilia and flagella. **Cilia** are hair-like projections on the surface of some cells. Their function is to sweep back and forth, creating movement around the cell. Cells with cilia can be found in the respiratory and reproductive tracts. In contrast, a **flagellum** is a long, whiplike extension from a cell that is used to move the cell itself. The only human cells with flagella are sperm cells.

CELL DIVISION

In order for an organism to grow, repair damage, and reproduce, its cells must be able to increase their numbers through a process known as *cell division*. The two forms of cell division, mitosis and meiosis, serve very different purposes.

Mitosis

Mitosis is the division of a single parent cell into two genetically identical daughter cells (Figure 10-2 ◆). Before the parent cell can divide, the genetic material or DNA must be replicated. This replication of DNA occurs during *interphase*, which is the period of time between one cell division (*mitotic event*) and the next. Once the DNA has been duplicated, the cell can enter the first of the four stages of mitosis.

Prophase is the first stage of mitosis. In this stage, the doubled DNA is actually visible as short rods if viewed through a microscope. It is at this point that the centrioles move towards opposite ends of the cell and begin to organize the spindle fibers. The organelles not necessary for division disappear.

In the next stage, *metaphase*, the chromosomes line up across the equator of the cell. The chromosomes attach to the spindle fibers at the centromeres.

Beginning in *anaphase*, the third stage, the duplicated chromosomes separate and are pulled toward opposite ends of the cell by the spindle fibers.

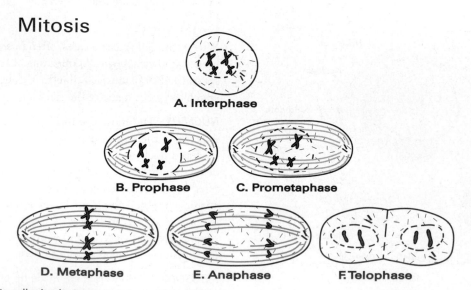

Mitosis

A. Interphase

B. Prophase   C. Prometaphase

D. Metaphase   E. Anaphase   F. Telophase

Figure 10-2. ◆ Steps in cell mitosis. *Source:* Drawing by Thomas Ramont.

During *telophase,* the fourth stage of mitosis, the cell begins to form around each set of chromosomes. The cell begins to pinch in the middle and continues until it splits into two identical daughter cells.

Once the cell division has occurred, the organelles that disappeared in the beginning reappear in the two daughter cells and the centrioles are duplicated in preparation for the next episode of mitosis.

While all the cells in the human body are capable of mitosis, the rate at which it occurs varies widely. For example, skin cells and the cells of the stomach lining are in almost constant mitosis due to the continuous stress they are under. At the opposite extreme are nerve cells (neurons) and most muscle cells. In an adult, these cells do not experience mitosis and if they are damaged, they are not repaired. This is why, when a person's spinal cord is severed, permanent paralysis occurs below the point of injury.

There is also a general tendency for mitosis to occur more slowly as a person ages. As a result, bone fractures and lacerations take longer to heal in the elderly than in a young person.

Meiosis

The second, more complex form of cell division, **meiosis,** is responsible for the formation of sex cells, or **gametes** (sperm and egg cells). Each human cell contains 46 chromosomes, except for the gametes formed during meiosis (Figure 10-3 ◆).

Prior to the start of meiosis, the cell's chromosomes are duplicated. Once DNA replication has occurred, meiosis begins. The cell begins its first division. A brief rest period follows, called interkinesis. After interkinesis is completed, the two cells resulting from the first division divide again. The result of this final division is four separate cells, each containing 23 chromosomes. These are gametes.

When an egg cell is fertilized by a sperm cell, 23 chromosomes from each cell pair up, and the resulting zygote contains the proper 46 chromosomes associated with human beings.

◆ Tissues

When cells with similar structures and functions come together, they are known as **tissue.** There are many different types of tissue in the human body. Just as it takes a variety of materials to construct a building, so it is with tissue and the human body.

There are four main classifications of tissue: epithelial, connective, muscle, and nervous tissue.

EPITHELIAL TISSUE

The type of tissue that forms a covering or lining is known as epithelial tissue, or **epithelium.** This type of tissue includes the outer layer of the skin; the lining of the respiratory, intestinal, and urinary tracts; the blood vessels; the uterus; and the other body cavities.

Meiosis

A. Interphase

B. Prophase I

C. Metaphase I

D. Anaphase I

E. Telophase I
Prophase II

F. Metaphase II

G. Anaphase II

H. Telophase II
4 Daughter Cells

Figure 10-3. ◆ Steps in cell meiosis. *Source:* Drawing by Thomas Ramont.

The shape of the cells and the number of cell layers are used to classify epithelial tissue further.

There are three general cell shapes:

◆ *Squamous* cells are thin, flat, and irregular in shape.
◆ *Cuboidal* cells are square or cube-shaped.
◆ *Columnar* cells are longer than they are wide (like columns).

The next criterion is the number of cell layers. If there is only a single layer of cell, the term used is *simple.* When there are two or more layers, the tissue is said to be *stratified.*

The shape and the number of layers of cells are used together to describe epithelial tissue. So a single layer of flat, irregular cells is said to be simple squamous. Several layers of flat, irregular cells are said to be stratified squamous.

There is one type of epithelial tissue that does not fit into this classification system. *Transitional epithelium* varies in shape from squamous to round and tends to be stratified. This tissue is found in the urinary bladder. These cells change shape depending on the bladder's fullness.

In addition to being a covering or lining, several kinds of epithelium produce secretions. These secretions include mucus, sweat, digestive juices, and hormones. When tissue produces some form of secretion, it is considered a **gland.**

Glands are divided into two categories: exocrine and endocrine glands. Exocrine glands have ducts that carry the secretions away from the gland. Examples include sweat, sebaceous (oil), and lacrimal (tear) glands. **Endocrine glands** do not have ducts. Their secretions, known as **hormones,** are transported away from the gland by blood flowing through the gland. The pituitary, thyroid, and adrenal glands are examples of endocrine glands.

CONNECTIVE TISSUE

Connective tissue is the supporting fabric of the body. It is classified according to its hardness. These classifications include liquid, soft, fibrous, and hard connective tissues. At first, it may seem that these different forms have little in common. The characteristic that they all share, besides being cellular, is a **matrix,** a network of nonliving, intracellular material, which contains water, fibers, and hard minerals.

Liquid Connective Tissue

Blood and lymph fluid are examples of liquid connective tissue. Both of them have cells suspended in a liquid environment with varying amounts of dissolved salts, nutrients, and waste products. In blood, the matrix is *plasma,* which makes up about 50 to 60 percent of total blood volume. Plasma's primary function is to transport material through the circulatory system. The cellular component of blood consists of red blood cells, white blood cells, and platelets. *Lymph fluid,* the transport medium of the lymphatic system, consists mainly of water with proteins, salts, urea, digested fats, and glucose.

Soft Connective Tissue

Soft connective tissue is found around vessels and organs, between muscles, and under the skin. It is loosely held together with semiliquid material and includes *areolar* (loose) connective tissue and *adipose* (fat) tissue.

The matrix of areolar connective tissue consists of collagen and elastic protein fibers, and tissue fluid. It is found beneath the epithelial tissue of all the body systems. It is the most common type of connective tissue in the body.

Adipose tissue is predominantly used to store excess energy supplies as fat, to retain heat (insulator), and to cushion and protect organs and joints. The amount of matrix material adipose tissue contains is limited. It consists mainly of tissue fluid and collagen fibers.

Fibrous Connective Tissue

As the name implies, fibrous connective tissue contains a large number of fibers that give it strength and flexibility. It is made predominantly of a flexible white protein known as *collagen.* The varying component in the different types of fibrous connective tissue is the number of elastic fibers present in the tissue. Where it is necessary for the tissue to stretch, more elastic fibers are present. Where strength and support are necessary, there are fewer elastic fibers and more collagen fibers.

Fibrous connective tissue is found in the vocal cords, respiratory tract, and the walls of arteries. It forms capsules around organs such as the liver, kidneys, and glands. Fibrous connective tissue is also present in *tendons* (which connect muscles to bones) and *ligaments* (which connect bones to other bones). In tendons and ligaments, the fibers are all arranged in the same direction.

Hard Connective Tissue

The last type of connective tissue is hard connective tissue. As the name implies, it is more solid than the other types and includes cartilage and bone.

There are three types of cartilage found in the body. The most prevalent is hyaline cartilage. It is used by the body to reduce friction between moving parts such as bones, to attach the ribs to the sternum (breastbone), and to form the structure of the larynx.

The other two types of cartilage are fibrocartilage and elastic cartilage. Fibrocartilage, due to its highly compressible nature, is used by the body as a shock absorber and is found in the disks between the vertebrae of the spinal column. Elastic cartilage is more flexible than the other two types of cartilage and is found in the external ear.

Cartilage has no blood vessels of its own, which means repair by the body takes a long time if it is damaged. In some cases, repair may not take place at all.

Bone or *osseous* tissue is similar to cartilage in its cellular structure, but it is harder and not flexible. The matrix consists of collagen fibers impregnated with calcium and phosphorous salts, which give bone its characteristic hardness.

In addition to providing the framework of the body, bone is the site of blood cell production.

MUSCLE TISSUE

Movement of material in the body and of the body itself is generally due to the contraction of muscle tissue. There are three types of muscle tissue: skeletal, smooth, and cardiac. Each serves a very different purpose.

Skeletal muscle is attached to the bones by tendons. It moves the bones and thus the body. It is sometimes called *voluntary muscle,* because it can be made to contract by conscious thought. At the cellular level, skeletal muscle has large, cylinder-shaped cells with striations (lines) and multiple nuclei.

Smooth (or visceral) muscle is found in the walls of the digestive organs, in tubular structures such as blood vessels, and at the base of each body hair. Because this type of muscle contracts without conscious thought, it is said to be *involuntary*. Some functions include moving food and waste through the digestive tract and regulating blood pressure by contracting and relaxing blood vessels. The cells of smooth muscle are small and tapered, have no striations, and contain a single nucleus for each cell.

Cardiac muscle, as the name implies, involves the heart. It forms the walls of the chambers of the heart and is also known as myocardium. It is another type of involuntary muscle. Its function is to pump blood throughout the body. Its contractions produce what we refer to as heartbeats. Cardiac muscle is characterized by branching cells, slight striations, and a single nucleus per cell.

NERVOUS TISSUE

Nervous tissue is a highly specialized tissue composed of neurons. It is capable of generating and transmitting electrochemical impulses. These impulses are information that the brain uses to control all of the systems of the human body. *Neurons,* the basic unit of nervous tissue, consist of a cell body, axon, and dendrite. The cell body is the central portion of the neuron, which contains the nucleus. It regulates the function of the neuron. The axon is a single fiber that carries impulses or information away from the cell body. Dendrites, on the other hand, are fibers that carry impulses to the nerve cell body. Special support cells in nervous tissue produce myelin sheaths around axons (neuroglia) and protect neurons from foreign organisms (Schwann cells). These special cells do not conduct nerve impulses (Figure 10-4 ◆).

◆ Body Systems

When organs function together for the same general purpose, they are said to be part of an **organ system.** The human body contains eleven major organ systems: integumentary,

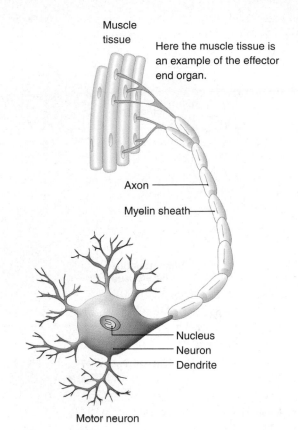

Muscle tissue

Here the muscle tissue is an example of the effector end organ.

Axon

Myelin sheath

Nucleus
Neuron
Dendrite

Motor neuron

Figure 10-4. ◆ Neuron.

skeletal, muscular, nervous, endocrine, circulatory, lymphatic, respiratory, digestive, urinary, and reproductive.

INTEGUMENTARY SYSTEM

The skin is the body's largest organ and the only organ that can be inspected in its entirety without special equipment or surgery. The skin and its associated structures (including the hair, nails, oil and sweat glands, blood vessels, nerves, and sensory organs) make up the **integumentary system** (Figure 10-5 ◆). Nursing care of the integumentary system is discussed in detail in Chapter 12. ⊖⊘ The primary functions of this system are the following:

1. Protect the body from infection by preventing pathogens from entering.
2. Protect against dehydration by preventing fluid loss.
3. Regulate body temperature. This involves dilation and constriction of blood vessels and perspiration.
4. Collect sensory information by special receptors. This information includes pain, touch, pressure, and temperature.

NERVOUS SYSTEM

In order for the systems of the body to work together, there has to be a control center and a method of sending and receiving information. This is accomplished by the nervous system

Figure 10-5. ◆ Cross-section of skin.

Hair shaft

Nerve fibers

Arrector pili muscle

Epidermis

Dermis

Subcutaneous fatty tissue

Sweat gland

Sweat pore

Sebaceous (oil) gland

Nerve ending

Hair root

Bulb

Papilla

Vein

Artery

Deep fascia

Fatty lobule

Muscle

Brain

Spinal cord

Spinal nerves

Nervous system

Figure 10-6. ◆ Nervous system.

Pineal

Pituitary

Parathyroids

Thyroid

Thymus

Pancreas

Adenals

Ovaries (in women)

Testes (in men)

Figure 10-7. ◆ Endocrine system.

THE SKELETON

Skull (cranium)
Orbit (eye socket)
Zygomatic bone

Frontal bone
Parietal bone
Occipital bone
Temporal bone
Temporomandibular joint
Maxilla
Mandible

Cervical vertebra (neck)

Acromioclavicular joint
Glenohumeral joint

Clavicle (collarbone)

Sternum (breast bone)

Scapula (shoulder blade)

Xiphoid process

Ribs

Humerus (arm bone)

Costal cartilage

Elbow
Forearm
Ulna
Radius
Sacrum

Lumbar vertebra

Illiac crest
Illium (hip)
Pelvic girdle

Ischium

Greater trochanter

Coccyx (tail bone)

Lesser trochanter

Carpals (wrist)

Symphysis pubis

Metacarpals (hand)
Phalanges (fingers)
Femur (thigh bone)
Patella (knee cap)

Lower leg bones
Tibia
Fibula
Tarsals (ankle)

Axial

Appendicular

Metatarsals (foot)
Phalanges (toes)

Calcaneus (heel)

Figure 10-8. ◆ Skeletal system.

(Figure 10-6 ◆). The human nervous system consists of two divisions: the central nervous system (CNS) and the peripheral nervous system (PNS). The central nervous system includes the brain and spinal cord. This is where information or stimuli are analyzed and responses are generated. The CNS is also the site of thought, reasoning, and memory.

The information that the CNS receives comes from the PNS, which consists of all nervous tissue not included in the CNS. The PNS has a vast number of receptors, which are used to gather information pertaining to the outside world.

ENDOCRINE SYSTEM

The endocrine system (Figure 10-7 ◆) is made up of all of the hormone secreting glands used by the body to regulate such activities as growth, metabolism, and reproduction. The endocrine system works in conjunction with the nervous system to regulate the body's systems.

SKELETAL SYSTEM

There are 206 bones in the human body. Together, they form the skeletal system (Figure 10-8 ◆). The skeleton serves five major functions:

Frontalis
Temporalis
Orbicularis Oculi

Masseter
Orbicularis Oris

Sternocleidomastoid
Trapezius

Deltoid

Pectoralis

Triceps
Serratus
Anterior
Biceps
Lattisimus
Dorsi
Rectus
Abdominis
Exterior
Oblique

Sartorius

Rectus Femoris

Vastus Lateralis

Vastus Medialis

Gastrocnemius

Gluteus
Maximus

How a Muscle Attaches to a Bone

Periosteum

Muscle Body Fibers

Bone

Tendon

Figure 10-9. ◆ Musculoskeletal system.

1. Serves as the body's framework.
2. Protects delicate structures like the brain and spinal cord.
3. Works with muscles as levers to produce movement.
4. Acts as a storehouse for calcium that can be used if calcium levels in the blood drop too low. Calcium is a very important component in muscle contractions and blood clotting.

5. Bones produce the blood cells in the red bone marrow. The cells produced are red blood cells, white blood cells, and platelets.

MUSCULAR SYSTEM

The muscles of the body are responsible for producing movement (Figure 10-9 ◆). Muscles move the body when muscles

Figure 10-11. ◆ Lymphatic system in torso.

attached to bone contract. They also move food through the digestive tract, when smooth muscle present there contracts. When the heart muscle contracts, it moves blood through the body. The contraction of skeletal muscle produces heat, helping to keep the body warm.

CIRCULATORY SYSTEM

The body's tissues need a steady supply of oxygen and nutrients. In addition, the waste products of metabolism must be removed from these same tissues. These materials are transported by the blood, which is pumped throughout the body by the heart (Figure 10-10 ◆ see page 190). The circulatory system includes the heart and all the vasculature that carries oxygenated blood to, and deoxygenated blood away from, the body.

LYMPHATIC SYSTEM

The tissues of the body contain a large amount of fluid. This fluid needs to be removed from the tissues so it does not accumulate and cause the tissues to swell. The lymphatic system works to remove the fluid from the tissues and return it to the blood (Figure 10-11 ◆). A second function of the lymphatic system is to protect the body from pathogens. When fluid enters the lymphatic system, it is filtered through lymph nodes. There, foreign materials are removed and destroyed by white blood cells.

RESPIRATORY SYSTEM

The respiratory system (Figure 10-12 ◆) consists of the lungs and the passages that lead to them. The purpose of this system is to bring oxygen into the body so that it can enter the blood

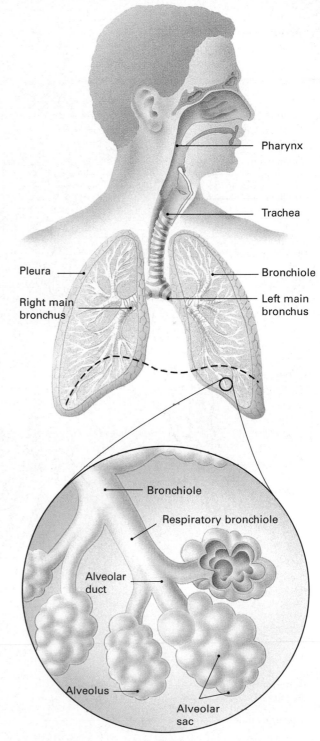

Figure 10-12. ◆ Respiratory system.

and be transported to all the tissues of the body. Additionally, the respiratory system removes carbon dioxide, a waste product of cellular metabolism, from the body. See Chapter 16. ∞

DIGESTIVE SYSTEM

The cells of the human body need a constant supply of energy in order to function properly. This energy comes from the food we

MAJOR ARTERIES

MAJOR VEINS

Internal carotid
External carotid
Common carotid

Subclavian
Innominate

Axillary
Pulmonary

Aorta

Brachial

Radial
Ulnar
Common iliac

Palmar
arches

Digital

Deep femoral
Femoral

Popliteal

Anterior tibial
Peroneal

Posterior tibial

Dorsal pedis
Arcuate

External jugular
Internal jugular
Innominate
Brachial

Cephalic

Axillary

Basilic   Antecubital

Volar digital

Subclavian
Venae cavae
Splenic artery and vein
Right gastric artery and vein
Hepatic artery and vein

Renal artery and vein
Mesenteric arteries and veins
Common iliac

Great saphenous

Femoral

Popliteal

Peroneal

Posterior tibial

Anterior tibial

Dorsal venous arch

Figure 10-10. ◆ Circulatory system.

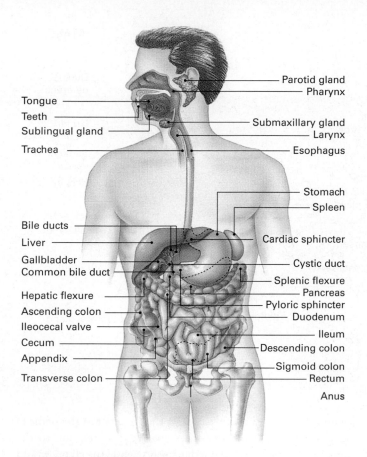

Figure 10-13. ◆ Digestive system.

Figure 10-14. ◆ Urinary system.

eat. Since food cannot directly enter the bloodstream, it needs to be broken down by the digestive system (Figure 10-13 ◆). Food is broken down through mechanical and chemical processes to a form that can enter the blood. The organs of the digestive system include the mouth, pharynx, esophagus, stomach, small intestine, and large intestine. Additionally, the salivary glands, liver, gallbladder, and pancreas play accessory roles in the process of digestion. See Chapters 17 and 19. ⌖

URINARY SYSTEM

The main purpose of the urinary system is to eliminate waste products and excess water from the body (Figure 10-14 ◆). The organs of this system include the kidneys, ureters, urinary bladder, and the urethra. Additionally, the urinary system aids in acid–base balance and electrolyte composition of body fluids. See Chapter 18. ⌖

REPRODUCTIVE SYSTEM

The purpose of the male and female reproductive systems (Figure 10-15 ◆) is to produce offspring to allow for continuation of the human species. Both male and female systems produce gametes. When an egg cell is fertilized by a sperm cell, the resulting zygote becomes implanted in the woman's uterus

and stays there until it is sufficiently developed to survive outside the womb.

Despite obvious differences between males and females, the reproductive organs of each system can be divided into two groups: primary and accessory organs.

The *primary reproductive organs* (gonads) are responsible for producing the gametes. The gonads of the male are the testes and of the female are the ovaries.

The *accessory reproductive organs* are those structures that transport, protect, and nourish the gametes after they leave the gonads. In the male, the accessory organs include the epididymis, ductus deferens, seminal vesicles, prostate gland, bulbourethral glands, scrotum, and penis. In the female they are the uterine tubes (fallopian tubes), uterus, vagina, and vulva.

Hormones control the production of gametes in both the male and female. In males, follicle-stimulating hormone (FSH) and interstitial cell-stimulating hormone (ICSH) (which stimulates the testes to produce testosterone) are the major hormones. Testosterone is also responsible for the development of **secondary sex characteristics** (traits associated with gender but not directly necessary for reproduction in males). These characteristics include a deeper voice, broader shoulders, more muscle mass, and more body hair than in females.

The hormones that control the female reproductive cycle are follicle-stimulating hormone (FSH), estrogen, leutinizing hormone (LH), and progesterone. If fertilization occurs, the embryo produces a hormone known as human chorionic gonadotropin (hCG). (See also Chapter 29). ⌖

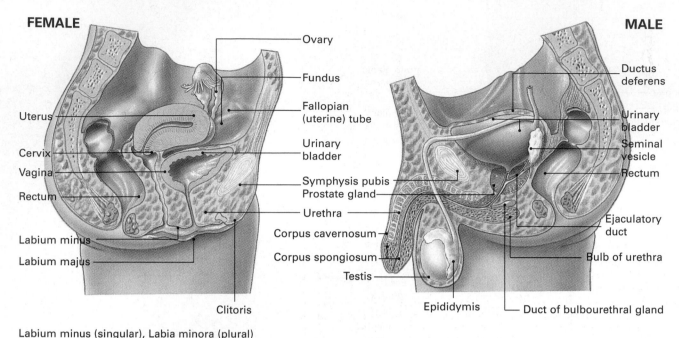

FEMALE **MALE**

Labium minus (singular), Labia minora (plural)
Labium majus (singular), Labia majora (plural)

Figure 10-15. ◆ Reproductive system.

◆ Anatomic Positions

When discussing the human body, it is important to use terminology that accurately identifies the area that is being viewed. This section provides basic terminology.

The starting position is known as the **anatomic position.** In this position the body is upright with the face front, arms at the sides with the palms facing forward, and feet parallel (Figure 10-16 ◆). Anatomic terms for direction are listed in Box 10-1 ◆. For example, the hand is farther from the

shoulder than is the elbow. Using the shoulder as the point of origin, the term that describes the hand in relation to the shoulder would be *distal* (farther away), while the elbow would be *proximal* (nearer).

Figure 10-16. ◆ Anatomic positions.

BOX 10-1
ANATOMICAL TERMS FOR DIRECTION

◆ **Anterior** or ventral—toward the front of the body or the belly

◆ **Posterior** or dorsal—toward the back of; opposite of ventral

◆ **Superior**—above or in a higher position

◆ **Inferior**—a point lower than or below a reference point

◆ **Superficial**—a point that is pertaining to or situated near the surface of an object

◆ **Deep**—a point or area that is below the surface of an object

◆ **Medial**—closer to the middle of the body

◆ **Lateral**—the opposite of medial, or toward the side

◆ **Proximal**—a point nearer the origin of a structure

◆ **Distal**—farther away from the origin of a structure

Frontal
(coronal) plane

Sagittal plane

Transverse
(horizontal) plane

Figure 10-17. ◆ Body planes (frontal or coronal, sagittal, and transverse or horizontal).

BODY PLANES

When studying anatomy, it is often necessary to picture the body as being divided by planes. A **plane** is an imaginary flat surface that divides a structure into two portions. Three planes are used most often in anatomy (Figure 10-17 ◆).

The *sagittal plane* runs from front to back, separating the body into left and right portions. If the portions are equal, the plane is said to be *midsagittal*.

The *frontal plane* runs from one side of the body to the other, separating the body into front and back portions.

The *transverse plane* cuts the body horizontally, creating a *superior* (higher) and *inferior* (lower) portion.

◆ Body Cavities

The body contains two large internal spaces or cavities in which various organs are located. These spaces are the dorsal and ventral cavities (Figure 10-18 ◆).

The dorsal cavity can be divided into the cranial and spinal cavities. The cranial cavity is the space inside the skull and is where the brain is located. The spinal cavity is where the spinal cord is housed. These two cavities form one continuous space.

The ventral cavity is much larger than the dorsal cavity. The ventral cavity can be divided into two smaller cavities, the thoracic and abdominopelvic cavities. The muscle known as the diaphragm divides the two cavities. The abdominopelvic cavity is sometimes further divided into the upper (abdominal) cavity and the lower (pelvic) cavity.

The thoracic cavity, above the diaphragm, contains the heart, lungs, and the major blood vessels that are attached to

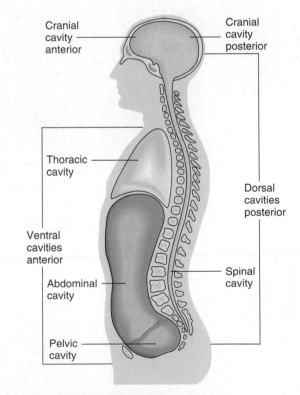

Figure 10-18. ◆ Major body cavities.

the heart. The organs located in the thoracic cavity are protected by the rib cage.

The abdominal portion of the abdominopelvic cavity is located below the diaphragm and extends downward to the top of the hipbones. Contained within the abdominal cavity are the stomach, kidneys, liver, spleen, gallbladder, and most of the intestines. Unlike the thoracic cavity, there is no protective skeletal structure over the abdominal cavity.

The pelvic cavity is below the abdominal cavity and contains the urinary bladder, rectum, and internal parts of both the male and female reproductive systems.

Because the abdominal cavity is so large, it is often divided even further to clarify which region is being discussed. This is especially helpful if a client reports "abdominal pain." It is very difficult to diagnose the cause of the pain if a region is not specified.

There are two methods of subdividing the abdominal cavity. The first one divides the cavity into four quadrants: the right upper quadrant (RUQ), the left upper quadrant (LUQ), the right lower quadrant (RLQ), and the left lower quadrant

(LLQ). Figure 10-19 ◆ shows the placement of these quadrants.

A more precise method is to divide the abdominal cavity into nine regions. The upper three regions begin below the sternum and include the right hypochondriac region, epigastric region, and the left hypochondriac region. The middle three regions cover the navel and the area of the abdomen to the right and left of the navel. They are called the right lumbar region, umbilical region, and the left lumbar region. The final three regions cover the pelvis and are known as the right iliac region, hypogastric region, and the left iliac region. See Figure 10-20 ◆ for proper placement of these regions.

Note: The bibliography listings for this and all chapters have been compiled at the back of the book.

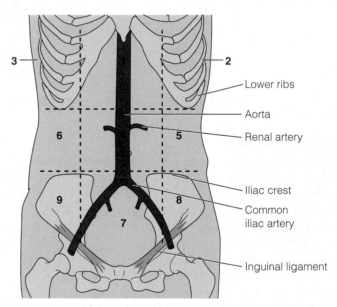

Figure 10-19. ◆ The four abdominal quadrants and the underlying organs: *1,* right upper quadrant; *2,* left upper quadrant; *3,* right lower quadrant; *4,* left lower quadrant.

Labels (Figure 10-19):
- Xiphoid process
- Liver
- Stomach
- Transverse colon
- Descending colon
- Umbilicus
- Small intestine
- Ascending colon
- Sigmoid colon
- Bladder
- Pubic symphysis

Figure 10-20. ◆ Nine abdominal regions: *1,* epigastric; *2, 3,* left and right hypochondriac; *4,* umbilical; *5, 6,* left and right lumbar; *7,* suprapubic and hypogastric; *8, 9,* left and right inguinal or iliac.

Labels (Figure 10-20):
- Lower ribs
- Aorta
- Renal artery
- Iliac crest
- Common iliac artery
- Inguinal ligament

Chapter Review

Key Terms by Topics

Use the audio glossary feature of either the CD-ROM or the Companion Website to hear the correct pronunciation of the following key terms.

Introduction
anatomy, physiology

Cells
cell, homeostasis, cell membrane, receptors, enzymes, channels, transporters, anti-

gens, cytoplasm, nucleus, endoplasmic reticulum, mitochondria, adenosine triphosphate (ATP), Golgi apparatus, cilia, flagellum, mitosis, meiosis, gametes

Tissues
tissue, epithelium, gland, endocrine glands, hormones, connective tissue, matrix

Body Systems
organ system, integumentary system, secondary sex characteristics

Anatomic Positions
anatomic position, planes (frontal, sagittal, midsagittal, transverse)

Key Points

* Anatomy is the study of body structures, while physiology is the study of body functions.

* The cell is the basic unit of life. It consists of a limiting boundary known as a plasma membrane, a nucleus surrounded by cytoplasm, and numerous structures called organelles.

* There are two types of cell division: mitosis and meiosis. Mitosis is involved in growth and repair of an organism. Meiosis is responsible for sperm and egg cells.

* The four main classifications of tissue are epithelial, connective, muscle, and nervous tissue.

* The human body consists of 11 major organ systems: integumentary, skeletal, muscular, nervous, endocrine, circulatory, lymphatic, respiratory, digestive, urinary, and reproductive.

* The anatomic position is achieved when the body is upright, face front, arms at the sides, palms facing forward, and the feet parallel.

* The planes of division of the body are sagittal, frontal, and transverse.

* The two main body cavities are the dorsal and ventral cavities.

EXPLORE MediaLink

Additional interactive resources for this chapter can be found on the Companion Website at www.prenhall.com/ramont. Click on Chapter 10 and "Begin" to select the activities for this chapter.

For chapter-related NCLEX-style questions and an audio glossary, access the accompanying CD-ROM in this book.

Animations:
* Introduction to body systems
* Normal heart hemodynamics
* Head and neck
* Skeleton
* Exploded skull
* Cell structure
* Head and face
* Heart
* Skull

⌘ For Further Study

Nursing care of the integumentary system is discussed in detail in Chapter 12.

Further information about the cardiovascular and respiratory systems is in Chapter 16.

For more about the digestive system, see Chapters 17 and 19.

For further study of the urinary system, see Chapter 18.

For more information on sexuality, see Chapter 29.

NCLEX-PN Exam Preparation

1. The basic unit of all living organisms is the:
   a. Respiratory system
   b. Brain
   c. Cell
   d. Heart

2. When all the components of the body are working properly and are in equilibrium, the body is said to be experiencing:
   a. A disease
   b. Homeostasis
   c. Physiology
   d. Prophase

3. The ventral cavity has two subdivisions. They are:
   a. Cranial and spinal
   b. Superior and inferior
   c. Thoracic and cranial
   d. Thoracic and abdominopelvic

4. The main body system that provides oxygen to and carries carbon dioxide away from the body is the:
   a. Respiratory system
   b. Urinary system
   c. Skeletal system
   d. Nervous system

5. The correct order of the stages in mitosis is:
   a. Prophase, anaphase, metaphase, telophase
   b. Metaphase, anaphase, prophase, telophase
   c. Prophase, telophase, anaphase, metaphase
   d. Prophase, metaphase, anaphase, telophase

6. The body plane that divides the body into left and right portions is the:
   a. Frontal plane
   b. Sagittal plane
   c. Transverse plane
   d. Coronal plane

7. A band of connective tissue that connects bone to bone is:
   a. A ligament
   b. A tendon
   c. Cartilage
   d. A fascia

8. The term for many layers of cells is:
   a. Squamous
   b. Columnar
   c. Stratified
   d. Simple

9. Endocrine glands are often referred to as ductless glands and they secrete:
   a. Oil
   b. Hormones
   c. Tears
   d. Blood

10. Within the cell, ribosomes are attached to the:
    a. Golgi apparatus
    b. Lysosomes
    c. Endoplasmic reticulum
    d. Centrioles

Answers for Review Questions appear in Appendix IV.

Health Assessment

LEARNING outcomes

After completing this chapter, you will be able to:

- Discuss the LPN/LVN's role in health assessment.
- Identify the purposes of the physical health examination.
- List three types of physical assessment.
- Discuss preparation of client and environment.
- Explain the three methods of examination.
- Explain the significance of selected physical findings.
- Describe suggested sequencing to conduct a physical health assessment in an orderly fashion.
- Discuss variations in assessment techniques that are appropriate for clients of different ages.

Assessing a client's health status is a major component of nursing care. There are two aspects of assessment: the nursing health history and the physical examination. The physical examination or assessment is the focus of this chapter. A **physical assessment** can be any of three types:

1. A *complete assessment* (see Figure 8-1)
2. A *focused assessment by body systems* (Figure 11-1 ◆)
3. A *focused assessment of a body part*. Box 11-1 ◆ (see page 000) provides some guidelines for assessment by body systems.

◆ Physical Health Assessment

COMPLETE ASSESSMENT

A complete assessment is conducted by an RN when the client is admitted to the health care facility. The LPN/LVN may be asked to collect some data for this. It includes a full head-to-toe assessment as well as information that pertains to the client's level of functioning. Information collected may include allergies; client's level of ambulation; personal property brought to the facility by the client, and people with whom any valuables are sent home; chronic health conditions and any medications taken for these conditions; past medical history; fall risk assessment; dietary habits; impairments and disabilities (see Figure 8-1). This complete assessment should remain in the client's chart so that all staff involved in the client's care may refer to it. This assessment also provides baseline information about the client to all staff members.

FOCUSED ASSESSMENT

A focused assessment may be conducted by the LPN/LVN at the beginning and end of the shift. It may be conducted in several ways. One efficient method is by starting at the head and proceeding in a systematic manner downward to the toes. The procedure can vary according to the age of the individual, the severity of the illness, the method preferences of the nurse, the location of the examination, and the agency's priorities and required procedures. Regardless of what type of procedure is used, the client's

energy and time need to be considered. The physical health assessment is always conducted in a systematic and efficient manner that requires the fewest position changes for the client.

The sequence of the assessment differs with children and adults. Box 11-2 ◆ (see page 000) discusses age-related differences and considerations. Frequently, nurses assess a specific system's body part or area instead of the entire body. These specific (or focused) assessments are made in relation to client complaints, the nurse's own observation of problems, the client's presenting problem, the nursing interventions provided, and medical therapies. Examples of these situations and assessments are presented in Table 11-1 ◆.

PREPARING THE CLIENT

Most people need an explanation of the physical health assessment. The nurse should explain when and where it will take place, why it is important, and what will happen during the assessment. The nurse assists the client as needed to undress and put on an examination gown.

Clients should be instructed to empty their bladders before the examination. Doing so helps them feel more relaxed and facilitates palpation of the abdomen and pubic area. If a urinalysis is required, the urine should be collected at this time. Often, clients are anxious about what the nurse will find. They can be reassured during the assessment by explanations at each step.

> **clinical ALERT**
>
> Health assessments are usually painless. However, it is important to determine, in advance, any positions that are contraindicated for a particular client.

Positioning

Frequently, several positions are required during the physical assessment. It is important to consider the client's ability to assume a position. The client's physical condition, energy level, and age should also be taken into consideration. The

TABLE 11-1	SELECTED CLIENT SITUATIONS AND FOCUSED ASSESSMENTS
SITUATION	**PHYSICAL ASSESSMENT**
Client complains of abdominal pain.	Inspect, auscultate, and palpate the abdomen; assess vital signs.
Client is admitted with a head injury.	Assess level of consciousness using Glasgow Coma Scale (see Table 11-2); assess pupils for reaction to light and accommodation; assess vital signs.
The nurse prepares to administer a cardiotonic drug to a client.	Assess apical pulse and compare with baseline data.
The nurse administers postural drainage.	Auscultate lungs before and after the procedure.
The client has just had a cast applied to the lower leg.	Assess peripheral perfusion of toes, capillary blanch test, pedal pulse if able, and vital signs.
The client's fluid intake is minimal.	Assess tissue turgor, fluid intake and output, and vital signs.

PeaceHealth
ST. JOHN MEDICAL CENTER
LONGVIEW, WASHINGTON

MED / SURG / TELE / ONC - DAILY CARE RECORD

Symbol Key
Empty box = Not assessed
✓ = Assessment matches normal parameters
X = Variation, describe in Comments
→ = Variations same as last assessment
* = See progress notes
Initial each assessment block on line
Use right box for reassessment or daily care (dc) assessment

Date:	NOC - Time: /		DAY - Time: /		EVE - Time: /	
SYSTEMS ASSESSMENTS	Comments	Reassess ☐ D/C ☐	Comments	Reassess ☐ D/C ☐	Comments	Reassess ☐ D/C ☐
Neurological LEVEL OF CONSCIOUSNESS: alert SPEECH: coherent, clearly understandable speech, symmetry of facial expression SWALLOWING: handles oral secretions ORIENTATION: aware of time, place, person; short-term memory intact BEHAVIOR: interactions appropriate to situation	☐	☐	☐	☐	☐	☐
Cardiovascular VITAL SIGNS: HR reg, BP & temp WNL for pt. RADIAL PULSE: easily palpated and regular SKIN: warm, dry, natural color for patient CIRCULATION: no peripheral edema or calf pain	☐	☐	☐	☐	☐	☐
Respiratory RATE: regular pattern, rate WNL for patient EFFORT: unlabored at rest on room air BREATH SOUNDS: no audible wheeze, stridor, rattles or other adventitious sounds COUGH: none reported or observed SPUTUM: absent or reported clear	☐	☐	☐	☐	☐	☐
Gastrointestinal PALPATION: soft, non-tender AUSCULTATION: normally active bowel sounds INTAKE: tolerating at least half of prescribed diet without nausea/vomiting BM: continent of soft, formed stool within past 48°	☐	☐	☐	☐	☐	☐
Genitourinary URINATION: observed/reported continent voiding of clear urine in sufficient quantity; no dysuria BLADDER DISTENTION: none visible GENITALIA: no observed/reported genital discharge or swelling	☐	☐	☐	☐	☐	☐
Musculoskeletal EXTREMITIES: functional, non-painful ROM x4 MOVEMENT: independent gait, transfers and ambulates without use of assistive devices	☐	☐	☐	☐	☐	☐
Integumentary/Wounds PRESSURE: no blanching or redness at boney prominences. No skin breakdown. HYDRATION: normal skin turgor; moist mucosa WOUND: well-approximated edges, no redness, swelling, drainage OR dressing clean, dry, intact	☐	☐	☐	☐	☐	☐
Psych/Soc SUPPORT: fam/soc support sys evident/ reported AFFECT: calm, cooperative, normal eye contact (within cultural context) SLEEP PATTERNS: able to sleep at night if undisturbed; absence of unusual fatigue	☐	☐	☐	☐	☐	☐

Safety Risk Factors
☐ Patient concerned about falling
☐ Family concerned about falling
☐ History of falls within last few months

☐ Bladder/bowel urgency
☐ Impaired mobility
☐ Cognitive impairment
☐ In RN assessment patient is fall risk

☐ If yes to any, Implement Fall Prevention
☐ If yes to cognitive impairment, bed alarm placed
☐ No safety risk factors identified

Initials	Signature - NOC	Initials	Signature - NOC	Initials	Signature - NOC

Figure 11-1. ◆ Focused assessment by body system. Source: Courtesy of PeaceHealth St. John Medical Center, Longview, WA. Used with permission.

BOX 11-1
NURSING CARE CHECKLIST

ASSESSMENT BY BODY SYSTEMS

Neurologic

☑ LOC (level of consciousness)
  ◆ A/O ✕3 (alert and oriented to name, time, and place)
☑ Verbal Response
  ◆ Clear
  ◆ Incoherent, rambling, slurred, stuttering
  ◆ Dysphasia, aphasia
☑ Motor Response (<, = bilaterally, >)
  ◆ Grips (note strength)
  ◆ Obeys commands, localizes pain, withdrawal, flexion, extension, none
  ◆ Pain—sharp, burning, intense, sudden, agonizing, throbbing, stabbing
  ◆ Pain level 1–10
☑ Assess Pupils
  ◆ Note shape
  ◆ Pupils equally round and react to light, and accommodate (PERRLA)
    1. 1 mm after surgery
    2. 2–3 mm normal
    3. 6–9 mm "blown"; if permanent, possible herniation

Integumentary

☑ General Appearance
  ◆ Pale, flushed, cyanotic, discolored, freckled
  ◆ Moist, diaphoretic, clammy
  ◆ Hot, warm, cold
  ◆ Dry, scaly, oily
  ◆ Rash, abrasion, laceration, incisions, broken, sores, lesions, scars, calloused, contusions
  ◆ Tanned, glossy, tatoos
  ◆ Swollen, coarse or fine texture
☑ Turgor
  ◆ Normal
  ◆ Loose
  ◆ Tight
  ◆ Tenting
☑ Integrity
  ◆ Intact
  ◆ Impaired
☑ Mucous membranes
  ◆ Color
  ◆ Condition

Cardiovascular (normal pulse 60–100)

☑ Ap, B/P, Radial PP (present <, = bilaterally, >)
  ◆ Rate/rhythm
    • Regular

  • Irregular
  • Strong
  • Rapid
  • Weak
  • Absent
  • Thready
  ◆ Intensity
    • 1, 2 (hypo)
    • 3, 4 (hyper or bounding)
  ◆ Doppler
☑ Skin—pale, flushed, cyanotic, discolored, moist, cold, clammy
☑ Edema—pitting, nonpitting
☑ Capillary refill < 3 sec
☑ Homan's sign +/−

Respiratory (18–20 normal respirations)

☑ Breathing
  ◆ Dyspnea
  ◆ Apnea
  ◆ Deep/shallow
☑ SOB (shortness of breath)
  ◆ With which activities?
☑ Chest
  ◆ Excursion symmetrical/asymmetrical
☑ Lung Sounds (audible all lobes)
  ◆ Rales
  ◆ Crackles
  ◆ Rhonchi
  ◆ Wheezes
☑ Sputum
  ◆ Clear
  ◆ Thin/Thick
  ◆ Tenacious
  ◆ Note color
☑ Measure O_2 Saturation
  ◆ Pulse Oximeter

Gastrointestinal

☑ Abdomen
  ◆ Soft, firm, rigid, tender, sensitive to touch
  ◆ Enlarged, distended, flat, round
  ◆ Note any rebound tenderness
☑ Bowel sounds (listen all 4 quads—2 to 5 min)
  ◆ Normal, faint, hypo, absent, hyper
☑ BM size (sm, med, lg)
☑ N/V (nausea/vomiting)—amount/color/frequency
  ◆ cc's, small, large
  ◆ Blood tinged, fecal
  ◆ Projectile
☑ Diarrhea (amt/color/freq)

☑ Appetite (tolerance to prescribed diet)
◆ Percentage

Genitourinary (30 cc/hr normal output)

☑ Urination: independent, catheter, incontinent
◆ Amount
◆ Color—yellow, amber, bloody, brown, dark red
◆ Appearance—clear, cloudy, sediment
◆ Odor—offensive, foul, musty, aromatic, ammonia-like, odorless

☑ I/O (intake/output)—all fluids should be balanced with output

☑ Bladder distention
◆ Check, feel, palpate

Musculoskeletal

☑ ROM (range of motion)
☑ Gait
☑ Deformities

Psychosocial

☑ Mental and spiritual
◆ Moods, affect, judgment, abilities, lifestyle, patterns, age

assessment is organized so that several body areas can be assessed in one position. The LPN/LVN most frequently assesses the client in (a) the prone or supine position in bed (Figure 11-2 ◆) or (b) sitting in bed or in a chair.

Draping

Drapes, usually the client's bed linens, should be arranged so that the area to be assessed is exposed while other body areas are covered. Exposure of the body is frequently embarrassing to clients. Drapes provide not only a covering but also warmth.

Preparing the Environment

It is important to prepare the environment before starting the assessment. The time for the physical assessment should be convenient for both the client and the nurse. The environment should be well lighted and the equipment should be organized for use.

Providing privacy is important. Curtains should be drawn. Most people are embarrassed if others can overhear or view them during the assessment. Family and friends should not be present during the examination unless the client specifically requests their presence.

A

B

Figure 11-2. ◆ Two most common client positions for assessment in bed. **A.** Prone. **B.** Supine.

The room temperature should be warm enough to be comfortable for the client. A well-prepared environment affects the client's response to the examination. The client who is physically relaxed usually experiences little discomfort.

Methods of Examination

Three primary techniques used by the practical/vocational nurse in the physical examination are: inspection, auscultation, and palpation. A fourth technique, percussion, is learned in later training and is used in specific procedures. These techniques are defined below and discussed throughout this chapter as they apply to each body system.

INSPECTION

Inspection is visual examination, that is, assessing by using the sense of sight. Inspection should be deliberate, purposeful, and systematic. In addition to visual observations, *olfactory* (smelling) and *auditory* (hearing) cues are noted. Nurses frequently use visual inspection to assess moisture, color, and texture of body surfaces, as well as shape, position, size, color, and symmetry of the body. Lighting must be sufficient for the nurse to see clearly; either natural or artificial light can be used. When using the auditory senses, it is important to have a quiet environment for accurate hearing. Inspection can be combined with the other assessment techniques.

AUSCULTATION

Auscultation is the process of listening to sounds produced within the body. Auscultation may be direct or indirect. *Direct auscultation* is the use of the unaided ear, for example, to listen to a respiratory wheeze or the grating of a moving joint. *Indirect auscultation* (shown in the procedure at the end of the chapter) is done with the use of a stethoscope. The stethoscope amplifies the sounds and conveys them to the nurse's ears. A stethoscope is used primarily to listen to sounds from within the body, such as bowel sounds in the abdomen or valve sounds of the heart.

PALPATION

Palpation is the examination of the body using the sense of touch. The pads of the fingers are used because their concen-

BOX 11-2

POPULATION FOCUS

ASSESSMENT DIFFERENCES BY AGE OR CONDITION

Infants and Children

Skin

- *Jaundice* (yellowish skin) possible in newborns for several weeks after birth.
- May have increased pigmentation in sacral area of infants and young children of dark-skinned races.
- Possible *milia* (whiteheads) over the nose and face, and *vernix caseosa* (white, greasy, protective material) on skin of newborns.

Head

- Shape altered by delivery for about 1 week in most newborns.
- Posterior *fontanel* (soft spot) generally closes by 8 weeks and anterior fontanel by 18 months.
- Voluntary head control by 6 months of age.

Eyes, Ears, Nose, Mouth

- Horizontal line from eye to top of the ear is normal. Auricle should angle no more than 10 degrees from vertical. (*Note:* Variation may indicate mental retardation or renal abnormalities.)
- Infants may blink at a sharp sound. (*Note:* To assess gross hearing, ring a bell from behind the infant or have the parent call the child's name to check for a response. At 3 to 4 months, the infant will turn head and eyes toward the sound.)
- Tooth development should be appropriate for age; permanent teeth are darker than deciduous teeth.
- Inspect the palate for a cleft.

Chest, Heart, and Lungs

- Infants and children up to age 6 tend to breathe more from abdomen than from chest.
- Chest circumference measurements at delivery and up to 9 months rule out birth injuries, congenital anomalies, or other dysfunction.
- Auscultated sounds are louder and harsher because of thinner chest wall.
- A third heart sound, best heard at the apex, is present in about one third of all children.
- Palpation of pulses in the lower extremities (particularly the femoral pulses) can be used to screen for certain heart abnormalities.

Gastrointestinal

- Abdomen of the newborn and infant is round. Characteristic "pot belly" appearance of toddlers persists until about age 5.
- Peristaltic waves usually more visible than in adults.

- Children may not be able to pinpoint areas of tenderness. Observe facial expressions to determine areas of maximum tenderness.
- Liver is relatively larger than in adults, and can be palpated 1 to 2 cm below the right costal margin.

Musculoskeletal

- *Lordosis* (swayback) is common in young children.
- *Pronation* (in-turning) of the feet is common between 12 and 30 months of age.
- *Genu varum* (bowleg) is normal for 1 year after beginning to walk.
- Asymmetric gluteal folds, asymmetric abduction of the legs, or apparent shortening of the femur suggest developmental dysplasia of the hip (congenital dislocation).

Pregnant Women

- Breast, areola, and nipple size increase.
- Areolae and nipples darken. Nipples may become more erect. Areolae contain small, scattered, elevated Montgomery's glands.
- Superficial veins become more prominent. Stretch marks may develop.
- *Colostrum* (thick yellow fluid) may be expressed from the nipples after the first trimester.

Older Adults

Skin, Hair, and Nails

- Skin loses elasticity, appears thin, translucent, more wrinkled.
- Skin often dry and flaky, takes longer to return to its natural shape after being tented between the thumb and finger.
- Increased number of discolorations and skin lesions.
- Scalp and facial hair grays.
- Toenails grow more slowly and thicken.
- Longitudinal bands commonly develop on fingernails in older adults, and the nails tend to split.

Eyes, Ears, Nose, and Mouth

- Ears may appear dry, with increased coarse hair growth.
- Tympanic membrane is more translucent and less flexible.
- Earwax is drier.
- Hearing loss (presbycusis) occurs.
- Oral mucosa may be drier because of decreased salivary gland activity or dehydration.
- Gums recede, giving an appearance of increased toothiness.
- Taste sensations diminish due to atrophy of the taste buds and a decreased sense of smell.
- Tooth loss may occur as a result of gum disease.

Chest, Heart, and Lungs

◆ Anteroposterior diameter of the chest deepens, giving the person barrel-chested appearance due to loss of skeletal muscle strength in the thorax and diaphragm and constant lung inflation (from excessive expiratory pressure on the alveoli).
◆ Breathing rate and rhythm are unchanged at rest; heart rate after activity may take longer to return to the resting rate.
◆ Inspiratory muscles become less powerful, and depth of respiration decreases.
◆ Expiration may require the use of accessory muscles. The amount of air remaining in the lungs at the end of a normal breath increases.
◆ Cilia in the airways become fewer and are less effective in removing mucus.
◆ Heart size remains the same (if no disease is present).
◆ Cardiac output and strength of contraction decrease, so activity tolerance is less.
◆ Sudden emotional and physical stresses may result in cardiac arrhythmias and heart failure.
◆ Overall effectiveness of blood vessels decreases; lower extremities are more likely to show signs of impairment.
◆ Systolic and diastolic blood pressures may increase.

clinical ALERT

Clients with a blood pressure reading above 140/90 should be referred for follow-up assessments.

◆ Peripheral edema is frequently observed.

Gastrointestinal

◆ Abdomen may appear round due to increase in *adipose* (fatty) tissue and decreased muscle tone. Abdominal wall is slacker and thinner, so palpation is easier and more accurate.
◆ Side effects of drugs are often manifested by nausea, vomiting, and diarrhea.
◆ Pain threshold is often higher; major abdominal problems such as appendicitis or other acute emergencies may therefore go undetected.

◆ Gastrointestinal pain needs to be differentiated from cardiac pain. (*Note:* Gastrointestinal pain may be located in the chest or abdomen, whereas cardiac pain is usually located in the chest. Factors aggravating gastrointestinal pain are usually related to either ingestion or lack of food intake; gastrointestinal pain is usually relieved by antacids, food, or an upright position. Common factors that can aggravate cardiac pain are activity or anxiety; cardiac pain is relieved by rest or nitroglycerin.)
◆ Emptying time of the stomach is slower because gastric acid secretion is decreased, resulting in indigestion and intolerance of certain foods. Decreases in the production of pancreatic enzymes also contribute to complaints of indigestion and anorexia.
◆ Stool passes through the intestines at a slower rate, and the perception of stimuli that produce the urge to defecate often diminishes.
◆ Fecal incontinence may occur in confused or neurologically impaired older adults.

clinical ALERT

Absence of a daily bowel movement does not signify constipation. When assessing for constipation, the nurse must consider the client's diet, activity, and medications; the characteristics of feces and ease or difficulty in defecating; as well as the frequency of bowel movements.

◆ Decreased absorption of oral medications.
◆ In the liver, impaired metabolism of certain drugs may occur.

Musculoskeletal

◆ Muscle mass decreases progressively with age, but there are wide variations among different individuals.
◆ Decreases in speed, strength, resistance to fatigue, reaction time, and coordination occur.
◆ Bones become more fragile. Osteoporosis leads to a loss of total bone mass, predisposition to fractures, and compressed vertebrae.
◆ Osteoarthritic changes in joints may be observed.

tration of nerve endings makes them highly sensitive and able to detect small differences or changes. Palpation is used to determine (a) texture (e.g., of the hair); (b) temperature (e.g., of a skin area); (c) vibration (e.g., of a joint); (d) position, size, consistency, and mobility of organs or masses; (e) distention (e.g., of the urinary bladder); (f) pulsation; and (g) the presence of pain upon pressure.

There are two types of palpation: light and deep. The LPN/LVN is trained in light palpation (Figure 11-3 ◆). Deep palpation is not usually done by the LPN/LVN, because pressure can damage internal organs. It is usually avoided in clients who have acute abdominal pain or who have pain that is not yet diagnosed.

Figure 11-3. ◆ The position of the hand for light palpation.

PERCUSSION

Percussion is the act of striking a part with short, sharp blows (a) to help gather data about internal organs; (b) to assist in massage; or (c) to help a client to clear the respiratory tract.

NURSING CARE

ASSESSING

General Survey

Physical assessment begins with a general survey that involves observation of the client's general appearance and behavior, and measurement of vital signs, height, and weight.

Many components of the general survey are assessed when the RN takes the client's health history, such as the client's body build, posture, hygiene, and mental status. These data can be used by the LPN/LVN as a baseline with which to compare future assessment findings. Procedure 11-1 describes how to perform a focused physical assessment by body systems.

The general appearance and behavior of an individual must be assessed in relationship to current circumstances. For example, an individual who has recently experienced a personal loss may appropriately appear depressed. Also, the client's age, sex, and race are useful factors in interpreting findings that suggest increased risk for known conditions.

Neurological Status

Level of Consciousness. **Level of consciousness (LOC)** can lie anywhere along a continuum from a state of alertness to coma. A fully alert client responds to questions spontaneously; a comatose client may not respond at all to verbal stimuli. The Glasgow Coma Scale was originally developed to predict recovery from a head injury; however, it is used by many professionals to assess LOC. It tests in three major areas: eye response, motor response, and verbal response. An assessment totaling 15 points indicates the client is alert and completely oriented. A comatose client scores 7 or less (Table 11-2 ◆).

Orientation. The nurse determines the client's orientation to time, place, and person by tactful questioning. **Orientation** is easily assessed by asking the client the city and state of residence, time of day, date, day of the week, duration of illness, and names of family members. More direct questioning may be necessary for some people; for example, "Where are you now?" "What day is it today?" Most people readily respond and accept these questions. The nurse listens for *quantity* of speech (amount and pace), *quality* (loudness, clarity, and inflection), and *organization* (coherent thought, connection to what was asked, overgeneralization, or vagueness).

Pupil Reaction. Pupils are normally black, are equal in size (about 3 to 7 mm in diameter), and have round, smooth bor-

TABLE 11-2	LEVELS OF CONSCIOUSNESS: GLASGOW COMA SCALE	
FACULTY MEASURED	**RESPONSE**	**SCORE**
Eye Opening	Spontaneous	4
	To verbal command	3
	To pain	2
	No response	1
Motor Response	To verbal command	6
	To localized pain	5
	Flexes and withdraws	4
	Flexes abnormally	3
	Extends abnormally	2
	No response	1
Verbal Response	Oriented, converses	5
	Disoriented, converses	4
	Uses inappropriate words	3
	Makes incomprehensible sounds	2
	No response	1

ders. Cloudy pupils often indicate cataracts. Unequal pupils (*anisocoria*) may result from a central nervous system disorder; however, slight variations may be normal. The reactions a nurse must check are discussed in Procedure 11-1. They include:

1. **Direct response**—In a semi-darkened room, a pupil should constrict or tighten when a bright light is shone into it.
2. **Consensual response**—When the bright light is shone on the same pupil a second time, the pupil of the other eye should also constrict.
3. **Accommodation**—A person alternates looking from a near object (about 10 cm or 4 in from the bridge of the nose) to a distant object (such as a point on the far wall). Accommodation is the alternating change in pupil size (constricts when looking at the near object, dilates when looking at the distant one).

A normal assessment of the pupils is recorded using the abbreviation **PERRLA** (pupils equally round and react to light and accommodation).

Skull. The skull of an adult client is not usually directly assessed. However, if the client has had head trauma or a procedure involving this area, the skull is assessed.

Part A of Procedure 11-1 focuses on assessing general appearance and mental status.

Vital Signs

Vital signs are measurements of temperature, pulse, respirations, and blood pressure. They are measured (a) to establish baseline data against which to compare future measurements and (b) to detect actual and potential health problems.

Normal adult vital signs are T 98.6°F (37°C); P 60 to 100 per minute, average 80 beats per minute; R 12 to 20 per minute, average 16 per minute; BP 120/80. See Chapter 14 for full information and instructions related to taking vital signs. 🔗

Height and Weight

In adults, the ratio of weight to height provides a general measure of health. It is also important that the nurse and client be aware of any significant unintentional weight gain or loss. The height and weight are usually measured when a client is admitted to a health care agency. Measurement of height and weight is discussed in Chapter 17. 🔗

Weight may also be measured regularly, for example, each morning before breakfast. When accuracy is essential, the nurse should use the same scale each time (because every scale weighs differently). The weight should be measured at the same time each day, making sure the client wears the same kind of clothing and no shoes. The client usually stands on a platform, and the weight is read from a digital display panel or a balancing arm. Clients who cannot stand are weighed on bed or chair scales.

Integumentary System

The integumentary system includes the skin, hair, and nails. In most documentation paperwork, condition of hair would be documented as a narrative note only in the event of a problem. Examination begins with a generalized inspection using a good source of lighting, preferably indirect natural daylight.

Skin. Assessment of the skin involves inspection and palpation. The nurse may also need to use the nose (*olfactory* sense) to detect unusual skin odors. These odors are usually most evident in the skin folds or in the axillae. Pungent body odor is frequently related to poor hygiene, *hyperhidrosis* (excessive perspiration), or *bromhidrosis* (foul-smelling perspiration). The entire skin surface may be assessed at one time or as each aspect of the body is assessed.

Pallor occurs when there is too little circulating blood or hemoglobin, which results in reduced amounts of oxygen being carried to body tissues. It is usually characterized by the absence of underlying red tones in the skin and may be most readily seen in the buccal mucosa. In brown-skinned clients, pallor may appear as a yellowish brown tinge; in black-skinned clients, the skin may appear ashen gray. Pallor in all people is usually most evident in areas with the least pigmentation such as the conjunctiva, oral mucous membranes, nail beds, palms of the hand, and soles of the feet.

The integument can also be characterized as cyanotic, erythematous, or edematous. **Cyanosis** (a bluish tinge) is most evident in the nail beds, lips, and buccal mucosa. Bruised areas normally blanch when pressure is applied. Cyanotic skin does not blanch to the same degree as bruised skin.

Erythema is a redness associated with a variety of rashes. **Edema** is the presence of excess interstitial fluid (see Procedure 11-1B). Elasticity or **turgor** (fullness) of the skin is also observed.

A skin **lesion** is an alteration in a client's normal skin appearance. Nurses are responsible for describing skin lesions accurately in terms of *location* (e.g., face), *distribution* (i.e., body regions involved), and *configuration* (the arrangement or position of several lesions). They also note the color, shape, size, firmness, texture, and characteristics of individual lesions.

Assessment of the feet is an important consideration. This is especially important for clients with diabetes or peripheral vascular disease (see Table 11-3 ◆).

Nails. Nails are inspected for nail plate shape, nail texture, nail bed color, the intactness of the tissues around the nails, and the angle between the nail and the nail bed (Figure 11-4 ◆).

Nail texture is normally smooth. Excessively thick nails can appear in the elderly, in the presence of poor circulation, or

TABLE 11-3	ASSESSMENT OF THE FEET	
METHOD	**NORMAL FINDINGS**	**DEVIATIONS FROM NORMAL**
Inspect all skin surfaces, particularly between the toes, for cleanliness, odor, dryness, inflammation, swelling, abrasions, or other lesions	Intact skin Absence of swelling or inflammation	Excessive dryness Areas of inflammation or swelling (e.g., corns, calluses) Fissures Scaling and cracking of skin (e.g., athlete's foot) Plantar warts
Palpate anterior and posterior surfaces of ankles and feet for edema	No swelling	Swelling or pitting edema (see Procedure 11-1)
Palpate dorsalis pedis pulse on dorsal surface of foot	Strong, regular pulses in both feet	Weak or absent pulses
Compare skin temperatures of the two feet	Warm skin temperature	Cool skin temperature in one or both feet

Figure 11-4. ◆ **A.** A normal nail, showing the convex shape and the plate angle of about 160 degrees. **B.** A spoon-shaped nail, which may be seen in clients with iron deficiency anemia. **C.** Early clubbing. **D.** Late clubbing (may be caused by long-term oxygen lack). **E.** Beau's line on nail (may result from severe injury or illness).

in relation to a chronic fungal infection. A bluish or purplish tint to the nail bed may reflect cyanosis. Pallor in the nail bed may reflect poor arterial circulation.

A blanch test can be carried out to test the **capillary refill** time (the time the nail bed takes to return to its usual color after being pressed), to assess peripheral circulation. Normal nail bed capillaries blanch when pressed but quickly turn pink or their usual color when pressure is released. A capillary refill rate of more than 3 seconds may indicate circulatory problems.

Procedure 11-1 Part B describes how to assess the skin and nails.

Cardiovascular System

Heart. In every physical assessment, it is important to listen to and count the apical **pulse** (heartbeat) for 1 full minute. Note pulse quality (bounding, normal, thready). Also note extra or skipped beats.

Associated with these sounds are systole and diastole. **Systole** is the period in which the ventricles contract. It begins with the first heart sound and ends at the second heart sound. Systole is normally shorter than diastole. **Diastole** is the period in which the ventricles relax. It starts with the second sound and ends at the following first sound. Both sounds are low in pitch and heard best at the apical site, with the bell of the stethoscope, and with the client lying on the left side.

Peripheral Vascular System. The **peripheral vascular system** includes all the blood vessels that carry oxygenated blood to body tissues and organs and return deoxygenated blood to the heart and lungs. When palpating peripheral pulses, note quality of pulses; document as *bounding* (palpable, forceful), *normal, weak* (difficult to palpate and easily stopped by pressure), or *absent* (not palpable). Assessing the peripheral vascular system also includes measuring the blood pressure; inspecting, palpating, and auscultating the carotid pulse; inspecting the jugular and peripheral veins; and inspecting the skin and tissues to determine **perfusion** (blood supply to an area) to the extremities. Certain aspects of peripheral vascular assessment are often incorporated into other parts of the assessment procedure. For example, blood pressure is usually measured at the beginning of the physical examination (see Chapter 14, the section on pulse sites and Procedure 14-2; see also Procedure 14-4 on assessing blood pressure). ⨋⨋ Procedure 11-1 Part C describes how to assess the cardiovascular and peripheral vascular systems.

Respiratory System

Thorax and Lung Assessment. Abnormal breath sounds, called **adventitious breath sounds,** occur when air passes through narrowed airways or airways filled with fluid or mucus, or when pleural linings are inflamed. Adventitious sounds—*crackles* (referred to as rales or crepitations), *gurgles, pleural friction rub,* and *wheezes*—are often superimposed over normal sounds. Table 11-4 ◆ describes normal sounds and adventitious breath sounds. *Absence of breath sounds* over some lung areas is also a significant finding; it is associated with collapsed and surgically removed lobes. Oxygenation is discussed in depth in Chapter 16. ⨋⨋

Assessing the lungs is frequently critical to assessing the client's aeration status. Changes in the respiratory system can come about slowly or quickly. In clients with chronic obstructive pulmonary disease (COPD), such as chronic bronchitis, emphysema, and asthma, changes often occur gradually as the body attempts to increase lung expansion.

Auscultation. To hear the breath sounds accurately, the nurse performs auscultation with the stethoscope on the skin, not through clothing. For efficiency, the nurse usually examines the posterior chest first, then the anterior chest. For posterior and lateral chest examinations, the client is uncovered to the waist and is in a sitting position. A sitting or lying position may be used for anterior chest examination. The sitting position is preferred because it maximizes chest expansion. However, if the client is unable to sit up, the examination can be performed with the client lying on his or her side.

Ask the client to take slow, deep breaths through the mouth while the exam is performed. This allows the client to move a greater amount of air through the lungs, which helps the nurse detect abnormal sounds. It can sometimes be helpful to have the client cough two or three times before the nurse begins auscultation. Coughing clears the lung fields, which in turn clears airway secretions.

To auscultate the anterior chest, begin just above the clavicle starting on the client's right side. Move to the left side. Move to each lobe in a right-to-left pattern. When auscultating the anterior chest of a female client, it may be necessary to have her lie down so that her breasts fall to the side, allowing more accurate auscultation of the lung fields.

Respirations should also be counted at this time. Respirations normally range from 18 to 20 breaths per

TABLE 11-4 NORMAL AND ADVENTITIOUS BREATH SOUNDS

TYPE/NAME	DESCRIPTION	CHARACTERISTICS/CAUSES	LOCATION
Normal Breath Sounds			
Vesicular	Soft-intensity, low-pitched, "gentle sighing" sounds created by air moving through smaller airways (bronchioles and alveoli)	Best heard on inspiration, which is about 2.5 times longer than the expiratory phase (5:2 ratio)	Over peripheral lung; best heard at base of lungs
Bronchovesicular	Moderate-intensity and moderate-pitched "blowing" sounds created by air moving through larger airways (bronchi)	Equal inspiratory and expiratory phases (1:1 ratio)	Between the scapulae and lateral to the sternum at the first and second intercostal spaces
Bronchial (tubular)	High-pitched, loud, "harsh" sounds created by air moving through the trachea	Louder than vesicular sounds; have a short inspiratory phase and long expiratory phase (1:2 ratio)	Anteriorly over the trachea; not normally heard over lung tissue
Adventitious Breath Sounds			
Crackles (rales)	Fine, short, interrupted crackling sounds; alveolar rales are high-pitched. Sound can be simulated by rolling a lock of hair near the ear. Best heard on inspiration but can be heard on both inspiration and expiration. May not be cleared by coughing.	Air passing through fluid or mucus in any air passage	Most commonly heard in the bases of the lower lung lobes
Gurgles (rhonchi)	Continuous, low-pitched, coarse, gurgling, harsh, louder sounds with a moaning or snoring quality. Best heard on expiration but can be heard on both inspiration and expiration. May be altered by coughing.	Air passing through narrowed air passages as a result of secretions, swelling, tumors	Loud sounds can be heard over most lung areas but predominate over the trachea and bronchi
Friction rub	Superficial grating or creaking sounds heard during inspiration and expiration. Not relieved by coughing.	Rubbing together of inflamed pleural surfaces	Heard most often in areas of greatest thoracic expansion (e.g., lower anterior and lateral chest)
Wheeze	Continuous, high-pitched, squeaky musical sounds. Best heard on expiration. Not usually altered by coughing.	Air passing through constricted bronchi as a result of secretions, swelling, tumors	Heard over all lung fields

minute. Respirations should be described as present, absent, deep, shallow, and with or without difficulty. A procedure called pulse oximetry is frequently conducted on clients with respiratory impairment (see Procedure 16-1 for explanation of use of oximeter). ⊖⊘

The nurse should also note any sputum, its appearance and amount. See Box 11-1 for suggestions. It is also important to note if the client is short of breath and which activity, if any, produces shortness of breath. Procedure 11-1 Part D describes how to assess the lungs.

Gastrointestinal System

Upper GI. When assessing the mouth and oropharynx, the nurse should observe for the following: inflammation of the tongue and oral mucosa; accumulation of food, microorganisms, and epithelial elements on the teeth and gums (referred

to as *sordes*); or bleeding of the gums (which may be due to disease process or medication).

The mouth is the beginning of the gastrointestinal system (digestive system) and should be assessed carefully. The Centers for Disease Control and Prevention (CDC) recommends that nurses wear gloves when in contact with the buccal mucosa (Figure 11-5A, B ◆). A tongue blade can be used to aid inspection.

The nurse should note any difficulty swallowing and obtain further information about the cause. The nurse also notes any subjective indications of discomfort or nausea and records the client's statement of when these manifestations began and how long they have persisted. Any abnormal findings or change in client condition should be reported to the team leader.

Abdomen. To assist in obtaining valid observations and to enhance client comfort, as mentioned previously, the nurse

Figure 11-5. ◆ **A.** Inspecting the mucosa of the lower lip. **B.** Inspecting the buccal mucosa using a tongue blade.

asks the client to urinate before beginning the assessment. If necessary, the nurse assists the client to a supine position, with arms placed comfortably at the sides. The nurse also places small pillows beneath the knees and the head. This position and an empty bladder prevent tension in the abdominal muscles. By contrast, the abdominal muscles tense when the client is sitting or when the client is supine with knees and arms extended and hands clasped behind the head.

The nurse exposes only the client's abdomen from chest line to the pubic area to avoid chilling and shivering, which can also tense the abdominal muscles.

The nurse locates and describes abdominal findings in a client by dividing the abdomen into quadrants, imagining a vertical line from the xiphoid process to the pubic symphysis, and a horizontal line across the umbilicus (see Figure 10-19). ⊂⊃ These quadrants are labeled (1) right upper quadrant (RUQ), (2) left upper quadrant (LUQ), (3) right lower

quadrant (RLQ), and (4) left lower quadrant (LLQ). Assessment of the abdomen involves all four methods of examination (inspection, auscultation, palpation, and percussion). As mentioned above, inspection, auscultation, and light palpation are the skills first practiced by LPNs/LVNs.

The nurse performs inspection first, followed by auscultation, and palpation last. Auscultation is done before palpation because palpation causes movement or stimulation of the bowel. This can increase bowel motility and heighten bowel sounds, creating false results.

Thus, the order of abdominal assessment should be:

1. **Look.** While standing at the side of the supine client, inspect the abdomen for contour and symmetry. Is it flat, rounded, or concave? If rounded, is it *distended* (stretched out)? When distention is present, measure the abdominal girth by placing a tape around the abdomen at the level of the umbilicus (Figure 11-6 ◆). Look for movement associated with peristalsis or pulsations.

2. **Listen.** Place the diaphragm of your stethoscope lightly on the client's abdomen and listen for bowel sounds in all four quadrants (see Figure 10-19). ⊂⊃ Landmarks for identifying abdominal areas are shown in Figure 11-7 ◆. Are sounds normal, increased, decreased, or absent? If you suspect absent bowel sounds, listen for 5 minutes. Be sure that the client's bladder is empty before reporting absent bowel sounds. A full bladder may obscure sounds.

3. **Feel.** Light palpation is used mainly for determining areas of tenderness. Palpate in all four quadrants (Figure 11-8 ◆). The best indicator of tenderness is the client's facial expression. Voluntary or involuntary guarding may be present. Procedure 11-1 Part E describes how to assess the abdomen.

Figure 11-6. ◆ Measuring abdominal girth at the level of the umbilicus.

- Xiphoid process
- Costal margins
- Midline
- Anterior superior iliac spines
- Umbilicus
- Inguinal (Poupart's) ligaments
- Superior margin of pubic bone

Figure 11-7. ◆ Landmarks commonly used to identify abdominal areas.

Figure 11-9. ◆ Palpating the bladder.

Genitourinary System

Note whether the client is continent or incontinent of urine or if an indwelling catheter is present. The amount, color, frequency, and odor of the urine should be described. This is a good opportunity to check the client's intake and output.

In some clients, it may be necessary to palpate the bladder to determine whether the client has emptied it completely (Figure 11-9 ◆). Locate the edge of the bladder by pressing in the midline about 1 to 2 inches above the symphysis pubis. If the bladder is palpable, the nurse will feel a smooth, firm, slightly bouncy area. The client may indicate the urge to empty the bladder when it is palpated. During the postpartum period, the bladder can be easily palpated by first identifying the fundus of the uterus and then creeping the fingers down toward the symphysis pubis.

Procedure 11-1 Part F describes how to assess the bladder and urine.

Musculoskeletal System

The musculoskeletal system encompasses the muscles, bones, and joints (see Figure 10-7). 🔗

Figure 11-8. ◆ Light palpation used in all four quadrants to check for areas of tenderness.

Range of Motion. There are two types of range of motion (ROM), active and passive.

In **active range of motion**, the extremities and joints are moved by the client through a systematic series of movements. The nurse asks the client to move each joint through a full range of motion. The nurse notes the degree and type of pain or weakness, or any limitation of movement. Each movement is compared with the same movement on the other side. The nurse proceeds to passive ROM if the client is unable to perform active ROM.

In **passive range of motion**, the client's extremities and joints are supported and moved by the nurse. The same series of movements are made as in active ROM. Any pain or increased limitation of movement is noted, and each movement is compared with the other side. If client is able to stand or walk, observe his or her ability. Also describe any deformities. (See Procedure 20-5 for passive ROM exercises.) 🔗

Procedure 11-1 Part G describes how to assess the extremities, joints,z and movement.

Psychosocial Status

Psychosocial status should be considered. The client's mental and spiritual status can have significant effects on physical recovery. Much can be discovered about the client through an assessment of mood, affect, judgment, abilities, and lifestyle patterns. Refer to Chapters 24, 26, 28, and 30 for more about psychosocial aspects of care. 🔗

◆ DIAGNOSING, PLANNING, and IMPLEMENTING

Data from focused assessments are used to shape the plan of care and provide appropriate interventions to suit the client's needs. The nurse learns to assess using all the senses and is always alert to changes in the client's condition.

An accurate picture of the client's health can be achieved by thorough, organized assessment of all the body systems and by regular communication of all findings to the team leader. Assessment serves as a tool to all members of the healthcare team who care for the client.

 EVALUATING

The LPN/LVN performs focused assessment as ordered. Usually at the end of a shift, a focused assessment is done. The results are shared in an end-of-shift report. During a shift, changes in status are reported to the charge nurse as needed and according to institutional policy.

Nursing Process Case Study:
CLIENT WITH POSTPARTUM BLEEDING

Stephanie Franklin is a 35-year-old lawyer who gave birth to her first baby 3 hours ago. Her labor and delivery were uneventful and she is now on the postpartum floor. Her vaginal bleeding has increased in the past hour.

Assessment Janet Rodriguez, Ms. Franklin's day shift nurse, assists her to the bathroom and notices that she has bled through two pads in the past hour. Ms. Franklin passes an orange-sized, bright red clot of blood; she complains of dizziness. Ms. Rodriguez assists Ms. Franklin back to bed. On palpation of the uterus, Ms. Rodriguez notes that it is boggy. Two more orange-sized blood clots are expressed as Ms. Rodriguez firmly massages the *fundus* (top of the uterus). Ms. Rodriguez continues fundal massage; however, the bleeding remains heavy.

Ms. Rodriguez collects the following assessment data: T 98.6, BP 80/50, P 120, quick hemoglobin & hematocrit (Hemocue®) result 6. Complains of dizziness and nausea. Increased blood loss is discussed with RN and reported to physician.

Diagnosis The current nursing diagnoses for Ms. Franklin are as follows:

◆ *Risk for Deficient Fluid Volume* related to blood loss

◆ *Activity Intolerance* related to dizziness secondary to blood loss
◆ *Risk for Infection* related to possible retained placenta
◆ *Risk for Interrupted Family Processes*

Expected Outcomes The expected outcomes specify that Ms. Franklin will:

◆ Regain fluid balance as evidenced by normal BP and pulse, and no further drop in hemoglobin level
◆ Be able to ambulate without dizziness
◆ Maintain a normal temperature
◆ Have a fluid intake of at least 2,000 mL/day
◆ Breast-feed baby according to baby's feeding needs

Planning and Implementation The following nursing interventions are planned and implemented:

◆ Monitor vital signs according to doctor's orders
◆ Monitor condition of fundus q 30 minutes
◆ Encourage fluid intake
◆ Provide perineal care q 2 hours
◆ Bring baby to mother for feedings and remain with mother and baby throughout feeding
◆ Intake and output q 4 hours

Evaluation After being transported to the labor and delivery unit for manual removal of remaining placenta, Ms. Franklin is returned to the postpartum unit. At the end of the shift, Ms. Franklin is sitting up in bed, breast-feeding her baby. She complains of "a little dizziness if I sit up too fast." BP 110/68, Temp 98.5, Hemocue® remains at 6. 1,000 mL urine output in 4 hours. Oral intake 400 mL, IV intake 1,000 mL in 4 hours.

Critical Thinking in the Nursing Process

1. Why was Ms. Franklin's blood pressure low and pulse elevated?
2. Why did Ms. Franklin complain of dizziness?
3. Why would the nursing diagnosis Risk for Interrupted Family Processes with Baby be appropriate?

(*Note:* The bibliography listings for this and all chapters have been compiled at the back of the book.)

PROCEDURE 11-1

Focused Physical Assessment by Body Systems*

PURPOSE

- To obtain measurements to compare to baseline data.
- To obtain information to assess effect of medications.
- To determine health and comfort status of the client before or after a procedure or at the end of shift.

EQUIPMENT

- Stethoscope or DUS
- Penlight or flashlight
- Thermometer
- Sphygmomanometer and cuff

Part A: General Appearance and Mental Status

GENERAL APPEARANCE

INSPECTION

1. Observe body build, height, and weight in relation to the client's age, lifestyle, and health.

2. Observe the client's posture and gait, standing, sitting, and walking.

3. Observe the client's overall hygiene and grooming. Relate these to the person's activities prior to the assessment.

4. Note body and breath odor in relation to activity level.

5. Observe for signs of distress in posture (e.g., bending over because of abdominal pain) or facial expression (e.g., wincing or labored breathing).

6. Note obvious signs of health or illness (e.g., in skin color or breathing).

BEHAVIOR

1. Assess the client's attitude.

2. Note the client's affect/mood; assess the appropriateness of the client's response and level of orientation to time, place, and persons.

3. Listen for quantity of speech (amount and pace), quality (loudness, clarity, inflection), and organization (coherence of thought, overgeneralization, vagueness).

4. Listen for relevance and organization of thoughts.

Normal Findings

- Varies with lifestyle
- Relaxed, erect posture; coordinated movement

- Clean, neat
- No body odor or minor body odor relative to work or exercise; no breath odor
- Healthy appearance
- Cooperative
- Appropriate to situation
- Understandable, moderate pace
- Exhibits thought association
- Logical sequence
- Makes sense; has sense of reality

Deviations from Normal

- Excessively thin or obese
- Tense, slouched, bent posture; uncoordinated movement; tremors
- Dirty, unkempt
- Foul body odor; ammonia odor; acetone breath odor; foul breath
- Pallor; weakness; obvious illness
- Negative, hostile, withdrawn
- Inappropriate to situation
- Rapid or slow pace
- Uses generalizations; lacks association
- Illogical sequence
- Flight of ideas; confusion

NEUROLOGICAL

LEVEL OF CONSCIOUSNESS (LOC)

1. Ask client to give name; present location; and date or time of day

---

*This is an abbreviated assessment that can be conducted by the LPN/LVN at the beginning and/or end of the shift. A complete physical assessment is done by the RN on admission. Although vital signs could be done along with the appropriate body system, they are usually done at the beginning or the end of this procedure. (See full discussion of vital signs in Chapter 14. ∞)

Normal Findings

◆ Alert and oriented ×3: able to give correct name, location and/or time of day or date.

Deviations from Normal

◆ Inability to correctly name one or more items

VERBAL RESPONSE

1. Assess how the client communicates rather than what is communicated, through normal conversation.

Normal Findings

◆ Clear
◆ Rate consistent with overall psychomotor status
◆ Volume audible, normal conversational tone
◆ Modulation and flow—fluid and expressive
◆ Production—able to produce words

Deviation from Normal

◆ Incoherent, rambling, slurred, stuttering
◆ Monotone
◆ Dysphasia, aphasia

MOTOR RESPONSE ASSESSMENT
Grips

1. Ask the client to grasp your index and middle finger while you try to pull the fingers out.

Pushes/Pulls

1. Have the client hold arm up and resist while you try to push it down.
2. Have the client fully extend each arm and try to flex it while you attempt to hold arm in extension.
3. Have the client resist while you attempt to dorsiflex the foot and again while you attempt to flex the foot.

Walking Gait

1. Ask the client to walk across the room and back with eyesight focused ahead; assess the client's gait.

Normal Findings

◆ Bilateral/equal 100% normal strength; normal full movement; against gravity and against full resistance
◆ Has upright posture and steady gait with opposing arm swing; walks unaided, maintaining balance

Deviations from Normal

◆ Unequal strength
◆ 10% of normal strength; no movement, contraction of muscle is palpable or visible
◆ Has poor posture and unsteady, irregular, staggering gait with wide stance; bends legs only from hips; has rigid or no arm movements

ASSESSING PUPIL REACTIONS
Direct and Consensual Reaction to Light

1. Partially darken the room.
2. Ask the client to look straight ahead.
3. Using a penlight or flashlight and approaching from the side, shine a light on the pupil.
4. Observe the response of the illuminated pupil. It should constrict (direct response).
5. Shine the light on the pupil again, and observe the response of the other pupil. It should also constrict (consensual response).

Reaction to Accommodation

1. Hold an object (a penlight or pencil) about 10 cm (4 in) from the bridge of the client's nose.
2. Ask the client to look first at the top of the object and then at a distant object (e.g., the far wall) behind the penlight. Alternate the gaze from the near to the far object.
3. Observe the pupil response. The pupils should constrict when looking at the near object and dilate when looking at the far object.
4. Next, move the penlight or pencil toward the client's nose. The pupils should converge.
5. To record normal assessment of the pupils, use the abbreviation *PERRLA* (pupils equally round and react to light and accommodation).
6. Assess each pupil's reaction to accommodation.

Normal Findings

◆ Pupils constrict when looking at near object; pupils dilate when looking at far object; pupils converge when near object is moved toward nose.

Deviations from Normal

◆ One or both pupils fail to constrict, dilate, or converge.

Part B: Integumentary Assessment

ASSESSING THE SKIN

1. Inspect skin color (best assessed under natural light and on areas not exposed to the sun).
2. Inspect uniformity of skin color.
3. Assess edema, if present (i.e., location, color, temperature, and the degree to which the skin remains indented or pitted when pressed by a finger). See Figure 11-10 ◆.

4. Inspect and describe skin lesions.

clinical ALERT

Assess skin turgor over the sternum in older adults. Loss of subcutaneous tissue in aging makes the skin of the arms a less reliable indicator of fluid status.

Figure 11-10. ◆ Assess edema by pressing your finger firmly against client's skin for several seconds (especially in ankle area). After removing your finger, observe for lasting impression or indentation.

5. Observe and palpate skin moisture.

6. Palpate skin temperature. Compare the two feet and the two hands, using the backs of your fingers. *Backs of fingers pick up temperature differences more readily*.

7. Note skin turgor (fullness or elasticity) by lifting and pulling the skin on an extremity into a tent position.

Normal Findings

◆ Varies from light to deep brown; from ruddy pink to light pink; from yellow overtones to olive
◆ Generally uniform except in areas exposed to the sun; areas of lighter pigmentation (palms, lips, nail beds) in dark-skinned people

Scale for Describing Edema
1 = Barely detectable
2 = Indentation of less than 5 mm
3 = Indentation of 5 to 10 mm
4 = Indentation of more than 10 mm

◆ Freckles, some birthmarks, some flat and raised nevi (moles); no abrasions or other lesions
◆ Moisture in skin folds and the axillae (varies with environmental temperature and humidity, body temperature, and activity)
◆ Uniform; within normal range
◆ When tented, skin springs back to previous state

Deviations from Normal

◆ Pallor, cyanosis, jaundice, erythema
◆ Areas of either hyperpigmentation or hypopigmentation (e.g., vitiligo, albinism, edema)
◆ Various interruptions in skin integrity
◆ Excessive moisture (e.g., in hyperthermia); excessive dryness (e.g., in dehydration)
◆ Generalized hyperthermia (e.g., in fever); generalized hypothermia (e.g., in shock); localized hyperthermia

(e.g., in infection); localized hypothermia (e.g., in arteriosclerosis)
◆ Skin stays tented or moves back slowly (e.g., in dehydration)

ASSESSING MUCOUS MEMBRANES

1. Inspect and palpate the inner lips and buccal mucosa for color, moisture, texture, and the presence of lesions. Uniform pink color (darker, e.g., bluish hue, in dark-skinned clients)

Normal Findings

◆ Soft, moist, smooth texture
◆ Uniform pink color (freckled brown pigmentation in dark-skinned clients)
◆ Moist, smooth, soft, glistening, and elastic texture

Deviations from Normal

◆ Pallor; cyanosis
◆ Blisters; generalized or localized swelling; fissures, crusts, or scales (may result from excessive moisture, nutritional deficiency, or fluid deficit)
◆ Inability to purse lips (indicative of facial nerve damage)
◆ Pallor; white patches (leukoplakia)
◆ Excessive dryness

ASSESSING TEETH AND GUMS

1. Inspect the teeth and gums while examining the inner lips and buccal mucosa.

Normal Findings

◆ 32 adult teeth
◆ Smooth, white, shiny tooth enamel
◆ Pink gums (bluish or dark patches in dark-skinned clients)
◆ Moist, firm texture to gums
◆ No retraction of gums (pulling away from the crown of the tooth)

Deviations from Normal

◆ Missing teeth
◆ Ill-fitting dentures
◆ Brown or black discoloration of the enamel (may indicate staining or the presence of caries)
◆ Excessively red gums
◆ Spongy texture; bleeding; tenderness (may indicate periodontal disease)
◆ Receding, atrophied gums; swelling that partially covers the teeth
◆ Dry, furry tongue (associated with fluid deficit)
◆ Nodes, ulcerations, discolorations (white or red areas); areas of tenderness
◆ Restricted mobility
◆ Swelling, ulceration
◆ Swelling, nodules
◆ Inflammation (redness and swelling)
◆ Discoloration (e.g., jaundice or pallor)

◆ Palates the same color
◆ Irritations
◆ Bony growths (exostoses) growing from the hard palate
◆ Deviation to one side from tumor or trauma; immobility (may indicate damage to trigeminal {fifth cranial} nerve or vagus {tenth cranial} nerve)
◆ Reddened or edematous; presence of lesions, plaques, or exudate

◆ Inflamed
◆ Presence of discharge
◆ Swollen

ASSESSING THE NAILS

1. Note the color of the nailbed. *Bluish nails suggest cyanosis.*
2. Perform a capillary refill test if necessary. *A capillary refill time of more than 3 seconds may indicate circulatory problems.*

Part C: Cardiovascular Assessment

ASSESSING HEART SOUNDS

1. Auscultate the heart in all four anatomic sites: aortic, pulmonic, tricuspid, and apical (mitral). Auscultation need not be limited to these areas. However, the nurse may need to move the stethoscope to find the most audible sounds for each client.
2. Eliminate all sources of room noise. *Heart sounds are of low intensity, and other noise hinders the nurse's ability to hear them.*
3. Keep the client in a supine position with head elevated 30 to 45 degrees.
4. Use both the flat-disc diaphragm and the bell-shaped diaphragm to listen to all areas.
5. In every area of auscultation, distinguish both S_1 and S_2 sounds.
6. When auscultating, concentrate on one particular sound at a time in each area: the first heart sound, followed by systole, then the second heart sound, then diastole. Systole and diastole are normally silent intervals.
7. Later, reexamine the heart while the client is in the upright sitting position. *Certain sounds are more audible in this position.*

Normal Findings

◆ S_1: Usually heard at all sites. Usually louder at the apical and tricuspid areas
◆ S_2: Usually heard at all sites. Usually louder at base of heart and aortic and pulmonic areas
◆ Systole: Silent interval. Slightly shorter duration than diastole at normal heart rate (60–90 beats/min)
◆ Diastole: Silent interval. Slightly longer duration than systole at normal heart rates
◆ S_3 in children and young adults
◆ S_4 in many older adults

Deviations from Normal

◆ Increased or decreased intensity
◆ Varying intensity with different beats
◆ Increased intensity at aortic area
◆ Increased intensity at pulmonic area
◆ Sharp-sounding ejection clicks
◆ S_3 in older adults
◆ S_4 may be a sign of hypertension

ASSESSING THE PERIPHERAL VASCULAR SYSTEM

PERIPHERAL PULSES

1. Palpate the peripheral pulses (except the carotid pulse) on both sides of the client's body simultaneously and systematically to determine the symmetry of pulse volume. *This helps determine symmetry of pulse volume.*
2. Assess radial pulses and compare. Check capillary refill. Ask client to wiggle fingers. Ask client not to look at his/her feet. Touch the client's feet one at a time, asking the client if he/she is able to feel your touch. *This will determine level of touch perception.*
3. Assess pedal pulses and compare one side to the other. Note strength of pulse. If pedal pulses are not palpable, palpate posterior tibial pulse and compare one side to the other. Check capillary refill in toes. Ask client to wiggle toes. Ask client if he/she experiences numbness or tingling in extremities or sensation of cold. *Tibial pulse should be more palpable because it is closer to the heart.*
4. Palpate skin temperature. Compare the two feet and two hands, using the backs of your fingers. *Coolness may indicate lack of tissue perfusion.*
5. Note color of feet and toes and edema of the lower extremities.
6. Check for Homan's sign. To perform this test, the nurse supports the leg while flexing the foot in dorsiflexion. Ask the client if pain is felt as the foot is flexed. Palpate muscles of calf for tender, hot areas. *A positive Homan's sign indicates venous thrombosis.*

Normal Findings

◆ Symmetric pulse volumes
◆ Full pulsations
◆ In dependent position, distention and nodular bulges at calves are present
◆ When limbs are elevated, veins collapse (veins may appear tortuous or distended in older people)
◆ Limbs not tender
◆ Symmetric in size

Deviations from Normal

◆ Asymmetric volumes (indicate impaired circulation)
◆ Absence of pulsation (indicates arterial spasm or occlusion)

◆ Decreased, weak, thready pulsations (indicate impaired cardiac output)

◆ Increased pulse volume (may indicate hypertension, high cardiac output, or circulatory overload)

◆ Distended veins in the anteromedial part of thigh and/or lower leg or on posterolateral part of calf from knee to ankle

◆ Tenderness on palpation

◆ Pain in calf muscles with passive dorsiflexion of the foot (Homan's sign)

◆ Warmth and redness over vein

◆ Swelling of one calf or leg

PERIPHERAL PERFUSION

1. Inspect the skin of the hands and feet for color, temperature, edema, and skin changes. *These factors can identify poor blood perfusion.*

clinical ALERT

Report
If signs of arterial insufficiency occur, report findings to charge nurse.

2. Assess the adequacy of arterial flow if arterial insufficiency is suspected.

Normal Findings

◆ Natural skin color

◆ Skin temperature not excessively warm or cold

◆ No edema

◆ Skin texture resilient and moist

◆ Buerger's test: Original color returns in 10 seconds; veins in feet or hands fill in about 15 seconds

◆ Capillary refill test: Immediate return of color

Deviations from Normal

◆ Cyanosis, pallor

◆ Skin cool

◆ Marked edema

◆ Skin thin and shiny or thick, waxy, shiny, and fragile, reduced hair, ulceration

◆ Delayed color return or mottled appearance; delayed venous filling; marked redness of arms or legs (indicates arterial insufficiency)

◆ Delayed return of color (arterial insufficiency)

Part D: Respiratory Assessment

ASSESSING THE THORAX AND LUNGS

POSTERIOR THORAX

1. Inspect the shape and symmetry of the thorax from posterior and lateral views.

2. Palpate the posterior thorax.

3. For clients who have no respiratory complaints, rapidly assess the temperature and integrity of all chest skin.

4. For clients who do have respiratory complaints, palpate all chest areas for bulges, tenderness, or abnormal movements. Do not perform deep palpation. Observe caution when palpating (lightly). *If rib is fractured, deep palpation could lead to displacement of the bone fragment against the lungs.*

Normal Findings

◆ Chest symmetric

Deviations from Normal

◆ Chest asymmetric

◆ Bulges, tenderness, or abnormal movements in chest area

ANTERIOR THORAX

1. Auscultate the chest using the flat-disc diaphragm of the stethoscope. *Flat-disc side is best for transmitting the high-pitched breath sounds.* Use the systematic zigzag procedure used in percussion (Figure 11-11 ◆). *This ensures that no areas are missed.*

2. Ask the client to take slow, deep breaths through the mouth. Listen at each point to the breath sounds during a complete inspiration and expiration. Compare findings at each point with the corresponding point on the opposite

Figure 11-11. ◆ Systematic zigzag pattern.

side of the chest. *Slow, deep breaths move more air and allow abnormalities to be heard.*

Normal Findings

◆ Quiet, rhythmic, and effortless respirations

◆ Full symmetric respiratory effort

Deviations from Normal

◆ Adventitious breath sounds (e.g., crackles, rhonchi, wheeze, friction rub

◆ Absence of breath sounds (associated with collapsed and surgically removed lung lobes)

◆ Asymmetric and/or decreased respiratory exchange

Part E. Abdominal Assessment

ASSESSMENT

INSPECTION

1. Inspect the abdomen for skin integrity (refer to the discussion of skin assessment earlier in this chapter).

2. Inspect the abdomen for contour and symmetry.

3. Observe the abdominal contour (profile line from the rib margin to the pubic bone) while standing at the client's side when the client is supine.

4. Ask the client to take a deep breath and to hold it (makes any abnormality such as an enlarged liver or spleen more obvious).

5. Assess the symmetry of contour while standing at the foot of the bed.

6. If distention is present, measure the abdominal girth by placing a tape around the abdomen at the level of the umbilicus. *Distention may indicate hidden fluid imbalances.*

Normal Findings

- ◆ Unblemished skin
- ◆ Uniform color
- ◆ Silver-white striae or surgical scars
- ◆ Flat, rounded (convex), or *scaphoid* (concave or boat-shaped)
- ◆ No evidence of enlargement of liver or spleen
- ◆ Symmetric contour

Deviations from Normal

- ◆ Presence of rash or other lesions
- ◆ Tense, glistening skin (may indicate ascites, edema)
- ◆ Purple striae (associated with Cushing's disease)
- ◆ Generalized distention (associated with gas retention, obesity, ascites, or tumors)
- ◆ Lower abdominal distention (may indicate bladder distention, pregnancy, or ovarian mass)
- ◆ Markedly scaphoid abdomen (associated with malnutrition)
- ◆ Evidence of enlargement of liver or spleen
- ◆ Asymmetric contour, such as localized protrusions around umbilicus, inguinal ligaments, or scars (possible hernia or tumor)

AUSCULTATION

1. Auscultate the abdomen for bowel sounds and vascular sounds.

2. Warm the hands and the stethoscope diaphragms. *Cold hands and a cold stethoscope may cause the client to contract the abdominal muscles, and these contractions may be heard during auscultation.*

For Bowel Sounds

1. Use the flat-disc diaphragm (Figure 11-12 ◆). *Intestinal sounds are relatively high-pitched and best accentuated by the*

Figure 11-12. ◆ Auscultating the abdomen for bowel sounds.

flat-disc diaphragm. Light pressure with the stethoscope is adequate to detect sounds.

2. Ask when the client last ate. *The frequency of sounds relates to the state of digestion or the presence of food in the gastrointestinal tract. Shortly after or long after eating, bowel sounds may normally increase. They are loudest when a meal is long overdue. Four to seven hours after a meal, bowel sounds in the RLQ may be heard continuously over the ileocecal valve area while the digestive contents from the small intestine empty through the valve into the large intestine.*

3. Place the flat-disc diaphragm of the stethoscope in each of the four quadrants of the abdomen (see Figure 10-19). 🔗 Many nurses begin in the right lower quadrant in the area of the cecum.

4. Listen for active bowel sounds—irregular gurgling noises occurring about every 5 to 20 seconds. *The duration of a single sound may range from less than a second to more than several seconds.*

5. Normal bowel sounds are described as audible. Alterations in sounds are described as absent or hypoactive, that is, extremely soft and infrequent (e.g., one per minute), and hyperactive or increased, that is, high-pitched, loud, rushing sounds that occur frequently (e.g., every 3 seconds), also known as borborygmi. *Absence of sounds indicates a cessation of intestinal motility. Hypoactive sounds indicate decreased motility and are usually associated with manipulation of the bowel during surgery, inflammation, paralytic ileus, or late bowel obstruction. Hyperactive sounds indicate increased intestinal motility and are usually associated with diarrhea, an early bowel obstruction, or the use of laxatives.*

Absent, Hypoactive, or Hyperactive Bowel Sounds

1. If bowel sounds appear to be absent, listen for 3 to 5 minutes before concluding that they are absent. *Because bowel sounds are so irregular, a longer time and more sites are used to confirm absence of sounds.*

Normal Findings

◆ Audible bowel sounds

Deviations from Normal

◆ Limited movement due to pain or disease process
◆ Visible peristalsis in nonlean clients (with bowel obstruction)

PALPATION

1. Perform light palpation first to detect areas of tenderness and/or muscle guarding. Systematically explore all four quadrants. *Palpation is used to detect tenderness, the presence of masses or distention, and the outline and position of abdominal organs (e.g., the liver, spleen, and kidneys). Two types of palpation are used: light and deep. In some practice settings, palpation is limited to light abdominal palpation to assess tenderness and bladder palpation to assess for distention.*

2. Before palpation, ensure that the client's position is appropriate for relaxation of the abdominal muscles, and (b) warm the hands. *Cold hands can elicit muscle tension and thus impede palpatory evaluation.*

3. For light palpation, hold the palm of your hand slightly above the client's abdomen, with your fingers parallel to the abdomen.

4. Depress the abdominal wall lightly, about 1 cm or to the depth of the subcutaneous tissue, with the pads of your fingers (Figure 11-13 ◆).

5. Move the finger pads in a slight circular motion.

6. Note areas of slight tenderness or superficial pain, large masses, and muscle guarding. To determine areas of tenderness, ask the client to tell you about them, watch for

Figure 11-13. ◆ For light palpation of the abdomen, depress the abdominal wall lightly, about 1 cm or to the depth of the subcutaneous tissue, with the pads of your fingers.

changes in the client's facial expressions, and note areas of muscle guarding.

Normal Findings

◆ No tenderness; relaxed soft abdomen with smooth, consistent tension; pain free
◆ As for light palpation

Deviations from Normal

◆ Tenderness and hypersensitivity
◆ Superficial masses
◆ Localized areas of increased tension
◆ Generalized or localized areas of tenderness

Part F: Genitourinary Assessment

URINATION

1. Assess client for continence and independent urination.

Normal Findings

◆ Continent

Deviation from Normal

◆ Incontinent

INDWELLING CATHETER

1. Assess amount, color, odor, clarity, sediment, and frequency

Normal Findings / Deviation from Normal

Refer to Table 18-4 for normal characteristics of urine. ⌾

PALPATION OF THE BLADDER

1. Palpate the area above the pubic symphysis if the client's history indicates possible urinary retention

Normal Findings

◆ Not palpable

Deviation from Normal

◆ Distended and palpable as smooth, round, tense mass (indicates urinary retention)

Part G: Musculoskeletal System

MUSCLES

1. Inspect the muscles for size. Compare the muscles on one side of the body (e.g., of the arm, thigh, and calf) to the same muscle on the other side. For any discrepancies, measure the muscles with a tape.

2. Inspect the muscles and tendons for contractures (shortening).

3. Inspect the muscles for fasciculations and tremors. Inspect any tremors of the hands and arms by having the client hold the arms in front of the body.

BONES

1. Inspect the skeleton for normal structure and deformities.

2. Examine for scoliosis in persons over age 12. Client stands facing away from the nurse and bends over to touch the toes.

JOINTS

1. Inspect the joints for swelling.

2. Palpate each joint for tenderness, smoothness of movement, swelling, crepitation, or presence of nodules.

3. Assess joint range of motion.

Normal Findings

◆ Equal size on both sides of the body
◆ No contractures
◆ No fasciculations or tremors
◆ Normally firm
◆ Smooth coordinated movements
◆ Equal strength on each body side
◆ No deformities
◆ Straight spine
◆ No tenderness or swelling
◆ No swelling
◆ No tenderness, swelling, crepitation, or nodules
◆ Joints move smoothly
◆ Varies to some degree in accordance with person's genetic makeup and degree of physical activity

Deviations from Normal

◆ Atrophy (a decrease in size) or hypertrophy (an increase in size)

◆ Malposition of body part (e.g., a foot fixed in dorsiflexion)
◆ Presence of fasciculation or tremor
◆ Atonic (lacking tone)
◆ Flaccidity (weakness or laxness) or spasticity (sudden involuntary muscle contraction)
◆ 25% or less of normal strength
◆ Bones misaligned
◆ A hump in the thoracic spine indicating a lateral curve
◆ Presence of tenderness or swelling (may indicate fractures, neoplasms, or osteoporosis)
◆ One or more swollen joints
◆ Presence of tenderness, swelling, crepitation, or nodules
◆ Limited range of motion in one or more joints

◆ SAMPLE DOCUMENTATION

9/13/03	Client alert and oriented x3, eyes
1200	PERRLA, I+O 700 mL in 6 h; BP
	130/80; R 16; P 80; breath sounds
	clear; bowel sounds present and active
	in all quadrants. Abdominal incision open
	to air, without redness or swelling,
	staples intact. Complained of incision
	pain with a stated pain level of 7. PRN
	Pain meds given 1100. Pain level 1 at
	1145. Barbara Cook, LPN

Chapter Review

Key Terms by Topics

Use the audio glossary feature of either the CD-ROM or the Companion Website to hear the correct pronunciation of the following key terms.

Introduction
physical assessment

Methods of examination
inspection, auscultation, palpation, percussion

Assessing
level of consciousness (LOC), orientation, direct response, consensual response, accommodation, PERRLA, vital signs, pallor, cyanosis, erythema, edema, turgor, lesion, capillary refill, pulse, systole, diastole, peripheral vascular system, perfusion, adventitious breath sounds, active range of motion, passive range of motion

Key Points

- The health examination is conducted to assess the function and integrity of the client's body parts.
- The health examination may entail a complete head-to-toe assessment or focused assessment of one or more body systems or a body part. If the head-to-toe assessment is performed during the admission process, it is carried out by the RN. Findings by the LPN/LVN during the focused assessment should be brought to the attention of the RN.
- The health assessment is conducted in a systematic manner that requires the fewest position changes for the client.
- Aspects of the physical assessment procedures should be incorporated in the assessment, intervention, and evaluation phases of the nursing process.
- Data obtained in the physical health examination are reported to the charge nurse. They are used to help establish nursing diagnoses and are helpful to all nursing staff in planning the client's care and evaluating nursing care outcomes.
- Initial assessment findings provide baseline data about the client's functional abilities. Subsequent assessment findings are compared to them.

EXPLORE MediaLink

Additional interactive resources for this chapter can be found on the Companion Website at www.prenhall.com/ramont. Click on Chapter 11 and "Begin" to select the activities for this chapter.

For chapter-related NCLEX-style questions and an audio glossary, access the accompanying CD-ROM in this book.

Animation:
- ear abnormalities
- mouth
- cavities
- ear frequencies
- tonsils
- nervous system

For Further Study

For detailed instruction related to vital signs (body temperature, pulse, respirations, and blood pressure), see Chapter 14, Procedures 14-1 to 14-4.

For more discussion of oxygenation and assessing respirations, see Chapter 16.

See Procedure 16-4 for using a pulse oximeter.

For additional information on measurement of height and weight, and for more about fluid balance, see Chapter 17.

For further study of urinary and bowel elimination, see Chapters 18 and 19, respectively.

See Table 18-4 for characteristics of urine.

See Procedure 20-1 for passive range of motion exercises.

Refer to Chapters 24, 26, 28, and 30 for more about psychosocial aspects of care.

Critical Thinking Care Map

Caring for a Client with Activity Intolerance

NCLEX-PN Focus Area: Physiological Integrity

Case Study: Theresa Harris, 88, was admitted from a long-term care facility yesterday to rule out pneumonia. Theresa states, "I get dizzy when I get out of bed." Theresa has a history of cerebral vascular accident with some residual weakness of the left hand.

Nursing Diagnosis: Activity Intolerance

COLLECT DATA

Subjective	Objective
_____	_____
_____	_____
_____	_____
_____	_____
_____	_____
_____	_____

Would you report this data? Yes/No

If yes, to: _____

Nursing Care

_____
_____
_____
_____
_____
_____
_____
_____
_____
_____
_____
_____
_____
_____
_____

How would you document this? _____
_____
_____
_____
_____

Data Collected

(use those that apply)

- Weight 135
- BP 128/80—110/72—90/50: lying/sitting/standing
- Pulse 89
- Respiratory rate at rest 18 and shallow; 26 and shallow on exertion
- Temp 99.0°F
- Skin is pale and client is diaphoretic
- Complains of dizziness on standing
- Skin dry and flaky
- Oral mucosa dry
- Taking oral antibiotics q 4 hours
- Pitcher of water is on the left side of the bed and is full
- Family not present, uninvolved in care of client
- Saline lock in place and patent
- Complains of loss of appetite over the past week
- Crackles noted in lower lobes of lungs, bilaterally
- Nonproductive cough
- Blood oxygen level 98%
- Client unmotivated to get better
- Pupils PERRLA

Nursing Interventions

(use those that apply)

- Place water pitcher on client's right side, within reach.
- Determine cause of activity intolerance: physical, psychological, motivational.
- State, "You need to eat your meals to get better."
- Encourage client to change positions slowly.
- Instruct client to sit up in bed for a few minutes before standing.
- Put a bed alarm in place according to agency policy.
- Slow pace of care, allowing client extra time to carry out activities.
- Check physician's orders for IV fluid administration and discuss with RN.
- When mobilizing client, monitor for orthostatic hypotension accompanied by dizziness and/or fainting.
- Encourage client to deep breathe and cough.
- Encourage client to increase clear fluid intake.
- Instruct client to call for assistance before ambulating.
- Use a walking belt when ambulating client.

NCLEX-PN Exam Preparation

TEST-TAKING TIP

Remember that collecting data is the first step of the nursing process. When you are asked to select your first or initial nursing action, follow the steps of the nursing process.

1. You are assigned to care for a 19-year-old female client who has been brought to the hospital by her parents. They are concerned that she may be seriously ill because of noticeable weight loss and frequent vomiting and diarrhea. The physician suspects that she may be suffering from an eating disorder. Which of the following signs would help to confirm a diagnosis of an eating disorder?
   a. Headaches, confusion, and lack of concentration
   b. Dental caries and skin excoriations on knuckles
   c. Yellow skin and sclera
   d. Excessive bruising and petechiae

2. The nurse's observation of the problem, the client's presenting problem, nursing interventions provided, and medical therapies are specific assessments made in relationship to:
   a. The nursing diagnosis
   b. The client's complaints
   c. Physician's orders
   d. Nursing orders

3. A client is admitted through the ER with a complaint of severe right lower quadrant abdominal pain of 5 hours' duration. Lab work reveals elevated WBCs; vital signs are T 101.2; P 98, R 24, BP 120/78. Which of the following data collected during the focused assessment would help to confirm a diagnosis of appendicitis?
   a. A palpable mass in the right upper quadrant
   b. Report of black tarry stools
   c. Rebound tenderness at McBurney's point
   d. Projectile vomiting

4. You are setting up for a focused assessment for a client with tonsillitis. Of the following choices, which pieces of equipment would be required?
   a. Stethoscope and sphygmomanometer
   b. Tongue depressor and flashlight
   c. Ophthalmoscope and split-lamp
   d. Thermometer and scale

5. Your primary nurse requests that you assess peripheral perfusion of toes, capillary blanch test, pedal pulse if able, and vital signs. This assessment would be carried out for a client with which of the following conditions?
   a. Deep vein thrombosis (DVT)
   b. Hip fracture with Buck's traction application
   c. Femur fracture with long leg cast
   d. Total knee replacement leg in continuous passive motion (CPM) machine

6. You have been assigned to take a client's blood pressure. The reading is 100/60. Which would be the most appropriate action for you to take?
   a. Retake the blood pressure in 1 hour.
   b. Chart the blood pressure reading.
   c. Report the findings immediately.
   d. Administer antihypertensive medication immediately.

7. Breath sounds that are continuous, low-pitched, coarse, gurgling, harsh, louder sounds with a moaning or snoring quality, which may be altered by coughing are known as:
   a. Crackles (rales)
   b. Gurgles (rhonchi)
   c. Friction rub
   d. Wheeze

8. You are assigned to assist with the admission assessment of a client who has been living alone and is unable to provide for his/her own hygiene needs. As you examine the integumentary system you notice numerous red lesions, which appear as "red tracks" under the skin. Which of the following would be an appropriate nursing action?
   a. Don gloves prior to continuing your assessment.
   b. Postpone your assessment until the nursing assistant has bathed the client.
   c. Place the client in isolation.
   d. Proceed with the assessment but do not touch the client.

9. You are assigned to work the night shift. As you are completing your assessment for a client who had surgery today, the client begins to yell, "Get them off of me! There are rats crawling all over the bed." Your best nursing action would be to:
   a. Turn on the light and tell her there are no rats.
   b. Stop the pain medication.
   c. Check her chart for a history of mental illness.
   d. Inform the charge nurse or the physician immediately.

10. Moods, affect, judgment, abilities, and lifestyle are part of what type of assessment?
    a. History and physical
    b. Psychosocial assessment
    c. Focus assessment
    d. Family health history

Answers for Review Questions, as well as discussion of Case Study and Critical Thinking Care Map questions, appear in Appendix IV.

Chapter 12

Skin Integrity and Wound Care

SHARING experiences

"The first time I held and comforted a child, it was a heartfelt moment. Helping others in need brings me great satisfaction. Being an LPN is truly rewarding."

Tina Banzhof, LPN, Lancaster, PA.

LEARNING outcomes

After completing this chapter, you will be able to:

- Describe factors affecting skin integrity.
- Describe the four stages of pressure ulcer development.
- Describe the three phases of wound healing.
- Describe factors that affect wound healing.
- Identify data pertinent to skin integrity, pressure sites, and wounds.
- Discuss measures to prevent and treat pressure ulcer formation.
- Identify purposes of commonly used dressing materials and binders.
- Describe methods of applying dry and moist heat and cold.
- Identify essential steps of obtaining wound specimens, applying transparent and hydrocolloid dressings, and irrigating a wound.

MediaLink

www.prenhall.com/ramont

Use the address above to access the free, interactive Companion Website created for this textbook. Get hints, instant feedback, and textbook references to chapter-related NCLEX-style questions. Link to other interesting sites.

Audio Glossary:
Use the Companion Website, or the CD-ROM disk enclosed with your textbook, to hear the pronunciation of key terms in the chapter.

The skin is the largest organ in the body. It protects the body and helps to maintain health. Factors that increase risk for impaired skin integrity are: aging, restricted mobility, chronic illnesses, trauma, and invasive health care procedures. Nursing care of the skin includes maintaining skin integrity and promoting wound healing. Nurses must be aware of risk factors and specific measures that promote optimal skin conditions. They must also understand the physiology of wound healing.

 ## Skin Integrity

Intact skin is normal skin and skin layers, uninterrupted by wounds. Genetics and heredity determine many aspects of a person's skin, including skin color, sensitivity to sunlight, and allergies. Age influences skin integrity in both young and old populations. Aging skin is more fragile and susceptible to injury. Wounds tend to heal more rapidly in infants and children.

Many chronic illnesses and their treatments affect skin integrity. People with impaired peripheral arterial circulation may have loss of leg hair and skin on the legs that appears shiny and damages easily. Some medications, such as steroids, cause thinning of the skin and allow it to be much more readily harmed. Certain antibiotics increase sensitivity to sunlight and can predispose a person to severe sunburns. Poor nutrition can interfere with the appearance and function of normal skin, as well as with healing.

Types of Wounds

Body wounds may be intentional or unintentional. *Intentional traumas* occur during therapy. Operations and venipunctures are intentional traumas that break skin integrity. *Unintentional wounds* are accidental; for example, a person may fracture an arm in an automobile collision. If the tissues are traumatized without a break in the skin, there is a *closed wound*. An *open wound* occurs when the skin or mucous membrane surface is broken.

Wounds are frequently described according to how they are acquired (Table 12-1 ◆). They also can be described according to the likelihood and degree of wound contamination.

Clean wounds are uninfected wounds in which minimal inflammation is encountered. Clean wounds are primarily closed wounds.

Contaminated wounds include open, fresh, accidental wounds and surgical wounds involving a major break in sterile technique. Contaminated wounds show evidence of inflammation.

Dirty or infected wounds include both old, accidental wounds containing dead tissue and wounds with evidence of a clinical infection, such as purulent drainage.

Wounds are also classified by depth, that is, the tissue layers involved in the wound. *Partial-thickness wounds* are confined to the skin (dermis and epidermis). *Full-thickness wounds* involve the dermis, epidermis, subcutaneous tissue, and possibly muscle and bone.

Pressure ulcers are a type of wound (usually preventable) that progress from closed to open. They are a great concern in hospitals, in long-term care facilities, and in clients with impaired mobility. Pressure ulcers are discussed separately later in this chapter.

Wound Healing

Wound healing is the regeneration (renewal) of tissues. There are two types of healing, distinguished by the amount of tissue

TABLE 12-1	TYPES OF WOUNDS	
TYPE	**CAUSE**	**DESCRIPTION AND CHARACTERISTICS**
Incision	Sharp instrument (e.g., knife or scalpel)	Open wound; painful; deep or shallow
Contusion	Blow from a blunt instrument	Closed wound, skin appears ecchymotic (bruised) because of damaged blood vessels
Abrasion	Surface scrape, either unintentional (e.g., scraped knee from a fall) or intentional (e.g., dermal abrasion to remove pockmarks)	Open wound involving the skin; painful
Puncture	Penetration of the skin and often the underlying tissues by a sharp instrument, either intentional or unintentional	Open wound
Laceration	Tissues torn apart, often from accidents (e.g., with machinery)	Open wound; edges are often jagged
Penetrating wound	Penetration of the skin and the underlying tissues, usually unintentional (e.g., from a bullet or metal fragments)	Open wound

loss. *Primary intention healing* (or first intention healing) occurs where the tissue surfaces have been *approximated* (closed) and there is minimal or no tissue loss. It characteristically has minimal granulation tissue and scarring. A closed surgical incision is an example of primary intention healing (Figure 12-1 ◆).

A wound that is extensive and involves considerable tissue loss, and in which the edges cannot or should not be approximated, heals by *secondary intention healing*. A pressure ulcer is an example of a wound that heals by secondary intention. Secondary intention healing differs from primary intention healing in three ways: (1) the repair time is longer; (2) the scarring is greater; and (3) the risk of infection is greater.

PHASES OF WOUND HEALING

The phases of healing are the steps in the body's natural processes of tissue repair. The rate of healing varies depending on factors such as the type of healing, wound location and size, and the health of the client. Wound healing can be broken down into three phases: inflammatory, proliferative, and maturation.

Inflammatory Phase

The inflammatory phase starts immediately after injury and lasts 3 to 6 days. Two major processes (hemostasis and phagocytosis) occur during this phase.

Hemostasis (the arrest or cessation of bleeding) results from vasoconstriction, *retraction* (drawing back) of injured blood vessels, the deposition of fibrin (connective tissue), and blood clot formation. The blood clots become the framework for cell repair. A scab, made of clots and dead or dying tissue, also forms on the surface of the wound. This scab aids hemostasis and helps prevent contamination of the wound by microorganisms.

During the inflammatory phase, vascular and cellular responses promote removal of foreign substances and dead or dying tissue. The blood supply to the wound increases, bringing with it substances and nutrients needed in the healing process. The area appears reddened and edematous as a result.

Macrophages (certain white blood cells) engulf microorganisms and cellular debris by a process known as **phagocytosis.** This inflammatory response is essential to healing. Measures that impair inflammation, such as use of steroid medications, can slow or prevent the healing process.

Proliferative Phase

The proliferative phase, the second phase in healing, extends from day 3 to about day 21 postinjury. *Fibroblasts* (connective tissue cells) migrate into the wound about 24 hours after injury. There they begin to synthesize collagen, a whitish protein substance that adds strength to the wound and gradually decreases the wound's chance of reopening.

Capillaries grow across the wound, increasing the blood supply, which brings oxygen and nutrients. Fibroblasts move from the bloodstream into the wound, depositing fibrin. As the capillary network develops, the tissue becomes a translucent red color. This tissue, called **granulation tissue,** is fragile and bleeds easily.

When the skin edges of a wound are not sutured, the area fills in with granulation tissue. If the wound does not close by *epithelialization* (skin formation), the area becomes covered with dried plasma proteins and dead cells. This is called **eschar** (black, leathery formation). Initially, wounds that heal by secondary intention seep blood-tinged (**serosanguineous**) drainage.

Maturation Phase

The maturation phase begins about day 21 and can extend 1 or 2 years after the injury. Fibroblasts continue to synthesize collagen. The collagen fibers reorganize into a more orderly structure. During maturation, the wound is remodeled and contracted. The scar becomes stronger, but the repaired area is never as strong as the original tissue. In some individuals, particularly dark-skinned persons, an abnormal amount of collagen is laid down. This can result in a hypertrophic scar (or **keloid**).

KINDS OF WOUND DRAINAGE

Exudate is material, such as fluid and cells, that has escaped from blood vessels during the inflammatory process and is deposited in tissue or on tissue surfaces. The nature and amount of exudate vary according to the tissue involved, the intensity and duration of the inflammation, and the presence of microorganisms.

There are three major types of exudate: serous, purulent, and sanguineous (hemorrhagic). A *serous* exudate consists

First intention

Second intention (contraction and epithelialization)

Figure 12-1. ◆ Classification of wound healing. **A.** First intention: A clean incision is made with primary closure: there is minimal scarring. **B, C.** Second intention: The wound is left open so that granulation can result (B), or the wound is intentially left open and later closed when there is no further evidence of infection.

chiefly of serum (the clear portion of the blood) derived from blood. It looks watery and has few cells.

A *purulent exudate* is thicker than serous exudate because it contains pus. Pus consists of leukocytes, liquefied dead tissue debris, dead and living bacteria. The process of pus formation is referred to as **suppuration.** Purulent exudates may have tinges of blue, green, or yellow. The color may depend on the causative organism. However, not all microorganisms are *pyogenic* (pus-producing).

A **sanguineous** *(hemorrhagic) exudate* consists of large amounts of red blood cells. This type of exudate indicates damage to capillaries that allows escape of red blood cells from the plasma. It is frequently seen in open wounds. Nurses often need to distinguish whether the sanguineous exudate is dark or bright. A bright sanguineous exudate indicates fresh bleeding. Dark sanguineous exudate denotes older bleeding. Mixed types of exudates are often observed.

COMPLICATIONS OF WOUND HEALING

Hemorrhage

Some escape of blood from a wound is normal. However, *hemorrhage* (persistent bleeding) is abnormal. It may be caused by a dislodged clot, a slipped suture, or erosion of a blood vessel.

Internal hemorrhage may often be detected by swelling or distention in the area of the wound or by sanguineous drainage from a surgical drain. Some clients have a hematoma, a localized collection of blood underneath the skin, that may appear as a reddish-blue swelling.

External hemorrhage either appears under a dressing or escapes from the dressing and pools under the client. The risk of hemorrhage is greatest during the first 48 hours after surgery. Hemorrhage is an emergency that requires the application of extra sterile pressure dressings to the area, monitoring the client's vital signs, and notifying the physician.

Infection

A wound can be infected with microorganisms at the time of injury, during surgery, or postoperatively during open wound healing (see Chapter 7). 🔗 Wounds that occur as a result of injury (bullet and knife wounds) are most likely to be contaminated at the time of injury. Surgery involving the intestines can also result in infection from the microorganisms inside the intestine. Surgical infection is most likely to become apparent 2 to 11 days postoperatively.

Dehiscence with Possible Evisceration

Dehiscence is the partial or total rupturing of a sutured wound. Dehiscence usually involves an abdominal wound in which the layers below the skin also separate. **Evisceration** is the protrusion of the internal viscera through an incision. A number of factors, including obesity, poor nutrition, multiple trauma, suture failure, excessive coughing, vomiting, and dehydration, heighten a client's risk of wound dehiscence.

FACTORS AFFECTING WOUND HEALING

Age and Lifestyle

Healthy children and adults often heal more quickly than older people. See Box 12-1 ◆ for factors inhibiting wound healing in older adults.

People who exercise regularly tend to have good circulation. Because blood brings oxygen and nourishment to the wound, people who exercise are more likely to heal quickly. Smoking reduces the amount of functional hemoglobin in the blood, thus limiting the oxygen-carrying capacity of the blood.

Nutrition

Wound healing requires a diet rich in protein, carbohydrates, lipids, vitamins A and C, and minerals, such as iron, zinc, and copper. Malnourished clients may require time to improve their nutritional status before surgery. Obese clients are at increased risk of wound infection and slower healing because *adipose* (fatty) tissue usually has a minimal blood supply.

Medications

Anti-inflammatory drugs (e.g., steroids and aspirin), heparin, and antineoplastic agents interfere with healing. Prolonged

BOX 12-1

POPULATION FOCUS

FACTORS THAT INHIBIT WOUND HEALING IN OLDER ADULTS

- Vascular changes associated with aging, such as atherosclerosis and atrophy of capillaries in the skin, can impair blood flow to the wound.
- Collagen tissue is less flexible.
- Changes in the immune system may reduce the formation of antibodies and monocytes necessary for wound healing.
- Nutritional deficiencies may reduce the numbers of red blood cells and leukocytes, thus impeding the delivery of oxygen and the inflammatory response essential for wound healing. Oxygen is needed for the synthesis of collagen and the formation of new epithelial cells.
- Scar tissue is less elastic.

use of antibiotics may make a person susceptible to wound infection by resistant organisms.

Contamination and Infection

Contamination of a wound surface with pathogenic microorganisms usually results in infection. These organisms compete with new cells for oxygen and nutrition and can impair wound healing. When the microorganisms multiply, infection occurs. Clients who are immunosuppressed are especially susceptible to wound infections.

COLLABORATIVE CARE

Wound Cleaning

Wound cleaning has traditionally involved the removal of *debris* (i.e., foreign materials, excess slough, necrotic tissue, bacteria, and other microorganisms). Formerly, antimicrobial solutions such as povidone–iodine (Betadine), hydrogen peroxide, alcohol, and Dakin's solution were commonly used. However, these solutions have caustic effects on granulation tissue and the skin. The choices of cleaning agent and method depend largely on agency protocol and the physician's preference.

WOUND IRRIGATION AND PACKING. An *irrigation (lavage)* is the washing or flushing out of an area. Sterile technique is required for a wound irrigation, because there is a break in the skin integrity.

Using piston syringes instead of bulb syringes to irrigate a wound reduces the risk of aspirating drainage and provides safe, effective pressure. For deep wounds with small openings, a sterile straight catheter may also be necessary. Frequently used irrigation solutions are sterile normal saline, lactated Ringer's solution, and antibiotic solutions.

Gauze packing is placed in wounds to facilitate the formation of granulation tissue and healing by secondary intention. Generally, moistened 4 × 4 non–cotton-filled gauze dressings are used. Cotton fibers are contraindicated because they can pull loose and remain in the wound, encouraging bacterial growth and contamination.

The wet-to-damp technique is generally used to pack wounds. In this technique, moist gauzes are packed in the wound to absorb exudate, but they are not allowed to dry before removal.

Wound Dressings

Dressings are applied to wounds for the following purposes:

- To protect the wound from mechanical injury
- To protect the wound from microbial contamination
- To provide or maintain high humidity of the wound
- To provide thermal insulation
- To absorb drainage or debride a wound or both
- To prevent hemorrhage (when applied as a pressure dressing or with elastic bandages)
- To splint or immobilize the wound site and thereby facilitate healing and prevent injury
- To provide psychologic comfort

Various dressing materials are available to cover wounds. The type of dressing used depends on several factors:

- The location, size, and type of the wound
- The amount of exudate
- Whether the wound requires debridement, is infected, or has sinus tracts
- Such considerations as frequency of dressing change, ease or difficulty of dressing application, and cost.

Table 12-2 ◆ describes materials for dressing wounds. Common gauze dressings (Figure 12-2 ◆) may be applied in several ways to achieve different goals. Other dressing materials are used for specific types and conditions of wounds. Methods of applying gauze dressings are described in Table 12-3 ◆.

TRANSPARENT WOUND BARRIERS. Transparent dressings are often applied to wounds including ulcerated or burned skin areas (Figure 12-3 ◆). These dressings offer several advantages:

- They act as temporary skin.
- They are nonporous, self-adhesive dressings that do not require changing as other dressings do.
- Because they are transparent, the wound can be assessed through them.
- Because they are occlusive, the wound remains moist and retains the serous exudate, which promotes epithelial growth, hastens healing, and reduces the risk of infection.
- Because they are elastic, they can be placed over a joint without disrupting the client's mobility.
- They adhere only to the skin area around the wound and not to the wound itself because they keep the wound moist.
- They allow the client to shower or bathe without removing the dressing.
- They can be removed without damaging wound tissues.

Figure 12-2. ◆ Some frequently used dressing materials (clockwise from bottom left): surgipad or abdominal pad, 2 × 2 gauze, 2-in roller gauze, 4 × 4 gauze, 4-in roller. *Source:* © Elena Dorfman.

TABLE 12-2 **SELECTED TYPES OF WOUND DRESSINGS**

DRESSING	DESCRIPTION	PURPOSE	EXAMPLES
Transparent adhesive films/ wound barriers	Adhesive plastic semipermeable *nonabsorbent* dressings that allow exchange of oxygen between the atmosphere and wound bed. They are impermeable to bacteria and water.	To provide protection against contamination and friction; to maintain a clean moist surface that facilitates cellular migration; to provide insulation by preventing fluid evaporation; and to facilitate wound assessment	Op-Site, Tegaderm, Bio-occlusive, ACU-derm
Impregnated nonadherent dressings	Woven or nonwoven cotton or synthetic materials that are impregnated with petrolatum, saline, zinc-saline, antimicrobials, or other agents. Require secondary dressings to secure them in place, retain moisture, and provide wound protection.	To cover, soothe, and protect partial- and full-thickness wounds without exudate	Vaseline gauze, Carragauze, Dermagran Wet Dressing, Xeroform
Hydrocolloids	Waterproof adhesive wafers, pastes, or powders. Wafers, designed to be worn for up to 7 days, consist of two layers. The inner adhesive layer has particles that absorb exudate and form a hydrated gel over the wound; the outer film provides a seal.	To absorb exudate; to produce a moist environment that facilitates healing but does not cause maceration of surrounding skin; to protect the wound from bacterial contamination, foreign debris, and urine or feces; and to prevent shearing	DuoDERM, Comfeel, Tegasorb, Restore, Replicare
Hydrogels	Glycerin or water-based *nonadhesive* jellylike sheets, granules, or gels that are oxygen permeable, unless covered by a plastic film. May require secondary occlusive dressing.	To liquefy necrotic tissue or slough, rehydrate the wound bed, and fill in dead space	Aquasorb, ClearSite, Elasto-Gel, Intrasite, Vigilon
Polyurethane foams	*Nonadherent* hydrocolloid dressings that need to have their edges taped down or sealed. Require secondary dressings to obtain an occlusive environment. Surrounding skin must be protected to prevent maceration.	To absorb light to moderate amounts of exudate; to debride wounds	Lyofoam, Allevyn, Nuderm, Flexan
Exudate absorbers	Nonadherent dressings of powder, beads or granules, or paste that conform to the wound surface and absorb up to 20 times their weight in exudate; require a secondary dressing.	To provide a moist wound surface by interacting with exudate; to form a gelatinous mass; to absorb exudate; to eliminate dead space or pack wounds, and to support debridement	Debrisan, Triad paste, Sorbsan

Procedure 12-1 Part A describes how to apply a moist transparent wound barrier.

HYDROCOLLOID DRESSINGS. Hydrocolloid dressings (see Table 12-2) are frequently used over venous stasis leg ulcers and pressure ulcers. These dressings offer several advantages:

◆ They can last 5 to 7 days.
◆ They do not need a "cover" dressing and are water resistant.
◆ They can be molded to uneven body surfaces.
◆ They act as temporary skin and provide an effective bacterial barrier.
◆ They decrease pain and thus reduce the need for analgesics.
◆ They absorb some drainage and therefore can be used on draining wounds.

◆ They contain wound odor.

These dressings have certain limitations, however. Some of their disadvantages include the following:

◆ They are opaque and obscure wound visibility.
◆ They have a limited absorption.
◆ They can facilitate anaerobic bacterial growth.
◆ They can soften and wrinkle at the edges with wear and movement.
◆ They can be difficult to remove and may leave a residue on the skin.

Hydrocolloid dressings should not be used for infected wounds or those with deep tracts or **fistulas** (abnormal passage that develops between a hollow organ and the skin or

TABLE 12-3	METHODS OF APPLYING GAUZE DRESSINGS	
DRESSING	**DESCRIPTION**	**PURPOSE**
Dry-to-dry	A layer of wide-mesh cotton gauze lies next to the wound surface. A second layer of dry absorbent cotton or Dacron is on top.	Protect the wound. If the wound is open or draining, necrotic debris and exudate are trapped in the interstices of the gauze layer and are removed when the dressing is removed.
Wet-to-dry	Next to the wound surface is a layer of wide-mesh cotton gauze saturated with saline or an antimicrobial solution. This layer is covered by a moist absorbent material that is moistened with the same solution.	Debride the wound. Necrotic debris is softened by the solution and then adheres to the mesh gauze as it dries. It is removed when the dressing is removed. Also, moisture helps dilute viscous exudate.
Wet-to-damp	A variation of the wet-to-dry dressing, this dressing is removed before it has completely dried.	The wound is debrided when the gauze is removed.
Wet-to-wet	A layer of wide-mesh gauze saturated with antibacterial solution lies next to the wound surface. Above is a second layer of absorbent material saturated with the same solution. The entire dressing is kept moist with a wetting agent.	The wound surface is continually bathed. Moisture dilutes viscous exudate.

between two hollow organs). Procedure 12-1 Part B describes how to apply hydrocolloid dressings.

MEANS OF SECURING DRESSINGS. Dressings over wounds must cover the entire wound in order to protect it. They must also be secured so that they do not become dislodged, exposing the healing wound. The correct type of tape must be selected. For example, elastic tape can provide pressure; nonallergenic tape can be used when a client is allergic to other tape.

Montgomery straps (tie tapes) are commonly used for wounds that require frequent dressing changes (Figure 12-4 ◆). These straps prevent skin irritation and discomfort caused by removing the adhesive each time the dressing is changed. The nurse can protect the skin by applying tincture of benzoin to the site where the adhesive is to be placed.

Supporting and Immobilizing Wounds

Bandages and binders serve various purposes:

- ◆ Supporting a wound (e.g., a fractured bone)
- ◆ Immobilizing a wound (e.g., a strained shoulder)

Nonadhesive portion

Adhesive portion

Figure 12-4. ◆ Montgomery straps, or tie tapes, are used to secure large dressings that require frequent changing.

Figure 12-3. ◆ A transparent wound dressing. *Source:* © Jenny Thomas.

- Applying pressure (e.g., elastic bandages on the lower extremities to improve venous blood flow)
- Securing a dressing (e.g., for an extensive abdominal surgical wound)
- Retaining warmth (e.g., a flannel bandage on a rheumatoid joint)

There are several types of bandages and binders and several ways in which they are applied. When correctly applied, they promote healing, provide comfort, and can prevent injury. Clinical guidelines for bandaging are discussed in the Nursing Care section.

BANDAGES. A *bandage* is a strip of cloth used to wrap some part of the body. Bandages are available in various widths, most commonly 1.5 to 7.5 cm (0.5 to 3 in), and are usually supplied in rolls for easy application to a body part.

Many types of materials are used for bandages. Gauze is one of the most commonly used; it is light and porous and readily molds to the body. It is also relatively inexpensive, so it is generally discarded when soiled. Gauze is frequently used to retain dressings on wounds and to bandage the fingers, hands, toes, and feet. It supports dressings and at the same time permits air to circulate. It can also be saturated with petroleum jelly or other medications for application to wounds.

Many kinds of elasticized bandages are applied to provide pressure to an area. They are commonly used as tensor bandages or as partial stockings (TEDS). They provide support and improve the venous circulation in the legs.

The width of the bandage used depends on the size of the body part to be bandaged. The greater the circumference of a part, the wider the bandage. Padding (e.g., abdominal pads and gauze squares) is frequently used to cover bony prominences (e.g., the elbow) or to separate skin surfaces (e.g., the fingers).

Before applying a bandage, the nurse needs to know its purpose and to assess the area requiring support. See Box 12-2 ◆ for assessment guidelines. When bandages are used to secure dressings, the nurse wears gloves to prevent contact with body fluids.

BINDERS. A *binder* is a type of bandage designed for a specific body part; for example, the triangular binder (sling) fits the arm. Binders are used to support large areas of the body, such as the abdomen, arm, or chest.

A triangular arm binder or *sling* is usually applied as a full triangle to support the arm, elbow, and forearm of the client or to reduce or prevent swelling of a hand. Most agencies use commercial strap slings.

Straight abdominal binders are used to support the abdomen. A straight binder is also used to support the chest. Chest binders often have shoulder straps.

Heat and Cold Applications

Heat and cold are applied to the body for local and systemic effects. They can be useful in the healing process for closed wounds.

BOX 12-2 ASSESSING CLIENTS BEFORE APPLYING BANDAGES OR BINDERS

- Inspect and palpate the area for swelling.
- Inspect for the presence of and status of wounds. (Open wounds will require a dressing before a bandage or binder is applied.)
- Note the presence of drainage (amount, color, odor, viscosity).
- Inspect and palpate for adequacy of circulation (skin temperature, color, and sensation). Pale or cyanotic skin, cool temperature, tingling, and numbness can indicate impaired circulation.
- Ask the client about any pain experienced (location, intensity, onset, quality).
- Assess the ability of the client to reapply the bandage or binder when needed.
- Assess the capabilities of the client regarding activities of daily living (e.g., to eat, dress, comb hair, bathe) and assess the assistance required during the convalescence period.

EFFECTS OF HEAT AND COLD. Heat causes vasodilation and increases blood flow to the affected area, bringing oxygen, nutrients, antibodies, and leukocytes. Table 12-4 ◆ describes the physiologic effects of heat and cold. Application of heat

TABLE 12-4 PHYSIOLOGIC EFFECTS OF HEAT AND COLD

HEAT	COLD
Vasodilation	Vasoconstriction
Increases capillary permeability	Decreases capillary permeability
Increases cellular metabolism	Decreases cellular metabolism
Relaxes muscles	Relaxes muscles
Increases inflammation; increases blood flow to an area	Slows bacterial growth, decreases inflammation
Decreases pain by relaxing muscles	Decreases pain by numbing the area, slowing the flow of pain impulses, and by increasing the pain threshold
Sedative effect	Local anesthetic effect
Reduces joint stiffness by decreasing viscosity of synovial fluids	Decreases bleeding

promotes soft tissue healing and increases suppuration. Heat is often used for clients with musculoskeletal problems such as joint stiffness from arthritis, contractures, and low back pain.

A possible disadvantage of heat is that it increases capillary permeability, allowing extracellular fluid and substances such as plasma proteins to pass through the capillary walls. This may result in edema. Also, when heat is applied to a large body area, it may cause excessive peripheral vasodilation and a drop in blood pressure. A significant drop in blood pressure can cause fainting.

Cold lowers the temperature of the skin and underlying tissues and causes vasoconstriction, which reduces blood flow to the affected area. It reduces the supply of oxygen and metabolites, decreases the removal of wastes, and produces skin pallor and coolness. Cold applications are most often used for sports injuries (e.g., sprains, strains, fractures) to limit postinjury swelling and bleeding.

Prolonged exposure to cold results in impaired circulation, cell deprivation, and subsequent damage to the tissues from lack of oxygen and nourishment. The signs of tissue damage due to cold are a bluish-purple mottled appearance of the skin, numbness, and sometimes blisters and pain.

Shivering is an initial, normal response to systemic cold, as the body attempts to warm itself (see also Chapter 14). 🔗 With extensive cold applications, a client's blood pressure can increase because vasoconstriction causes blood to be shunted from the cutaneous circulation to the internal blood vessels.

THERMAL TOLERANCE. Variables such as extremes of age, length of exposure, and intactness of the skin affect tolerance to heat and cold. Some body parts (like the back of the hand and the foot) are not very temperature sensitive. Others (the neck, the inside of the wrist, the perineal area) are very sensitive to temperature. Certain conditions require added caution in the use of hot or cold applications:

◆ *Neurosensory impairment.* People who cannot perceive heat or cold normally are at risk for burns or tissue injury.
◆ *Impaired mental status.* People who are confused or have an altered level of consciousness need monitoring during applications to ensure safe therapy.
◆ *Impaired circulation.* People with peripheral vascular disease, diabetes, or congestive heart failure lack the normal ability to dissipate heat via the blood circulation. This puts them at risk for tissue damage with heat and cold applications.
◆ *Recent injury or surgery.* Immediately after injury or surgery, heat increases bleeding and swelling.
◆ *Open wounds.* Cold can decrease blood flow to the wound, thereby inhibiting healing.

Methods for Applying Heat and Cold

Heat can be applied to the body in both dry and moist forms. Dry heat is applied locally by means of a hot water bottle,

electric pad, aquathermia pad, or disposable heat pack. Moist heat can be provided by compress, hot pack, soak, or sitz bath. Guidelines for nurses to follow for local applications of heat or cold are discussed in the Nursing Care section later in the chapter.

AQUATHERMIA PAD. The aquathermia or aquamatic pad (also referred to as a K-pad) is a pad constructed with tubes containing water. The pad is attached by tubing to an electrically powered control unit that has an opening for water and a temperature gauge (Figure 12-5 ◆). Some aquathermia pads have an absorbent surface through which moist heat can be applied. The other surface of the pad is waterproof. These pads are disposable.

HOT AND COLD PACKS. Commercially prepared packs provide heat or cold for a designated time. Directions on the package tell how to initiate the heating or cooling process, such as by striking, squeezing, or kneading the pack.

ICE BAG, ICE GLOVE, ICE COLLAR. Ice bags, ice gloves, and ice collars are filled either with ice chips or with an alcohol-based solution. They are applied to the body to provide cold to a localized area (e.g., a collar is often applied to the throat following a tonsillectomy).

COMPRESSES. Compresses can be either warm or cold. A *compress* is a moist gauze dressing applied to a wound. When hot compresses are ordered, the solution is heated to the temperature indicated by the order or according to agency protocol, for example, 40.5°C (105°F). When there is a break in the skin or when the body part (e.g., an eye) is vulnerable to microbial invasion, sterile technique is necessary. Sterile gloves are needed to apply the compress, and all materials must be sterile.

SOAKS. A *soak* refers to immersing a body part (e.g., an arm) in a solution or to wrapping a part in gauze dressings and then

Figure 12-5. ◆ An aquathermia heating unit.

saturating the dressing with a solution. Sterile technique is generally indicated for open wounds, such as a burn or an unhealed surgical incision. Determine agency protocol regarding the temperature of the solution. Hot soaks are frequently done to soften and remove encrusted secretions and dead tissue.

SITZ BATH. A **sitz bath** is used to soak a client's pelvic area. The client sits in a special tub or chair and is usually immersed from the mid-thighs to the iliac crests or umbilicus. Special tubs or chairs are preferred, because a regular bathtub decreases blood circulation to the perineum or pelvic area. Disposable sitz baths are also available.

The temperature of the water should be from 40 to 43°C (105 to 110°F), unless the client is unable to tolerate the heat. Determine agency protocol. Some sitz tubs have temperature indicators attached to the water taps. The duration of the bath is generally 15 to 20 minutes, depending on the client's health.

COOLING SPONGE BATH. The purpose of a cooling sponge bath is to reduce a client's fever by promoting heat loss through conduction and vaporization. The bath consists of water or a combination of alcohol and water that is below body temperature. Alcohol evaporates at a low temperature and therefore removes body heat rapidly. However, alcohol-and-water sponge baths are less frequently used than in the past because alcohol has a drying effect on the skin. The temperatures for cooling sponge baths range from 18 to 32°C (65 to 90°F). A tepid sponge bath generally refers to one in which the water temperature is 32°C (90°F) throughout the bath.

The decision to give a tepid sponge bath is generally made only when there is a marked fever or when a temperature increase is noted. Some agencies require a physician's order; others permit a decision by the primary nurse.

HYPERTHERMIA AND HYPOTHERMIA BLANKETS. Hyperthermia and hypothermia blankets are used to increase or decrease a client's body temperature. The blanket has an associated control panel on which the desired temperature is set and the client's core temperature registers. Follow institutional policy for further details.

Laboratory Data

Laboratory data often supports the nurse's clinical assessment of the wound's progress in healing. A decreased leukocyte count can delay healing and increase the possibility of infection. Blood coagulation studies are also significant. Prolonged coagulation times can result in excessive blood loss and prolonged clot absorption. Serum protein analysis provides an indication of the body's nutritional reserves for rebuilding cells. Wound cultures can either confirm or rule out the presence of infection. Sensitivity studies are helpful in the selection of appropriate antibiotic therapy.

NURSING CARE

ASSESSING

The nurse examines the integument as part of a routine observation and assessment during regular care. During the review of systems as part of the nursing history, the nurse collects information about skin diseases, previous bruising, general skin condition, skin lesions, and usual healing of sores. Inspection and palpation of the skin focus on skin color distribution, skin turgor, presence of edema, and characteristics of any lesions. Box 12-3 ◆ describes assessment of common pressure sites.

Untreated Wounds

Untreated wounds usually are seen shortly after an injury (e.g., at the scene of an accident or in an emergency center). The following steps are important when assessing an untreated wound:

- Note size and severity of wound and check for associated injuries. Call for help to treat severe wounds.
- Inspect the wound for foreign bodies (soil, glass, etc.).
- If wound is contaminated with foreign material, assess need for tetanus immunuzation or booster.

BOX 12-3 ASSESSING COMMON PRESSURE SITES

- Be sure there is good lighting, preferably natural or fluorescent.
- Regulate the environment before beginning the assessment so that the room is neither too hot nor too cold. Heat can cause the skin to flush; cold can cause the skin to blanch or become cyanotic.
- Inspect pressure areas for any whitish or reddened spots; discoloration can be caused by impaired blood circulation to the area. It should disappear in a few minutes when rubbing restores circulation.
- Inspect pressure areas for abrasions and excoriations. An abrasion (wearing away of the skin) can occur when skin rubs against a sheet (e.g., when the client is pulled). Excoriations (loss of superficial layers of the skin) can occur when the skin has prolonged contact with body secretions or excretions or with dampness in skinfolds.
- Palpate the surface temperature of the skin over the pressure areas. Normally, the temperature is the same as that of the surrounding skin. Increased temperature is abnormal and may be due to inflammation or blood trapped in the area.
- Palpate over bony prominences and dependent body areas for the presence of edema, which feels spongy.

Treated Wounds

Treated wounds, or sutured wounds, are usually assessed to determine the progress of healing. These wounds may be inspected during a dressing change unless a transparent dressing has been applied. If the wound itself cannot be inspected directly, the dressing is inspected and other data regarding the wound (e.g., the presence of pain) are assessed. Many treated wounds are covered with a transparent occlusive dressing that permits observation of the wound without exposure to the air.

Assessment of a treated wound includes observation of its appearance, size, and drainage; the presence of swelling or pain; and status of drains or tubes.

 DIAGNOSING, PLANNING, and IMPLEMENTING

Nursing diagnoses that relate to clients who have skin wounds or who are at risk for skin breakdown are:

◆ Risk for Impaired Skin Integrity
◆ Impaired Skin Integrity: commonly applies to superficial wounds extending through the epidermis but not through the dermis

◆ Impaired Tissue Integrity: applies to wounds extending into subcutaneous tissue, muscle, or bone
◆ Risk for Infection
◆ Pain related to nerve involvement
◆ Disturbed Body Image

In planning nursing care, the primary goals are maintaining skin integrity and avoiding potential risks. For clients with Impaired Skin Integrity or Impaired Tissue Integrity, the goal is to achieve progressive wound healing and regain intact skin.

Nursing interventions for maintaining skin integrity and providing wound care involve supporting wound healing, preventing pressure ulcers, treating pressure ulcers, cleaning and dressing wounds, supporting and immobilizing wounds, and applying heat and cold.

Examples of nursing interventions for maintaining intact skin follow.

◆ Inspect skin at regular intervals.
◆ Keep skin clean, dry, and moisturized.
◆ Provide appropriate pressure-relieving devices and measures (Table 12-5 ◆).

TABLE 12-5	MECHANICAL DEVICES FOR REDUCING PRESSURE ON BODY PARTS
DEVICE	**DESCRIPTION/COMMENTS**
Gel flotation pads	Polyvinyl, silicone, or Silastic pads filled with a gelatinous substance similar to fat.
Sheepskins (natural and artificial)	Some manufacturers produce mixed natural and synthetic pads; artificial pads are less likely to be damaged by washing but are more likely to make the client hot than natural skins.
Pillows and wedges (foam, gel and air, foam and fluid)	Can raise a body part (e.g., heels) off the bed surface.
Heel protectors (sheepskin boots, padded splints, foam wedges)	Limit pressure on heels when the client is in bed.
Egg crate mattress	Polyurethane foam mattress resembling an egg crate; some types are flammable.
Foam mattress	Foam molds to the body.
Alternating pressure mattress	Composed of a number of cells in which the pressure alternately increases and decreases; uses a pump.
Water bed	Special mattress filled with water; controls temperature of water.
Air-fluidized (AF) bed (static high air loss [HAL] bed)	Forced temperature-controlled air is circulated around millions of tiny silicone-coated beads, producing a fluidlike movement. Provides uniform support to body contours. Decreases skin maceration by its drying effect. Moisture from the client penetrates the bedsheet and soaks the beads. Air flow forces the beads away from the client and rapidly dries the sheet. A major disadvantage is that the head of the bed cannot be elevated.
Static low air loss (LAL) bed	Consists of many air-filled cushions divided into four or five sections. Separate controls permit each section to be inflated to a different level of firmness; thus pressure can be reduced on bony prominences but increased under other body areas for support.
Active or second-generation low air loss (LAL) bed	Like the static LAL, but in addition greatly pulsates or rotates from side to side, thus stimulating capillary blood flow and facilitating movement of pulmonary secretions.

For clients with untreated wounds, the nurse performs the following interventions:

◆ Control severe bleeding, apply direct pressure to the wound, and elevate the extremity.
◆ Prevent infection by cleansing or flushing abrasions or lacerations with water. Box 12-4 ◆ provides guidelines for cleaning wounds.
◆ If bleeding is severe or if internal bleeding is suspected, assess the client and report any signs of shock (rapid, thready pulse; cold, clammy skin; pallor; lowered blood pressure).
◆ Cover the wound with a clean dressing (a sterile dressing is preferred). If the first layer of dressing becomes saturated with blood, apply a second layer. *Removing the first layer of dressing might disturb blood clots, resulting in more bleeding.*

BOX 12-4
NURSING CARE CHECKLIST

CLEANING WOUNDS

☑ Use physiologic solutions, such as isotonic saline or lactated Ringer's solution, to clean or irrigate wounds. If antimicrobial solutions are used, make sure they are well diluted.
☑ When possible, warm the solution to body temperature before use. This prevents lowering of the wound temperature, which slows the healing process.
☑ If a wound is grossly contaminated by foreign material, bacteria, slough, or necrotic tissue, clean the wound at every dressing change. Foreign bodies and devitalized tissue act as a focus for infection and can delay healing.
☑ If a wound is clean, has little exudate, and reveals healthy granulation tissue, avoid repeated cleaning. Unnecessary cleaning can delay wound healing by traumatizing newly produced, delicate tissues, reducing the surface temperature of the wound, and removing exudate which itself may have bactericidal properties.
☑ Use gauze squares. Avoid using cotton balls and other products that shed fibers onto the wound surface. The fibers become embedded in granulation tissue and can act as foci for infection. They may also stimulate "foreign body" reactions, prolonging the inflammatory phase of healing and delaying the healing process.
☑ Clean superficial noninfected wounds by irrigating them with normal saline. The hydraulic pressure of an irrigating stream of fluid dislodges contaminating debris and reduces bacterial colonization.
☑ To retain wound moisture, avoid drying a wound after cleaning it.

Supporting Wound Healing

There are three major areas in which nurses can support wound healing: obtaining sufficient nutrition and fluids, preventing wound infections, and positioning the client properly.

◆ Assist the client to take in at least 2,500 mL of fluids a day unless conditions contraindicate this amount. The nurse should ensure that clients receive sufficient protein; vitamins C, A, B_1, and B_5; and zinc. *Although there is no evidence that excessive doses of vitamins or minerals enhance wound healing, adequate amounts are extremely important.*
◆ Provide excellent infection control: (1) prevent microorganisms from entering the wound, and (2) prevent transmission of bloodborne pathogens to or from the client to others. (See Chapter 7 for more information about infection control. ⌘)
◆ With physician order, obtain a wound culture whenever an infection is suspected. Procedure 12-2 provides guidelines for obtaining a specimen of wound drainage.
◆ Position clients to keep pressure off the wound. Changes of position and transfers must be accomplished without shear or friction damage.
◆ Encourage the client to be as mobile as possible. *Activity enhances circulation.* If the client cannot move independently, implement range-of-motion exercises and a turning schedule.

Cleaning, Irrigating, and Dressing Wounds

◆ Wear gloves and follow standard precautions to prevent transmission of bloodborne pathogens.
◆ Wash hands before and after caring for wounds.
◆ Follow recommended guidelines for cleaning wounds (see Box 12-4). A major principle of cleaning wounds is always to clean from "clean to dirty."
◆ Touch an open or fresh surgical wound only when wearing sterile gloves or using sterile forceps. *Irrigate* (wash or flush out) the wound using sterile technique. *Sterile technique is required because of the break in skin integrity.* See Procedure 12-3 for the steps involved in irrigating a wound.
◆ Pack the wound as ordered. Clinical guidelines for applying wet-to-damp dressings are described on page 240.

Securing Dressings

◆ Ensure that the dressing covers the entire wound, and select the appropriate tape to secure it.
◆ Place the tape so that the dressing cannot be folded back to expose the wound. Place strips at the ends of the dressing, and space tapes evenly in the middle (Figure 12-6 ◆).
◆ Ensure that the tape is long and wide enough to adhere to several inches of skin on each side of the dressing, but not so long or wide that the tape loosens with activity.
◆ Place the tape in the opposite direction from expected body action (Figure 12-7 ◆).

Figure 12-6. ◆ The strips of tape should be placed at the ends of the dressing and must be sufficiently long and wide to secure the dressing. The tape should adhere to intact skin.

Applying Bandages and Binders

General guidelines for bandaging include the following interventions:

◆ Bandage the part in its normal position, with the joint flexed slightly. *This avoids putting strain on the ligaments and muscles of the joint.*
◆ Pad between skin surfaces and over bony areas. *This prevents friction and abrasion of the skin.*
◆ Bandage body parts from the distal to the proximal end. *This aids the return of venous blood.*
◆ If possible, leave the end of the body part (e.g., a toe) exposed. *This allows visual assessment of blood circulation to the extremity.*

Figure 12-7. ◆ Dressings over moving parts must remain secure in spite of the movement. Place the tape over a joint at a right angle to the direction the joint moves.

◆ Cover the dressings with bandages at least 5 cm (2 in) beyond the edges of the dressing. *This prevents dressing and wound from becoming contaminated.*
◆ Face the client when applying the bandage. *This maintains uniform tension and alignment of the bandage.*

Circular turns are used chiefly to anchor bandages or to bandage certain areas, such as the proximal aspect of a finger or a wrist. Circular turns for roller bandages are done as follows:

◆ Apply the end of the bandage to the part of the body to be bandaged.
◆ Wrap the bandage around the body part a few times or as often as needed, each turn directly covering the previous turn (Figure 12-8 ◆). *This provides even support to the area.*
◆ Secure the end of the bandage with tape, metal clips, or a safety pin over an uninjured area. Clips and pins can be uncomfortable when situated over an injured area.

Figure-eight turns are used to bandage an elbow, knee, or ankle, because they permit some movement after application. To apply a figure-eight turn with a roller bandage, follow these steps:

◆ Anchor the bandage with two circular turns.
◆ Carry the bandage above the joint, around it, and then below it, making a figure eight (Figure 12-9 ◆).
◆ Continue above and below the joint, overlapping the previous turn by two thirds the width of the bandage.
◆ End the bandage above the joint with two circular turns, and secure the end appropriately.

Binders are also sometimes called slings. To apply a large arm sling:

◆ Place one end of the unfolded triangular binder over the shoulder of the uninjured side so that the binder falls down the front of the chest of the client with the point of the triangle (apex) under the elbow of the injured side.
◆ Take the upper corner, and carry it around the neck until it hangs over the shoulder on the injured side (Figure 12-10 ◆).

Figure 12-8. ◆ Starting a bandage with two circular turns. *Source:* © Elena Dorfman.

Figure 12-9. ◆ Applying a figure-eight bandage.

- Bring the lower corner of the binder up over the arm to the shoulder of the injured side. Using a square knot, secure this corner to the upper corner at the side of the neck on the involved side.
- Fold the sling neatly at the elbow, and secure it with safety pins or tape. It may be folded and fastened at the front.

Straight abdominal binders are also useful. To apply straight abdominal binders, follow these steps:

- With the client in a supine position, place the abdominal binder smoothly under the client, with the upper border of the binder at the waist and the lower border at the level of the gluteal fold. *A binder placed above the waist can interfere with respiration. One placed too low can interfere with elimination and walking.*
- Apply padding over the iliac crests if the client is thin.
- For a straight abdominal binder, bring the ends around the client, overlap them, and secure them with pins or Velcro.

Heat and Cold Applications

Heat and cold applications can assist the healing process. Nursing care guidelines for selected heat and cold therapies are provided in Box 12-5 ◆.

A   B

Figure 12-10. ◆ Large arm sling.

BOX 12-5
NURSING CARE CHECKLIST

SELECTED HEAT AND COLD APPLICATIONS

Aquathermia Pad

- ☑ Fill the reservoir of the unit two-thirds full of distilled water.
- ☑ Set the desired temperature. Check the manufacturer's instructions. Most units are set at 40.5°C (105°F) for adults.
- ☑ Cover the pad and plug in the unit. Some manufacturers suggest warming the pad before applying it.
- ☑ Apply the pad to the body part. The treatment is usually continued for 10 to 15 minutes. Check orders and agency protocol.

Ice Bag, Glove, or Collar

- ☑ Always wrap the container in a cloth or towel before applying.

Sitz Bath

- ☑ Assist the client into the tub. Provide support for the client's feet; a footstool can prevent pressure on the backs of the thighs.
- ☑ Provide a bath blanket for the client's shoulders, and eliminate drafts to prevent chilling.
- ☑ Observe the client closely during the bath for signs of faintness, dizziness, weakness, accelerated pulse rate, and pallor.
- ☑ Maintain the water temperature.
- ☑ Following the sitz bath, assist the client out of the tub. Help the client to dry.

Cooling Sponge Bath

- ☑ Determine the client's vital signs (i.e., TPR).
- ☑ Protect the client's bed with moistureproof material.
- ☑ Sponge the face, arms, legs, back, and buttocks. The chest and abdomen are not usually sponged. Each area is sponged slowly and gently. Rubbing may increase heat production.
- ☑ Leave each area wet, and cover with a damp towel.
- ☑ Place ice bags and cold packs, if used, or a cool cloth on the forehead for comfort and in each axilla and at the groin. These areas contain large superficial blood vessels that help the transfer of heat.
- ☑ Sponge one body part and then another. The sponge bath should take about 30 minutes. A bath given more quickly tends to increase the body's heat production by causing shivering.
- ☑ Discontinue the bath if the client becomes pale or cyanotic or shivers, or if the pulse becomes rapid or irregular.
- ☑ Pat each area dry.
- ☑ Reassess the vital signs at 15 minutes and after completing the sponge bath.

For all local applications of heat or cold, the following guidelines apply:

♦ Determine the client's ability to tolerate the therapy.
♦ Identify conditions that might contraindicate treatment (e.g., bleeding, circulatory impairment).
♦ Explain the application to the client.
♦ Assess the skin area to which the heat will be applied.
♦ Ask the client to report any discomfort.
♦ Return to the client 15 minutes after starting the heat, and observe the local skin area for any untoward signs (e.g., redness). Stop the heat if any problems occur.
♦ Remove the equipment at the designated time, and dispose of it appropriately.
♦ Examine the area to which the heat was applied, and record the client's response.

EVALUATING

To judge whether client outcomes have been achieved, the nurse uses data collected during care, such as skin status over bony prominences and perineal area, nutritional and fluid intake, mental status, signs of healing if an ulcer is present, and so on. If outcomes are not achieved, the nurse should explore the reasons why:

♦ Has the client's physical condition changed?
♦ Were risk factors correctly identified?
♦ Were appropriate lifting devices and techniques used?
♦ Was the repositioning schedule followed?
♦ Are the client's nutritional and fluid intake adequate?

DISCHARGE CONSIDERATIONS

Prior to discharge, the nurse must ensure that clients have an understanding of wound care. Clients should know how to change a dressing and how frequent. They should understand what normal healing looks like. They should be given a list of signs that might indicate an infection or other complication and when to notify the physician.

Pressure Ulcers

Pressure ulcers (also called decubitus ulcers, pressure sores, or bedsores) are lesions caused by unrelieved pressure that results in damage to underlying tissue. Pressure ulcers are a problem in both acute care settings and long-term care settings, including homes.

Pressure ulcers are caused by localized **ischemia,** a deficiency in the blood supply to the tissue. The tissue is caught between two hard surfaces, usually the surface of the

bed and the bony skeleton. When blood cannot reach the tissue, the cells are deprived of oxygen and nutrients, and waste products accumulate in the cells. Prolonged, unrelieved pressure damages the small blood vessels, and the tissue eventually dies.

Pressure ulcers usually occur over bony prominences. After the skin has been compressed, it appears pale. When pressure is relieved, the skin takes on a bright red flush, called **reactive hyperemia.** The flush is due to vasodilation; extra blood floods to the area to compensate for the impeded blood flow. If the redness disappears, no tissue damage can be anticipated. If the redness does not disappear, then tissue damage has occurred.

Besides pressure, two other factors often produce pressure ulcers: friction and shearing force. **Friction** is a force acting parallel to the skin surface. For example, sheets rubbing against skin create friction. Friction can remove the superficial layers, making the skin more prone to breakdown.

Shearing force is a combination of friction and pressure. It occurs commonly when a client assumes a Fowler's position in bed. The body slides down toward the foot of the bed, but the skin over the sacrum tends not to move. The skin and superficial tissues are held by the bed surface, but the deeper tissues attached to the skeleton move downward. The shearing force occurs where the deeper tissues and the superficial tissues meet. The force damages blood vessels and tissues in this area.

RISK FACTORS

Several factors contribute to the formation of pressure ulcers:

♦ *Immobility.* Immobility and inactivity are important risk factors for pressure ulcers. Immobility refers to a reduction in the amount of movement a person has. Paralysis, extreme weakness, or any cause of decreased activity can hinder a person's ability to change positions independently and relieve the pressure.

♦ *Inadequate nutrition.* Nutritional factors are crucial in the development of pressure ulcers. Generally, prolonged inadequate nutrition causes weight loss, muscle atrophy, and the loss of subcutaneous tissue. Reduction in padding between the skin and the bones increases the risk of pressure sore development. Inadequate intake of protein, carbohydrates, fluids, and vitamin C specifically contributes to pressure ulcer formation.

♦ *Edema* (presence of excess fluid in the tissues) makes skin more prone to injury by decreasing its elasticity and resilience.

♦ *Fecal and urinary incontinence.* Moisture from incontinence promotes skin ***maceration*** (softening of tissue by prolonged wetting) and makes the epidermis susceptible to injury. Digestive enzymes in feces also contribute to skin excoriation. Any accumulation of secretions or excretions is irritating to the skin, harbors microorganisms, and makes an individual prone to skin breakdown and infection.

◆ *Decreased mental status*. Individuals with a reduced level of awareness and those who are unconscious or heavily sedated are at risk for pressure ulcers. They are less able to recognize and respond to pain associated with prolonged pressure.

◆ *Diminished sensation*. Paralysis, or other neurologic disease causing loss of sensation, reduces a person's ability to respond to damaging levels of heat and cold and to feel the tingling ("pins and needles") that signals loss of circulation.

◆ *Excessive body heat*. Body heat is another factor in the development of pressure sores. An elevated body temperature increases the body's metabolic rate, increasing the need for cellular oxygen. This increased need is severe in the cells of an area under pressure, which are already oxygen deficient. Severe infections with accompanying elevated body temperatures may affect the body's ability to deal with the effects of tissue compression.

◆ *Advanced age*. The aging process can make older people more prone to impaired skin integrity. Older adults may be prone to loss of lean body mass, generalized thinning and dryness of the epidermis, and decreased strength and elasticity of the skin. They may have diminished pain perception due to decreased sensation of pressure and light touch. (See also Box 12-1.)

◆ *Other factors*. Poor lifting techniques, incorrect positioning, repeated injections in the same area, hard support surfaces, and incorrect application of pressure-relieving devices also contribute to the formation of pressure sores.

STAGES OF PRESSURE ULCER FORMATION

The four stages in pressure ulcer formation relate to observable tissue damage. See Figures 12-11 ◆ and 12-12 ◆.

Stage I: Nonblanchable erythema of intact skin.

Stage II: Partial-thickness skin loss involving epidermis, dermis, or both. The ulcer is superficial and presents as an abrasion, blister, or shallow crater.

Stage III: Full-thickness skin loss involving damage or necrosis of subcutaneous tissue that may extend down to, but not through, underlying fascia. The ulcer presents as a deep crater with or without undermining of adjacent tissue.

Stage IV: Full-thickness skin loss with extensive destruction, tissue necrosis, or damage to muscle, bone, or supporting structures, such as a tendon or joint capsule. Undermining and sinus tracts may also be associated with stage IV pressure ulcers.

COLLABORATIVE CARE

Supportive Devices

For clients confined to bed, special support surfaces and positioning devices can be used to protect bony prominences. Three types of support surfaces can be used to relieve pressure.

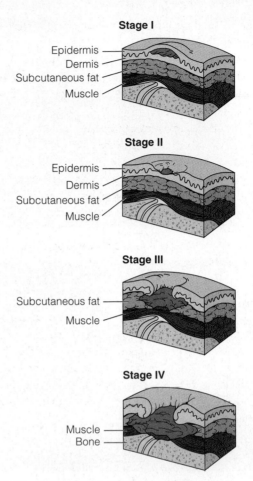

Figure 12-11. ◆ Four stages of pressure ulcers.

The overlay mattress or eggcrate mattress (Figure 12-13 ◆) is applied on top of the standard bed mattress. A replacement mattress is a mattress that replaces the standard mattress; most are made of foam and gel combinations. Specialty beds replace hospital beds. They provide pressure relief, eliminate shearing and friction, and decrease moisture. See Table 12-5 for selected mechanical devices for reducing pressure on body parts.

When a client is confined to bed or to a chair, pressure-reducing devices, such as pillows made of foam, gel, air, or a combination of these, can be used. When the client is sitting, weight should be distributed over the entire seating surface so that pressure does not center on just one area. To protect a client's heels in bed, supports such as wedges or pillows can be used to raise the heels completely off the bed. Doughnut-type devices should not be used (PPPPUA, 1994).

Risk Assessment Tools

Several risk assessment tools are available that help the nurse identify clients at high risk for pressure ulcer development. Data collection includes the areas of immobility, incontinence, nutrition, and level of consciousness. Two validated assessment tools are the Braden scale (Figure 12-14 ◆) and the

Figure 12-12. ◆ The four stages of a decubitus ulcer: **A.** Stage I: Nonblanchable erythema signaling potential ulceration. **B.** Stage II: Abrasion, blister, or shallow crater involving the epidermis and possibly the dermis. **C.** Stage III: Deep ulcer exhibiting necrotic tissue and extending through the subcutaneous layer. **D.** Stage IV: Tissue necrosis and damage involving muscle, bone, or supporting structures. *Source:* 12-12D © Custom Medical Stock Photo, Inc. Used with permission.

Figure 12-13. ◆ An eggcrate mattress provides comfort and helps to distribute the body weight evenly, thus helping to reduce pressure on bony prominences. *Source:* © Elena Dorfman.

Norton scale (Table 12-6 ◆). These scales include subscales and categories that are assigned points. Scores of 16 or lower may be indicators of potential risk.

THE RYB COLOR CODE. To guide wound care, the nurse can use the RYB color code of wounds developed by Marion Laboratories (Stotts, 1990). This concept is based on the color of an open wound—red, yellow, or black (RYB)—rather than the depth or size of a wound. On this scheme, the goals of wound care are to:

◆ *Protect (cover) red.* Wounds that are red are usually in the late regeneration phase of tissue repair (i.e., developing granulation tissue). They need to be protected to avoid disturbance to regenerating tissue.

◆ *Cleanse yellow.* Yellow wounds are characterized primarily by liquid to semiliquid "slough" that is often accompanied by purulent drainage. The nurse cleanses yellow wounds to remove nonviable tissue.

◆ *Debride black.* Black wounds are covered with thick necrotic tissue, or eschar. Black wounds require **debridement**

BRADEN SCALE FOR PREDICTING PRESSURE SORE RISK

Patient's Name _____ Evaluator's Name _____ Date of Assessment _____

	1	2	3	4
SENSORY PERCEPTION Ability to respond meaningfully to pressure-related discomfort	**1. Completely Limited:** Unresponsive (does not moan, flinch, or grasp) to painful stimuli, due to diminished level of consciousness or sedation, OR limited ability to feel pain over most of body surface.	**2. Very Limited:** Responds only to painful stimuli. Cannot communicate discomfort except by moaning or restlessness, OR has a sensory impairment which limits the ability to feel pain or discomfort over 1/2 of body.	**3. Slightly Limited:** Responds to verbal commands but cannot always communicate discomfort or need to be turned, OR has some sensory impairment which limits ability to feel pain or discomfort in 1 or 2 extremities.	**4. No Impairment:** Responds to verbal commands. Has no sensory deficit which would limit ability to feel or voice pain or discomfort.
MOISTURE Degree to which skin is exposed to moisture	**1. Constantly Moist:** Skin is kept moist almost constantly by perspiration, urine, etc. Dampness is detected every time patient is moved or turned.	**2. Moist:** Skin is often but not always moist. Linen must be changed at least once a shift.	**3. Occasionally Moist:** Skin is occasionally moist, requiring an extra linen change approximately once a day.	**4. Rarely Moist:** Skin is usually dry; linen requires changing only at routine intervals.
ACTIVITY Degree of physical activity	**1. Bedfast:** Confined to bed.	**2. Chairfast:** Ability to walk severely limited or nonexistent. Cannot bear own weight and/or must be assisted into chair or wheelchair.	**3. Walks Occasionally:** Walks occasionally during day but for very short distances, with or without assistance. Spends majority of each shift in bed or chair.	**4. Walks Frequently:** Walks outside the room at least twice a day and inside room at least once every 2 hours during waking hours.
MOBILITY Ability to change and control body position	**1. Completely Immobile:** Does not make even slight changes in body or extremity position without assistance.	**2. Very Limited:** Makes occasional slight changes in body or extremity position but unable to make frequent or significant changes independently.	**3. Slightly Limited:** Makes frequent though slight changes in body or extremity position independently.	**4. No Limitations:** Makes major and frequent changes in position without assistance.
NUTRITION Usual food intake pattern	**1. Very Poor:** Never eats a complete meal. Rarely eats more than 1/3 of any food offered. Eats 2 servings or less of protein (meat or dairy products) per day. Takes fluids poorly. Does not take a liquid dietary supplement, OR is NPO and/or maintained on clear liquids or IVs for more than 5 days.	**2. Probably Inadequate:** Rarely eats a complete meal and generally eats only about 1/2 of any food offered. Protein intake includes only 3 servings of meat or dairy products per day. Occasionally will take a dietary supplement, OR receives less than optimum amount of liquid diet or tube feeding.	**3. Adequate:** Eats over half of most meals. Eats a total of 4 servings of protein (meat, dairy products) each day. Occasionally will refuse a meal, but will usually take a supplement if offered, OR is on a tube feeding or TPN regimen, which probably meets most of nutritional needs.	**4. Excellent:** Eats most of every meal. Never refuses a meal. Usually eats a total of 4 or more servings of meat and dairy products. Occasionally eats between meals. Does not require supplementation.
FRICTION AND SHEAR	**1. Problem:** Requires moderate to maximum assistance in moving. Complete lifting without sliding against sheets is impossible. Frequently slides down in bed or chair, requiring frequent repositioning with maximum assistance. Spasticity, contractures, or agitation leads to almost constant friction.	**2. Potential Problem:** Moves feebly or requires minimum assistance. During a move skin probably slides to some extent against sheets, chair, restraints, or other devices. Maintains relatively good position in chair or bed most of the time but occasionally slides down.	**3. No Apparent Problem:** Moves in bed and in chair independently and has sufficient muscle strength to lift up completely during move. Maintains good position in bed or chair at all times.	

Total Score _____

Figure 12-14. ◆ Braden Scale for Predicting Pressure Sore Risk. *Source:* US Department of Health and Human Services, Clinical practice guideline, *Pressure Ulcers in Adults: Prediction and Prevention*, Pub. no. 92-0047 (Rockville, MD: Public Health Service, 1992), pp. 16–17. Copyright © Barbara Braden and Nancy Bergstrom, 1988. Reprinted with permission.

TABLE 12-6   NORTON'S PRESSURE AREA RISK ASSESSMENT FORM (SCORING SYSTEM)

A GENERAL PHYSICAL CONDITION		B MENTAL STATE		C ACTIVITY		D MOBILITY		E INCONTINENCE	
Good	4	Alert	4	Ambulatory	4	Full	4	Absent	4
Fair	3	Apathetic	3	Walks with help	3	Slightly limited	3	Occasional	3
Poor	2	Confused	2	Chairbound	2	Very limited	2	Usually urinary	2
Very bad	1	Stuporous	1	Bedfast	1	Immobile	1	Double	1

Source: Norton, D., McLaren, R., & Exton-Smith, A.N. (1962). *An investigation of geriatric nursing problems in hospital.* Edinburgh: Churchill Livingstone. Reissued, 1975. Used by permission.

(removal of the necrotic material). Removal of nonviable tissue from a wound must occur before the wound can heal. The physician can perform sharp debridement with a scalpel or scissors to remove dead tissue. Mechanical debridement is accomplished through scrubbing force or wet-to-damp dressings. Box 12-6 ◆ provides information about applying wet-to-damp dressings.

Chemical debridement uses an enzyme agent to breakdown eschar. In autolytic debridement, dressings that contain wound moisture facilitate the body's own enzymatic breakdown of necrotic tissue. This method takes longer but causes the least damage to healthy tissues. When the eschar is removed, the wound is treated as yellow, then red.

clinical ALERT

When more than one color is present in a pressure ulcer, the nurse treats the most serious color first.

NURSING CARE

ASSESSING

Particular attention is paid to skin condition in areas most likely to break down: in skinfolds (such as under the breasts);

BOX 12-6
NURSING CARE CHECKLIST

APPLYING WET-TO-DAMP DRESSINGS

☑ Open the packages of the sterile dressing set, fine-mesh gauze, and sterile solution container.

☑ Pour the ordered solution into the solution container.

☑ Don gloves.

☑ Place the fine-mesh gauze dressings into the solution container, and thoroughly saturate them with solution. The entire gauze must be moistened to enhance its absorptive abilities.

☑ If agency protocol indicates, clean the wound.

☑ Wring out the packing material so that it is slightly moist. Avoid packing that is too wet. An excessively wet wound bed increases the risk for bacterial growth and may macerate the surrounding skin.

☑ Pack the moistened dressings into all depressions and grooves of the wound, ensuring that all exposed surfaces are covered. If necessary, use forceps to feed the gauze gradually into deep depressed areas. Necrotic

tissue is usually more prevalent in depressed wound areas and needs to be covered with gauze.

☑ Avoid applying packing too tightly. A tight application inhibits wound edges from contracting and compresses capillaries.

☑ To prevent maceration of the surrounding skin, pack only to the edge of the wound without overlapping the skin.

☑ If necessary, protect surrounding skin with a skin barrier (e.g., hydrocolloid dressing).

☑ Apply a secondary dressing (e.g., 4 × 4 gauze) over the wet dressings to absorb excess exudate.

☑ Cover all the dressings with a surgipad or abdominal pad. The pad protects the wound from external contaminants.

☑ Remove gloves inside out and discard them.

☑ To remove dressings, wear disposable gloves. If packing material adheres to any tissue during removal, soak it with normal saline. This facilitates removal and preserves new granulation tissue.

in areas that are frequently moist (such as the perineum); and in areas that receive extensive pressure (such as the coccyx and trochanters) (Figure 12-15 ◆; see also Box 12-3, assessing the common pressure sites).

When a pressure ulcer is present, the nurse notes:

- Location of the lesion
- Size of lesion in centimeters. (Measure length, width, and depth, beginning with length [head to toe] and then width [side to side]. To measure depth, gently insert a sterile

Q tip at the deepest part of the wound, and then measure against a measuring guide.)

- Stage of the ulcer (see Figure 12-11)
- Color of the wound bed and location of necrosis or eschar
- Condition of the wound margins
- Integrity of surrounding skin
- Clinical signs of infection, such as redness, warmth, swelling, pain, odor, and exudate (note color of exudate)

◆ DIAGNOSING, PLANNING, and IMPLEMENTING

Nursing diagnoses that are common in clients with pressure ulcers are:

- Impaired Skin Integrity: commonly applies to stage I and II pressure ulcers
- Impaired Tissue Integrity: applies to stage III and IV pressure ulcers
- Pain

Preventing Pressure Ulcers

To prevent pressure ulcers, the LPN/LVN, in collaboration with RN, implements meticulous skin care as described earlier in the chapter.

- Provide nutritional supplements for nutritionally compromised clients. *An inadequate intake of calories, protein, and iron is believed to be a risk factor for pressure ulcer development.*
- Keep the client's skin clean, dry, and free of irritation from urine, feces, and sweat. When bathing the client, avoid using hot water and apply minimal force and friction. Use mild cleansing agents that do not disrupt the skin's "natural barriers," and apply moisturizing lotions as needed. Also, minimize dryness by not exposing clients to cold and low humidity.
- Avoid massaging over bony prominences. *Nurses have used massage to stimulate blood circulation, with the intention of preventing pressure sores. Scientific evidence does not support this belief; in fact, massage may lead to deep tissue trauma.*
- Provide the client with a smooth, firm, and wrinkle-free foundation on which to sit or lie down. Position, transfer, and turn clients correctly. For bedridden clients, reduce shearing force by elevating the head of the bed to no more than 30 degrees, if this position is not contraindicated by the client's condition.
- Encourage or assist the client to shift weight every 15 to 30 minutes and, whenever possible, exercise or ambulate to stimulate blood circulation. *Frequent shifts in position, even if only slight, effectively change pressure points.*
- When lifting a client to change position, use a lifting device such as a trapeze rather than dragging the client across or up in bed. *The friction that results from dragging the skin against a sheet can cause blisters and abrasions, which may contribute to more extensive tissue damage.*

A Heels (calcaneus) Sacrum Elbows (olecranon process) Scapulae Back of head (occipital bone)

B Malleolus (medial and lateral) Knee (medial and lateral condyles) Greater trochanter Ilium Shoulder (acromial process) Ear Side of head (parietal and temporal bones)

C Toes (phalanges) Knees (patellas) Genitalia (men) Breasts (women) Shoulder (acromial process) Cheek and ear (zygomatic bone)

D Heels (calcaneus) Vertebrae (spinal processes) 30° Pelvis (ischial tuberosity) Sacrum

Figure 12-15. ◆ Body pressure areas in **A.** supine position; **B.** lateral position; **C.** prone position; **D.** Fowler's position.

◆ At least every 2 hours, reposition any at-risk client who is confined to bed—even when a special support mattress is used. Establish a written schedule for turning and repositioning. This allows another body surface to bear the weight. Six body positions, can be used: prone, supine, right and left lateral (side-lying), and right and left Sims' positions.

Treating Pressure Ulcers

To treat clients with pressure ulcers, the following interventions are performed:

◆ Follow the agency protocols and the physician's orders, if any.
◆ Protect red wounds (like those developing granulation tissue). Clean them gently, apply a topical antimicrobial agent, cover with a transparent film or hydrocolloid dressing, and disturb the dressing as infrequently as possible). *This will allow the healing process to continue uninterrrupted.* Box 12-7 ◆ provides guidelines for treating pressure ulcers.
◆ Clean yellow wounds to remove nonviable tissue. See Irrigating a Wound, Procedure 12-3.
◆ Report any signs of infection and obtain a wound specimen with a physician order (see Procedure 12-2).
◆ Provide supportive care of the client during removal of black (nonviable) tissue. Once the necrotic tissue has been removed, treat the wound as yellow, then as red.

 ## EVALUATING

Pressure sores are a challenge for nurses because of the number of variables involved (e.g., risk factors, types of ulcers, and

---

BOX 12-7
NURSING CARE CHECKLIST

TREATING PRESSURE ULCERS

☑ Minimize direct pressure on the ulcer. Reposition the client at least every 2 hours. Use a schedule, and record position changes on the client's chart.
☑ Clean the pressure ulcer daily. The method of cleaning depends on the stage of the ulcer and agency protocol. For example, a whirlpool bath may be indicated for a stage II ulcer and a wound irrigation for a stage IV ulcer (see Procedure 12-3).
☑ Clean and dress the ulcer using surgical asepsis.
☑ If the pressure ulcer is infected, obtain a sample of the drainage for culture and sensitivity, with physician order (see Procedure 12-2).
☑ If the client cannot keep weight off the pressure ulcer, use pressure-relieving devices such as an eggcrate mattress.
☑ Teach the client to move, if only slightly, to relieve pressure.
☑ Provide range-of-motion (ROM) exercises as the client's condition permits.

---

degrees of impairment) and the many treatment measures that are advocated. Existing and potential infections are the most serious complications of pressure sores.

Evaluation of a client with pressure ulcers includes documentation of location, size, depth, stage, color, status of wound margins and surrounding skin, and specific signs of infection. Include care provided and client response to treatment.

DISCHARGE CONSIDERATIONS

Clients and their support people often need teaching in order to carry out measures to prevent pressure ulcers. The following information should be provided:

◆ Causes of pressure ulcers
◆ Skin care plan to keep the skin clean, lubricated, and protected from secretions and excretions
◆ Importance of maintaining or increasing correct activity level
◆ Avoidance of massage, "doughnuts," and heat lamps
◆ Need to contact the physician when there is skin reddening, blister formation, or breakdown

---

Nursing Process Case Study:
CLIENT WITH PRESSURE ULCER

Jamie Lee, a 73-year-old female, was admitted to the hospital for a decubitus ulcer on her left hip. Jamie lives in a skilled nursing center and is being treated for diabetes. She takes insulin twice a day. Mrs. Lee is unhappy with the restrictions on her diabetic diet. The staff must remind her about the dangers of eating candy bars, which they frequently find in her bedside table. Her mobility is limited, and she complains when the staff encourages her to sit up. She favors her left side because she can watch the television from that angle easily.

Assessment VS: T 99, apical pulse 76, R 22. BP 146/90; blood sugar 320, hemoglobin 10, hematocrit 36, WBC 12,000.

The decubitus ulcer is described having full-thickness skin loss, measuring 2 × 2 across and 1/2 inch deep. No undermining noted.

Diagnosis

◆ Impaired Skin Integrity
◆ Risk for Infection related to decubitus ulcer
◆ Activity Intolerance
◆ Powerlessness related to illness related regimen
◆ Deficient Knowledge related to diabetes

Expected Outcomes

◆ Skin integrity effectively managed.
◆ Wound is maintained without evidence of infection.

- Expresses an understanding of need to balance rest and activity.
- Participates in planning care; makes decision regarding care and treatments when possible.
- Expresses a basic understanding of the principles in diabetes care and treatment.

Planning and Implementation

- Monitor wound healing, measurements and documentation taken when dressing is changed.
- Maintain glucose levels with insulin adjustments.
- Observe for signs and symptoms of infection.
- Encourage the client to be independent in activities when possible.
- Determine the client's perception of level and strength.
- Refer to physical therapy to help increase activity level and strength.
- Reinforce diabetes teaching and understanding to family and client.

Evaluation Mrs. Lee returns to her skilled nursing center after 5 days of hospitalization. Her vital signs are stable and glucose level has steadily dropped to 150. Wound cultures are negative for infection. Granulation tissue is apparent as evidence of healing progresses. Dressing changes will continue with nursing supervision. The client expresses understanding about mobility and position changes. She has been sitting up three times for meals and extends the time with each sitting. The client and family members understand the diabetic diet calorie restriction and the need to control blood sugars. She states she has a better understanding of diabetes and how it affects healing. She wants to take a more active role in her care and management.

Critical Thinking in the Nursing Process

1. How will you reinforce Mrs. Lee's understanding of diabetes and wound healing?
2. Compare treatment for a Stage III and Stage IV decubitus ulcer.

Note: The bibliography listings for this and all chapters have been compiled at the back of the book.

PROCEDURE 12-1

Wound Dressings

Part A: Moist Transparent Barrier Dressing

Before applying or changing a moist transparent wound barrier, (a) verify the physician's order regarding frequency and type of dressing change, and (b) determine agency protocol about solutions used to clean the wound and whether clean or sterile technique is to be used. Many agencies recommend clean rather than sterile technique for chronic wounds such as a decubitus ulcer.

Assessment Focus Appearance and size of the wound; the amount and character of exudate; complaints of discomfort; signs of systemic infection (e.g., elevated body temperature, diaphoresis, malaise; leukocytosis)

PURPOSES

◆ To provide a moist wound environment and promote wound healing
◆ To protect the wound from trauma and infectious agents
◆ To facilitate assessment of wound healing
◆ To prevent the entrance of microorganisms into the wound
◆ To minimize wound discomfort
◆ To promote autolysis of necrotic material by white blood cells
◆ To decrease the frequency of dressing changes

EQUIPMENT

◆ Disposable gloves
◆ Hair scissors or clippers
◆ Alcohol or acetone
◆ Moistureproof bag
◆ Sterile gloves (optional)
◆ Sterile gauze and the wound-cleaning agents specified by the physician or agency (e.g., sterile saline)
◆ Wound barrier dressing
◆ Scissors
◆ Paper tape
◆ Dressing set
◆ Sterile normal saline or other cleaning agent used by the agency
◆ Hydrocolloid dressing at least 3–4 cm (1.5 in) larger than wound on all four sides

INTERVENTIONS

1. Obtain assistance as needed.
  ◆ If the size of the wound requires it, acquire the assistance of a coworker to help apply the dressing.
2. Thoroughly clean the skin area around the wound.
  ◆ Put on disposable gloves.
  ◆ Clean the skin well with normal saline or a mild cleansing agent. Always rinse the adjacent skin well prior to applying a dressing.
  ◆ Clip the hair about 5 cm (2 in) around the wound area if indicated.
  ◆ If adherence of the dressing is a concern, clean the area adjacent to the wound with alcohol or acetone, and allow it to dry. *Alcohol or acetone defats the skin. Defatted, clean, dry skin ensures better adhesion of the dressing.*
  ◆ Remove gloves, and dispose of them in the moistureproof bag.

3. Clean the wound if indicated.
  ◆ Put on clean disposable or sterile gloves in accordance with agency practice.
  ◆ Clean the wound with the prescribed solution. Either (a) pour the sterile solution directly on the wound and collect drainage with an emesis basin, or (b) use a moist sterile gauze and hold it so that the area that touches the wound remains sterile.
  ◆ Dry the surrounding skin with a dry gauze.
4. Assess the wound.
5. Apply the wound barrier.
  ◆ Remove part of the paper backing on the dressing. If you have an assistant, remove all of the paper backing; the two of you should hold the colored tabs attached to the dressing.
  ◆ Apply the dressing at one edge of the wound site, allowing at least 2.5-cm (1-in) coverage of the skin surrounding the wound.

◆ Gently lay or press the barrier over the wound. Keep it free of wrinkles, but avoid stretching it too tightly. *A stretched dressing restricts mobility.*

◆ Cut off the colored tabs after the wound is completely covered.

◆ Remove and dispose of gloves appropriately.

6. Reinforce the dressing only if absolutely needed.

◆ Apply paper or other porous tape to the edges of the dressing.

7. Assess the wound at least daily.

◆ Determine the extent of serous fluid accumulation under the dressing, wound healing, and the need to repair the dressing.

◆ If excessive serum has accumulated, consider replacing the transparent wound barrier with a more absorbent type of dressing, such as hydrocolloid.

◆ If the dressing is leaking, remove it and apply another dressing.

8. Document the procedure and all nursing assessments.

Part B: Hydrocolloid Dressing

A hydrocolloid dressing should be changed whenever it becomes dislodged, leaks, or develops an odor. If the wound has substantial drainage or yellow slough, the dressing may need to be changed every 24 to 72 hours. When drainage subsides, the dressing may be left in place for 3 to 7 days.

INTERVENTIONS

1. Remove the old dressing.

◆ Put on disposable gloves.

◆ Pull the dressing off gradually in the direction of hair growth. *This minimizes skin irritation.*

◆ Dispose of the soiled dressing in the moistureproof bag.

2. Clean the skin area around the wound.

◆ Gently wash the skin surrounding the wound with a mild cleansing agent or with normal saline and dry it thoroughly with gauze squares.

◆ Leave the residue that is difficult to remove on the skin.

◆ Remove gloves and dispose of them in the moisture-proof bag.

3. Clean the wound if indicated.

◆ Open the sterile dressing supplies.

◆ Pour saline or other cleaning agent into the sterile container.

◆ Put on disposable or sterile gloves in accordance with agency protocol.

◆ Clean the wound with the prescribed solution.

4. Assess the wound.

◆ Observe the appearance and the size of the wound and the amount and character of exudate.

◆ Determine presence of pain.

5. Apply the dressing.

◆ Follow the manufacturer's instructions.

◆ Remove and dispose of the gloves.

◆ Optional: Tape all four sides of the dressing as required or according to agency protocol. *Taping prevents the dressing from sticking to bed linens and keeps the edges from lifting.*

6. Assess and change the dressing as indicated.

◆ Inspect the dressing at least daily for leakage, dislodgement, odor, and wrinkling.

◆ Change the dressing if any of these signs are present.

7. Document the technique and all nursing assessments.

◆ SAMPLE DOCUMENTATION

6/9/04	1300 Stage II superficial reddened wound 2 × 2 to coccyx cleansed with saline, hydrocolloid wafer applied and windowed with tape. Client complained of 3/10 on pain scale, medicated prior to procedure. D. Haus LVN

PROCEDURE 12-2

Obtaining a Specimen of Wound Drainage

PURPOSES

◆ To identify the microorganisms potentially causing an infection and the antibiotics to which they are sensitive
◆ To evaluate the effectiveness of antibiotic therapy

EQUIPMENT

◆ Disposable gloves
◆ Sterile gloves
◆ Moisture-resistant bag
◆ Sterile dressing set
◆ Normal saline and irrigating syringe
◆ Culture tube with swab and culture medium (aerobic and anaerobic tubes are available) and/or sterile syringe with needle for anaerobic culture
◆ Completed labels for each container
◆ Completed requisition to accompany the specimens to the laboratory

INTERVENTIONS

1. Remove any dressings that cover the wound.
   ◆ Put on disposable gloves.
   ◆ Remove the dressing, observe any drainage on it. Hold the dressing so that the client does not see the drainage. *The appearance of the drainage could upset the client.*
   ◆ Determine the amount of the drainage, for example, one 2 × 2 gauze saturated with pale yellow drainage.
   ◆ Discard the dressing in the moisture-resistant bag. Handle it carefully so that the dressing does not touch the outside of the bag. *Touching the outside of the bag will contaminate it.*
   ◆ Remove gloves and dispose of them properly.

2. Open the sterile dressing set using sterile technique.

3. Assess the wound.
   ◆ Put on sterile gloves.
   ◆ Assess the appearance of the tissues in and around the wound and the drainage. *Infection can cause reddened tissues with a thick discharge, which may be foul-smelling, whitish, or colored.*

4. Clean the wound.
   ◆ Irrigate the wound with normal saline until all visible exudate has been washed away. See Procedure 12-3.
   ◆ After irrigating, apply a sterile gauze pad to the wound. *This absorbs excess saline.*
   ◆ If a topical antimicrobial ointment or cream is being used to treat the wound, use a swab to remove it. *Residual antiseptic must be removed prior to culture.*
   ◆ Remove and discard sterile gloves.

5. Obtain the culture.
   ◆ Open a specimen tube and place the cap upside down on a firm, dry surface so that the inside will not become contaminated, or if the swab is attached to the lid, twist the cap to loosen the swab. Hold the tube in one hand, and take out the swab in the other (Figure 12-16 ◆).
   ◆ Rotate the swab back and forth over clean areas of granulation tissue from the sides or base of the wound. *Microorganisms most likely to be responsible for a wound infection reside in viable tissue.*
   ◆ Do not use pus or pooled exudate to culture. *These secretions contain a mixture of contaminants that are not the same as those causing the infection.*
   ◆ Avoid touching the swab to intact skin at the wound edges. *This prevents the introduction of superficial skin organisms into the culture.*

Figure 12-16. ◆ A culturette tube for a wound specimen. *Source:* © Elena Dorfman.

◆ Return the swab to the culture tube, taking care not to touch the top or the outside of the tube.

◆ Crush the inner ampule containing the medium for organism growth at the bottom of the tube. *This ensures that the swab with the specimen is surrounded by culture medium.*

◆ Twist the cap to secure it.

◆ If a specimen is required from another site, repeat the preceding steps. Specify the exact site (e.g., inferior drain site or lower aspect of incision) on the label of each container. Be sure to put each swab in the appropriately labeled tube. *This ensures that tests can be carried out as intended.*

6. Dress the wound.

◆ Apply any ordered medication to the wound.

◆ Cover the wound with a sterile moist transparent wound dressing. See Procedure 12-1A.

7. Arrange for the specimen to be transported to the laboratory immediately. Be sure to include the completed requisition. *This prevents specimen from being lost or mislabeled.*

8. Document all relevant information.

◆ Record on the client's chart the taking of the specimen and source.

◆ Include the date and time; the examination requested; the appearance of the wound; the color, consistency, amount, and odor of any drainage; and any discomfort experienced by the client. *Complete documentation supports continuity of care.*

VARIATION: OBTAINING A SPECIMEN FOR ANAEROBIC CULTURE, USING A STERILE SYRINGE AND NEEDLE

◆ Insert a sterile 10-mL syringe (without needle) into the wound, and aspirate 1 to 5 mL of drainage into the syringe.

◆ Attach the 21-gauge needle to the syringe, and expel all air from the syringe and needle.

◆ Immediately inject the drainage into the anaerobic culture tube.

or

If a rubber stopper or cork is available, insert the needle into the rubber stopper or cork to prevent the entry of air.

◆ Label the tube or syringe appropriately.

◆ Send the syringe of drainage to the laboratory immediately. *This ensures that the specimen will be fresh when it reaches the laboratory.*

◆ **SAMPLE DOCUMENTATION**

7/30/05	1200 Anaerobic Culture of Lt. hip wound obtained and sent to the lab.
	Ⓓ Haus LVN

PROCEDURE 12-3

Irrigating a Wound

Before irrigating a wound, determine (a) the type of irrigating solution to be used, (b) the frequency of irrigations, and (c) the temperature of the solution.

PURPOSES

◆ To clean the area

◆ To apply heat and hasten the healing process

◆ To apply an antimicrobial solution

EQUIPMENT

◆ Sterile dressing equipment and dressing materials

◆ Sterile irrigating syringes (e.g., a 30- to 50-mL piston syringe) with a catheter of an appropriate size (e.g. #18 or #19) attached or a 250-mL squeezable bottle with irrigating tip

◆ Sterile basin for the irrigating solution

◆ Moistureproof bag

◆ Sterile basin to receive the irrigation returns

◆ Irrigating solution, usually 200 mL (6.5 oz) of solution warmed to body temperature, according to the agency's or physician's choice

◆ Clean disposable gloves

◆ Sterile gloves

◆ Moistureproof sterile drape

◆ Sterile straight catheter or irrigating tip, if needed

INTERVENTIONS

1. Verify the physician's order.
   - Confirm the type and strength of the solution.
2. Prepare the client.
   - Assist the client to a position in which the irrigating solution will flow by gravity from the upper end of the wound to the lower end and then into the basin.
   - Place the waterproof drape over the client and the bed.
   - Put on disposable gloves and remove and discard the old dressing.
   - Clean from the center of the wound outward, using circular strokes.
   - Use a separate swab for each stroke, and discard each swab after use. *This prevents the introduction of microorganisms to other wound areas.*
   - Assess the wound and drainage.
   - Remove and discard disposable gloves.
3. Prepare the equipment.
   - Open the sterile dressing set and supplies.
   - Pour the ordered solution into the solution container.
   - Put on sterile gloves.
   - Position the sterile basin below the wound to receive the irrigating fluid.
4. Irrigate the wound.
   - Instill a steady stream of irrigating solution into the wound. Make sure all areas of the wound are irrigated.
   - Use either a syringe with a catheter attached or a 250-mL squeezable bottle with irrigating tip to flush the wound. *Effective irrigation requires 4 to 15 pounds per square inch of pressure. These devices provide this pressure; bulb syringes do not.*
   - If you are using a catheter, insert the catheter into the wound until resistance is met. Do not force the catheter. *Forcing the catheter can cause tissue damage.*

- Continue irrigating until the solution becomes clear (no exudate is present). *The irrigation washes away tissue debris and drainage so that later returns are clearer.*
- Dry the area around the wound. *Moisture left on the skin promotes the growth of microorganisms and can cause skin irritation and breakdown.*

5. Assess and dress the wound.
   - Assess the appearance of the wound, noting in particular the type and amount of exudate and the presence and extent of granulation tissue.
   - Pack the wound if ordered.
   - Apply a sterile dressing to the wound as described in Procedure 12-1.
6. Document all relevant information.
   - Document the irrigation, the solution used, the appearance of the irrigation returns, and nursing assessments. Note the presence of any exudate and sloughing tissue.

◆ SAMPLE DOCUMENTATION

1/3/05	lt. hip wound, Stage IV measured 2 X
1600	4, 1 inch in depth. Drainage consists of
	yellow purulent material, no necrosis
	noted. Wound irrigated with saline
	solution and packed with ½-inch gauze,
	covered with gauze dressing. No sinus
	tract detected. Client complained of
	minimal pain, 4/10 on pain scale. Client
	medicated prior to procedure. ——
	D. Haus LVN

Chapter Review

Key Terms by Topics

Use the audio glossary feature of either the CD-ROM or the Companion Website to hear the correct pronunciation of the following key terms.

Wound healing
hemostasis, phagocytosis, granulation tissue, eschar, serosanguineous, keloid, exudate, suppuration, sanguineous, dehiscence, evisceration

Nursing Care
fistula, sitz bath

Pressure ulcers
pressure ulcer, ischemia, reactive hyperemia, friction, shearing force, maceration, debridement

Key Points

- Skin integrity is the body's first line of defense.
- The wound-healing process has three phases: inflammatory, proliferative, and maturation.
- Major types of wound exudate are serous, purulent, and sanguineous (hemorrhagic). The main complications of wound healing are hemorrhage, infection, dehiscence, and evisceration.
- A pressure ulcer is caused by unrelieved pressure resulting in damage to underlying tissues. Friction and shearing forces can also produce a pressure ulcer. Frequent change of position and care when moving a client can help prevent pressure ulcers.
- The nurse describes a pressure ulcer in terms of location, size, depth, stage, color, status of wound margins and surrounding skin, and specific signs of infection.
- Wound assessment continually requires visual inspection, palpation, and the sense of smell. Essential data for wounds include wound appearance, size, drainage, swelling, pain, and the presence of tubes and drains.
- Nurses are usually responsible for obtaining specimens of wound drainage for culture. Laboratory data support wound assessment.
- Nurses must wash hands before and after providing wound care to prevent infection and transmission of bloodborne pathogens.
- Major nursing responsibilities related to wound care include preventing infection, preventing further tissue damage, preventing hemorrhage, promoting healing, and preventing skin excoriation around draining wounds.
- Wound care may involve cleaning wounds, changing dressings, maintaining drains, irrigating, inserting packing, applying heat and cold, and applying bandages and binders.
- In the RYB color code, the nurse protects red, cleanses yellow, and debrides black (with permission from physician or RN).
- Nurses must use extra precautions when applying heat or cold to clients with neurosensory or circulatory impairment.

EXPLORE MediaLink

Additional interactive resources for this chapter can be found on the Companion Website at www.prenhall.com/ramont. Click on Chapter 12 and "Begin" to select the activities for this chapter.

For chapter-related NCLEX-style questions and an audio glossary, access the accompanying CD-ROM in this book.

Animation:
- cell structure flythrough
- pressure ulcers
- integumentary repair
- penicillin

∞ For Further Study

For more information about infection control, see Chapter 7.

For further information about the body's normal responses to heat and cold, see Chapter 14.

Critical Thinking Care Map

Caring for a Debilitated Client

NCLEX-PN Focus Area: Physiological Integrity

Case Study: Mr. Johns is an 84-year-old client being treated for a urinary tract disorder. Mr. Johns suffered a cerebrovascular accident (stroke) 6 months ago and has difficulty ambulating and attending to his own needs because of right-sided weakness. While assessing Mr. Johns you note that he is thin for his 6-foot frame, weighing 135 lbs, is incontinent of foul-smelling urine, and has deeply reddened areas on his right hip, coccyx, and entire peritoneal area. He is alert and oriented to person, place, and time, but he has decreased sensation on his entire right side. He spends most of his time in bed or sitting at his bedside chair due to his difficulty with ambulation.

Nursing Diagnosis: Risk for Impaired Skin Integrity

COLLECT DATA

Subjective

_____
_____
_____
_____
_____
_____

Objective

_____
_____
_____
_____
_____
_____

Would you report this data? Yes/No

If yes, to: _____

Nursing Care

_____
_____
_____
_____
_____
_____
_____
_____
_____
_____

How would you document this? _____
_____
_____
_____
_____

Data Collected
(use those that apply)

- Difficulty ambulating
- Height 6′
- Weight 135 lbs
- Client states, "I'm not hungry most of the time"
- Weakened
- BP 150/88
- Incontinent of urine
- Deeply reddened coccyx, right hip, and peritoneal area
- Alert and oriented
- Decreased sensation to his entire right side
- Right-sided weakness
- Negative for fecal blood
- TSH 5μIU/mL

Nursing Interventions
(Use all that apply)

- Monitor urine output.
- Turn client q2h.
- Steadily increase ambulation.
- Monitor reddened area.
- Offer urinal frequently.
- Refer to dietitian.
- Daily weights.
- Vital signs q2h.

NCLEX-PN Exam Preparation

TEST-TAKING TIP

Utilize the process of elimination. Eliminate the incorrect options before selecting an answer.

1. In some clients, pressure can cause the beginning of a decubitus ulcer within a matter of hours. When you observe the first sign of pressure, you should immediately do which of the following?
   a. Make sure the skin is warm and dry.
   b. Reposition and turn the client at least q2h.
   c. Put on an airflow mattress.
   d. Apply protective pads and adhesive dressings.

2. The purpose of a wet to damp dressing is:
   a. Cooling
   b. Antipruritic
   c. Nevus
   d. Debridement

3. When intact skin surface has been injured or broken the client has lost some ability to:
   a. Resist infection
   b. Take in Vitamin D
   c. Eliminate waste products
   d. Lubricate the skin

4. A client has a decubitus ulcer exposing the bone in the hip. The nurse identifies this type of ulcer as a:
   a. Stage I
   b. Stage II
   c. Stage III
   d. Stage IV

5. A danger seen in closed wet dressings is:
   a. Maceration
   b. Frequent dressing changes
   c. Debridement
   d. Ischemia

6. In the second phase of healing, a wound will show evidence of a red tissue that is fragile and bleeds easily. It is called:
   a. Granulation tissue
   b. Phagocytosis
   c. Necrosis
   d. Exudates

7. There are many factors involved in the development of pressure ulcers. A combination of friction and pressure occurs when a client slides down in bed but the skin does not move. This is known as:
   a. Evisceration
   b. Hematoma
   c. Reactive hyperemia
   d. Shearing force

8. A surgical wound infection can be reduced by:
   a. Leaving incisions open to air
   b. Changing dressings using surgical technique
   c. Adhering to the principles of handwashing
   d. Cleansing incisions from the least contaminated to the most contaminated area

9. Diabetes is a predisposing condition for decubitus ulcer formation. Which factor may be involved?
   a. Peripheral vascular disease
   b. Kidney disease
   c. Immune disorder
   d. Hepatic disease

10. A disadvantage of using alcohol as a cooling measure is:
    a. It blisters the skin.
    b. It dries the skin.
    c. Maceration
    d. Suppuration

Answers for Review Questions, as well as discussion of Case Study and Critical Thinking Care Map questions, appear in Appendix IV.

Chapter 13

Hygiene

SHARING experiences

"Find the place in nursing where you are happy and do that job to the best of your ability. The LPN/LVN role is very broad nowadays. You can find an area that you like and excel in that area. Being an LPN/LVN is very rewarding. Where else do you find a family member say- ing thank you for being so nice to my Mom or Dad? It is the little things in the profession that make it all worth while. I love this profession because you can be happy about making a person's day go better. There is room in this profession for each and every one of us."

Jane Pond, LPN, President LPN Association of Indiana; Practicing LPN, Lewis Memorial Christian Home, Springfield, IL.

LEARNING outcomes

After completing this chapter, you will be able to:
- Describe the kinds of hygienic care the LPN/LVN provides to clients.
- Identify factors influencing personal hygiene.
- Identify normal and abnormal findings obtained during inspection and palpation of the skin, feet, nails, mouth, hair, eyes, ears, and nose.
- Describe nursing interventions for the skin, feet, nails, mouth, hair, eyes, ears, and nose.
- Explain specific ways in which the LPN/LVN assists clients with self-care deficits in maintaining personal hygiene.
- Describe methods of making an unoccupied and an occupied bed.
- Identify safety and comfort measures that are part of bed-making procedures.

MediaLink

www.prenhall.com/ramont

Use the address above to access the free, interactive Companion Website created for this textbook. Get hints, instant feedback, and textbook references to chapter-related NCLEX-style questions. Link to other interesting sites.

Audio Glossary:
Use the Companion Website, or the CD-ROM disk enclosed with your textbook, to hear the pronunciation of key terms in the chapter.

Hygiene is the science of health and its maintenance. Personal hygiene is the self-care by which people attend to such functions as bathing, toileting, general body hygiene, and grooming. Hygiene is a highly personal matter determined by individual values and practices. Culture plays a role in how often a person bathes and how much privacy a person needs when bathing. Economics also plays a role, since access to warm water, soap, shampoo, and other hygiene items may be limited.

Hygiene involves care of the skin (including perineal and genital areas), hair, nails, teeth, oral and nasal cavities, eyes, and ears. Nursing assistance with hygiene also includes bedmaking and changing clients' clothes.

It is important for the LPN/LVN to know exactly how much assistance a client needs for hygienic care. Clients may require help after urinating or defecating, after vomiting, and whenever they become soiled, such as from wound drainage or profuse perspiration. Box 13-1 ◆ lists factors that influence hygiene practices.

The following terms are commonly used to describe types of hygienic care. **Early morning care** is provided to clients as they awaken in the morning. This care consists of

providing a urinal or bedpan to the client confined to bed, washing the face and hands, and giving oral care. **Morning care** is provided after clients have breakfast. It usually includes the provision of a urinal or bedpan (to clients who are not ambulatory), a bath or shower, perineal care, back massages, and oral, nail, and hair care. It also includes making the client's bed. **Afternoon care** often includes providing a bedpan or urinal, washing the hands and face, and assisting with oral care to refresh clients' mouths. **Hour of sleep (HS) care** is provided to clients before they retire for the night. It usually involves providing for elimination needs, washing face and hands, giving oral care, and giving a back massage. **As-needed (prn) care** is provided as required by the client. For example, a client who is *diaphoretic* (sweating profusely) may need frequent bathing and changes of clothes and linen.

◆ Skin, Foot, and Nail Care

The skin is the largest organ of the body. As described in Chapter 12, the skin protects underlying tissues from injury. ᏀᎧ It regulates body temperature. (See Chapter 14 for a detailed discussion of body heat losses and gains ᏀᎧ .) Skin secretes an oily substance called **sebum** that softens and lubricates the hair and skin. (Sebum decreases water loss from the skin when the external humidity is low. Because fat is a poor conductor of heat, sebum lessens the amount of heat lost from the skin. Sebum also has a *bactericidal* [bacteria-killing] action). Skin transmits sensations through nerve receptors, which are sensitive to pain, temperature, touch, and pressure. It also produces and absorbs vitamin D in conjunction with ultraviolet rays from the sun. The normal skin of a healthy person has transient and resident microorganisms that are not usually harmful (see Table 7-1). ᏀᎧ

TYPES OF BATHS

Two categories of baths are given to clients: cleaning and therapeutic. **Cleaning baths** are given chiefly for hygiene purposes and include these types:

- *Complete bed bath.* The LPN/LVN washes the entire body of a dependent client in bed.
- *Self-help bed bath.* Clients confined to bed are able to bathe themselves with assistance for the back and perhaps the feet.
- *Partial bath.* Only the parts of the client's body that might cause discomfort or odor, if neglected, are washed: the face, hands, axillae, perineal area, and back. The arms, chest, abdomen, legs, and feet are omitted. The LPN/LVN provides this care for dependent clients and assists self-sufficient clients confined to bed by washing their backs. Some ambulatory clients prefer to take a partial bath at the sink. The client can be assisted with washing the back.
- *Bag bath.* The equipment needed consists of: a plastic bag, 10 to 12 washcloths, and a nonrinsable cleaner and water mixture. The solution and washcloths are warmed in a microwave. The warming time is about 1 minute, but the

BOX 13-1 ▶

POPULATION FOCUS

INFLUENCES ON INDIVIDUAL HYGIENIC PRACTICES

Culture: North American culture places a high value on cleanliness. Many North Americans bathe or shower once or twice a day, whereas people from some other cultures bathe once a week. Some cultures consider privacy essential for bathing, whereas others practice communal bathing. Body odor is offensive in some cultures and accepted as normal in others.

Religion: Ceremonial washings are practiced by some religions.

Environment: Finances may affect the availability of facilities for bathing. For example, homeless people may not have warm water available; soap, shampoo, shaving lotion, and deodorants may be too expensive for people who have limited resources.

Developmental level: Children learn hygiene in the home. Practices vary according to the individual's age; for example, preschoolers can carry out most tasks independently with encouragement.

Health and energy: Ill people may not have the motivation or energy to attend to hygiene. Some clients who have neuromuscular impairments may be unable to perform hygienic care.

Personal preferences: Some people prefer a shower or a tub bath.

LPN/LVN needs to determine how long it takes to attain a desirable temperature. Each area of the body is cleaned with a different cloth and then air dried. Because the body is not rubbed dry, the emollient in the solution remains on the skin. Some agencies may provide commercially prepared, disposable bag baths. Each pack usually contains enough wipes to bathe the entire body. These are warmed in the microwave according to directions on the packaging.

◆ *Tub bath.* Tub baths are preferred to bed baths because it is easier to wash and rinse in a tub. Tubs are also used for therapeutic baths. The amount of assistance offered depends on the abilities of the client. There are specially designed tubs for dependent clients. These tubs greatly reduce the work and potential for injury in lifting clients in and out of the tub and offer greater benefits than a sponge bath in bed.

◆ *Shower.* Many ambulatory clients are able to use shower facilities and require only minimal assistance.

Therapeutic baths are given for physical effects, such as to soothe irritated skin or to treat an area (e.g., the perineum). Medications may be placed in the water. A therapeutic bath is generally taken in a tub one-third or one-half full, about 114 L (30 gal). The client remains in the bath for a designated time, often 20 to 30 minutes. If the client's back, chest, and arms are to be treated, these areas need to be immersed in the solution. The bath temperature is generally included in the order; 37.7 to 46°C (100 to 115°F) may be ordered for adults and 40.5°C (105°F) is usually ordered for infants. Procedure 13-1 provides guidelines for bathing clients.

Purposes of Baths

Bathing removes accumulated oil, perspiration, dead skin cells, and some bacteria. The LPN/LVN will understand the quantity of oil and dead skin cells produced upon observing the removal of a cast that has been on someone for 6 weeks. The skin underneath the cast is crusty, flaky, and dry. Applications of oil over several days are usually necessary to remove the debris.

Excessive bathing, however, can interfere with the intended lubricating effect of the sebum, causing dryness of the skin. This is an important consideration, especially for older adults, who produce less sebum.

In addition to cleaning the skin, bathing stimulates circulation. A warm or hot bath dilates superficial arterioles, bringing more blood and nourishment to the skin. Vigorous rubbing has the same effect. Rubbing with long, smooth strokes from the distal to proximal parts of extremities (from the point farthest from the body to the point closest) is particularly effective in facilitating venous blood flow.

Bathing also produces a sense of well-being. It is refreshing and relaxing and frequently improves morale, appearance, and self-respect. Some people take a morning shower for its refreshing, stimulating effect. Others prefer an evening bath because it is relaxing. These effects are more evident when a person is ill. For example, it is not uncommon for clients who have had a restless or sleepless night to feel relaxed, comfortable, and sleepy after a morning bath.

Bathing offers an excellent opportunity for the LPN/LVN to assess ill clients. During the bath it is easy to observe the condition of the client's skin and physical conditions such as sacral edema or rashes. While assisting a client with a bath, the LPN/LVN can also assess the client's psychosocial needs, such as orientation to time and ability to cope with the illness. Learning needs, such as a diabetic client's need to learn foot care, can also be assessed.

FEET

The feet are essential for ambulation. They need attention even when people are confined to bed. Children's feet are easily damaged by tight, binding stockings and ill-fitting shoes. They should be well supported, and the bony structure and the feet should grow without restrictions. Feet are not fully grown until about age 20. Healthy feet remain relatively unchanged during life. However, the elderly often require special attention for their feet. Reduced blood supply and accompanying arteriosclerosis can make a foot prone to infection following trauma. Common foot problems include calluses, corns, unpleasant odors, plantar warts, fissures between the toes, and fungal infections such as athlete's foot.

NAILS

Nails are normally present at birth. They continue to grow throughout life and change very little until people are elderly. At that time, the nails tend to be tougher, more brittle, and in some cases thicker. The nails of an older person normally grow less quickly than those of a younger person and may be ridged and grooved.

NURSING CARE

 ASSESSING

The LPN/LVN checks the nursing history for the client's skin care practices, self-care abilities, and past or current skin problems. Data about the client's skin care practices enable the LPN/LVN to incorporate the client's needs and preferences as much as possible in the plan of care and to determine necessary learning needs. Clients may have difficulty performing bathing activities. They may not be able to wash the body or body parts, to obtain or get to a water source, or to regulate water temperature or flow. Clients may also have difficulties in dressing and grooming. They may not be able to obtain, put on, take off, fasten, or replace articles of clothing; and to maintain appearance at a satisfactory level. They may have difficulties with toileting, such as getting to the toilet or commode, or sitting on and rising from it. Also, clients may have trouble manipulating their clothes for toileting, cleaning themselves after using the toilet, flushing the toilet, or emptying the *commode* (portable toilet, often used at the bedside by people who have limited mobility).

The client's self-care abilities determine the amount of nursing assistance and the kind of bath (bed, tub, or shower) the client requires. The client's balance, coordination, and strength are important factors. The confused or very ill client will lack the motivation and energy to provide self-care. It is important to determine the client's functional level, so the nurse can maintain and promote as much client independence as possible. This also enables the LPN/LVN to identify the client's potential for growth and rehabilitation.

A physical assessment of the skin is performed, and clients who are at risk for developing skin impairment are identified (Box 13-2 ◆). The presence of past or current skin problems alerts the LPN/LVN to specific nursing interventions or referrals the client may require. Common skin problems and implications for nursing interventions are shown in Table 13-1 ◆. Refer to Chapter 12 for types and descriptions

---

BOX 13-2 RISK FACTORS FOR SELF-CARE DEFICIT

Visual impairment
Activity intolerance or weakness
Pain or discomfort
Mental impairment
Neuromuscular or skeletal impairment
Psychologic or motivation impairment
Medically prescribed restriction
Therapeutic procedure restraining mobility (e.g., intravenous infusion, cast)
Environmental barriers

---

of skin lesions. ⊂⊃ Nursing implications for common skin problems are discussed below.

Physical assessment of the skin, feet and nails, which involves inspection and palpation, is discussed in Chapter 11 (see Table 11-3 and Figures 11-4 and 11-13) and is described further in Chapter 12. ⊂⊃ A systematic head-to-toe assess-

---

TABLE 13-1 COMMON SKIN PROBLEMS AND NURSING IMPLICATIONS

PROBLEM AND APPEARANCE	NURSING IMPLICATIONS
Abrasion Superficial layers of the skin are scraped or rubbed away. Area is reddened and may have localized bleeding or serous weeping.	1. Prone to infection; therefore, wound should be kept clean and dry. 2. Do not wear rings or jewelry when providing care to avoid causing abrasions to clients. 3. Lift, do not pull, a client across a bed. See Chapter 20. ⊂⊃
Excessive Dryness Skin can appear flaky and rough.	1. Prone to infection if the skin cracks; therefore, provide alcohol-free lotions to moisturize the skin and prevent cracking. 2. Bathe client less frequently; use no soap, or limit use of nonirritating soap. Rinse skin thoroughly because soap can be irritating and drying. 3. Encourage increased fluid intake if health permits to prevent dehydration.
Ammonia Dermatitis (Diaper Rash) Caused by skin bacteria reacting with urea in the urine. The skin becomes reddened and is sore.	1. Keep skin dry and clean by applying protective ointments containing zinc oxide to areas at risk (e.g., buttocks and perineum). 2. Boil an infant's diapers or wash them with an antibacterial detergent to prevent infection. Rinse diapers well because detergent is irritating to an infant's skin.
Acne Inflammatory condition with papules and pustules.	1. Keep the skin clean to prevent secondary infection. 2. Treatment varies widely.
Erythema Redness associated with a variety of conditions, such as rashes, exposure to sun, elevated body temperature.	1. Wash area carefully to remove excess microorganisms. 2. Apply antiseptic spray or lotion to prevent itching, promote healing, and prevent skin breakdown.
Hirsutism Excessive hair on a person's body and face, particularly in women.	1. Remove unwanted hair by using depilatories, shaving, electrolysis, or tweezing. 2. Enhance client's self-concept. See Chapter 27. ⊂⊃

ment includes collection of data about skin color, uniformity of color, texture, turgor, temperature, intactness, and lesions.

Attention is paid to risk factors for foot problems (such as diabetes) and foot discomfort. The feet are assessed at the beginning and end of each shift, unless otherwise ordered. Changes are reported to the RN.

DIAGNOSING, PLANNING, and IMPLEMENTING

For clients who have problems performing hygiene care, "Self-Care Deficit" diagnoses are used in collaboration with the LPN/LVN. Three Self-Care Deficit diagnoses are discussed in this chapter:

Self-Care Deficit: Bathing/Hygiene
Self-Care Deficit: Dressing/Grooming
Self-Care Deficit: Toileting

Associated diagnoses commonly include Deficient Knowledge (e.g., related to lack of experience with skin condition and treatment) and Situational Low Self-Esteem (e.g., related to body odor). The diagnoses "Risk for Impaired Skin Integrity" and "Impaired Skin Integrity" are discussed in Chapter 12. ⟷

In planning care, the LPN/LVN identifies nursing interventions that will assist the client to maintain or improve skin cleanliness, maintain circulation to the skin, and improve or maintain a sense of well-being. Nursing activities for hygiene include assisting dependent clients with bathing, skin and nail care, and perineal care, providing back massages to promote circulation (discussed in Chapter 20), and providing instruction to clients about ways to promote good hygiene and prevent skin lesions. ⟷

When planning to assist a client with personal hygiene, the nurse considers the client's personal preferences, health, and limitations; the best time to give the care; and the equipment, facilities, and personnel available. A client's personal preferences about when and how to bathe should be followed as long as they are compatible with the client's health and the equipment available. The LPN/LVN provides whatever assistance the client requires, either directly or by delegating this task to other personnel.

Examples of desired outcomes for clients with self-care deficits might be:

◆ Client bathes in tub twice weekly with assistance.
◆ Client participates in self-care (foot-hygiene) to optimal level of capacity (specify).
◆ Client reports satisfaction with appearance.
◆ Client demonstrates nail care as instructed.

Nursing guidelines for providing skin care to clients are listed in Box 13-3 ◆.

Bathing

Sponge baths are suggested for the newborn to prevent hypothermia. An infant's ability to regulate body temperature

---

has not yet fully developed. Body surface area is very large in relation to body mass, contributing to heat loss. Infants perspire minimally, and shivering starts at a lower temperature. Therefore, significant heat loss occurs before shivering begins. After the bath, the infant should be immediately dried and wrapped (swaddled) for warmth.

Caution is needed when bathing clients who are receiving intravenous therapy. Easy-to-remove gowns that have Velcro or snap fasteners along the sleeves may be used. If a special gown is not available, the LPN/LVN must pay special attention when changing the client's gown after the bath (or whenever the gown becomes soiled). These guidelines are provided in Box 13-4 ◆. These guidelines do not apply if the client has an IV pump or controller. In this situation, use a special gown or do not put the sleeve of a gown over the client's involved arm.

The water for a bath should feel comfortably warm to the client. People vary in their sensitivity to heat; generally, the temperature should be 43 to 46°C (110 to 115°F). Most clients can verify a comfortable temperature. The water for a bed bath should be changed at least once.

Perineal–Genital Care.
Perineal–genital care is also referred to as perineal care or peri-care. Perineal care as part of the bed bath is embarrassing for many clients. LPN/LVNs also may find it embarrassing initially, particularly with clients of the opposite sex. Most clients who require a bed bath are able to clean their own genital areas with minimal assistance. The LPN/LVN may need to hand a moistened washcloth and soap to the client, rinse the washcloth, and provide a towel.

Because some clients are unfamiliar with terminology for the genitals and perineum, it may be difficult to explain what is expected. Most clients, however, understand what is meant if the LPN/LVN simply says, "I'll give you a washcloth to finish your bath." Older clients may be familiar with the term *private parts*. Whatever expression is used, it needs to be one that the client understands and one that is comfortable for the LPN/LVN to use.

The LPN/LVN needs to provide perineal care efficiently and matter-of-factly. Nurses wear gloves while providing this care, both for the comfort of the client and to protect themselves from infection. Procedure 13-1B explains how to provide perineal–genital care.

Foot.
Interventions may include teaching the client about correct nail and foot care, proper footwear, and ways to prevent potential foot problems (e.g., infection, injury, and decreased circulation). For clients with self-care difficulties, the LPN/LVN plans a schedule for soaking the client's feet and assisting with regular cleaning and trimming of nails (if not contraindicated and within agency policy). Foot and nail care is often provided during the client's bath but may be provided at any time in the day to accommodate the client's preference or schedule. The frequency of foot care is determined by the LPN/LVN and client. It is based on objective assessment data and the client's specific problems. For some clients, the feet need to be bathed daily; for those whose feet perspire excessively, bathing more than once a day may be necessary.

Procedure 13-1C describes how to provide foot care. (See also discussion of nails.) During these procedures, the LPN/LVN has the opportunity to teach the client appropriate methods for foot care (see Discharge Considerations on page 258). Clients with reduced peripheral circulation to the feet, such as clients with diabetes or peripheral vascular disease, may require specialized care by a physician or podiatrist. These clients should be discouraged from attempting some aspects of personal foot care and cautioned about "commercial" pedicures, such as at salons or spas.

Nails.
One hand or foot is soaked, if needed, and dried. Then the nail is cut or filed straight across beyond the end of the finger or toe (Figure 13-1 ◆). Avoid trimming or digging into nails at the lateral corners. (This predisposes the client to ingrown toenails.) File rather than cut the nails of clients who have diabetes or circulatory problems. Inadvertent injury to tissues can occur if scissors are used. After the initial cut or filing, file the nail to round the corners, and clean under the nail. Push the cuticle back gently, taking care not to injure it. Care for the next finger or toe in the same manner. Record and report any abnormality, such as inflammation of the tissue around the nail, to the RN.

BOX 13-4
NURSING CARE CHECKLIST

CHANGING A HOSPITAL GOWN FOR A CLIENT WITH AN IV INFUSION

☑ Slip the gown completely off the arm without the infusion and onto the tubing connected to the arm with the infusion.

☑ Holding the container above the client's arm, slide the sleeve up over the container to remove the used gown.

☑ Place the clean gown sleeve for the arm with the infusion over the container as if it were an extension of the client's arm, from the inside of the gown to the sleeve cuff.

☑ Rehang the container. Slide the gown carefully over the tubing toward the client's hand.

☑ Guide the client's arm and tubing into the sleeve, taking care not to pull on the tubing.

☑ Assist the client to put the other arm into the second sleeve of the gown, and fasten as usual.

☑ Count the rate of flow of the infusion to make sure it is correct before leaving the bedside. Immediately report an incorrect rate of flow to RN.

Figure 13-1. ◆ Fingernails are trimmed straight across.

EVALUATING

Using data collected during care, the LPN/LVN judges whether desired outcomes have been achieved, and documents changes in self-care. The nurse determines whether the client maintains skin cleanliness, reports satisfaction with appearance, states that feet are not as sore, and so on.

If the outcomes are not achieved, the LPN/LVN explores reasons why. For example:

◆ Did the LPN/LVN overestimate the client's functional abilities (physical, mental, emotional) for self-care?
◆ Were instructions not clear?
◆ Were appropriate assistive devices or supplies not available to the client?
◆ Did the client's condition change?
◆ Were required analgesics provided before hygienic care?
◆ What currently prescribed medications and therapies could affect the client's abilities or tissue integrity?
◆ Is the client's fluid and food intake adequate or appropriate to maintain skin and mucous membrane moisture and integrity?

 DISCHARGE CONSIDERATIONS

To provide for continuity of care when a client is to be discharged, the nurse assesses the client's and family's abilities for care. Referrals and home health services may be required. Also, the nurse determines the client's learning needs and provides written or verbal instructions as needed. Use the guidelines listed in Box 13-3 to provide client teaching on general skin care. Clients with impaired circulation or diabetes are especially in need of teaching about foot care (Box 13-5 ◆).

Nursing Process Case Study: CLIENT WITH DIABETES

Gerard Bucholz is a 52-year-old divorced man who was admitted to the hospital with a nonhealing cut on his left great toe. The cut occurred when Mr. Bucholz trimmed his toenails a month ago. He is an insulin-dependent diabetic and was diagnosed 6 years ago. It has taken him most of the 6 years to begin managing his diabetes well and to comply with his prescribed diet. Although his blood sugars have been in good control over the last 1½ years, the high blood sugar in the past has resulted in poor peripheral circulation. His lower extremities are mainly affected, but he does complain of decreased sensation in his fingertips. Mr. Bucholz states, "Nobody ever told me I shouldn't cut my nails."

Assessment T 98.6°F, apical pulse 72, R 18, BP 130/72. Pedal pulses weak, bilaterally, radial pulses palpable. Feet cold to touch, client denies feeling in toes when touched. Hands cool, client states he has feeling in the tips of fingers when

BOX 13-5

TEACHING FOR DISCHARGE

FOOT CARE
◆ Wash the feet daily, and dry them well, especially between the toes.
◆ When washing, inspect the skin of the feet for breaks or red or swollen areas. Use a mirror if needed to visualize all areas.
◆ To prevent burns, check the water temperature before immersing the feet.
◆ Use creams or lotions to moisten the skin, or soak the feet in warm water with Epsom salts to avoid excessive drying of the skin of the feet. Lotion will also soften calluses. A lotion that reduces dryness effectively is a mixture of lanolin and mineral oil.
◆ To prevent or control an unpleasant odor due to excessive foot perspiration, wash the feet frequently and change socks and shoes at least daily. Special deodorant sprays or absorbent foot powders are also helpful.
◆ File the toenails rather than cutting them to avoid skin injury. File the nails straight across the ends of the toes. If the nails are too thick or misshapen to file, consult a podiatrist.
◆ Wear clean stockings or socks daily. Avoid socks with holes or darns that can cause pressure areas.
◆ Wear correctly fitting shoes that neither restrict the foot nor rub on any area; rubbing can cause corns and calluses. Check worn shoes for rough spots in the lining. Break in new shoes gradually by increasing the wearing time 30 to 60 minutes each day.
◆ Avoid walking barefoot, because injury and infection may result. Wear slippers in public showers and in change areas to avoid contracting athlete's foot or other infections.
◆ Several times each day exercise the feet to promote circulation. Point the feet upward, point them downward, and move them in circles.
◆ Avoid wearing constricting garments such as knee-high elastic stockings and avoid sitting with the legs crossed at the knees, which may decrease circulation.
◆ When the feet are cold, use extra blankets and wear warm socks rather than using heating pads or hot water bottles, which may cause burns. Test bathwater before stepping into it.
◆ Wash any cut on the foot thoroughly, apply a mild antiseptic, and notify the physician.
◆ Avoid self-treatment for corns or calluses. Pumice stones and some callus and corn applications are injurious to the skin. Consult a podiatrist or physician first.
◆ Notify the physician if you notice abnormal sores or drainage, pain, or changes in temperature, color, and sensation of the foot.

touched. Ulcerated area on left great toe, approximately 2 cm × 2 cm. Skin around and inside ulcer is black, client denies pain. The bone is visible.

Diagnosis The following nursing diagnoses have been established for Mr. Bucholz:

♦ Impaired Skin Integrity related to nonhealing skin injury
♦ Deficient Knowledge (diabetic nail care) related to possible lack of exposure to information

Expected Outcome The expected outcomes for the plan of care are that Mr. Bucholz will:

♦ Demonstrate proper nail care.
♦ Have no further injuries to the extremities as a result of improper nail care.

Planning and Implementation The following nursing interventions are implemented for Mr. Bucholz:

♦ Discuss with client the relationship between diabetes and decreased peripheral circulation.
♦ Discuss with client other activities that may cause impaired skin integrity (e.g., possible burn related to use of a heating pad on areas with impaired circulation, going without proper footwear outside).
♦ Demonstrate proper nail care techniques to client.
♦ Supply client with handouts explaining proper nail care techniques and encourage him to keep them in an accessible area at home.

Evaluation Mr. Bucholz is able to repeat information given him regarding proper nail care. He has made a monthly appointment with a podiatrist near his home.

Critical Thinking in the Nursing Process

1. What might have helped Mr. Bucholz to avoid cutting himself in the first place?
2. Why is it important to note in the evaluation that Mr. Bucholz has contacted a podiatrist and has a standing appointment?

Hair Care

The appearance of the hair often reflects a person's feelings or general state of health. A person who feels ill may neglect grooming. Changes in hair texture and volume can result from disease or medication. For example, hypothyroidism may cause excessively thin, dry, or brittle hair. Chemotherapy or radiation to treat cancer often causes hair loss (**alopecia**).

Newborns may have **lanugo** (the fine hair on the body of the fetus, also referred to as down or woolly hair) over their shoulders, back, and sacrum. This generally disappears, and the hair distribution on the eyebrows, head, and eyelashes of

young children becomes noticeable. Some newborns have hair on their scalps. Others grow hair over the scalp during the first year.

Pubic hair usually appears in early puberty followed in about 6 months by the growth of axillary hair. Boys develop facial hair in later puberty. In adolescence, sebaceous gland activity increases. Hair follicle openings enlarge to accommodate increased sebum, which can make the adolescent's hair more oily.

In older adults, the hair is generally thinner, grows more slowly, and loses its color as a result of aging tissues and diminishing circulation. Men often lose their scalp hair and may become completely bald. Male baldness is influenced by genetics; it may occur even when a man is relatively young. The older person's hair also tends to become drier. Axillary and pubic hair becomes finer and scanter, but eyebrows become bristly and coarse. Many women develop some facial hair.

NURSING CARE

ASSESSING

During the nursing history, data about usual hair care, self-care abilities, history of hair or scalp problems, and conditions (like hypothyroidism) that affect the hair are obtained. Questions about medications, hair dyes, and curling or straightening preparations can provide more information to assess dry and brittle hair. Common hair problems follow.

Often accompanied by itching, **dandruff** appears as a diffuse scaling of the scalp. In severe cases it involves the auditory canals and the eyebrows. Dandruff can usually be treated effectively with a commercial shampoo. In severe or persistent cases, the client may need the advice of a physician.

Hair loss and growth are continual processes. By middle age some permanent thinning of hair normally occurs. Baldness, common in men, is thought to be a hereditary problem. Hairpieces, surgical hair transplantation, and various medications address the issue of baldness.

Ticks are small, gray-brown parasites that bite into tissue and suck blood. Ticks transmit several diseases to people, including Rocky Mountain spotted fever, Lyme disease, babesiosis, and tularemia. Ticks should never be forcibly pulled from the skin because the sucking apparatus remains and may become infected. To ease removal, cover the tick with mineral oil or a lubricating jelly such as petroleum jelly. This deprives the tick of oxygen and allows it to be removed more easily.

Lice are parasitic insects that infest mammals. They are very small, grayish white, and difficult to see. The crab louse in the pubic area has red legs. Lice may be contracted from infested clothes and direct contact with an infested person.

Infestation with lice is called **pediculosis.** Hundreds of varieties of lice can infest humans. Three common kinds are *Pediculus capitis* (the head louse), *Pediculus corporis* (the body louse), and *Pediculus pubis* (the crab louse).

Pediculus capitis tends to stay hidden in scalp hair; similarly, *Pediculus pubis* stays in pubic hair. Head and pubic lice lay their eggs on the hairs. The eggs are oval, similar in appearance to dandruff, although they cling to the hair. Bites and pustular eruptions may be noticed at the hairline and behind the ears. *Pediculus corporis* tends to cling to clothing, so when a client undresses, the lice may not be seen on the body. These lice suck blood from the person and lay their eggs on the clothing. The nurse can suspect their presence in the clothing if (a) the person habitually scratches, (b) there are scratches on the skin, and (c) there are hemorrhagic spots on the skin where the lice have sucked blood.

Gamma benzene hexachloride (Kwell) was widely used for treatment of pediculosis, but serious side effects with its use were reported. It is more common now to use an over-the-counter preparation such as pyrethrin. If the client has head lice, the hair is washed with the shampoo and the bed linens are changed. This treatment is repeated 12 to 24 hours later if needed. A client with pubic or body lice takes a bath or shower, dries, and applies the lotion or cream—to the entire body surface for body lice, and to the pubic area and adjacent areas for pubic lice. After 12 to 24 hours the lotion is washed off, and clean clothing and linens are supplied.

Scabies is a contagious skin infestation by the itch mite. The characteristic lesion is the burrow produced by the female mite as it penetrates into the upper layers of the skin. Burrows are short, wavy, brown or black threadlike lesions, usually seen between the webs of the fingers and the folds of the wrists and elbows. The mites cause intense itching. Itching is more pronounced at night, because the increased warmth of the skin stimulates the parasites. Secondary lesions caused by scratching include vesicles, papules, pustules, excoriations, and crusts. Treatment involves thorough cleansing of the body with soap and water to remove scales and debris from crusts, and then an application of a scabicide lotion. All bed linens and clothing are washed in very hot or boiling water.

clinical ALERT

Because some conditions of the scalp are highly contagious, the nurse should always don gloves for the initial physical assessment of the scalp and hair.

The growth of excessive body hair is called **hirsutism.** The acceptance of body hair in the axillae and on the legs is largely dictated by culture. In North American media, well-groomed women are depicted with no hair on legs or under axillae. In many other cultures, it is customary for women not to remove this hair. Excessive facial hair on a woman is thought unattractive in most Western and Asian cultures.

The cause of excessive body hair is not always known. Older women may have some on their faces, and women in menopause may also experience the growth of facial hair. These conditions may be due to hormonal changes. Heredity also influences the pattern of hair distribution and the production of androgens by the adrenal glands.

Inflammation, flaking, and itching may also be produced by a fungal infection of the skin. When it appears on the upper body, it is sometimes called "ringworm." When it appears in the groin it is commonly called "jock itch." A fungal infection of the feet produces redness, peeling, and cracking of the skin and is commonly known as "athlete's foot."

 DIAGNOSING, PLANNING, and IMPLEMENTING

Nursing diagnoses related to hair hygiene and hair and scalp problems include:

Self-Care Deficit: Grooming
Impaired Skin Integrity
Risk for Infection
Disturbed Body Image

Factors like imposed immobility (bed rest), pain in upper extremities, and insect bite can contribute to these diagnosis. Examples of desired outcomes might be:

◆ Client performs hair grooming with assistance (specify)
◆ Client has reduced or absent scalp lesions or infestations
◆ Client uses preventive measures for specific hair problem (e.g., dandruff)

Plans for assisting the client should take into account the client's personal preferences, health, and energy resources as well as the time, equipment, and personnel available. Often, clients like to receive hair care after a bath, before receiving visitors, and before retiring. At some agencies, shampoos can be given to clients only after a physician's order.

Shampooing the Hair

Hair should be washed as often as needed to keep it clean. There are several ways to shampoo clients' hair, depending on their health, strength, and age. The client who is well enough to take a shower can shampoo there. The client who is unable to shower may be given a shampoo while sitting on a chair in front of a sink. The client who must remain in bed can be given a shampoo with water brought to the bedside. Shampoo basins to catch the water and direct it to the washbasin or other receptacle are usually made of plastic or metal. A pail or large washbasin can be used to catch the shampoo water. If possible, the receptacle should be large enough to hold all the shampoo water so that it does not have to be emptied during the shampoo.

Water used for the shampoo should be 40.5°C (105°F) for an adult or child to be comfortable and not injure the scalp. Usually, the client will supply a liquid or cream shampoo. If the shampoo is being given to destroy lice, a medicated shampoo should be used. Dry shampoos are also available. They will remove some of the dirt, odor, and oil. Their main disadvantage is that they dry the hair and scalp. Another option available for shampoo for bed rest clients is commercial "bag shampoo." The shampoo solution is in a shower cap. It can be warmed in the microwave, in the same manner as the "bag bath." After warming, the cap is placed on the client's head for 20 minutes. The nurse massages the client's head through the cap prior to removing. The hair is towel dried and then styled.

How often a person needs a shampoo is highly individual, depending largely on the person's activities and the amount of sebum secreted by the scalp. Oily hair tends to look stringy and dirty, and it feels unclean to the person.

Procedure 13-2A explains how to provide a shampoo for a client confined to bed.

Brushing and Combing Hair

To be healthy, hair needs to be brushed daily. Brushing stimulates the circulation of blood in the scalp, distributes the oil along the hair shaft, and helps to arrange the hair.

For clients confined to bed, hair should be combed and brushed at least once a day to prevent matting. A brush with stiff bristles provides the best stimulation to the scalp, but bristles should not be sharp enough to injure the client's scalp. A comb with dull, even teeth is advisable. Some clients are pleased to have their hair tied neatly in the back or braided until other assistance is available or until they feel better and can look after it themselves.

African-American people often have thicker, drier, curlier hair than many Caucasian people. Spiraled or very curly hair may stand out from the scalp and has less strength than straight hair. If straightened, it tends to tangle and mat easily, especially at the back and the sides if the client is confined to bed. Some African-Americans style their hair in small braids (Figure 13-2 ◆). These braids do not have to be unbraided for shampooing and washing. The LPN/LVN should obtain the client's permission before any such unbraiding. Some people with spiraled hair need to oil their hair daily to prevent hair strands from breaking and the scalp from becoming too dry. Procedure 13-3B describes how to provide hair care for African American clients.

Beard and Mustache Care

Beards and mustaches also require daily care. The most important aspect of the care is to keep them clean. Food particles tend to collect in beards and mustaches, and they need washing and combing periodically. Clients may also wish a beard or mustache trim to maintain a well-groomed appearance. A beard or mustache should not be shaved off without the client's consent.

Male clients often shave or are shaved after a bath. Frequently clients supply their own electric or safety razors. Box 13-6 ◆ provides steps involved in shaving facial hair with a safety razor.

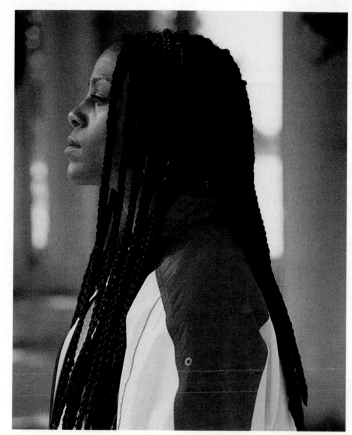

Figure 13-2. ◆ An African American's hair styled with braids.
Source: © Elena Dorfman/Addison Wesley/Longman.

 EVALUATING

The nurse collects data to determine whether desired outcomes have been reached.

 Mouth Care

Teeth begin to appear 5 to 8 months after birth; by age 2 years, children usually have all 20 temporary teeth (Figure 13-3A ◆). These are gradually replaced by the 32 permanent teeth (Figure 13-3B) by age 25.

The incidence of periodontal disease increases during pregnancy. Many pregnant women experience more bleeding during brushing and increased redness and swelling of the *gingiva* (the gums).

Older adults may lose permanent teeth; some have dentures. Loss of permanent teeth is usually due to periodontal disease (gum disease) rather than to dental *caries* (cavities). However, caries are also common in middle-aged adults.

Some receding of the gums and a brownish pigmentation of the gums occur with age. Saliva production decreases with age, so dryness of the oral mucosa is a common finding in older people.

 MediaLink Cavities

Figure 13-3. ◆ **A.** Temporary teeth and their times of eruption (stated in months). **B.** Temporary teeth and their times of eruption (stated in years).

Poor oral hygiene, dry mouth, and poor nutrition are common causes of oral problems. Poor oral hygiene may be the result of a lack of knowledge or illness. Confused, depressed, physically weak (or comatose) clients generally have poor oral hygiene. Clients who have nasogastric tubes, are on oxygen or breathe through their mouths, experience increased oral dryness. Dry mouth is also caused by aging and medication. Older adults experience decreased saliva production and thinning of the oral mucosa. Medications that cause dry mouth include diuretics, laxatives (if used excessively), tranquilizers such as chlorpromazine (Thorazine) and diazepam (Valium), and chemotherapeutic agents to treat cancer. Dry mouth is aggravated by anxiety, poor fluid intake (dehydration), high salt intake, and smoking. Poor eating habits, such as excessive intake of salt and refined sugars, can erode tooth enamel, increasing risk. Recent mouth injury or surgery increases the risk of infection. Clients with impaired immune systems (such as those on chemotherapy or with HIV) and those who wear dental appliances (such as retainers) are at increased risk of developing mouth lesions.

NURSING CARE

◆ ASSESSING

Assessment of the client's mouth and hygiene practices includes (a) a nursing history, (b) physical assessment of the mouth, and (c) identification of clients at risk for developing oral problems.

During the nursing history, data are obtained about the client's oral hygiene practices, including dental visits, self-care abilities, and past or current mouth problems. Learning needs, client preferences, and self-care abilities are also determined. Clients whose hand coordination is impaired, whose cognitive function is impaired, whose illness alters energy levels and motivation, or whose therapy imposes restrictions on activities will need assistance. Common problems of the mouth and nursing implications are detailed in Table 13-2 ◆. For more information about mouth assessment, see also Chapter 11. ⊗

 DIAGNOSING, PLANNING, and IMPLEMENTING

Three nursing diagnoses related to problems with oral hygiene and the oral cavity are Self-Care Deficit, Impaired Oral Mucous Membrane, and Deficient Knowledge. The North American Nursing Diagnosis Association (NANDA) includes oral hygiene in the diagnostic label Self-Care Deficit: Bathing/Hygiene. In this book, the diagnosis Self-Care Deficit: Oral Hygiene is used for clients who cannot perform oral care independently. This includes the inability to brush or floss teeth or clean dentures.

The diagnosis Impaired Oral Mucous Membrane refers to the state in which an individual experiences disruptions in the tissue layers of the oral cavity. Manifestations include a coated tongue; dry mouth; dental caries; *halitosis* (bad breath); gingivitis; oral plaque, pain, discomfort, erythema, lesions, or ulcers; and lack of or decreased salivation. These may be the result of inadequate oral hygiene; physical injury or drying effect (e.g., mouth breathing, oxygen therapy); mechanical trauma (e.g., surgery; injury from oral tube, broken teeth, or ill-fitting dentures); chemical trauma (e.g., side effects of medications); or radiation injury. The diagnosis Deficient Knowledge is discussed in detail in Chapter 23. ⊗

A major goal for clients with oral hygiene or oral problems is to maintain or restore the integrity of the oral tissues and to prevent associated risks.

Examples of desired outcomes include:

◆ Gums are firm, well hydrated, uniform in color, and do not bleed.
◆ Brushes teeth after meals and at bedtime.
◆ Mucosa, tongue, and lips are pink, moist, and intact.

Good oral hygiene includes daily stimulation of the gums, mechanical brushing and flossing of the teeth, and flushing of the mouth. The LPN/LVN is often in a position to help people maintain oral hygiene by helping or teaching them to clean the teeth and oral cavity, and by inspecting whether clients (especially children) have done so. They can provide special oral hygiene for clients who are debilitated, unconscious, or have lesions of the mucous membranes or other oral tissues. (See Procedure 13-3.) The LPN/LVN can also be instrumental

TABLE 13-2	COMMON PROBLEMS OF THE MOUTH AND NURSING IMPLICATIONS	
PROBLEM	**DESCRIPTION**	**NURSING IMPLICATIONS**
Halitosis	Bad breath	Teach or provide regular oral hygiene.
Glossitis	Inflammation of the tongue	As above
Gingivitis	Inflammation of the gums	As above
Periodontal disease	Gums appear spongy and bleeding	As above
Reddened or excoriated mucosa		Check for ill-fitting dentures.
Excessive dryness of the buccal mucosa		Increase fluid intake as health permits.
Cheilosis	Cracking of lips	Lubricate lips, use antimicrobial ointment to prevent infection.
Dental caries	Teeth have darkened areas, may be painful	Advise client to see a dentist.
Sordes	Accumulation of foul matter (food, microorganisms, and epithelial elements) in the mouth	Teach or provide regular cleaning.
Stomatitis	Inflammation of the oral mucosa	Teach or provide regular cleaning.
Parotitis	Inflammation of the parotid salivary glands	Teach or provide regular oral hygiene.

in identifying problems that require the intervention of a dentist or oral surgeon and in arranging a referral. These problems should be discussed with the RN before conferring with the physician.

Promoting Oral Health Through the Life Span

A major role of the LPN/LVN in promoting oral health is to teach clients about specific oral hygiene measures. Most dentists recommend that dental hygiene should begin when the first tooth erupts and be practiced after each feeding. Cleaning can be accomplished by using a wet washcloth or a cotton ball or small gauze moistened with water.

Dental caries (cavities) occur frequently during the toddler period, often as a result of the excessive intake of sweets or a prolonged use of the bottle during naps and at bedtime. The LPN/LVN should give parents the following instructions to promote and maintain dental health:

◆ Beginning at about 18 months of age, brush the child's teeth with a soft toothbrush. Use only a toothbrush moistened with water. Introduce toothpaste later; use one that contains fluoride.

◆ Give a fluoride supplement daily or as recommended by the physician or dentist, unless the drinking water is fluoridated.

◆ Schedule an initial dental visit for the child at about 2 or 3 years of age, as soon as all 20 primary teeth have erupted.

◆ Some dentists recommend an inspection type of visit when the child is about 18 months old to provide an early pleasant introduction to the dental examination.

◆ Seek professional dental attention for any problems such as discoloring of the teeth, chipping, or signs of infection such as redness and swelling.

Because deciduous teeth guide the entrance of permanent teeth, dental care for preschoolers and school-age children is essential to keep these teeth in good repair. Abnormally placed or lost deciduous teeth can cause misalignment of permanent teeth. Fluoride helps prevent dental caries. Preschoolers need to be taught to brush their teeth after eating, and parents should limit the child's intake of refined sugars. Regular dental checkups are required during these years when permanent teeth appear.

Proper diet and tooth and mouth care should be taught to adolescents and adults.

Care of Teeth

Brushing and Flossing the Teeth.
Thorough brushing of the teeth is important in preventing tooth decay. The mechanical action of brushing removes food particles that can harbor and incubate bacteria. It also stimulates circulation in the gums, maintaining their healthy firmness. Fluoride toothpaste is often recommended because of its antibacterial protection. An effective toothpaste can also be made by combining two parts table salt to one part baking soda. (However, this paste is not to be used by clients on sodium restricted diets.) Procedure 13-3A provides instruction in brushing and flossing the client's teeth.

Caring for Dentures.
Dentures (a "plate" of artificial teeth for one jaw) may be worn to replace upper or lower teeth or both. When only a few artificial teeth are needed, a "bridge" may be worn. Bridges may be fixed or removable. Clients should always be encouraged to wear their dentures (or other oral prostheses) to prevent gum shrinkage and further tooth loss.

Like natural teeth, dentures collect microorganisms and food. They need to be cleaned at least once a day. Dentures may be removed, scrubbed with a toothbrush, rinsed, and reinserted. Some people use toothpaste; others use commercial cleaning compounds or soaking solutions for plates. Always rinse dentures thoroughly before inserting into the mouth, especially after soaking. Procedure 13-3B describes how to clean dentures.

Assisting Clients with Oral Care.
When providing mouth care for partially or totally dependent clients, the LPN/LVN should wear gloves. Required equipment includes a curved basin that fits snugly under the client's chin (e.g., a kidney basin) to receive the rinse water and a towel to protect the client and the bedclothes. (See Procedure 13-3A). Foam swabs are often used in health care agencies to clean the mouths of dependent clients. These swabs are convenient and effective in removing excess debris from the teeth and mouth but should be used infrequently and for short periods (i.e., less than 3 days). Foam swabs are not as effective as a toothbrush in removing plaque from "sheltered" areas of the teeth and gingival crevices.

Most people prefer privacy when they take their artificial teeth out to clean them. Many do not like to be seen without their teeth. One of the first requests of many postoperative clients is, "May I have my teeth in, please?"

For the client who is debilitated or unconscious or who has excessive dryness, sores, or irritations of the mouth, it may be necessary to clean the oral mucosa and tongue in addition to the teeth. Agency practices differ in regard to special mouth care and the frequency with which it is provided. Depending on the health of the client's mouth, special care may be needed every 2 to 8 hours. Mouth care for unconscious or debilitated people is important because their mouths tend to become dry and consequently predisposed to infections. Dryness occurs because the client cannot take fluids by mouth, is often breathing through the mouth, or is receiving oxygen, which tends to dry the mucous membranes.

The LPN/LVN can use commercially prepared applicators of lemon oil juice and oil glycerine to clean the mucous membranes. If these are unavailable, a gauze square wrapped around a tongue blade and dipped into lemon juice and oil or into mouthwash usually suffices. Most commercial mouthwashes contain alcohol, which can lead to further dryness of the mucosa. An alcohol-free mouthwash is usually available from agency pharmacies or central supply units. Mineral oil is contraindicated because aspiration could cause an infection. Hydrogen peroxide is not recommended for use in oral care. It can be irritating to healthy oral mucosa and may affect the microflora of the mouth. Normal saline solution is recommended for oral hygiene for the dependent client.

Procedure 13-3C focuses on oral care for the unconscious person but may be adapted for conscious persons who are seriously ill or have mouth problems.

 ## EVALUATING

To evaluate care of the mouth, data are collected on the status of oral mucosa, lips, tongue, and teeth. The nursing team determines whether desired outcomes have been achieved. If they are not achieved, the RN, LPN/LVN, and client explore the reasons. The care plan may be modified.

 # Eye Care

Normally, eyes require no special hygiene, because *lacrimal fluid* (tears) continually washes the eyes, and because the eyelids and lashes prevent the entrance of foreign particles. However, special interventions are needed for unconscious clients and for clients recovering from eye surgery or having eye injuries, irritations, or infections. In unconscious clients, the blink reflex may be absent, and excessive drainage may accumulate along eyelid margins. In clients with eye trauma or eye infections, excessive discharge or drainage is common. Excessive secretions on the lashes need to be removed before they dry on the lashes as crusts. Clients who wear eyeglasses, contact lenses, or an artificial eye also may require instruction and care by the LPN/LVN.

NURSING CARE

 ## ASSESSING

During the nursing history, the RN obtains data about the client's eyeglasses or contact lenses, recent examination by an ophthalmologist, and any history of eye problems and related treatments. In the physical assessment, all external eye structures are inspected for signs of inflammation, excessive drainage, encrustations, or other obvious abnormalities. Inspection of the external eye structures is detailed in Chapter 11.

 ## DIAGNOSING, PLANNING, and IMPLEMENTING

Nursing diagnoses related to eye problems may include:

◆ Self-Care Deficit (such as contact lens insertion, removal, and cleaning)

◆ Risk for Infection (as with accumulation of secretions on eyelids)
◆ Risk for Injury (e.g., related to absence of blink reflex associated with unconsciousness)

Nursing activities are identified that will assist the client to maintain the integrity of the eye structures or a prosthesis and to prevent eye injury and infection. Nursing activities may include teaching clients about how to insert, clean, and remove contact lenses or a prosthesis, and ways to protect the eyes from injury and strain. Examples of desired outcomes to evaluate the effectiveness of nursing interventions include:

◆ Eyelids free of secretions
◆ No eye discomfort
◆ Demonstrates appropriate methods of caring for contact lenses

Eye Care
When giving eye care, always wear clean gloves.

Dried secretions that have accumulated on the lashes need to be softened and wiped away. Soften dried secretions by placing a sterile cotton ball moistened with sterile water or normal saline over the lid margins. Wipe the loosened secretions from the inner canthus of the eye to the outer canthus to prevent the particles and fluid from draining into the lacrimal sac and nasolacrimal duct.

If the client is unconscious and lacks a blink reflex or cannot close the eyelids completely, drying and irritation of the cornea must be prevented. Lubricating eye drops may be ordered. See Box 13-7 ◆ for eye care for the comatose client.

BOX 13-7
NURSING CARE CHECKLIST

EYE CARE FOR THE COMATOSE CLIENT

When a comatose client's corneal reflex is impaired, eye care is essential to keep moist the areas of the cornea that are exposed to air.

☑ Administer moist compresses to cover the eyes every 2 to 4 hours.
☑ Clean the eyes with saline solution and cotton balls. Wipe from the inner to outer canthus. This prevents debris from being washed into the nasolacrimal duct.
☑ Use a new cotton ball for each wipe. This prevents extending infection in one eye or to the other eye.
☑ Instill ophthalmic ointment or artificial tears into the lower lids as ordered. This keeps the eyes moist.
☑ If the client's corneal reflex is absent, keep the eyes moist with artificial tears and protect the eye with a protective shield. These should be ordered by a physician.
☑ Monitor the eyes for redness, exudate, or ulceration.

Eyeglass Care

It is essential to exercise caution when cleaning eyeglasses to prevent breaking or scratching the lenses. Glass lenses can be cleaned with warm water and dried with a soft tissue that will not scratch the lenses. Plastic lenses are more easily scratched; they may require special cleaning solutions and drying tissues. When not being worn, all glasses should be placed in a case that is labeled appropriately. They should be stored in the client's bedside table drawer.

Contact Lens Care

Contact lenses, thin curved discs of hard or soft plastic, fit on the cornea of the eye directly over the pupil. They float on the tear layer of the eye. For some people, contact lenses offer several advantages over eyeglasses. They cannot be seen and thus have cosmetic value. They are highly effective in correcting some astigmatisms. They are safer than glasses for some physical activities. They do not fog, as eyeglasses do. They provide better vision in many cases.

Contact lenses may be either hard or soft or a compromise between the two types—gas-permeable lenses. Hard contact lenses are made of a rigid, unwettable, airtight plastic that does not absorb water or saline solutions. They usually cannot be worn for more than 12 to 14 hours and are rarely recommended for first-time wearers.

Soft contact lenses cover the entire cornea. Because they are more pliable and soft, they mold to the eye for a firmer fit. The duration of extended wear varies by brand from 1 to 30 days or more. Eye specialists recommend that long-wear brands be removed and cleaned at least once a week. These lenses require very careful care and handling.

Gas-permeable lenses are rigid enough to provide clear vision but are more flexible than the traditional hard lens. They permit oxygen to reach the cornea, thus providing greater comfort, and will not cause serious damage to the eye if left in place for several days.

Most clients normally care for their own contact lenses. In general, each lens manufacturer provides detailed cleaning instructions. Depending on the type of lens and cleaning method, warm tap water, normal saline, or special rinsing or soaking solutions may be used.

clinical ALERT

Never substitute saline marked "for injection" as a wetting or cleansing solution. Injectable saline may harm soft lenses or the client's eye.

All users should have a special container for their lenses. Each lens container has a slot with a label indicating whether it is for the right or left lens. Lenses must be stored in the appropriate slot so that they are placed in the correct eye.

Removing Contact Lenses. Hard contact lenses must be positioned directly over the cornea for proper removal. If the lens is displaced, the LPN/LVN asks the client to look straight ahead, and gently exerts pressure on the upper and lower lids to move the lens back onto the cornea. Figure 13-4 A–C ◆ shows the steps needed to remove a hard lens. To avoid lens mix-ups, always place the first lens in its designated storage cup before removing the second lens.

Soft lenses can be removed in two ways. First, after separating the eyelids with the nondominant hand, move the lens down to the inferior part of the sclera using the pad of the dominant index finger (Figure 13-5A ◆). This reduces the risk of damage to the cornea. Second, remove the lens by gently pinching it between the pads of the thumb and index finger of your dominant hand (Figure 13-5B). Pinching causes the lens to double up, so that air entering under the lens overcomes the suction and allows removal. Use the pads of the fingers to prevent scratching the eye or the lens with the fingernails.

A   B   C

Figure 13-4. ◆ Removing hard contact lenses: **A.** Separate the eyelids until they are beyond the edge of the lens. **B.** Hold the top eyelid stationary at the edge to the lens, and lift the bottom edge of the contact lens by pressing the lower lid at its margin. **C.** After the lens is slightly tipped, slide the lens out of the eye by moving both eyelids toward each other.

A

B

Figure 13-5. ◆ **A.** Moving a soft lens down to the inferior part of the sclera. **B.** Remove a soft lens by pinching it between the pads of the thumb and index finger.

Inserting Contact Lenses. Seriously ill clients whose contact lenses have been removed do not need them reinserted until they become more active in their care and require the lenses to see properly. Contact lenses need to be lubricated in a sterile, nonirritating wetting solution (usually a saline solution) before they are inserted. The wetting solution helps the lens glide over the cornea and reduces the risk of injury. Most clients, when well, will reinsert the lenses independently.

Artificial Eyes

Artificial eyes are usually made of glass or plastic. Some are permanently implanted; others are removed regularly for cleaning. Most clients who wear a removable artificial eye follow their own care regimen. Even for an unconscious client, daily removal and cleaning are not necessary.

To remove an artificial eye, the LPN/LVN dons clean gloves and uses the dominant thumb to pull the client's lower eyelid down over the infraorbital bone, exerting slight pres-

sure below the eyelid to overcome the suction in the eye socket (Figure 13-6A ◆). An alternate method is to compress a small rubber bulb and apply the tip directly to the eye. As the pressure on the bulb is gradually released, the suction of the bulb counteracts the suction of the socket and draws the eye out of the socket.

The eye is cleaned with warm normal saline and placed in a container filled with water or saline solution. The socket and tissues around the eye are usually cleaned with cotton wipes and normal saline. To reinsert the eye, the thumb and index finger of one hand are used to retract the eyelids, exerting pressure on the supraorbital and infraorbital bones. The nurse holds the eye between the thumb and index finger of the other hand and slips the eye gently into the socket (Figure 13-6B).

◆ EVALUATING

Assessing the eyes is part of a regular head-to-toe or body systems assessment. Any unusual redness, discharge, or pain should be documented and reported to the team leader.

◆ DISCHARGE CONSIDERATIONS

Many clients may need to learn specific information about care of the eyes. The nurse can provide these general guidelines:

◆ Avoid home remedies for eye problems. Eye irritations or injuries at any age should be treated medically and immediately.

A

B

Figure 13-6. ◆ **A.** Removing an artificial eye by retracting the lower eyelid and exerting slight pressure below the eyelid. **B.** Hold an artificial eye between the thumb and index finger for insertion.

- If dirt or dust gets into the eyes, clean them copiously with clean, tepid water as an emergency treatment.
- Take measures to guard against eyestrain and to protect vision, such as maintaining adequate lighting for reading and obtaining shatterproof lenses for glasses.
- Schedule regular eye examinations, particularly after age 40, to detect problems such as cataracts and glaucoma.

Ear Care

Normal ears require minimal hygiene. Clients who have excessive **cerumen** (earwax) and dependent clients who have hearing aids may require assistance. Hearing aids are usually removed before surgery.

CLEANING THE EARS

The auricles of the ear are cleaned during the bed bath. The LPN/LVN or client removes excessive cerumen that is visible or that causes discomfort or hearing difficulty. Visible cerumen may be loosened and removed by retracting the auricle downward. If this measure is ineffective, irrigation is necessary (see the section on otic irrigation in Chapter 21, "Medications"). Clients should be advised never to use bobby pins, toothpicks, or cotton-tipped applicators to remove cerumen. Bobby pins and toothpicks can injure the ear canal and rupture the tympanic membrane. Cotton-tipped applicators can cause wax to become impacted within the canal.

CARE OF HEARING AIDS

A **hearing aid** is a battery-powered, sound-amplifying device used by hearing-impaired persons (Figure 13-7 A and B ◆). It consists of a microphone that picks up sound and converts it to electric energy, an amplifier that magnifies the electric energy electronically, a receiver that converts the ampli-

fied energy back to sound energy, and an earmold that directs the sound into the ear. There are several types of hearing aids. They may be positioned in or behind the ear or on the body.

Procedure 13-4 describes how to remove, clean, and insert a hearing aid.

Nose Care

The LPN/LVN usually does not need to provide special care for the nose. Clients can ordinarily clear nasal secretions by blowing gently into a soft tissue. When the external nares are encrusted with dried secretions, they should be cleaned with a cotton-tipped applicator or moistened with saline or water. The applicator should not be inserted beyond the length of the cotton tip; inserting it further may cause injury to the mucosa.

Supporting a Hygienic Environment

Because ill people are usually confined to bed, often for long periods, the bed becomes an important element in the client's life. A place that is clean, safe, and comfortable contributes to the client's ability to rest and sleep and to a sense of well-being. Basic furniture in a health care facility includes the bed, bedside table, overbed table, one or more chairs, and a storage space for clothing. Most bed units also have a call light, light fixtures, electric outlets, and hygienic equipment on the bedside table. Three types of equipment that are often installed in an acute care facility are a suction outlet for several kinds of suction, an oxygen outlet for most oxygen equipment, and a sphygmomanometer (blood pressure cuff and gauge) to measure the client's blood pressure. Some long-term care agencies also permit clients to have personal furniture,

Earmold

Connecting tube

Ear hook

On/off (TM) switch

Microphone

Volume control

Battery compartment

A

Combined on/off switch and volume control

Sound tube

Battery compartment

Microphone

B

Figure 13-7. ◆ **A.** A behind-the-ear hearing aid. **B.** An in-the-ear hearing aid.

such as a television, a chair, and lamps, at the bedside. In the home a client often has personal and medical equipment.

To provide a comfortable environment, it is important to consider the client's age, severity of illness, and level of activity. The very young, the very old, and the acutely ill frequently need a room temperature higher than normal. A room temperature between 20 and 23°C (68 and 74°F) is comfortable for most clients.

Good ventilation is important to remove unpleasant odors and stale air. For example, odors caused by urine, draining wounds, or vomitus can be offensive. Room deodorizers can help eliminate odors, but good hygienic practices are the best way to prevent offensive body and breath odors. Hospitals are required to restrict smoking. Hospitals often have a smoking area for clients and prohibit smoking in client rooms.

Certain clients may benefit from specially ventilated rooms. Infection can be contained by using special rooms with different types of air pressure, depending on the type of infection. A negative pressure room is used for clients with highly communicable disease. This negative pressure filters the contamination without allowing it to pass out of the room into other areas. Positive pressure rooms keep the contamination out; they are used for clients who are vulnerable to infection, such as those who have just undergone transplant surgery.

Ill persons are usually sensitive to noise such as clanging of metal equipment, loud talking, and laughter. The nursing staff should always try to control noise in health care settings. (See Chapter 20, "Activity, Exercise, Rest & Sleep.") ◉

HOSPITAL BEDS

The frame of a hospital bed is divided into three sections. This permits the head and the foot to be elevated separately. Most hospital beds have electric motors to operate the movable joints. The motor is activated by pressing a button or by moving a small lever, located either at the side of the bed or on a small panel separate from the bed but attached to it by a cable, which the client can readily use. Common bed positions are shown in Table 13-3 ◆.

Hospital beds are usually narrower than the average single bed, so that the nursing staff can reach the client from either side of the bed without undue stretching. The length is usually 1.9 m (6.5 ft). Some beds can be extended in length to accommodate very tall clients. Long-term care facilities for ambulatory clients usually have low beds to facilitate movement in and out of bed. Most hospital beds have "high" and "low" positions that can be adjusted either mechanically or electrically by a button or lever. The high position permits the nursing staff to reach the client without undue stretching or stooping. The low position allows the client to step easily to the floor.

Mattresses

Mattresses are usually covered with a water-repellent material that resists soiling and can be cleaned easily. Most mattresses have handles on the sides, called "lugs," by which the mattress can be moved. Many special mattresses are also used in hospitals to relieve pressure on the body's bony prominences, such as the heels. They are particularly helpful for clients confined

TABLE 13-3 COMMONLY USED BED POSITIONS		
POSITION	**DESCRIPTION**	**INDICATIONS FOR USE**
Flat	Mattress is completely horizontal.	Client sleeping in a variety of bed positions, such as back-lying, side-lying, and prone (face down) To maintain spinal alignment for clients with spinal injuries To assist clients to move and turn in bed Bed-making by LPN/LVN
Fowler's position	Semisitting position in which head of bed is raised to angle of at least 45°. Knees may be flexed or horizontal.	Convenient for eating, reading, visiting, watching TV Relief from lying positions To promote lung expansion for client with respiratory problem To assist a client to a sitting position on the edge of the bed
Semi-Fowler's position	Head of bed is raised only to 30° angle.	Relief from lying position To promote lung expansion
Trendelenburg's position	Head of bed is lowered and the foot raised in a straight incline.	To promote venous circulation in certain clients To provide postural drainage of basal lung lobes
Reverse Trendelenburg's position	Head of bed raised and the foot lowered. Straight tilt in direction opposite to Trendelenburg's position	To promote stomach emptying and prevent esophageal reflex in client with hiatal hernia

to bed for a long time. For additional information about mattresses, see Chapter 12, Table 12-4. 🔗

Side Rails

Side rails, or safety sides, are used on both hospital beds and stretchers. They are of various shapes and sizes and are usually made of metal. Devices to raise and lower them differ. When side rails are being used, it is crucial that the client's bedside is never left while the rail is lowered. Some agencies have a release form that the client can sign if the use of side rails is refused.

Footboard or Footboot

Footboards are used to support the client's foot in a normal right angle to the legs to prevent plantar flexion contractures.

Bed Cradles

A **bed cradle,** sometimes called an Anderson frame, is a device designed to keep the top bedclothes off the feet, legs, and even abdomen of a client. The bedclothes are arranged over the device and may be pinned in place. There are several types of bed cradles. One of the most common is a curved metal rod that fits over the bed. Part of the cradle fits under the mattress, and small metal brackets press down on each side of the mattress to keep the cradle in place. The frame of some cradles extends over half of the width of the bed, above one leg.

INTRAVENOUS RODS

Intravenous (IV) rods (poles, stands, standards), usually made of metal, support IV infusion containers while fluid is being administered to a client. These rods were traditionally freestanding on the floor beside the bed. Now, IV rods are often attached to the hospital beds. Some hospital units have overhead hanging rods on a track for IVs. The nurse will frequently encounter free-standing IV poles when IVs or PCA (patient controlled analgesia) pumps are being used.

MAKING BEDS

The LPN/LVN needs to be able to prepare hospital beds in different ways for specific purposes. In most instances, beds are made after the client receives certain care and when beds are unoccupied. However, at times it may be necessary to make an occupied bed or prepare a bed for a client who is having surgery (an anesthetic, postoperative, or surgical bed). Certain guidelines apply no matter what type of bed equipment is available, whether the bed is occupied or unoccupied, or why the bed is being prepared. The guidelines for bedmaking are summarized in Box 13-8 ◆.

An unoccupied bed can be either closed or open. Generally, the top covers of an *open bed* are folded back (thus the term open bed) to make it easier for a client to get in. Open and closed beds are made the same way, except that the top sheet, blanket, and bedspread of a *closed bed* are drawn up to the top of the bed and under the pillows.

Beds are often changed after bed baths. The linen can be collected before the bath. The linen is not usually changed unless it is soiled. Check the policy at each clinical agency.

BOX 13-8
NURSING CARE CHECKLIST

BED MAKING AND CHAIN OF INFECTION

☑ Wash hands thoroughly after handling a client's bed linen. Linens and equipment that have been soiled with secretions and excretions harbor microorganisms that can be transmitted to others directly or by the LPN/LVN's hands or uniform.

☑ Hold soiled linen away from uniform.

☑ Linen for one client is never (even momentarily) placed on another client's bed.

☑ Place soiled linen directly in a portable linen hamper or tucked into a pillow case at the end of the bed before it is gathered up for disposal.

☑ Do not shake soiled linen in the air because shaking can disseminate secretions and excretions and the microorganisms they contain.

☑ When stripping and making a bed, conserve time and energy by stripping and making up one side as much as possible before working on the other side.

☑ To avoid unnecessary trips to the linen supply area, gather all linen before starting to strip a bed.

Unfitted sheets, blankets, and bedspreads are *mitered* (folded at a fitted angle) at the corners of the bed. The purpose of mitering is to secure the bedclothes while the bed is occupied. Figure 13-8 ◆ shows how to miter the corner of a bed.

Procedure 13-5A explains how to change an unoccupied bed.

Changing an Occupied Bed

Some clients may be too weak to get out of bed because of the nature of their illness. Others may be restricted in bed by the presence of traction or other therapies. When changing an occupied bed, the LPN/LVN works quickly and disturbs the client as little as possible. To conserve the client's energy, use the following guidelines:

◆ Maintain the client in good body alignment. Never move or position a client in a manner that is contraindicated by the client's health. Obtain help if necessary to ensure safety.

◆ Move the client gently and smoothly. Rough handling can cause the client discomfort and abrade the skin.

◆ Throughout the procedure, explain what you plan to do before you do it. Use terms that the client can understand.

◆ Use the bedmaking time, like the bed bath time, to assess and meet the client's needs.

Procedure 13-5B describes how to change an occupied bed.

Note: The bibliography listings for this and all chapters have been compiled at the back of the book.

These two lines parallel

These two lines parallel

Figure 13-8. ◆ Mitering the corner of a bed: **A.** Tuck in the bedcover (sheet, blanket, and/or spread) firmly under the mattress at the bottom or top of the bed. **B.** Lift the bedcover at point 1 so that it forms a triangle with the side edge of the bed and the edge of the bedcover is parallel to the end of the bed. **C.** Tuck the part of the cover that hangs below the mattress under the mattress while holding the cover against the side of the mattress. **D.** Bring point 1 down toward the floor while the other hand holds the fold of the cover against the side of the mattress. **E.** Remove the hand and tuck the remainder of the cover under the mattress, if appropriate. The side of the top sheet, blanket, and bedspread may be left hanging freely rather than being tucked in. If the bedspread is mitered separately it may be left hanging freely, but the top sheet and blanket would be tucked in.

PROCEDURE 13-1

Bathing Clients

PURPOSES

◆ To remove transient microorganisms, body secretions and excretions, and dead skin cells and remove normal secretions and odors
◆ To stimulate circulation to the skin
◆ To produce a sense of well-being
◆ To promote relaxation and comfort
◆ To prevent or eliminate unpleasant body odors
◆ To maintain skin integrity

EQUIPMENT

◆ Bedpan or urinal
◆ Changing table
◆ Bath blanket
◆ Gloves (if giving perineal care)
◆ Washcloth

◆ Soap
◆ Washbasin
◆ Water between 43 and 46°C (110 and 115°F) for adults, 38 and 40°C (100 and 105°F) for children
◆ Two bath towels
◆ Additional bed linen and towels, if required
◆ Hygiene supplies such as lotion and deodorant
◆ Clean gown or pajamas as needed
◆ Cotton balls or swabs
◆ Solution bottle, pitcher, or container filled with warm water or a prescribed solution
◆ Bedpan to receive rinse water
◆ Moisture-resistant bag or receptacle for used cotton swabs
◆ Moisture-resistant disposable pad
◆ Pillow (optional)

Part A: Bathing an Adult or Pediatric Client

INTERVENTIONS

1. Prepare the client and the environment.
   ◆ Invite a parent or family member to participate if desired.
   ◆ Close the windows and doors to make sure that the room is free from drafts. *Air currents increase loss of heat from the body by convection.*
   ◆ Provide privacy by drawing the curtains or closing the door. *Hygiene is a personal matter. Some agencies provide signs indicating the need for privacy.*
   ◆ Offer the client a bedpan or urinal or ask whether the client wishes to use the toilet or commode. *The client will be more comfortable after voiding, and voiding before cleaning the perineum is advisable.*
   ◆ During the bath, assess each area of the skin carefully.

FOR A BED BATH

2. Prepare the bed, and position the client appropriately.
   ◆ Place the bed in the high position. Place an infant or small child on a changing table or elevated crib. *This avoids undue strain on the LPN/LVN's back.*
   ◆ Remove the top bed linen and replace it with the bath blanket. If the bed linen is to be reused, place it over the

bedside chair. If it is to be changed, place it in the linen hamper.
   ◆ Assist the client to move near you. *This helps prevent undue reaching and straining.*
   ◆ Remove the client's gown.

3. Make a bath mitt with the washcloth (Figure 13-9 ◆). *A bath mitt retains water and heat better than a cloth loosely held.*
   ◆ Triangular method: (1) Lay your hand on the washcloth; (2) fold the top corner over your hand; (3, 4) fold the side corners over your hand; (5) tuck the second corner under the cloth on the palmar side to secure the mitt.
   ◆ Rectangular method: (1) Lay your hand on the washcloth and fold one side over your hand; (2) fold the second side over your hand; (3) fold the top of the cloth down; and (4) tuck it under the folded side against your palm to secure the mitt.

4. Wash the face.
   ◆ Place one towel across the client's chest.
   ◆ Wash the client's eyes with water only and dry them well. Use a separate corner of the washcloth for each eye. *Using separate corners prevents transmitting microorganisms from one eye to the other.* Wipe from the inner to the outer

Figure 13-9. ◆ Making a bath mitt: **A.** Triangular method:
B. Rectangular method.

canthus. *Cleaning from the inner to the outer canthus prevents secretions from entering the nasolacrimal ducts.*

◆ Ask whether the client wants soap used on the face. *Soap has a drying effect, and the face, which is exposed to the air more than other body parts, tends to be drier.*

◆ Wash, rinse, and dry the client's face, neck, and ears.

5. Wash the arms and hands. (Omit the arms for a partial bath.)

◆ Place the bath towel lengthwise under the arm. *It protects the bed from becoming wet.*

◆ Wash, rinse, and dry the arm, using long, firm strokes from distal to proximal areas (from the point farthest from the body to the point closest). *Firm strokes from distal to proximal areas increase venous blood return.*

◆ Wash the axilla well. Repeat for the other arm. Exercise caution if an intravenous infusion is present, and check its flow after moving the arm. Immediately report any problems with the IV to the RN.

◆ Place a towel directly on the bed and put the basin on it. Place the client's hands in the basin. *Many clients enjoy immersing their hands in the basin and washing themselves.* Assist the client as needed to wash, rinse, and dry the hands, paying particular attention to the spaces between the fingers.

6. Wash the chest and abdomen. (Omit the chest and abdomen for a partial bath. However, the areas under a woman's breast may require bathing if they are irritated.)

◆ Fold the bath blanket down to the client's pubic area, and place the towel alongside the chest and abdomen.

◆ Wash, rinse, and dry the chest and abdomen, giving special attention to the skinfold under breasts. Keep chest and abdomen covered with the towel between the wash and rinse. *This provides warmth and privacy.*

◆ Replace the bath blanket when the areas have been dried. Avoid undue exposure when washing the chest and abdomen. For some clients, it may be preferable to wash the chest and the abdomen separately. In that case, place the bath towel horizontally across the abdomen first and then across the chest.

7. Wash the legs and feet. (Omit legs and feet for a partial bath.)

◆ Wrap one of the client's legs and feet with the bath blanket, ensuring that the pubic area is well covered.

◆ Place the bath towel lengthwise under the other leg, and wash that leg. Use long, smooth, firm strokes, washing from the ankle to the knee to the thigh. *Washing from distal to proximal areas stimulates venous blood flow.*

◆ Rinse and dry that leg, reverse the coverings, and repeat for the other leg.

◆ Wash the feet by placing them in the basin of water.

◆ Dry each foot. Pay particular attention to the spaces between the toes. If you prefer, wash one foot after that leg, before washing the other leg.

◆ Obtain fresh, warm bathwater now or when necessary. *Water may become dirty or cold. Because surface skin cells are removed with washing, the bathwater from dark-skinned clients may be dark; however, this does not mean the client is dirty.*

8. Wash the back and then the perineum.

◆ Assist the client to turn to a prone position or side-lying position facing away from you, and place the bath towel lengthwise alongside the back and buttocks.

◆ Wash and dry the back, buttocks, and upper thighs, paying particular attention to the gluteal folds. Avoid undue exposure of the client, as for the abdomen and chest in step 6.

◆ Assist the client to the supine position, and determine whether the client can wash the perineal-genital area independently. If the client cannot do so, drape the client as shown in Figure 13-10 ◆ and wash the area. See also Procedure 13-1B.

9. Assist the client with grooming aids such as lotion or deodorant.

◆ Help the client to put on a clean gown or pajamas.

◆ Assist the client to care for hair, mouth, and nails. *Some people prefer or need mouth care prior to the bath.*

Figure 13-10. ◆ Draping the client for perineal–genital care.

10. Document pertinent data.
- Record assessments, such as excoriation in the folds beneath the breasts or reddened areas over bony prominences and report changes to the RN.
- Record the type of bath given (i.e., complete, partial, or self-help). *This is usually recorded on a flowsheet.*

FOR A TUB BATH OR SHOWER

11. Prepare the client and the tub.
- Fill the tub about one-third to one-half full of water at 43 to 46°C (110 to 115°F). *Sufficient water is needed to cover the perineal area.*
- Cover all intravenous catheters or wound dressings with plastic coverings, and instruct client to prevent wetting these areas if possible.
- Obtain assistance with holding a pediatric client as indicated. *Holding minimizes contamination of open skin areas.*
- Apply a rubber bath mat or towel to the floor of the tub if safety strips are not on tub floor. *These prevent slippage of the client during the bath or shower.*
- Use a small basin or large sink for a small child. *Smaller containers decrease the danger of slippage of an active child and possible drowning.*

12. Assist the client into the shower or tub.
- Assist the client taking a standing shower with the initial adjustment of the water temperature and water flow pressure, as needed. *Some clients need a chair to sit in the shower because of weakness. Elderly people often feel faint under hot water.*
- If the client requires considerable assistance with a tub bath, additional staff may be needed. To provide support as the client sits down in the tub, fold a towel lengthwise and place it around the chest under both axillae; then hold the ends securely at the back as the client sits. It may be helpful to seat the client on the edge of the tub or on a chair beside the tub before transferring the client into the tub.
- Explain how the client can signal for help, leave the client for 2 to 5 minutes, and place an "occupied" sign on the door.
- Never leave an infant or small pediatric client unattended in a tub. *Slippage and drowning can occur in a matter of seconds and in very little water.*

13. Assist the client with washing and getting out of the tub.
- Wash the client's back, lower legs, and feet, if necessary.
- Assist the client out of the tub. If the client is unsteady, place a bath towel over the client's shoulders and drain the tub of water before the client attempts to get out of it. *Draining the water first lessens the likelihood of a fall. The towel prevents chilling.*

14. Dry the client, and assist with follow-up care.
- Follow step 9.
- Assist the client back to the room.
- Clean the tub or shower in accordance with agency practice, discard used linen in the laundry hamper, and place the "unoccupied" sign on the door.

15. Document pertinent data.
- Follow step 10.

Part B: Providing Perineal–Genital Care

INTERVENTIONS

1. Prepare the client.
- Offer the client an appropriate explanation, being particularly sensitive to any embarrassment felt by the client.
- Determine whether the client is experiencing any discomfort in the perineal–genital area.
- Fold the top bed linen to the foot of the bed, and fold the gown up to expose the genital area.
- Place a bath towel under the client's hips. *The bath towel prevents the bed from becoming soiled.*

2. Position and drape the client, and clean the upper inner thighs.

FOR FEMALES

- Position the female in a back-lying position, with the knees flexed and spread well apart (abducted).
- Cover her body and legs with the bath blanket. Drape the legs by tucking the bottom corners of the bath blanket under the inner sides of the legs (see Figure 13-10). *Minimum exposure lessens embarrassment and helps to provide warmth.* Bring the middle portion of the base of the blanket up over the pubic area.
- Don gloves, and wash and dry the upper inner thighs.

3. Inspect the perineal area.

4. Wash and dry the perineal–genital area.

FOR FEMALES

◆ Clean the labia majora. Then spread the labia to wash the folds between the labia majora and the labia minora. Note areas of inflammation, excoriation, or swelling. (Figure 13-11A ◆). *Secretions that tend to collect around the labia minora facilitate bacterial growth.*

◆ Use separate quarters of the washcloth for each stroke, and wipe from the pubis to the rectum. For menstruating women and clients with indwelling catheters, use disposable wipes, cotton balls, or gauze. Take a clean ball for each stroke. *Using separate quarters of the washcloth or new cotton balls or gauzes prevents the transmission of microorganisms from one area to the other.* Wipe from the area of least contamination (the pubis) to that of greatest (the rectum).

◆ Rinse the area well. You may place the client on a bedpan and use a periwash or solution bottle to pour warm water over the area. Dry the perineum thoroughly, paying

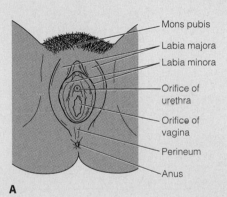

Mons pubis
Labia majora
Labia minora
Orifice of urethra
Orifice of vagina
Perineum
Anus

A

Prostate gland
Glans penis
Prepuce
Urethral meatus
Testes
Scrotum

B

Figure 13-11. ◆ A. Female genitals. **B.** Male genitals.

particular attention to the folds between the labia. *Moisture supports the growth of many microorganisms.*

FOR MALES

◆ Position the male client in a supine position with knees slightly flexed and hips slightly externally rotated.

◆ Don gloves, and wash and dry the upper inner thighs.

◆ Note particular areas of inflammation, excoriation, or swelling, especially between the scrotal folds.

◆ Also note excessive discharge or secretions from the orifices and the presence of odors.

◆ Wash and dry the penis, using firm strokes. *Handling the penis firmly may prevent an erection.*

◆ If the client is uncircumcised, retract the prepuce (foreskin) to expose the glans penis (the tip of the penis) for cleaning. Replace the foreskin after cleaning the glans penis (Figure 32–11B). *Retracting the foreskin is necessary to remove the smegma that collects under the foreskin and facilitates bacterial growth.*

◆ Wash and dry the scrotum. The posterior folds of the scrotum may need to be cleaned in step 6 with the buttocks. *The scrotum tends to be more soiled than the penis because of its proximity to the rectum; thus, it is usually cleaned after the penis.*

5. Inspect perineal orifices for intactness.

◆ Inspect particularly around the urethra in clients with indwelling catheters. *A catheter may cause excoriation around the urethra.*

6. Clean between the buttocks.

◆ Assist the client to turn onto the side facing away from you.

◆ Pay particular attention to the anal area and posterior folds of the scrotum in males. Clean the anus with toilet tissue before washing it, if necessary.

◆ Dry the area well.

◆ For postdelivery or menstruating females, apply a perineal pad as needed from front to back. *This prevents contamination of the vagina and urethra from the anal area.*

7. Document any assessments (redness, swelling, discharge) and report findings to RN.

Part C: Providing Foot Care

INTERVENTIONS

1. Prepare the equipment and the client.

◆ Fill the washbasin with warm water at about 40 to 43°C (105 to 110°F). *Warm water promotes circulation, comforts, and refreshes.*

◆ Assist the ambulatory client to a sitting position in a chair, or the bed client to a supine or semi Fowler's position.

◆ Place a pillow under the bed client's knees. *This provides support and prevents muscle fatigue.*

◆ Place the washbasin on the moisture-resistant pad at the foot of the bed for a bed client or on the floor in front of the chair for an ambulatory client.

◆ For a bed client, pad the rim of the washbasin with a towel. *The towel prevents undue pressure on the skin.*

2. Wash the foot and soak it as required (Figure 13-12 ◆).

◆ Place one of the client's feet in the basin, and wash it with soap, paying particular attention to the interdigital areas. *Prolonged soaking is generally not recommended for diabetic clients or individuals with peripheral vascular disease.*

Figure 13-12. ◆ Soaking a foot in a basin. *Source:* © Jenny Thomas.

Prolonged soaking may remove natural skin oils, thus drying the skin and making it more susceptible to cracking and injury.

◆ Rinse the foot well to remove soap. *Soap irritates the skin if not properly removed.*

◆ Rub callused areas of the foot with the washcloth. *This helps remove dead skin layers.*

◆ If the nails are brittle or thick and require trimming, replace the water and allow the foot to soak for 10 to 20 minutes. *Soaking softens the nails and loosens debris under them.* Clean the nails as required with an orange stick or the blunt end of a toothpick. *This removes excess debris that harbors microorganisms.*

◆ Remove the foot from the basin and place it on the towel.

3. Dry the foot thoroughly and apply lotion or foot powder.

◆ Blot the foot gently with the towel to dry it thoroughly, particularly between the toes. *Harsh rubbing can damage the skin. Thorough drying reduces the risk of infection.*

◆ Apply lotion or lanolin cream. *This lubricates dry skin.*

4. *If agency policy permits,* trim the nails of the first foot while the second foot is soaking.

◆ See the discussion on nails for the appropriate method to trim nails. Note that in many agencies toenail trimming requires a physician's order or is contraindicated for clients with diabetes mellitus, toe infections, and peripheral vascular disease, unless performed by a podiatrist or general practice physician.

5. Document any foot problems observed and report them to the RN.

◆ Foot care is not generally recorded unless problems are noted.

◆ Record any signs of inflammation, infection, breaks in the skin, corns, troublesome calluses, bunions, and pressure areas. *This is of particular importance for clients with peripheral vascular disease and diabetes.*

◆ **SAMPLE DOCUMENTATION**

10:15 A.M.,	Self-help, bed bath given. Client
12/08/2005	tolerated bath without complaint.
	Client able to complete bath with
	assistance only for back. Skin intact,
	no redness or inflammation noted. —
	Lisa Patel, LPN

PROCEDURE 13-2

Providing Hair Care

PURPOSES

◆ To stimulate the blood circulation to the scalp through massage

◆ To clean the hair and increase the client's sense of well-being

◆ To distribute hair oils and provide a healthy sheen

◆ To assess or monitor hair or scalp problems (e.g., matted hair or dandruff)

EQUIPMENT

◆ Comb and brush

◆ Plastic sheet or pad

◆ Two bath towels

◆ Shampoo basin

◆ Washcloth or pad

◆ Bath blanket

◆ Receptacle for the shampoo water

◆ Cotton balls (optional)
◆ Pitcher of water
◆ Bath thermometer
◆ Liquid or cream shampoo

◆ Hair dryer
◆ Large, open-toothed or long-toothed comb (a pick)
◆ Lubricant (optional)

Part A: Shampooing the Hair

INTERVENTIONS

1. Verify agency policy and the physician's order.
   ◆ Determine whether a physician's order is needed before a shampoo can be given. *Some agencies require an order.*
   ◆ Determine the type of shampoo to be used (e.g., medicated shampoo).

2. Prepare the client.
   ◆ Determine the best time of day for the shampoo. Discuss this with the client. *A person who must remain in bed may find the shampoo tiring.* Choose a time when the client is rested and can rest after the procedure.
   ◆ Assist the client to the side of the bed from which you will work.
   ◆ Remove pins and ribbons from the hair, and brush and comb it to remove any tangles.

3. Arrange the equipment.
   ◆ Put the plastic sheet or pad on the bed under the head. *The plastic keeps the bedding dry.*
   ◆ Remove the pillow from under the client's head, and place it under the shoulders. *This hyperextends the neck.*
   ◆ Tuck a bath towel around the client's shoulders. *This keeps the shoulders dry.*
   ◆ Place the shampoo basin under the head (Figure 13-13 ◆), putting a folded washcloth or pad where the client's neck rests on the edge of the basin. *If the client is on a stretcher, the neck can rest on the edge of the sink with the washcloth as padding. Padding supports the muscles of the neck and prevents undue strain and discomfort.*
   ◆ Fanfold the top bedding down to the waist, and cover the upper part of the client with the bath blanket. *The folded bedding will stay dry, and the bath blanket, which can be discarded after the shampoo, will keep the client warm.*
   ◆ Place the receiving receptacle on a table or chair at the bedside. Put the spout of the shampoo basin over the receptacle.

4. Protect the client's eyes and ears.
   ◆ Place a damp washcloth over the client's eyes. *The washcloth protects the eyes from soapy water. A damp washcloth will not slip.*
   ◆ Place cotton balls in the client's ears if indicated. These keep water from collecting in the ear canals.

Figure 13-13. ◆ Shampooing the hair of a client confined to bed. Note the shampoo basin and the receptacle below. *Source:* © Jenny Thomas.

5. Shampoo the hair.
   ◆ Wet the hair thoroughly with the water.
   ◆ Apply shampoo to the scalp. Make a good lather with the shampoo while massaging the scalp with the pads of your fingertips. Massage all areas of the scalp systematically, for example, starting at the front and working toward the back of the head. *Massaging stimulates the blood circulation in the scalp.* The pads of the fingers are used so that the fingernails will not scratch the scalp.
   ◆ Rinse the hair briefly, and apply shampoo again.
   ◆ Make a good lather and massage the scalp as before.
   ◆ Rinse the hair thoroughly this time to remove all the shampoo. *Shampoo remaining in the hair may dry and irritate the hair and scalp.*
   ◆ Squeeze as much water as possible out of the hair with your hands.

6. Dry the hair thoroughly.

◆ Rub the client's hair with a heavy towel.
◆ Dry the hair with the dryer. Set the temperature at "warm."
◆ Continually move the dryer to prevent burning the client's scalp.

7. Ensure client comfort.
◆ Assist the person confined to bed to a comfortable position.

◆ Arrange the hair using a clean brush and comb.

8. Document the shampoo and any assessments.
◆ Report any problems noted to the RN.

Part B: Providing Hair Care for African-American Clients

INTERVENTIONS

1. Position and prepare the client appropriately.
◆ Assist the client who can sit to move to a chair. *Hair is more easily brushed and combed when the client is in a sitting position.* If health permits, assist a client confined to a bed to a sitting position by raising the head of the bed. Otherwise, assist the client to alternate side-lying positions, and do one side of the head at a time.
◆ If the client remains in bed, place a clean towel over the pillow and the client's shoulders. Place it over the sitting client's shoulders. *The towel collects any removed hair, dirt, and scaly material.*
◆ Remove any pins or ribbons in the hair.

2. Comb the hair.
◆ Apply a lubricant as the client indicates or as needed.
◆ Using a large and open-toothed comb, start at the neckline and lift and fluff the hair outward, moving upward toward the forehead (Figure 13-14A ◆).
◆ Continue fluffing the hair outward and upward until all of the hair is combed on one half of the head. Repeat the procedure for the other half.

3. Remove tangles gradually.
◆ After the hair has been lubricated, weave and lift your opened fingers through the hair to ease the tangles free.
or

Support the hair securely at the base of the scalp, if possible, to prevent pulling and discomfort. Insert a long-toothed comb into the ends of the hair and carefully comb out the ends of the tangles (Figure 13-14B).
◆ Repeat this step, each time working the comb farther up the hair shaft toward the scalp, until the hair is untangled.

4. Document assessments and special nursing interventions.
◆ Daily combing and brushing of hair are not normally recorded.
◆ Record problems such as excessive dandruff, very dry or very oily hair, or the presence of lice.

◆ SAMPLE DOCUMENTATION

9/21/2004.	Client's hair shampooed with client in
11:30 A.M.	bed using shampoo basin. Scalp
	intact. No dryness or flaking noted.
	Client tolerated procedure without
	complaint of discomfort. Client able to
	comb and style hair without assistance.
	Jeanette Rusch, LPN.

Figure 13-14. ◆ **A.** Removing tangles with a long-toothed comb **B.** Using a large open toothed comb to comb an African-American client's hair from the neckline upward toward the forehead. *Source:* © Jenny Thomas.

PROCEDURE 13-3

Providing Oral Care

PURPOSES

◆ To remove food particles and microorganisms from around and between the teeth and artificial teeth
◆ To remove dental plaque
◆ To enhance the client's feelings of well-being
◆ To prevent sores and infection of the oral tissues
◆ To maintain the continuity of the lips, tongue, and mucous membranes of the mouth
◆ To clean and moisten the membranes of the mouth and lips

EQUIPMENT

◆ Towel
◆ Disposable gloves
◆ Curved basin (emesis basin)
◆ Toothbrush (or stiff-bristled brush for dentures)

◆ Cup of tepid water
◆ Toothpaste or denture cleaner
◆ Mouthwash
◆ Dental floss, at least two pieces 20 cm (8 in) in length
◆ Floss holder (optional)
◆ Tissue or piece of gauze
◆ Denture container
◆ Clean washcloth
◆ Bite-block to hold the mouth open and teeth apart
◆ Rubber-tipped bulb syringe
◆ Suction catheter with suction apparatus (optional)
◆ Applicators and cleaning solution for cleaning the mucous membranes
◆ Petroleum jelly (Vaseline)

Part A: Brushing and Flossing the Teeth

INTERVENTIONS

1. Prepare the client.
   ◆ Explain the procedure.
   ◆ Assist the client to a sitting position in bed, if health permits. If not, assist the client to a side-lying position with the head on a pillow so that the client can spit out the rinse water.

2. Prepare the equipment.
   ◆ Place the towel under the client's chin.
   ◆ Don gloves. *Wearing gloves while providing mouth care prevents the LPN/LVN from acquiring infections. Gloves also prevent transmission of microorganisms to the client.*
   ◆ Moisten the bristles of the toothbrush with tepid water, and apply the toothpaste to the toothbrush.
   ◆ Use a soft toothbrush (a small one for a child) and the client's choice of toothpaste. For the person who does not have toothpaste, use a mixture of salt and baking soda.
   ◆ For the client who must remain in bed, place or hold the curved basin under the client's chin, fitting the small curve around the chin or neck.
   ◆ Inspect the mouth and teeth.

3. Brush the teeth.
   ◆ Hand the toothbrush to the client, or brush the client's teeth as follows:
   a. Hold the brush against the teeth with the bristles at a 45-degree angle (Figure 13-15A ◆).
      The tips of the outer bristles should rest against and penetrate under the gingival sulcus (Figure 13-15B). *The brush will clean under the sulcus of two or three teeth at one time. This sulcular technique removes plaque and cleans under the gingival margins.*
   b. Move the bristles back and forth using a vibrating or jiggling motion, from the sulcus to the crowns of the teeth.
   c. Repeat until all outer and inner surfaces of the teeth and sulci of the gums are cleaned.
   d. Clean the biting surfaces by moving the brush back and forth over them in short strokes (Figure 13-15C).
   e. If the tongue is coated, brush it gently with the toothbrush. *Brushing removes accumulated materials and coatings. A coated tongue may be caused by poor oral hygiene and low fluid intake.* Brushing gently and carefully helps prevent gagging or vomiting.

A B C

Figure 13-15. ◆ **A.** The sulcular technique: placing the bristles at a 45 angle against the teeth. **B.** Directing the tips of the outer bristles under the gingival margins. **C.** Brushing the biting surface.

◆ Hand the client the water cup or mouthwash to rinse the mouth vigorously. Then ask the client to spit the water and excess toothpaste into the basin. Some agencies supply a standard mouthwash. Alternatively, a mouth rinse of normal saline can be an effective cleaner and moisturizer. *Vigorous rinsing loosens food particles and washes out already loosened particles.*

◆ Repeat the preceding steps until the mouth is free of toothpaste and food particles.

◆ Remove the curved basin, and help the client wipe the mouth.

4. Floss the teeth.

◆ Assist the client to floss independently, or floss the teeth as follows. Waxed floss is less likely to fray than unwaxed floss; particles between the teeth attach more readily to unwaxed floss than to waxed floss. Some believe that waxed floss leaves a residue on the teeth and that plaque then adheres to the wax.

a. Wrap one end of the floss around the third finger of each hand (Figure 13-16A ◆).

b. To floss the upper teeth, use your thumb and index finger to stretch the floss (Figure 13-16B). Move the floss up and down between the teeth from the tops of the crowns to the gum and along the gum lines as far as possible. Make a "C" with the floss around the tooth edge being flossed. Start at the back on the right side and work around to the back of the left side, or work from the center teeth to the back of the jaw on either side.

c. To floss the lower teeth, use your index fingers to stretch the floss (Figure 13-16C).

◆ Give the client tepid water or mouthwash to rinse the mouth and a curved basin in which to spit the water.

◆ Assist the client in wiping the mouth.

5. Remove and dispose of equipment appropriately.

◆ Remove and clean the curved basin.

◆ Remove and discard the gloves.

6. Document assessment of the teeth, tongue, gums, and oral mucosa. Include any problems such as sores or inflammation and swelling of the gums and report findings to RN. *Brushing and flossing teeth are not usually recorded.*

A B C

Figure 13-16. ◆ **A.** Stretching the floss between the third finger of each hand. **B.** Flossing the upper teeth by using the thumbs and index fingers to stretch the floss. **C.** Flossing the lower teeth by using the index finger to stretch the floss.

Part B: Cleaning Dentures

Before beginning to clean dentures, determine (a) areas in the mouth that require ongoing assessment, and (b) whether the client has upper and lower dentures.

INTERVENTIONS

1. Place denture solution in denture container according to directions.

2. Prepare the client.
 ◆ Assist the client to a sitting or side-lying position.

3. Remove the dentures.
 ◆ Don gloves. Wearing gloves protects the LPN/LVN and client from infection.
 ◆ If the client cannot remove the dentures, take the tissue or gauze, grasp the upper plate at the front teeth with your thumb and second finger, and move the denture up and down slightly (Figure 13-17 ◆). The slight movement breaks the suction that holds the plate on the roof of the mouth.
 ◆ Lower the upper plate, move it out of the mouth, and place it in the denture container.
 ◆ Lift the lower plate, turning it so that the left side, for example, is slightly lower than the right, to remove the plate from the mouth without stretching the lips. Place the lower plate in the denture container.

4. Inspect the dentures and the mouth.
 ◆ Observe the dentures for any rough, sharp, or worn areas that could irritate the tongue or mucous membranes of the mouth, lips, and gums.
 ◆ Inspect the mouth for any redness, irritated areas, or indications of infection.
 ◆ Assess the fit of the dentures. People who have them should see a dentist at least once a year to check the fit

and the presence of any irritation to the soft tissues of the mouth. *Clients who need repairs to their dentures or new dentures may need a referral for financial assistance.*

5. Return the dentures to the mouth.
 ◆ Offer some mouthwash and a curved basin to rinse the mouth. If the client cannot insert the dentures independently, insert the plates one at a time. Hold each plate at a slight angle while inserting it, to avoid injuring the lips (Figure 13-18 ◆).

6. Assist the client as needed.
 ◆ Wipe the client's hands and mouth with the towel.
 ◆ If the client does not want to or cannot wear the dentures, store them in a denture container with water. Label the cup with the client's name and identification number.

7. Remove and discard gloves.

8. Document all relevant information.
 ◆ Document all assessments, and include any problems, such as an irritated area on the mucous membrane and report findings to RN.
 ◆ Once dentures are clean, replace them in client's mouth unless client prefers them to be left out.

Figure 13-17. ◆ Removing the top dentures by first breaking the suction.

Figure 13-18. ◆ Inserting the denture at a slight angle.

Part C: Providing Special Oral Care

INTERVENTIONS

1. Prepare the client.
 ◆ Position the unconscious client in a side-lying position, with the head of the bed lowered. *In this position, the saliva automatically runs out by gravity rather than being aspirated into the lungs. This position is the one of choice for the unconscious client receiving mouth care. If the client's head cannot be lowered, turn it to one side. The fluid will readily run out of the mouth or pool in the side of the mouth, where it can be suctioned.*
 ◆ Place the towel under the client's chin.

 ◆ Place the curved basin against the client's chin and lower cheek to receive the fluid from the mouth (Figure 13-19 ◆).
 ◆ Don gloves.

2. Clean the teeth and rinse the mouth.
 ◆ If the client has natural teeth, brush the teeth as described in Procedure 13-3A. Brush gently and carefully to avoid injuring the gums. If the client has artificial teeth, clean them as described in Procedure 13-3B.
 ◆ Rinse the client's mouth by drawing about 10 mL of water or mouthwash into the syringe and injecting it

Figure 13-19. ◆ Position of the client and placement if curved basin when providing special mouth care. *Source:* © Elena Dorfman.

gently into each side of the mouth. *If the solution is injected with force, some of it may flow down the client's throat and be aspirated into the lungs.*

◆ Watch carefully to make sure that all the rinsing solution has run out of the mouth into the basin. If not, suction the fluid from the mouth. See the section on oropharyngeal suctioning in Chapter 16. ⊂⊃ *Fluid remaining in the mouth may be aspirated into the lungs.*

◆ Repeat rinsing until the mouth is free of toothpaste, if used.

3. Inspect and clean the oral tissues.

◆ If the tissues appear dry or unclean, clean them with the applicators or gauze and cleaning solution following agency policy.

◆ Picking up one applicator, wipe the mucous membrane of one cheek. If no commercially prepared applicators are available, wrap a small gauze square around a tongue blade and moisten it. Discard the applicator or tongue blade in a waste container, and with a fresh one clean the next area. *Using separate applicators for each area of the*

mouth prevents the transfer of microorganisms from one area to another.

◆ Clean all the mouth tissues in an orderly progression, using separate applicators: the cheeks, roof of the mouth, base of the mouth, and tongue.

◆ Observe the tissues closely for inflammation and dryness.

◆ Rinse the client's mouth as described in step 2.

◆ Remove and discard gloves.

4. Ensure client comfort.

◆ Remove the basin, and dry around the client's mouth with the towel. Replace artificial dentures, if indicated.

◆ Lubricate the client's lips with petroleum jelly. *Lubrication prevents cracking and subsequent infection.*

5. Document pertinent data.

◆ Record special oral hygiene and pertinent observations.

◆ Report problems to the RN in charge.

◆ **SAMPLE DOCUMENTATION**

0930, 11/10/2003.	Assisted client with oral care. Client able to brush and floss teeth. Partial denture soaked and replaced in client's mouth. Oral mucosa intact without signs and symptoms of irritation or infection. Client states dentures fit comfortably without slipping. Daniel Fortune, LPN.

PROCEDURE 13-4

Removing, Cleaning, and Inserting a Hearing Aid

PURPOSE
◆ To maintain proper hearing aid function

EQUIPMENT
◆ Client's hearing aid
◆ Soap, water, and towels or a damp cloth
◆ Pipe cleaner or toothpick (optional)
◆ New battery (if needed)

INTERVENTIONS

1. Remove the hearing aid.
- Turn the hearing aid off and lower the volume. The on/off switch may be labeled "O" (off), "M" (microphone), "T" (telephone), or "TM" (telephone/microphone). *The batteries continue to run if the aid is not turned off.*
- Remove the earmold by rotating it slightly forward and pulling it outward.
- If the aid is not to be used for several days, remove the battery. *Removal prevents corrosion of the aid from battery leakage.*
- Store the hearing aid in a safe place. Avoid exposure to heat and moisture. *Proper storage prevents loss or damage.*

2. Clean the earmold.
- Detach the earmold if possible. Disconnect the earmold from the receiver of a body hearing aid or from the hearing aid case of behind-the-ear and eyeglasses aids where the tubing meets the hook of the case. Do not remove the earmold if it is glued or secured by a small metal ring. *Removal facilitates cleaning and prevents inadvertent damage to the other parts.*
- If the earmold is detachable, soak it in a mild soapy solution. Rinse and dry it well. Do not use isopropyl alcohol. *Alcohol can damage the hearing aid.*
- If the earmold is not detachable or is for an in-the-ear aid, wipe the earmold with a damp cloth.
- Check that the earmold opening is patent. Blow any excess moisture through the opening or remove debris (e.g., earwax) with a pipe cleaner or toothpick.
- Reattach the earmold if it was detached from the rest of the hearing aid.

3. Insert the hearing aid.
- Determine from the client if the earmold is for the left or the right ear.
- Check that the battery is inserted in the hearing aid. Turn off the hearing aid, and make sure the volume is turned all the way down. *A volume that is too loud is distressing.*
- Inspect the earmold to identify the ear canal portion. Some earmolds are fitted for only the ear canal and concha; others are fitted for all the contours of the ear. *The canal portion, common to all, can be used as a guide for correct insertion.*
- Line up the parts of the earmold with the corresponding parts of the client's ear.
- Rotate the earmold slightly forward, and insert the ear canal portion.
- Gently press the earmold into the ear while rotating it backward.
- Check that the earmold fits snugly by asking the client if it feels secure and comfortable.
- Adjust the other components of a behind-the-ear or body hearing aid.
- Turn the hearing aid on, and adjust the volume according to the client's needs.

4. Correct problems associated with improper functioning.
- If the sound is weak or there is no sound:
  a. Ensure that the volume is turned high enough.
  b. Ensure that the earmold opening is not clogged.
  c. Check the battery by turning the aid on, turning up the volume, cupping your hand over the earmold, and listening. A constant whistling sound indicates the battery is functioning. If necessary, replace the battery. Be sure that the negative (−) and positive (+) signs on the battery match those on the aid.
  d. Ensure that the ear canal is not blocked with wax. *Wax can obstruct sound waves.*
- If the client reports a whistling sound or squeal after insertion:
  a. Turn the volume down.
  b. Ensure that the earmold is properly attached to the receiver.
  c. Reinsert the earmold.

5. Document pertinent data.
- The removal and the insertion of a hearing aid are not normally recorded.
- Record any problems the client has with the hearing aid and report findings to the RN.

◆ SAMPLE DOCUMENTATION:

5/18/2006, 0730.	No wax buildup in external ear canal noted. Client denies ear discomfort. Hearing aid inserted and volume adjusted by client. Client denies discomfort upon insertion and states adequacy of hearing acuity. Alfred Donofrio, LPN.

PROCEDURE 13-5

Changing a Bed

PURPOSE

- ◆ To promote the client's comfort
- ◆ To provide a clean, neat environment for the client
- ◆ To provide a smooth, wrinkle-free bed foundation, thus minimizing sources of skin irritation
- ◆ To conserve the client's energy and maintain current health status

EQUIPMENT

- ◆ Two large sheets (some agencies may use fitted bottom sheets)
- ◆ Cloth drawsheet (optional)
- ◆ One blanket
- ◆ One bedspread (some agencies do not use bedspreads)
- ◆ Waterproof drawsheet or waterproof pads (optional)
- ◆ Pillowcase(s) for the head pillow(s)
- ◆ Portable linen hamper, if available

Part A: Changing an Unoccupied Bed

INTERVENTIONS

1. Place the fresh linen on the client's chair or overbed table; do not use another client's bed. *This prevents cross-contamination (the movement of microorganisms from one client to another) via soiled linen.*

2. Assess and assist the client out of bed.
   - ◆ Make sure that this is an appropriate and convenient time for the client to be out of bed.
   - ◆ Assess the client's health status to determine that the person can safely get out of bed. *In some hospitals it is necessary to have a written order if the client has been in bed continuously.*
   - ◆ Assess the client's pulse and respirations if indicated.
   - ◆ Assist the client to a comfortable chair.

3. Strip the bed.
   - ◆ Check bed linens for any items belonging to the client, and detach the call bell or any drainage tubes from the bed linen.
   - ◆ Loosen all bedding systematically, starting at the head of the bed on the far side and moving around the bed up to the head of the bed on the near side. *Moving around the bed systematically prevents stretching and reaching and possible muscle strain.*
   - ◆ Remove the pillowcases, if soiled, and place the pillows on the bedside chair near the foot of the bed.
   - ◆ Fold reusable linens, such as the bedspread and top sheet on the bed, into fourths. First, fold the linen in half by bringing the top edge even with the bottom

edge, and then grasp it at the center of the middle fold and bottom edges (Figure 13-20 ◆). *Folding linens saves time and energy when reapplying the linens on the bed.*
- ◆ Remove the waterproof pad and discard it if soiled.
- ◆ Roll all soiled linen inside the bottom sheet, hold it away from your uniform, and place it directly in the linen hamper. These actions are essential to prevent the transmission of microorganisms to the LPN/LVN and others.
- ◆ Grasp the mattress securely, using the lugs if present, and move the mattress up to the head of the bed.

4. Apply the bottom sheet and drawsheet.
   - ◆ Place the folded bottom sheet with its center fold on the center of the bed. Make sure the sheet is hemside down

Figure 13-20. ◆ Folding reusable linens into fourths when removing them from the bed.

for a smooth foundation. Spread the sheet out over the mattress, and allow a sufficient amount of sheet at the top to tuck under the mattress. The top of the sheet needs to be well tucked under to remain securely in place, especially when the head of the bed is elevated. Place the sheet along the edge of the mattress at the foot of the bed and do not tuck it in (unless it is a contour sheet).

◆ If the bottom sheet is not fitted miter the sheet at the top corner on the near side (see Figure 13-8) and tuck the sheet under the mattress, working from the head of the bed to the foot.

◆ If a waterproof drawsheet is used, place it over the bottom sheet so that the center fold is at the center line of the bed and the top and bottom edges will extend from the middle of the client's back to the area of the midthigh or knee. Fanfold the uppermost half of the folded drawsheet at the center or far edge of the bed and tuck in the near edge.

◆ Lay the cloth drawsheet over the waterproof sheet in the same manner.

◆ Optional: Before moving to the other side of the bed, place the top linens on the bed hemside up, unfold them, tuck them in, and miter the bottom corners. *Completing the entire side of the bed saves time and energy.*

5. Move to the other side and secure the bottom linens.
   ◆ Tuck the bottom sheet in under the head of the mattress, pull the sheet firmly, and miter the corner of the sheet if a fitted sheet is not being used.
   ◆ Pull the remainder of the sheet firmly so that there are no wrinkles. *Wrinkles can cause discomfort for the client.* Tuck the sheet in at the side.
   ◆ Complete this same process for the drawsheet(s).

6. Apply or complete the top sheet, blanket, and spread.
   ◆ Place the top sheet, hemside up, on the bed so that its center fold is at the center of the bed and the top edge is even with the top edge of the mattress.
   ◆ Unfold the sheet over the bed.
   ◆ Optional: Make a vertical or a horizontal toe pleat in the sheet to provide additional room for the client's feet.
   a. Vertical toe pleat: Make a fold in the sheet 5 to 10 cm (2 to 4 in) perpendicular to the foot of the bed (Figure 13-21A ◆).
   b. Horizontal toe pleat: Make a fold in the sheet 5 to 10 cm (2 to 4 in) across the bed near the foot (Figure 13-21B). *Loosening the top covers around the feet after the client is in bed is another way to provide additional space.*
   ◆ Follow the same procedure for the blanket and the spread, but place the top edges about 15 cm (6 in) from the head of the bed to allow a cuff of sheet to be folded over them.
   ◆ Tuck in the sheet, blanket, and spread at the foot of the bed, and miter the corner, using all three layers of linen. Leave the sides of the top sheet, blanket, and spread hanging freely unless toe pleats were provided.

A

B

Figure 13-21. ◆ **A.** A vertical toe pleat. **B.** A horizontal toe pleat.

◆ Fold the top of the top sheet down over the spread, providing a cuff. *The cuff of sheet makes it easier for the client to pull the covers up.*

◆ Move to the other side of the bed and secure the top bedding in the same manner.

7. Put clean pillowcases on the pillows as required.
   ◆ Grasp the closed end of the pillowcase at the center with one hand.
   ◆ Gather up the sides of the pillowcase and place them over the hand grasping the case. Then grasp the center of one short side of the pillow through the pillowcase (Figure 13-22 ◆).
   ◆ With the free hand, pull the pillowcase over the pillow.

Figure 13-22. ◆ Method for putting a clean pillowcase on a pillow.

◆ Adjust the pillowcase so that the pillow fits into the corners of the case and the seams are straight. *A smoothly fitting pillowcase is more comfortable than a wrinkled one.*
◆ Place the pillows appropriately at the head of the bed.

8. Provide for client comfort and safety.
   ◆ Attach the signal cord so that the client can conveniently use it. Some cords have clamps that attach to the sheet or pillowcase. Others are attached by a safety pin.
   ◆ If the bed is currently being used by a client, either fold back the top covers at one side or fanfold them down to the center of the bed. *This makes it easier for the client to get into the bed.*

◆ Place the bedside table and the overbed table so that they are available to the client.
◆ Leave the bed in the high position if the client is returning by stretcher, or place in the low position if the client is returning to bed after being up.

9. Document and report pertinent data.
   ◆ Bedmaking is not normally recorded.
   ◆ Record any nursing assessments, such as the client's physical status and pulse and respiratory rates before and after being out of bed, as indicated. Report any changes in client's status to the RN.

Part B: Changing an Occupied Bed

INTERVENTIONS

1. Remove the top bedding.
   ◆ Remove any equipment attached to the bed linen, such as a signal light.
   ◆ Loosen all the top linen at the foot of the bed, and remove the spread and the blanket.
   ◆ Leave the top sheet over the client (the top sheet can remain over the client if it is being changed and if it will provide sufficient warmth), or replace it with a bath blanket as follows:
   a. Spread the bath blanket over the top sheet.
   b. Ask the client to hold the top edge of the blanket.
   c. Reaching under the blanket from the side, grasp the top edge of the sheet and draw it down to the foot of the bed, leaving the blanket in place.
   d. Remove the sheet from the bed and place it in the soiled linen hamper.

2. Move the mattress up on the bed.
   ◆ Place the bed in the flat position, if the client's health permits.
   ◆ Grasp the mattress lugs and, using good body mechanics, move the mattress up to the head of the bed. Ask the client to assist, if permitted, by grasping the head of the bed and pulling as you push. If the client is heavy, you may need help another staff member.

3. Change the bottom sheet and drawsheet.
   ◆ Assist the client to turn on the side facing away from the side where the clean linen is.
   ◆ Raise the side rail nearest the client. This protects the client from falling. If there is no side rail, have another staff member support the client at the edge of the bed.
   ◆ Loosen the foundation of the linen on the side of the bed near the linen supply.
   ◆ Fanfold the drawsheet and the bottom sheet at the center of the bed (Figure 13-23 ◆), as close to the client as possible. *Doing this leaves the near half of the bed free to be changed.*

Figure 13-23. ◆ Fanfolding soiled linen as close to the client as possible.

◆ Place the new bottom sheet on the bed, and vertically fanfold the half to be used on the far side of the bed as close to the client as possible. Tuck the sheet under the near half of the bed and miter the corner if a fitted sheet is not being used.
◆ Place the clean drawsheet on the bed with the center fold at the center of the bed. Fanfold the uppermost half vertically at the center of the bed and tuck the near side edge under the side of the mattress.
◆ Assist the client to roll over toward you onto the clean side of the bed. The client rolls over the fanfolded linen at the center of the bed.
◆ Move the pillows to the clean side for the client's use. Raise the side rail before leaving the side of the bed.
◆ Move to the other side of the bed and lower the side rail.
◆ Remove the used linen and place it in the portable hamper.
◆ Unfold the fanfolded bottom sheet from the center of the bed.
◆ Facing the side of the bed, use both hands to pull the bottom sheet so that it is smooth and tuck the excess under the side of the mattress.

◆ Unfold the drawsheet fanfolded at the center of the bed and pull it tightly with both hands. Pull the sheet in three sections: (a) face the side of the bed to pull the middle section; (b) face the far top corner to pull the bottom section; and (c) face the far bottom corner to pull the top section.

◆ Tuck the excess drawsheet under the side of the mattress.

4. Reposition the client in the center of the bed.

◆ Reposition the pillows at the center of the bed.

◆ Assist the client to the center of the bed. Determine what position the client requires or prefers and assist the client to that position.

5. Apply or complete the top bedding.

◆ Spread the top sheet over the client and either ask the client to hold the top edge of the sheet or tuck it under the shoulders. *The sheet should remain over the client when the bath blanket or used sheet is removed.*

◆ Complete the top of the bed.

6. Ensure continued safety of the client.

◆ Raise the side rails. Place the bed in the low position before leaving the bedside.

◆ Attach the signal cord to the bed linen within the client's reach.

◆ Put items used by the client within easy reach.

◆ SAMPLE DOCUMENTATION

2/3/2005,	Bed linens changed with client
1145.	occupying bed. Client able to turn in
	bed with assistance and denies
	discomfort during procedure. Indwelling
	catheter patent and draining. IV tubing
	patent. Client sitting up in bed with
	side rails up, call light within reach. ———
	Tari Heiland, LPN.

Chapter Review

Use the audio glossary feature of either the CD-ROM or the Companion Website to hear the correct pronunciation of the following key terms.

Introduction
hygiene, early morning care, morning care, afternoon care, hour of sleep (HS) care, as-needed (prn) care

Skin, foot, and nail care
sebum, cleaning baths, therapeutic baths

Hair care
alopecia, lanugo, dandruff, ticks, pediculosis, scabies, hirsutism

Ear care
cerumen, hearing aid

Supporting a hygienic environment
bed cradle

Key Points

* Clients' hygienic practices are influenced to a large degree by their sociocultural background.

* When clients cannot meet their own hygiene needs, the LPN/LVN assists them. While providing care, the nurse has an excellent opportunity to observe the client's condition, build the nurse–client relationship, and provide some teaching.

* Nursing care of the skin takes into account the client's age and functional ability, as well as the condition of the skin.

* When planning hygiene care the LPN/LVN must consider client preferences.

* The LPN/LVN provides perineal–genital care for clients who are unable to do so for themselves.

* The LPN/LVN can often teach clients how to prevent foot problems. Foot assessment should be done at least at the beginning and end of each shift.

* Oral hygiene should include daily dental flossing and mechanical brushing of the teeth.

* Regular dental checkups and fluoride supplements are recommended to maintain healthy teeth.

* The LPN/LVN provides special oral care to clients who are helpless (e.g., unconscious) and who have oral problems.

* Hair care includes daily combing and brushing and regular shampooing.

* African-American clients' hair may require special care.

* The LPN/LVN may need to assist helpless clients with their artificial eyes, eyeglasses, and contact lenses.

* Clients with a hearing aid may require nursing assistance with the device.

* Changing bed linens is a part of maintaining hygiene.

* It is important to keep beds clean and comfortable for clients.

EXPLORE MediaLink

Additional interactive resources for this chapter can be found on the Companion Website at www.prenhall.com/ramont. Click on Chapter 13 and "Begin" to select the activities for this chapter.

For chapter-related NCLEX-style questions and an audio glossary, access the accompanying CD-ROM in this book.

Animation:
* cavities

∞ For Further Study

For detailed information about physical assessment, see Chapter 11.

For discussion of skin integrity, skin impairment, and heat and cold applications, see Chapter 12.

For a detailed discussion of body heat losses and gains, see Chapter 14.

Oropharyngeal suctioning is discussed in Chapter 16.

Back massages to promote circulation are discussed in Chapter 20.

For additional information on medications, see Chapter 21.

The diagnosis Deficient Knowledge is discussed in detail in Chapter 23.

Critical Thinking Care Map

Caring for a Client with Oral Cavity Problems

NCLEX Focus Area: Health Promotion and Maintenance: Prevention and Early Detection of Disease

Case Study: Joe Kwan, 46 years old, was admitted with a fractured femur. He is on bed rest and is in Buck's traction. He is scheduled for an ORIF at 11:00 A.M. Maureen Stiffel, LVN, has been assigned to assist him with his bath and oral hygiene. Mr. Kwan is NPO; a Foley catheter is in place. He is receiving intravenous D_5W in NSS; it is infusing at 100 cc/hr. VS: 99.2/78/20, BP 134/82, pulse ox 98% on room air.

Nursing Diagnosis: Impaired Oral Mucous Membrane

COLLECT DATA

Subjective	Objective
_____	_____
_____	_____
_____	_____
_____	_____
_____	_____
_____	_____

Would you report this data? Yes/No

If yes, to: _____

Nursing Care

_____

_____

_____

_____

_____

_____

_____

_____

_____

_____

_____

How would you document this? _____

_____

_____

_____

_____

Data Collected
(use those that apply)

- Teeth stained from heavy smoking.
- One large cavity evident in second lower left molar.
- Tartar buildup along gum margins.
- Pronounced halitosis.
- Gums are reddened in some area and bleed when flossed.
- States, "I can't remember when I last saw a dentist."

Nursing Interventions
(use those that apply)

- Inspect oral cavity at least once daily and note any discoloration, lesions, edema, bleeding, exudate, or dryness.
- Encourage client to take deep breaths and cough at intervals.
- Thoroughly orient the client to environment. Place call light within reach and show how to call for assistance. Answer call light promptly.
- Determine client's usual method of oral care and address any concerns related to oral care.
- Use tap water or normal saline to provide oral care; do not use commercial mouthwash containing alcohol or hydrogen peroxide.
- Plan care activities around periods of greatest comfort whenever possible.
- Identify reasons client has not seen a dentist regularly.
- Use foam sticks to moisten the oral mucous membrane, clean out debris and swab while client is NPO.
- Keep lips well lubricated using petroleum jelly or a similar product.

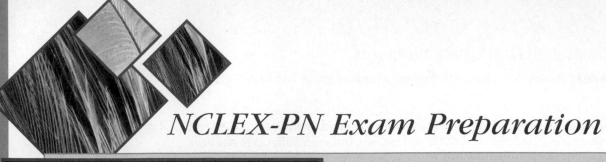

NCLEX-PN Exam Preparation

1. A client's primary nurse asks you if your assigned client has had early A.M. care. The primary nurse wants to know if you (or someone else) has done which of the following things with or for the client?
   a. Taken the client's vital signs
   b. Completed the initial assessment
   c. Helped the client with oral care and face and handwashing
   d. Given the client a shower or bath and ambulated the client

2. When working with a client who needs assistance with personal hygiene and who has a number of personal preferences about how and when it should be done, the best action on your part would be to:
   a. Follow client's preferences as long as compatible with client's health and equipment available
   b. Tell client you are a professional nurse and you will determine when and how to do these tasks
   c. Determine the most efficient way to carry out the personal hygiene tasks and do it this way
   d. Ignore the client's preferences and quietly do hygiene tasks the way you have been taught

3. You are assigned to care for a client with impaired circulation of the lower extremities. You assess the client's feet and find that the skin is very dry and the heels have reddened areas. Of the following, which is the appropriate intervention?
   a. Be sure that the bottom sheet is taut and free of wrinkles.
   b. Massage the feet with alcohol and allow to air dry.
   c. After bathing the client, dry the client's feet briskly.
   d. Tuck top sheet and blanket in tightly to keep feet warm.

4. The incidence of skin breakdown in the elderly in a long-term care facility can most be reduced through which of the following actions on the part of the nursing staff?
   a. Offering a wider variety of pureed foods
   b. Restricting the use of caffeine drinks
   c. Offering water throughout the day to ensure hydration
   d. Reducing the amount of pain medication

5. When doing oral hygiene on an unconscious client, the position of choice is which of the following positions?
   a. Head elevated
   b. Side-lying
   c. Prone
   d. Supine

6. The long-term care facility nursing staff has scheduled the elderly clients to be showered or bathed every other day. Younger clients are being showered or bathed daily. The best reason for showering or bathing the elderly clients every other day is:
   a. Showering and bathing tires the elderly more.
   b. It takes longer to shower or bathe the elderly.
   c. There is not enough staff to give everyone daily showers or baths.
   d. Less frequent bathing prevents removal of sebum from the skin, which would cause dryness.

7. When a client is not going to be using her hearing aid for several days, the nurse needs to:
   a. Turn the volume down
   b. Plug hearing aid into a charger
   c. Remove the batteries
   d. Store hearing aid in refrigerator

8. The school nurse is working with students and the physical education director in order to prevent tinea pedis. The nurse will evaluate that a student understands prevention of tinea pedis if the student:
   a. Washes her body well with an antiseptic soap in the gym shower
   b. Wears shower shoes in the shower and the dressing room
   c. Dries her feet well after leaving the shower room
   d. Wears stockings and changes these stockings daily

9. You are bathing a client whose corneal reflex is impaired. Which of the following actions is most important when providing eye care?
   a. Wipe from the outer to inner canthus
   b. Use a different cotton ball for each wipe
   c. Cover the eyes with an eye shield
   d. Use fresh water to cleanse the eyes

10. When changing a client's bed linens, the nurse should:
    a. Shake each of the client's bed linens before putting them in the hamper
    b. Wrap soiled linen in bottom sheet, hold away from you, and put it in the hamper
    c. Put the dirty linen on the floor until you have finished changing the bed linens
    d. Take the dIrty linen out of the room before putting the clean linen on the bed

Answers for Review Questions, as well as discussion of Case Study and Critical Thinking Care Map questions, appear in Appendix IV.

Vital Signs

SHARING experiences

During my first days in clinical passing meds, I was so nervous about knowing everything [I needed to know] about my meds. I had to give a lot of blood pressure lowering medications. I discovered that one client's BP was already low, *so I had to hold most of the meds. I learned that it is not just identifying the meds that is important, but knowing what they are, what they can do, and why your client is receiving them.*

Michelle Marshall, LVN student, North Orange County Regional Occupational Program, Anaheim, CA.

LEARNING outcomes

After completing this chapter, you will be able to:

- Describe factors that affect the vital signs and their accurate measurement.
- Identify normal ranges for each vital sign and variations by age.
- Describe ways in which the body produces and loses heat.
- Describe the body's temperature-regulating system.
- Discuss the advantages and disadvantages of oral, tympanic, rectal, and axillary methods for measuring body temperature.
- Describe appropriate nursing care for alterations in body temperature.
- Identify nine sites commonly used to assess the pulse and state the reasons for their use.
- Explain how to measure the apical pulse and apical–radial pulse.
- Describe the mechanics of breathing and identify the characteristics that should be included in a respiratory assessment.
- Differentiate systolic from diastolic blood pressure and describe five phases of Korotkoff's sounds.
- Describe various methods and sites used to measure blood pressure.

MediaLink

www.prenhall.com/ramont

Use the address above to access the free, interactive Companion Website created for this textbook. Get hints, instant feedback, and textbook references to chapter-related NCLEX-style questions. Link to other interesting sites.

Audio Glossary:
Use the Companion Website, or the CD-ROM disk enclosed with your textbook, to hear the pronunciation of key terms in the chapter.

Together, the vital or cardinal signs—body temperature, pulse, respirations, and blood pressure—reflect changes in function that otherwise might not be observed. Monitoring a client's vital signs should be a thoughtful, scientific assessment. Vital signs must be evaluated with reference to the client's present and prior health status and be compared to accepted normal standards. (See Table 14-1 ◆.) The "fifth vital sign," pain, is discussed in the following chapter. ◎

Some medical facilities have policies about how often to take the clients' vital signs. Physicians may also order a vital sign (e.g., "blood pressure q2h") to be taken at specific times. Ordered assessments, however, should be considered the minimum. A nurse should measure vital signs more often if the client's health status requires it. Vital signs are routinely assessed in the following order: temperature first; pulse and respirations are taken while the thermometer is in place, if possible. Respirations should be assessed while your fingers are still touching the pulse point, so that the client will be unaware and not alter the breathing pattern. The blood pressure should follow the other vital signs.

◆ Body Temperature

Body temperature reflects the balance between the heat produced and the heat lost from the body, measured in heat units called degrees.

The normal body temperature (temperature of deep tissues of the body) is actually a range of temperatures. When measured orally, the average body temperature of an adult is between 36.7°C (98°F) and 37°C (98.6°F) (Figure 14-1 ◆). Rectal temperature is one degree higher, 37.5°C (99.6°F); axillary is one degree lower, 35.4°C (97.6°F); and tympanic is 37.6°C (99.7°F).

Figure 14-1. ◆ Estimated ranges of body temperatures in normal persons. *Source:* E. F. DuBois, *Fever and the regulation of body temperature* (Springfield, IL: Charles C. Thomas, 1948). Courtesy of Charles C. Thomas, Publisher.

The body continually produces heat as a by-product of metabolism. When the amount of heat produced by the body exactly equals the amount of heat lost, the person is in heat balance.

A number of factors affect the body's heat production. The most important are these five:

1. *Basal metabolic rate (BMR).* The basal metabolic rate is the rate of energy utilization in the body required to maintain essential activities such as breathing. Metabolic rates decrease with age. In general, the younger the person, the higher the BMR.
2. *Muscle activity.* Muscle activity, including shivering, increases the metabolic rate.
3. *Thyroxine output.* Increased thyroxine output increases the rate of cellular metabolism throughout the body and increases heat.

TABLE 14-1 VARIATIONS IN NORMAL VITAL SIGNS BY AGE

AGE	TEMPERATURE IN DEGREES CELSIUS	PULSE (AVERAGE AND RANGES)	RESPIRATIONS (AVERAGE AND RANGES)	BLOOD PRESSURE (MM HG)
Newborns	36.8 (axillary)	130 (80–180)	35 (30–80)	73/55
1–3 years	37.7 (rectal)	120 (80–140)	30 (20–40)	90/55
6–8 years	37 (oral)	100 (75–120)	20 (15–25)	95/57
10 years	37 (oral)	70 (50–90)	19 (15–25)	102/62
Teen years	37 (oral)	70 (50–90)	18 (15–20)	120/80
Adult	37 (oral)	80 (60–100)	16 (12–20)	120/80
Older Adult (> 70 years)	36 (oral)	80 (60–100)	16 (15–20)	Possible increased diastolic

4. *Epinephrine, norepinephrine, and sympathetic stimulation.* These hormones immediately increase the rate of cellular metabolism in many body tissues.
5. *Fever.* Fever increases the cellular metabolic rate and thus increases the body's temperature further.

REGULATION OF BODY TEMPERATURE

When the skin becomes chilled over the entire body or when cold sensors in the brain are stimulated, three physiologic processes take place to increase the body temperature:

1. *Shivering* increases heat production.
2. Sweating is inhibited to decrease heat loss.
3. Vasoconstriction decreases heat loss.

When the sensors in the hypothalamus of the brain detect heat, they send out signals intended to reduce the temperature. The body decreases heat production and increases heat loss by:

1. Sweating, which increases evaporation and cooling.
2. Peripheral vasodilatation, which facilitates cooling.

Also, when sensors are stimulated, the person consciously makes appropriate adjustments, such as putting on additional clothing in response to cold or turning on a fan in response to heat.

Factors Affecting Body Temperature

Nurses should be aware of the factors that can affect a client's body temperature. They should recognize normal temperature variations and understand the significance of body temperature measurements that deviate from normal. Among the factors that affect body temperature are the following:

◆ *Age.* The infant is greatly influenced by the temperature of the environment and must be protected from extreme changes. Children's temperatures continue to fluctuate more than those of adults until puberty. Older people, particularly those over 75 years, are sensitive to extremes in temperature, and are at risk of hypothermia (temperatures below 36°C, or 96.8°F). Some of the reasons for this include inadequate diet, loss of subcutaneous fat, lack of activity, and reduced efficiency of the temperature regulating system (see Table 14-1).
◆ *Diurnal variations (circadian rhythms).* Body temperatures normally change throughout the day, varying as much as 1.0°C (1.8°F) between the early morning and the late afternoon. The point of highest body temperature is usually reached between 1600 and 2000 hours (4:00 P.M. and 8 P.M.), and the lowest point is reached during sleep between 0400 and 0600 hours (4:00 and 6:00 A.M.) (Figure 14-2 ◆).
◆ *Exercise.* Hard work or strenuous exercise can increase body temperature to as high as 38.3 to 40°C (101 to 104°F) measured rectally.
◆ *Hormones.* Women usually experience more hormonal fluctuations than men. In women, progesterone secretion at the

Figure 14-2. ◆ Range of oral temperatures during 24 hours for a healthy young adult.

time of ovulation raises body temperature by about 0.3 to 0.6°C (0.5 to 1.0°F) above basal temperature.
◆ *Stress.* Stimulation of the sympathetic nervous system can increase the production of epinephrine and norepinephrine, thereby increasing metabolic activity and heat production. Nurses may anticipate that a highly stressed or anxious client could have an elevated body temperature for that reason.
◆ *Environment.* Extremes in environmental temperatures can affect a person's temperature regulatory systems. If the temperature is assessed in a very warm room the temperature may be elevated. Similarly, if the client has been outside in extremely cold weather without suitable clothing, the body temperature may be low.

ALTERATIONS IN BODY TEMPERATURE

Pyrexia

A body temperature above the usual range is called **pyrexia, hyperthermia,** or fever. A very high fever, such as 41°C (105.8°F), is called *hyperpyrexia* (Figure 14-3 ◆). The client who has a fever is referred to as *febrile;* one who does not have a fever is referred to as **afebrile.**

Four common types of fevers are intermittent, remittent, relapsing, and constant. During an *intermittent fever,* the body temperature alternates at regular intervals between periods of fever and periods of normal or subnormal temperatures. During a *remittent fever,* a wide range of temperature fluctuations (more than 2°C [3.6°F]) occurs over the 24-hour period, all of which are above normal. In a *relapsing fever,* short febrile periods of a few days are interspersed with periods of 1 or 2 days of normal temperature. During a *constant fever,* the body temperature fluctuates minimally but always remains above normal. The manifestations of fever vary with the onset, course, and abatement stages of the fever (Box 14-1 ◆).

Very high temperatures, such as 41 to 42°C (106 to 108°F), damage cells throughout the body, particularly in the brain where destruction of neuronal cells is irreversible. Damage to the liver, kidneys, and other body organs can also be great enough to disrupt functioning and eventually cause death.

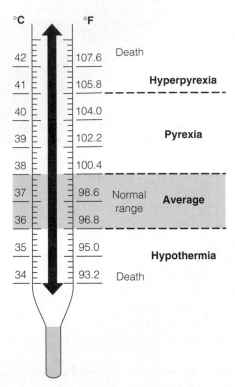

Figure 14-3. ◆ Terms used to describe alterations in body temperature (oral measurements) and ranges in Celsius (centigrade) and Fahrenheit scales.

When the cause of the high temperature is suddenly removed, the body's thermostat is reduced to a lower value, perhaps even back to the original normal level. In this instance, the hypothalamus now attempts to lower the temperature to 37°C (98.6°F). Heat loss responses cause a reduction of the body temperature to occur; manifestations are excessive sweating and a hot, flushed skin due to sudden vasodilation. This sudden change of events is known as the **crisis** of a pyrexic condition. A more gradual return of the body temperature to normal is referred to as a *resolution by lysis.* Nursing interventions for a client who has a fever are designed to support the body's normal physiologic processes, provide comfort, and prevent complications. During the course of fever, the nurse needs to monitor the client's vital signs closely (Box 14-2 ◆).

Nursing measures during the chill phase are designed to help the client decrease heat loss and raise the core body temperature. During the flush or crisis phase, body processes are attempting to lower the core temperature to normal. At this time, the nurse takes measures to increase heat loss and decrease heat production.

Hypothermia

Hypothermia is core body temperature below the lower limit of normal. The three physiologic mechanisms of hypothermia are (a) excessive heat loss; (b) inadequate heat production to counteract the heat loss; and (c) impaired hypo-

---

BOX 14-1
MANIFESTATIONS OF FEVER

Onset (Cold or Chill Stage)
◆ Increased heart rate
◆ Increased respiratory rate and depth
◆ Shivering
◆ Pallid, cold skin
◆ Complaints of feeling cold
◆ Cyanotic nail beds
◆ "Gooseflesh" appearance of the skin
◆ Cessation of sweating

Course
◆ Absence of chills
◆ Skin that feels warm
◆ Photosensitivity
◆ Glassy-eyed appearance
◆ Increased pulse and respiratory rates
◆ Increased thirst
◆ Mild to severe dehydration
◆ Drowsiness, restlessness, delirium, or convulsions
◆ Herpetic lesions of the mouth
◆ Loss of appetite (if the fever is prolonged)
◆ Malaise, weakness, and aching muscles

Defervescence (Fever Abatement)
◆ Skin that appears flushed and feels warm
◆ Sweating
◆ Decreased shivering
◆ Possible dehydration

---

thalamic temperature regulation. The manifestations of hypothermia are given in Box 14-3 ◆.

Hypothermia may be accidental or induced. Accidental hypothermia can occur as a result of (a) exposure to a cold environment (i.e., below 16°C [60.8°F]), (b) immersion in cold water, and (c) lack of adequate clothing, shelter, or heat. In older people the problem can be compounded by a decreased metabolic rate and the use of sedatives, which depress the metabolic rate further.

Managing the hypothermia involves removing the client from the cold and rewarming the client's body. For the client with mild hypothermia, the body is rewarmed by applying blankets. For the client with severe hypothermia, a hyperthermia blanket (an electronically controlled blanket that provides a specified temperature) is applied, and warm intravenous fluids are given. Wet clothing, which increases heat loss because of the high conductivity of water, should be replaced with dry clothing. See Box 14-4 ◆ for nursing interventions for clients who have hypothermia.

Induced hypothermia is the deliberate lowering of the body temperature to decrease the need for oxygen by the body

---

BOX 14-2
NURSING CARE CHECKLIST

CLIENTS WITH FEVER

☑ Monitor vital signs.
☑ Assess skin color and temperature.
☑ Monitor white blood cell count, hematocrit value, and other pertinent laboratory reports for indications of infection or dehydration.
☑ Remove excess blankets when the client feels warm, but provide extra warmth when the client feels chilled.
☑ Provide adequate nutrition and fluids (e.g., 2,500–3,000 mL per day) to meet the increased metabolic demands and prevent dehydration. Clients who sweat profusely can become dehydrated.

☑ Measure intake and output.
☑ Reduce physical activity to limit heat production, especially during the flush stage.
☑ Administer antipyretics (drugs that reduce the level of fever) as ordered.
☑ Provide oral hygiene to keep the mucous membranes moist. They can become dry and cracked as a result of excessive fluid loss.
☑ Provide a tepid sponge bath to increase heat loss through conduction.
☑ Provide dry clothing and bed linens.

---

tissues. Induced hypothermia can involve the whole body or a body part. It is sometimes indicated prior to surgery (e.g., cardiac and brain surgery).

TEMPERATURE ASSESSMENT METHODS

The four most common sites for measuring body temperature are oral, rectal, axillary, and the tympanic membrane. Each of the sites has advantages and disadvantages (Table 14-2 ◆).

The *tympanic membrane* (see photo in Procedure 14-1), is becoming the preferred site for taking body temperature. Tympanic membrane temperature readings average 1.1 to 1.5°F higher than oral temperature readings. Like the sublingual oral site, the tympanic membrane has an abundant arterial blood supply. The tympanic infrared method is quickly becoming the method of choice in clients over 3 months of age. The oral site is an equally preferred site. This method reflects

TABLE 14-2 COMPARISON OF FOUR SITES FOR MEASURING BODY TEMPERATURE

SITE	ADVANTAGES	DISADVANTAGES
Oral	Most accessible and convenient	Mercury-in-glass thermometers can break if bitten; therefore they are contraindicated for children under 6 years and clients who are confused or who have convulsive disorders. Inaccurate if client has just ingested hot or cold food or fluid or smoked. Could injure the mouth following oral surgery.
Rectal	Most reliable measurement	Inconvenient and more unpleasant for clients; difficult for client who cannot turn to the side. Could injure the rectum following rectal surgery. Placement of the thermometer at different sites within the rectum yields different temperatures, yet placement at the same site each time is difficult. A rectal glass thermometer does not respond to changes in arterial temperatures as quickly as an oral thermometer, a fact that may be potentially dangerous for febrile clients because misleading information may be acquired. Presence of stool may interfere with thermometer placement. If the stool is soft, the thermometer may be embedded in stool rather than against the wall of the rectum. If the stool is impacted, the depth of the thermometer insertion may be insufficient. In newborns and infants, insertion of the rectal thermometer has resulted in ulcerations and rectal perforations. *Many agencies advise against using rectal thermometers on neonates.*
Axillary	Safest and most noninvasive	The thermometer must be left in place a long time to obtain an accurate measurement.
Tympanic membrane	Readily accessible; reflects the core temperature. Very fast.	Can be uncomfortable and involves risk of injuring the membrane if the probe is inserted too far. Repeated measurements may vary. Right and left measurements can differ. Presence of cerumen can affect the reading.

BOX 14-3
MANIFESTATIONS OF HYPOTHERMIA

◆ Decreased body temperature, pulse, and respirations
◆ Severe shivering (initially)
◆ Feelings of cold and chills
◆ Pale, cool, waxy skin
◆ Hypotension
◆ Decreased urinary output
◆ Lack of muscle coordination
◆ Disorientation
◆ Drowsiness progressing to coma

BOX 14-4
NURSING CARE CHECKLIST

CLIENTS WITH HYPOTHERMIA

☑ Provide a warm environment (room temperature).
☑ Provide dry clothing.
☑ Apply warm blankets.
☑ Keep limbs close to body.
☑ Cover the client's scalp with a cap or turban.
☑ Supply warm oral or intravenous fluids.
☑ Apply warming pads.

---

changing body temperature more quickly than the rectal method. Rectal temperature readings are considered to be the most accurate. The axilla is the preferred site for measuring temperature in newborns because it is accessible and offers no possibility of rectal perforation. Nursing students should check facility protocol when taking the temperature of newborns, infants, toddlers, and children. Clients for whom the axillary method of temperature assessment is appropriate include adult clients with oral inflammation or wired jaws, clients recovering from oral surgery, clients who are breathing through their mouths (e.g., following nasal surgery), irrational clients, and clients for whom other temperature sites are contraindicated.

In addition to the four common sites for measuring temperature, the forehead may also be used. Body temperature is measured by using a chemical thermometer. Forehead temperature measurements are most useful for infants and children where a more invasive measurement is not necessary. If the forehead indicates a temperature elevation, a glass or electronic thermometer should be used to obtain a more accurate measurement.

Types of Thermometers

Traditionally, body temperatures have been measured using mercury-in-glass thermometers. Oral thermometers may have long, slender tips or short, rounded tips (Figure 14-4 ◆). The rounded thermometer can be used at the rectal as well as other sites. In some medical facilities, thermometers may be color coded (red thermometers for rectal temperatures, silver blue for oral and axillary temperatures).

Many facilities have discontinued use of mercury-in-glass thermometers due to breakage and potential for hazardous contamination from spilled mercury.

Electronic thermometers offer another method of assessing body temperatures. They can provide a reading in only 2 to 60 seconds, depending on the model. The equipment consists of a battery-operated portable electronic unit, a probe that the nurse attaches to the unit, and a probe cover, which is usually disposable (Figure 14-5 ◆).

Chemical disposable thermometers are also used to measure body temperatures. Chemical thermometers using liquid crystal dots, bars, or heat-sensitive tape or patches applied to the forehead change color to indicate temperature. Some of these are single use and others may be reused several times. One type that has small chemical dots at one end is shown in

Figure 14-4. ◆ Two types of thermometer tips for glass thermometers. *Source:* © Elena Dorfman.

Figure 14-5. ◆ An electronic thermometer. Note the probe and probe cover. *Source:* © Elena Dorfman.

Figure 14-6. ◆ A chemical thermometer showing a reading of 99.2°F.

Figure 14-6 ◆. To read the temperature, the nurse notes the highest reading among the dots that have changed color.

Temperature-sensitive tape may also be used to obtain a general indication of body surface temperature. The tape contains liquid crystals that change color according to temperature. When applied to the skin, usually of the forehead or abdomen, the temperature digits on the tape respond by changing color (Figure 14-7 ◆). The skin area should be dry. After the length of time specified by the manufacturer (e.g., 15 seconds), a color appears on the tape. The tape is removed and discarded after the color has been compared to the scale provided by the manufacturer. This method is particularly useful at home and for infants whose temperatures are to be monitored for any reason.

Temperature Scales

The body temperature is measured in degrees on two scales: Celsius (centigrade) and Fahrenheit. On a glass thermometer the Celsius scale normally extends from 34.0° to 42.0°C. The Fahrenheit scale usually extends from 94° to 108°F. Body temperatures rarely extend beyond these scales (see Figure 14-3).

Sometimes a nurse needs to convert a Celsius reading to Fahrenheit, or vice versa. To convert from Fahrenheit to Celsius, deduct 32 from the Fahrenheit reading and then multiply by the fraction 5/9, that is:

$$C = (\text{Fahrenheit temperature} - 32) \times 5/9$$

For example, when the Fahrenheit reading is 100:

$$C = (100 - 32) \times 5/9 = (68) \times 5/9 = 37.7$$

Figure 14-7. ◆ A temperature-sensitive skin tape. *Source:* © Jenny Thomas.

To convert from Celsius to Fahrenheit, multiply the Celsius reading by the fraction 9/5 and then add 32; that is:

$$F = (\text{Celsius temperature} \times 9/5) + 32$$

For example, when the Celsius reading is 40:

$$F = (40 \times 9/5) + 32 = (72) + 32 = 104$$

NURSING CARE

ASSESSING

Times for assessing vital signs are listed in Box 14-5 ◆. See Box 14-1 for manifestations of fever and Box 14-3 for manifestations of hypothermia. Refer to Table 14-1 for normal temperature range by age.

DIAGNOSING, PLANNING, and IMPLEMENTING

The most common nursing diagnosis for clients with alterations of temperature beyond normal limits is Ineffective Themoregulation. Refer to Table 14-2 for selecting an appropriate site for measuring body temperature. Procedure 14-1 explains how to measure body temperature.

EVALUATING

The temperature measurement is compared to baseline data or normal range. Client's age, time of day, and any other influencing factors are considered. Temperature readings are reviewed in relation to other vital signs.

Safety Precautions

Safety is a major consideration when assessing temperature due to the disadvantages of the various sites and equipment.

BOX 14-5
TIMES TO ASSESS VITAL SIGNS

- ◆ On admission to a health care agency to obtain baseline data
- ◆ When a client has a change in health status or reports symptoms such as chest pain or feeling hot or faint
- ◆ Before and after surgery or an invasive procedure
- ◆ Before and/or after the administration of a medication that could affect the respiratory or cardiovascular systems (e.g., before giving a digitalis preparation)
- ◆ Before and after any nursing intervention that could affect the vital signs (e.g., ambulating a client who has been on bed rest)

Never force any type of thermometer into place. If it does not enter easily, reassess the site and consider using a different location or type of thermometer.

The oral site should not be used if the client cannot cooperate or there is a risk that he or she may bite a glass thermometer. The rectal thermometer should always be held in place and never be left unattended. Severe injury could occur if the client rolled onto the thermometer. Glass thermometers must be handled carefully since they pose a safety hazard if broken. If a glass thermometer does not shake down easily or has any signs of cracks, it should be disposed of according to facility policy.

Electronic thermometers and other electrical equipment should not be used if damaged, since malfunctioning equipment can present a shock hazard to both the client and the nurse.

DISCHARGE CONSIDERATIONS

* Teach the client accurate use and reading of the type of thermometer to be used. Reinforce the importance of reporting the site and type of thermometer used and the value of using one consistently. Provide a recording chart or table if indicated.
* Discuss means of keeping the thermometer clean, such as warm water and soap, and avoiding cross-contamination.
* Ensure that the client has water-soluble lubricant if using a rectal thermometer.
* Have the client or family member demonstrate use of the thermometer so proper technique can be reinforced.
* Instruct the client or family member to notify the health care provider if the temperature is 37.7°C (100°F) or higher.

Pulse

The pulse is a wave of blood created by contraction of the left ventricle of the heart. The heart is a pulsating pump, and the blood enters the arteries with each contraction, causing pressure pulses or pulse waves. Generally, the pulse wave represents the stroke volume output and the amount of blood that enters the arteries with each ventricular contraction. *Compliance* of the arteries is their ability to contract and expand. When a person's arteries lose their ability to expand, as can happen in old age, greater pressure is required to pump the blood into the arteries because the rigid arterial walls offer resistance.

When an adult is resting, the heart pumps about 5 liters of blood each minute. This volume is called the cardiac output.

In a healthy person, the pulse reflects the heartbeat. In other words, the pulse rate is the same as the rate of the ventricular contractions of the heart. However, in some types of cardiovascular disease, the heartbeat and pulse rates can differ. For example, a client's heart may produce very weak or small

pulse waves that are not detectable in a peripheral pulse far from the heart. In these instances, the nurse should assess the heartbeat and the peripheral pulse. See the section on assessing the apical pulse later in this chapter. A **peripheral pulse** is a pulse located in the periphery of the body, for example, in the foot, hand, or neck. The *apical pulse,* in contrast, is a central pulse; that is, it is located at the apex of the heart.

FACTORS AFFECTING PULSE RATE

The rate of the pulse is expressed in beats per minute (BPM). A pulse rate varies according to a number of factors. The nurse should consider each of the following factors when assessing a client's pulse:

* *Age.* As age increases, the pulse rate gradually decreases. See Table 14-1 for specific variations in pulse rates from birth to adulthood.
* *Sex.* After puberty, the average male's pulse rate is slightly lower than the female's.
* *Exercise.* The pulse rate normally increases with activity. The rate of increase in the professional athlete is often less than in the average person because of greater cardiac size, strength, and efficiency.
* *Fever.* The pulse rate increases (a) in response to the lowered blood pressure that results from peripheral vasodilation associated with elevated body temperature and (b) because of the increased metabolic rate.
* *Medications.* Some medications decrease the pulse rate, and others increase it. For example, cardiotonics (e.g., digitalis preparations) decrease the heart rate, whereas epinephrine causes an increase.
* *Hemorrhage.* Loss of blood from the vascular system (hemorrhage) normally increases pulse rate. In adults the loss of a small amount of blood (e.g., 500 mL, the amount lost after a blood donation) results in a temporary adjustment of the heart rate as the body compensates for the lost blood volume. An adult has about 5 liters of blood in the system and can usually lose up to 10 percent without adverse effects.
* *Stress.* In response to stress, sympathetic nervous stimulation increases the overall activity of the heart. Stress increases the rate as well as the force of the heartbeat. Fear and anxiety as well as the perception of severe pain stimulate the sympathetic system.
* *Position changes.* When a person assumes a sitting or standing position, blood usually pools in dependent vessels of the venous system. Pooling results in a transient decrease in the venous blood return to the heart and a subsequent reduction in blood pressure and increase in heart rate.

PULSE SITES

Nine of the sites where a pulse is commonly taken (Figure 14-8 ◆) are the following:

1. *Temporal,* where the temporal artery passes over the temporal bone of the head. The site is superior (above) and lateral to (away from the midline of) the eye.

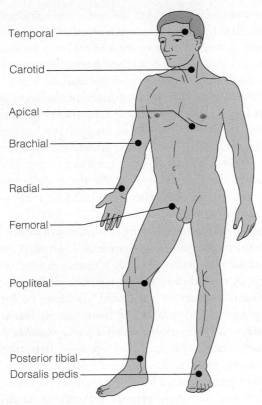

Temporal
Carotid
Apical
Brachial
Radial
Femoral
Popliteal
Posterior tibial
Dorsalis pedis

Figure 14-8. ◆ Nine sites commonly used for assessing a pulse.

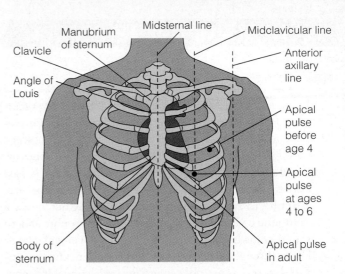

Clavicle
Angle of Louis
Manubrium of sternum
Midsternal line
Midclavicular line
Anterior axillary line
Apical pulse before age 4
Apical pulse at ages 4 to 6
Body of sternum
Apical pulse in adult

Figure 14-9. ◆ Location of the apical pulse for a child under 4 years, a child 4 to 6 years, and an adult.

an imaginary line drawn from the middle of the ankle to the space between the big and second toes.

The radial site is most commonly used. It is easily found in most people and is readily accessible. The reasons for use of each site are given in Table 14-3 ◆.

2. *Carotid,* at the side of the neck where the carotid artery runs between the trachea and the sternocleidomastoid muscle. Never press both carotids at the same time as this can cause a reflex drop in blood pressure or pulse rate.
3. **Apical,** at the apex of the heart. In an adult this is located on the left side of the chest, no more than 8 cm (3 in) to the left of the sternum (breastbone) and at the fourth, fifth, or sixth intercostal space (area between the ribs). For a child 7 to 9 years of age, the apical pulse is located at the fourth or fifth intercostal spaces. Before 4 years of age, it is left of the midclavicular line (MCL); between 4 and 6 years, it is at the MCL (Figure 14-9 ◆).
4. *Brachial,* at the inner aspect of the biceps muscle of the arm (especially in infants) or medially in the antecubital space (elbow crease).
5. *Radial,* where the radial artery runs along the radial bone, on the thumb side of the inner aspect of the wrist.
6. *Femoral,* where the femoral artery passes alongside the inguinal ligament.
7. *Popliteal,* where the popliteal artery passes behind the knee. This point is difficult to find, but it can be palpated if the client flexes the knee slightly (see Figure 14-8).
8. *Posterior tibial,* on the medial surface of the ankle where the posterior tibial artery passes behind the medial malleolus.
9. *Pedal* (dorsalis pedis), where the dorsalis pedis artery passes over the bones of the foot. This artery can be palpated by feeling the *dorsum* (upper surface) of the foot on

TABLE 14-3	REASONS FOR USING SPECIFIC PULSE SITES
PULSE SITE	**REASONS FOR USE**
Radial	Readily accessible
Temporal	Used when radial pulse is not accessible
Carotid	Used for infants Used in cases of cardiac arrest Used to determine circulation to the brain
Apical	Routinely used for infants and children up to 3 years of age Used to determine discrepancies with radial pulse Used in conjunction with some medications
Brachial	Used to measure blood pressure Used during cardiac arrest for infants
Femoral	Used in cases of cardiac arrest Used for infants and children Used to determine circulation to a leg
Popliteal	Used to determine circulation to the lower leg
Posterior tibial	Used to determine circulation to the foot
Pedal	Used to determine circulation to the foot

NURSING CARE

◆ ASSESSING

A pulse is commonly assessed by palpation (feeling) or auscultation (hearing). The middle three fingertips are used for palpating all pulse sites except the apex of the heart. A stethoscope is used for assessing apical pulses and fetal heart tones. A Doppler ultrasound stethoscope (DUS; Figure 14-10 ◆) is used for pulses that are difficult to assess. The DUS headset has earpieces similar to standard stethoscope earpieces, but it has a long cord attached to a volume-controlled audio unit and an ultrasound transducer. The DUS detects movement of red blood cells through a blood vessel. In contrast to the conventional stethoscope, it excludes environmental sounds. It cannot detect blood flow in deep vessels or in blood vessels underlying bone, such as the vessels in the abdomen, thorax, or skull.

A pulse is normally palpated by applying moderate pressure with the three middle fingers of the hand. The pads on the most distal aspects of the finger are the most sensitive areas for detecting a pulse. With excessive pressure one can obliterate a pulse, whereas with too little pressure one may not be able to detect it. Before the nurse assesses the resting pulse, the client should assume a comfortable position. The nurse should also be aware of the following:

◆ Whether the client has taken any medication that could affect the heart rate.
◆ Whether the client has been physically active. If so, wait 10 to 15 minutes until the client has rested and the pulse has slowed to its usual rate.
◆ Whether any baseline data exists about the normal heart rate for the client. For example, a physically fit athlete may have a heart rate below 60 beats per minute.
◆ Whether the client should assume a particular position (e.g., sitting). In some clients, the rate changes with the position because of changes in blood flow volume and autonomic nervous system activity.

When assessing the pulse, the nurse collects the following data: the rate, rhythm, volume, arterial wall elasticity, and presence or absence of bilateral equality. The normal pulse rates are shown in Table 14-1. An excessively fast heart rate (e.g., over 100 beats per minute in an adult) is referred to as *tachycardia*. A heart rate in an adult of 60 beats per minute or less is called *bradycardia*. If a client has either tachycardia or bradycardia, the apical pulse should be assessed.

The pulse rhythm is the pattern of the beats and the intervals between the beats. Equal time elapses between beats of a normal pulse. A pulse with an irregular rhythm is referred to as a *dysrhythmia* or *arrhythmia*. It may consist of random, irregular beats or a predictable pattern of irregular beats. When a dysrhythmia is detected, the apical pulse should be assessed. An electrocardiogram (ECG or EKG) is necessary to define the dysrhythmia further.

Pulse volume, also called the pulse strength or amplitude, refers to the force of blood with each beat. Usually, the pulse volume is the same with each beat. It can range from absent to bounding. A normal pulse can be felt with moderate pressure of the fingers and can be obliterated (unable to be felt) with greater pressure. A forceful or full blood volume that is obliterated only with difficulty is called a *full or bounding pulse*. A pulse that is readily obliterated with pressure from the fingers is referred to as weak, feeble, or *thready*. A pulse volume is usually measured on a scale of 0 to 3 (Table 14-4 ◆).

The elasticity of the arterial wall reflects its ability to expand or its deformities. A healthy, normal artery feels straight, smooth, soft, and pliable. Older people often have inelastic arteries that feel twisted (*tortuous*) and irregular on palpation.

When assessing a peripheral pulse to determine the adequacy of blood flow to a particular area of the body, the nurse should also assess the corresponding pulse on the other side of the body. The second assessment gives the nurse data with which to compare the pulses. For example, when assessing the blood flow to the right foot, the nurse assesses the right dorsalis pedis pulse and then the left dorsalis pedis pulse. If the client's right and left pulses are the same, the client's dorsalis pedis pulses are bilaterally equal.

Peripheral Pulse Assessment

A peripheral pulse, usually the radial pulse, is assessed by palpation in all individuals except:

Figure 14-10. ◆ An ultrasound (Doppler or DUS) stethoscope. *Source:* © Elena Dorfman.

TABLE 14-4	SCALE FOR MEASURING PULSE VOLUME
SCALE	DESCRIPTION OF PULSE
0	Absent, not discernible
1	Thready or weak, difficult to feel
2	Normal, detected readily, obliterated by strong pressure
3	Bounding, difficult to obliterate

- Newborns and children up to 2 or 3 years. Apical pulses are assessed in these clients.
- Very obese or elderly clients, whose radial pulse may be difficult to palpate. Doppler equipment may be used for these clients, or the apical pulse is assessed.
- Individuals with a heart disease, who require apical pulse assessment.
- Individuals in whom the circulation to a specific body part must be assessed; for example, following leg surgery, the pedal (dorsalis pedis) pulse is assessed.

Apical–Radial Pulse Assessment

An apical–radial pulse may need to be assessed for clients with certain cardiovascular disorders. Normally, the apical and radial rates are identical. An apical pulse rate greater than a radial pulse rate can indicate that the thrust of the blood from the heart is too feeble for the wave to be felt at the peripheral pulse site, or it can indicate that vascular disease is preventing impulses from being transmitted. Any differences between the two pulse rates (called a **pulse deficit**) needs to be reported promptly. In no instance is the radial pulse greater than the apical pulse.

An apical–radial pulse can be taken by two nurses or one nurse, although the two-nurse technique may be more accurate.

DIAGNOSING, PLANNING, and IMPLEMENTING

A possible nursing diagnosis would be Decreased Cardiac Output. Refer to Table 14-3 for selection of appropriate site. Procedure 14-2 provides guidelines for various methods of assessing pulse.

EVALUATING

Evaluate pulse in relationship to baseline data or normal range for age of client, relationship of pulse rate and volume to other vital signs, and health status. Compare peripheral pulses; equality, rate, and volume in corresponding extremities.

DISCHARGE CONSIDERATIONS

- Teach the client or family member to monitor the pulse prior to taking medications that affect the heart rate.
- Tell the client to report any notable changes in heart rate or rhythm (regularity) to the health care provider.
- Ensure that the client or family member is aware of what pulse findings should be reported and to whom.

Nursing Process Case Study: CLIENT WITH LEFT-SIDED HEART FAILURE

Naomi Munson, a 75-year-old female, has been a resident at Knight's Bridge Road Retirement Center since her husband died 6 months ago. She was admitted through the ER for left-sided heart failure. Mrs. Munson expresses a dislike for her low-sodium diet. She admits to taking no medication except "natural" therapy prescribed by her herbalists.

She is presently taking multivitamins and dried English hawthorne to decrease her blood pressure and decrease her oxygen needs. She states, "I don't want to take drugs because they gave them to my husband and he died anyway."

Assessment VS: T 97.4, apical pulse 102 and irregular, 28 and labored, BP 148/90, pulse ox 94%; orthopnea; inspiratory crackles and wheezes base of lungs; nonproductive cough; states, "I have to sleep sitting up in a chair." +3 edema ankles bilaterally, abdomen distended. ECG–atrial fib.; chest x-ray revealed cardiomegaly.

Diagnosis

- Excess Fluid Volume related to impaired excretion of sodium and water
- Activity Intolerance related to weakness, fatigue
- Powerlessness related to illness-related regimen

Expected Outcomes

- Maintains clear lung sounds, no evidence of dyspnea or orthopnea
- Expresses an understanding of need to balance rest and activity
- Participates in planning care; makes decision regarding care and treatments when possible

Planning and Implementation

- Monitor location and extent of edema, using a millimeter tape in the same area at the same time each day to measure edema in extremities and abdomen.
- Monitor lung sounds for crackles; monitor respirations for effort and determine the presence and severity of orthopnea.
- Recognize that the presence of risk factors for excessive fluid volume is particularly serious in the elderly.
- Slow the pace of care. Allow client extra time to carry out activities.
- Encourage family and/or caretaker to help/allow elder to be independent in whatever activities possible.
- Refer client to physical therapy to help increase activity level and strength.
- Establish therapeutic relationship by listening; give the client choices and accept her statement of limitations.
- Help client identify factors not under her control.
- Validate client's feelings regarding the impact of health status on current lifestyle.

Evaluating Mrs. Munson is being discharged to the skilled nursing center in her retirement community, after 4 days of hospitalization. Her respirations are unlabored at rest and edema in ankles reduced to +2. Lungs clear, able to sleep in low Fowler's position. Mrs. Munson referred to dietitian at the care facility to develop an eating plan that she can live with; stated, "I will take my meals in the dining room after I return to my own apartment so that I can follow my prescribed diet." Participating in PT 3 days per week, can ambulate 25 feet without difficulty or shortness of breath. Taking Lasix 20 mg qd and still refusing other medications. BP 140/80. Mrs. Munson expresses fear of having a stroke.

Critical Thinking in the Nursing Process

1. Mrs. Munson expressed a wish to return to her own apartment as soon as possible. Design an activity program that will help her regain her strength and mobility
2. Mrs. Munson wants to continue her natural medicine. What would be your response to her desire?

Respirations

Respiration is the act of breathing. **External respiration** refers to the interchange of oxygen and carbon dioxide between the alveoli of the lungs and the pulmonary blood. **Internal respiration** is the interchange of these same gases between the circulating blood and the cells of the body tissues.

Inhalation or inspiration refers to the intake of air into the lungs. *Exhalation* or expiration refers to breathing out or the movement of gases from the lungs to the atmosphere. *Ventilation* is also used to refer to the movement of air in and out of the lungs. Hyperventilation refers to very deep, rapid respirations; hypoventilation refers to very shallow respirations.

There are basically two types of breathing. *Costal* (thoracic) breathing involves external intercostal and accessory muscles. It can be observed by the movement of the chest upward and outward. *Diaphragmatic* (abdominal) breathing involves contraction and relaxation of the diaphragm. The abdomen moves with the diaphragm's contraction and downward movement.

MECHANICS AND REGULATION

During inhalation, the diaphragm contracts, the ribs move upward and outward, and the sternum moves outward (Figure 14-11 ◆). During exhalation, the diaphragm relaxes, the ribs move downward and inward, and the sternum moves inward, decreasing the size of the thorax as the lungs are compressed. Normal breathing is automatic and effortless. An inspiration lasts 1 to 1.5 seconds, and an expiration lasts 2 to 3 seconds.

Respiration is controlled by (a) respiratory centers in the medulla oblongata and the pons of the brain and (b) by chemoreceptors located centrally in the medulla and peripherally in the carotid and aortic bodies. These centers and receptors respond to changes in the concentrations of oxygen (O_2),

carbon dioxide (CO_2), and hydrogen (H^+) in the arterial blood. See Chapter 16 for details.

NURSING CARE

ASSESSING

Resting respirations should be assessed when the client is relaxed. Both exercise and anxiety affect respiratory rate and depth. Respirations may also need to be assessed after exercise to identify the client's tolerance to activity. Before assessing a client's respirations, a nurse should be aware of:

◆ The client's normal breathing pattern
◆ The influence of health problems on respirations
◆ Any medications or therapies that might affect the client's respirations
◆ Relationship of respirations to cardiovascular function

The rate, depth, rhythm, and special characteristics of respirations should always be assessed. Box 14-6 ◆ provides terms for breathing patterns, sounds, and movements. For the respiratory rates for different age groups, see Table 14-1. Several factors influence respiratory rate; major factors are listed in Table 14-5 ◆.

The depth of a person's respirations can be established by watching the movement of the chest. Respiratory depth is generally described as normal, deep, or shallow. During a normal inspiration and expiration, an adult takes in about 500 mL of air. Body position also affects the amount of air that can be inhaled. People in a supine position experience two physiologic processes that suppress respiration: an increase in the volume of blood inside the thoracic cavity, and compression of the chest. So, clients lying on their back have poorer lung aeration. This predisposes them to the stasis of fluids and subsequent infection. Certain medications also affect the respiratory depth. For exam-

TABLE 14-5	MAJOR FACTORS INFLUENCING RESPIRATORY RATE	
FACTOR		**INFLUENCE**
Exercise: increases metabolism		Increase
Stress: readies the body for "fight or flight"		Increase
Environment: increased temperature		Increase
Environment: decreased temperature		Decrease
Increased altitude: lower oxygen concentration		Increase
Certain medications (e.g., narcotic, analgesic)		Decrease
Increased intracranial pressure		Decrease

MediaLink ● Respiratory System

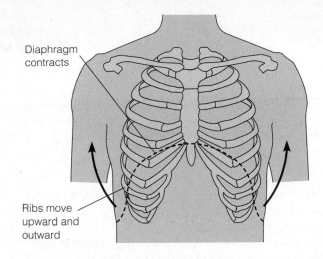

Sternum moves outward

Diaphragm contracts

Diaphragm contracts

Ribs move upward and outward

A

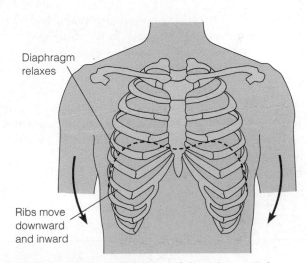

Sternum moves inward

Diaphragm relaxes

Diaphragm relaxes

Ribs move downward and inward

B

Figure 14-11. ◆ **A.** Respiratory inhalation. Left: lateral view; Right: anterior view. **B.** Respiratory exhalation. Left: lateral view; Right: anterior view.

ple, barbiturates in large doses depress the respiratory centers in the brain, thereby depressing the respiratory rate and depth.

Respiratory rhythm or pattern refers to the regularity of expirations and inspirations. Normally, respirations are evenly spaced. Respiratory rhythm can be described as regular or irregular. An infant's respiratory rhythm may be less regular than an adult's.

Respiratory quality or character refers to those aspects of breathing that are different from normal, effortless breathing. Two of these are the amount of effort a client must exert to breathe and the sound of breathing. Usually, breathing does not require noticeable effort; some clients, however, breathe only with decided effort, referred to as *labored breathing*.

The sound of breathing is also significant. Normal breathing is silent. Many sounds occur as a result of the presence of fluid in the lungs, and are most clearly heard with a stethoscope (see Box 14-6).

The effectiveness of respirations is measured in part by the uptake of oxygen from the air into the blood and the release of carbon dioxide from the blood into expired air. The amount of hemoglobin in arterial blood that is saturated with oxygen can be measured indirectly through pulse oximetry. (See Chapter 16 for illustration of pulse oximeter.)

DIAGNOSING, PLANNING, and IMPLEMENTING

A common nursing diagnosis for clients with respiratory difficulty is Ineffective Breathing Pattern. Procedure 14-3 provides guidelines for assessing respirations.

EVALUATING

Respirations are evaluated in relationship to the client's baseline data or normal range for age. The nurse documents the rate, volume, rhythm, and effort of respirations.

BOX 14-6 ALTERED BREATHING PATTERNS AND SOUNDS

Breathing Patterns

Rate

◆ **Tachypnea**—rapid respiration marked by quick, shallow breaths
◆ **Bradypnea**—abnormally slow breathing
◆ **Apnea**—cessation of breathing

Volume

◆ **Hyperventilation**—an increase in the amount of air in the lungs characterized by prolonged and deep breaths; may be associated with anxiety
◆ **Hypoventilation**—a reduction in the amount of air in the lungs, characterized by shallow respirations

Rhythm

◆ **Cheyne–Stokes breathing**—rhythmic waxing and waning of respirations, from very deep to very shallow breathing and temporary apnea; often associated with cardiac failure, increased intracranial pressure, or brain damage

Ease or Effort

◆ **Dyspnea**—difficult and labored breathing during which the individual has a persistent, unsatisfied need for air and feels distressed
◆ **Orthopnea**—ability to breathe only in upright sitting or standing positions

Breath Sounds

Audible without Amplification

◆ **Stridor**—a shrill, harsh sound heard during inspiration with laryngeal obstruction
◆ **Stertor**—snoring or sonorous respiration, usually due to a partial obstruction of the upper airway
◆ **Wheeze**—continuous, high-pitched musical squeak or whistling sound occurring on expiration and sometimes on inspiration when air moves through a narrowed or partially obstructed airway
◆ **Bubbling**—gurgling sounds heard as air passes through moist secretions in the respiratory tract

Chest Movements

◆ **Intercostal retraction**—indrawing between the ribs
◆ **Substernal retraction**—indrawing beneath the breastbone
◆ **Suprasternal retraction**—indrawing above the clavicles
◆ **Flail chest**—the ballooning out of the chest wall through injured rib spaces; results in paradoxical breathing, during which the chest wall balloons on expiration but is depressed or sucked inward on inspiration

Secretions and Coughing

◆ **Hemoptysis**—the presence of blood in the sputum
◆ **Productive cough**—a cough accompanied by expectorated secretions
◆ **Nonproductive cough**—a dry, harsh cough without secretions

◆ Blood Pressure

Arterial **blood pressure** is a measure of the pressure exerted by the blood as it flows through the arteries. Because the blood moves in waves, there are two blood pressure measures. The **systolic pressure** is the pressure of the blood as a result of contraction of the ventricles (the pressure of the height of the blood wave). The **diastolic pressure** is the pressure when the ventricles are at rest; it is the lower pressure that is present at all times within the arteries. The difference between the diastolic and the systolic pressures is called the *pulse pressure*.

Blood pressure is measured in millimeters of mercury (mm Hg) and recorded as a fraction. The systolic pressure is written over the diastolic pressure. The average blood pressure

clinical ALERT

Because BP varies among individuals, the nurse must know a client's baseline BP. If a client's usual BP is 180/100 mm Hg, but after surgery is 120/80 mm Hg, report this drop in pressure to the physician.

of a healthy adult is 120/80 mm Hg. A number of conditions are reflected by changes in blood pressure.

DETERMINANTS OF BLOOD PRESSURE

Arterial blood pressure is the result of several factors: the pumping action of the heart, the *peripheral vascular resistance* (the resistance supplied by the blood vessels through which the blood flows), and the blood volume and viscosity.

Pumping Action of the Heart

Cardiac output is the volume of blood pumped into the arteries by the heart. When the pumping action of the heart is weak, less blood is pumped into arteries, and the blood pressure decreases. When the heart's pumping action is strong and the volume of blood pumped into the circulation increases, the blood pressure increases.

Peripheral Vascular Resistance

Peripheral resistance can increase blood pressure. The diastolic pressure especially is affected. Some factors that create resistance in the arterial system are the size of the arterioles and capillaries, the compliance of the arteries, and the viscosity of the blood.

The size of the arterioles and the capillaries determines in great part the peripheral resistance to the blood in the body. A lumen is a channel within a tube. The smaller the lumen of a vessel, the greater the resistance. Normally, the arterioles are in a state of partial constriction. Increased vasoconstriction raises the blood pressure, whereas decreased vasoconstriction lowers the blood pressure.

The arteries account for most of the peripheral resistance. The major factor reducing arterial compliance is pathologic change affecting the arterial walls. When elastic and muscular tissues of the arteries are replaced with fibrous tissue, the arteries lose much of their compliance. This condition, most common in middle-aged and elderly adults, is known as *arteriosclerosis*.

Blood Volume

When the blood volume decreases (e.g. from hemorrhage or dehydration), the blood pressure decreases because of decreased fluid in the arteries. When the volume increases (e.g., with an intravenous infusion), the blood pressure increases because of the greater fluid volume within the circulatory system.

Blood Viscosity

Viscosity is a physical property that results from friction of molecules in a fluid. In a viscous (or "thick") fluid, there is a great deal of friction among the molecules as they slide by each other. The blood pressure is higher when the blood is highly viscous, that is, when the proportion of red blood cells to the blood plasma is high. This proportion is referred to as the *hematocrit*. The viscosity increases markedly when the hematocrit is more than 60 to 65 percent.

FACTORS AFFECTING BLOOD PRESSURE

Among the factors influencing blood pressure are:

◆ *Age*. Newborns have a mean systolic pressure of about 75 mm Hg. The pressure rises with age, reaching a peak at the onset of puberty, and then tends to decline somewhat. One quick way to determine the normal systolic blood pressure of a child is to use the following formula:

Normal systolic BP = 80 + (2 × child's age in years)

In older people, elasticity of the arteries is decreased—the arteries are more rigid and less yielding to the pressure of the blood. This produces an elevated systolic pressure. Because the walls no longer retract as flexibly with decreased pressure, the diastolic pressure is also higher. (See Table 14-1.)

◆ *Exercise*. Physical activity increases the cardiac output and the blood pressure. So, 20 to 30 minutes of rest following exercise is indicated before the resting blood pressure can be reliably assessed.

◆ *Stress*. Stimulation of the sympathetic nervous system increases cardiac output and vasoconstriction of the arteri-

oles, increasing the blood pressure reading. However, severe pain can decrease blood pressure greatly and cause shock by inhibiting the vasomotor center and producing vasodilation.

◆ *Race*. African-American males over 35 years have higher blood pressures than European-American males of the same age.

◆ *Obesity*. Pressure is generally higher in some overweight and obese people than in people of normal weight.

◆ *Sex*. After puberty, females usually have lower blood pressures than males of the same age; this difference is thought to be due to hormonal variations. Women generally have higher blood pressures after menopause than before.

◆ *Medications*. Many medications may increase or decrease the blood pressure; nurses should be aware of the specific medications a client is receiving and consider their possible impact when interpreting blood pressure readings.

◆ *Diurnal variations*. Pressure is usually lowest early in the morning, when the metabolic rate is lowest, then rises throughout the day and peaks in the late afternoon or early evening.

◆ *Disease process*. Any condition affecting the cardiac output, blood volume, blood viscosity, and/or compliance of the arteries has a direct effect on the blood pressure.

HYPERTENSION

A blood pressure that is persistently above normal is called *hypertension*. It is usually asymptomatic and is often a contributing factor to myocardial infarctions (heart attacks). An elevated blood pressure of unknown cause is called *primary hypertension*. An elevated blood pressure of known cause is called *secondary hypertension*. Hypertension is a widespread health problem. The diagnosis is made when the average of two or more diastolic readings on two visits following the initial assessment is 90 mm Hg or higher, or when the average of multiple systolic blood pressure readings is higher than 140 mm Hg. Categories of hypertension have been identified and are described in Table 14-6 ◆. Factors associated with hypertension include thickening of the arterial walls, which reduces the size of the arterial lumen; inelasticity of the arteries; as well as such lifestyle factors as cigarette smoking, obesity, heavy alcohol consumption, lack of physical exercise, high blood cholesterol levels, and continued exposure to stress. Follow-up care should include lifestyle changes conducive to lowering the blood pressure as well as monitoring the pressure itself.

HYPOTENSION

Hypotension is a blood pressure that is below normal (a systolic reading consistently between 85 and 110 mm Hg in an adult). **Orthostatic hypotension** is a blood pressure that falls when the client sits or stands. It is usually the result of peripheral vasodilation in which the blood flow leaves the central body organs, especially the brain, and moves to the periphery,

TABLE 14-6 FOLLOW-UP RECOMMENDATIONS FOR BLOOD PRESSURE MEASUREMENT FOR ADULTS > 18 YEARS

INITIAL SCREENING BLOOD PRESSURE (MM HG)[a]

SYSTOLIC	DIASTOLIC	FOLLOW-UP RECOMMENDED[b]
<130	<85	Recheck in 2 years.
130–139	85–89	Recheck in 1 year.[c]
140–159	90–99	Confirm within 2 months.
160–179	100–109	Evaluate or refer to source of care within 1 month.
180–209	110–119	Evaluate or refer to source of care within 1 week.
≥210	≥120	Evaluate or refer to source of care immediately.

[a]If the systolic and diastolic categories are different, follow recommendation for the shorter time to follow up (e.g., 160/85 mm Hg should be evaluated or referred to source of care within 1 month).
[b]The scheduling of follow-up should be modified by reliable information about past blood pressure measurements, other cardiovascular risk factors, or target-organ disease.
[c]Consider providing advice about lifestyle modifications.

Source: From the fifth report of the Joint National Committee for the Detection, Evaluation, and Treatment of High Blood Pressure, National Heart, Lung, and Blood Institute, National Institutes of Health, 1993, Archives of Internal Medicine, 329, 1912.

often causing the person to feel faint. Hypotension can also be caused by analgesics such as meperidine hydrochloride (Demerol), bleeding, severe burns, and prolonged diarrhea and vomiting. It is important to monitor hypotensive clients carefully to prevent falls. See Box 14-7 ◆ for instructions for measuring blood pressure for clients with orthostatic hypotension.

BLOOD PRESSURE EQUIPMENT

Blood pressure is measured with a blood pressure cuff, a sphygmomanometer, and a stethoscope. The blood pressure cuff consists of a rubber bag that can be inflated with air. It is called the *bladder* (Figure 14-12 ◆). It is covered with cloth and has two tubes attached to it. One tube connects to a rub-

ber bulb that inflates the bladder. A small valve on the side of this bulb releases the air in the bladder. When the valve is closed, air pumped into the bladder remains there. The other tube is attached to a sphygmomanometer.

The sphygmomanometer indicates the pressure of the air within the bladder. There are two types of sphygmomanometers: aneroid and mercury (Figure 14-13 ◆). The

BOX 14-7 MEASURING BLOOD PRESSURE FOR ORTHOSTATIC HYPOTENSION

When measuring the blood pressure of a client who has orthostatic hypotension:

◆ Place the client in a supine position for 2 to 3 minutes. This allows the blood pressure and pulse to stabilize in this position.
◆ Record the client's pulse and blood pressure.
◆ Assist the client to sit or stand slowly. Support the client in case of faintness.
◆ After 1 minute in the upright position, recheck the client's pulse and blood pressure in the same sites as previously.

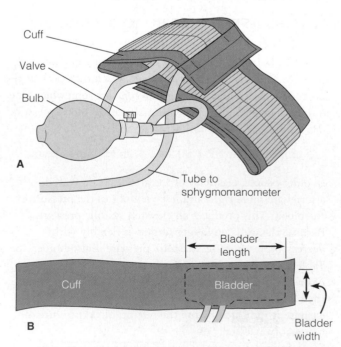

Figure 14-12. ◆ Blood pressure equipment: **A.** Aneroid manometer and cuff; **B.** Mercury manometer and cuff.

A

B

Figure 14-13. ◆ **A.** Blood pressure cuff and bulb; **B.** Bladder inside the cuff. *Source:* © Elena Dorfman.

aneroid sphygmomanometer is a calibrated dial with a needle that points to the calibrations.

The mercury sphygmomanometer is a calibrated cylinder filled with mercury. The pressure is indicated at the point to which the rounded curve (the base) of the meniscus rises (Figure 14-14 ◆). The blood pressure reading should be made with the eye at the level of the rounded curve in order to be accurate. If the eye is looking up or down, a distortion in the reading can occur. A distortion that occurs as a result of the angle of view is called *parallax*.

Some medical facilities use electronic sphygmomanometers (Figure 14-15 ◆), which eliminate the need to listen to the sounds of the client's systolic and diastolic blood pressures through a stethoscope. Electronic blood pressure devices should be calibrated against a mercury sphygmomanometer to check accuracy. Automated electronic devices have been shown to give higher values than manual cuffs.

Doppler ultrasound stethoscopes (DUSs) are also used to assess blood pressure (see Figure 14-10 ◆). These are of particular value when blood pressure sounds are difficult to hear, such as in infants, obese clients, and clients in shock. A systolic blood pressure assessed with a DUS is recorded with a large D, for example, 85D. Systolic pressure may be the only blood pressure obtainable with some ultrasound models.

Blood pressure cuffs come in various sizes because the bladder must be the correct width and length for the client's arm (Figure 14-16 ◆). If the bladder is too narrow, the blood pressure reading will be erroneously elevated; if it is too wide, the reading will be erroneously low. The arm circumference, not the age of the client, should always be used to determine bladder size (Figure 14-17 ◆).

Figure 14-14. ◆ In order to obtain an accurate reading from a mercury manometer, position the meniscus at eye level.

Figure 14-15. ◆ Automatic blood pressure monitors register systolic, diastolic, and mean blood pressures. *Source:* © Jenny Thomas.

Figure 14-16. ◆ Three standard cuff sizes: a small cuff for an infant, small child, or frail adult; a normal adult-size cuff; and a large cuff for measuring the blood pressure on the leg or on the arm of an obese adult. *Source:* © Elena Dorfman.

Figure 14-17. ◆ The nurse must determine that the bladder of a blood pressure cuff is 40 percent of the arm circumference or 20 percent wider than the diameter of the midpoint of the limb, in order to ensure an accurate reading. To do this, the nurse lays the cuff lengthwise at the midpoint of the upper arm, holding the outermost side of the bladder edge laterally on the arm. With the other hand, the nurse wraps the width of the cuff around the arm to ensure that it covers 40 percent of the arm's circumference.

The length of the bladder also affects the accuracy of measurement. The bladder should be sufficiently long to cover at least two thirds of the limb's circumference.

Blood pressure cuffs are made of nondistensible material so that an even pressure is exerted around the limb. Most cuffs are held in place by hooks, snaps, or Velcro.

BLOOD PRESSURE ASSESSMENT SITES

The blood pressure is usually assessed in the client's arm using the brachial artery and a standard stethoscope. If the arm is very large or grossly misshapen and the conventional cuff cannot be properly applied, leg or forearm measurements can be taken. See Procedure 14-4 for directions for measuring blood pressure on the thigh.

Assessing the blood pressure on a client's thigh is usually indicated in these situations:

◆ The blood pressure cannot be measured on either arm (e.g., because of burns or other trauma).
◆ The blood pressure in one thigh is to be compared with the blood pressure in the other thigh.

Blood pressure is not measured on a client's arm or thigh in the following situations:

◆ The shoulder, arm, or hand (or the hip, knee, or ankle) is injured or diseased.
◆ A cast or bulky bandage is on any part of the limb.
◆ The client has had removal of axillary (or hip) lymph nodes on that side.
◆ The client has an intravenous infusion in that limb.
◆ The client has an arteriovenous fistula (e.g., for renal dialysis) in that limb.

To obtain a forearm blood pressure, apply an appropriate-sized cuff to the forearm 14 cm (5 in) below the elbow. Blood pressure sounds then can be heard from the radial artery.

METHODS

Blood pressure can be assessed directly or indirectly. Direct (invasive monitoring) measurement involves the insertion of a catheter into the brachial, radial, or femoral artery. Arterial pressure is represented as wavelike forms displayed on an oscilloscope. With correct placement, this pressure reading is highly accurate.

Two noninvasive indirect methods of measuring blood pressure are the auscultatory and palpatory methods. The auscultatory method is most commonly used in hospitals, clinics, and homes. When carried out correctly, the auscultatory method is relatively accurate.

When taking a blood pressure using a stethoscope, the nurse identifies five phases in the series of sounds called Korotkoff's sounds (Figure 14-18 ◆). Box 14-8 ◆ describes Korotkoff's phases.

Figure 14-18. ◆ Korotkoff's sounds can be differentiated into 5 phases. In the illustration the blood pressure is 138/90 or 138/102/90.

BOX 14-8
KOROTKOFF'S SOUNDS

- ◆ **Phase 1:** The pressure level at which the first faint, clear tapping or thumping sounds are heard. These sounds gradually become more intense. To ensure that they are not extraneous sounds, the nurse should identify at least two consecutive tapping sounds. The first tapping sound heard during deflation of the cuff is the systolic blood pressure.
- ◆ **Phase 2:** The period during deflation when the sounds have a muffled, whooshing, or swishing quality.
- ◆ **Phase 3:** The period during which the blood flows freely through an increasingly open artery and the sounds become crisper and more intense and again assume a thumping quality but softer than in Phase 1.
- ◆ **Phase 4:** The time when the sounds become muffled and have a soft, blowing quality.
- ◆ **Phase 5:** The pressure level when the last sound is heard. This is followed by a period of silence. The pressure at which the last sound is heard is the diastolic blood pressure in adults.[a]

[a]For children, the AHA (1987, p. 4) recommends that the onset of Phase 4, where the sounds become muffled, be considered the diastolic pressure. In agencies in which the fourth phase is considered the diastolic pressure of adults, three measures are recommended (systolic pressure, diastolic pressure, and phase 5). These may be referred to as systolic, first diastolic, and second diastolic pressures. The phase 5 (second diastolic pressure) reading may be zero; that is, the muffled sounds are heard even when there is no air pressure in the blood pressure cuff. In some instances, muffled sounds are never heard, in which case a dash is inserted where the reading would normally be recorded (e.g., 190/–/110).

NURSING CARE

ASSESSING

The palpatory method is sometimes used when Korotkoff's sounds cannot be heard and electronic equipment to amplify the sounds is not available, or when an auscultatory gap occurs. An *auscultatory gap,* which occurs particularly in hypertensive clients, is the temporary disappearance of sounds normally heard over the brachial artery when the cuff pressure is high followed by the reappearance of the sounds at a lower level. This temporary disappearance of sounds occurs in the latter part of phase 1 and phase 2 and may cover a range of 40 mm Hg. Instead of listening for the blood flow sounds, the nurse palpates the pulsations of the artery as the pressure in the cuff is released. The systolic pressure is read from the sphygmomanometer when the first pulsation is felt. A single whiplike vibration, felt in addition to the pulsations, identifies the point at which the pressure in the cuff nears the diastolic pressure. This vibration is no longer felt when the cuff pressure is below the diastolic pressure. To palpate the diastolic pressure, the nurse applies light to moderate pressure over the pulse point.

Common Errors in Assessing Blood Pressure

The importance of the accuracy of blood pressure assessments cannot be overemphasized. Many judgments about a client's health are made on the basis of blood pressure. It is an important indicator of the client's condition and is used extensively as a basis for nursing interventions. Some reasons for erroneous blood pressure readings are given in Table 14-7 ◆.

DIAGNOSING PLANNING and IMPLEMENTING

A frequent nursing diagnosis for clients with problems of blood pressure is Ineffective Therapeutic Regimen Management. Procedure 14-4 gives guidelines for assessing blood pressure.

Vital signs are documented in a flow sheet (see Figure 9-5) or in graphic form in most facilities. This type of documentation provides easy access for the physician and other members of the health care team. Occasionally, a nurse will insert vital signs in a nurse's note. See Box 14-9 ◆ for an example of this.

EVALUATING

Vital signs individually as well as in combination tell the nurse and ultimately the physician what is happening with

TABLE 14-7	BLOOD PRESSURE ASSESSMENT ERRORS
ERROR	**EFFECT**
Bladder cuff too narrow	Erroneously high
Bladder cuff too wide	Erroneously low
Arm unsupported	Erroneously high
Insufficient rest before the assessment	Erroneously high
Repeating assessment too quickly	Erroneously high systolic or low diastolic readings
Cuff wrapped too loosely or unevenly	Erroneously high
Deflating cuff too quickly	Erroneously low systolic and high diastolic readings
Deflating cuff too slowly	Erroneously high diastolic reading
Failure to use the same arm consistently	Inconsistent measurements
Arm above level of the heart	Erroneously low
Assessing immediately after a meal or while client smokes or has pain	Erroneously high
Failure to identify auscultatory gap	Erroneously low systolic pressure and erroneously low diastolic pressure

BOX 14-9 SAMPLE NURSE'S NOTES CONTAINING VITAL SIGNS

Focus

CVS	D	0835	VS 99.8/100/24 158/90 c/o chest pain 5/10. Sitting in chair.
	A		PRN ms given as prescribed. Assisted to return to bed. K. Turner LVN
	R	0915	Client resting comfortably chest pain resolved. 0/10. VS 98.8/86/20 140/88. K. Turner LVN

the client. The nurse knows that a low blood pressure (hypotension) in the presence of a rapid pulse (tachycardia) can be signs of hemorrhage and impending shock. Widening pulse pressure—a separation of more than 40 mm between the systolic and diastolic blood pressure readings—should alert the nurse to possible increased intracranial pressure. In the presence of pain, vital signs may also be elevated. It is important to consider not only the vital sign readings, but also the whole assessment. The data obtained from vital signs measurement will aid you in making sound judgments regarding the client's care.

Note: The bibliography listings for this and all chapters have been compiled at the back of the book.

PROCEDURE 14-1

Assessing Body Temperature

PURPOSES

◆ To establish baseline data for follow-up evaluation

◆ To identify whether the core temperature is within normal range

◆ To monitor clients at risk for change in temperature (e.g., clients at risk for infection or diagnosis of infection; those who have been exposed to temperature extremes; those with a leukocyte count below 5,000 or above 12,000)

EQUIPMENT

◆ Oral, rectal, axillary, thermometer

◆ Towel, if the axillary site is used

◆ Lubricant and tissue, if the rectal site is used

◆ Disposable gloves, if the rectal site is used

INTERVENTIONS

1. Prepare client.

For an Oral Temperature

◆ Determine the time the client last took hot or cold food or fluids or smoked. *To obtain an accurate oral temperature reading, allow 15 to 30 minutes to elapse between a client's intake or smoking and the measurement.*

For a Rectal Temperature

◆ Assist the client to assume a lateral position. Place newborn in a lateral or prone position. Place a young child in a lateral position with knees flexed, or prone across the lap.

For Comfort and Safety

◆ Provide privacy before folding the bedclothes back to expose the buttocks. *Privacy is essential because exposure of the buttocks embarrasses most people.*

For an Axillary Temperature

◆ Expose the client's axilla. If the axilla is moist, dry it with the towel, using a patting motion. *Friction created by rubbing can raise the temperature of the axilla.*

2. Prepare the equipment.

◆ Remove the thermometer from its storage container, and check the temperature reading on the thermometer.

◆ Shake down the mercury (if necessary) by holding the thermometer between the thumb and forefinger at the end farthest from the bulb. Snap the wrist downward. Repeat until the mercury is below 35°C (95°F). *For Accurate Assessment of Subnormal Temperature*

◆ Place the thermometer in a plastic sheath according to agency policy. *Disposable sheaths prevent spread of infections.*

3. Take the temperature.

For an Oral Temperature

◆ Place the thermometer or probe at the base of the tongue to the right or left of the frenulum, in the posterior sublingual pocket (Figure 14-19 ◆). *The thermometer needs to reflect the core temperature of the blood in the larger blood vessels of the posterior pocket.*

◆ Ask the client to close the lips, not the teeth, around the thermometer. *A client who bites a glass thermometer can break it and injure the mouth.*

◆ Leave the thermometer in place a sufficient time for the temperature to register or for the length of time recommended by the agency. *The recommended time is generally 2 minutes.*

For a Rectal Temperature

◆ Place some lubricant on a piece of tissue. Then apply lubricant to the thermometer. *The lubricant facilitates insertion of the thermometer without irritating the mucous membrane.*

Frenulum of tongue
Tip of thermometer

Figure 14-19. ◆ The tip of the oral thermometer is placed beside the frenulum below the tongue.

◆ Put on disposable gloves. With the nondominant hand, raise the client's upper buttock to expose the anus.

◆ Ask the client to take a deep breath, and insert the thermometer into the anus anywhere from 1.5 to 4 cm (0.5 to 1.5 in), depending on the age and size of the client (for example, 1.5 cm [0.5 in] for an infant, 2.5 cm [0.9 in] for a child, and 3.7 cm [1.5 in] for an adult). *Taking a deep breath often relaxes the external sphincter muscle, thus easing insertion.*

◆ Do not force insertion of the thermometer. *Inability to insert the thermometer into a newborn could indicate the rectum is not patent.*

◆ Hold the thermometer in place for 3 minutes or for the length of time recommended by the agency (Figure 14-20 ◆). For neonates hold the thermometer in place for 5 minutes or according to agency protocol. Hold the young child firmly while the probe is in the rectum. *The thermometer may become displaced inside or outside the anus if not held in place.*

For an Axillary Temperature

◆ Place the thermometer in the center of the client's axilla (Figure 14-21 ◆). *In order for the thermometer to come in contact with axillary blood supply*

◆ Assist the client to place the arm tightly across the chest to keep the thermometer in place. *This maintains the proper position.*

◆ Leave the thermometer in place for 9 minutes or according to agency protocol. For infants and children, leave the thermometer in place 5 minutes. *Device must stay in position long enough to ensure an accurate temperature.*

◆ Remain with the client, and hold the thermometer in place if the client is irrational or very young. *This provides safety for the client and prevents breakage.*

4. Remove the thermometer.

◆ Remove the plastic sheath, or if a sheath is not used, wipe the thermometer with a tissue. Wipe in a rotating

Figure 14-21. ◆ Placing the bulb of the thermometer in the center of the axilla. *Source:* © Elena Dorfman.

manner toward the bulb. *The thermometer is wiped from the area of least contamination to that of greatest contamination.*

◆ Discard the tissue or sheath in a receptacle used for contaminated items. *This prevents spread of infection.*

5. Read the temperature.

◆ Hold the thermometer at eye level and rotate it until the mercury column is clearly visible. The upper end of the mercury column registers the client's body temperature. On the Fahrenheit thermometer, each long line reflects 1 degree, and each short line 0.2 degree. On the Celsius (centigrade) thermometer, each long line reflects 0.5 degree, and each short line 0.1 degree.

6. Clean and shake down the thermometer.

◆ Wash the thermometer in tepid, soapy water. Rinse the thermometer in cold water, dry it, and store it dry. *Organic material, such as mucus, must be removed before the thermometer can be stored. Organic materials on the thermometer can harbor microorganisms. Hot water expands the mercury and may break the thermometer.*

◆ Shake down the thermometer and return it to its container or discard it. *Some agencies also have special equipment for spinning down the mercury levels.*

◆ If the thermometer is to be disinfected before storage, follow agency policy.

7. Document the temperature.

◆ Record the temperature to the nearest indicated tenth (for example, 37.1°C, 98.4°F,) on a designated flowsheet. See Figure 9–5. *Recording the temperature immediately ensures it is not forgotten.*

VARIATION: USING AN ELECTRONIC THERMOMETER

◆ Remove the electronic unit from the battery charging area.

◆ Remove the temperature probe. If the probe is not attached, attach it to the appropriate circuit (oral, rectal, or axillary) in models that have separate circuits for each.

Figure 14-20. ◆ Inserting a rectal thermometer. *Source:* © Elena Dorfman.

- Place a disposable cover securely on the probe.
- Warm up the machine by switching it on if removal of the probe does not automatically prepare the machine for functioning.
- Take the temperature as indicated in step 3.
- Listen for a sound indicating that the maximum measurement has been reached, and read the temperature on the dial or readout.
- Remove the thermometer.
- Record the temperature.
- Remove and discard the probe cover.
- Return the unit to the charging base.

VARIATION: USING A TYMPANIC (INFRARED) THERMOMETER

- Apply a disposable sheath to the probe. Different sheaths fit adults and infants. They can be applied without being touched.
- Select the ear opposite the side on which the client may have been lying. The ear against a surface can build up heat.
- Use your right hand to hold the thermometer when using the client's right ear, left hand for the left ear. This helps achieve the proper angle for a good seal.
- Gently pull the pinna upward and back for children over age 3 and adults (Figure 14-22 ◆), straight back for children under age 3. This straightens the ear canal.
- Place the probe tip into the outer position of the ear canal just at the opening. The probe tip seals the opening of the canal.
- Press the button on the electronic thermometer. Do not wait too long to do this. The presence of the probe can "draw down" the temperature reading.

Figure 14-22. ◆ Pull the pinna of the ear up and back while inserting the tympanic thermometer. *Source:* © Jenny Thomas.

- Remove the thermometer.
- Read the temperature on the screen. In 1 to 2 seconds, the temperature is displayed on the screen.
- Remove and discard the probe cover. Covers can be ejected without being touched.
- Return the unit to the charging base.

◆ SAMPLE DOCUMENTATION

> See Figure 9-5 for a common documentation of temperature.

PROCEDURE 14-2
Assessing Pulse

PURPOSES

- To establish baseline data for subsequent evaluation
- To identify whether the pulse rate is within normal range
- To determine whether the pulse rhythm is regular and the pulse volume is appropriate
- To compare the equality of corresponding peripheral pulses on each side of the body
- To monitor and assess changes in the client's health status
- To monitor clients at risk for pulse alterations (e.g., those with a history of heart disease or experiencing cardiac arrhythmias, hemorrhage, acute pain, infusion of large volumes of fluids, fever)
- To obtain the heart rate of newborns, infants, and children 2 to 3 years old or of an adult with an irregular peripheral pulse
- To determine whether the cardiac rate is within normal range and the rhythm is regular
- To monitor clients with cardiac disease and those receiving medications to improve heart action
- To determine adequacy of peripheral circulation or presence of pulse deficit

A   **B**

Figure 14-23. ◆ A. Stethoscope with both a bell-shaped and flat-disc amplifier. **B.** Close-up of a flat-disc amplifier (left) and a bell amplifier (right). *Source:* © Elena Dorfman.

EQUIPMENT

- Watch with a second hand or indicator
- If using Doppler ultrasound stethoscope, the transducer in the DUS probe, a stethoscope headset, and transmission gel
- Antiseptic wipes
- Stethoscope with a bell-shaped or flat disc (Figure 14-23 ◆)
- Stethoscope

Part A: Peripheral Pulse

INTERVENTIONS

1. Prepare the client.
- Select the pulse point. *Normally, the radial pulse is taken unless it cannot be exposed or circulation to another body area is to be assessed.*
- Assist the client to a comfortable resting position. When the radial pulse is assessed, the client's arm can rest alongside the body, the palm facing downward. Or the forearm can rest at a 90-degree angle across the chest with the palm downward. For the client who can sit, the forearm can rest across the thigh, with the palm of the hand facing downward or inward. Position a child comfortably in the parent's arms, or have the parent remain close by. *Having the parent close or holding the child may decrease anxiety and yield more accurate results.*

2. Palpate and count the pulse (Figure 14-24 ◆).
- Place two or three middle fingertips lightly and squarely over the pulse point (Figure 14-24B). *Using the thumb is contraindicated because the thumb has a pulse that the nurse could mistake for the client's pulse.*
- If the pulse is regular, count for 30 seconds and multiply by 2. If it is irregular, count for 1 minute. When taking a client's pulse for the first time or obtaining baseline data, count the pulse for a full minute. *An irreg-*

ular pulse requires a full minute's count for a correct assessment and indicates the need to take the apical pulse.

3. Assess the pulse rhythm and volume.
- Assess the pulse rhythm by noting the pattern of the intervals between the beats. *A normal pulse has equal time periods between beats.* If this is an initial assessment, assess for 1 minute.
- Assess the pulse volume. *A normal pulse can be felt with moderate pressure, and the pressure is equal with each beat. A forceful pulse volume is full; an easily obliterated pulse is weak.*

4. Document and report to the nurse in charge, pertinent assessment data.
- Record the pulse rate, rhythm, and volume on the appropriate records.
- Report to the nurse in charge pertinent data such as (a) pale skin color and cool skin temperature, (b) a pulse rate faster or slower than normal for the client, (c) a full, bounding, or weak pulse volume, and (d) an irregular pulse rhythm.

VARIATION: USING A DUS

- Plug the stethoscope headset into one of the two output jacks located next to the volume control. DUS units may have two jacks so that a second person can listen to the signals (see Figure 14-10).

Figure 14-24. ◆ Assessing the pulses: **A.** Brachial; **B.** Radial; **C.** Carotid; **D.** Femoral; **E.** Popliteal; **F.** Posterior tibial; **G.** Pedal (dorsalis pedis).

◆ Apply transmission gel either to the probe at the narrow end of the plastic case housing the transducer or to the client's skin. Ultrasound beams do not travel well through air. *The gel makes an airtight seal, which then promotes optimal ultrasound wave transmission.*
◆ Press the "on" button.
◆ Hold the probe against the skin over the pulse site. Use a light pressure, and keep the probe in contact with the skin. *Too much pressure can stop the blood flow and obliterate the signal.*
◆ Distinguish artery sounds from vein sounds. The artery sound (signal) is distinctively pulsating and has a pumping quality. The venous sound is intermittent and varies with respirations. *Both artery and vein sounds are heard simultaneously through the DUS because major arteries and veins are situated close together throughout the body.*
◆ If arterial sounds cannot be easily heard, reposition the probe.
◆ After assessing the pulse, remove all the gel from the probe to prevent damage to its surface. Clean the transducer with aqueous solutions. *Alcohol or other disinfectants may damage the face of the transducer. Remove all gel from the client.*

Part B: Apical Pulse

INTERVENTIONS

1. Prepare client. Position the client appropriately.
◆ Assist an adult or young child to a comfortable supine position or to a sitting position.
◆ Place a baby in a supine position, and offer a pacifier if the baby is crying or restless. *Crying and physical activity will increase the pulse rate.* Take the apical pulse rate of infants and small children before assessing body temperatures.
◆ Demonstrate the procedure to the child using a stuffed animal or doll, and allow the child to handle the stethoscope before beginning the procedure. *This will decrease anxiety and promote cooperation.*
◆ Expose the area of the chest over the apex of the heart. *Clothing may interfere with ability to assess heartbeat.*

2. Locate the apical impulse.
◆ This is the point over the apex of the heart where the apical pulse can be most clearly heard. It is also referred to as the point of maximal impulse (PMI).

- Palpate the angle of Louis (the angle between the manubrium, the top of the sternum, and the body of the sternum). It is palpated just below the suprasternal notch and is felt as a prominence (see Figure 14-9).
- Slide your index finger just to the left of the client's sternum, and palpate the second intercostal space.
- Place your middle or next finger in the third intercostal space, and continue palpating downward until you locate the apical impulse, usually about the fifth intercostal space if the client is an adult or a child 7 years or older. If the client is a young child, palpate downward to the fourth intercostal space. *The apex of the heart is normally located in the fifth intercostal space in individuals who are 7 years of age and over; it is in the fourth intercostal space in young children, and one or two spaces above the adult apex during infancy.*
- Palpate the apical impulse. If the client is an adult, move your index finger laterally along the fifth intercostal space to the MCL. *Normally, the apical impulse is palpable at or just medial to the MCL.* For a young child, move your finger along the fourth intercostal space to a position between the MCL and the anterior axillary line (see Figure 14-9).

3. Auscultate and count heartbeats.
- Use antiseptic wipes to clean the earpieces and diaphragm of the stethoscope if their cleanliness is in doubt. *The diaphragm needs to be cleaned and disinfected if soiled with body substances.*
- Warm the diaphragm of the stethoscope by holding it in the palm of the hand for a moment. *The metal of the diaphragm is usually cold and can startle the client when placed immediately on the chest.*
- Insert the earpieces of the stethoscope into your ears in the direction of the ear canals, or slightly forward. *This facilitates hearing.*
- Tap your finger lightly on the diaphragm to be sure it is the active side of the head. If necessary, rotate the head to select the diaphragm side.
- Place the diaphragm of the stethoscope over the apical impulse (Figure 14-25 ◆) and listen for the normal S1 and S2 heart sounds, which are heard as "lub-dub." Each lub-dub is counted as one heartbeat. The heartbeat is normally loudest over the apex of the heart. The two

Figure 14-25. ◆ Taking an apical pulse using the flat disc of the stethoscope. Note how the amplifier is held against the chest. *Source:* © Elena Dorfman.

heart sounds are produced by closure of the valves of the heart. The S1 heart sound (lub) occurs when the atrioventricular valves close after the ventricles have been sufficiently filled. The S2 heart sound (dub) occurs when the semilunar valves close after the ventricles empty.
- If the rhythm is regular, count the heartbeats for 30 seconds and multiply by 2. If the rhythm is irregular or if the apical impulse is being taken on an infant or child, count the beats for 60 seconds. *A 60-second count provides a more accurate assessment of an irregular pulse than a 30-second count.*

4. Assess the rhythm and the strength of the heartbeat.
- Assess the rhythm of the heartbeat by noting the pattern of intervals between the beats. *A normal pulse has equal time periods between beats.*
- Assess the strength (volume) of the heartbeat. *Normally, the heartbeats are equal in strength and can be described as strong or weak.*

5. Document and report pertinent assessment data.
- Record the pulse site and rate, rhythm, and volume on the appropriate records.
- Report to the nurse in charge any pertinent data such as pallor, cyanosis, dyspnea, tachycardia, bradycardia, irregular rhythm, and reduced strength of the heartbeat.

Part C: Apical–Radial Pulse

INTERVENTIONS

1. Position the client appropriately.
- Assist the client to assume the position described for taking the apical pulse above.
- If previous measurements were taken, determine what position the client assumed and use the same position. *This ensures an accurate comparative measurement.*

2. Locate the apical and radial pulse sites.

3. Count the apical and radial pulse rates.

Two-Nurse Technique
- In the two-nurse technique, one nurse locates the apical impulse by palpation or with the stethoscope while the other nurse palpates the radial pulse site.

◆ Place the watch where both nurses can see it. The nurse who is taking the radial pulse may hold the watch.

◆ Decide on a time to begin counting. *A time when the second hand is on 12, 3, 6, or 9 is usually selected to help in obtaining an accurate reading.* The nurse taking the radial pulse says "Start" at the designated time. *This ensures that simultaneous counts are taken.*

◆ Each nurse counts the pulse rate for 60 seconds. Both nurses end the count when the nurse taking the radial pulse says "Stop." *A full 60-second count is necessary for accurate assessment of any differences between the two pulse sites.*

◆ The nurse who assesses the apical rate also assesses the apical pulse rhythm and volume (i.e., whether the heartbeat is strong or weak). If the pulse is irregular, note whether the irregular beats come at random or at predictable times.

◆ The nurse assessing the radial pulse rate also assesses the radial pulse rhythm and volume.

One-Nurse Technique (Not Recommended for Clients with Irregular Heartbeat)

◆ Assess the apical pulse for 60 seconds.

◆ Assess the radial pulse for 60 seconds.

4. Document and report pertinent assessment data.

◆ Promptly report any notable changes from previous measurements or any difference between the two pulses.

◆ Document the apical and radial (AR) pulse rates, rhythm, volume, and any pulse deficit.

◆ Record any other pertinent observations, such as pallor, cyanosis, or dyspnea.

◆ Check the physician's orders for any directions related to a difference in the AR pulse rates.

◆ **SAMPLE DOCUMENTATION**

5/06/05	Apical-radial pulse taken: 80 apical,
0830	65 radial at left wrist and weak.
	Edema left arm +2.
	S. Markham, LPN

PROCEDURE 14-3

Assessing Respirations

PURPOSES

◆ To acquire baseline data against which future measurements can be compared

◆ To monitor abnormal respirations and respiratory patterns and identify changes

◆ To assess respirations before the administration of a medication such as morphine (an abnormally slow respiratory rate may warrant withholding the medication)

◆ To monitor respirations following the administration of a general anesthetic or any medication that influences respirations

◆ To monitor clients at risk for respiratory alterations (e.g., those with fever, pain, acute anxiety, chronic obstructive pulmonary disease, respiratory infection, pulmonary edema or emboli, chest trauma or constriction, brain stem injury)

EQUIPMENT

◆ Watch with a second hand or indicator

INTERVENTIONS

1. Determine the client's activity schedule.

◆ Choose a suitable time to monitor the respirations. *A client who has been exercising will need to rest for a few minutes to permit the accelerated respiratory rate to return to normal. An infant or child who is crying will have an abnormal respiratory rate and will need quieting before respirations can be accurately assessed.*

2. Observe or palpate and count the respiratory rate.

◆ Place a hand against the client's chest to feel the client's chest movements, or place the client's arm across the chest and observe the chest movements while appearing to take the radial pulse. Because young children are diaphragmatic breathers, observe the rise and fall of the abdomen. *Awareness of respiratory rate assessment could cause the client voluntarily to alter the respiratory pattern.*

◆ Count the respiratory rate for 30 seconds if the respirations are regular. Count for 60 seconds if they are irregular. An inhalation and an exhalation count as one respiration.

3. Observe the depth, rhythm, and character of respirations.

◆ Observe the respirations for depth by watching the movement of the chest. *During deep respirations a large volume of air is exchanged; during shallow respirations a small volume is exchanged.*

◆ Observe the respirations for regular or irregular rhythm. *Normally, respirations are evenly spaced.*

◆ Observe the character of respirations—the sound they produce and the effort they require. *Normally, respirations are silent and effortless.*

4. Document and report pertinent assessment data.

◆ Document the respiratory rate, depth, rhythm, and character on the appropriate records.

◆ Report:
   a. Respiratory rate significantly above or below the normal range and any notable change in respirations from previous assessments
   b. Irregular respiratory rhythm
   c. Inadequate respiratory depth
   d. Abnormal character of breathing—orthopnea, wheezing, stridor, or bubbling
   e. Any complaints of dyspnea

◆ **SAMPLE DOCUMENTATION**

06/04/05	Client c/o difficulty breathing. R 26.
2:30 PM	Wheezing noted. Encouraged huff
	coughing. Expelled thick yellow sputum.
	R 20. Resting in semi-Fowler. ————
	Erin McClellan, LVN

PROCEDURE 14-4

Assessing Blood Pressure

PURPOSES

◆ To obtain a baseline measure of arterial blood pressure for subsequent evaluation

◆ To determine the client's hemodynamic status (e.g., stroke volume of the heart and blood vessel resistance)

◆ To identify and monitor changes in blood pressure resulting from a disease process and medical therapy (e.g., presence or history of cardiovascular disease, renal disease, circulatory shock, or acute pain; rapid infusion of fluids or blood products)

EQUIPMENT

◆ Stethoscope or DUS

◆ Blood pressure cuff of the appropriate size (newborn, infant, child, small adult, adult, large adult, thigh)

◆ Sphygmomanometer

INTERVENTIONS

1. Prepare and position the client appropriately.

◆ Make sure that the client has not smoked or ingested caffeine within 30 minutes prior to measurement. *Nicotine and caffine can elevate BP.*

◆ Make sure that the bladder of the cuff encircles at least two thirds of the arm and that the width of the cuff is appropriate (see Figure 14-17). *Inappropriate size can result in altered readings.*

◆ Position the client in a sitting position unless otherwise specified. The elbow should be slightly flexed with the palm of the hand facing up and the forearm supported at heart level. *Readings in any other position should be specified. The blood pressure is normally similar in sitting, standing, and lying positions, but it can vary significantly by position in certain people. The blood pressure increases when the arm is below heart level and decreases when the arm is above heart level.*

◆ Expose the upper arm.

2. Wrap the deflated cuff evenly around the upper arm.

◆ Locate the brachial artery (Figure 14-26 ◆).

◆ Apply the center of the bladder directly over the artery. *The bladder inside the cuff must be directly over the artery to be compressed if the reading is to be accurate.*

◆ For an adult, place the lower border of the cuff approximately 2.5 cm (1 in) above the antecubital space. The lower edge can be closer to the antecubital space of an infant.

◆ If this is the client's initial examination, perform a preliminary palpatory determination of systolic pressure. *The initial estimate tells the nurse the maximal pressure to which the manometer needs to be elevated in subsequent determinations. It also prevents underestimation of the systolic pressure or overestimation of the diastolic pressure should an auscultatory gap occur.*

Blood pressure cuff

Brachial artery

Ulnar artery

Radial artery

Figure 14-26. ◆ Location of the brachial artery and application of the cuff.

◆ Palpate the brachial artery with the fingertips.

◆ Close the valve on the pump by turning the knob clockwise.

◆ Pump up the cuff until you no longer feel the brachial pulse. *At that pressure the blood cannot flow through the artery.*

◆ Note the pressure on the sphygmomanometer at which the pulse is no longer felt. *This gives an estimate of the maximum pressure required to measure the systolic pressure.*

◆ Release the pressure completely in the cuff, and wait 1 to 2 minutes before making further measurements. *A waiting period gives the blood trapped in the veins time to be released.*

3. Position the stethoscope appropriately.

◆ Clean the earpieces with alcohol or recommended disinfectant. *Infection control measures are necessary unless nurse is using personal stethoscope.*

◆ Insert the ear attachments of the stethoscope in your ears so that they tilt slightly forward. *Sounds are heard more clearly when the ear attachments follow the direction of the ear canal.*

◆ Ensure that the stethoscope hangs freely from the ears to the diaphragm. *Rubbing the stethoscope against an object can obliterate the sounds of the blood within an artery.*

◆ Place the bell side of the stethoscope (see Figure 14-23) over the brachial pulse. *Because the blood pressure is a low-frequency sound, it is best heard with the bell-shaped diaphragm* (Bates, 1995, p. 278). Hold the diaphragm with the thumb and index finger.

4. Auscultate the client's blood pressure.

◆ Pump up the cuff until the sphygmomanometer registers about 30 mm Hg above the point where the brachial pulse disappeared.

◆ Release the valve on the cuff carefully so that the pressure decreases at the rate of 2 to 3 mm Hg per second. *If the rate is faster or slower an error may occur.*

◆ As the pressure falls, identify the manometer reading at each of the five phases.

◆ Deflate the cuff rapidly and completely.

◆ Wait 1 to 2 minutes before making further determinations. *This permits blood trapped in the veins to be released.*

◆ Repeat the preceding steps once or twice as necessary to confirm the accuracy of the reading.

5. Remove the cuff.

◆ Wipe the cuff with an approved disinfectant. *Cuffs can become significantly contaminated.*

◆ If this is the client's initial examination, repeat the procedure on the client's other arm.

◆ There should be a difference of no more than 5 to 10 mm Hg between the arms.

◆ The arm found to have the higher pressure should be used for subsequent examinations.

6. Document and report pertinent assessment data.
- ◆ Document the blood pressure according to agency policy. Record two pressures in the form "130/80" where "130" is the systolic (phase 1) and "80" is the diastolic (phase 5) pressure. Record three pressures in the form "130/110/90," where "130" is the systolic, "110" is the first diastolic (phase 4), and "90" is the second diastolic (phase 5) pressure. Use the abbreviations RA for right arm and LA for left arm. Record a difference of greater than 10 mm Hg in the arms.
- ◆ Report any significant change in the client's blood pressure. Also report these findings:
  - **a.** Systolic blood pressure (of an adult) above 140 mm Hg
  - **b.** Diastolic blood pressure (of an adult) above 90 mm Hg
  - **c.** Systolic blood pressure (of an adult) below 100 mm Hg

VARIATION: TAKING A THIGH BLOOD PRESSURE

- ◆ Help the client to assume a prone position. If the client cannot assume this position, measure the blood pressure while the client is in a supine position with the knee slightly flexed. *Slight flexing of the knee will facilitate placing the stethoscope on the popliteal space.*
- ◆ Expose the thigh, taking care not to expose the client unduly.
- ◆ Locate the popliteal artery (Figure 14-27 ◆).
- ◆ Wrap the cuff evenly around the midthigh with the compression bladder over the posterior aspect of the thigh and the bottom edge above the knee. The bladder must be directly over the posterior popliteal artery if the reading is to be accurate.
- ◆ If this is the client's initial examination, perform a preliminary palpatory determination of systolic pressure by palpating the popliteal artery (see Figure 14-24E). The systolic pressure in the popliteal artery is usually 20 to 30 mm Hg higher than that in the brachial artery because of use of a larger bladder; the diastolic pressure is usually the same.
- ◆ Auscultate the pressure as for the arm.

VARIATION: USING AN ELECTRONIC INDIRECT BLOOD PRESSURE MONITORING DEVICE

- ◆ Unplug the electronic unit from the electrical outlet.
- ◆ Place the blood pressure cuff on the extremity according to the manufacturer's guidelines.
- ◆ Turn on the blood pressure switch.
- ◆ When the device has determined the blood pressure reading, note the digital results.
- ◆ Record the blood pressure according to agency policy.

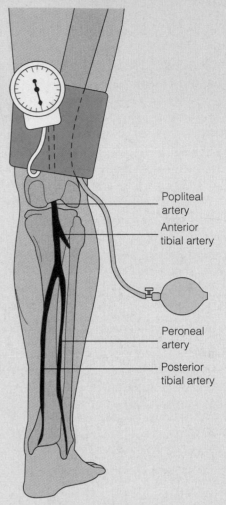

Popliteal artery
Anterior tibial artery
Peroneal artery
Posterior tibial artery

Figure 14-27. ◆ Location of the popliteal artery and application of the cuff.

◆ SAMPLE DOCUMENTATION

4/14/06	T 38 rectal, P 95, R 22, BP 145/95.
1530	Client confused, not oriented to time and place. Team leader notified. ————
	S. Lopez, LPN

Chapter Review

Key Terms by Topics

Use the audio glossary feature of either the CD-ROM or the Companion Website to hear the correct pronunciation of the following key terms.

Body temperature
basal metabolic rate (BMR), pyrexia, hyperthermia, afebrile, crisis, hypothermia

Pulse
peripheral pulse, apical, pulse deficit

Respirations
respiration, external respiration, internal respiration

Blood pressure
blood pressure, systolic pressure, diastolic pressure, cardiac output, viscosity, orthostatic hypotension

Key Points

◆ Vital signs reflect changes in body function that otherwise might not be observed.

◆ Various sites and methods can be used to assess vital signs. The nurse selects the site and method that is safe for the client and that will provide the most accurate measurement possible.

◆ The most accurate values are obtained when the client is at rest and comfortable.

◆ Changes in one vital sign can trigger changes in other vital signs.

◆ Vital signs are assessed when a client is admitted to a health care agency to establish baseline data and when there is a change or possibility of a change in the client's condition.

◆ Data obtained from measurements of vital signs are used to plan and implement appropriate nursing interventions and to evaluate a client's response to these interventions or prescribed medical therapy.

◆ Body temperature is the balance between heat produced by the body and heat lost from the body.

◆ Knowledge of factors affecting heat production and heat loss helps the nurse to implement appropriate interventions when the client has a fever or hypothermia.

◆ Factors affecting body temperature include age, diurnal variations, exercise, hormones, stress, and environmental temperatures.

◆ Pyrexia (fever) is a common sign of disease. Four common types of fever are intermittent, remittent, relapsing, and constant. Clinical signs of fever vary during the onset, course, and abatement stages.

◆ Hypothermia involves three mechanisms: excessive heat loss, inadequate heat production by body cells, and increasing impairment of hypothalamic temperature regulation.

◆ Body temperature can be measured orally, tympanically, rectally, or by axilla. The nurse selects the most appropriate site according to the client's age and condition.

◆ Normally a peripheral pulse reflects the client's heartbeat, but it may differ from the heartbeat in clients with certain cardiovascular diseases; in these instances, the nurse takes an apical pulse and compares it to the peripheral pulse.

◆ Many factors affect a person's pulse rate: age, sex, exercise, presence of fever, certain medications, hemorrhage, stress, and (in some situations) position changes.

◆ Respirations are normally quiet, effortless, and automatic and are assessed by observing respiratory rate, depth, rhythm, and sound.

◆ Blood pressure reflects cardiac output, peripheral vascular resistance, blood volume, and blood viscosity. Peripheral vascular resistance varies according to the size of the arterioles and capillaries, and the elasticity of the arteries.

EXPLORE MediaLink

Additional interactive resources for this chapter can be found on the Companion Website at www.prenhall.com/ramont. Click on Chapter 14 and "Begin" to select the activities for this chapter.

For chapter-related NCLEX-style questions and an audio glossary, access the accompanying CD-ROM in this book.

Animation:
◆ Cardiac cycle
◆ Chambers of the human heart
◆ Atrial contraction
◆ Blood flow to atria
◆ Ventricular contraction
◆ Oxygen transport
◆ Gas exchange in lung
◆ Carbon dioxide transport
◆ Systole and diastole
◆ Endocrine system
◆ Propranolol

For Further Study

See Figure 9–5 for documenting vitals signs on a graphic flowsheet.

For more information about regulation of breathing and about pulse oximetry, see Chapter 16.

For in-depth discussion of pain, see Chapter 15.

Critical Thinking Care Map

Caring for a Client after a Heart Attack

NCLEX–PN Focus Area: Physiological Adaptation

Case Study: Edgar Wilson, a 50-year-old African-American, was brought to the ER after chest pain of 1 hour's duration. He was admitted to rule out myocardial infarction (MI). He described the pain as radiating to his back and down his left arm, 9/10. He was given morphine sulfate 4 mg IV × 3. His pain is now 5/10. He has a history of hypertension (treated with Verapamil) and a family history of cardiovascular disease. His father died of a heart attack at 56. His mother had a disabling stroke at age 60.

Vital signs: BP 158/90, P 100, R 24, T 99.8 oral. Height 5'10", weight 295 lbs. Cardiac monitoring showed sinus tachycardia with occasional PVC. Twelve-lead ECG and cardiac enzymes obtained in ER.

Mr. Wilson was in a motor vehicle accident 1 week ago in which he sustained a head injury. He lives with his wife; a son lives nearby. He is a history teacher at the local community college. Mr. Wilson states, "I probably won't live to an old age. I have bad genes for heart attack and stroke."

Nursing Diagnosis: Health-Seeking Behaviors Related to Lack of Knowledge

COLLECT DATA

Subjective	Objective
_____	_____
_____	_____
_____	_____
_____	_____
_____	_____
_____	_____
_____	_____

Would you report this data? Yes/No

If yes, to: _____

Nursing Care

_____
_____
_____
_____
_____
_____
_____

How would you document this? _____
_____
_____
_____
_____

Data Collected
(use those that apply)

- 50-year old African-American male
- Chest pain, radiating to back and left arm 9/10. Morphine Sulfate 4 mg IV ×3; pain now 5/10.
- Verapamil E.R. 180 mg bid for hypertension
- Father died of a heart attack age 56
- Mother stroke at 60; now 69, disabled
- VS: T 99.8, P 100, R 24, BP 158/90
- Height 5' 10", weight 295 lbs
- Diet—"I normally eat fast food for lunch. My wife does make healthy dinners."
- Sinus tachycardia with occassional PVC
- 12-lead ECG and cardiac enzymes obtained in ER (no report)
- MVA 1 week ago sustained a head injury
- Lives with wife; one son nearby
- History teacher at local college
- "I probably won't live to an old age. I have bad genes for heart attack and stroke."

Nursing Interventions
(use all that apply)

- Assess client's feelings, values, and reasons for not following prescribed plan of care.
- Discuss client's beliefs about health and his ability to maintain health.
- Identify barriers and benefits to being healthy.
- Help client to choose healthly lifestyle and to have appropriate diagnostic tests.
- Compare client's height and weight to standards for age and height.
- Encourage client to eat a diet with fresh foods, low saturated fat, and no added salt.
- Teach stress-relieving techniques.
- Assess for the influences of culture and values on the client's beliefs about health.
- Identify support groups related to the disease process.

NCLEX-PN Exam Preparation

1. You are assigned to take morning vital signs on several clients on a medical surgical unit. Of the following vital signs, which would you report immediately to the RN?
   a. 99.6 (R), 86, 24, 140/88
   b. 97.2 (O), 110, 18, 110/78
   c. 101.8 (A), 72, 18, 90/60
   d. 98 (O), 100, 26, 148/80

2. Your assigned client has a history of mastectomy of right breast, one year ago. She has been admitted with a fracture of her left humerus. You need to assess her blood pressure. Using your knowledge of her condition and your critical thinking skills, what method would you use to assess the blood pressure?
   a. Apply the cuff to her right arm, being careful not to pump it up above 150 mm.
   b. Obtain a large cuff and assess her blood pressure using her thigh.
   c. Place the the cuff below her left elbow and palpate her radial pulse.
   d. Take her other vital signs and chart that you were unable to assess the blood pressure.

3. It is important to use the appropriate size of cuff when assessing blood pressure. When a cuff that is too narrow is used, you expect the result to be a blood pressure that is an:
   a. Erroneously high reading
   b. Erroneously low reading
   c. Erronously low diastolic reading
   d. Erronously high systolic

4. Phase five of Korotkoff's sounds is considered to be:
   a. The systolic blood pressure
   b. The diastolic blood pressure in an adult
   c. The diastolic blood pressure in a child
   d. The period of silence at the end of the blood pressure

5. Your primary nurse tells you that your client needs to have Tylenol administered for a fever. The temperature is recorded as 38.6°C. The physician has written an order for Tylenol for a temperature above 101°F. You will need to convert the temperature to Fahrenheit in order to determine if client should be medicated. Of the following readings, which is closest to 38.6°C?
   a. 100.6
   b. 104
   c. 103.2
   d. 101.5

6. You are assigned to admit clients in the pediatric urgent care unit. Using your knowledge of the cardiovascular system, which of the peripheral pulse sites would you normally select for a 30-month-old child?
   a. Radial
   b. Carotid
   c. Brachial
   d. Apical

7. Your neighbor asks you what is the normal blood pressure for her 6-year-old child. Which of the following would be the most appropriate answer?
   a. Systolic blood pressure of 92
   b. 100/70
   c. Diastolic blood pressure of 80
   d. 72/40

8. Standing, sitting, and lying blood pressures are taken to assess for:
   a. Orthostatic hypotension
   b. Orthostatic hypertension
   c. Pulse deficit
   d. Auscultatory gap

9. Your client has a physician's order for digoxin. Prior to administering the medication the nurse should:
   a. Assess the blood pressure and give medication if systolic pressure is greater than 140.
   b. Assess the radial pulse and hold if it is greater than 100.
   c. Assess the apical pulse and hold if less than 60.
   d. Assess the apical pulse and give if less than 60.

10. Your client is being discharged home. The physician has ordered MS Contin for pain control. Of the following discharge instructions, which one should be considered when administering morphine?
    a. Take blood pressure prior to administration.
    b. Take blood pressure 20 minutes after administration.
    c. Assess respirations following administration.
    d. Assess apical pulse prior to administration.

Answers for Review Questions, as well as discussion of Case Study and Critical Thinking Care Map questions, appear in Appendix IV.

Chapter 15

Pain, The Fifth Vital Sign

SHARING experiences

" While working as a CNA, I found how reward-ing it was to care for people. I wanted to be able to do more, know more. This desire to be of more help and gain more knowledge of what I could do, inspired me to apply for the LPN program. "

LaReta Gugelman, PN student, Idaho State University, Pocatello, ID.

LEARNING outcomes

After completing this chapter, you will be able to:

- Identify types and categories of pain according to location, eti-ology, and duration.
- Differentiate pain threshold from pain tolerance.
- Describe pain transmission, perception, interpretation, and modulation.
- Describe the gate control theory and its application to nurs-ing care.
- Identify subjective and objective data to collect and analyze when assessing pain.
- Identify examples of nursing diagnoses for clients with pain.
- State outcome criteria by which to evaluate a client's response to interventions for pain.
- Identify barriers to effective pain management.
- Describe pharmacologic interventions for pain.
- Define tolerance, dependence, and addiction.
- Describe the World Health Organization's three-step ladder approach to cancer pain.
- Identify rationales for using various analgesic delivery routes.
- Describe nonpharmacologic pain control interventions.

MediaLink

www.prenhall.com/ramon

Use the address above to access the free, interactive Companion Website created for this textbook. Get hints, instant feedback, and textbook references to chapter-related NCLEX-style questions. Link to other interesting sites.

Audio Glossary:
Use the Companion Website, or the CD-ROM disk enclosed with your textbook, to hear the pronunciation of key terms in the chapter.

Pain is a highly unpleasant and very personal sensation. Pain can consume a person's thoughts and take over daily activities. Yet pain is a difficult concept for a client to communicate. A nurse can neither feel nor see a client's pain.

No two people experience pain in exactly the same way. Because of the differences in how individuals perceive and react to pain, as well as the many causes of pain, the nurse is faced with a complex situation when developing a plan to relieve pain and provide comfort. Effective pain management is an important aspect of care.

As we have learned more about pain, we have seen a shift in focus toward pain control and pain management independent of the cause of the pain. Severe pain is now being viewed as an emergency situation deserving anticipation and prompt treatment. Pain is more than a symptom of a problem; it is a high-priority problem in itself. Pain presents both physiologic and psychologic dangers to health and recovery. Pain increases morbidity and mortality. Unresolved pain has been shown to prolong hospital stays, delay the healing process, and contribute to depression.

◆ Types of Pain

Although pain is a universal experience, its exact nature remains a mystery. There are a number of definitions of pain. It is known that **pain** is sensation that is highly subjective and individual; it is one of the body's defense mechanisms indicating that there is a problem.

McCaffery (1979, p. 11) defines pain as "whatever the experiencing person says it is, existing whenever he (or she) says it does." The most vital part of this definition is the care provider's willingness to believe that the client is experiencing pain and that the client is the real authority about that pain.

Pain may be described in terms of its duration, location, or etiology. When pain lasts only through the expected recovery period, it is described as **acute pain,** whether it has a sudden or slow onset and regardless of the intensity. **Chronic pain** lasts beyond the typical healing time period. Pain is generally labeled chronic after 3 to 6 months. Chronic pain can be further classified as chronic malignant pain, when associated with cancer or other life-threatening conditions, or as chronic nonmalignant pain when the etiology is a nonprogressive disorder, such as damage from trauma. Chronic pain that persists despite therapeutic interventions is classified as **intractable pain.** Acute and chronic pain result in different physiologic and behavioral responses, shown in Table 15-1 ◆.

Pain can be categorized according to its origin as cutaneous, deep somatic, or visceral. **Cutaneous pain** originates in the skin or subcutaneous tissue. A paper cut causing a sharp pain with some burning is an example of cutaneous pain. **Somatic pain** arises from ligaments, tendons, bones, blood vessels, and nerves. It is diffuse and tends to last longer than cutaneous pain. An ankle sprain is an example of deep somatic pain. **Visceral pain** results from stimulation of pain recep-

TABLE 15-1	COMPARISON OF ACUTE AND CHRONIC PAIN	
ACUTE PAIN	**CHRONIC PAIN**
Mild to severe	Mild to severe
Sympathetic nervous system responses: 　Increased pulse rate 　Increased respiratory rate 　Elevated blood pressure 　Diaphoresis 　Dilated pupils	Parasympathetic nervous system responses: 　Vital signs normal 　Dry, warm skin 　Pupils normal or dilated
Related to tissue injury; resolves with healing	Continues beyond healing
Client appears restless and anxious	Client appears depressed and withdrawn
Client reports pain	Client often does not mention pain unless asked
Client exhibits behavior indicative of pain: crying, rubbing area, holding area	Pain behavior often absent

tors in the abdominal cavity, cranium, and thorax. Visceral pain tends to appear diffuse and often feels like deep somatic pain, that is, burning, aching, or creating a feeling of pressure. Visceral pain is frequently caused by stretching of the tissues, ischemia, or muscle spasms. For example, an obstructed bowel will result in visceral pain.

Pain may also be described according to where it is experienced in the body. **Radiating pain** is perceived at the source of the pain and extends to nearby tissues. For example, cardiac pain may be felt not only in the chest but also along the left shoulder and down the arm. **Referred pain** is pain felt in a part of the body that is considerably removed from the tissues causing the pain. The pain is felt along the nerve pathways for the tissue of origin. For example, pain from one part of the abdominal viscera may be perceived in an area of the skin remote from the organ causing the pain (Figure 15-1 ◆).

Intractable pain is pain that is highly resistant to relief. One example is the pain from an advanced malignancy. Often, nurses are challenged to use a number of methods, such as imagery and patient-controlled analgesia (PCA), to provide a client with pain relief.

Neuropathic pain is the result of a disturbance of the nerve pathways either from past or continuing tissue damage that results in pain. Neuropathic pain is described as shooting or stabbing and is often severe. Clients with conditions such as AIDS and diabetes often suffer from neuropathic pain.

Phantom pain, which is a painful sensation perceived in a body part that is missing (e.g., an amputated leg) or para-

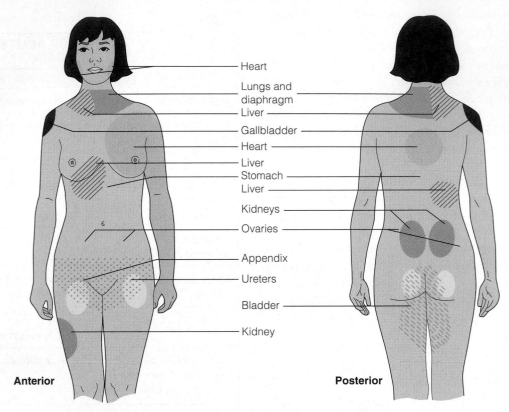

Anterior		Posterior
	Heart	
	Lungs and diaphragm	
	Liver	
	Gallbladder	
	Heart	
	Liver	
	Stomach	
	Liver	
	Kidneys	
	Ovaries	
	Appendix	
	Ureters	
	Bladder	
	Kidney	

Figure 15-1. ◆ Common sites of referred pain from various body organs.

lyzed by a spinal cord injury, is also an example of neuropathic pain. This can be distinguished from phantom sensation, that is, the feeling that the missing body part is still present.

Concepts Associated with Pain

When an individual perceives pain from injured tissue, the **pain threshold** is reached. An individual's pain threshold is the amount of pain stimulation a person requires in order to feel pain. People's pain threshold is generally fairly uniform; however, it can change. For example, the same stimuli that once produced mild pain can at another time produce intense pain.

Two additional terms used in the context of pain are pain reaction and tolerance. **Pain reaction** includes the autonomic nervous system and behavioral responses to pain. The *autonomic nervous system response* is the automatic reaction of the body that often protects the individual from further harm, such as the automatic withdrawal of the hand from a hot stove. The *behavioral response* is a learned response used as a method of coping with the pain. Behavioral responses can be related to the anticipation of pain, the sensation of pain, or the aftermath of pain. For example, explaining to a client what he or she will feel prior to administering an injection may reduce the behavioral reaction to the injection.

Pain tolerance is the maximum amount and duration of pain that an individual is willing to endure. Some clients are unable to tolerate even the slightest pain, whereas others are willing to endure severe pain rather than be treated for it. Thus, pain tolerance varies greatly among people and is widely influenced by psychological and sociocultural factors. Pain tolerance may increase with age.

Physiology of Pain

How pain is transmitted and perceived is still incompletely understood. Whether pain is perceived and to what degree depend on the interaction between the body's analgesia system and the nervous system's transmission and interpretation of stimuli.

TRANSMISSION AND PERCEPTION

The peripheral nervous system includes primary sensory neurons specialized to detect tissue damage and to evoke the sensation of touch, heat, cold, pain, and pressure. The receptors that transmit pain sensation are called **nociceptors** (Figure 15-2 ◆). These pain receptors or nociceptors can be excited by mechanical, thermal, or chemical stimuli (Table 15-2 ◆). When there are sufficient noxious stimuli, biochemical mediators are released that sensitize or activate the nociceptors. These chemicals cause the cardinal signs and symptoms we see

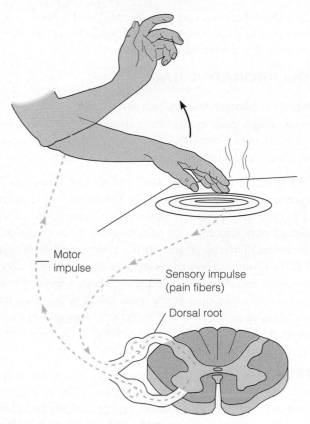

Motor impulse

Sensory impulse
(pain fibers)

Dorsal root

Figure 15-2. ◆ Proprioceptive reflex to a pain stimulus.

when tissue damage has occurred. The release of inflammatory chemicals causes vasodilation (redness) and increased capillary permeability (swelling); it also contributes to the conduction of nociception. (See also Chapter 12. ⊙)

Pain impulses are transmitted via two types of fibers. The A-delta (large-diameter) fibers are *myelinated* (they conduct electrical impulses rapidly). These fibers are associated with the sensation of sharp, pricking pain. The C fibers (small-diameter, unmyelinated fibers) transmit the impulse

more slowly and mediate long-lasting, burning pain. The fast A fibers primarily conduct impulses from mechanical and thermal pain. The slow, type C fibers conduct impulses from mechanical, thermal, and chemical stimuli.

As pain impulses stimulate the brain, nerve fibers conduct impulses from the brain to the spinal cord, where the pain impulses are inhibited in the spinal cord by the release of **endogenous opioids.** The three classes of endogenous opioids are enkephalins, dynorphins, and beta endorphins. These substances bind to opiate receptor sites in the central and peripheral nervous system, decreasing or blocking any pain impulse. The opiate binding sites are the same sites where **exogenous opioid** analgesics (e.g., morphine) bind to provide pain relief.

GATE CONTROL THEORY

In 1965, Melzack and Wall proposed the **gate control theory.** According to this theory, peripheral nerve fibers carrying pain to the spinal cord can have their message modified at the spinal cord level before transmission to the brain. Synapses in the spinal cord act as gates that close to keep messages from reaching the brain or open to permit messages to ascend to the brain.

According to the gate control theory, small-diameter nerve fibers carry pain stimuli through a gate, but large-diameter nerve fibers going through the same gate can inhibit the transmission of those pain messages—that is, close the gate (Figure 15-3 ◆). Because a limited amount of sensory information can reach the brain at any given time, certain cells can interrupt the pain messages. The brain also appears to influence whether the gate is open or closed. For example, previous experiences with pain are known to affect how an individual responds to pain. The involvement of the brain helps explain why painful stimuli are interpreted differently by people. Although the gate control theory is not unanimously accepted, it does help explain why electrical and mechanical

MediaLink ● Composition of Reflex Arc

TABLE 15-2	TYPES OF PAIN STIMULI	
STIMULUS TYPE	**PHYSIOLOGIC BASIS OF PAIN**
Mechanical	
1. Trauma to body tissues (e.g., surgery)	Tissue damage; direct irritation of the pain receptors; inflammation
2. Alterations in body tissues (e.g., edema)	Pressure on pain receptors
3. Blockage of a body duct	Distention of the lumen of the duct
4. Tumor	Pressure on pain receptors; irritation of nerve endings
5. Muscle spasm	Stimulation of pain receptors (also see chemical stimuli)
Thermal	
Extreme heat or cold (e.g., burns)	Tissue destruction; stimulation of thermosensitive pain receptors
Chemical	
1. Tissue ischemia (e.g., blocked coronary artery)	Stimulation of pain receptors because of accumulated lactic acid (and other chemicals, such as bradykinin and enzymes) in tissues
2. Muscle spasm	Tissue ischemia secondary to mechanical stimulation (see above)

Figure 15-3. ◆ A schematic illustration of the gate control theory.

interventions as well as heat and pressure can relieve pain. The gate control theory, simply put, suggests that a nerve pathway can only carry a few messages at a time. To inhibit the pain message we must send another message on the nerve pathway for the brain to interpret. For example, a back massage may stimulate impulses in large nerves, which in turn close the gate to back pain allowing only the message of tactile stimulation to reach the brain, not the message of pain.

RESPONSES TO PAIN

The body's response to pain is a complex process rather than a specific action. It involves physiologic and psychosocial aspects. Initially the sympathetic nervous system responds, resulting in the fight-or-flight response. As pain continues, the body adapts; the parasympathetic nervous system takes over, reversing many of the initial physiologic responses. This adaptation to the pain occurs after several hours or days of pain. The actual pain receptors adapt very little and continue to transmit the pain message. This serves the purpose of keeping the person continually aware of the damaging stimuli causing the pain (Guyton & Hall, 2000). The person may learn to cope with the pain through cognitive and behavioral activities, such as diversions, imagery, and excessive sleeping. The individual may respond to pain by seeking out physical interventions to manage the pain, such as analgesics, massage, and exercise.

FACTORS AFFECTING THE PAIN EXPERIENCE

Numerous factors can affect a person's perception of and reaction to pain. These include the person's ethnic and cultural

values, developmental stage, environment and support people, previous pain experiences, and the meaning of the current pain, as well as anxiety and stress (Box 15-1 ◆).

COLLABORATIVE CARE

Pharmacologic Management

Pharmacologic pain management involves the use of opioids (narcotics), nonopioids/NSAIDs (nonsteroidal anti-inflammatory drugs), and adjuvants, or coanalgesic drugs.

WHO THREE-STEP LADDER APPROACH. The World Health Organization (WHO) recommends a sequential or three-step ladder approach to manage cancer pain (Figure 15-4 ◆). This approach may also apply to pain resulting from causes other than cancer. Therapy begins with a nonopioid/NSAID (step 1). If the client receives the maximum recommended dose of nonopioids and continues to experience pain, a weak opioid is given (step 2). The dose of the weak opioid is increased until the ceiling dose is reached. If the client continues to experience pain, a stronger opioid is given (step 3). Adjuvant drugs may also be given at any stage of therapy.

OPIOID ANALGESICS. Opioid (narcotic) analgesics include opium derivatives, such as morphine and codeine. Narcotics relieve pain and provide a sense of euphoria largely by binding to opiate receptors and activating endogenous pain suppression in the central nervous system.

When administering any analgesic, the nurse must review side effects. All opioids result in some initial drowsiness when first administered, but with regular administration, this side effect tends to decrease. Opioids also may cause

Figure 15-4. ◆ The WHO three-step analgesic ladder. *Source:* World Health Organization.

BOX 15-1 FACTORS AFFECTING PAIN EXPERIENCE

Ethnic and Cultural Values

◆ Ethnic background and cultural heritage. Behavior related to pain is a part of the socialization process.

◆ There appears to be little variation in pain threshold, but cultural background can affect the level of pain that an individual is willing to tolerate. In some Middle Eastern and African cultures, self-infliction of pain is a sign of mourning or grief. In other groups, pain may be anticipated as part of the ritualistic practices, and therefore tolerance of pain signifies strength and endurance. Additionally, studies have shown that individuals of northern European descent tend to be more stoic and less expressive of their pain than people from southern European backgrounds.

Developmental Stage

◆ Behavioral observation is recommended for pain assessment in infants since physiologic responses vary greatly.

◆ Children are less able to articulate their experience or needs related to pain; therefore, their pain is often undertreated.

◆ The prevalence of pain in the older population is generally higher due to both acute and chronic disease conditions.

◆ Pain threshold does not appear to change with aging, although the effect of analgesics may increase due to physiologic changes related to drug metabolism.

Environment and Support People

◆ A strange environment such as a hospital, with its noises, lights, and activity, can compound pain.

◆ A person who is without a support network may perceive pain as severe, whereas the person who has supportive people around may perceive less pain.

◆ Some people prefer to withdraw when they are in pain, whereas others prefer the distraction of people and activity around them.

◆ Family caregivers can be a significant support for a person in pain. With the increase in outpatient and home care, families are assuming an increased responsibility for the management of pain.

◆ Education related to the assessment and management of pain can positively affect the perceived quality of life for both clients and their caregivers.

◆ Expectations of significant others can affect a person's perceptions of and responses to pain (e.g., girls may be permitted to express pain more openly than boys).

◆ Family role can also affect how a person perceives or responds to pain (e.g., a single mother supporting three children may ignore pain because of her need to stay on the job).

◆ The presence of support people often changes a client's reaction to pain (e.g., toddlers often tolerate pain more readily when supportive parents or nurses are nearby).

Past Pain Experiences

◆ Previous pain experiences alter a client's sensitivity to pain. People who have personally experienced pain or who have been exposed to the suffering of someone close are often more threatened by anticipated pain than people without a pain experience.

◆ The success or lack of success of pain relief measures influence a person's expectations for relief (e.g., a person who has tried several pain relief measures without success may have little hope about the helpfulness of nursing interventions).

Meaning of Pain

◆ Some clients may accept pain more readily than others, depending on the circumstances and the client's interpretation of its significance.

◆ A client who associates the pain with a positive outcome may withstand the pain amazingly well (e.g., a woman giving birth to a child or an athlete undergoing knee surgery to prolong his career may tolerate pain better because of the benefit associated with it).

◆ Clients with unrelenting chronic pain may suffer more intensely. They may respond with despair, anxiety, and depression because they cannot attach a positive significance or purpose to the pain. In this situation, the pain may be looked upon as a threat to body image or lifestyle and as a sign of possible impending death.

Anxiety and Stress

◆ Anxiety often accompanies pain. Threat of the unknown and the inability to control the pain or the events surrounding it often augment the pain perception. See Chapter 30 for more on effects of stress. ⊖⊃

◆ Fatigue also reduces a person's ability to cope, thereby increasing pain perception. When pain interferes with sleep, fatigue and muscle tension often result and increase the pain; thus, a cycle of pain, fatigue, pain develops.

◆ People in pain who believe that they have control of their pain have decreased fear and anxiety, which decreases their pain perception.

◆ A perception of lacking control or a sense of helplessness tends to increase pain perception.

◆ The expression of pain to an attentive listener and the participation in pain management decisions can increase the sense of control.

nausea, vomiting, constipation, and respiratory depression. The most common and most troubling side effect of opioids is constipation. If a client requires long-term opioid therapy, a laxative should be prescribed along with the opioid.

Opioids must be used cautiously in clients with respiratory problems. If the client experiences significant respiratory depression (e.g., a drop from 18 to 12) or is overly sedated, the dosage is excessive.

clinical ALERT

Before administering narcotics, the nurse needs to assess a client's level of alertness and respiratory rate for baseline data. An increased sedation level can be an early warning sign of impending respiratory depression.

See the sedation rating scale in Box 15-2 ◆. Often clients will manifest an increase in sedation before they manifest a decrease in respiratory rate and depth. The nurse should assess and document the client's level of sedation at the same time that respiratory status is checked. Early recognition of an increasing level of sedation or respiratory depression will enable the nurse to implement appropriate measures promptly (e.g., obtaining an order to decrease the opioid dosage). Health care providers should never allow the fear of respiratory depression to inhibit adequate pain control. Box 15-3 ◆ provides common side effects of, and preventive measures for, opioid analgesics.

Older clients are particularly sensitive to the analgesic properties of opioids and often require less medication than younger clients. This sensitivity may be related to reduced excretion of the drug in elderly clients.

NONOPIOIDS/NSAIDS. Nonopioids (nonnarcotic analgesics) include NSAIDs such as aspirin and ibuprofen. These analgesics have anti-inflammatory, analgesic, and antipyretic effects. Acetaminophen has only analgesic and antipyretic effects. They relieve pain by acting on peripheral nerve endings at the injury site and decreasing the level of inflammatory mediators generated at the site of injury.

BOX 15-2
SEDATION RATING SCALE

S = sleeping, easily aroused; requires no action
1 = awake and alert; requires no action
2 = occasionally drowsy, easy to arouse; requires no action
3 = frequently drowsy, arousable, drifts off to sleep during conversation; decrease the opioid dose
4 = somnolent, minimal or no response to stimuli; discontinue opioid and consider use of naloxone (Narcan)

Source: McCaffery, M., Pasero, C. (1999). *Pain clinical manual,* p. 267. St. Louis, MO: Mosby. Reprinted by permission.

BOX 15-3 COMMON OPIOID SIDE EFFECTS AND PREVENTIVE MEASURES

Constipation
◆ Increase fluid intake (e.g., to 8 glasses daily).
◆ Increase fiber and bulk-forming agents to the diet (e.g., fresh fruits and vegetables).
◆ Increase exercise regimen.
◆ Administer stool softeners and provide a mild laxative if necessary.

Nausea and Vomiting
◆ Inform client that tolerance to this emetic effect generally develops after several days of opiate therapy.
◆ Provide an antiemetic as required.
◆ Change the analgesic as indicated.

Sedation
◆ Inform client that tolerance usually develops over 3 to 5 days.
◆ Administer a stimulant, such as dextroamphetamine sulfate (Dexedrine) or methylphenidate hydrochloride (Ritalin) each morning to clients who receive opiate therapy for chronic pain and do not develop tolerance.

Respiratory Depression
◆ Administer an opioid antagonist, such as naloxone hydrochloride (Narcan) until respirations return to an acceptable rate. Administer the medication slowly by intravenous route with 10 mL of saline. Monitor the client, and repeat the procedure as required.
◆ If the client is receiving intravenous patient-controlled analgesia (PCA), stop or slow the infusion.

Pruritus
◆ Apply cool packs, lotion, and diversional activity.
◆ Administer an antihistamine (e.g., diphenhydramine hydrochloride [Benadryl]).
◆ Inform the client that tolerance also develops to pruritus.

Urinary Retention
◆ May need to catheterize client.
◆ Administer narcotic antagonist (naloxone hydrochloride [Narcan]).

Individual drugs in this category vary widely in their analgesic properties, metabolism, excretion, and side effects. In addition, the analgesic activity of these drugs has a ceiling effect—the level at which increasing the dose results in no further increase in analgesia.

The most common side effect of nonopioid analgesics is indigestion, which can be prevented by taking the medication with antacid or food. Stomach ulcers and gastric bleeding have also been reported. NSAIDs reduce the dose of opioids needed when the drugs are given together and provide better pain relief than use of either type separately. These drugs must be ordered by the physician; they all have a maximum daily dose limit.

Pharmacologic management of mild to moderate pain should begin with NSAIDs, unless there is a specific contraindication (Pinnell, 1996, p.646). NSAIDs are contraindicated, for example, in clients with impaired blood clotting, gastrointestinal bleeding or ulcer risk, renal disease, thrombocytopenia, and possibly infection (because NSAIDs will obscure fever).

ADJUVANT ANALGESICS. Adjuvant analgesics are medications that were developed for uses other than analgesia but have been found to reduce certain types of chronic pain in addition to their primary action. For example, mild sedatives or tranquilizers, such as diazepam (Valium), may help reduce painful muscle spasms as well as anxiety, stress, and tension so that the client can obtain a good night's sleep. Antidepressants, such as amitriptyline hydrochloride (Elavil), are used to treat underlying depression or mood disorders but may also enhance other pain strategies. Anticonvulsants, such as carbamazepine (Tegretol) and clonazepam (Klonopin), usually prescribed to treat seizures, can be useful in controlling painful neuropathies such as herpes zoster (shingles) and diabetic neuropathies.

Nonpharmacologic Pain Management

Nonpharmacologic pain management consists of a variety of physical and cognitive–behavioral pain management strategies. Physical interventions include cutaneous stimulation, immobilization, transcutaneous electrical nerve stimulation (TENS), and acupuncture. Mind–body (cognitive–behavioral) interventions include distraction activities, relaxation techniques, imagery, meditation, biofeedback, hypnosis, and therapeutic touch. See Box 15-4 ◆ for a detailed description of these interventions.

◆ Key Factors in Pain Management

ACKNOWLEDGING AND ACCEPTING

Basic to all strategies for reducing pain is that nurses convey to clients that they believe the client is having pain. Four ways of communicating this belief follow:

1. Verbally acknowledge the presence of the pain. "I understand your leg is very painful. How do you feel about the pain?"
2. Listen attentively to what the client says about the pain.
3. Convey that you are assessing the client's pain to understand it better, not to determine whether the pain is real, for example, "How does your pain feel now?" or "Tell me how it feels compared to an hour ago."
4. Attend to the client's needs promptly.

ASSISTING SUPPORT PERSONS

Support persons often need assistance to respond positively to the client experiencing pain. Enlisting the aid of support persons in the provision of pain relief to the client, such as massaging the client's back, may diminish his or her feelings of helplessness and foster a more positive attitude toward the client's pain experience. Support persons also may need the nurse's verbal recognition of their concern and participation in the client's care.

REDUCING MISCONCEPTIONS ABOUT PAIN

Reducing a client's misconceptions about the pain and its treatment will often avoid intensifying the pain. The nurse should explain to the client that pain is a highly individual experience and that it is only the client who really experiences the pain, although others can understand and empathize. Misconceptions are also dealt with when nurse and client discuss why the pain has increased or decreased at certain times. For example, a client whose pain increases in the evening may mistakenly think this is the result of eating dinner rather than the result of fatigue.

REDUCING FEAR AND ANXIETY

It is important to help relieve the emotional component, that is, anxiety or fear, associated with the pain. When clients have no opportunity to talk about their pain and associated fears, their perceptions and reactions to the pain can be intensified. The client may become angry or complain about the nurse's care when the problem really is a belief that the pain is not being attended to. If the nurse is honest and sincere and promptly attends to the client's needs, the client is much more likely to know that the nurse does believe the client is in pain.

By providing accurate information, the nurse can also reduce many of the client's fears, such as a fear of addiction or a fear that the pain will always be present. It also helps many clients to have privacy when they are experiencing pain.

PREVENTING PAIN

A preventive approach to pain management involves the provision of measures to treat the pain before it occurs or before it is severe. **Preemptive analgesia** is the administration of analgesics prior to an invasive or operative procedure. Nurses can also use a preemptive approach by providing analgesic around-the-clock (ATC), rather than as needed (prn). For clients who routinely feel pain, for example with diseases such as cancer, administering pain medication at scheduled intervals maintains the level of analgesia without allowing the peaks and valleys associated with metabolism of the medication given on a prn basis. Client or patient-controlled analgesia (PCA) pumps allow clients to self-administer medication to lessen breakthrough pain (Figure 15-5 ↑).

BOX 15-4 NONPHARMACOLOGIC PAIN INTERVENTIONS

Cutaneous Stimulation

Cutaneous stimulation can provide effective temporary pain relief. It distracts the client and focuses attention on the tactile stimuli, away from the painful sensations, thus reducing pain perception. Cutaneous stimulation can be applied directly to the painful area, proximal to the pain, distal to the pain, and contralateral (opposite side) to the pain. Cutaneous stimulation techniques include the following:

Massage

Massage is a comfort measure that can aid relaxation, decrease muscle tension, and may ease anxiety. Massage can also decrease pain intensity by increasing superficial circulation to the area. Massage can involve the back and neck, hands and arms, or feet. The use of ointments or liniments may provide localized pain relief with joint or muscle pain.

Heat and Cold Applications

A warm bath, heating pads, ice bags, ice massage, hot or cold compresses, and warm or cold sitz baths in general relieve pain and promote healing of injured tissues.

Acupressure

Acupressure developed from the ancient Chinese healing system of acupuncture. The therapist applies finger pressure to points that correspond to many of the points used in acupuncture.

Contralateral Stimulation

Contralateral stimulation can be accomplished by stimulating the skin in an area opposite to the painful area (e.g., stimulating the left knee if the pain is in the right knee). The contralateral area may be scratched for itching, massaged for cramps, or treated with cold packs or analgesic ointments. This method is particularly useful when the painful area cannot be touched because it is hypersensitive, inaccessible by a cast or bandages, or when the pain is felt in a missing part (phantom pain).

Transcutaneous Electrical Nerve Stimulation (TENS)

TENS is a method of applying low-voltage electrical stimulation directly over identified pain areas, at an acupressure point, along peripheral nerve areas that innervate the pain area, or along the spinal column. The TENS unit consists of a portable, battery-operated device with lead wire and electrode pads that are applied to the chosen area of skin. Cutaneous stimulation from the TENS unit is thought to activate large-diameter fibers that modulate the transmission of the nociceptive impulse in the peripheral and central nervous system (closing the pain "gate"), resulting in pain relief. This stimulation may also cause a release of endorphins from the central nervous system centers.

Distraction

Distraction draws the person's attention away from the pain and lessens the perception of pain. In some instances, distraction can make a client completely unaware of pain. For example, a client recovering from surgery may feel no pain while watching a football game on television, yet feel pain again when the game is over.

Visual Distraction

◆ Reading or watching TV
◆ Watching a baseball game
◆ Guided imagery

Auditory Distraction

◆ Humor
◆ Listening to music

Tactile Distraction

◆ Slow, rhythmic breathing
◆ Massage
◆ Holding or stroking a pet or toy

Intellectual Distraction

◆ Crossword puzzles
◆ Card games (e.g., bridge)
◆ Hobbies (e.g., stamp collecting, writing a story)

Nonpharmacologic Invasive Therapies

A **nerve block** is a chemical interruption of a nerve pathway, effected by injecting a local anesthetic into the nerve. Nerve blocks are widely used during dental work. The injected drug blocks nerve pathways from the painful tooth, thus stopping the transmission of pain impulses to the brain. Nerve blocks are often used to relieve the pain of whiplash injury, lower-back disorders, bursitis, and cancer.

Pain conduction pathways can be interrupted surgically. Because this disruption is permanent, surgery is performed only as a last resort, generally for intractable pain. Several surgical procedures may be performed and depend on area of pain origin.

MediaLink ❖ Heat, Cold, Touch, Pressure, Pain

◆ Barriers to Pain Management

Misconceptions and biases can affect pain management. Some of these involve attitudes of the nurse or the client as well as knowledge deficits. Clients respond to pain experiences based on their culture, personal experiences, and the meaning the pain has for them. For many people, pain is expected and accepted as a normal aspect of illness. Clients and families may lack knowledge of the adverse effects of pain and may have misinformation regarding the use of analgesics. Clients may not report pain because they expect nothing can be done, they think it is not severe enough, or because they feel it would distract or prejudice the health care provider. Other common misconceptions are shown in Table 15-3 ◆.

Figure 15-5. ◆ A continuous subcutaneous PCA infusion device.

ROUTES FOR OPIATE DELIVERY

Opioids have traditionally been administered by oral, subcutaneous, intramuscular, and intravenous routes. In addition, newer methods of delivering opiates have been developed to circumvent potential obstacles that occur with these traditional routes. Examples are transnasal and transdermal drug therapy, continuous subcutaneous infusions, and intraspinal infusion See Table 15-4 ◆ for routes and their benefits.

NURSING CARE

◆ ASSESSING

Accurate pain assessment is essential for effective pain management. Because pain is subjective and experienced uniquely by each individual, nurses need to assess all factors affecting the pain experience—physiologic, psychological, behavioral, emotional, and sociocultural.

Pain is considered the fifth vital sign, and should be assessed at least every 4 hours. Pain is also assessed following pain management interventions. Pain intensity should be reassessed at an interval appropriate for the intervention. For example, following the intravenous administration of morphine, the severity of pain should be reassessed in 20 to 30 minutes.

> ### clinical **ALERT**
>
> A quick pain assessment rubric is:
>
> P—Precipitation/Palliation: What causes your pain? What relieves (or helps) your pain?
> Q—Quality: What does your pain feel like (sharp, dull, shooting, etc.)?
> R—Region/Radiation: Where did the pain start? Does it radiate (travel to another location)?
> S—Severity: How bad is the pain on a pain scale with zero meaning no pain and 10 meaning the worst pain imaginable?
> T—Timing: When did the pain start? How long does it last?

Because many people will not voice their pain unless asked about it, pain assessments *must* be initiated by the nurse. Some of the many reasons clients may be reluctant to report pain are listed in Box 15-5 ◆. Nurses must listen to and rely on the client's perceptions of pain. Believing the person experiencing and conveying the perceptions is crucial in establishing a sense of trust. (See Client Communication, Chapter 25. ⬚)

TABLE 15-3	COMMON MISCONCEPTIONS ABOUT PAIN	
MISCONCEPTION	**CORRECTION**
Clients experience severe pain only when they have had major surgery.	Even after minor surgery, clients can experience intense pain.
The nurse or other health care professionals are the authorities about a client's pain.	The person who experiences the pain is the only authority about its existence and nature.
Administering analgesics regularly for pain will lead to addiction.	Clients are unlikely to become addicted to an analgesic provided to treat pain.
The amount of tissue damage is directly related to the amount of pain.	Pain is a subjective experience, and the intensity and duration of pain vary considerably among individuals.
Visible physiologic or behavioral signs accompany pain and can be used to verify its existence.	Even with severe pain, periods of physiologic and behavioral adaptation can occur.

TABLE 15-4 ROUTES OF ADMINISTRATION FOR PAIN MEDICATIONS AND THEIR BENEFITS

ROUTE OF ADMINISTRATION	BENEFITS
Oral	Oral administration of opiates remains the preferred route of delivery because of ease of administration. Because the duration of action of most opiates is approximately 4 hours, people with chronic pain have had to awaken several times during the night to medicate themselves for pain. To circumvent this problem, long-acting forms of morphine with a duration of 8 or more hours have been developed. Two examples of long-acting morphine are MS Contin and Oramorph SR. Clients receiving long-acting morphine also may need prn rescue doses of immediate-release analgesics (e.g., short-acting morphine) for acute breakthrough pain. Another new method of oral opiate delivery is high-concentration liquid morphine. This formulation enables clients who can swallow only small amounts to continue taking the drug orally.
Nasal	Transnasal administration has the advantage of rapid action of the medication because of direct absorption through the vascular nasal mucosa. A commonly used agent is butorphanol (Stadol) for acute headaches.
Transdermal	Transdermal drug therapy is advantageous in that it delivers a relatively stable plasma drug level and is noninvasive. Fentanyl (Duragesic) is an opioid currently available as a skin patch with various dosages. It provides drug delivery for up to 72 hours.
Rectal	Several opiates are now available in suppository form. The rectal route is particularly useful for clients who have dysphagia (difficulty swallowing) or nausea and vomiting. Oral analgesics, with the exception of sustained release analgesics, may be crushed, dissolved in water, and given rectally (McCaffery & Beebe, 1989, p. 92).
Subcutaneous	Although the subcutaneous (SC) route has been used extensively to deliver opioids, a new technique uses subcutaneous catheters and infusion pumps to provide continuous subcutaneous infusion (CSCI) of narcotics. CSCI is particularly helpful for clients (a) whose pain is poorly controlled by oral medications, (b) who are experiencing dysphagia or gastrointestinal obstruction, or (c) who have a need for prolonged use of parenteral narcotics. CSCI involves the use of a small, light, battery-operated pump that administers the drug through a 23- or 25-gauge butterfly needle. The needle can be inserted into the anterior chest, the subclavicular region, the abdominal wall, the outer aspects of the upper arms, or the thighs. Client mobility is maintained with the application of a shoulder bag or holster to hold the pump. The frequency of site change ranges from 3 to 7 days.
Intramuscular	The intramuscular (IM) route is the least desirable route for opioid administration because of variable absorption, pain involved with administration, and the need to repeat administration every 3 to 4 hours.
Intravenous	The intravenous (IV) route provides rapid and effective pain relief with few side effects. The analgesic can be administered by IV bolus or by continuous infusion controlled by the client using a patient-controlled analgesia (PCA) machine at the bedside.
Intraspinal	Another recent method of delivery is the infusion of opiates into the epidural or intrathecal (subarachnoid) space. Intraspinal analgesics act directly on opiate receptors in the spinal cord. Two commonly used medications are preservative-free morphine sulfate and fentanyl. The major benefit of intraspinal drug therapy is that it exerts a lesser sedative effect than do systemic opiates. The epidural space is most commonly used because the dura mater acts as a protective barrier against infection, including meningitis.
Patient-Controlled Analgesia	Patient-controlled analgesia (PCA) is the self-administration of an analgesic by a client who has been instructed regarding the process (Carr et al., 1992). The physician prescribes the analgesic dose, route, and frequency, with the client administering the medication. With the parenteral routes, an infusion pump is used to deliver the medication. Whether in an acute hospital setting, an ambulatory clinic, or with home care, the nurse is responsible for the initial instruction regarding use of the PCA and for the ongoing monitoring of the therapy. The client's pain must be assessed at regular intervals and analgesic use is documented in the client's record. PCA can be effectively used for clients with acute pain related to a surgical incision, traumatic injury, or labor and delivery, and for chronic pain, as with cancer. In some settings PCAs are used even if the client is unable to initiate a dose by pushing the button, as long as a caregiver is willing to accept the responsibility; for example, when the client is an infant or toddler or is physically or cognitively impaired (Pasero & McCaffery, 1996). The benefits of this mode of administration include ◆ Self-control over pain relief ◆ More stable analgesic blood level for sustained pain relief ◆ Tendency for the client to need less medication for pain relief

TABLE 15-4	ROUTES OF ADMINISTRATION FOR PAIN MEDICATIONS AND THEIR BENEFITS
ROUTE OF ADMINISTRATION	**BENEFITS**
Patient-Controlled Analgesia *(continued)*	PCA pumps usually have a chamber or cartridge that contains the analgesic, a mechanism for setting the ordered dose, and a control for client activation (Figure 15-5). When clients want a dose of analgesic they can push a button attached to the infusion pump and the preset dose is delivered. A programmable lockout interval (usually 10 to 15 minutes) follows the dose, when an additional dose cannot be given even if the client activates the button. It is also possible to program the maximum dose that can be delivered over a period of hours (usually 4). Many pumps are capable of delivering a low continuous infusion, or basal rate, to provide sustained analgesia during times of rest and sleep.

Pain assessments consist of a pain history to obtain facts from the client and direct observation of behavioral and physiologic responses of the client. The goal of assessment is to gain an objective understanding of a subjective experience.

While taking pain histories, the nurse must provide an opportunity for clients to express in their own words how they view the pain and the situation. This will help the nurse understand what the pain means to the client and how the client is coping with it. Remember that each person's pain experience is unique and that the client is the best interpreter of the pain experience. The initial pain assessment for someone in severe acute pain may consist of only a few questions before intervention occurs, such as location, intensity, and quality. For the person with chronic pain, the nurse may focus on the client's coping mechanisms, effectiveness of current pain management, and ways in which the pain has affected activities of daily living (ADLs).

BOX 15-5 WHY CLIENTS MAY BE RELUCTANT TO REPORT PAIN

- Unwillingness to trouble staff who are perceived as busy
- Fear of the injectable route of analgesic administration (children in particular)
- Belief that pain is to be expected as part of the recovery process
- Belief that pain is a normal part of aging or a necessary part of life (older adults in particular)
- Belief that expressions of pain reveal weakness
- Difficulty expressing personal discomfort
- Concern about risks associated with opioid drugs (e.g., addiction)
- Fear about the cause of pain or that reporting pain will lead to further tests and expenses
- Concern about unwanted side effects, especially of opioid drugs
- Concern that use of drugs now will render the drug inefficient if or when the pain becomes worse

Location

To identify the specific location of the pain, ask the individual to point to the site of the discomfort. A chart consisting of drawings of the body can assist in identifying pain locations. The client marks the location of pain on the chart. This tool can be especially effective with clients who have more than one source of pain.

When assessing the location of a child's pain, the nurse needs to understand the child's vocabulary. For example, "tummy" might mean the abdomen or part of the chest. Asking the child to point to the pain helps clarify the child's word usage to identify location. Again, the use of figure drawings can assist in identifying pain locations. (See also Chapter 23. ◷) Parents can also be helpful in interpreting the meaning of a child's words.

Intensity

The single most important indicator of the intensity of pain is the client's report of pain. Studies have shown that health care providers may underrate or overrate the pain intensity. The use of pain intensity scales is an easy and reliable method of determining pain intensity. Such scales provide consistency for nurses to communicate with the client and other health care providers. Most scales use either a 0 to 5 or 0 to 10 range with 0 indicating "no pain" and the highest number indicating the "worst pain possible" for that individual. A 10-point rating scale is shown in Figure 15-6 ◆. It is important for the nurse to understand the pain scale is intended to compare the client to him/herself, not to other individuals. A nurse should never compare one client's rating of pain with another client's rating of pain. The scale is intended to gauge the amount of relief or

Figure 15-6. ◆ A 10-point pain intensity scale with word modifiers.

distress the client is in at any given time. It should not be used to compare levels of pain perception.

When noting pain intensity it is important to determine any related factors that may be affecting the pain. When the intensity changes the nurse needs to consider the possible cause. For example, the abrupt cessation of acute abdominal pain may indicate a ruptured appendix. Several factors affect the perception of intensity: (1) the amount of distraction, or the client's concentration on another event; (2) the client's state of consciousness; (3) the level of activity; and (4) the client's expectations.

Not all clients can understand or relate to numerical pain intensity scales. These include children who are unable to communicate discomfort verbally, elderly clients with impairments in cognition or communication, and people who do not speak English. For these clients the Wong/Baker Faces Rating Scale (Figure 15-7 ◆) may be easier to use (Pasero, 1997b). The face scale includes a number scale in relation to each expression so that the pain intensity can be documented. When it is not possible to use any kind of rating scale with a client, the nurse must rely on observation of behavior and the physiologic cues discussed later in this section. The input of the client's significant others, such as parents or caregivers, can assist the nurse in interpreting the observations. An objective description of the behavior and physiologic data are then documented.

For effective use of pain rating scales clients need to not only understand the use of the scale but also be educated about how the information will be used to determine changes in their condition and the effectiveness of pain management interventions. Clients should also be asked to indicate what level of comfort is acceptable so that they can perform specific activities. This will ensure that adequate pain management is achieved.

Quality

Descriptive adjectives help people communicate the quality of pain. A headache may be described as "hammerlike" or an abdominal pain as "piercing like a knife." Sometimes clients have difficulty describing pain because they have never experienced any sensation like it. Terms commonly used to describe pain can be classiffed as sensory words and affective words. Examples of sensory words are *searing, scalding, sharp, piercing, drilling, wrenching, shooting, splitting, crushing, penetrating, numb, radiating, dull, aching,* and *cramping.* Examples of affective words are *unbearable, killing, intense, torturing, agonizing, terrifying, grueling, suffocating, frightful, punishing, miserable, annoying, nagging, tiring,* and *troublesome.*

Nurses need to record the exact words clients use to describe pain. A client's words are more accurate and descriptive than an interpretation in the nurse's words. Exact information can be significant in both the diagnosis of the pain etiology and in the treatment choices made. For example, pain described as hot, electrical, and sharp tends to be neuropathic in origin and will be more responsive to anticonvulsants (e.g., Tegretol) than to an opioid (e.g., morphine).

Pattern

The pattern of pain includes time of onset, duration, and recurrence or intervals without pain. The nurse therefore determines when the pain began; how long the pain lasts; whether it recurs and, if so, the length of the interval without pain; and when the pain last occurred.

Precipitating Factors

Certain activities sometimes precede pain; for example, physical exertion may precede chest pain, or abdominal pain may

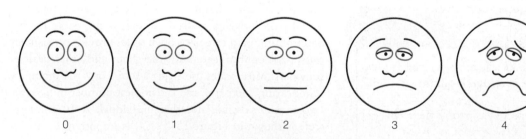

| 0 | 1 | 2 | 3 | 4 | 5 |

1. Explain to the child that each face is for a person who feels happy because he or she has no pain (hurt, or whatever word the child uses) or feels sad because he or she has some or a lot of pain.

2. Point to the appropriate face and state, "This face..." :
   0—"is very happy because he (or she) doesn't hurt at all."
   1—"hurts just a little bit."
   2—"hurts a little more."
   3—"hurts even more."
   4—"hurts a whole lot."
   5—"hurts as much as you can imagine, although you don't have to be crying to feel this bad."

3. Ask the child to choose the face that best describes how he or she feels. Be specific about which pain (eg. "shot" or incision) and what time (eg. Now? Earlier before lunch?)

Figure 15-7. ◆ The Wong/Baker Faces Rating Scale. *Source:* Wong, D. L. (2001). *Wong's essentials of pediatric nursing* (6th ed.). St. Louis, MO: Mosby. Reprinted with permission.

occur after eating. These observations can help prevent pain and determine its cause.

Environmental factors such as extreme cold or heat and extremes of humidity can affect some types of pain. For example, sudden exercise on a hot day can cause muscle spasm.

Physical and emotional stressors can also precipitate pain. Emotional tension frequently brings on a migraine headache. Intense fear or physical exertion can cause angina.

Alleviating Factors

Nurses must ask clients to describe anything that they have done to help alleviate the pain (e.g., home remedies such as herbal teas, or medications, rest, applications of heat or cold, prayer, or distractions like TV). It is important to explore the effect any of these measures had on the pain, whether or not relief was obtained, or whether the pain became worse.

Associated Symptoms

Also included in the clinical appraisal of pain are other associated symptoms, such as nausea, vomiting, dizziness, and diarrhea. These symptoms may relate to the onset of the pain or they may result from the presence of the pain.

Effect on Activities of Daily Living

When caring for clients with chronic pain, knowing how activities of daily living (ADLs) are affected helps the nurse understand the client's perspective on the pain's severity. The nurse asks the client to describe how the pain has affected the following aspects of life:

◆ Sleep
◆ Appetite
◆ Concentration
◆ Work/school
◆ Interpersonal relationships
◆ Marital relations/sex
◆ Home activities
◆ Driving/walking
◆ Leisure activities
◆ Emotional status (mood, irritability, depression, anxiety)

A rating scale of none, a little, or a great deal or another range can be used to determine the degree of alteration.

Coping Resources

Each individual will exhibit personal ways of coping with pain. Strategies may relate to past pain experiences or the specific meaning of the pain; some may reflect religious or cultural influences. Nurses can encourage and support the client's use of methods known to have helped in modifying pain. Strategies may include withdrawal, use of distraction, prayer or other religious practices, and support from significant others.

Affective Responses

Affective responses vary according to the situation, the degree and duration of pain, the interpretation of it, and many other factors. The nurse needs to explore the client's feelings, for example, anxiety, fear, exhaustion, depression, or a sense of failure. Because many people with chronic pain become depressed and potentially suicidal, it may also be necessary to assess the client's suicide risk. In such situations, the nurse needs to ask the client, "Do you ever feel so bad that you want to die? Do you feel that way now?"

Observation of Behavioral and Physiologic Responses

There are wide variations in nonverbal responses to pain. For clients who are very young, aphasic, confused, or disoriented, nonverbal expressions may be the only means of communicating pain. Facial expression is often the first indication of pain, and it may be the only one. Clenched teeth, tightly shut eyes, open somber eyes, biting of the lower lip, and other facial grimaces may be indicative of pain. Vocalizations like moaning and groaning or crying and screaming are also associated with pain.

Immobilization of the body or a part of the body may also indicate pain. The client with chest pain often holds the left arm across the chest. A person with abdominal pain may assume the position of greatest comfort, often with the knees and hips flexed, and moves reluctantly.

Purposeless body movements can also indicate pain—for example, tossing and turning in bed or flinging the arms about. Involuntary movements such as a reflexive jerking away from a needle inserted through the skin indicate pain. An adult may be able to control this reflex; however, a child may be unable or unwilling to do so.

Rhythmic body movements or rubbing may indicate pain. An adult or child may assume a fetal position and rock back and forth when experiencing abdominal pain. During labor a woman may massage her abdomen rhythmically with her hands.

It is important to note that behavioral responses can be controlled and so may not be very revealing. When pain is chronic there are rarely overt behavioral responses as the individual develops personal coping styles for dealing with pain, discomfort, or suffering. Therefore, it is imperative that nurses believe clients when they report they are in pain. It is unacceptable for the nurse to doubt a client who reports pain because "he did not look like he was hurting."

Physiologic responses vary with the origin and duration of the pain. Early in the onset of acute pain the sympathetic nervous system is stimulated, resulting in increased blood pressure, pulse rate, respiratory rate, pallor, diaphoresis, and pupil dilation. However, in clients with chronic pain, the sympathetic nervous system adapts to the stimulus, making the physiologic responses less evident or even absent. When people experience visceral pain, signs of parasympathetic stimulation may be observed, such as decreased blood pressure and pulse rate; pupil constriction; and warm, dry skin.

Daily Pain Diary. For clients who experience chronic pain, a daily diary may help the client and nurse identify pain patterns and factors that exacerbate or mediate the pain experience. In home care, the family or other caregiver can be taught to complete the diary. The record can include time or onset of pain, activity before pain, pain-related positions or behaviors, pain intensity level, use of analgesics or other relief measures, duration of pain, and time spent in relief activities. Recorded data can provide the basis for developing or modifying the plan for care. For this tool to be effective it is important that the nurse educate the client and family about the value and use of the diary in achieving effective pain control. Determining the client's abilities to use the diary is essential.

DIAGNOSING, PLANNING, and IMPLEMENTING

The North American Nursing Diagnosis Association (NANDA) includes the following diagnostic labels for clients experiencing pain or discomfort:

◆ Acute Pain
◆ Chronic Pain

Goals and interventions for clients should be individualized for the client, the particular pain process, and developmental level (Table 15-5 ◆).

Because the presence of pain can affect so many areas of a person's functioning, pain may be the etiology of other nursing diagnoses. Examples of such nursing diagnoses follow:

◆ Ineffective Airway Clearance related to postoperative incisional chest pain
◆ Powerlessness related to past experiences of poor control of pain (See also Chapter 31. ⟨⟩)
◆ Ineffective Coping related to prolonged continuous back pain, ineffective pain management, and inadequate support systems
◆ Impaired Physical Mobility related to arthritic pain in knee and ankle joints
◆ Disturbed Sleep Pattern related to increased pain perception at night

Preventing Pain

Review the section Key Factors in Pain Management on pages 331–332. As mentioned, the nurse provides measures to treat the pain before it occurs or before it is severe. Preemptive analgesia is appropriate before an invasive or operative procedure. It is often appropriate for clients with chronic pain. Administering pain medication at scheduled intervals maintains the level of analgesia without allowing the peaks and valleys in pain relief. Box 15-6 ◆ lists guidelines for individualizing care for clients with pain.

Supporting the Client and Significant Others

Nurses assist the client who is in pain by assessing pain regularly. Open-ended questions that allow the client to describe the type, location, or level of pain are much more useful than

TABLE 15-5	SELECTED NURSING INTERVENTIONS BY DEVELOPMENTAL LEVEL
DEVELOPMENTAL LEVEL	SELECTED NURSING INTERVENTIONS
Infant	Give a glucose pacifier. Use tactile stimulation. Play music or tapes of a heartbeat.
Toddler/ preschooler	Distract the child with toys, books, pictures. Involve the child in blowing bubbles as a way of "blowing away the pain." Appeal to the child's belief in magic by using a "magic" blanket or glove to take away pain. Hold the child to provide comfort. Explore misconceptions about pain.
School-age child	Use imagery to turn off "pain switches." Provide a behavioral rehearsal of what to expect and how it will look and feel. Provide support and nurturing.
Adolescent	Provide opportunities to discuss pain. Provide privacy. Present choices for dealing with pain. Encourage music or TV for distraction.
Adult	Deal with any misconceptions about pain. Focus on the client's control in dealing with the pain. Allay fears and anxiety when possible.
Older adult	Spend time with the client, and listen carefully. Clarify misconceptions. Encourage independence whenever possible.

closed questions. For example, "How is your side feeling now?" encourages the client to answer more fully than, "Did that medication work?" An attentive attitude and prompt attention to the client's needs help to build trust and reduce the anxiety that often accompanies severe or unremitting pain. The nurse can also help the client analyze when and why the pain worsens. Understanding more about the pain can sometimes help the client feel more in control.

The nurse's attitude of respect for the client in pain is important. Nurses can help family members by giving them accurate information about medications and about expected resolution of pain (e.g., period of recovery after surgery). Explaining when pain is likely to be the worst, when pain medication begins to take effect, and when the effect of medication wears off will enable support persons to organize their time and efforts to help the client. Providing accurate information about possible side effects, as well as reassurance that

BOX 15-6
NURSING CARE CHECKLIST

INDIVIDUALIZING CARE FOR CLIENTS WITH PAIN

☑ Establish a trusting relationship. Convey your concern, and acknowledge that you believe that the client is experiencing pain. A trusting relationship promotes expression of the client's thoughts and feelings and enhances effectiveness of planned pain therapies.

☑ Consider the client's ability and willingness to participate actively in pain relief measures. Some clients who are excessively fatigued, are sedated, or have altered levels of consciousness are less able to participate actively. For example, a client with an altered level of consciousness or altered thought processes may not be able to deal with patient-controlled analgesia (PCA). In contrast, a fatigued client may express a willingness to use pain-relief measures that require little effort, such as listening to music or performing relaxation techniques.

☑ Use a variety of pain relief measures. It is thought that using more than one measure has an additive effect in relieving pain. Two measures that should always be part of any pain relief plan are (a) establishing a client–nurse relationship and (b) client teaching. Because a client's pain may vary throughout a 24-hour period, different types of pain relief are often indicated during that time.

☑ Provide measures to relieve pain before it becomes severe. For example, providing an analgesic before the onset of pain is preferable to waiting for the client to complain of pain, when a larger dose may be required.

☑ Use pain-relieving measures that the client believes are effective. It has been recognized that clients are usually the authorities about their own pain. Thus, incorporating the client's measures into a pain relief plan is sensible unless they are harmful.

☑ Base the choice of pain relief measure on the client's report of the severity of the pain. If a client reports mild pain, an analgesic such as aspirin may be indicated, whereas a client who reports severe pain often requires a more potent relief measure.

☑ If a pain relief measure is ineffective, encourage the client to try it once or twice more before abandoning it. Anxiety may diminish the effects of a pain measure, and some approaches, such as distraction strategies, require practice before they are effective.

☑ Maintain an unbiased attitude (open mind) about what may relieve the pain. New ways to relieve pain are continually being developed. It is not always possible to explain pain relief measures; however, measures should be supported unless they are harmful.

☑ Keep trying. Do not ignore a client because pain persists in spite of measures. In these circumstances, reassess the pain, and consider other relief measures.

☑ Prevent harm to the client. Pain therapy should not increase discomfort or harm the client. Some pain relief measures may have adverse untoward effects, such as fatigue, but they should not disable the client.

☑ Educate the client and support people about pain. Clients and support people need to be informed about possible causes of pain, precipitating and alleviating factors, and alternatives to drug therapy. Misconceptions also need to be corrected.

medications used appropriately will not cause addiction, is also a part of client teaching. The nurse can encourage family to participate in client care and to provide distractions they know the client would enjoy.

Chronic pain is debilitating and frustrating. When chronic pain exists, the nurse can serve an important role in reminding support people that only the client really knows the pain. The client is the source about the client's pain. However, family and significant others can provide caring, encouragement, distraction, and empathy, all of which support the client.

◆ EVALUATING

The nurse reviews client goals and outcomes to determine whether they have been achieved. Both subjective data (physical stance and facial expression) and objective data (heart rate and respirations) are collected to evaluate client comfort.

To assist in the evaluation process, flowsheet records or a client diary may be helpful. A weekly log or diary can be structured in a similar fashion for the individual client. For example, columns including day, time, onset of pain, activity before pain, pain relief measure, and duration of pain can be devised to help the client and nurse determine the effectiveness of pain relief strategies.

If outcomes are not achieved, the nurse and client might consider the following:

◆ Would the client benefit from a change in dose or in the time interval between doses?
◆ Did the client understate the pain experience for some reason?
◆ Did the client and support people understand the instructions about pain management techniques?
◆ Is the client receiving adequate support from significant others?
◆ Has the client's physical condition changed?

Nursing Process Case Study: CLIENT WITH PAIN

Mrs. Lundahl underwent abdominal surgery approximately 6 hours ago. She has a 15-cm midline incision that is covered with a dry and intact surgical dressing.

Assessment Mrs. Lundahl is perspiring, lying in a rigid position, holding her abdomen, and grimacing. Her blood pressure is 150/90, heart rate 100, and respiratory rate 32. When asked to rate her pain on a scale of 1 to 10, Mrs. Lundahl rates her pain as 5.

Diagnosis The priority nursing diagnosis for Mrs. Lundahl is Acute Pain related to surgical incision.

Expected Outcomes

◆ States postoperative discomfort is relieved within 20 to 30 minutes of verbalized pain
◆ Practices one relaxation technique for relief of pain by end of second postop day
◆ Turns, coughs, and deep breathes with minimum of discomfort by second postop day

Planning and Implementation The following interventions are implemented for Mrs. Lundahl:

◆ Teach Mrs. Lundahl about her medications, as well as side effects and how to treat them.

◆ Encourage Mrs. Lundahl to request PRN analgesics before pain becomes unmanageable.
◆ Teach Mrs. Lundahl relaxation and distraction techniques.

Evaluation Mrs. Lundahl c/o dizziness following 2 tabs Vicodin ES; 1 tab adequately relieved pain without noticeable side effects in 30 minutes. Able to space PRN pain meds to 5 to 6 hours by using relaxation technique (deep breathing and muscle group relaxation). Mrs. Lundahl using pillow to splint during coughing, able to change position and transfer to chair from bed without discomfort.

Critical Thinking in the Nursing Process

1. What conclusions, if any, can be drawn about Mrs. Lundahl's pain status?
2. Does Mrs. Lundahl's rating her pain as 5 mean that she is not experiencing pain severe enough to warrant intervention?
3. What type of pain is Mrs. Lundahl experiencing?
4. What interventions, in addition to pain medication, may be useful in reducing Mrs. Lundahl's pain?
5. How will you know if your interventions have been effective in reducing Mrs. Lundahl's pain?

Note: The bibliography listings for this and all chapters have been compiled at the back of the book

Chapter Review

Key Terms by Topics

Use the audio glossary feature of either the CD-ROM or the Companion Website to hear the correct pronunciation of the following key terms.

Types of pain
pain, acute pain, chronic pain, intractable pain, cutaneous pain, somatic pain, visceral

pain, radiating pain, referred pain, neuropathic pain, phantom pain

Concepts associated with pain
pain threshold, pain reaction, pain tolerance

Physiology of pain
nociceptors, endogenous opioids, exogenous opioids, gate control theory

Key factors in pain management
preemptive analgesia, nerve block

Key Points

- Pain is a subjective sensation. Pain can directly impair health and prolong recovery from surgery, disease, and trauma.
- Ethnic and cultural values, age, environment and support people, anxiety, and stress all influence a person's perception and reaction to pain.
- The overall client goal is to increase a client's functional capacity by preventing, modifying, or eliminating pain.
- The most reliable indicator of the presence or intensity of pain is the client's self-report.
- Nurses must acknowledge and convey belief in the client's report of pain and reduce fear and anxiety associated with the pain. Nurses should also assist support people and reduce misconceptions about pain.
- Do not allow fear of potential side effects to inhibit full and aggressive treatment of a client's pain.
- The nurse's evaluation of the client's pain therapy is multifaceted and should include the response of the client, changes in the pain, and the client's perceptions of the effectiveness of therapy.

EXPLORE MediaLink

Additional interactive resources for this chapter can be found on the Companion Website at www.prenhall.com/ramont. Click on Chapter 15 and "Begin" to select the activities for this chapter.

For chapter-related NCLEX-style questions and an audio glossary, access the accompanying CD-ROM in this book.

∞ For Further Study

For more information about thermal injury and use of heat and cold applications to relieve pain, see Chapter 12.

For further discussion of listening skills, see Chapters 23 and 25.

For effects of anxiety and stress, see Chapter 30.

For more about helplessness in relation to pain, see Chapter 31.

Critical Thinking Care Map

Caring for a Client with Postoperative Pain

NCLEX Focus Area: Physiological Adaptation

Case Study: Mr. Lee Chin is a 57-year-old Chinese businessman who was admitted to the surgical unit for treatment of a possible strangulated inguinal hernia. Two days ago he had a partial bowel resection.

Nursing Diagnosis: Acute Pain related to surgical incision

COLLECT DATA

Subjective	Objective
_____	_____
_____	_____
_____	_____
_____	_____
_____	_____
_____	_____
_____	_____

Would you report this data? Yes/No

If yes, to: _____

Nursing Care

_____
_____
_____
_____
_____
_____
_____
_____
_____
_____
_____
_____
_____
_____
_____

How would you document this? _____
_____
_____
_____
_____
_____

Data Collected

(use those that apply)

- Height: 188 cm (6'3")
- Weight: 90.0 kg (200 lbs)
- Temperature: 37° C (98.6°F)
- Pulse: 90 bpm
- Respirations: 24/min
- Blood pressure: 158/82 mm Hg
- Lying in dorsal recumbent position with legs drawn up
- Skin pale and moist, pupils dilated
- NPO, intravenous infusion of D5 ½NS at 125 cc/hr left arm, nasogastric tube to low intermittent suction restless
- Complaint of pain (7 on a scale of 1–10)
- "I am cold and tired, I wish I could sleep"
- Complaint of being thirsty
- Midline abdominal incision, sutures dry and intact
- Chest x-ray and urinalysis negative
- WBC 12,000
- Complaint of nausea but no vomiting

Nursing Interventions

(use those that apply)

- Medicate before an activity to increase participation.
- Teach client to use incentive spirometer.
- Evaluate the effectiveness of the pain control measures used through ongoing assessment.
- Assess wound drainage at each dressing change.
- Provide extra blanket for warmth.
- Determine analgesic selections (narcotic, nonnarcotic, or NSAID) based on type and severity of pain.
- Institute safety precautions as appropriate if receiving narcotic analgesics.
- Encourage coughing and deep breathing.
- Instruct client to request prn pain medication before the pain is severe.
- Create a quiet, nondisruptive environment with dim lights and comfortable temperature when possible.

NCLEX-PN Exam Preparation

1. The nurse is faced with a complex situation when developing a plan to relieve pain and provide comfort because:
   a. Most clients have very low pain tolerance and request medication too frequently.
   b. Physicians are reluctant to order adequate pain control.
   c. Pain is a sensation that is highly subjective and individual.
   d. The client does not have enough knowledge to be an authority about pain.

2. You are assigned to do postsurgical checks on a client returning to the surgical unit. The client is complaining of incisional pain. Which of the following statements by the nurse would be most effective in determining the severity of the pain?
   a. "Can you describe your pain for me?"
   b. "Please rate your pain on a scale of 0 to 10, with 10 being the worst pain."
   c. "Your facial expression appears pained. Are you in pain?"
   d. "Would you describe your pain as mild, moderate, or severe?"

3. Pain that lasts only through the expected recovery period, regardless of its intensity, is described as:
   a. Chronic pain
   b. Intractable pain
   c. Referred pain
   d. Acute pain

4. The most common and most troubling side effect of opioids is:
   a. Constipation
   b. Respiratory depression
   c. Rash
   d. Anaphylaxis

5. Pain described as hot, electrical, and sharp tends to be neuropathic in origin and will be more responsive to a(n):
   a. Nonsteroidal anti-inflammatory
   b. Nonopioid analgesic
   c. Anticonvulsant
   d. Opioid

6. Time of onset, duration, and recurrence or intervals without pain are known as the pain:
   a. Intensity
   b. Pattern
   c. Duration
   d. Severity

7. Fentanyl (Duragesic) is an opioid analgesic available as a skin patch. It provides drug delivery for up to 72 hours. Which of the following is the appropriate label for the form of this drug?
   a. Patient-controlled analgesic
   b. Intraspinal analgesic
   c. Transdermal analgesic
   d. Intravenous analgesic

8. Level 4 of the sedation rating scale is characterized by:
   a. Easily arousable sleep
   b. Being awake and alert
   c. Frequent drowsiness, arousability, drifting off to sleep during conversation
   d. Minimal or no response to stimuli

9. Which of the following is a chemical type of pain stimuli?
   a. Trauma to body tissues (e.g., surgery)
   b. Tissue ischemia
   c. Blockage of a body duct
   d. Tumor

10. Which of the following could be described as an invasive, nonpharmacological pain control?
    a. Transcutaneous electrical nerve stimulation (TENS)
    b. Nerve block
    c. Distraction
    d. Guided imagery

Answers for Review Questions, as well as discussion of Case Study and Critical Thinking Care Map questions, appear in Appendix IV.

Chapter 16

Oxygenation

SHARING experiences

"It was my second rotation as a student. I was at Garden Grove Hospital and the client I was assigned to was an old frail lady with pneumonia. When I walked in to do my assessment on her, she was choking on her own thick secretions and I had to suction her right away.

I was scared at first but once I got in and suctioned and saw her being able to breathe again, I got this feeling that I could help and make things better. So ever since then, I've had this drive to help any and everyone that I can."

Jessica Thielmann, VN student, North Orange County Regional Occupational Program, Anaheim, CA.

LEARNING outcomes

After completing this chapter, you will be able to:
- Outline the structure and function of the respiratory system.
- Outline the structure and function of the cardiovascular system.
- Describe the processes of breathing (ventilation) and gas exchange (respiration).
- Identify factors influencing respiration and circulatory function.
- Identify common signs of impaired respiratory function.
- Identify and describe nursing measures to promote cardiorespiratory function and oxygenation.
- Explain the use of therapeutic measures such as artificial airways, medications, oxygen therapy, inhalation therapy, pharyngeal suction, and chest drainage to promote cardiorespiratory function.

MediaLink

  www.prenhall.com/ramont

Use the address above to access the free, interactive Companion Website created for this textbook. Get hints, instant feedback, and textbook references to chapter-related NCLEX-style questions. Link to other interesting sites.

Audio Glossary:
Use the Companion Website, or the CD-ROM disk enclosed with your textbook, to hear the pronunciations of key terms in the chapter.

Oxygen, a clear, odorless gas that constitutes about 21 percent of the air we breathe, is necessary for all living cells. The absence of oxygen can lead to death. Although the delivery of oxygen to body tissues is affected at least indirectly by all body systems, the respiratory system and the cardiovascular system are directly involved in this process. Impaired function of either system can significantly affect our ability to breathe, transport gases, and participate in everyday activities. Respiration is the process of gas exchange between the individual and the environment. The process of respiration involves several components:

1. Pulmonary **ventilation** (breathing)—the movement of air between the atmosphere and the alveoli of the lungs
2. Diffusion of oxygen and carbon dioxide between the alveoli and pulmonary capillaries
3. Transport of oxygen and carbon dioxide via the blood to and from tissues
4. Diffusion of oxygen and carbon dioxide between the capillaries and the cells of body tissues

Structure and Function of the Respiratory System

The primary function of the respiratory system is gas exchange. Structures of the respiratory system function to move air, eliminate waste products, maintain acid–base balance, and protect the airway from infection.

STRUCTURE OF THE RESPIRATORY SYSTEM

The respiratory system (Figure 16-1A ◆) is divided structurally into the upper respiratory system and the lower respiratory system. The mouth, nose, pharynx, and larynx compose the upper respiratory system. The lower respiratory system includes the trachea and lungs, with the bronchi, bronchioles, alveoli, pulmonary capillary network, and pleural membranes. See also Figure 10-12.

Air enters through the nose, where it is warmed, humidified, and filtered. Large particles in the air are trapped by the hairs at the entrance of the *nares* (nostrils), and smaller particles are filtered and trapped by the nasal turbinates and septum inside the nose. The sneeze reflex is initiated by irritants in nasal passages. During a sneeze, a large volume of air exits rapidly through the nose and mouth, helping to clear nasal passages.

Inspired air passes from the nose through the *pharynx*, commonly known as the throat. The pharynx is a shared pathway for air and food. It is richly supplied with lymphoid tissue that traps and destroys pathogens entering with the air.

The *larynx* can be identified externally (the Adam's apple). In addition to its role in speech, the larynx is important for maintaining airway patency and protecting the lower airways from swallowed food and fluids. During swallowing,

the inlet to the larynx (the **epiglottis**) closes, routing food to the esophagus. The epiglottis is open during breathing, allowing air to move freely into the lower airways.

Below the larynx, the trachea leads to the right and left main bronchi (primary bronchi) and the airways of the lungs. Within the lungs, the primary bronchi divide repeatedly into smaller and smaller bronchi, ending with the terminal bronchioles. Together these airways are known as the *bronchial tree*. The trachea and bronchi are lined with cells that produce a thin layer of mucus to trap pathogens and microscopic matter. These foreign particles are then swept upward toward the larynx and throat by *cilia*, tiny hairlike projections on the epithelial cells. The cough reflex is triggered by irritants in the larynx, trachea, or bronchi.

The respiratory zone of the lungs includes the respiratory bronchioles, the alveolar ducts, and the alveoli (Figure 16-1B). Until air enters the respiratory bronchioles and alveoli, no gas exchange occurs. Alveoli have very thin walls, composed of a single layer of epithelial cells covered by a thick mesh of pulmonary capillaries. The alveolar and capillary walls form the membrane where gas exchange occurs (see Figure 16-1B).

The outer surface of the lungs is covered by a thin, double layer of tissue known as the *pleura*. The pleura has two parts:

1. The parietal pleura lines the thorax and surface of the diaphragm.
2. The visceral pleura covers the external surface of the lungs.

Between these pleural layers is a space that contains a small amount of pleural fluid, a serous lubricating solution. This fluid prevents friction during the movements of breathing and keeps the layers adherent, much as a film of water can cause two glass slides to cling to each other.

PULMONARY VENTILATION

Ventilation (breathing) is accomplished through **inspiration** (inhalation) when air flows into the lungs and **expiration** (exhalation) when air moves out of the lungs. When inflammation, edema, and excessive mucus production occur, small airways become clogged, impairing ventilation of the alveoli.

The respiratory centers of the medulla and pons in the brain stem control breathing. Severe head injury or drugs that depress the central nervous system (e.g., opiates or barbiturates) can affect the respiratory centers, impairing the drive to breathe.

The degree of chest expansion during normal breathing is minimal and requires little energy. However, when a client has **chronic obstructive pulmonary disease (COPD),** persistent obstruction of bronchial air flow, chest expansion requires greater effort. This client must use accessory muscles of respiration, including the anterior neck muscles, intercostal muscles, and muscles of the abdomen, to move air into and out of the chest.

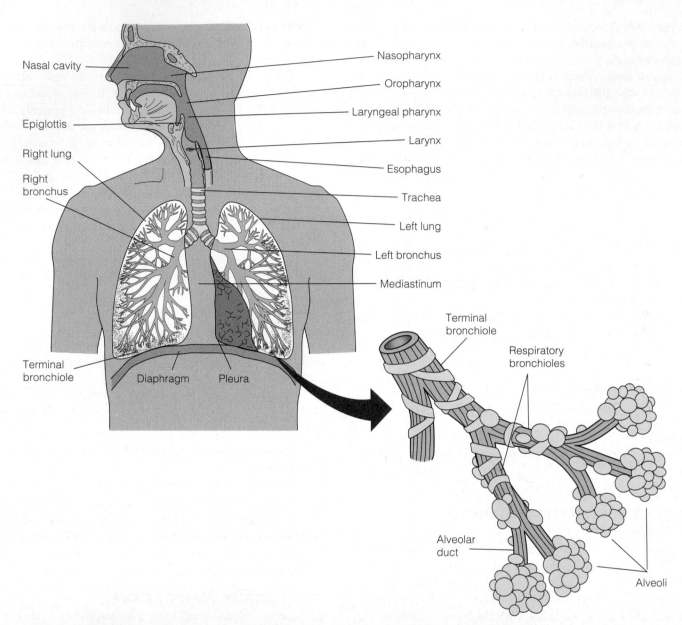

Figure 16-1. ◆ **A.** Organs of the respiratory tract. **B.** Respiratory bronchioles, alveolar ducts, and alveoli.

When a client has diseases or trauma such as spinal cord injury that affect the muscles of respiration, the thoracic cavity may not be able to expand and contract effectively. When trauma occurs to the chest wall, the pressure within the chest cavity changes, causing the lung to collapse. If the thin, double-layered pleural membrane is disrupted by lung disease, surgery, or trauma, negative pressure between the pleural layers may be lost and the lung may collapse. Air in the pleural space is known as a **pneumothorax.** Blood (**hemothorax**) or fluid (**pleural effusion**) in the pleural space places pressure on lung tissue and also interferes with lung expansion.

ALVEOLAR GAS EXCHANGE

The second phase of the respiratory process is the diffusion of oxygen from the alveoli into the pulmonary blood vessels. **Diffusion** is the movement of gases or other particles from an area of greater pressure or concentration to an area of lower pressure or concentration.

Pressure differences in the gases on each side of the respiratory membrane affect diffusion. When the pressure of oxygen is greater in the alveoli than in the blood, oxygen diffuses into the blood. Likewise, when the pressure of carbon dioxide in venous blood is greater than the pressure of carbon dioxide in the alveoli, carbon dioxide diffuses from the blood into the alveoli, where it can be eliminated with expired air.

TRANSPORT OF OXYGEN AND CARBON DIOXIDE

The third part of the respiratory process involves the transport of respiratory gases. Oxygen needs to be transported from the lungs to the tissues, and carbon dioxide must be transported from the tissues back to the lungs. Normally, 97 percent of the oxygen combines loosely with **hemoglobin** (an oxygen-carrying red pigment) in the red blood cells. It is carried to the tissues as *oxyhemoglobin* (the compound of oxygen and hemoglobin). The remaining oxygen is dissolved and transported in the fluid of the plasma and cells.

Several factors affect the rate of oxygen transport from the lungs to the tissues: cardiac output, number of **erythrocytes** (red blood cells), and exercise.

The amount of blood pumped by the heart is called cardiac output. Normally, it is approximately 5 liters per minute. Any pathologic condition that decreases cardiac output (e.g., damage to the heart muscle, blood loss, or pooling of blood in the peripheral blood vessels) diminishes the amount of oxygen delivered to the tissues. The heart compensates for inadequate output by increasing its pumping rate. However, with severe damage or blood loss, this may not restore adequate blood flow and oxygen to the tissues.

Another factor influencing oxygen transport is the number of erythrocytes. **Hematocrit** is a measurement of the percentage of *erythrocytes* (red blood cells, or RBCs) in the blood. (In men, the number of circulating erythrocytes normally averages about 5 million per cubic milliliter of blood, and in women, about 4.5 million per cubic milliliter. Normally, the hematocrit is about 40 to 54 percent in men and 37 to 47 percent in women.) Excessive increases in the blood hematocrit raise the blood *viscosity* (thickness), reducing the cardiac output and oxygen transport. Excessive reductions in the blood hematocrit, such as occur in anemia, reduce oxygen transport.

Exercise also has a direct influence on oxygen transport. In well-trained athletes, oxygen transport can be increased up to 20 times the normal rate, due in part to an increased cardiac output and to efficient use of oxygen by the cells.

RESPIRATORY REGULATION

Respiratory rate and depth are controlled by nerves and the concentration of certain gases in the blood. The brain regulates respirations to maintain correct concentrations of oxygen, carbon dioxide, and hydrogen ions in the body fluids. An area in the medulla of the brain is highly responsive to increases in blood carbon dioxide (CO_2). When CO_2 or hydrogen ion concentration increases, the brain increases the rate and depth of respirations. In addition, special nerve receptors are sensitive to decreases in oxygen (O_2) concentration in the blood. When they sense decreases in the amount of oxygen in the arteries, they stimulate the respiratory center to increase respirations. Of the three blood gases (hydrogen, oxygen, and carbon dioxide), increased carbon dioxide concentration normally stimulates respiration most strongly.

ALTERATIONS IN RESPIRATORY FUNCTION

Respiratory function can be altered by conditions that affect:

◆ The movement of air into or out of the lungs
◆ The diffusion of oxygen and carbon dioxide between the alveoli and the pulmonary capillaries

◆ The transport of oxygen and carbon dioxide through the blood to and from the tissue cells

clinical **ALERT**

In clients with certain lung ailments such as emphysema or COPD, oxygen concentration (not carbon dioxide) determines regulation of respiration. For such clients, decreased oxygen concentration is the main stimulus for respiration. This is called the *hypoxic drive*. If the concentration of oxygen is increased, it will depress the respiratory rate, causing the client to go into respiratory distress. Oxygen must be administered to these clients only in low concentrations to avoid causing severe respiratory problems or death. See Box 16-1 ◆ for O_2 guidelines in clients with COPD.

Three major alterations in respiration are hypoxia, altered breathing patterns, and obstructed or partially obstructed airway.

Hypoxia

Hypoxia is a condition of insufficient oxygen anywhere in the body. The inhaled air may lack enough oxygen, or an insufficient amount of oxygen may be delivered to the tissues. It can be related to ventilation, diffusion of gases, or transport of gases by the blood. It can be caused by any condition that alters one or more parts of the respiratory process.

Hypoventilation, or inadequate exchange of gases through the alveoli, can lead to hypoxia. Hypoventilation may be due to respiratory diseases, drugs, or anesthesia. It often causes carbon dioxide to accumulate in the blood; this is a condition called **hypercarbia** or **hypercapnia.**

Hypoxia can also develop when oxygen does not diffuse effectively into the arterial blood (as in pulmonary edema). Hypoxia can also result from problems in the delivery of oxygen to the tissues. This occurs with anemia, heart failure, and pulmonary embolism. The term *hypoxemia* refers to reduced oxygen in the blood. Box 16-2 ◆ lists manifestations of hypoxia.

Cyanosis (bluish discoloration of the skin, nailbeds, and mucous membranes, due to reduced hemoglobin–oxygen sat-

BOX 16-1

POPULATION FOCUS

CLIENTS WITH COPD

Low-flow oxygen systems are essential for clients with COPD. People with COPD may have a chronically high carbon dioxide level. Their stimulus to breathe is not high levels of carbon dioxide but low levels of oxygen *(hypoxemia)*. High flows of oxygen can potentially relieve this hypoxemia, but they may also remove the stimulus to breathe. Low flows maintain a slightly hypoxemic state, thus maintaining the respiratory drive. Clients who have COPD and are receiving oxygen therapy should be observed carefully (especially when therapy is first initiated) for respiratory depression or arrest.

uration) may be present with hypoxia. The brain can tolerate hypoxia for only 4 to 6 minutes before permanent damage occurs. The face of the acutely hypoxic person usually appears anxious, tired, and drawn. The person usually assumes a sitting position, often leaning forward slightly to permit greater expansion of the thoracic cavity.

With chronic hypoxia, the client often appears fatigued and is lethargic. The client's fingers and toes may be clubbed as a result of long-term lack of oxygen. With *clubbing*, the base of the nail becomes swollen and the ends of the fingers and toes increase in size. The angle between the nail and the base of the nail increases to more than 180 degrees (see Figure 11-4D). 🔗

Altered Breathing Patterns

Breathing patterns refer to the rate, volume, rhythm, and relative ease or effort of respiration. Normal respiration **(eupnea)** is quiet, rhythmic, and effortless. **Tachypnea** (rapid breathing rate) is seen with fevers, metabolic acidosis, pain, hypercapnia, or hypoxemia. **Bradypnea** is an abnormally slow respiratory rate, which may be seen in clients who have taken narcotics, who have metabolic alkalosis, or who have increased intracranial pressure (e.g., from brain injuries). **Apnea** is defined as periods of no breathing. (For further information see Box 14-6. 🔗)

Hyperventilation is an increased rate and depth of respirations. In this situation, more CO_2 is eliminated than is produced. One particular type of hyperventilation that accompanies metabolic acidosis is called **Kussmaul's breathing.** The body attempts to rid itself of excess body acids by blowing off the carbon dioxide through deep and rapid breathing. Hyperventilation also often occurs as a response to stress.

Normal breathing is effortless, with evenly spaced respirations that vary little in depth. Abnormal respiratory rhythms create an irregular breathing pattern. Review the different respiratory rhythms in Box 14-6. 🔗

Difficult or labored breathing is called **dyspnea.** The dyspneic person often appears anxious and may experience **shortness of breath (SOB),** a feeling of being unable to get enough air. When a person is dyspneic, the nostrils may be flared because of the increased effort of inspiration. The skin may appear dusky; heart rate is increased.

Obstructed Airway

A completely or partially obstructed airway can occur anywhere along the upper or lower respiratory passageways. An obstruction of the nose, pharynx, or larynx is an *upper airway obstruction*. It can be caused by a foreign object such as food, by the tongue blocking the oropharynx when a person is unconscious, or by secretions collecting in the passageways. In the last instance, the respirations sound gurgly or bubbly as the air attempts to pass through the secretions. *Lower airway obstruction* involves partial or complete blockage of the passageways in the bronchi and lungs. This can be caused by bronchospasm; increased production of secretions; thick, sticky secretions; or bronchial inflammation.

Maintaining an open *(patent)* airway is a nursing responsibility that requires immediate action. A low-pitched snoring sound during inhalation indicates partial obstruction of the upper airways. Complete obstruction is indicated by extreme inspiratory effort that produces no chest movement. *Intercostal retractions* (the drawing of skin and muscle against the ribs) indicate this extreme effort. Lower airway obstruction is not always as easy to observe. **Stridor** (a harsh, high-pitched sound) may be heard during inspiration. The client may have altered arterial blood gas levels, restlessness, dyspnea, and *adventitious* (abnormal) breath sounds. (See Chapter 11 on assessment and Box 14-6. 🔗)

◆ Structure and Function of the Cardiovascular System

The respiratory and cardiovascular systems are closely linked and depend on each other to deliver oxygen to the tissues of the body. Alterations in function of either system can affect the other and lead to hypoxia, or lack of oxygen.

The heart, blood vessels, and blood form the major transport system of the body, bringing oxygen and nutrients to the cells and removing wastes for disposal (see Figure 10-10) . The heart serves as the system pump, moving blood through the vessels to the tissues.

THE HEART

The heart is a hollow, cone-shaped organ about the size of a fist. It is located in the mediastinum (between the lungs and below the sternum). The heart is made of three layers:

1. The *endocardium* lining the inside of the heart's chambers and great vessels
2. The *myocardium*, cardiac muscle cells that form the bulk of the heart and contract with each beat
3. The *epicardium*, which forms the outer layer. It is enclosed by a double-layered membrane known as the *pericardium*. The parietal, or outermost, pericardium protects the heart and anchors it to surrounding structures. The visceral pericardium adheres to the surface of the heart and forms the epicardium.

The heart contains four hollow chambers: two upper atria and two lower ventricles. They are separated by a septum, or wall, that forms two parallel pumps (Figure 16-2 ◆). The atria and ventricles are separated from one another by the atrioventricular valves. The tricuspid valve is on the right and the bicuspid or mitral valve is on the left. The ventricles, in turn, are separated from the *great vessels* (the pulmonary arteries and aorta) by the semilunar valves. The pulmonic valve is on the right and the aortic valve is on the left. The valves direct the flow of blood from the atria to the ventricles, and the ventricles to the great vessels. The valves act as one-way doors, allowing the blood to flow in one direction and preventing backflow.

Deoxygenated blood returns to the heart from the veins. It enters the right atrium through the superior and inferior venae cavae. From there it flows into the right ventricle, which pumps it through the pulmonary artery into the lungs for gas exchange. Freshly oxygenated blood enters the pulmonary veins and returns to the left atrium. From here the blood enters the left ventricle to be pumped out through the aorta to the body.

Coronary Circulation

The heart pumps blood to the lungs and peripheral tissues but receives no oxygen or nourishment from the blood within its chambers. Instead, it is supplied by a network of vessels known as the *coronary circulation*. The coronary arteries start at the base of the aorta, branching out to encircle and penetrate the myocardium. The coronary arteries bring oxygen-rich blood to the myocardium. If these arteries become clogged with **atherosclerotic plaque** (fat deposits within the blood vessels) or if the arteries are obstructed by a blood clot, oxygenated blood cannot reach the myocardium. The client may develop chest pain (**angina pectoris**) or experience a **myocardial infarction (MI)** (heart attack).

Cardiac Output

Cardiac output, the amount of blood pumped by the ventricles in 1 minute, is an important indicator of how well the heart is functioning as a pump. If the cardiac output is poor, tissue perfusion suffers and oxygen and nutrients do not reach the cells as needed.

BLOOD VESSELS

With each cardiac contraction, blood is ejected into a closed system of blood vessels that transport blood to the tissues and return it to the heart. The heart supports two circulatory systems: the low-pressure pulmonary system and the higher-pressure systemic circulatory system.

Pulmonary Circulation

Deoxygenated blood from the right ventricle enters the pulmonary vascular system through the pulmonary arteries. The pulmonary arteries subdivide into lobar arteries that branch out to form arterioles and the dense capillary networks that encompass the alveoli. Oxygen diffuses into the blood from the alveoli, and carbon dioxide diffuses into the alveoli from the blood. The blood then returns to the left side of the heart via venules and the pulmonary veins.

Systemic Circulation

The muscular left ventricle of the heart pumps oxygenated blood into the aorta. The blood then moves into major arteries that branch from the aorta, and into successively smaller arteries, arterioles, and finally the thin-walled capillary beds of

Figure 16-2. ◆ The heart and blood vessels. The left side of the heart pumps oxygenated blood into the arteries. Deoxygenated blood returns via the venous system into the right side of the heart.

Labels in figure:
- Capillary beds of lungs where gas exchange occurs
- Pulmonary Circulation
- Pulmonary arteries
- Pulmonary veins
- Aorta and branches
- Venae cavae
- Left atrium
- Right atrium
- Left ventricle
- Right ventricle
- Systemic Circulation
- Capillary beds of all body tissues where gas exchange occurs
- Oxygen-poor, CO_2-rich blood
- Oxygen-rich, CO_2-poor blood

MediaLink ECG Rhythm Strip

MediaLink Normal Heart Hemodynamics

organs and tissues. Capillary walls contain only one thin layer of cells. Gases and molecules can diffuse easily between the blood and the tissues. In the capillary beds, oxygen and nutrients are exchanged for metabolic waste products. The deoxygenated blood then returns to the heart through a series of venules and veins that become progressively larger until they empty into the superior and inferior venae cavae.

BLOOD

Blood transports oxygen via the lungs and nutrients from the gastrointestinal system to the cells. Blood is a mixture of cells suspended in fluid *(plasma)*. Its primary functions are:

◆ Transporting oxygen, nutrients, and hormones to the cells
◆ Transporting metabolic wastes from the tissues for elimination through the lungs, liver, and kidneys
◆ Regulating body temperature, pH, and fluid volume
◆ Controlling infection and blood loss

As previously noted, most oxygen is transported bound to hemoglobin. Hemoglobin is a major component of erythrocytes, the predominant cells present in blood. Hemoglobin binds easily with oxygen, releasing it in the body tissues. **Anemia** is a condition of too few RBCs that contain too little or abnormal hemoglobin. This condition interferes with oxygen delivery to the tissues, causing fatigue and activity intolerance.

ALTERATIONS IN CARDIOVASCULAR FUNCTION

Cardiovascular function can be altered by conditions that affect:

1. The function of the heart as a pump (cardiac output)
2. Blood flow to organs and peripheral tissues (tissue perfusion)
3. The composition of the blood and its ability to transport oxygen and carbon dioxide (blood alterations)

Decreased Cardiac Output

Although the heart normally is able to increase its rate and force of contraction to increase cardiac output during exercise, fever, or other times of need, some conditions interfere with these mechanisms. Heart attack (MI), congestive heart failure (CHF), and certain infections of the heart *(myocarditis)* cause damage to the heart muscle. When this occurs, the heart can no longer pump effectively.

Very irregular or excessively rapid or slow heart rates can decrease the cardiac output. Abnormalities of the heart rate and rhythm are known as **dysrhythmias** and can be identified on an electrocardiogram (ECG).

Alterations in the structure of the heart can affect cardiac output. Congenital heart defects and infectious heart disorders such as bacterial endocarditis and rheumatic fever can both cause decreased cardiac output.

Impaired Tissue Perfusion

Ischemia is a lack of blood supply to tissues and organs due to obstructed circulation. **Atherosclerosis** (narrowing and

obstruction of circulatory vessels) is by far the most common cause of ischemia. Any artery in the body may be affected by atherosclerosis. Risk factors for atherosclerosis include:

◆ Cigarette smoking
◆ High fat intake
◆ Obesity
◆ Sedentary lifestyle
◆ Hypertension
◆ Uncontrolled diabetes mellitus

Obstruction of the coronary arteries causes myocardial ischemia. Ischemia of the cerebral vessels may cause a *transient ischemic attack (TIA)* or *cerebral vascular accident* (CVA or stroke). Peripheral vascular disease leads to ischemia of distal tissues such as the legs and feet. Gangrene and amputation may result.

Veins that do not function properly can cause impaired tissue perfusion. When heart valves do not open and close correctly, blood may pool in veins, causing edema and decreasing venous return to the heart. Veins also can become inflamed, reducing blood flow and increasing the risk of **thrombosis** (clot formation) (see "Preventing Venous Stasis" in the Diagnosing, Planning, and Implementing Section of this chapter). The thrombus may then break loose, becoming an **embolus** (plural: emboli). Emboli tend to travel as far as the pulmonary circulation, where they become trapped in small vessels *(pulmonary emboli),* blocking blood supply to the alveolar–capillary membrane. Although alveolar ventilation to the affected area often remains adequate, no gas exchange occurs there because of impaired blood flow.

Blood Alterations

When blood is unable to transport oxygen to tissues effectively, impaired tissue perfusion results. Lack of RBCs, low hemoglobin levels, and abnormal hemoglobin structure all affect tissue oxygenation. Anemia may be caused by: acute or chronic bleeding, a diet deficient in iron or folic acid, malfunction in the formation of hemoglobin and RBCs, or disorders that cause RBCs to break down excessively. People with sickle cell disease produce an abnormal form of hemoglobin and may experience tissue ischemia during **exacerbations** (flare-ups) of the disease.

Blood volume also affects tissue oxygenation. If the blood volume is inadequate as in hemorrhage or severe dehydration **(hypovolemia),** the blood pressure and cardiac output fall, and tissues may become ischemic. **Hypervolemia** (excess blood volume) can result from fluid retention or kidney failure and may lead to tissue ischemia.

Factors That Affect Oxygenation

In the healthy person, the cardiovascular and respiratory systems can provide sufficient oxygen to meet the body's needs. However, certain factors can affect oxygen delivery and oxygen entering the bloodstream:

◆ Diseases of the cardiovascular and/or respiratory systems (e.g., anemia)

- Medications. Narcotics such as morphine and meperidine (Demerol) depress the respiratory center in the medulla, causing decreased respiratory depth and rate.
- Stress. When stressed, some people hyperventilate. Oxygen levels in arterial blood rise and carbon dioxide levels fall. This causes symptoms of dizziness, numbness of fingers and toes, and numbness around the mouth.
- Anger may be connected to heart disease. Recent studies indicate that people who repress their anger or become hostile appear to have a higher incidence of heart disease.
- Gender may affect cardiopulmonary function. Through middle adulthood (until menopause), estrogen has a protective effect in women, slowing the progress of atherosclerosis and reducing the risk of cardiovascular disease. This effect is lost at menopause, but hormone replacement therapy may be beneficial in reducing this risk later in life. Among people in their 40s and 50s, men have a higher incidence of hypertension than women.

Figure 16-3. ◆ A finger clip sensor for a pulse oximeter. *Source:* © Jenny Thomas.

 Treatment of Oxygenation Problems

COLLABORATIVE CARE

Pulse Oximetry

A pulse oximeter is a noninvasive device that measures oxygen saturation (SaO_2, or O_2 Sat). The pulse oximeter is connected to a sensor attached to the client's finger (Figure 16-3 ◆), toe, nose, earlobe, or forehead (or around the hand or foot of a neonate). The sensor detects hypoxemia before clinical signs and symptoms develop.

The pulse oximeter uses infrared light and a process known as spectrophotometry to measure the amount of oxygenated hemoglobin in arterial blood. Normal SaO_2 is 95 to 100 percent. An SaO_2 below 70 percent is life threatening. Measurement of SaO_2 may be taken intermittently, often as an aspect of vital sign measurement, but it also may be continuously monitored. The procedure for using a pulse oximeter is described in Procedure 16-1.

clinical ALERT

Pulse oximetry measures only the amount of hemoglobin that is bound with oxygen. Results can be misleading if the client's hemoglobin is bound to another substance, such as carbon monoxide.

Cardiac Monitoring

Cardiac monitoring allows continuous observation of the client's cardiac rhythm. It is used in many instances, such as during and after surgery, and in clients who have known or suspected cardiovascular disease. Electrodes placed on the client's chest may be attached to a monitor cable and bedside monitor. The monitor is equipped with alarms used to warn

of potential problems such as very fast or very slow heart rates.

Diagnostic Studies

The physician may order various diagnostic tests to assess respiratory and cardiovascular status, function, and oxygenation. These tests include sputum specimens, throat cultures, skin testing for allergies, venous and arterial blood specimens, pulmonary and cardiac function tests, and visualization procedures. Check the facility's policy for specimens that the LPN/LVN is responsible for collecting.

SPECIMENS. Sputum is the mucous secretion from the lungs, bronchi, and trachea. It is important to differentiate it from saliva, the clear liquid secreted by the salivary glands in the mouth, sometimes referred to as "spit."

Healthy individuals do not produce sputum. Clients need to cough to bring sputum up from the lungs, bronchi, and trachea into the mouth in order to *expectorate* it (spit it out) into a collecting container (Figure 16-4 ◆).

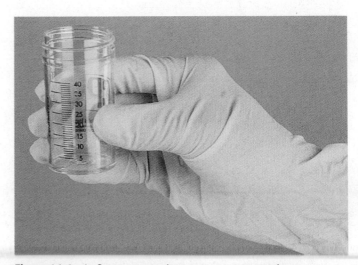

Figure 16-4. ◆ Sputum container. *Source:* © Elena Dorfman.

A throat culture sample is collected from the mucosa of the oropharynx and tonsillar regions using a culture swab (Figure 16-5 ◆). The sample is then cultured and examined for the presence of disease-producing microorganisms. Guidelines for obtaining a client sputum sample and a throat culture are provided in Box 16-3 ◆.

BLOOD TESTS. Specimens of venous blood are taken for a complete blood count (CBC), which includes hemoglobin and hematocrit measurements, erythrocyte (RBC) count, leukocyte (WBC) count, RBC indices, and a differential white cell count.

A number of other tests may be performed on blood serum (the liquid portion of the blood). These tests are often referred to as blood chemistries. Common chemistry examinations include serum electrolytes (sodium, potassium, chloride, calcium, and bicarbonate), cardiac enzymes, serum glucose, hormones such as thyroid hormone, metabolic waste products like creatinine and blood urea nitrogen (BUN), and other substances like cholesterol and triglycerides. These tests provide valuable diagnostic cues. Nurses often obtain venous blood samples for testing. Arterial blood gases give information about oxygen levels, carbon dioxide levels, and pH of the blood. Arterial samples are usually obtained by health care staff who have had additional training.

ELECTROCARDIOGRAPHY. Electrocardiography provides a graphic recording of the heart's electrical activity. Electrodes placed on the skin transmit the electrical impulses to an oscilloscope or graphic recorder. The electrocardiogram (ECG) can then be examined to detect dysrhythmias and alterations in conduction, which may indicate myocardial damage, enlargement of the heart, or drug effects.

Stress electrocardiography uses ECGs to assess the client's response to an increased cardiac workload during exercise. As the body's demand for oxygen increases with exercise, the cardiac workload increases, as does the oxygen demand of the heart muscle itself. Clients with coronary artery disease may develop chest pain and characteristic ECG changes during exercise.

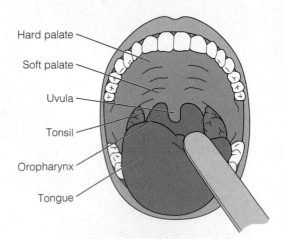

Hard palate

Soft palate

Uvula

Tonsil

Oropharynx

Tongue

Figure 16-5. ◆ Taking a throat culture.

BOX 16-3
NURSING CARE CHECKLIST

COLLECTING A SPUTUM SPECIMEN OR A THROAT SWAB SPECIMEN

Collecting a Sputum Specimen

☑ Offer mouth care so that the specimen will not be contaminated with microorganisms from the mouth.

☑ Ask the client to breathe deeply and then cough up 15 to 30 mL (1 or 2 tablespoons) of sputum.

☑ Wear gloves to avoid direct contact with the sputum. Follow special precautions if tuberculosis is suspected, obtaining the specimen in a room equipped with a special airflow system or ultraviolet light, or outdoors. If these options are not available, wear a mask capable of filtering droplet nuclei.

☑ Ask the client to *expectorate* (spit out) the sputum into the specimen container. Make sure the sputum does not contact the outside of the container (see Figure 16-4). If the outside of the container does become contaminated, wash it with a disinfectant.

☑ Following sputum collection, offer mouthwash to remove any unpleasant taste.

☑ Document the amount of sputum collected, color, odor, consistency (thick, tenacious, watery), and presence of **hemoptysis** (blood in sputum).

Collecting a Throat Culture Specimen

☑ Don clean gloves.

☑ Insert the swab into the oropharynx, and run the swab along the tonsils and areas on the pharynx that are reddened or contain exudate. (The gag reflex is active in some clients. It may be decreased by having the client sit upright if health permits, open the mouth, extend the tongue, and say "ah," and by taking the specimen quickly.)

☑ If the posterior pharynx cannot be seen, use a light and depress the tongue with a tongue blade (see Figure 16-5).

☑ Carefully place the swab with culture into the culture container, being sure not to contaminate the outside of the container.

PULMONARY FUNCTION TESTS. Pulmonary function tests measure lung volume and capacity. Clients undergoing pulmonary function tests, which are usually carried out by a respiratory therapist, do not require an anesthetic. The client breathes into a tube attached to a machine and a computer. The tests are painless but often tiring, especially for clients with pulmonary or cardiac conditions. The test requires the client's full cooperation.

VISUALIZATION PROCEDURES. A number of visualization procedures can be done to examine the respiratory tract and cardiovascular system. Roentgenography (x-ray), lung scan, endoscopy (bronchoscopy and laryngoscopy), angiography, and echocardiography are a few visualization procedures.

OXYGEN THERAPY

Clients who have difficulty ventilating all areas of their lungs, those whose gas exchange is impaired, or people with heart failure may require oxygen therapy to prevent hypoxia.

Oxygen therapy is prescribed by the physician, who specifies the concentration, method of delivery, and liter flow per minute. The nurse may initiate oxygen therapy in an emergency situation. As mentioned earlier, a low-flow oxygen system is essential for clients who have chronic obstructive pulmonary disease (COPD). Safety precautions are essential during oxygen therapy. Box 16-4 ◆ provides instructions for oxygen safety.

Because oxygen is colorless, odorless, and tasteless, people are often unaware of its presence. Although oxygen by itself will not burn or explode, it does facilitate combustion and burning. For example, a bed sheet ordinarily burns slowly when ignited in the atmosphere. However, if the sheet is saturated with oxygen and ignited by a spark, it will burn rapidly. The greater the concentration of the oxygen, the more rapidly fires start and burn, and the harder they are to extinguish.

Oxygen is supplied in several different ways. In hospitals and some long-term care facilities, it is usually piped into wall outlets at the client's bedside, making it readily available for use at all times (Figure 16-6 ◆). Tanks or cylinders of oxygen under pressure are also frequently available for use when wall oxygen either is unavailable or impractical.

Clients who require oxygen therapy in the home, or in facilities without piped-in oxygen, may use small cylinders of oxygen, oxygen in liquid form, or an oxygen concentrator. Portable oxygen delivery systems are available to increase the client's independence. Home oxygen therapy services are readily available in most communities. These services generally supply the oxygen and delivery devices, training for the client and family, equipment maintenance, and emergency services should a problem occur.

Oxygen administered from a cylinder or wall-outlet system is dry. Dry gases dehydrate the respiratory mucous membranes. Humidifying devices that add water vapor to inspired air are thus an essential adjunct of oxygen therapy, particularly for liter flows over 2 L per minute (Figure 16-7 ◆). These devices provide 20 to 40 percent humidity. The oxygen passes through distilled water and then along a line to the device through which the moistened oxygen is inhaled (e.g., a nasal cannula or oxygen mask). Liter flows of 2 L per minute or less by nasal cannula do not require humidification.

OXYGEN DELIVERY SYSTEMS. Oxygen is most often delivered via cannula or face mask. When it is important to regulate the percentage of oxygen received by the client more precisely, a Venturi mask may be used. Refer to Procedure 16-2 for descriptions of equipment and interventions.

BOX 16-4
NURSING CARE CHECKLIST

OXYGEN THERAPY SAFETY PRECAUTIONS

☑ Place cautionary signs reading "No Smoking: Oxygen in Use" on the client's door, at the foot or head of the bed, and on the oxygen equipment.

☑ Handle and store oxygen cylinders with caution, and strap them securely in wheeled transport devices or stands to prevent possible falls and outlet breakages. Place them away from traffic areas and heaters.

☑ Instruct the client and visitors about the hazard of smoking with oxygen in use. Teach family members and roommates to smoke only outside or in provided smoking rooms away from the client.

☑ Make sure that electric devices (e.g., razors, hearing aids, radios, televisions, and heating pads) are in good working order to prevent the occurrence of short-circuit sparks.

☑ Avoid materials that generate static electricity, such as woolen blankets and synthetic fabrics. Advise clients and caregivers to wear cotton fabrics and use cotton blankets.

☑ Avoid the use of volatile, flammable materials, such as oils, greases, alcohol, ether, and acetone (e.g., nail polish remover), near clients receiving oxygen.

Figure 16-6. ◆ An oxygen flow meter attached to a wall outlet.
Source: © Jenny Thomas.

Figure 16-7. ◆ An oxygen humidifier. *Source:* © Elena Dorfman.

Artificial Airways

Artificial airways are inserted to maintain a patent air passage for clients whose airway has become or may become obstructed. Three of the more common types of artificial airways are:

1. Oropharyngeal and nasopharyngeal airways (Figure 16-8A and B ◆) are used to keep the upper air passages open when they may become obstructed by secretions or the tongue. These airways are easy to insert and have a low risk of complications.

2. Endotracheal tubes (Figure 16-8C) are most commonly inserted for clients who have had general anesthetics or for those in emergency situations where mechanical ventilation is required. An endotracheal tube is inserted by the physician or RN with specialized education. Because an endotracheal tube passes through the epiglottis and glottis, the client is unable to speak while it is in place.

3. Clients who need long-term airway support may have a **tracheostomy** (Figure 16-9 ◆), a surgical incision in the trachea just below the larynx through which a tracheostomy tube is inserted.

Tracheostomy tubes may be either plastic or metal and are available in different sizes. Tracheostomy tubes (Figure 16-10 ◆) have an outer *cannula* that is inserted into the trachea and a *flange* that rests against the neck and allows the tube to be secured in place with tape or ties. All tubes also have an *obturator*, which is used to insert the outer cannula and is then removed. The obturator is kept at the client's bedside in case the tube becomes dislodged and needs to be reinserted. Some tracheostomy tubes have an inner cannula that may be removed for periodic cleaning.

Cuffed tracheostomy tubes (Figure 16-11 ◆) are surrounded by an inflatable cuff that produces an airtight seal between the tube and the trachea. Procedure 16-3 describes tracheostomy care.

Chest Tubes and Drainage Systems

Chest tubes may be inserted into the pleural cavity to restore negative pressure and drain collected fluid or blood. Because air rises, chest tubes for pneumothorax often are placed in the upper anterior thorax. Chest tubes used to drain blood or fluid are usually placed in the lower lateral chest wall.

When chest tubes are inserted, they must be connected to a sealed drainage system or a one-way valve that allows air and fluid to be removed from the chest cavity but prevents air from entering from the outside. Water-seal drainage systems are used to prevent outside air from entering the chest tube. Sterile disposable systems commonly are used. These systems typically have a closed collection chamber for drainage that is connected to the water-seal chamber (Figure 16-12 ◆). When the client inhales, the water prevents air from entering the sys-

A

B

C

Figure 16-8. ◆ **A.** An oropharyngeal airway. **B.** A nasopharyngeal airway. **C.** An endotracheal tube.

Figure 16-9. ◆ A tracheostomy tube in place.

Figure 16-11. ◆ A tracheostomy tube with a low-pressure cuff. *Source:* © Elena Dorfman.

tem from the atmosphere. During exhalation, however, air can exit the chest cavity, bubbling up through the water. Suction can be added to the system to facilitate removing air and secretions from the chest cavity.

NURSING CARE

ASSESSING

A nursing history and physical exam give valuable information about past health problems and current oxygenation status. During the physical exam, it is very important to evaluate the blood pressure in both arms to detect deficits (see Chapter 14). There should be no more than 10 mm Hg difference between the arms.

Variations in the shape of the thorax may indicate adaptation to chronic respiratory conditions. For example, clients with emphysema frequently develop a barrel chest.

The nursing assessment specific to oxygenation includes pulse oximetry, cardiac monitoring, and the review of results of diagnostic tests. Nurses obtain sputum or throat swab cultures for culturing (see Box 16-3).

DIAGNOSING, PLANNING, and IMPLEMENTING

Some of the NANDA diagnoses that may be appropriate for clients with oxygenation problems are:

◆ Impaired Gas Exchange
◆ Ineffective Breathing Patterns
◆ Impaired Tissue Perfusion

It is important to be familiar with the NANDA diagnoses; a complete list can be found in Appendix I.

Outer cannula with flange

Inner cannula

Obturator

Figure 16-10. ◆ Components of a tracheostomy tube.

Figure 16-12. ◆ A disposable chest drainage system. Fluid and blood collect in the white calibrated chambers. The red chamber provides the water seal, and the blue chamber is a suction-control chamber. *Source:* © Elena Dorfman.

Promoting Oxygenation

Respiratory Function. Most people in good health give little thought to their respiratory and cardiovascular function. Changing position frequently, ambulating, and exercising usually maintain adequate ventilation, gas exchange, and cardiovascular function in healthy people.

When people become ill, however, pain and immobility may cause shallow respirations or inadequate chest expansion. Respiratory secretions may pool in the lungs and promote infection. This situation is often compounded when clients are given narcotics for pain.

Interventions by the nurse to maintain the normal respirations of clients include:

◆ Positioning the client in semi-Fowler's or high-Fowler's to allow for maximum chest expansion
◆ Encouraging or providing frequent changes in position, especially from side to side to promote lung expansion and mobilization of pulmonary secretions. Orthopneic position helps relieve pressure on the diaphragm from abdominal organs.
◆ Encouraging ambulation
◆ Implementing measures that promote comfort, such as giving pain medications

Cardiovascular Function. Immobility is detrimental to cardiovascular function. Without exercise of the calf and leg muscles, blood pools in the veins of the lower extremities and *thrombi* (blood clots) may form. Interventions by the nurse to maintain cardiovascular function in clients include:

◆ Positioning with the legs elevated to promote venous return to the heart
◆ Avoiding pillows under the knees or more than 15 degrees of knee flexion to improve blood flow to the lower extremities and reduce venous stagnation
◆ Encouraging leg exercises (such as flexion and extension of the feet, active contraction and relaxation of calf muscles) for a client on bed rest, and promoting ambulation as soon as possible
◆ Encouraging or providing frequent position changes

Oxygenation. Deep breathing exercises and coughing help remove secretions from the lungs. Breathing exercises are frequently indicated for clients with restricted chest expansion, such as people with COPD or clients recovering from thoracic surgery.

Commonly employed breathing exercises are abdominal (diaphragmatic) breathing and pursed-lip breathing. Abdominal (diaphragmatic) breathing permits deep full breaths with little effort. Pursed-lip breathing helps the client develop control over breathing. The pursed lips create a resistance to the air flowing out of the lungs, prolong exhalation, and prevent airway collapse by maintaining positive airway pressure. Box 16-5 ◆ provides instructions for performing abdominal (diaphragmatic) and pursed-lip breathing.

BOX 16-5 ▶

CLIENT TEACHING

BREATHING AND COUGHING TECHNIQUES
Abdominal (Diaphragmatic) and Pursed-Lip Breathing

Teach client to:

◆ Assume a comfortable semi-sitting position in bed or a chair or a lying position in bed with one pillow.
◆ Flex the knees to relax the muscles of the abdomen.
◆ Place one or both hands on the abdomen, just below the ribs.
◆ Breathe in deeply through the nose, keeping the mouth closed.
◆ Concentrate on feeling the abdomen rise as far as possible; stay relaxed, and avoid arching the back. If it is difficult to raise the abdomen, take a quick, forceful breath through the nose.
◆ Then purse lips as if about to whistle, and breathe out slowly and gently, making a slow whooshing sound without puffing out the cheeks. This pursed-lip breathing creates a resistance to air flowing out of the lungs, increases pressure within the bronchi (main air passages), and minimizes collapse of smaller airways, a common problem for people with chronic obstructive pulmonary disease.
◆ Concentrate on feeling the abdomen fall or sink, and tighten (contract) the abdominal muscles while breathing out to enhance effective exhalation. Count to 7 during exhalation.
◆ Use this exercise whenever feeling short of breath, and increase gradually to 5 to 10 minutes four times a day. Regular practice will help you do this type of breathing without conscious effort. The exercise, once learned, can be performed when sitting upright, standing, and walking.

Controlled and Huff Coughing

◆ After using a bronchodilator treatment (if prescribed), inhale deeply and hold your breath for a few seconds.
◆ Cough twice: The first cough loosens the mucus; the second expels secretions.
◆ For huff coughing, lean forward and exhale sharply with a huff sound. This technique helps keep airways open while moving secretions up and out of the lungs.
◆ Inhale by taking rapid short breaths in succession (sniffing) to prevent mucus from moving back into smaller airways.
◆ Rest.
◆ Try to avoid prolonged episodes of coughing as these may cause fatigue and hypoxia.

Forceful coughing often is less effective than using controlled or huff coughing techniques. Instructions for coughing techniques are also provided in Box 16-5.

Incentive Spirometry. Incentive spirometers, also referred to as sustained maximal inspiration devices (SMIs), are used to:

- Improve pulmonary ventilation
- Counteract the effects of anesthesia or hypoventilation
- Loosen respiratory secretions
- Facilitate respiratory gaseous exchange
- Expand collapsed alveoli

Incentive spirometers measure the flow of air inhaled through the mouthpiece. They therefore offer an incentive to improve inhalation (Figure 16-13 ◆).

The client should be assisted into a position, preferably an upright sitting position in bed or a chair. As stated, this position facilitates maximum ventilation. Box 16-6 ◆ lists instructions for clients in the use of incentive spirometers.

Hydration of Inspired Air. Adequate hydration maintains the moisture of the respiratory mucous membranes. Normally, respiratory tract secretions are thin and therefore moved readily by ciliary action. However, when the client is dehydrated or when the environment has a low humidity, the respiratory secretions can become thick and tenacious. Fluid intake should be as great as the client can tolerate.

Humidifiers are devices that add water vapor to inspired air. Room humidifiers provide cool mist to room air. *Nebulizers* (atomizers, devices for throwing spray) are used to deliver humidity and medications. They also are used with oxygen

Figure 16-13. ◆ Client using a plastic disposable volume-oriented incentive spirometer, or SMI.

BOX 16-6

CLIENT TEACHING

USING AN INCENTIVE SPIROMETER

- Hold or place the spirometer in an upright position. A tilted flow-oriented device requires less effort to raise the ball or disc; a volume-oriented device will not function correctly unless upright.
- Exhale normally.
- Seal the lips tightly around the mouthpiece.
- Take in a slow, deep breath to elevate the ball or cylinder, and then hold the breath for 2 seconds initially, increasing to 6 seconds (optimum), to keep the ball or cylinder elevated if possible.
- For a flow-oriented device, avoid brisk, low-volume breaths that snap the ball to the top of the chamber. Greater lung expansion is achieved with a very slow inspiration than with a brisk, shallow breath, even though it may not elevate the ball or keep it elevated while you hold your breath. Sustained elevation of the ball or cylinder ensures adequate ventilation of the alveoli (lung air sacs).
- If you have difficulty breathing only through the mouth, a nose clip can be used.
- Remove the mouthpiece, and exhale normally.
- Cough after the incentive effort. Deep ventilation may loosen secretions, and coughing can facilitate their removal.
- Relax, and take several normal breaths before using the spirometer again.
- Do five to ten repetitions. Repeat the procedure. Practice increases inspiratory volume, maintains alveolar ventilation, and prevents atelectasis (collapse of the air sacs).
- Clean the mouthpiece with water and shake it dry. Change disposable mouthpieces every 24 hours.

---

delivery systems to provide moistened air directly to the client. Their purposes are to prevent mucous membranes from drying and becoming irritated and to loosen secretions for easier expectoration.

Percussion, Vibration, and Postural Drainage. Percussion, vibration, and postural drainage (PVD) are dependent nursing functions performed according to a physician's order. These procedures help loosen thick, tenacious secretions. The positions in postural drainage facilitate the removal of secretions. Nurses who work in areas where they are expected to assist with these procedures will receive additional training.

Suctioning. When clients have difficulty expectorating their secretions or when an airway is in place, suctioning may be necessary to clear air passages. **Suctioning** means aspirating secretions through a catheter connected to a suction machine or wall suction outlet. Even though the upper airways (the oropharynx and nasopharynx) are not sterile, sterile technique is recommended for all suctioning to avoid introducing pathogens into the airways.

Suction catheters may be either open-tipped or whistle-tipped (Figure 16-14 ◆). The whistle-tipped catheter is less irritating to respiratory tissues, although the open-tipped catheter may be more effective for removing thick mucus plugs. Most suction catheters have a thumb port on the side to control the suction. The catheter is connected to suction tubing, which in turn is connected to a collection chamber and suction control gauge (Figure 16-15 ◆).

Oropharyngeal or nasopharyngeal suctioning removes secretions from the upper respiratory tract. Refer to Procedure 16-4 for steps in suctioning.

Monitoring Chest Tubes and Drainage Systems

Nurses are responsible for the care of clients with chest tubes and drainage systems in the pleural cavity. Nursing responsibilities regarding drainage systems include the following:

◆ Assist with the insertion and removal of the tube.
◆ Maintain the water seal and patency of the drainage system.
◆ Assess the client's vital signs, cardiovascular status, and respiratory status.
◆ Monitor the patency and integrity of the drainage system.
◆ Always keep the drainage system below the level of the client's chest to prevent fluid and drainage from being drawn back into the chest cavity.
◆ Keep rubber-tipped clamps and a sterile occlusive dressing near the client. The chest tube will need to be clamped quickly, close to the insertion site, if connections are broken or an air leak develops in the drainage system. If the chest tube is inadvertently pulled out, the wound should be immediately covered with a sterile occlusive dressing.

Preventing Venous Stasis

When clients have limited mobility or are confined to bed, venous return to the heart is impaired and the risk of venous

Figure 16-14. ◆ Types of suction catheters. **A.** open-tipped. **B.** whistle-tipped.

Figure 16-15. ◆ A wall suction unit. *Source:* © Jenny Thomas.

stasis increases. Immobility is a problem not only for ill or debilitated clients but also for some travelers who sit with legs dependent for long periods in a motor vehicle or an airplane. Venous stasis can lead to thrombus formation and edema of the extremities.

Preventing venous stasis is an important nursing intervention to reduce the risk of complications following surgery, trauma, or major medical problems. Positioning and leg exercises are discussed in Chapter 20. ⊖⊘ Antiembolism stockings and sequential compression devices are additional measures to help prevent venous stasis.

Antiemboli Stockings. Antiemboli stockings are tightly fitting elastic hosiery that provide varying degrees of leg compression. They frequently are used for clients with limited mobility. When obtaining antiemboli stockings for a client, follow the manufacturer's recommendation for measuring and fitting the stockings.

Sequential Compression Devices. Clients who are undergoing surgery or who are immobilized because of illness or injury may benefit from a sequential compression device (SCD) to promote venous return from the legs. SCDs consist of plastic sleeves wrapped around the legs that inflate and deflate to promote venous return. The plastic sleeves are attached by tubing to an air pump that alternately inflates and deflates portions of the sleeve to a specified pressure. The ankle area inflates first, followed by the calf region, and then the thigh area. This sequential inflation and deflation assists the leg muscles in moving blood toward the heart.

Antiembolism stockings are worn under the SCD to provide added support and protect the skin from irritation by the plastic. The SCD is removed for ambulation and is usually discontinued when the client resumes activities. SCDs are useful in preventing thrombi and edema from venous stasis, but they are not used for clients who have arterial insufficiency, cellulitis, infection of the extremity, or preexisting venous thrombosis. Procedure 16-5 outlines how to apply a sequential compression device.

Cardiopulmonary Resuscitation

Cardiopulmonary resuscitation (CPR) is a combination of oral resuscitation (mouth-to-mouth breathing), which supplies oxygen to the lungs; and external cardiac massage (chest compression), which is intended to reestablish cardiac function and blood circulation. CPR is also referred to as basic life support (BLS). Training in CPR is provided by some facilities, by the Red Cross, and by the American Heart Association. See more about CPR in Chapter 6.

A *cardiac arrest* is the cessation of cardiac function; the heart stops beating. Often, a cardiac arrest is unexpected and sudden. When it occurs, the heart no longer pumps blood to any of the organs of the body. Breathing then stops and the person becomes unconscious and limp. Within 20 to 40 seconds of a cardiac arrest the victim is clinically dead. After 4 to 6 minutes the lack of oxygen supply to the brain can cause permanent and extensive damage.

A *respiratory arrest* (pulmonary arrest) is the cessation of breathing. It often occurs as a result of a blocked airway, but it can occur following a cardiac arrest and for other reasons. A respiratory arrest may occur abruptly or be preceded by short, shallow breathing that becomes increasingly labored.

It is vital that all nurses be trained to perform CPR so that resuscitation measures can be initiated immediately when a cardiac or respiratory arrest occurs. Nurses also can be instrumental in increasing community awareness of the need for CPR training and ensuring its availability. Most health care agencies have established practices and policies governing CPR.

EVALUATING

Using the goals and desired outcomes identified in the planning stage of the nursing process, the nurse collects data to evaluate the effectiveness of interventions. If outcomes are not achieved, the nurse, client, and support person, if appropriate, need to explore the reasons before modifying the care plan. Outcomes for clients with alterations in oxygenation might include:

◆ Maintaining a patent airway with breath sounds clear/clearing and absence of dyspnea
◆ Demonstrating behaviors to improve airway clearance (e.g., cough effectively and expectorate secretions)
◆ Demonstrating improved ventilation and adequate oxygenation of tissues by arterial blood gases (ABGs) within patient's normal range and be free of symptoms of respiratory distress

◆ Establishing a normal/effective respiratory pattern within patient's normal range
◆ Be free of cyanosis and other signs/symptoms of hypoxia

DISCHARGE CONSIDERATIONS

The nurse provides client education regarding:

◆ Behaviors/lifestyle changes to regain and/or maintain appropriate weight
◆ Identifying interventions to prevent/reduce risk of infection
◆ Verbalization of condition/disease process and treatment
◆ Identification of relationship of current signs/symptoms to the disease process and correlation of these with causative factors

Nursing Process Case Study
CLIENT WITH HEMOTHORAX

Jerry Markert, age 21, was admitted to the acute care facility following a biking accident in which he received multiple injuries, including a hemothorax. He is receiving 6 L of oxygen by nasal cannula, has a chest tube connected to a closed drainage system.

Assessment The client is alert, stable, and progressing well. Pulse oximeter indicates an oxygen saturation level of 98 percent, BP 110/60; pulse 120. C/o difficulty breathing. Multiple bruises left side of torso, breath sounds decreased. Lacerations on forehead and legs, no evidence of extremity fracture. Chest x-ray revealed hemothorax.

Diagnosis The following nursing diagnoses are identified for Mr. Markert:

◆ Impaired Gas Exchange
◆ Risk for Injury

Expected Outcomes The expected outcomes specify that Mr. Markert will:

◆ Demonstrate improved ventilation and adequate oxygenation as evidenced by blood gases within client's normal parameters
◆ Maintain clear lung fields and remain free of signs of respiratory distress
◆ Remain free of injury as evidenced by chest tube in place and closed drainage system functioning properly.

Planning and Implementation The following interventions are planned and implemented:

◆ Document vital signs, oxygen saturation, and respiratory status every 4 hours.
◆ Place in Fowler's position.
◆ Administer oxygen as ordered.

◆ Provide rest.

◆ Assess chest tube and drainage system at least every 2 hours.

◆ Secure chest tube to chest wall and prevent tension during care.

◆ Prevent kinking or occlusion of drainage or chest tube.

◆ Keep drainage system below chest when sitting or ambulating.

◆ Observe for redness, swelling, drainage, or pain at insertion site.

◆ If tube is inadvertently dislodged/removed, promptly seal with sterile occlusion dressing.

Evaluation Chest tube in place connected to closed drainage, secured to chest wall, 200 cc of bloody drainage. O_2 sat 98% on 2 L. Diminished breaths sounds on left. 20, HR 86, and BP 120/78.

Critical Thinking in the Nursing Process

1. If Mr. Markert is stable and progressing well, why is his oxygen saturation being monitored?

2. What precautions need to be taken when caring for Mr. Markert while his chest tube is in place?

3. Offer suggestions that would help Mr. Markert, or any person with a respiratory problem, to establish healthy breathing after his chest tube is removed.

Note: The bibliography listings for this and all chapters have been compiled at the back of the book.

PROCEDURE 16-1
Measuring Pulse Oximetry

PURPOSES

◆ To measure the arterial blood oxygen saturation (SaO_2)
◆ To detect the presence of hypoxemia before visible signs develop

EQUIPMENT

◆ Pulse oximeter
◆ Nail polish remover as needed
◆ Sheet or towel

INTERVENTIONS

1. Select an appropriate sensor.
◆ Choose a sensor appropriate for the client's weight and size. *Because weight limits of infant, pediatric, and adult sensors overlap, a neonatal sensor could be used for an infant or a pediatric sensor for a small adult.* See the manufacturer's directions for weight limits.
◆ If the client is allergic to adhesive, use a clip or reflectance sensor without adhesive.

2. Select an appropriate site.
◆ Use a location appropriate for the type of sensor.
◆ If using an extremity, assess the proximal pulse and capillary refill at the point closest to the site. *Decreased circulation can alter the SaO_2 measurements.*
◆ If the client has low tissue perfusion due to peripheral vascular disease or therapy using vasoconstrictive medications, use a nasal sensor or a reflectance sensor on the forehead.
◆ Avoid using lower extremities that have a compromised circulation and extremities that are used for infusions or other invasive monitoring.

3. Prepare the site.
◆ Remove a female client's nail polish or acrylic nails. *These items can interfere with accurate measurements.*

4. Apply the sensor, and connect it to the pulse oximeter.
◆ Make sure the LED and photodetector are accurately aligned, that is, opposite each other on either side of the finger, toe, nose, or earlobe. Many sensors have markings to facilitate correct alignment of the LED and photodetector. *Correct alignment is essential for accurate SaO_2 measurement.*
◆ Attach the sensor cable to the connection outlet on the oximeter. Appropriate connection will be confirmed by an audible beep indicating each arterial pulsation. Turn on the machine according to the manufacturer's

directions. Some devices have a wheel that can be turned clockwise to increase the signal volume and counterclockwise to decrease it.
◆ Ensure that the bar of light or waveform on the face of the oximeter fluctuates with each pulsation and reflects the pulse volume or strength. *A signal that is too weak will not produce an accurate SaO_2 measurement.*

5. Set and turn on the alarm.
◆ Check the preset alarm limits for high and low oxygen saturation and high and low pulse rates.
◆ Change these alarm limits according to the manufacturer's directions as indicated.
◆ Ensure that the audio and visual alarms are on before you leave the client. A tone will be heard and a number will blink on the faceplate.

6. Ensure client safety.
◆ Inspect the location of an adhesive toe or finger sensor every 4 hours and a spring-tension sensor every 2 hours. Move it slightly or change the location as needed. *Movement prevents tissue necrosis due to prolonged pressure.*
◆ Inspect the sensor site tissues for irritation from adhesive sensors.

7. Ensure the accuracy of measurement.
◆ Minimize motion artifacts by using an adhesive sensor, or immobilize the client's monitoring site. *Movement of the client's finger or toe may be misinterpreted by the oximeter as arterial pulsations.*
◆ Cover a sensor with a sheet or towel to block large amounts of light from external sources (e.g., sunlight, procedure lamps, or bilirubin lights in the nursery). *Large amounts of outside light may be sensed by the photodetector and alter the SaO_2 value.*
◆ Verify that the client's hemoglobin level is normal. *An SaO_2 measurement may register normal when the client's hemoglobin is low because the available hemoglobin to carry oxygen is fully saturated.*

8. Document all relevant information.
   ◆ Record the application of the pulse oximeter, its type and size, and all nursing assessments.

◆ SAMPLE DOCUMENTATION

6/12/05 8:30 AM	Oxygen saturation 91. Client complained of discomfort on rt second finger. Moved tester to rt third finger. Expressed comfort. T 36°C, P 62, R 15, BP 128/85.
	R. Parks, LVN

PROCEDURE 16-2

Administering Oxygen by Nasal Cannula or Face Mask

PURPOSES

◆ Nasal cannula: To deliver a relatively low concentration of oxygen when only minimal O_2 support is required
◆ To allow uninterrupted delivery of oxygen while the client ingests food or fluids
◆ Face mask: To provide moderate O_2 support and a higher concentration of oxygen and/or humidity than is provided by cannula

EQUIPMENT

◆ Oxygen supply with a flow meter
◆ Humidifier with sterile, distilled water or tap water according to agency protocol
◆ Nasal cannula or prescribed face mask and tubing
◆ Gauze pads as needed

INTERVENTIONS

1. Determine the need for oxygen therapy, and verify the order for the therapy.
   ◆ Perform a respiratory assessment. *This determines the need for O_2 therapy and develops baseline data if not already available.*
2. Prepare the client and support people.
   ◆ Assist the client to a semi-Fowler's position if possible. *This position permits easier chest expansion and breathing.*
   ◆ Explain that oxygen is not dangerous when safety precautions are observed and that it will ease the discomfort of dyspnea. Inform the client and support people about the safety precautions connected with oxygen use.
3. Set up the oxygen equipment and the humidifier.
4. Turn on the oxygen at the prescribed rate, and ensure proper functioning.
   ◆ Check that the oxygen is flowing freely through the tubing. *There should be no kinks in the tubing, and the connections should be airtight. There should be bubbles in the humidifier as the oxygen flows through the water. You should feel the oxygen at the outlets of the cannula or mask.*
   ◆ Set the oxygen at the flow rate ordered, for example, 2 to 6 L/min.
5. Apply the appropriate oxygen delivery device.

Cannula

◆ Put the cannula over the client's face, with the outlet prongs fitting into the nares and the elastic band around the head (Figure 16-16 ◆). Some models have a strap that adjusts under the chin.
◆ If the cannula will not stay in place, tape it at the sides of the face.
◆ Pad the tubing and band over the ears and cheekbones as needed. *This helps prevent skin breakdown.*

Face Masks (Figure 16-17A ◆ to D).

◆ Guide the mask toward the client's face, and apply it from the nose downward.

Figure 16-16. ◆ **A.** Nasal cannula. **B.** The cannula in place.

Figure 16-17. ◆ **A.** A simple oxygen mask. *Source:* © Jenny Thomas. **B.** A partial rebreather mask. *Source:* © Elena Dorfman. **C.** A nonrebreather mask. *Source:* © Jenny Thomas. **D.** A Venturi oxygen mask. *Source:* © Elena Dorfman.

◆ Fit the mask to the contours of the client's face. *The mask should mold to the face, so that very little oxygen escapes into the eyes or around the cheeks and chin.*

◆ Secure the elastic band around the client's head so that the mask is comfortable but snug.

◆ Pad the band behind the ears and over bony prominences. *Padding will prevent irritation from the mask.*

6. Assess the client regularly. *This allows early response to any changes or problems.*

   ◆ Assess the client's level of anxiety, color, ease of respirations, and pulse oximeter reading (if available). Provide support while the client adjusts to the device.

   ◆ Assess the client in 15 to 30 minutes, depending on the client's condition, and regularly thereafter. Assess vital signs, color, breathing patterns, and chest movements.

   ◆ Assess the client regularly for clinical signs of hypoxia, tachycardia, confusion, dyspnea, restlessness, and cyanosis. Obtain arterial blood gas results if they are available.

Nasal Cannula

◆ Assess the client's nares for encrustations and irritation. Apply a water-soluble lubricant as required. *Lubricants soothe the mucous membranes.*

Face Mask

◆ Inspect the facial skin frequently for dampness or chafing, and dry and treat it as needed.

7. Inspect the equipment on a regular basis.

   ◆ Check the liter flow and the level of water in the humidifier in 30 minutes and whenever providing care to the client.

   ◆ Maintain the level of water in the humidifier.

   ◆ Make sure that safety precautions are being followed.

8. Document relevant data.

   ◆ Record the initiation of the therapy and all nursing assessments.

◆ **SAMPLE DOCUMENTATION: FOCUS CHARTING**

Date	Time	Data Action Response
11/6/05	0800	D: Client is anxious, resp rate 32, labored and shallow. Use of accessory muscles noted. c/o SOB. O₂ Sat 86% on room air. No history of COPD. A: Assisted client to semi-Fowler's and applied O₂ @ 4 L/min via nasal cannula per MD order. Distilled water humidification added. Assured patency of tubing/O₂ flowing freely w/ bubbling in humidifier. Nasal prongs positioned properly in nares; gauze placed under tubing on ears. ———— N. Nurse, LPN
11/6/05	0900	R: Decreased anxiety, RR 26, resp less labored. O₂ sat 91% on 4 L/min. Client states, "It's easier to breathe." N. Nurse, LPN

PROCEDURE 16-3
Providing Tracheostomy Care

PURPOSES

◆ To maintain airway patency
◆ To maintain cleanliness and prevent infection at the tracheostomy site
◆ To facilitate healing and prevent skin excoriation around the tracheostomy incision
◆ To promote comfort

EQUIPMENT

◆ Sterile disposable tracheostomy cleaning kit or supplies including sterile containers, sterile nylon brush and/or pipe cleaners, sterile applicators, gauze squares
◆ Towel or drape to protect bed linens
◆ Hydrogen peroxide and sterile normal saline

- ◆ Sterile gloves (1 pair)
- ◆ Clean gloves
- ◆ Moisture-proof bag
- ◆ Commercially prepared sterile tracheostomy dressing or sterile 4 × 4 gauze dressing

- ◆ Cotton twill ties or commercially prepared self-closing ties
- ◆ Clean scissors

INTERVENTIONS

1. Prepare the client and the equipment.
   - ◆ Assist the client to a semi-Fowler's or Fowler's position. *This promotes lung expansion.*
   - ◆ Explain the procedure to the client and provide for a means of communication, such as eye blinking or raising a finger to indicate pain or distress. *This reduces client anxiety.*
   - ◆ Don clean gloves, remove the soiled tracheostomy dressing, and discard the glove and the dressing.
   - ◆ Open the tracheostomy kit or sterile basins. Pour sterile normal saline into both basins. Pour hydrogen peroxide into one basin only.
   - ◆ Establish a sterile field.
   - ◆ Don sterile gloves; place sterile towel on client's chest and under tracheostomy area.
   - ◆ Open other sterile supplies as needed including sterile applicators, and tracheostomy dressing.

2. Remove inner cannula.
   - ◆ Using one part of a fully opened 4 × 4 gauze, stabilize the flange with one hand. With the other end of the 4 × 4, use the other gloved hand, to unlock the inner cannula (if present) and remove it by gently pulling it out toward you in line with its curvature. Place the inner cannula in the hydrogen peroxide solution to soak. *This moistens and loosens dried secretions.*

3. Clean the incision site and tube flange.
   - ◆ Using sterile applicators or gauze dressings moistened with normal saline, clean the stoma site (Figure 16-18 ◆). Use each applicator or gauze dressing only once, then discard. *This avoids contaminating a clean area with a soiled gauze dressing or applicator.*
   - ◆ The hydrogen peroxide/saline solution may be used to remove encrustations. Thoroughly rinse the cleaned area, using gauze squares moistened with sterile normal saline. *Hydrogen peroxide can be irritating to the skin and inhibit healing if not thoroughly removed.*
   - ◆ Clean the flange of the tube in the same manner.
   - ◆ Thoroughly dry the client's skin and tube flanges with dry gauze squares.

4. Clean the inner cannula.
   - ◆ Remove the inner cannula from the soaking solution.
   - ◆ Clean the lumen and entire inner cannula thoroughly, using the brush or pipe cleaners moistened with sterile normal saline (Figure 16-19 ◆). Inspect the cannula for cleanliness by holding it at eye level and looking through it into the light.
   - ◆ Rinse the inner cannula thoroughly in sterile normal saline. *Thorough rinsing is important to remove the hydrogen peroxide from the inner cannula.*
   - ◆ After rinsing, use a pipe cleaner folded in half to dry only the inside of the cannula; do not dry the outside. *This removes excess liquid from the cannula and prevents possible aspiration by the client, while leaving a film of moisture on the outer surface to lubricate the cannula for reinsertion.*

5. Replace the inner cannula, securing it in place.
   - ◆ Insert the inner cannula by grasping the outer flange and inserting the cannula in the direction of its curvature.
   - ◆ Lock the cannula in place by turning the lock (if present) into position to secure the flange of the inner cannula to the outer cannula.

6. Apply a sterile dressing
   - ◆ Use a commercially prepared tracheostomy dressing of nonraveling material, or open and refold a 4 × 4 gauze dressing into a V shape as shown in Figure 16-20 ◆. Avoid using cotton-filled gauze squares or cutting the 4

Figure 16-18. ◆ Using an applicator stick to clean the tracheostomy site. *Source:* © Jenny Thomas.

Figure 16-19. ◆ Cleaning the inner cannula with a brush. *Source:* © Elena Dorfman.

Figure 16-20. ◆ Folding a 4 × 4 gauze to make a tracheostomy dressing.

× 4 gauze. *Cotton lint or gauze fibers can be aspirated by the client, potentially creating a tracheal abscess.*
- ◆ Place the dressing under the flange of the tracheostomy tube.
- ◆ While applying the dressing, ensure that the tracheostomy tube is securely supported. *Excessive movement of the tracheostomy tube irritates the trachea.*

7. Change the tracheostomy ties.

One-Strip Method

- ◆ Cut a length of twill tape 2.5 times the length needed to go around the client's neck from one tube flange to the other.
- ◆ Thread one end of the tape into the slot on one side of the flange.
- ◆ Bring both ends of the tape together, and take them around the client's neck, keeping them flat and untwisted.
- ◆ Thread the end of the tape next to the client's neck through the slot from the back to the front.
- ◆ Have the client flex the neck. Tie the loose ends with a square knot at the side of the client's neck, allowing for

Figure 16-21. ◆ Placing a finger underneath the tie tape before tying it. *Source:* © Jenny Thomas.

slack by placing one finger under the ties as shown in Figure 16-21 ◆. Cut off long ends.

8. Check the tightness of the ties.
- ◆ Frequently check the tightness of the tracheostomy ties. *Neck movement may cause the ties to become too taut, interfering with coughing and circulation. Ties can loosen in restless clients, allowing the tracheostomy tube to extrude from the stoma.*

9. Document all relevant information.
- ◆ Record tracheostomy care, and the dressing change, noting your assessments.

◆ SAMPLE DOCUMENTATION: FOCUS CHARTING

Date	Time	Data Response Action
11/6/05	1100	D: Encrustations noted around
		stoma; due for routine trach care.
		Breath sounds clear; no distress
		noted. A: Using aseptic technique,
		removed soiled trach dressing. Set up
		sterile field per P+P and removed inner
		cannula for cleaning. Cleansed stoma
		site + flange. Reinserted inner cannula
		+ locked into place. Applied clean ties
		using the one-strip method; 2 fingers fit
		tightly under ties. Applied clean dressing
		around stoma and under flange. R:
		Patient tolerated procedure without
		SOB or distress noted. Tracheal
		stoma pink, free of encrustations, and
		skin dry. Trach ties secure and inner
		cannula locked. ————————
		N. Nurse, L.V.N.

PROCEDURE 16-4

Suctioning

PURPOSES

◆ To remove secretions that obstruct the airway
◆ To facilitate ventilation
◆ To obtain secretions for diagnostic purposes
◆ To prevent infection that may result from accumulated secretions

EQUIPMENT

◆ Towel or moisture-resistant pad (sterile towel for tracheal or endotracheal suctioning)
◆ Portable or wall suction machine with tubing and collection receptacle
◆ Sterile disposable container for fluids
◆ Sterile normal saline or water

◆ Sterile gloves
◆ Sterile suction catheter kit (12 to 18 Fr for adults; 8 to 10 Fr for children, and 5 to 8 Fr for infants); if both the oropharynx and the nasopharynx are to be suctioned, one sterile catheter is required for each
◆ Water-soluble lubricant (for nasopharyngeal suctioning)
◆ Y-connector
◆ Sterile gauzes
◆ Moisture-resistant disposal bag
◆ Sputum trap, if specimen is to be collected
◆ Resuscitation bag (Ambu bag) connected to 100 percent oxygen for tracheal or endotracheal care
◆ Goggles and mask if necessary
◆ Gown (if necessary)

Part A. Oropharyngeal and Nasopharyngeal Cavities

INTERVENTIONS

1. Prepare the client.
◆ Explain to the client that suctioning will relieve breathing difficulty and that the procedure is painless but may be uncomfortable and stimulate the cough, gag, or sneeze reflex. *Knowing that the procedure will relieve breathing problems is often reassuring and enlists the client's cooperation.*
◆ Position a conscious person who has a functional gag reflex in the semi-Fowler's position with the head turned to one side for oral suctioning or with the neck hyperextended for nasal suctioning. *These positions facilitate the insertion of the catheter and help prevent aspiration of secretions.*
◆ Position an unconscious client in the lateral position, facing you. *This position allows the tongue to fall forward, so that it will not obstruct the catheter on insertion. Lateral position also facilitates drainage of secretions from the pharynx and prevents the possibility of aspiration.*
◆ Place the towel or moisture-resistant pad over the pillow or under the chin.

2. Prepare the equipment.
◆ Set the pressure on the suction gauge, and turn on the suction. Many suction devices are calibrated to three pressure ranges:

Wall unit

Adult: 100 to 120 mm Hg
Child: 95 to 110 mm Hg
Infant: 50 to 95 mm Hg

Portable unit

Adult: 10 to 15 mm Hg
Child: 5 to 10 mm Hg
Infant: 2 to 5 mm Hg

◆ Open the lubricant if performing nasopharyngeal suctioning
◆ Open the sterile suction package.
  a. Set up the cup or container, touching only its outside.
  b. Pour sterile water or saline into the container.
  c. Don sterile gloves and attach the catheter to the suction unit. (Figure 16-22 ◆) (The hand that touched the suction unit is no longer sterile.) *The sterile gloved hand maintains the sterility of the suction catheter, and the unsterile glove prevents the transmission of the microorganisms to the nurse.*

3. Make an approximate measure of the depth for the insertion of the catheter and test the equipment.
◆ Measure the distance between the tip of the client's nose and the earlobe, or about 13 cm (5 in) for an adult.

Figure 16-22. ◆ Attaching the catheter to the suction unit.

◆ Mark the position on the tube with the fingers of the sterile gloved hand.
◆ Test the pressure of the suction and the patency of the catheter by applying your nonsterile gloved thumb to the port or open branch of the Y-connector (the suction control) to create suction.

4. Lubricate and introduce the catheter.

◆ For nasopharyngeal suction, lubricate the catheter tip with sterile water, saline, or water-soluble lubricant; for oropharyngeal suction, moisten the tip with sterile water or saline. *This reduces friction and eases insertion.*

For an Oropharyngeal Suction

◆ Pull the tongue forward, if necessary, using gauze.
◆ Do not apply suction (i.e., leave your thumb off the port) during insertion. *Applying suction during insertion causes trauma to the mucous membrane.*
◆ Advance the catheter about 10 to 15 cm (4 to 6 in) along one side of the mouth into the oropharynx. *Directing the catheter along the side prevents gagging.*

For a Nasopharyngeal Suction

◆ Without applying suction, insert the catheter the premeasured or recommended distance into either nares, and advance it along the floor of the nasal cavity. *This avoids the nasal turbinates.*
◆ Never force the catheter against an obstruction. If one nostril is obstructed, try the other.

5. Perform suctioning.

◆ Apply your thumb to the suction control port to start suction, and gently rotate the catheter. *Gentle rotation of the catheter ensures that all surfaces are reached and prevents trauma to any one area of the respiratory mucosa due to prolonged suction.*
◆ Apply suction for 5 to 10 seconds while slowly withdrawing the catheter, then remove your finger from the control, and remove the catheter.

◆ A suction attempt should last only 10 to 15 seconds. During this time, the catheter is inserted, the suction is applied and discontinued, and the catheter removed. (Keep in mind that the client is deprived of oxygen during the suction procedure.)
◆ It may be necessary during oropharyngeal suctioning to apply suction to secretions that collect in the vestibule of the mouth and beneath the tongue.

6. Clean the catheter, and repeat suctioning as above.

◆ Wipe off the catheter with sterile gauze if it is thickly coated with secretions. Dispose of the used gauze in a moisture-resistant bag.
◆ Flush the catheter with sterile water or saline.
◆ Relubricate the catheter, and repeat suctioning until the air passage is clear.
◆ Allow 20- to 30-second intervals between each suctions, and limit suction to 5 minutes in total. *Applying suction for too long may cause secretion to increase or decrease the clients oxygen supply.*
◆ Alternate nares for repeat suctionings. *This will decrease irritation to mucosal lining.*

7. Encourage the client to breathe deeply and to cough between suctionings. *Coughing and deep breathing help carry secretions from the trachea and bronchi into the pharynx, where they can be reached with the suction catheter.*

8. Promote client comfort.

◆ Offer to assist the client with oral or nasal hygiene.
◆ Assist the client to a position that facilitates breathing.

9. Dispose of equipment and ensure availability for the next suction.

◆ Dispose of the catheter, gloves, water, and waste container. Wrap the catheter around your sterile gloved hand, holding it as the glove is removed over it for disposal.
◆ Rinse the suction tubing as needed by inserting the end of the tubing into the used water container. Empty and rinse the suction collection container as needed or indicated by protocol. Change the suction tubing and container daily. *This provides good infection control.*
◆ Ensure that supplies are available for the next suctioning (suction kit, gloves, water or normal saline).

10. Assess the effectiveness of suctioning.

◆ Auscultate the client's breath sounds to ensure they are clear of secretions. Observe skin color, dyspnea, and level of anxiety.

11. Document relevant data.

◆ Record the procedure: the amount, consistency, color, and odor of sputum (e.g., foamy, white mucus; thick, green-tinged mucus; or blood-flecked mucus) and the client's breathing status before and after the procedure.
◆ If the technique is carried out frequently, for example, every hour, it may be appropriate to record only once, at the end of the shift; however, the frequency of the suctioning must be recorded.

Part B. Tracheostomy or Endotracheal Tube

INTERVENTIONS

1. Prepare the client.
- ◆ Inform the client that suctioning usually causes some intermittent coughing and that this assists in removing the secretions.
- ◆ If not contraindicated because of health, place the client in semi-Fowler's position to promote deep breathing, maximum lung expansion, and productive coughing. *Deep breathing oxygenates the lungs, counteracts the hypoxic effects of suctioning, and may induce coughing. Coughing helps to loosen and move secretions.*
- ◆ If necessary, provide analgesia prior to suctioning. *Endotracheal suctioning stimulates the cough reflex, which can cause pain for clients who have had thoracic or abdominal surgery or who have experienced traumatic injury. Premedication can increase the client's comfort during the suctioning procedure.*

2. Prepare the equipment.
- ◆ Open the sterile supplies in readiness for use.
- ◆ Place the sterile towel, if used, across the client's chest below the tracheostomy.
- ◆ Turn on the suction, and set the pressure in accordance with agency policy. For a wall unit, pressure of about 100 to 120 mm Hg is normally used for adults, 50 to 95 mm Hg for infants and children.
- ◆ Put on goggles, mask, and gown if necessary.
- ◆ Put on sterile gloves. Some agencies recommend putting a sterile glove on the dominant hand and a non-sterile glove on the nondominant hand to protect the nurse.
- ◆ Holding the catheter in the dominant hand and the connector in the nondominant hand, attach the suction catheter to the suction tubing (see Figure 16-22 ◆).

3. Flush and lubricate the catheter.
- ◆ Using the dominant hand, place the catheter tip in the sterile saline solution.
- ◆ Using the thumb of the nondominant hand, occlude the thumb control, and suction a small amount of the sterile solution through the catheter. *This determines that the suction equipment is working properly and lubricates the outside and the lumen of the catheter. Lubrication eases insertion and reduces tissue trauma during insertion. Lubricating the lumen also helps prevent secretions from sticking to the inside of the catheter.*

4. Quickly but gently insert the catheter without applying any suction.
- ◆ With your nondominant thumb off the suction port, quickly but gently insert the catheter into the trachea through the tracheostomy tube (Figure 16-23 ◆). *To prevent tissue trauma and oxygen loss, suction is not applied during insertion of the catheter.*

Figure 16-23. ◆ Inserting the catheter into the trachea through the tracheostomy tube. *Source:* © Jenny Thomas.

- ◆ Insert the catheter about 12.5 cm (5 in) for adults, less for children, or until the client coughs or you feel resistance. *Resistance usually means that the catheter tip has reached the carina (bifurcation of the trachea into the main bronchi). To prevent damaging the mucous membranes at the bifurcation, withdraw the catheter about 1 to 2 cm (0.4 to 0.8 in) before applying suction.*

5. Perform suctioning.
- ◆ Apply intermittent suction for 5 to 10 seconds by placing the nondominant thumb over the thumb port. *Suction time is restricted to 10 seconds or less to minimize oxygen loss.*
- ◆ Rotate the catheter by rolling it between your thumb and forefinger while slowly withdrawing it. *This prevents tissue trauma by minimizing the suction time against any part of the trachea.*
- ◆ Withdraw the catheter completely, and release the suction.
- ◆ Ventilate the client.
- ◆ Then suction again.

6. Reassess the client's oxygenation status, and repeat suctioning.
- ◆ Observe the client's respirations and skin color. Check the client's pulse if necessary, using your nondominant hand.
- ◆ Encourage the client to breathe deeply and to cough between suctions.
- ◆ Allow 2 to 3 minutes between suctions when possible. *This provides an opportunity for reoxygenation of the lungs.*
- ◆ Flush the catheter, and repeat suctioning until the air passage is clear and the breathing is relatively effortless and quiet.
- ◆ After each suction, pick up the resuscitation bag with your nondominant hand and ventilate the client with five breaths.

7. Dispose of equipment and ensure availability for the next suction.

◆ Flush the catheter and suction tubing.

◆ Turn off the suction, and disconnect the catheter from the suction tubing.

◆ Wrap the catheter around your sterile hand, and peel the glove off so that it turns inside out over the catheter.

◆ Discard the glove and the catheter in the moisture-resistant bag.

◆ Replenish the sterile fluid and supplies so that the suction is ready to be used again. *Clients who require suctioning often require it quickly, so it is essential to leave the equipment at the bedside ready for use.*

8. Provide for client comfort and safety.

◆ Assist the client to a comfortable, safe position that aids breathing. *If the person is conscious, a semi-Fowler's position is frequently indicated. If the person is unconscious, Sims' position aids in the drainage of secretions from the mouth.*

9. Document relevant data.

◆ Record the suctioning, including the amount and description of suction returns, the amount of sterile saline instilled, and any other relevant assessments.

◆ **SAMPLE DOCUMENTATION: FOCUS CHARTING**

Date	Time	Data Action Response
11/6/05	0830	D: Client w/ audibly moist breath sounds; RR 30 and labored. Weak, ineffective cough. Rhonchi and coarse crackles auscultated A+P. A: Positioned client in semi-Fowler's position. Maintaining sterile technique + following P+P, performed nasopharyngeal suctioning. R: Copious amounts of thick, yellow secretions removed. RR 26 and less labored. Breath sounds with minimal coarse crackles @ bases bilaterally. — N. Nurse, L.V.N.

Applying a Sequential Compression Device

PURPOSES

◆ To facilitate venous return in immobilized clients
◆ To prevent thrombus formation

EQUIPMENT

◆ Measuring tape
◆ Antiembolism stockings
◆ Sequential compression device (SCD) including disposable sleeves, air pump, and tubing

INTERVENTIONS

1. Prepare the client.

◆ Place the client in a dorsal recumbent or semi-Fowler's position. Provide for privacy and drape the client appropriately.

◆ Measure the client's legs as recommended by the manufacturer if a thigh-length sleeve is required. *Knee-length sleeves come in just one size; the thigh circumference determines the size needed for a thigh-length sleeve.*

◆ Apply antiembolism stockings. *Antiembolism stockings provide added support and reduce skin irritation from the compression sleeve.* (See Procedure 22-2 ⊙⊙)

2. Apply the sequential compression sleeves.

◆ Place a sleeve under each leg with the opening at the knee.

◆ Wrap the sleeve securely around the leg, securing the Velcro tabs (Figure 16-24 ◆). Allow two fingers to fit between the leg and the sleeve. *This amount of space*

Figure 16-24. ◆ Applying a sequential compression device to the leg. *Source:* © Jenny Thomas.

ensures that the sleeve does not impair circulation when inflated.

3. Connect the sleeves to the control unit and adjust the pressure as needed.

◆ Connect the tubing to the sleeves and control unit, ensuring that arrows on the plug and the connector are in alignment and that the tubing is not kinked or twisted. *Improper alignment or obstruction of the tubing by kinks or twists will interfere with operation of the SCD.*

◆ Turn on the control unit and adjust the alarms and pressures as needed. The sleeve cooling control and alarm should be "on"; ankle pressure is usually set at 35 to 55 mm Hg. *It is important to have the sleeve cooling control on for comfort and to reduce the risk of skin irritation from moisture under the sleeve. Alarms warn of possible control unit malfunctions.*

4. Document the procedure.

◆ Record baseline assessment data and application of the SCD. Note control unit settings.

◆ Assess and document skin integrity and neurovascular status at least every 8 hours while the SCD is in place. Remove the unit and notify the physician if the client complains of numbness and tingling or leg pain. *These may be symptoms of nerve compression.*

◆ **SAMPLE DOCUMENTATION: FOCUS CHARTING**

Date	Time	Data Action Response
3/9/04	1030	D: Client is 1 day post Rt. THR. Antiembolism stockings + SCDs removed for bath. A: Assessed pedal and popiteal pulses. Assessed CMS status. Assessed skin integrity before replacing thigh-high antiembolism stockings and SCDs. Instructed client to report any numbness, tingling or leg pain. R: CMS intact. The sleeve cooling control + alarm are "on" with sleeve pressure at 45 mm Hg. ——— N. Nurse, L.P.N.

Chapter Review

Key Terms by Topics

Use the audio glossary feature of either the CD-ROM or the Companion Website to hear the correct pronunciation of the following key terms.

Introduction
ventilation

Structure and function of the respiratory system
epiglottis, inspiration, expiration, chronic obstructive pulmonary disease (COPD),

Pneumothorax, hemothorax, pleural effusion, diffusion, hemoglobin, erythrocytes, hematocrit, hypoxia, hypercarbia, hypercapnia, eupnea, tachypnea, bradypnea, apnea, hyperventilation, Kussmaul's breathing, dyspnea, shortness of breath (SOB), stridor

Structure and function of the cardiovascular system
atherosclerotic plaque, angina pectoris,

mycardial infarction (MI), anemia, dysrhythmias, atherosclerosis, thrombus, embolus, exacerbations, hypovolemia, hypervolemia

Treatment of oxygenation problems
sputum, electrocardiography, hemoptysis, pulmonary function tests, tracheostomy

Nursing care
suctioning, cardiopulmonary resuscitation

Key Points

- The respiratory system includes pulmonary ventilation (the movement of air between the atmosphere and the lungs) and the diffusion of oxygen and carbon dioxide across the pulmonary membrane.

- The cardiovascular system transports these gases in the blood to the tissues, facilitates the diffusion of gases between the capillaries and body tissues, and carries away waste products from the tissues.

- Ninety-Seven percent of oxygen is carried to the tissues loosely combined with hemoglobin in red blood cells (RBCs). Anemia, which is too few RBCs or low hemoglobin levels, impairs oxygen transportation.

- In most people, respirations are triggered by high carbon dioxide levels. However, people with COPD often have chronically high carbon dioxide levels, and their respirations are triggered by low oxygen (hypoxia). If they are given high levels of oxygen, they may stop breathing.

- Normal respirations are quiet and unlabored; altered respiratory patterns include tachypnea, bradypnea, hyperventilation, hypoventilation, and dyspnea. Shortness of breath is a subjective sensation of not getting enough air.

- A low-pitched snoring sound, stridor, and abnormal breath sounds may accompany partial airway obstruction.

EXPLORE MediaLink

Additional interactive resources for this chapter can be found on the Companion Website at www.prenhall.com/ramont. Click on Chapter 16 and "Begin" to select the activities for this chapter.

For chapter-related NCLEX-style questions and an audio glossary, access the accompanying CD-ROM in this book.

For Further Study

For further information regarding performing CPR, see Chapter 6.

For more illustrations of the circulatory and respiratory systems, see Figures 10-10 and 10-12.

For additional information about assessment of the respiratory system, see Chapter 11; for clubbing, see Figure 11-4D.

For more information about respiratory patterns and measuring blood pressure, see Box 14-6, and Chapter 14.

For steps in applying antiembolism stockings to clients, see Procedure 22-2.

For additional information about preventing venous stasis, see Chapter 20.

For more information on NANDA diagnoses, see Appendix I.

Critical Thinking Care Map

Caring for a Client with Pneumonia

NCLEX-PN Focus Area: Physiological Adaptation

Case Study: Johti Singh is a 39-year-old secretary who was admitted to the hospital with an elevated temperature, fatigue, and rapid labored respirations. Nursing history reveals that Ms. Singh has had a "bad cold" for several weeks that just wouldn't go away. She has been dieting for several months and skipping meals. In addition to her full-time job, she is attending college. She has smoked one pack of cigarettes per day since she was 18 years old. Chest x-ray confirms pneumonia.

Nursing Diagnosis: Ineffective Airway Clearance

COLLECT DATA

Subjective

_____
_____
_____
_____
_____

Objective

_____
_____
_____
_____
_____

Would you report this data? Yes/No

If yes, to: _____

Nursing Care

_____

How would you document this? _____

Data Collected
(use those that apply)

- Height 5'6"
- Weight 120 lbs
- VS: T-103 P-82 R-24 BP 118/70
- Skin pale; cheeks flushed; chills; nasal flaring; use of accessory muscles; inspiratory crackles with diminished breath sounds right base; thick, yellow sputum
- Chest x-ray: right lobar infiltration
- WBC 14,000
- pH 7.48
- $PaCO_2$: 33 mm Hg
- HCO_3: 20 mEq/L
- $PaCo_2$: 80 mm Hg

Nursing Interventions
(use those that apply)

- Assist Ms. Singh to a sitting position with head slightly flexed.
- Determine healthy body weight for age and height.
- Administer antipyretic medication for client comfort.
- Encourage client to relax the shoulders and flex the knees.
- Assess pain at least every 2 to 3 hours and administer analgesics as ordered.
- Provide written information as requested.
- Monitor intake, output, and daily weight.
- Arrange for dietary consult to determine calorie needs.
- Encourage her to take several deep breaths.
- Encourage her to take a deep breath, hold for 2 seconds, and cough two or three times in succession.
- Encourage use of incentive spirometry, as appropriate.
- Monitor rate, rhythm, depth, and effort of respirations.
- Auscultate breath sounds, noting area of decreased or absent ventilations and presence of adventitious sounds.
- Monitor respiratory secretions.
- Monitor increased restlessness, anxiety, and air hunger.

NCLEX-PN Exam Preparation

1. Your client is on strict bed rest. Which position facilitates the greatest expansion of the lungs?
   a. Trendelenburg
   b. Low-Fowler's
   c. Sims'
   d. High-Fowler's

2. A breathing pattern in which respirations increase and decrease in rate and depth with periods of apnea is known as:
   a. Kussmaul's
   b. Tachypnea
   c. Cheyne–Stokes
   d. Eupnea

3. Which of the following data will receive highest priority when assessing your 33-year-old client with pneumonia?
   a. Size of pupils, presence of sneezing, location of pain
   b. Presence of hiccups, amount of sweating, BP
   c. Capillary refill, amount of sputum, trembling
   d. Restlessness, chest wall movement, color of nails

4. A client is experiencing an asthma attack. Which of the following outcomes will receive the highest priority in the care of this client?
   a. The client will report a decrease in his anxiety level.
   b. The client will maintain an open airway with adequate gas exchange.
   c. The client will talk about how he feels about his disease.
   d. The client will maintain adequate fluid balance.

5. A client with emphysema has severe difficulty breathing and orthopnea. Orthopnea means that the client:
   a. Is in respiratory distress
   b. Has blood gases that indicate respiratory acidosis
   c. Has periods of apnea
   d. Has difficulty breathing unless he is sitting upright

6. Uses of a tracheostomy tube include:
   a. Promotion of nutrition
   b. Relief of flatus
   c. Achievement of an artificial airway
   d. Increasing dead space

7. An 87-year-old client with pneumonia has just been admitted. Which of the following assessments takes first priority?
   a. Rapid, irregular respiration of 32/min
   b. Skin warm, flushed, and dry
   c. Temperature of 99.4°F (37.4°C)
   d. Dry, nonproductive cough

8. Your client with pneumonia presents with dyspnea. This means:
   a. Respirations are shallow
   b. The client is breathing very rapidly
   c. The client cannot breathe in a supine position
   d. Breathing has become difficult and labored

9. The physician has ordered O_2 via nasal cannula at 3 L/min. Safety precautions when oxygen is in use include:
   a. Making sure that the room is well ventilated
   b. Placing "No Smoking" signs in prominent places in the client's room
   c. Keeping the flow rate < 4 L/min to prevent toxicity
   d. Avoiding use of any lotion for skin care

10. With early signs of hypoxia, the nurse would expect to assess a client with emphysema for:
    a. Dyspnea, neurologic changes, hypertension, diminished breath sounds
    b. Increased rate and depth of respirations, changes in behavior, decreased judgment, drowsiness
    c. Orthopnea, use of accessory muscles to breathe, cyanosis of nailbeds
    d. Labored breathing, crowing respirations, inspiratory wheezing

Answers for Review Questions, as well as discussion of Case Study and Critical Thinking Care Map questions, appear in Appendix IV.

Nutrition, Fluids and Electrolytes, and Acid–Base Balance

Chapter

17

SHARING experiences

I am from Liberia, West Africa. There was a very devastating civil war that went on for twelve years. It has ceased now, but infections in hospitals are very high because of the very many unsterile techniques used. There is also a shortage of nurses. Therefore, I told myself that becoming a nurse in the United States and learning the different ways of infection control, I could one day go back home and make a difference in my people's lives.

Margaret Kamara, LPN student, Idaho State University, Pocatello, ID.

LEARNING outcomes

After completing this chapter, you will be able to:
- Identify essential nutrients and the dietary sources of each.
- Describe normal digestion, absorption, and metabolism of carbohydrates, proteins, and fats.
- Explain essential aspects of energy balance.
- Discuss body weight and body mass standards.
- Identify developmental nutritional considerations.
- Describe nursing interventions to promote nutrition.
- Discuss the function, distribution, and regulation of fluids and electrolytes in the body.
- Identify factors affecting normal body fluids, electrolytes, and acid–base balance.
- Teach clients measures to maintain fluid and electrolyte balances.
- Identify nursing responsiblities in IV therapy.
- Identify nursing interventions for clients with acid-base disorders.

As health care providers, we work toward the goal that all people want to feel well, to enjoy good health. An essential part of this feeling of good health is to obtain the optimum nutrient supply for the body that is available. This chapter will introduce you to principles of nutrition, fluid and electrolyte balance, IV therapy, and other factors necessary for you to know, so that you can assist others in experiencing adequate nutrition.

Nutrition

MediaLink ● Digestive System Dissection and Tour

Nutrients

Nutrients are the organic, inorganic, and energy-producing substances found in foods. These nutrients are required for body functioning. The result of this interaction between nutrients and the human body is **nutrition.** Specific nutrients in food allow growth, maintenance of all body tissues, and normal functioning of all body processes.

Nutrients have three major functions. They provide energy for body processes and movement. They provide structural material for body tissues. They regulate body processes. When a person's food intake is adequate, there is a balance of these essential nutrients:

◆ Water
◆ Macronutrients: carbohydrates, proteins, and fats
◆ Micronutrients: vitamins and minerals

WATER

The body's most basic nutrient need is water. Water is vital to health and normal cellular function, serving as:

◆ A medium for metabolic reactions within cells
◆ A transporter for nutrients, waste products, and other substances
◆ A lubricant
◆ An insulator and shock absorber
◆ A means of regulating and maintaining body temperature

Age, body fat, and gender affect total body water. Infants have 70 to 80 percent of their body weight in water. The proportion of body water decreases with aging; in people over age 60, it is less than half of body weight. Fat tissue is essentially free of water; lean tissue contains a significant amount of water. So, water makes up a greater percentage of a lean person's body weight than an obese person's. Women have proportionally more body fat than men, and so have a lower percentage of body water.

MACRONUTRIENTS

Macronutrients provide fuel that converts to energy. These nutrients are found in carbohydrates, proteins, and fats.

Carbohydrates

Carbohydrates are composed of the elements carbon (C), hydrogen (H), and oxygen (O). There are two basic kinds: simple carbohydrates (sugars) and complex carbohydrates (starches and fiber).

Sugars, the simplest of all carbohydrates, are water soluble. Both plants and animals produce sugars. (Lactose is a sugar formed by combining glucose and galactose and is found in milk.) However, sugars are mostly produced naturally by plants, especially fruits, sugar cane, and sugar beets. Processed or refined sugars (e.g., table sugar, molasses, and corn syrup) are those that have been extracted and concentrated from natural sources. Processed sugars are added to foods such as soft drinks, cookies, candy, ice cream, and some cereals.

Starches are *insoluble* (they do not dissolve in water). Starches are nonsweet forms of carbohydrate. Like sugars, nearly all starches exist naturally in plants, such as grains, legumes, and potatoes. Starches are in foods such as cereals, breads, flour, and puddings.

Fiber is a complex carbohydrate derived from plants. It cannot be digested by humans but supplies roughage, or bulk, to the diet. This bulk satisfies the appetite and also helps the digestive tract to eliminate wastes.

It is important that carbohydrate intake include natural as well as processed foods. Natural sources of carbohydrates supply protein, vitamins, minerals, and dietary fiber; these are often missing in processed foods. Because processed carbohydrate foods are relatively low in nutrients and high in calories, they are often referred to as "empty calories."

The end products of carbohydrate digestion are monosaccharides (glucose, fructose, and galactose). Some simple sugars, therefore, require no digestion. After the body breaks carbohydrates down into glucose, some glucose continues to circulate in the blood to maintain blood glucose levels and to provide a readily available source of energy. The remainder is either used as energy or stored. In healthy persons, essentially all digested carbohydrate is absorbed by the small intestine (see Figure 10-13). ∞

Insulin, a hormone secreted by the pancreas, is needed for glucose to be transported into the cells. So, the body's use of glucose is controlled by the pancreas's ability to produce insulin. When the pancreas is unable to produce insulin, or to produce enough insulin, the resulting condition is diabetes mellitus. Diabetes can negatively affect almost every body system.

Digested carbohydrates are maintained either as **glycogen** (the stored form of glucose) or as fat. The process of glycogen formation is called *glycogenesis.* All body cells are capable of storing glycogen; however, most glycogen is stored in the liver and skeletal muscles. Glycogen can be converted back to glucose when needed to maintain blood levels or to provide energy. Glucose that cannot be stored as glycogen is converted to fat.

Proteins

Proteins are organic substances composed of amino acids. Like carbohydrates, proteins contain carbon, hydrogen, and oxygen, but proteins also contain nitrogen. **Amino acids,** the building blocks of proteins, are categorized as essential or nonessential. *Essential amino acids* are those that cannot be manufactured in the body and must be supplied by ingesting protein. *Nonessential amino acids* are those that the body can manufacture. The body takes apart amino acids from food and reconstructs new ones from their basic elements (carbohydrates and nitrogen). See also Chapter 12. ⚭

Proteins may be complete or incomplete. *Complete proteins* contain all of the essential amino acids plus many nonessential ones. Most animal proteins, including meats, poultry, fish, dairy products, and eggs, are complete proteins. *Incomplete proteins* lack one or more essential amino acids and are usually derived from vegetables. When an appropriate mixture of plant proteins is provided in the diet, a balance of essential amino acids can be achieved. For example, a combination of corn and beans is a complete protein. Specific combinations of two or more vegetables are called *complementary proteins.* Most protein is digested in the small intestine, where enzymes break it down into the end products of protein digestion, amino acids.

Amino acids are transported to the liver, where some are used to synthesize specific proteins such as albumin, globulin, and fibrinogen. Amino acids are also used to make protein for cell structures. In a sense, protein is "stored" as body tissue. The body cannot actually store excess amino acids for future use. However, a limited amount is available in the "metabolic pool" that exists as a result of the constant breakdown and buildup of the protein in body tissues.

Protein metabolism includes three activities: **anabolism** (building tissue), **catabolism** (breaking down tissue), and **nitrogen balance.** Because nitrogen is the element that distinguishes protein from lipids and carbohydrates, nitrogen balance reflects the status of protein nutrition in the body. Nitrogen balance is a measure of the intake and loss of nitrogen. When nitrogen intake equals nitrogen output, a state of nitrogen balance exists.

Lipids

Lipids are organic substances that are greasy and insoluble in water but soluble in alcohol or ether. *Fats* are lipids that are solid at room temperature; *oils* are lipids that are liquid at room temperature. In common use, the terms *fats* and *lipids* are used interchangeably. Lipids have the same elements (carbon, hydrogen, and oxygen) as carbohydrates, but they contain a higher proportion of hydrogen. Fatty acids, made up of carbon chains and hydrogen, are the basic structural units of most lipids. Based on their chemical structure, lipids are classified as simple or compound. Glycerides, the simple lipids, are the most common form of lipids. **Triglycerides** (which have three fatty acids) account for over 90 percent of the lipids in food and in the body. Triglycerides may be saturated or unsaturated. *Saturated triglycerides* are found in animal products, such as butter, and are usually solid at room temperature. The hardness of the fat at room temperature indicates the amount of saturated fats present, harder fats such as beef tallow are more saturated than chicken fat, a softer fat. These saturated fats contribute to elevated blood cholesterol in humans and are considered detrimental to health. *Unsaturated triglycerides* are usually liquid at room temperature and are found in plant products, such as olive oil and corn oil. The unsaturated fats do not elevate but lower the blood cholesterol. Fish and low-fat foods would be included in selecting a diet with unsaturated fats. Knowing how to select fats that are less saturated can reduce the risk of heart disease. Cholesterol is a fatlike substance that is both produced by the body and found in foods of animal origin. Most of the body's cholesterol is synthesized in the liver. However, some is absorbed from animal fats in the diet (e.g., from milk, egg yolk, and organ meats). Cholesterol is needed by the body to form bile acids and for the synthesis of steroid hormones. Cholesterol is also the primary lipid connected to heart disease. Testing for cholesterol levels is done to identify people at risk for developing coronary vessel disease. Lipids are digested mainly in the small intestine, where they are broken down to glycerol, fatty acids, and cholesterol. These are immediately reassembled inside the intestinal cells into triglycerides and cholesterol esters (cholesterol with a fatty acid attached to it), which are not water soluble. For these reassembled products to be transported and used, the small intestine and the liver must convert them into soluble compounds called lipoproteins. Lipoproteins are made up of various lipids and a protein. One of the roles of lipoproteins is to carry the cholesterol throughout the body. Cholesterol testing is ordered through *lipid profiles,* which test for lipoproteins and triglycerides. It is desirable to have a higher HDL (high-density lipoprotein) level and a lower LDL (low-density lipoprotein) level, because the risk of heart disease is greater when LDL is elevated. The LDL can be increased by the amount of saturated fats a person consumes.

MICRONUTRIENTS

Vitamins

A **vitamin** is an organic compound that cannot be manufactured by the body and is needed in small quantities to *catalyze* (or trigger) metabolic processes. Thus, when vitamins are lacking in the diet, metabolic deficits result. Vitamins are generally classified as fat soluble or water soluble. *Water-soluble vitamins* include C (ascorbic acid) and the B-complex vitamins: B_1 (thiamine), B_2 (riboflavin), B_3 (niacin or nicotinic acid), B_6 (pyridoxine), B_9 (folic acid), B_{12} (cobalamin), pantothenic acid, and biotin. The body cannot store water-soluble vitamins, so people must get a daily supply in the diet. Water-soluble vitamins can be affected by food processing, storage, and preparation. Vitamin content is highest in fresh foods that are consumed as soon as possible after harvest.

Fat-soluble vitamins include A, D, E, and K. The body can store these vitamins, though vitamins E and K can be stored only in limited amounts. Therefore, a daily supply of fat-soluble vitamins is not absolutely necessary.

Minerals

There are two categories of minerals. *Macrominerals* are those that people require daily in amounts over 100 mg. They include calcium, phosphorus, sodium, potassium, magnesium, chloride, and sulfur. *Microminerals* are those that people require daily in amounts less than 100 mg. They include iron, zinc, manganese, iodine, fluoride, copper, cobalt, chromium, and selenium. Both microminerals and macrominerals are found in vegetables, fruits, whole grains, and meats.

Nutritional needs are greatly affected by a person's age. Specific needs for macro- and micronutrients vary throughout the life span. Calorie requirements also rise and fall depending on the stage of life.

STANDARDS FOR A HEALTHY DIET

Various daily food guides have been developed to help healthy people meet the daily requirements of essential nutrients and to facilitate meal planning. Food group plans emphasize the gen-

eral types or groups of foods rather than the specific foods, because related foods are similar in composition and often have similar nutrient values. For example, all grains, whether wheat or oats, are significant sources of carbohydrates, iron, and the B vitamin thiamine. The Food Guide Pyramid (Figure 17-1 ◆) was developed by the U.S. Department of Agriculture as a graphic aid in making daily food choices. It divides foods into five groups of different sizes. Foods needed in the largest amounts (i.e., whole grains, cereal, rice, and pasta) appear in the largest block. Beside each block is the recommended number of daily servings. These are listed as ranges for meeting nutrient needs because individuals differ in size and activity level and therefore need different amounts of food. The USDA suggests that people eat a variety of whole foods to obtain the nutrients they need.

Energy Balance

Energy balance is the relationship between the energy obtained from food and the energy used by the body. The body gets energy in the form of **calories** (units of heat energy) from carbohydrates, protein, fat, and alcohol. The body uses energy for voluntary activities (like walking) and for involuntary activities (like breathing and growing). A person's energy balance is determined by comparing energy intake with energy output. See also Chapters 7 and 14. ☜

Metabolism is the term for all the biochemical and physiologic processes by which the body grows and maintains itself. The basal metabolic rate (BMR) is the rate at which the body metabolizes food to maintain the energy requirements of a person who is awake and at rest. Lean, active people have a higher BMR than overweight and inactive people. In other words, they burn calories faster even when at rest.

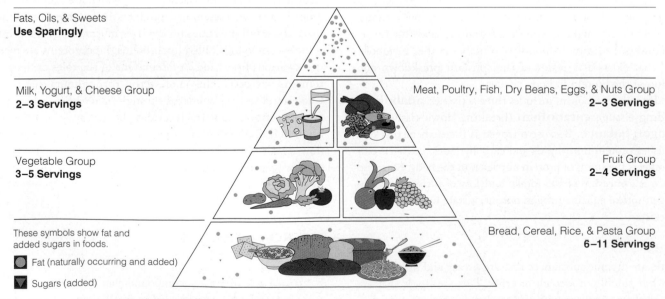

Figure 17-1. ◆ The Food Guide Pyramid. This pyramid is in process of revision. *Source:* U.S. Department of Agriculture. http://www.nal.usda.gov. June 2003.

NURSING CARE

 ASSESSING

Size and weight are factors we notice almost without thinking. If a client is very thin or very heavy, this will be one of the first things the nurse observes. The nurse collects data about the client's height and weight. The nurse selects the appropriate type of scale to be used (Figures 17-2 ◆ and 17-3 ◆). Box 17-1 ◆ provides guidelines about how to obtain a client's weight.

Ideal body weight (IBW) is the weight recommended for optimal health. A person is said to be overweight when body weight exceeds IBW by up to 20 percent. A person is said to be obese when body weight exceeds IBW by more than 20 percent. Standardized tables can provide approximate ideal weights, but they are not precise.

For people over 18 years old, the body mass index (BMI) may be a better indicator of whether a person's weight is appropriate for height. The BMI also may provide a useful estimate of malnutrition. However, the results must be used with caution in people who have fluid retention (e.g., ascites or edema).

To calculate an individual's BMI use this formula:

1. Measure the person's height in meters (1 meter = 3.3 ft, or 39.6 in). Divide number of inches by 39.6 to find height in meters.
2. Measure the weight in kilograms (1 kg = 2.2 pounds). Divide number of pounds by 2.2 to find the weight in kilograms.
3. Calculate the BMI using the following formula:

$$BMI = \frac{\text{Weight in kilograms}}{(\text{Height in meters})^2}$$

A Standing balance scale   **B** Mechanical lift scale   **C** Wheelchair platform scale

D

Figure 17-2. ◆ Types of scales: **A.** Standing balance scale. **B.** Mechanical lift scale. **C.** Wheelchair platform scale. **D.** Neonate balance scale.

A

B

Figure 17-3. ◆ Weighing the client. **A.** Client on standing balance scale. **B.** Client on bed scale.

4. Use the BMI number as follows: < 16, malnourished; 16–19, underweight; 20–25, normal; 26–30, overweight; 31–40, moderately to severely obese; and > 40, morbidly obese.

Problems of weight are among the most common health problems of adults. A person is said to be overweight when body weight exceeds IBW by 1 to 20 percent. **Obesity** is the term used when body weight exceeds IBW by more than 20 percent. Excess body weight causes stress on body organs and contributes to chronic health problems such as hypertension and diabetes mellitus. Morbid obesity is obesity that interferes

BOX 17-1
NURSING CARE CHECKLIST

OBTAINING A CLIENT'S WEIGHT

Adult Client

If client is able to stand

☑ Take measurement at the same time each day.
☑ Have the client wear the same kind and amount of clothing each day, and no shoes.
☑ Have client stand on the weighing platform while the nurse reads and records the weight (see Figure 17-3A).

If client cannot stand

☑ Weigh the client on a chair scale, *or*
☑ Weigh the client with a bed scale (canvas straps lift the client, and weight is recorded on a digital display or balance arm [see Figure 17-3B]).

Pediatric Client

☑ Lay neonates flat on the balance (see Figure 17-2D).
☑ Weigh infants without any clothing.
☑ Weigh young children in their underwear.

with mobility or breathing. Obese people may lack important nutrients even though they are eating excess calories.

Undernutrition means that nutrient intake is insufficient to meet daily energy requirements. It can occur because the person does not eat enough food, or because he or she cannot digest or absorb food. Risk factors for undernutrition are listed in Box 17-2 ◆.

Protein–calorie malnutrition (PCM), once associated mostly with the starving children of third-world countries, is now recognized as a significant problem of clients with cancer and chronic disease. Characteristics of PCM are weight loss and visible muscle and fat wasting.

◆ DIAGNOSING, PLANNING, and IMPLEMENTING

The most frequent nursing diagnoses related to nutrition are Imbalanced Nutrition: More than Body Requirements, Imbalanced Nutrition: Less than Body Requirements, and Risk for Imbalanced Nutrition. Nursing care of clients with imbalanced nutrition includes assisting with changes in diet, stimulating appetite, assisting with meals, monitoring blood glucose, and providing enteral nutrition.

Providing Therapeutic Diets

Alterations in the client's diet are often needed to treat a disease process such as diabetes mellitus, to prepare for a special examination or surgery, to increase or decrease weight, to

BOX 17-2
RISK FACTORS FOR UNDERNUTRITION

◆ Too few calories consumed
◆ Inability to digest or absorb food
◆ Inadequate production of hormones or enzymes
◆ Medical condition resulting in inflammation or obstruction of the gastrointestinal tract
◆ Inability to acquire and prepare food
◆ Lack of knowledge about essential nutrients and a balanced diet
◆ Discomfort during or after eating
◆ Dysphagia (difficulty swallowing)
◆ Nausea or vomiting
◆ Anorexia or bulimia

restore nutritional deficits, or to allow an organ to rest and promote healing. Diets may be modified in texture, calories, specific nutrients, seasonings, or consistency.

Clients who do not have special needs eat the *regular* (*standard* or *house*) *diet*. The house diet is a balanced diet that supplies the metabolic requirements of a sedentary person (about 2,000 kcal). Most agencies offer clients a daily menu from which to select their meals for the next day. Others provide standard meals to each client on the general diet. A variation of the regular diet is the *light diet,* designed for postoperative and other clients who are not ready for the regular diet. Foods in the light diet are plainly cooked; fat, bran, and high-fiber foods are usually omitted. Not all agencies provide a light diet.

Diets that are modified in consistency are often given to clients before and after surgery or to promote healing in clients with gastrointestinal distress. These diets include nothing by mouth (NPO, from the Latin *nil per os*), clear liquid, full liquid, soft, and diet as tolerated.

NPO or Nothing by Mouth.
On this diet, food and fluid are prohibited. This may be ordered before anesthesia or after surgery until bowel sounds return. IV fluids are often provided while a client is NPO to prevent dehydration. If a prolonged NPO diet is required, IV nutrition (TPN) is usually ordered.

Clear Liquid Diet.
This diet is limited to water, tea, coffee, clear broths, ginger ale or other carbonated beverages, strained and clear juices, and plain gelatin. This diet provides the client with fluid and carbohydrate (in the form of sugar) but does not supply adequate protein, fat, vitamins, minerals, or calories (no more than 600 kcal/day). It is a short-term diet (24 to 36 hours) provided for clients after certain types of surgery or when infection occurs in the gastrointestinal system. The major objectives of this diet are to relieve thirst, prevent dehydration, and minimize stimulation of the gastrointestinal tract.

Full Liquid Diet.
This diet contains only liquids or foods that turn to liquid at body temperature, such as ice cream. Full liquid diets are often eaten by clients who have gastrointestinal disturbances or are otherwise unable to tolerate solid or semisolid foods. This diet is not recommended for long-term use because it is low in iron, protein, and calories. In addition, its cholesterol content is high because of the amount of milk offered. If a client is on this diet for long periods, a nutritionally balanced oral supplement, such as Ensure, is usually ordered. Six or more feedings per day may work best for the client who must stay on this diet for a long period.

Soft Diet.
The soft diet is easily chewed and digested. It is often ordered for clients who have difficulty chewing and swallowing. It is a *low-residue* (low-fiber) diet with very few uncooked foods. The pureed diet is a modification of the soft diet. Liquid may be added to the food, which is then blended to a semisolid consistency.

Diet as Tolerated.
Diet as tolerated is ordered when the client's appetite, ability to eat, and tolerance for certain foods change. For example, on the first postoperative day a client may be given a clear liquid diet. If no nausea occurs, normal intestinal motility has returned, and the client feels like eating, the diet may be advanced to a full liquid, light, or regular diet.

Modification for Disease.
Many special diets may be prescribed to meet requirements for disease processes or altered metabolism. For example, a client with diabetes mellitus may need a diabetic diet recommended by the National Diabetic Association. An obese client may need a calorie-restricted diet. A cardiac client may need sodium and cholesterol restrictions. A client with allergies would need a nonallergenic diet. A client with diabetes would need a carbohydrate-controlled diet. Some clients must follow certain diets (e.g., the diabetic diet) for a lifetime. If the diet is long term, the client must not only understand the diet but also develop a healthy, positive attitude toward it. All dietary instructions must be individually designed to meet the client's intellectual ability, motivation level, lifestyle, culture, and economic status.

Monitoring Blood Glucose

Clients who have diabetes may need to monitor random blood glucose levels throughout the day. This can be accomplished in the home setting by the client or family member, as well as by persons formally trained in medical care. By testing a single drop of blood, the client can receive a reading of the blood glucose present at the moment. Clients who understand the significance of this reading will be more likely to participate successfully in their therapeutic diet for an optimum management of their diabetes. Procedure 17-1 describes the procedure for monitoring blood glucose.

Stimulating the Appetite

Physical illness, unfamiliar or unpalatable food, environmental and psychological factors, and physical discomfort or pain may depress a client's appetite. A short-term decrease in food intake usually is not a problem for adults. However, over time, it leads to weight loss, decreased strength and stamina, and other nutritional problems. A decreased food intake is often accompanied by a decrease in fluid intake, which may cause dehydration. The nurse must determine the reason for a client's lack of appetite and then take steps to intervene. Reducing unpleasant odors, positioning the client comfortably, and sometimes cooling the room slightly are interventions that may help stimulate appetite.

Assisting Clients with Meals

Certain groups of people frequently require help with their meals. These groups include older adults who are infirm; the physically impaired, such as blind clients; those who must remain in a back-lying position; and those who cannot use their hands.

When feeding a client, ask in which order the client would like to eat the food. If the client cannot see, tell the client which food is being given. Always allow ample time for the client to chew and swallow the food before offering more. Also, provide fluids as requested. If the client is unable to communicate, offer fluids after every three or four mouthfuls of solid food. It is important to make the time a pleasant one, choosing topics of conversation that are of interest to clients who want to talk.

Although normal utensils should be used whenever possible, special utensils may be needed to assist a client to eat. Many adaptive feeding aids are available to help clients maintain independence. A standard eating utensil with a built-up or widened handle helps clients who cannot grasp objects easily. Plates with rims and plastic or metal plate guards enable the client to pick up the food by first pushing it against this raised edge. A suction cup or damp sponge or cloth may be placed under the dish to keep it from moving while the client is eating. No-spill mugs and two-handled drinking cups are especially useful for persons with impaired hand coordination. Stretch terry cloth and knitted or crocheted glass covers enable the client to keep a secure grasp on a glass. Lidded tip-proof glasses are also available. Clients are more likely to participate in mealtime if their meal is set up for them as needed. The nursing staff may need to open packages and cartons to make the food accessible. Meat may need to be cut, a sugar packet opened, or tea bags placed in the hot water. These simple preparations encourage the client to begin eating. They also give a few moments for the nurse and client to engage in pleasant conversation, another stimulant for eating.

Providing Enteral Nutrition

Two types of alternative feeding methods are **enteral nutrition** (through the gastrointestinal system) and **parenteral nutrition** (intravenous) methods. Enteral nutrition (EN), also referred to as total enteral nutrition (TEN), is provided when the client is unable to ingest or absorb foods.

Enteral Access Devices. Enteral access is achieved by nasogastric or nasointestinal tubes, or gastrostomy or jejunostomy tubes.

A nasogastric tube is inserted through one of the nostrils, down the nasopharynx, and into the stomach or small intestine. Traditional *nasogastric tubes* are firm and larger than 12 Fr in diameter. They are passed through the nose and pharynx to the stomach. An example is the Levin tube, a flexible rubber or plastic, single-lumen tube with holes near the tip. The commonly used Salem Sump tube has two lumens, the smaller of the two for air entry to reduce the risk of a vacuum forming should the tube affix itself to the mucosal lining of the stomach. Softer tubes that are more flexible and smaller than 12 Fr in diameter are frequently used for TEN.

Nasogastric tubes are used for clients who have intact gag and cough reflexes, who have adequate gastric emptying, and who require short-term feedings. Procedure 17-2 provides guidelines for inserting and removing a nasogastric tube.

Nasogastric tubes may be inserted for reasons other than providing a route for feeding the client. These include:

◆ To prevent nausea, vomiting, and gastric distention following surgery. In this case, the tube is attached to a suction source.
◆ To remove stomach contents for laboratory analysis.
◆ To *lavage* (wash) the stomach in cases of poisoning or overdose of medications.

A *nasoenteric tube* is a longer tube than the nasogastric tube (at least 40 inches for an adult). It is inserted into one nostril and through the pharynx, esophagus, and stomach into the upper small intestine. Some agencies may require that specially trained nurses or physicians do this procedure. Nasoenteric tubes are used when risk for aspiration is high. Clients are at risk for aspiration if any of the following exist:

◆ Decreased level of consciousness
◆ Poor cough or gag reflexes
◆ Endotracheal intubation
◆ Recent extubation
◆ Inability to cooperate with the procedure
◆ Restlessness or agitation

Gastrostomy and *jejunostomy devices* are used for long-term nutritional support, generally more than 6 to 8 weeks. Conventional tubes may be placed surgically or by laparoscopy through the abdominal wall into the stomach (**gastrostomy**) or into the jejunum (**jejunostomy**). More commonly, though, the percutaneous endoscopic gastrostomy (PEG) is used.

Testing Feeding Tube Placement. Before feedings are introduced, tube placement is confirmed by radiography, particularly when a small-bore tube has been inserted or when the client is at risk for aspiration. After placement is confirmed, the nurse marks the tube with indelible ink or tape at its exit point from the nose and documents the length of visible tubing for baseline data.

clinical ALERT

> If a feeding tube accidentally becomes dislodged, formula could go into the lungs, causing aspiration or even death. Therefore, the nurse must verify that the tube is in the stomach before each intermittent feeding. In the case of continuous feedings, the nurse checks placement at least once per shift and before administering any medications through the tube.

Box 17-3 ◆ lists items for the nurse to check prior to tube feeding.

Enteral Feedings. The frequency of feedings and amounts to be administered are ordered by the physician. Liquid feeding mixtures are available commercially, for example, Ensure, Osmolite, or Jevity. Enteral feedings may be ordered as intermittent or continuous. An **intermittent feeding** is the administration of 300 to 500 mL of enteral formula several times per day. These feedings are usually administered through the tube into the stomach over at least 30 minutes. **Continuous feedings** are generally administered over a 24-hour period using an infusion pump that guarantees a constant flow. Continuous feedings are essential when feedings are administered in the small bowel. *Cyclic feedings* are continuous feedings that are administered in less than 24 hours (e.g., 12 to 16 hours). These feedings, often administered at night and referred to as nocturnal feedings, allow the client to attempt to eat regular meals through the day. Because nocturnal feedings may use higher nutrient densities and higher infusion rates than the standard continuous feeding, the client should be assessed for fluid volume excess.

Procedure 17-3 provides the essential steps for administering a tube feeding, and for administering and evaluating a gastrostomy or jejunostomy tube feeding.

Before administering a tube feeding, the nurse must check for any food allergies and assess tolerance to previous feedings. The nurse must also check the expiration date on a commercially prepared formula or the preparation date and time of agency-prepared solution. Any formula that has passed the expiration date or solution that has been at room temperature for more than 8 hours must be discarded.

 EVALUATING

To evaluate the client with imbalanced nutrition, the nurse would compare baseline weight with current data and determine the client's compliance with the recommended diet. Goals for activity would be assessed. The client's support system and sense of satisfaction with changes in weight would be reviewed. If necessary, plans and goals would be adjusted.

DISCHARGE CONSIDERATIONS

The nurse must be an educator in helping clients with nutritional imbalances. Positive effects of changes in diet must be emphasized. Negative effects of continued imbalances must also be addressed. Every effort must be made to have the client participate in the planned changes, because food choice is a central part of people's lifestyles. Discuss with the client what goals they have in mind, and point out how their therapeutic diet will help them reach those goals. If clients are involved and empowered, believing that they can make a difference, their chances for success are much improved. It is important to assess the support of family and friends available to the client.

Nursing Process Case Study: CLIENT WITH ALTERED NUTRITION

Andrea Brown is a 20-year-old single woman who has been diagnosed as having anorexia. She is underweight, 22% less than IBW, and weak. Despite her declining weight, she continues to make comments about being overweight such as, "I am still too fat for my body build. I have no control over my life no matter what I do." Her hair appears to be thinning and there are dark circles under her eyes. Upon collecting the meal tray one afternoon, the nurse notices that no food has been touched, and the client has requested soda crackers to go with her diet soda. Upon questioning, Ms. Brown states that she has had plenty to eat and is not hungry.

> ### BOX 17-3
> ### NURSING CARE CHECKLIST
>
> #### VERIFYING TUBE PLACEMENT FOR ENTERAL FEEDINGS
>
> ☑ Aspirate 20 to 30 mL of gastrointestinal secretions. *Note:* Small-bore tubes offer more resistance during aspirations than large-bore tubes and are more likely to collapse when negative pressure is applied.
>
> ☑ Measure the pH of aspirated fluid. This is the recommended method to determine tube placement. The pH of gastric fluid is normally 6 or lower, different from the pH of respiratory or intestinal fluids.
>
> ☑ Auscultate the epigastrium while injecting 5 to 20 mL of air. Air injected into the stomach produces whooshing, gurgling, or bubbling sounds over the epigastrium and the upper left quadrant. This method is less reliable than pH testing.
>
> ☑ Ensure initial radiographic verification of small-bore tubes.
>
> ☑ Closely observe the client for signs of obvious distress, and suspect tube dislodgment after episodes of coughing, sneezing, and vomiting.

Assessment. T 98, P 110, R 16, BP 110/74. Documentation of meals shows a poor intake, less than 25%, at each meal since admission. Skin turgor is poor and mucous membranes dry. Lab tests indicate protein is below normal levels.

Diagnosis. The following nursing diagnoses are established for Ms. Brown:

◆ Imbalanced Nutrition, Less than Body Requirements, related to anorexia.
◆ Adult Failure to Thrive related to inadequate nutritive intake.
◆ Risk for Impaired Skin Integrity related to alterations in nutritional state.

Expected Outcomes. The expected outcomes for the plan of care are that Ms. Brown will:

◆ Establish and maintain protein lab levels of normal value.
◆ Participate in psychiatric counseling program on a regular basis.
◆ Demonstrate stable weight without further losses in immediate future.

Planning and Implementation. The following nursing interventions are implemented for Ms. Brown. Assessments are done frequently to monitor her condition.

◆ Monitor weight daily.

◆ Record oral intake each meal.
◆ Dietitian consult to identify daily caloric intake necessary to stabilize weight loss and reach target weight.
◆ If client refuses to eat, notify physician.
◆ Work with health care team members and client to establish goals for weight gain and increased food intake.
◆ Establish an atmosphere of trust with the client.
◆ Request psychiatric consult order. Follow recommendations offered by mental health practitioner.
◆ Monitor skin for redness and breakdown daily during bath.

Evaluation. Although the client agrees to participate in the plan recommended by the health care team, progress is made slowly. Her weight loss is slowed, but continued monitoring and support of the health care team are necessary.

Critical Thinking in the Nursing Process

1. What possible interventions may need to be implemented to address a nutritional and fluid balance for Ms. Brown?
2. What would be the role of the psychiatric clinician when anorexia is demonstrated with physical characteristics?
3. Why would the diagnosis Disturbed Body Image be appropriate for Ms. Brown?

Fluid and Electrolytes, and Acid–Base Balance

In good health, homeostasis is maintained. Homeostasis is a delicate balance between fluids, electrolytes, and acids and bases in the body. Constant internal conditions such as chemistry, temperature, and blood pressure are maintained through homeostasis. Almost every illness has the potential to threaten this balance. Even in normal daily living, high temperatures or vigorous exercise without adequate water and salt intake can disturb homeostasis. Medical interventions such as diuretics or nasogastric suction without replacement of water and electrolytes can also cause fluid and electrolyte imbalances.

 ## Body Fluids and Electrolyte Balance

The body's fluid is divided into two major compartments, intracellular and extracellular. **Intracellular fluid (ICF)** is found within the cells of the body. It accounts for approximately two thirds of the total body fluid in adults and is vital to normal cell functioning. ICF contains oxygen, electrolytes, and glucose. **Extracellular fluid (ECF)** is found outside the cells and accounts for about one third of total body fluid. The ECF is subdivided into three compartments: intravascular, interstitial, and transcellular fluid (Figure 17-4 ◆). Extracellular fluid is the transport system that carries nutrients to, and waste products from, the cells. **Interstitial fluid** (three quarters of the ECF) surrounds the cells and includes lymph. Interstitial fluid transports wastes from the cells by way of the lymph system, as well as directly into the blood plasma through capillaries. Intravascular fluid (or *plasma*) is found within the blood. Transcellular fluid, which some consider to be distinct from intracellular and extracellular fluids, includes cerebrospinal, pleural, peritoneal, and synovial fluids.

COMPOSITION OF BODY FLUIDS

Extracellular and intracellular fluids contain oxygen, nutrients, carbon dioxide, and charged particles (called *ions*). Many salts break up into electrically charged ions when dissolved in water. These charged ions are called **electrolytes** because they are capable of conducting electricity. Ions that carry a

Cell fluid
25 liters

Total body fluid
40 liters

Plasma
3 liters

Interstitial and
Transcellular fluid
12 liters

Extracellular
fluid
15 liters

Figure 17-4. ◆ Total body fluid represents 40 L in adult males weighing 70 kg. Fluid amounts are indicated for different body compartments.

REGULATING BODY FLUIDS

In a healthy person, the volumes and chemical composition of the fluid compartments stay within narrow safe limits. Normally, fluid intake and fluid loss are balanced. Illness can upset this balance so that the body has too little or too much fluid.

Fluid Intake

During periods of moderate activity at moderate temperature, the average adult drinks about 1,500 mL per day but needs 2,500 mL per day, an additional 1,000 mL. This added volume is acquired from foods and as a by-product of food metabolism.

Fluid Output

Fluid losses from the body counterbalance the adult's 2,500-mL average daily intake of fluid. Fluid output occurs through several routes: urine, "insensible losses," and feces.

Urine formed by the kidneys and excreted from the urinary bladder is the major avenue of fluid output. Normal urine output for an adult is 1,400 to 1,500 mL per 24 hours, or at least 30 to 50 mL per hour. In healthy people, urine output may vary noticeably from day to day. Urine volume automatically increases as fluid intake increases. If fluid loss through perspiration is large, however, urine volume decreases to maintain fluid balance in the body.

Insensible losses occur through the skin and through the lungs. They are usually not noticeable and cannot be measured. Insensible fluid loss through the skin occurs in two ways: through diffusion and through perspiration. Water losses through diffusion are not noticeable but normally account for 350 to 400 mL per day. This loss can be significantly increased if the protective layer of the skin is damaged, as with burns or large abrasions. Perspiration varies depending on factors such as environmental temperature and metabolic activity. Fever and exercise increase metabolic activity and heat production, thereby increasing fluid losses through the skin.

Another type of insensible loss is the water in exhaled air. In an adult, this is normally 350 to 400 mL per day. When respiratory rate accelerates (as with exercise or an elevated body temperature), water loss can increase.

Loss through the intestines in feces usually amounts to 100 to 200 mL per day. The digested food that passes from the small intestine into the large intestine contains water and electrolytes. However, most fluid is reabsorbed in the proximal half of the large intestine.

Regulating Electrolytes

Electrolytes are present in all body fluids and fluid compartments. Just as maintaining the fluid balance is vital to normal body function, so is maintaining electrolyte balance. The concentration of specific electrolytes differs between fluid compartments, but a balance of *cations* (positively charged ions) and *anions* (negatively charged ions) should exist. Electrolytes are important for:

◆ Maintaining fluid balance
◆ Contributing to acid–base regulation

positive charge are called *cations*, and ions carrying a negative charge are called *anions*. Examples of cations are sodium, potassium, calcium, and magnesium. Anions include chloride, bicarbonate, phosphate, and sulfate. The composition of fluids varies from one body compartment to another.

In extracellular fluid, the principal electrolytes are sodium, chloride, and bicarbonate. Other electrolytes such as potassium, calcium, and magnesium are present, but in much smaller quantities. Plasma and interstitial fluid, the two primary components of ECF, contain essentially the same electrolytes and solutes, except for protein. Plasma is rich in protein, containing large amounts of albumin; interstitial fluid contains little or no protein.

Intracellular fluid (ICF) has a very different composition from ECF. Potassium and magnesium are the primary cations present in ICF; phosphate and sulfate are the major anions. Other electrolytes are present, but in much smaller concentrations. A balance of fluid volumes and electrolyte compositions in the fluid compartments of the body is essential to health. Normal and unusual fluid and electrolyte losses must be replaced if homeostasis is to be maintained.

Other body fluids, such as gastric and intestinal secretions, also contain electrolytes. When these fluids are lost from the body during severe vomiting, diarrhea, or gastric suctioning, electrolyte imbalance can result.

◆ Facilitating enzyme reactions
◆ Assisting neuromuscular reactions

Most electrolytes enter the body through dietary intake and are excreted in the urine. Some electrolytes, like sodium and chloride, are not stored and must be consumed daily to maintain normal levels. Table 17-1 ◆ lists important electrolytes of the body, their location, sources, and function.

 ## Acid–Base Balance

Body fluids are maintained within a narrow range that is *alkaline* (slightly above 7 on a scale from 0 to 14). The normal pH of arterial blood is between 7.35 and 7.45.

Acids are continually produced during metabolism. Buffers in the digestive tract, the respiratory system, and the renal system work constantly to maintain the narrow pH range necessary for optimal function.

ACID–BASE REGULATORS

Buffer Regulation

Buffers neutralize excess acids or bases. They are the body's first line of defense against acid–base balance changes in the body. The major buffer systems in extracellular fluids are bicarbonate and carbonic acid. As long as a ratio of 20 parts of bicarbonate to 1 part of carbonic acid is maintained, the pH remains within its normal range of 7.35 to 7.45. If bicarbonate is

TABLE 17-1	LOCATION, SOURCES, AND FUNCTION OF SELECTED ELECTROLYTES		
ELECTROLYTE	**LOCATION**	**SOURCES**	**FUNCTION**
Sodium	Extracellular fluid (most abundant cation)	Bacon, ham, processed cheese, table salt	Controls and regulates water balance
Potassium	Intracellular fluid (most abundant cation)	Fruits, vegetables, meat, fish, and other foods	Helps maintain ECF and ICF water balance and acid–base balance; vital for skeletal, cardiac, and smooth muscle activity; supports ICF enzyme reactions
Calcium	Mostly in skeletal system, small amount in ECF	Milk and milk products very high; dark green leafy vegetables, canned salmon	1% of total calcium outside bones and teeth regulates muscle contraction/relaxation, neuromuscular and cardiac function. With aging, less calcium absorbed in intestines and more excreted via kidneys; weight-bearing exercise and vitamin D protect against osteoporosis and fractures
Magnesium	Primarily in skeleton and ICF; only about 1% in ECF	Cereal grains; nuts; dried fruit; legumes; green, leafy vegetables; dairy products; meat; and fish	Aids intracellular metabolism, especially adenosine triphosphate (ATP) production; necessary for protein and DNA synthesis within cells. In ECF helps regulate neuromuscular and cardiac function
Chloride	Major anion of ECF; major component of gastric juice as hydrochloric acid (HCl)	Found in the same foods as sodium	Functions with sodium to regulate serum osmolality and blood volume; concentration in ECF is regulated by sodium; is usually reabsorbed with sodium in the kidney; helps regulate acid–base balance; acts as buffer in the exchange of oxygen and carbon dioxide in red blood cells
Phosphate	Major anion of intracellular fluids; also is found in ECF, bone, skeletal muscle, and nerve tissue. Much higher levels in children, probably due to higher growth hormone	Found in many foods such as meat, fish, poultry, milk products, and legumes	Involved in many chemical actions of the cell; essential for functioning of muscles, nerves, and red blood cells; also involved in protein, fat, and carbohydrate metabolism; absorbed from the intestine
Bicarbonate	ICF and ECF; excreted and reabsorbed by kidneys	Produced in metabolic process so dietary source unnecessary	Major body buffer involved in acid–base regulation

depleted while neutralizing a strong acid, the pH may drop below 7.35, resulting in a condition called *acidosis*. Likewise, if a strong base is added to ECF and depletes carbonic acid, the pH may rise over 7.45, resulting in a condition called *alkalosis*.

Bicarbonate is present in both intracellular and extracellular fluids. Extracellular bicarbonate levels are regulated by the kidneys. The kidneys excrete bicarbonate when too much is present. They regenerate and reabsorb bicarbonate ions if more is needed. Unlike other electrolytes that must be consumed in the diet, adequate amounts of bicarbonate are produced by the body to meet the body's needs.

In addition to the bicarbonate–carbonic acid buffer system, plasma proteins, hemoglobin, and phosphates also function as buffers in body fluids.

Respiratory System Regulation

The lungs help regulate acid–base balance by eliminating or retaining carbon dioxide, a potential acid. When carbon dioxide combines with water, it forms carbonic acid. This chemical reaction is reversible; carbonic acid breaks down into carbon dioxide and water. Working together with the buffer system, the lungs regulate acid–base balance and pH by altering the rate and depth of respirations. The response of the respiratory system to changes in pH is rapid, occurring within minutes.

Carbon dioxide is a powerful stimulator of the respiratory center. When blood levels of carbonic acid and carbon dioxide rise, respiratory center stimulation causes the rate and depth of respirations to increase. By contrast, when bicarbonate levels are excessive, the rate and depth of respirations are reduced.

Renal System Regulation

Although buffers and the respiratory system can compensate for changes in pH, the kidneys provide the primary long-term regulation of acid–base balance. However, their response is slower and more permanent and selective than that of the other systems. The kidneys maintain acid–base balance by selectively excreting or conserving bicarbonate and hydrogen ions. When excess hydrogen ion is present and the pH falls (*acidosis*), the kidneys reabsorb and regenerate bicarbonate and excrete hydrogen ion. When there is excess bicarbonate and a high pH (*alkalosis*), the kidneys excrete bicarbonate and retain hydrogen ions.

 ## Acid–Base Imbalances

When a deficiency occurs in the respiratory process, the acid–base balance is disturbed: The alveoli of the lungs are unable to reduce the carbon dioxide levels. Such a condition can be acute, as in excessive sedation, or chronic, as in chronic pulmonary disease.

RESPIRATORY ACIDOSIS

As carbon dioxide is retained, it creates carbonic acid that builds up in the blood; the pH drops, creating **respiratory**

acidosis. The changes in pH can be confirmed by an arterial blood gas (ABG) test showing a $PaCO_2$ (carbon dioxide measured in arterial blood) level above 45 mm Hg and a pH below 7.35. When the pH falls, hemoglobin is altered to make it give up its oxygen. This altered hemoglobin is alkaline and begins mopping up the excess carbonic acid. Oxygen saturation will drop. The increase in carbonic acid also causes changes in the respiratory center of the brain. Respirations become shallow and may even be ineffective. The client may exhibit headache, nausea and vomiting, and a change in mental status. If respiratory efforts fail to correct the imbalance, the $PaCO_2$ continues to rise. This triggers the kidneys to hold onto bicarbonate and sodium, which combine to form sodium bicarbonate, another buffer to mop up carbonic acid. If these compensatory mechanisms fail to right the imbalance, hydrogen ions move into the cells and force the potassium out. With the potassium now unchecked, the client develops resultant hyperkalemia, heart arrythmias, and a decreasing level of consciousness. The heart may experience such insult as to result in shock and even cardiac arrest. Treatment for respiratory acidosis is aimed at improving respiratory effort, including administration of oxygen.

RESPIRATORY ALKALOSIS

Respiratory alkalosis may develop when the opposite situation, hyperventilation, occurs. By breathing too rapidly, CO_2 (an acid) is blown off, causing a decrease in $PaCO_2$ and an elevated pH. This can occur when pain, anxiety reactions, or fever cause a client to hyperventilate. Arterial blood gases confirm this situation by showing a pH above 7.45 and $PaCO_2$ below 35 mm Hg. As the body defends itself, hydrogen ions leave the cells in exchange for potassium with resulting hypokalemia. The hydrogen ions join with the bicarbonate ions and lower the pH. As the $PaCO_2$ falls, the carotid and aortic bodies in the medulla are stimulated so the heart rate increases, but no change in the blood pressure occurs. There may be electrocardiographic (ECG) changes or chest pain, or the client may become restless and anxious. The blood vessels in the brain respond to the dropping $PaCO_2$ by constricting, reducing blood flow to the brain. The autonomic nervous system becomes overstimulated and the client may exhibit dizziness and numbness/tingling in the fingers or toes. The client could be encouraged to breathe into a paper bag, which increases the level of CO_2 in the blood. After about 6 hours of uncompensated alkalosis, the kidneys pour off the bicarbonate and hold back hydrogen ions. The client may show a decreased respiratory rate and hypoventilation. Eventually, the central nervous system and the heart are overcome by the alkalosis, resulting in a change in level of consciousness, hyper-reflexes, tetany, heart arrhythmias, seizures, and coma.

METABOLIC ACIDOSIS

Metabolic acidosis occurs when the bicarbonate is lost or acid is increased within the plasma. When fatty acids change to ketone bodies, perhaps from diabetes mellitus, starvation, or severe infection, metabolic acidosis may occur. Excessive loss of GI fluids may cause metabolic acidosis, as could renal insufficiency or failure. Arterial blood gases will confirm the imbalance with a pH below 7.35, a low bicarbonate level, and a low $PaCO_2$ level. The first clue is hyperventilation as the respiratory system tries to blow off the acid. Although this will correct the imbalance initially, it will not be enough compensation to correct the metabolic imbalance. Deep and rapid respirations (*Kussmaul's respirations*) may eventually develop. The central nervous system and the heart become depressed. Decreased cardiac function and hypotension may develop. The client develops weakness and headache as the blood vessels in the brain dilate. The client will show a change in the level of consciousness. Diminished muscle tone and deep tendon reflexes may be present. Nausea and vomiting are likely to occur. The kidneys try to correct the imbalance by secreting hydrogen, which combines with ammonia or phosphate and is excreted in the urine. Sodium and bicarbonate are held back by the kidneys to correct the acidosis. Hydrogen goes into the blood, forcing potassium out.

Signs of hyperkalemia may be seen, such as diarrhea, numbness and tingling of fingers or toes, weak or flaccid extremities, slowed heart rate, and ECG changes. The excess hydrogen ions cause further imbalance in the electrolytes, thereby reducing nervous system responses, resulting in central nervous system depression, lethargy, headache, confusion or stupor, and coma. To treat the acidosis the underlying cause must be found. Insulin needs to be given for the diabetic client. Insulin forces the potassium back into the cells, treating the hyperkalemia. A patent IV is necessary for effective reversal of this condition. Position the client to promote ventilation and record intake and output. Assess the level of consciousness frequently and make adaptations in the environment to promote the client's safety should confusion occur. In cases that fail to respond, the nurse should anticipate ventilatory support and possibly dialysis.

METABOLIC ALKALOSIS

Metabolic alkalosis occurs when the plasma loses hydrogen ions (acid) and gains bicarbonate. Arterial blood gases confirm this condition with a $PaCO_2$ greater than 45 mm Hg. The metabolic alkalosis often occurs from diuretics that fail to conserve potassium. Loss of gastric fluids, as in vomiting or NG tube suction, is another primary cause for alkalosis. The excessive bicarbonate ions that do not bind with the chemical buffers depress the vital sign center of the brain, and the client develops a decreased respiratory rate with slow and shallow respirations, thus increasing the $PaCO_2$. The kidneys let go of excess bicarbonate and hold on to the hydrogen ions to correct the imbalance. Sodium is thrown out by the kidneys, and the client shows polyuria followed by hypovolemia and thirst. To compensate for the hydrogen being thrown out by the kidneys, the potassium moves into the cells and the client shows

signs of hypokalemia such as anorexia, weakness, and diminished reflexes. Also in response to hydrogen being thrown out, sodium moves into the nerve cells and overstimulates them. The client shows tetany, irritability, disorientation, and seizures. The underlying condition must be treated to reverse the imbalance. Untreated, the client may develop arrythmias, and death may occur. A patent IV is required to treat this condition. Supplemental oxygen needs to be given when respiratory effort changes or oxygen saturations drop. NG suctioning should be discontinued, and nausea and vomiting treated with antiemetics. Seizure precautions need to be taken for client protection. As a precaution against this condition, NG tubes should be irrigated with normal saline instead of tap water.

NURSING CARE

 ## ASSESSING

In assessing the client's fluid balance it is important to consider unusual factors that may affect intake and output. If a client is extremely diaphoretic or has rapid, deep respirations, fluid loss is occurring even if it cannot be measured.

> ### clinical ALERT
>
> **Report**
>
> When there is a significant discrepancy between intake and output or when fluid intake or output is inadequate, report this information to the charge nurse, physician, or other care provider.

Fluid imbalances may be difficult to detect. Poor skin turgor, or a rapid weak pulse with low blood pressure, may indicate dehydration. Noisy, wet respirations and edema may indicate fluid excess.

Acid–base imbalances may be detected initially by changes in respiratory effort or rate. Other vital signs may be changing. The client may demonstrate a change in level of consciousness such as irritability/restlessness or lethargy, a change in muscle movement or reflexes, headache, nausea and vomiting, and a change in intake and output.

 ## DIAGNOSING, PLANNING, and IMPLEMENTING

Some common nursing diagnoses for clients with fluid and electrolyte or acid–base problems are: Deficient Fluid Volume, Excess Fluid Volume, and Impaired Gas Exchange (see Chapter 16 for information on monitoring oxygenation status). ⊖ Nursing interventions center on helping the client achieve and maintain homeostasis. Nurses assist clients by monitoring intake and output, monitoring intravenous infusions, and assisting with tubings, drains, and dressing changes.

Monitoring Intake and Output

Intake and output (I&O) is the measurement and recording of all fluid taken in and excreted during a 24-hour period (Figure 17-5 ◆). It provides important data about the client's fluid and electrolyte balance. Generally, intake and output are measured for hospitalized at-risk clients. The decision to place a client on intake and output can be an independent nursing measure.

Most agencies have a form for recording I&O, usually a bedside record on which the nurse lists all items measured and their quantities per shift. It is important to inform clients, family members, and all caregivers that accurate measurements of the client's fluid intake and output are required. Nursing staff should explain why the I&O is necessary and should emphasize the need to use a bedpan, urinal, commode, or in-toilet collection device. Clients who wish to be involved in recording fluid intake measurements need to be taught how to compute the values and what foods are considered fluids.

To measure fluid intake, the nurse records each item of fluid intake, specifying the time and type of fluid. All of the following fluids need to be recorded:

- *Oral fluids*. Include water, milk, juice, soft drinks, coffee, tea, cream, soup, and any other beverages. Include water taken with medications. To assess the amount of water taken from a water pitcher, measure what remains and subtract this amount from the volume of the full pitcher. Then refill the pitcher.
- *Ice chips*. Measure ice chips and record the amount of fluid intake as one half the amount of the ice chips.
- Foods that are or become liquid at room temperature. These include ice cream, sherbet, custard, and gelatin. Do not measure foods that are pureed, because purees are simply solid foods prepared in a different form.
- *Tube feedings*. Record the amount of formula infused during the shift. Remember to include the 30- to 60-mL water rinse at the end of intermittent feedings or during continuous feedings.
- *Parenteral fluids*. The exact amount of intravenous fluid administered is to be recorded, since some fluid containers may be overfilled. Blood transfusions are included.
- *Intravenous medications*. Intravenous medications that are prepared with solutions such as normal saline (NS) and are administered as an intermittent or continuous infusion must also be included.
- *Catheter or tube irrigants*. Fluid used to irrigate urinary catheters, nasogastric tubes, and intestinal tubes must be measured and recorded if not immediately withdrawn.

To measure fluid output, measure the following fluids (remember to observe appropriate infection control precautions):

EL CAMINO HOSPITAL					PATIENT LABEL				
INTAKE AND OUTPUT RECORD					PATIENT NAME _____				
					PATIENT # _____				
					PHYSICIAN _____				

INTAKE					OUTPUT				
TOTAL IV	INTRAVENOUS	TUBE FEED	ORAL	TIME	URINE	NG	EMESIS	BM	MISC.
				Date:					
				6-2					
				2-10					
				10-6					
				24°					
				Date:					
				6-2					
				2-10					
				10-6					
				24°					

Figure 17-5. ◆ Intake and output record. *Source:* Courtesy of El Camino Hospital, Mountain View, CA.

◆ *Urinary output*. After the client voids, pour the urine into a measuring container. Measure the amount, then record the time and amount on the I&O form. For clients with retention catheters, empty the drainage bag into a measuring container at the end of the shift (or at prescribed times if output is to be measured more often). Note and record the amount of urine output. In intensive care areas, urine output often is measured hourly.

◆ *Vomitus and liquid feces*. Measure in a graduated cylinder. Record the amount and type of fluid and the time.

◆ *Tube drainage*. Record the amount of drainage from gastric or intestinal drainage tubes.

◆ *Wound drainage and draining fistulas*. Wound drainage may be documented by the type and number of dressings saturated with drainage or by measuring the exact amount of drainage collected in a vacuum drainage or gravity drainage system.

When the nurse compares total intake and total output for a 24-hour period, fluid imbalance will be evident. If intake is greater than output, fluid volume excess is the problem. If intake is less than output, fluid volume deficit is the problem.

ASSISTING WITH IV THERAPY

When a client is unable to drink fluids, IV therapy is ordered to prevent fluid volume deficit and to provide necessary electrolytes.

Rules and regulations regarding the role of LPNs and LVNs in IV therapy vary from state to state. They are available from the Board of Nursing in each state. It is your responsibility to know what is legal for you to do; *always* perform duties within your scope of practice.

Intravenous Solutions. Intravenous solutions can be classified as isotonic, hypotonic, or hypertonic. Most IV solutions are **isotonic,** such as 0.9 percent sodium chloride (has the same concentration of solutes as blood plasma). Isotonic solutions are often used to restore vascular volume. **Hypertonic** solutions, such as 0.9 percent sodium chloride with 5 percent dextrose, have a greater concentration of solutes than plasma. **Hypotonic** solutions, such as 0.45 percent sodium chloride, have a lesser concentration of solutes.

IV solutions can also be categorized according to their purpose. *Nutrient solutions* contain carbohydrate in the form of dextrose. IV dextrose solution provide 3.4 calories per gram. For example, 1 L of 5 percent dextrose provides 170 calories. This amount of calories and fluid helps prevent dehydration and ketosis, but does not provide enough nutrients for body functions such as wound healing.

Electrolyte solutions contain varying amounts of cations and anions. Commonly used solutions are normal saline (0.9 percent sodium chloride solution), Ringer's solution (which contains sodium, chloride, potassium, and calcium), and lactated Ringer's solution (which contains sodium, chloride, potassium, calcium, and lactate). Saline and balanced electrolyte solutions commonly are used to restore va[?]ume, particularly after trauma or surgery. They al[?] used to replace fluid and electrolytes for clients wit[?] ing losses, for example, because of gastric suction [?] drainage.

Volume expanders are used to increase the bloo[?] following severe loss of blood (e.g., from hemorrha[?] of plasma (e.g., from severe burns, which draw large[?] of plasma from the bloodstream to the burn site).[?] volume expanders are dextran, plasma, and hum[?] albumin.

Assessing and Monitoring IV Infusion Sites

Monitoring IV infusion sites is a frequent responsibility of the LPN/LVN. Be aware and assess visually for redness and swelling at the infusion site. Make sure bedding is not crushing the tubing or slowing flow and that blood is not backing up in the tubing. Notify the team leader if problems are noted. Be aware of IV bags that are near empty. Report them to the team leader so that they can be changed by trained personnel. Many facilities have IV infusion pumps equipped with alarms. If the pump alarm sounds, notify the team leader. Do not just turn it off.

Discontinuing an IV

The physician may order an IV to be discontinued when it is no longer necessary or to be converted to a saline or heparin lock to provide a route for medication administration. Guidelines for discontinuing an IV infusion are outlined in Procedure 17-4.

Monitoring for Acid–Base Disorders

It may be impossible to determine the exact imbalance through signs and symptoms. Nurses work in collaboration with the physician and laboratory personnel to identify the problem. Laboratory results—arterial blood gases (ABGs)—will be the determinant of the client's imbalance. The LPN/LVN needs to be aware of normal values and should routinely check lab results to confirm clinical signs. The client should be monitored for changes in vital signs, especially in respiratory effort or rate. Lung sounds may be diminished or absent. The pulse oximeter recordings should be monitored for decreasing oxygen levels. (See Chapter 16 for more information about supporting oxygenation. ᴓᴑ) Level of consciousness and presence of seizures need to be followed to determine the extent of the imbalance. Reflexes may be hyperreflexive or absent, depending on the particular imbalance. The client may complain of numbness or tingling in fingers or toes, lethargy, or headache. A change in urinary output or NG output would be significant to report. The nurse performs regular assessment of mental status and vital signs. Any client who has an intake and output imbalance is at risk for acid–base imbalance, and should be monitored closely until balance is achieved.

EVALUATING

The client with fluid and electrolyte or acid–base disorders must be monitored regularly and carefully. Data on vital signs and I&O should be collected. IV and respiratory therapy must be monitored as ordered. Changes in level of consciousness, abnormal or worsening vital signs, and fluid imbalances should be reported to the charge nurse or physician.

 DISCHARGE CONSIDERATIONS

Teaching needs to take place addressing the underlying cause of imbalances. How the client should take their medications, especially new prescriptions, should be reviewed and the client's questions should be answered. The client needs to know what signs might indicate a respiratory compensation is beginning and what to report. Therapeutic dietary changes need to be reviewed.

Note: The bibliography listings for this and all chapters have been compiled at the back of the book.

PROCEDURE 17-1

Monitoring Blood Glucose

PURPOSES

◆ To determine the client's blood glucose level
◆ To provide data for administering insulin in clients with diabetes mellitus

EQUIPMENT

◆ Chemical strips for reading glucose measurement
◆ Glucose monitor
◆ Lancet mechanism for obtaining blood
◆ Gloves
◆ Insulin sliding scale

INTERVENTIONS

1. Prepare the client. Explain that a drop of blood is needed to determine the client's blood glucose level. *This promotes cooperation.*

2. Confirm the correct chemical strips with the machine code. *Matching the codes prevents a misreading.*

3. Remove chemical strip from container and place it in the machine.

4. Prepare the lancet for puncture.

5. Don gloves. *This supports infection control.*

6. Hold chosen finger downward and squeeze gently from base to fingertip. *This helps bring blood to the puncture site.*

7. Wipe intended puncture site (lateral pads of fingers) per hospital protocol.

8. Place lancet against side of finger and release spring or stick finger with darting motion.

9. Allow drop of blood to accumulate onto chemical strip.

10. Activate timing device if monitor is not equipped with automatic timer.

11. Apply pressure to puncture site.

12. Allow the appropriate time for a digital readout.

13. Obtain results from the digital reading.

14. Discard soiled materials and gloves in proper containers.

15. Position client for comfort with the call bell within reach.

16. Document appropriate dose of regular insulin from sliding scale if provided.

◆ SAMPLE DOCUMENTATION

3/3/05	BG: 250; 0740 Reg. Insulin 5 U given
0800	SC per sliding scale. ————————
	N. Agarwal, LPN

PROCEDURE 17-2

Inserting and Removing Nasogastric Tubes

Part A: Inserting a Nasogastric Tube

PURPOSES

◆ To administer tube feedings and medications directly into the GI tract for clients unable to eat by mouth or swallow a sufficient diet

◆ To establish a means for suctioning stomach contents to prevent gastric distention, nausea, and vomiting
◆ To remove stomach contents for laboratory analysis
◆ To *lavage* (wash) the stomach in case of poisoning, overdose of medications, or gastric bleeding

EQUIPMENT

- Nasogastric tube—Levine (single-lumen) or Salem Sump (double-lumen)
- Towels, tissue, and an emesis basis
- Nonallergenic adhesive tape, _ inch and 1 inch wide
- Disposable gloves
- Water-soluble lubricant
- Glass of water and drinking straw
- Irrigating set with 20-mL syringe or 30-mL syringe with catheter tip

- ◆ pH test strip
- ◆ Stethoscope
- ◆ Clamp or plug for tubing
- ◆ Suction equipment if required
- ◆ Tincture of benzoin
- ◆ Tongue blade and penlight
- ◆ Rubber band and safety pin
- ◆ Plastic disposable bag
- ◆ Oral care supplies

INTERVENTIONS

1. Prepare the client.
   - Explain to the client what you plan to do. *The passage of a gastric tube is not painful, but it is unpleasant because the gag reflex is activated during insertion.* Tell the client how to breathe and swallow upon your direction to facilitate insertion of the tube. Establish with the client what sign he or she could use (such as raising hand) to indicate for you to pause due to discomfort or gagging. *This form of communication gives client reassurance.*
   - Assist the client to a high-Fowler's position if health condition permits, and support the head on a pillow. *This facilitates passage of the tube into the esophagus.* Place a towel across the chest.
   - Remove the client's dentures so they do not become loose and interfere with insertion of the tube. Place tissues and emesis basin near client.

2. Assess the client's nares.
   - Ask the client if they have had nasal surgery, trauma, or a bleeding disorder. *An NG may be contraindicated in client's with such a history.*
   - Examine the nares for any obstructions or deformities by asking the client to breathe through one nostril while occluding the other.
   - Select the nostril that has the greater airflow.
   - Have client blow nose to clear.

3. Prepare the tube.
   - If needed, chill the tube for less flexibility, or warm the tube for increased flexibility. *A tube that is firm but not rigid will pass most easily and with the least amount of trauma.*

4. Determine how far to insert the tube.
   - Use the tube to mark off the distance from the tip of the client's nose to the tip of the earlobe and then from the tip of the earlobe to the tip of the sternum (Figure 17-6 ◆). This length approximates the distance from the nares to the stomach and may vary among individuals. Measuring the tube in this manner is more reliable and customizes

the placement for this client. Mark the measured length with adhesive tape.

5. Insert the tube.
   - Lubricate the tip of the tube well with water-soluble lubricant or water to ease insertion, avoiding covering the holes on the tube with lubricant. *The lubricant reduces friction, thus reducing trauma. A water-soluble lubricant dissolves if the tube accidentally enters the lungs. An oil-based lubricant, such as petroleum jelly, will not dissolve and could cause respiratory complications if it enters the lungs.*
   - Coil the tube's first 7 to 10 inches around your fingers to facilitate passage. Gently tip the client's head back and insert the tube, with its natural curve toward the client, into the selected nostril. Slowly advance the tube toward the nasopharynx by directing the tube towards the ear.

Figure 17-6. ◆ Measuring the appropriate length of NG tube. *Source;* © Elena Dorfman.

MediaLink ● Nasogastric Tube

- If the tube meets resistance, withdraw it, relubricate it, and insert it in the other nostril. *The tube should never be forced against resistance, because of the possibility of trauma.*
- Once the tube reaches the pharynx the client will feel the tube in the throat and may gag and retch. You may need to pause and have the client rest for a few moments. Have the client take sips of water to calm the gag reflex.
- Ask the client to tilt the head forward, and encourage the client to drink sips of water and swallow. *Tilting the head forward facilitates passage of the tube into the posterior pharynx and esophagus rather than into the larynx; swallowing moves the epiglottis over the opening to the larynx* (Figure 17-7 ◆).
- In cooperation with the client, pass the tube 5 to 10 cm (2 to 4 in) with each swallow, until the indicated length is inserted.
- Stop the procedure and immediately remove tube if the client shows signs of coughing or cyanosis. *This could indicate that the tube has slipped into the trachea.*
- If the client continues to gag and the tube does not advance with each swallow, withdraw it slightly, and inspect the throat by looking through the mouth. *The tube may be coiled in the throat. If so, withdraw it until it is straight, and try again to insert it.*

6. Ascertain correct placement of the tube.
   - Ask the client to speak or hum. *If unable to do so, the tube may be passed through the vocal cords or coiled in the back of the throat.*
   - Auscultate air insufflation. This is done by attaching a syringe with 10 to 20 mL of air in it to the end of the tube. Place your stethoscope over the left upper quadrant of the abdomen, and listen while the air is injected. *You will hear the movement of air if the placement is in the stomach. If the client belches, the tube may be in the esophagus.*
   - With the syringe in place, withdraw stomach contents to determine placement of the tube in the stomach. If unable to withdraw contents, turn client on left side, advance the tube 1 to 2 inches, and attempt again.
   - If the signs do not indicate placement in the stomach, advance the tube 5 cm (2 in), and repeat the tests.
   - Placement may be verified by x-ray. *It is unsafe to place the end of the tube in water to check placement, because it places the client at risk for aspiration.*

7. Connect the tube to suction or plug the tube end.
8. Apply tincture of benzoin to the bridge of the nose where tape will be placed. *Taping will improve the security of the tube.*
9. Prepare the tape by tearing it lengthwise halfway. Tape the unsplit end of tape to the nose and cross the split ends around the tubing (Figure 17-8 ◆). *Do not tape tube to forehead as it may cause trauma to the nostril.*
10. To allow for client movement, make a slip knot with a rubber band around the tube. Secure the tube by pinning the rubber band to the client's gown.
11. To connect to suction, attach the larger lumen of the Salem Sump. This begins intermittent or continuous suction (as ordered).
12. Document the insertion of the tube, including time, type of tube, size of tube, and client response.
13. Ensure the client's comfort.
14. Irrigate the tube every 2 hours or as ordered.
15. Specific care of the Salem Sump:
    - Inject 10 to 20 mL of air into the smaller lumen, the blue port. *This will clear the air vent, preventing gastric mucosal trauma if the tube adheres to the stomach lining. You can test for proper functioning of the air vent by putting the port near your ear. You will hear a hissing sound if patency exists.* Do not let the port hang downward or stomach contents may drain from it.

Figure 17-7. ◆ Swallowing closes the epiglottis and allows passage of the nasogastric tube.

Figure 17-8. ◆ Taping an NG tube to the bridge of the nose.

16. Clean the nares and provide oral care every shift and as needed to prevent infection and promote comfort. Assess nares for skin irritation.

- ◆ Apply water-soluble lubricant to the nostril if it appears dry or encrusted.
- ◆ Change the adhesive tape as required.
- ◆ Position Client in Semi-Fowler's position. *Head of bed must be elevated at least 30 degrees to minimize gastric reflux.*

17. Document placement checks and drainage amount, consistency, and color.

18. If suction is applied, ensure that the patency of both the nasogastric and suction tubes is maintained.

- ◆ Irrigations of the tube with 30 mL of normal saline may be required at regular intervals. In some agencies, irrigations must be ordered by the physician.
- ◆ Keep accurate records of the client's fluid intake and output, and record the amount and characteristics of the drainage. *This supports continuity of care.*
- ◆ For infants and young children, restraints may be necessary during tube insertion and throughout therapy. Restraints will prevent accidental dislodging of the tube.
- ◆ Place the infant in an infant seat, or position the infant with a rolled towel or pillow under the head and shoulders.
- ◆ When assessing the nares, obstruct one of the infant's nares, and feel for air passage from the other. If the nasal passageway is very small or is obstructed, an orogastric tube may be more appropriate.
- ◆ For infants and young children, measure appropriate NG tube length from the nose to the tip of the earlobe and then to the point midway between the umbilicus and the xiphoid process.
- ◆ If an orogastric tube is used, measure from the tip of the earlobe to the corner of the mouth to the xiphoid process.
- ◆ Do not hyperextend or hyperflex an infant's neck. *Hyperextension or hyperflexion of the neck could occlude the airway.*
- ◆ For infants or small children, tape the tube to the area between the end of the nares and the upper lip, as well as to the cheek.

SMALL-BORE FEEDING TUBE

1. Prepare the tube for insertion.

2. Do not ice the tube or it will be too stiff.

3. Insert the stylet (guidewire) into the tube. Lubricate tube with water to activate lubricant.

4. After tube is in the stomach, have the client lean forward or to the right to help in advancing the tube. Leave the stylet in.

5. X-ray must confirm proper placement before any feeding is introduced. The stylet is removed after placement is confirmed.

Part B: Removing a Nasogastric Tube

INTERVENTIONS

1. Confirm the physician's order to remove the tube.

2. Prepare the client.

- ◆ Assist the client to a sitting position if health permits.
- ◆ Place the towel or disposable pad across the client's chest to collect any spillage of mucous and gastric secretions from the tube.
- ◆ Provide tissues to the client to wipe the nose and mouth after tube removal.

3. Discontinue suction. Disconnect the NG tube from the suction and plug the end of the tube.

- ◆ Unpin the tube from the client's gown.
- ◆ Remove the adhesive tape securing the tube to the nose.

4. Wash your hands and don disposable gloves to protect yourself from body fluids.

5. Remove the tube.

- ◆ Ask the client to take a deep breath and to hold it. *This closes the glottis, thereby preventing accidental aspiration of any gastric contents.*
- ◆ Pinch the tube with the gloved hand. *Pinching the tube prevents any contents inside the tube from draining into the client's throat.*
- ◆ Slowly withdraw the tube for the first few inches, then quickly and smoothly withdraw the tube.
- ◆ Place the tube in the plastic bag. *Placing the tube immediately into the bag prevents the transference of microorganisms from the tube to other articles or people.*

6. Ensure client comfort.

- ◆ Provide oral care.
- ◆ Assist the client as required to blow the nose. *Excessive secretions may have accumulated in the nasal passages.*

7. Dispose of the equipment appropriately.

- ◆ Place the pad, bag with tube, and gloves in the receptacle designated by the agency. *Correct disposal prevents the transmission of microorganisms.*

8. Assess the nasogastric drainage if suction was used.

- ◆ Measure the amount of gastric drainage, and record it on the client's fluid output record.
- ◆ Inspect the drainage for appearance and consistency.

9. Document all relevant information.

- ◆ Record the removal of the tube, the amount and appearance of any drainage if connected to suction, and any relevant assessments of the client.

◆ **SAMPLE DOCUMENTATION**

04/02/06	20-gauge Salem Sump inserted through L nostril without difficulty. Low intermittent suction attached
0930	with immediate return of 200 mL green viscous fluid. Client tolerated procedure with minor discomfort.
	S. Norris, LPN
04/02/06	NG tube, Salem Sump, draining 50 mL of clear fluid during past 4 hours. Patency verified through
1330	irrigation with 20 mL NS. Placement confirmed. Oral care Q2H and upon request. Nares are free
	from irritation, with KY jelly applied. ————————————————
	S. Norris, LPN
04/03/06	Bowel sounds present, passed flatus. NG tube removed without difficulty. Client tolerated procedure
1000	well, relieved to have tube removed. No n/v or abdominal discomfort present. ———————
	D. Hernandez, LPN

PROCEDURE 17-3
Administering a Tube Feeding

Part A: Nasogastric or Orogastric Feeding

PURPOSE
◆ To restore or maintain nutritional status

EQUIPMENT
◆ Tube feeding formula
◆ 20- to 50-mL syringe with an adapter
◆ Emesis basin
◆ Large catheter-tip syringe with plunger
   or
◆ Calibrated plastic feeding bag with tubing that can be attached to the feeding tube
   or
◆ Prefilled bottle with a drip chamber, tubing, and a flow-regulator clamp
◆ pH test strip

◆ Measuring container from which to pour the feeding (if using open system)
◆ Water (60 mL unless otherwise specified) at room temperature
◆ Feeding pump as required
◆ Correct amount of feeding solution
◆ Graduated container to hold the feeding
◆ Graduated container with 60 mL of water to flush the tubing
◆ Graduated container to measure residual formula
◆ Four 3 × 4″ gauze squares to cover the end of the tube
◆ Elastic band
◆ Mild soap and water

INTERVENTIONS

1. Confirm physician order for specific type and amount of feeding.
2. Prepare the client.

◆ Assist the client to a Fowler's position in bed or a sitting position in a chair, the normal position for eating. If a sitting position is contraindicated, a slightly elevated right side-lying position is acceptable. The head of the bed should be raised 30 to 45 degrees. *These positions enhance the gravitational flow of the solution and prevent aspiration of fluid into the lungs.*

3. Assess tube placement.
   ◆ Auscultate placement of 20 to 30 mL of air into the tube with your stethoscope positioned over the epigastric area.
   ◆ Attach the syringe to the open end of the tube; aspirate alimentary secretions. Check the pH at least an hour after medications have been given. *Gastric content normal pH is 6 or below.*

4. Assess residual feeding contents.
   ◆ Aspirate all the stomach contents, and measure the amount prior to administering the feeding, the residual. *This is done to evaluate whether undigested formula from a previous feeding remains or the stomach is emptying properly.*
   ◆ If 75 to 150 mL (or more than half the last feeding) is withdrawn, check with the nurse in charge or refer to agency policy before proceeding. The precise amount to infuse is usually determined by the physician's order or by agency policy. *At some agencies, a feeding is withheld when the specified amount or more of formula remains in the stomach. In other agencies, the amount withdrawn is subtracted from the total feeding and that volume (less the undigested portion) is administered slowly.*
   or
   ◆ Reinstill the gastric contents into the stomach (to reduce fluid and electrolyte imbalance). Remove the syringe plunger, and pour the gastric contents via the syringe into the nasogastric tube. *Removal of the contents could disturb the client's electrolyte balance.*
   ◆ If the client is on a continuous feeding, check the gastric residual every 4 hours or according to agency protocol.

5. Administer the feeding.
   ◆ Before administering feeding:
   a. Check the expiration date of the feeding.
   b. Warm the feeding to room temperature. *An excessively cold feeding may cause cramps.*
   ◆ When an open system is used, clean the top of the feeding container before opening it. *This minimizes the risk of contaminants entering the feeding syringe or feeding bag.*

FEEDING BAG (OPEN SYSTEM)
   ◆ Hang the bag from an infusion pole about 30 cm (12 in) above the tube's point of insertion into the client.
   ◆ Clamp the tubing, and add the formula to the bag.
   ◆ Open the clamp, run the formula through the tubing, and reclamp the tube. *The formula will displace the air in the tubing, thus preventing the instillation of excess air into the client's stomach or intestine.*
   ◆ Attach the bag to the nasogastric tube (Figure 17-9 ◆). Regulate the drip by adjusting the clamp, or secure the tubing in the feeding pump for regulated administration.

SYRINGE (OPEN SYSTEM)
   ◆ Remove the plunger from the syringe, and connect the syringe to a pinched or clamped nasogastric tube. *Pinching*

Figure 17-9. ◆ Using a calibrated plastic bag to administer tube feeding.

or clamping the tube prevents excess air from entering the stomach and causing distention.
   ◆ Pour a small amount of feeding into the syringe barrel.
   ◆ Permit the feeding to flow in slowly at the prescribed rate. Raise or lower the syringe to adjust the flow as needed. Pinch or clamp the tubing to stop the flow for a minute if the client experiences discomfort. *If feeding is administered too quickly, flatus, crampy pain, and/or vomiting can occur.*

PREFILLED BOTTLE WITH DRIP CHAMBER (CLOSED SYSTEM)
   ◆ Remove the screw-on cap from the container, and attach the administration set with the drip chamber and tubing.
   ◆ Close the clamp on the tubing.
   ◆ Hang the container on an intravenous pole about 30 cm (12 in) above the tube's insertion point into the client. *At this height the formula should run at a safe rate into the stomach or intestine.*
   ◆ Squeeze the drip chamber to fill it to one third to one half of its capacity.
   ◆ Open the tubing clamp, run the formula through the tubing, and reclamp the tube. *The formula will displace the air in the tubing, thus preventing the instillation of excess air.*
   ◆ Attach the feeding set tubing to the feeding tube, and regulate the drip rate to deliver the feeding over the desired length of time. *Prefilled tube-feeding sets can be attached to a feeding pump to regulate the flow.*

6. Rinse the feeding tube immediately before all of the formula has run through the tubing.
   ◆ Instill 50 to 100 mL of water through the feeding tube. *Water flushes the lumen of the tube, preventing future blockage by sticky formula.*
   ◆ Be sure to add the water before the feeding solution has drained from the neck of a syringe or from the tubing of an administration set. Before adding water to a feeding

bag or prefilled tubing set, first clamp and disconnect both feeding and administration tubes. *Adding the water before the syringe or tubing is empty prevents the instillation of air into the stomach or intestine and thus prevents unnecessary distention.*

7. Clamp and cover the feeding tube.
   ◆ Clamp the feeding tube before all of the water is instilled. *Clamping prevents leakage of feeding or air from entering the tube.*
   ◆ Cover the end of the feeding tube with gauze held by an elastic band. *Covering the tube end prevents leakage from it.*

8. Ensure client comfort and safety.
   ◆ Pin the tubing to the client's gown by slip knotting a rubber band over the tube. *This minimizes pulling of the tube, thus preventing discomfort and dislodgment.*
   ◆ Ask the client to remain sitting upright in Fowler's position or in a slightly elevated right lateral position for at least 30 minutes. *These positions facilitate digestion and movement of the feeding from the stomach along the alimentary tract, and prevent potential aspiration of the feeding into the lungs. The head of the bed must remain elevated 30 to 45 degrees when a continuous feeding is taking place.*

9. Dispose of equipment appropriately.
   ◆ If the open system bag and connected tube are to be reused, wash it thoroughly with soap and water so that it is ready for reuse. Hang it to air dry.
   ◆ Change the open system bag and connected tube every 24 hours or according to agency policy, as well as any syringes or irrigation fluid/set being used.

10. Monitor the client for possible problems.
    ◆ Carefully assess clients receiving tube feedings for problems, particularly changes in lung sounds.
    ◆ To prevent dehydration, give the client supplemental water in addition to the prescribed tube feeding as ordered.

11. Document all relevant information.
    ◆ Document the feeding, including amount and kind of solution, duration of the feeding, and assessments of the client.

◆ Record the volume of the feeding and water administered on the client's intake and output record.

VARIATION: CONTINUOUS-DRIP FEEDING
   ◆ If the feeding is a continuous-drip tube feeding, place a label on the container. *The label should indicate when the new feeding bag was hung.*
   ◆ Check residual as ordered or indicated by agency protocol. Then flush the tubing with 30 to 50 mL of water. *This verifies correct placement of the tube. If placement of a small-bore tube is questionable, a repeat x-ray should be done.*
   ◆ Determine agency protocol regarding withholding a feeding based on residual obtained. *Many agencies withhold the feeding for more than 75 to 150 mL of residual feeding.*
   ◆ To prevent spoilage or bacterial contamination, do not allow the feeding solution to hang longer than 8 hours. Check agency policy or manufacturer's recommendations regarding time limits.
   ◆ Follow agency policy regarding how frequently to change the feeding bag and tubing. *Changing the feeding bag and tubing every 24 hours reduces the risk of contamination.*

PEDIATRIC CONSIDERATIONS
   ◆ Feeding tubes may be reinserted at each feeding to prevent irritation of the mucous membrane, nasal airway obstruction, and stomach perforation that may occur if the tube is left in place continuously. Check agency practice.
   ◆ Position a small child or infant in your lap, provide a pacifier, and hold and cuddle the child during feedings. *This promotes comfort, supports the normal sucking reflex of the infant, and facilitates digestion.*
   ◆ Check agency policy or physician's orders for acceptable amounts of stomach aspirates and reinstillation of residual feedings.

Part B: Gastrostomy or Jejunostomy Feeding

1. Follow steps for NG feeding, including the following: Check placement, pour 15 to 30 mL of water into the syringe, remove the tube clamp, and allow the water to flow into the tube. *This determines the patency of the tube. If water flows freely, the tube is patent.* If the water does not flow freely, notify the nurse in charge and/or physician.

2. Administer the feeding.
   ◆ Hold the syringe 7 to 15 cm (3 to 6 in) above the ostomy opening.
   ◆ Slowly pour the solution into the syringe and allow it to flow through the tube by gravity.

   ◆ Just before all the formula has run through and the syringe is empty, add 30 mL of water. *Water flushes the tube and preserves its patency.*
   ◆ If the tube is sutured in place, hold it upright, remove the syringe, and then clamp or plug the tube to prevent leakage. Cover the end of the tube with a 4 × 4 gauze, and secure the gauze with a rubber band.

3. Ensure client comfort and safety.
   ◆ Assess status of peristomal skin. *Gastric or jejunal drainage contains digestive enzymes that can irritate the skin.* Document any redness and broken skin areas. Check

orders about cleaning the peristomal skin, applying a skin protectant, and applying appropriate dressings. *Generally, the peristomal skin is washed with mild soap and water every shift and as needed.* Skin protectant may be applied around the stoma.
◆ Observe for common complications of enteral feedings: aspiration, hyperglycemia, abdominal distention, diarrhea, and fecal impaction. Report findings to physician. *Often, a change in formula or rate of administration can correct problems.*

VARIATION: PERCUTANEOUS ENDOSCOPIC GASTROSTOMY (PEG)

◆ A percutaneous endoscopic gastrostomy (PEG) is kept in place with a short crosspiece or bolster near the skin level at the stoma.
◆ Clean the stoma daily with soap and water using a cotton swab or small piece of gauze in a circular motion.
◆ Rotate the bolster and clean the skin under it. Rotate the tube in a full circle between the thumb and forefinger daily.

◆ After cleaning, allow the skin to air dry.
◆ Report any signs of redness, pain, soreness, swelling, or drainage to the health care provider.
◆ Do not apply a dressing over the PEG. *A dressing and tape may result in skin excoriation and breakdown.*

4. Document all assessments and interventions.

◆ SAMPLE DOCUMENTATION

4/10/05	PEG-tube site assessed and cleaned.
0730	Client denies pain or soreness. No skin
	irritation present. Skin barrier cream
	applied. N. Nurse, LPN

PROCEDURE 17-4
Discontinuing an Intravenous Infusion

EQUIPMENT

Nonsterile gloves
2 × 2 inch gauze pad (Alcohol is irritating and may sting.)
Adhesive sterile dressing (Band-Aid or sterile 2 × 2 gauze)

INTERVENTIONS

1. Prepare the equipment
◆ Don clean gloves.
◆ Clamp the infusion tubing. *This prevents the fluid from flowing out of the catheter onto the bed or the client.*
◆ Loosen the tape or transparent dressing at the venipuncture site while holding the needle firmly and applying countertraction to the skin. *Movement of the catheter can injure the vein and cause discomfort to the client. Countertraction prevents pulling the skin and causing discomfort or trauma.*
2. Withdraw the needle or catheter from the vein.
◆ While holding a sterile gauze above the venipuncture site, withdraw the catheter from the vein without

applying pressure over the site. Make this removal in one gentle movement. *Pull the catheter out in the direction of the vein to avoid trauma to the vein.*
◆ Immediately apply firm pressure to the site, using sterile guaze, for 2 to 3 minutes. *Pressure helps stop the bleeding and prevents hematoma formation.*
◆ Hold the client's limb above the level of the heart if bleeding persists. *Raising the limb decreases blood flow to the area.*
3. Examine the catheter removed from the client.
◆ Check the catheter to make sure it is intact. *If a piece of tubing remains in the client's vein, it could move centrally (toward the heart or lungs) and cause serious problems.*

clinical **ALERT**

If a broken piece of tubing can be palpated, apply a tourniquet above the insertion site to decrease the possibility of the piece moving.

Report

Report a broken catheter to the nurse in charge or physician immediately!

4. Cover the insertion site.
   ◆ Apply the sterile dressing to continue the pressure and cover the open area in the skin, preventing infection.
   ◆ An adhesive bandage may be applied to the insertion site once bleeding has stopped.
   ◆ Discard the IV solution container, if infusions are being discontinued, and discard the used supplies appropriately. *This prevents transmission of infection.*

5. Document relevant information.
   ◆ Record the amount of fluid infused on the intake and output record and on the chart according to agency practice. Include the container number, type of solution used, time of discontinuing the infusion, and the client's response.

◆ **SAMPLE DOCUMENTATION**

8/31/05	Bag #2 NS IV discontinued with
1950	catheter fully intact. Site without
	redness, swelling, or bruising. ————
	N. Nurse, LPN

Chapter Review

Key Terms by Topics

Use the audio glossary feature of either the CD-ROM or the Companion Website to hear the correct pronunciation of the following key terms.

Nutrition
nutrients, nutrition, glycogen, amino acids, anabolism, catabolism, nitrogen balance, lipids, triglycerides, vitamins, calories,

obesity, undernutrition, protein–calorie malnutrition, enteral nutrition, parenteral nutrition, gastrostomy, jejunostomy intermittent feeding, continuous feedings

Fluid and electrolytes, and acid–base balance
intracellular fluid (ICF), extracellular fluid (ECF), interstitial fluid, electrolytes, buffers,

respiratory acidosis, respiratory alkalosis, metabolic acidosis, metabolic alkalosis, intake and output (I&O), isotonic, hypertonic, hypotonic

Key Points

◆ For the body to grow, maintain body tissue, and perform all body functions normally, specific nutrients must be supplied. When a person is undernourished, carbohydrate reserves (stored as liver and muscle glycogen) meet energy requirements for a short time; then body protein is used. Over time, this may result in protein–calorie malnutrition.

◆ After a feeding tube is inserted, and before feedings are introduced, tube placement is confirmed by radiography. Tube placement must be confirmed anytime possible dislodgment may have occurred, before administering medication or feeding through the tube, and at least daily for continuous feedings.

◆ If diet therapy is long term, a client must not only understand the diet but also develop a healthy, positive attitude toward it. The client's belief that the diet will make a change is key to its success.

◆ Homeostasis depends on many physiologic processes. These processes regulate fluid intake and output. They also regulate the movement of water and dissolved substances between the body compartments. Fluid imbalances may signal the development of disease. Imbalances between fluid intake and fluid output need to be addressed without delay.

◆ Most electrolytes enter the body through dietary intake and are excreted in the urine. Some electrolytes, such as sodium and chloride, are not stored by the body and must be consumed daily to maintain normal levels.

◆ Changes in electrolyte levels and in acid–base balance can be life threatening. Clients with electrolyte or acid–base imbalances must be monitored often.

◆ If the flow of IV fluids is incorrect, problems such as hypervolemia, hypovolemia, or inadequate medication administration can result. The role of the LPN/LVN includes safe administration of such fluids. The LPN/LVN must consult a baseline assessment of the client's fluid status, in order to evaluate fluid balance.

◆ The role of the LPN/LVN includes collecting data on the IV site at each assessment and before delivering medicated infusions.

EXPLORE MediaLink

Additional interactive resources for this chapter can be found on the Companion Website at www.prenhall.com/ramont. Click on Chapter 17 and "Begin" to select the activities for this chapter.

For chapter-related NCLEX-style questions and an audio glossary, access the accompanying CD-ROM in this book.

Animations:
◆ Digestive system dissection and tour
◆ Mastication
◆ NG tube
◆ Fluid balance
◆ Acid balance

◆ Normal heart hemodynamics
◆ Glipizide
◆ Ranitidine
◆ Warfarin

For Further Study

See Chapter 7 for more about nutrition's role in maintaining homeostasis.

For more about visualizing the digestive track, see Figure 10-13.

For more about the role of nutrition in healing, see Chapter 12.

For information on assessing vital signs, see Chapter 14.

For more information about oxygenation, see Chapter 16.

Critical Thinking Care Map
Caring for a Client with Risk for Deficient Fluid Volume

NCLEX-PN Focus Area: Physiologic Integrity

Case Study: Patti Glove, a 40-year-old female, was admitted to an acute care hospital for treatment of intractable nausea/vomiting and diarrhea. Patti states that she has been experiencing the nausea and vomiting for the past 3 days, with the diarrhea beginning yesterday. She has not taken any medications at home for this condition. No fluids have been "kept down" for the 3 days. Patti states that she has been very weak and feels faint when she stands up.

Nursing Diagnosis: Deficient Fluid Volume

COLLECT DATA

Subjective

_____
_____
_____
_____
_____
_____

Objective

_____
_____
_____
_____
_____
_____

Would you report this data? Yes/No

If yes, to: _____

Nursing Care

_____
_____
_____
_____
_____
_____
_____
_____
_____
_____
_____
_____
_____
_____
_____
_____

How would you document this? _____
_____
_____
_____
_____
_____

Data Collected
(use those that apply)

- Weight: 145
- Blood pressure 98/62
- Pulse 110, regular
- Respirations, 16
- Mood: irritable, anxious
- States she is very thirsty
- Oxygen saturation: 93% on room air
- Nausea and vomiting present
- Mucous membranes dry
- Skin turgor poor
- Urine dark amber, 50 mL in last voiding

Nursing Interventions
(use those that apply)

- Monitor and report abnormal lab results.
- Monitor and document intake and output.
- Encourage fluid intake.
- Regularly monitor abdominal girth.
- Teach client to stand slowly.
- Monitor color, amount, and frequency of fluid loss.
- Assess for vertigo and hypotension.
- Take daily weights.
- Give and monitor effectiveness of antinausea medication as ordered.
- Give and monitor effectiveness of antidiarrheal medications as ordered.
- Monitor orthostatic blood pressure q4h.
- Administer IV therapy as ordered.
- Provide frequent oral care.
- Teach client about intake/output measurement.

NCLEX-PN Exam Preparation

1. A client who prefers vegetarian menus states that he has a greater need for carbohydrates and has not given thought to the amount of protein to consume. You would explain that the importance of eating at least the minimum daily requirements of protein is to allow the body to have:
   a. Adequate structural material for body tissues
   b. A limited amount of fat
   c. Adequate calories for maintaining blood glucose
   d. Adequate calcium for bone density

2. You are teaching a client about limiting fat intake to reduce undesirable cholesterol and triglyceride levels. Which statement by the client would indicate that he or she would be most likely to succeed in keeping with the dietary changes?
   a. "I think that if my spouse were here I would be sure to have the correct foods prepared for my meals."
   b. "I think that a person only lives once, and what one eats will not really make that much difference in the long run."
   c. "I think that I will be able to eat less fatty foods if I look at the food labels before I buy."
   d. "I think that my spouse will be upset if I don't eat the same foods along with him/her."

3. You are totaling the intake and output record for your shift. The client's IV fluid intake for the shift is 1,200 mL, and the output is 2,200 mL from a Foley catheter drainage bag. The client received 1,000 mL PO, and had emesis of 75 mL. What was the client's total output for your shift?
   a. 3,125 mL
   b. 2,275 mL
   c. 2,200 mL
   d. 2,125 mL

4. A client's spouse who has coronary vessel disease (heart disease) asks you how best to prepare the meals to keep from promoting the disease. What should you say?
   a. Cream sauces can be used to enhance the flavor of this diet.
   b. Serve fish for the meat choice often, instead of other meats.
   c. Seek assistance by shopping at health food stores.
   d. Substitute onion salt and celery salt for table salt to enhance flavor.

5. A client visiting the clinic has heard about the dangers of obesity and wants to know if she is considered to be obese. You could accurately answer that
   a. Anyone who is 10 percent or more above IBW is considered obese and at risk for health.
   b. Anyone who is 20 percent or less than IBW is considered to be obese and at risk for health.

   c. Anyone who is 20 percent or more above IBW is considered to be obese and at risk for health.
   d. Anyone who is 20 percent or more above IBW but is physically active is not considered to be obese.

6. A client is receiving tube feeding and has inadvertently pulled out the tube. The nurse has replaced the tube and is ready to restart the feeding. What step must be taken before starting the feeding?
   a. The client needs to be reweighed.
   b. The client needs to have tube placement verified, perhaps even by x-ray.
   c. The client should be tested on semisolid foods before returning to tube feeding.
   d. The client should receive bolus feedings until tube placement is confirmed by x-ray.

7. A client has been diagnosed recently as having diabetes mellitus. You will assist the client in learning how to adjust to her newly prescribed diet, instructing her that the primary function of carbohydrates is to:
   a. Furnish the body with energy
   b. Insulate the client to avoid loss of heat
   c. Provide building blocks to repair new tissue
   d. Supply client with adequate amounts of fiber

8. A client has undergone colon surgery today and will be receiving a clear liquid diet. Which of the following foods would you expect to be on the client's meal tray?
   a. Milkshake
   b. Cranberry juice
   c. Apricot nectar
   d. Creamed soups

9. When giving medications through a Salem Sump to a client, the proper procedure would be to:
   a. Administer the medications into the smaller blue port on the tube
   b. Administer the medications orally if they are liquid or crushed
   c. Administer the medications into the larger port on the tube
   d. Administer the medications only after the tube was removed

10. You are instructing a client on sodium restrictions about the purpose for the low-salt diet recently prescribed. You explain the importance of this diet, including the fact that the primary electrolyte for control and regulation of fluid balance in the body is
    a. Sodium
    b. Potassium
    c. Calcium
    d. Magnesium

Answers for Review Questions, as well as discussion of Case Study and Critical Thinking Care Map questions, appear in Appendix IV.

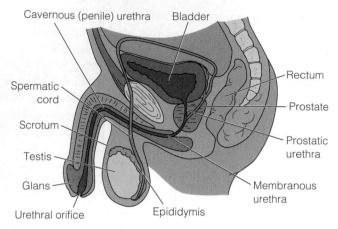

Figure 18-3. ◆ The male urogenital system.

gular area marked by the ureter openings at the posterior corners and the opening of the urethra at the anterior inferior corner. Urine exits the bladder through the urethra.

The bladder is able to stretch because of *rugae* (folds) in the mucous membrane lining and because of the elasticity of its walls. When full, the bladder may extend above the symphysis pubis. In extreme situations it may extend as high as the umbilicus.

URETHRA

The urethra extends from the bladder to the urinary meatus. The **meatus** is an opening in the external body that serves as a passageway for the elimination of urine. The female's urinary meatus is located between the labia minora, in front of the vagina and below the clitoris. The male urethra is about 10 cm (8 in) long and serves as a passageway for semen as well as urine (see Figure 18-3). The male's urinary meatus is located at the distal end of the penis.

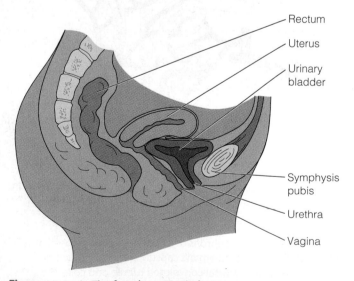

Figure 18-4. ◆ The female urogenital system.

The *internal sphincter* muscle situated at the base of the urinary bladder is under involuntary control. The *external sphincter* muscle is under voluntary control, allowing the individual to choose when urine is eliminated.

In both males and females the urethra has a mucous membrane lining that is continuous with the bladder and the ureters. This structure facilitates the spread of an infection of the urethra throughout the urinary tract to the kidneys. Women are particularly prone to urinary tract infections because of their short urethra and the proximity of the urinary meatus to the vagina and anus (see Figure 18-4).

URINATION

Micturition, voiding, and *urination* all refer to the process of emptying the urinary bladder. Urine collects in the bladder until pressure stimulates special sensory nerve endings in the bladder wall called *stretch receptors*. These receptors respond when the adult bladder contains between 250 and 450 mL of urine by transmitting impulses to the spinal cord, causing the internal sphincter to relax and stimulating the urge to void. The conscious portion of the brain relaxes the external urethral sphincter muscle, and urination takes place. If the time and place are inappropriate, voluntary controls allow the micturition reflex to subside until the bladder becomes more filled and the reflex is involuntarily stimulated again.

Voluntary control of urination is possible only if the nerves supplying the bladder and urethra, the neural tracts of the cord and brain, and the motor area of the cerebrum are intact. An individual must be able to sense that the bladder is full. Injury to any part of the nervous system above the level of the sacral region results in intermittent involuntary emptying of the bladder. Older people whose cognition is impaired may not be aware of the need to urinate or able to respond appropriately to nervous system stimulus.

◆ Factors Affecting Urinary Function

Numerous factors affect the volume and characteristics of the urine produced and the manner in which it is excreted.

See Table 18-1 ◆ for a summary of the developmental changes affecting urinary output.

PSYCHOSOCIAL FACTORS

Certain conditions that relate to comfort or relaxation help stimulate the micturition reflex. These conditions include privacy, normal position, sufficient time, and, occasionally, running water. Inability to relax abdominal and perineal muscles and the external urethral sphincter inhibits voiding. People also may voluntarily suppress urination (voluntary urinary retention) because of perceived time pressures. For example, nurses often ignore the urge to void until they are able to take a break, a behavior that can increase the risk of urinary tract infections.

TABLE 18-1	CHANGES IN URINARY ELIMINATION THROUGH THE LIFE SPAN
STAGE	VARIATIONS
Fetus	The fetal kidney begins to excrete urine between the 11th and 12th week of development.
Infant	Ability to concentrate urine is minimal; therefore, urine appears light yellow. Because of neuromuscular immaturity, voluntary urinary control is absent.
Child	Kidney function reaches maturity between the first and second year of life; urine is concentrated effectively and appears a normal amber color. Between 18 and 24 months of age, the child starts to recognize bladder fullness and is able to hold urine beyond the urge to void. At approximately 2½ to 3 years of age, the child can perceive bladder fullness, hold urine after the urge to void, and communicate the need to urinate. Full urinary control usually occurs at age 4 or 5 years; daytime control is usually achieved by age 3 years. The kidneys grow in proportion to overall body growth.
Adult	The kidneys reach maximum size between 35 and 40 years of age. After 50 years the kidneys begin to diminish in size and function. Most shrinkage occurs in the cortex of the kidney as individual nephrons are lost.
Older adult	An estimated 30% of nephrons are lost by age 80. Renal blood flow decreases because of vascular changes and a decrease in cardiac output. The ability to concentrate urine declines. Bladder muscle tone diminishes, causing increased frequency of urination and nocturia (awakening to urinate at night). Diminished bladder muscle tone and contractibility may lead to residual urine in the bladder after voiding, increasing the risk of bacterial growth and infection. Urinary incontinence may occur due to mobility problems or neurologic impairments.

FLUID AND FOOD INTAKE

The healthy body maintains a balance between the amount of fluid ingested and the amount of fluid eliminated. When the amount of fluid intake increases, the output normally increases. Certain fluids, such as alcohol, increase fluid output by inhibiting the production of antidiuretic hormone. Fluids that contain caffeine (e.g., coffee, tea, and cola drinks) also increase urine production. By contrast, food and fluids high in sodium can cause fluid retention.

Some foods and fluids can change the color of urine. For example, beets and blackberries can cause urine to appear red; carrots and other foods containing carotene can cause the urine to appear more yellow.

MEDICATIONS

Many medications, particularly those affecting the autonomic nervous system, interfere with the normal urination process and may cause retention. Included among the medications that may cause **urinary retention** (accumulation of urine in the bladder and inability of the bladder to empty itself) are: antispasmodics antidepressants, antihypertensives, and anti-histamines. **Diuretics** increase urine formation by preventing the reabsorption of water and electrolytes from the tubules of the kidney into the bloodstream. Diuretics are commonly prescribed for hypertension and cardiac disease to decrease fluid volume. Some medications also affect the color of urine.

MUSCLE TONE AND ACTIVITY

Regular exercise increases the muscle tone of the bladder and sphincters and also increases the metabolic rate. Clients who require a retention catheter for a long period may have poor bladder muscle tone because continuous drainage of urine prevents the bladder from filling and emptying normally. Abdominal muscle contraction assists in bladder emptying. Pelvic muscle tone is a factor in being able to retain urine voluntarily once the urge to urinate is perceived.

◆ Pathologic Conditions

Some diseases and pathologies can affect the formation and excretion of urine. Diseases of the kidneys may affect the ability of the nephrons to produce urine. Abnormal amounts of protein or blood cells may be present in the urine, or the kidneys may virtually stop producing urine altogether, a condition known as *renal failure*. Heart and circulatory disorders such as heart failure, shock, or hypertension can affect blood flow to the kidneys, interfering with urine production. If abnormal amounts of fluid are lost through another route (e.g., vomiting or high fever), water is retained by the kidneys and urinary output falls.

A urinary stone (**calculus**) may obstruct a ureter, blocking urine flow from the kidney to the bladder.

Hypertrophy of the prostate gland, a common condition affecting older men, may partially obstruct the urethra, impairing urination and bladder emptying.

ALTERED URINE PRODUCTION

Although patterns of urination are highly individual, most people void about five to seven times a day: usually upon awakening, before going to bed, and around mealtimes.

Polyuria

Polyuria refers to the production of abnormally large amounts of urine by the kidneys. Polyuria can follow excessive fluid intake (called polydipsia). It may be associated with diseases such as diabetes mellitus, diabetes insipidus, or chronic nephritis. **Diuresis** is another term for the production and excretion of large amounts of urine. This term is often used when medications are given to promote urine output. Polyuria or diuresis can cause excessive fluid loss, leading to intense thirst, dehydration, and weight loss.

Oliguria and Anuria

The terms *oliguria* and *anuria* are used to describe decreased urinary output. **Oliguria** is low urine output, usually less than 500 mL per day or 30 mL per hour. **Anuria** refers to a lack of urine production, with no effective urinary output. Although oliguria may occur as a result of abnormal fluid losses or a lack of fluid intake, it often indicates impaired blood flow to the kidneys or impending renal failure.

ALTERED URINARY ELIMINATION

Despite normal urine production, a number of factors or conditions can affect urinary elimination. Selected factors associated with altered patterns of urine elimination are identified in Table 18-2 ◆.

COLLABORATIVE CARE

Diagnostic Tests

Blood levels of urea and creatinine are routinely used to evaluate renal function. They are normally eliminated by the kidneys through filtration:

1. Urea, the end product of protein metabolism, is measured as *blood urea nitrogen (BUN)*.
2. Creatinine is produced in relatively constant quantities by the muscles. The *creatinine clearance test* uses 24-hour urine and serum creatinine levels to determine the glomerular filtration rate, a sensitive indicator of renal function.

Visualization procedures also may be used to evaluate urinary function. The KUB is an x-ray of the kidneys, ureters, and bladder. *Intravenous pyelography (IVP)* is a radiographic study used to evaluate the urinary tract. In intravenous pyelogram, contrast medium is injected intravenously. Following injection of the contrast medium, x-rays are taken to evaluate urinary tract structures. *Computed tomography (CT scan)* is a pain-

less, noninvasive x-ray procedure that distinguishes minor differences in the density of tissues. *Renal ultrasonography* is a noninvasive test that uses reflected sound waves to visualize the kidneys. During a *cystoscopy,* the bladder, ureteral orifices, and urethra can be visualized using a cystoscope, a lighted instrument inserted through the urethra.

Nurses are responsible for preparing clients for these studies and for follow-up care. There are several tests nurses perform on the unit. These are discussed under Diagnosing, Planning, and Implementing in the Nursing Care section that follows.

NURSING CARE

 ASSESSING

The LPN/LVN is responsible for assessing the client's urinary function by collecting data and collaborating with the RN. The nurse determines the client's normal voiding pattern and frequency, appearance of the urine and any recent changes, any past or current problems with urination, the presence of an ostomy, and factors influencing the elimination pattern.

Complete physical assessment of the urinary tract (completed by the RN) usually includes palpation of the kidneys to detect areas of tenderness and palpation of the bladder. The urethral meatus of both male and female clients may be inspected for swelling, discharge, and inflammation.

Because problems with urination can affect the elimination of wastes from the body, it is important that the LPN/LVN observe the skin for color, texture, and tissue turgor as well as for the presence of edema. If incontinence, dribbling, or dysuria is noted in the history, the skin of the perineum should be inspected for irritation, because contact with urine can excoriate the skin.

Urine Characteristics

Normal urine consists of 96 percent water and 4 percent solutes. Organic solutes include urea, ammonia, creatinine, and uric acid. Inorganic solutes include sodium, chloride, potassium, sulfate, magnesium, and phosphorus. Characteristics of normal and abnormal urine are shown in Table 18-3 ◆.

 DIAGNOSING, PLANNING, and IMPLEMENTING

The North American Nursing Diagnosis Association (NANDA) includes one general diagnostic label for urinary elimination problems and subcategories that are more specific. The broad label is Impaired Urinary Elimination. The goals established vary according to the diagnosis and related defining characteristics. Examples of overall goals for clients with urinary elimination problems may include:

TABLE 18-2	SELECTED FACTORS ASSOCIATED WITH ALTERED URINARY ELIMINATION
PATTERNS	**SELECTED ASSOCIATED FACTORS**
Polyuria (diuresis; eliminating abnormally large amounts of urine)	Ingestion of fluids containing caffeine or alcohol Prescribed diuretic Presence of thirst, dehydration, and weight loss History of diabetes mellitus, diabetes insipidus, or kidney disease
Oliguria, anuria (low amounts of urine or no urine)	Decrease in fluid intake Signs of dehydration (see Chapter 17 ☞) Presence of hypotension, shock, or heart failure History of kidney disease Signs of renal failure such as elevated blood urea nitrogen (BUN) and serum creatinine, edema, hypertension
Frequency or nocturia (voiding more than usual, nocturia—voiding two or more times at night)	Pregnancy Increase in fluid intake Urinary tract infection Any known contributing or initiating causes, such as stress Small quantities voided (50–100 mL)
Urgency (feeling that voiding must occur immediately)	Presence of psychological stress Urinary tract infection
Dysuria (painful or difficult urination)	Urinary tract inflammation, infection, or injury Presence of other signs that may accompany dysuria, such as hesitancy, hematuria, pyuria (pus in the urine), and frequency. Burning may accompany or follow voiding
Enuresis (involuntary discharge of urine after voluntary control has normally been reached)	Family history of enuresis Difficult access to toilet facilities Home stresses
Incontinence (inability to control excretion)	Bladder inflammation or other disease Difficulties in independent toileting (mobility impairment) Leakage when coughing, laughing, sneezing Cognitive impairment
Retention	Distended bladder on palpation and percussion Associated signs, such as pubic discomfort, restlessness, frequency, and small urine volume Recent anesthesia Recent perineal surgery Presence of perineal swelling Medications prescribed Lack of privacy or other factors inhibiting micturition
Neurogenic bladder (dysfunction of nerves supplying the bladder)	Lesions of the central nervous system or of nerves supplying the bladder

◆ Maintaining or restoring normal voiding pattern
◆ Regaining normal urine output
◆ Preventing associated risks such as infection, skin breakdown, fluid and electrolyte imbalance, and lowered self-esteem

Measuring Urinary Output

Normally, the kidneys produce urine at a rate of approximately 60 mL per hour or about 1,500 mL per day. Urine output is affected by many factors, including fluid intake, body fluid losses through other routes such as perspiration and breathing, and the cardiovascular and renal status of the individual.

Urine outputs below 30 mL per hour may indicate low blood volume or kidney malfunction and must be reported.

To measure fluid output the nurse follows these steps:

1. Wear clean gloves to prevent contact with body fluids.
2. Ask the client to void in a clean urinal, bedpan, commode, or toilet collection device ("hat").

TABLE 18-3	CHARACTERISTICS OF NORMAL AND ABNORMAL URINE		
CHARACTERISTIC	NORMAL	ABNORMAL	NURSING CONSIDERATIONS
Amount in 24 hours (adult)	1,200–1,500 mL	< 1,200 mL > 1,500 mL	Urinary output normally is approximately equal to fluid intake. Output of < 30 mL/hr may indicate decreased blood flow to the kidneys and should be immediately reported.
Color, clarity	Straw, amber Transparent	Dark amber Cloudy Dark orange Red or dark brown Mucus plugs, viscid, thick	Concentrated urine is darker in color. Dilute urine may appear almost clear, or very pale yellow. Some foods and drugs may color urine (e.g., beets, carrots, phenazopyridine, phenytoin). Red blood cells in the urine (hematuria) may be evident as pink, bright red, or rusty brown urine. Menstrual bleeding can also color urine but should not be confused with hematuria. White blood cells, bacteria, pus, or contaminants such as prostatic fluid, sperm, or vaginal drainage may cause cloudy urine.
Odor	Faint aromatic	Offensive	Some foods (e.g., asparagus) cause a musty odor; infected urine can have a fetid odor; urine high in glucose has a sweet odor.
Sterility	No micro-organisms present	Microorganisms present	Urine specimens may be contaminated by bacteria from the perineum during collection.
pH	4.5–8	< 4.5 > 8	Freshly voided urine is normally somewhat acidic. Alkaline urine may indicate a state of alkalosis, urinary tract infection, or a diet high in fruits and vegetables. More acidic urine (low pH) is found in acidosis, starvation, diarrhea, or with a diet high in protein foods or cranberries.
Specific gravity	1.010–1.025	< 1.010 > 1.025	Concentrated urine has a higher specific gravity; diluted urine has a lower specific gravity.
Glucose	Not present	Present	Glucose in the urine indicates high blood glucose levels (> 180 mg/dL), and may be indicative of undiagnosed or uncontrolled diabetes mellitus.
Ketone bodies (acetone)	Not present	Present	Ketones, the end product of the breakdown of fatty acids, are not normally present in the urine. They may be present in the urine of clients who have uncontrolled diabetes mellitus, are in a state of starvation, or who have ingested excessive amounts of aspirin.
Blood	Not present	Occult (microscopic) Bright red	Blood may be present in the urine of clients who have urinary tract infection, kidney disease, or bleeding from the urinary tract.

3. Instruct the client to keep urine separate from feces and to avoid putting toilet paper in the urine collection container.
4. Pour the voided urine into a calibrated container.
5. Holding the container at eye level, read the amount in the container.
6. If a specimen is required, pour some urine into the specimen container and discard the remainder, unless all urine is to be saved.
7. Record the amount on the fluid intake and output sheet, which may be at the client's bedside or in the bathroom.

8. Rinse the urine collection and measuring containers with cool water and store.
9. Remove gloves and wash hands.
10. Calculate and document the total output at the end of each shift and at the end of 24 hours on the client's chart.

Many clients can measure and record their own urine output when the procedure is explained to them.

When measuring urine from a client who has an indwelling catheter, the nurse follows these steps:

1. Wear clean gloves.
2. Take the calibrated container to the bedside.

3. Place the container under the urine collection bag so that the spout of the bag is above the container but not touching it. The calibrated container *is not* sterile. The inside of the collection bag *is* sterile.
4. Open the spout and permit the urine to flow into the container.
5. Close the spout, then proceed as described in the previous list.

Measuring Residual Urine

Residual urine (urine remaining in the bladder following the voiding) is normally not present or consists of only a few milliliters. A bladder outlet obstruction or loss of bladder muscle tone may interfere with complete emptying of the bladder during urination. Manifestations of urine retention may include frequent voiding of small amounts (e.g., less than 100 mL in an adult). Urinary stasis and urinary tract infection are possible consequences of incomplete bladder emptying. Residual urine is measured to assess the amount of retained urine after voiding and determine the need for interventions.

To measure residual urine, the nurse catheterizes the client immediately after voiding. The amount of urine voided and the amount obtained by catheterization are measured and recorded. An indwelling catheter may be inserted if the residual urine exceeds a specified amount.

Collecting Urine Specimens

The nurse is responsible for collecting urine specimens for a number of tests: clean voided specimens for routine urinalysis, clean-catch or midstream urine specimens for urine culture, and timed urine specimens for a variety of tests, depending on the client's specific health problem.

Clean Voided Specimen. Many clients are able to collect a clean voided specimen and provide the specimen independently with minimal instruction. Male clients generally are able to void directly into the specimen container. Female clients usually sit or squat over the toilet, holding the container between their legs during voiding. About 120 mL (4 oz) of urine is generally required for this specimen. Clients who are seriously ill, physically incapacitated, or disoriented may need to use a bedpan or urinal in bed; others may require supervision or assistance in the bathroom. Whatever the situation, explicit directions are required:

- Keep the specimen free of fecal contamination.
- Female clients should discard the toilet tissue in the toilet or in a waste bag rather than in the bedpan.
- Tighten the lid on the container to prevent spillage and contamination of other objects.

The nurse must make certain that the specimen label and the laboratory requisition contain the correct information and are securely attached to the specimen. Incorrect identification of the specimen can lead to errors in diagnosis or treatment.

Clean-Catch or Midstream Specimen. Clean-catch or midstream voided specimens are collected when urine culture is ordered to identify microorganisms causing urinary tract infection. In these specimens, the client allows some passage of urine to clear the urethra, then collects the specimen in the middle of the urinary flow (hence, the term **midstream**). Although some contamination by skin bacteria may occur with a clean-catch specimen, the risk of introducing microorganisms into the urinary tract through catheterization is more significant. Care is taken to ensure that the specimen is as free as possible from contamination by microorganisms around the urinary meatus. Clean-catch specimens are collected into a sterile specimen container with a lid. Disposable clean-catch kits are available (Figure 18-5 ◆). Procedure 18-1 explains how to collect a clean-catch urine specimen.

Timed Urine Specimen. Some urine examinations require collection of all urine produced and voided over a specific period of time, ranging from 1 to 2 hours to 24 hours. Timed specimens are generally refrigerated or contain a preservative to prevent bacterial growth or decomposition of urine components. To collect a timed urine specimen, follow these steps:

1. Obtain a specimen container with preservative (if indicated) from the laboratory. Label the container with identifying information for the client, the test to be performed, time started, and time of completion.
2. Provide a clean receptacle to collect urine (bedpan, commode, or toilet collection device).
3. Post signs in the client's chart, Kardex, room, and bathroom alerting personnel to save all urine during the specified time.
4. At the start of the collection period, have the client void and discard this urine.
5. Save all urine produced during the timed collection period in the container, refrigerating or placing the container on ice as indicated. Avoid contaminating the urine with toilet paper or feces.
6. At the end of the collection period, instruct the client to empty the bladder completely and save this voiding as part of the specimen. Take the entire amount of urine collected to the laboratory with the completed requisition.
7. Record collection of the specimen, time started and completed, and any pertinent observations of the urine on appropriate records.

Figure 18-5. ◆ Disposable clean-catch specimen equipment. Source: © Jenny Thomas.

MediaLink ◆ Intake and Output Chart

Indwelling Catheter Specimen. Sterile urine specimens can be obtained from closed drainage systems by inserting a sterile needle attached to a syringe through a drainage port in the tubing. Aspiration of urine from catheters can be done only with self-sealing rubber catheters. When self-sealing rubber catheters are used, the needle is inserted just above the place where the catheter is attached to the drainage tubing.

To collect a specimen from a Foley (retention) catheter or a drainage tube, follow these steps:

1. Wash hands.
2. Wear disposable gloves.
3. If there is no urine in the catheter, clamp the drainage tubing for about 30 minutes. This allows fresh urine to collect in the catheter.
4. Wipe the area where the needle will be inserted with a disinfectant swab. The site should be distal to the tube leading to the balloon to avoid puncturing this tube. Disinfecting the needle insertion site removes any microorganisms on the surface of the catheter.
5. Insert the needle at a 30- to 45-degree angle (Figure 18-6 ◆). This angle of entrance facilitates self-sealing of the rubber.
6. Unclamp the catheter.
7. Withdraw the required amount of urine, for example, 3 mL for a urine culture or 30 mL for a routine urinalysis.
8. Transfer the urine to the specimen container. Make sure the needle does not touch the outside of the container if a sterile culture tube is used.
9. Without recapping the needle, discard the syringe and needle in an appropriate sharps container.
10. Cap the container.
11. Remove gloves and discard appropriately and wash hands.
12. Label the container, and send the urine to the laboratory immediately for analysis or refrigeration.
13. Record collection of the specimen and any pertinent observations of the urine on the appropriate records.

Urine Testing

Several basic urine tests are often performed by nurses on the nursing units. These include tests for specific gravity, pH, and the presence of abnormal constituents such as glucose, ketones, protein, and occult blood.

Specific Gravity. The **specific gravity** of urine is a measure of its concentration, or the amount of solutes present in the urine. A urinometer or hydrometer in a cylinder of urine (Figure 18-7 ◆) or a spectrometer or refractometer may be used to measure the specific gravity. The specific gravity of distilled water is 1.000. The specific gravity of urine normally ranges from 1.010 to 1.025. As urine becomes more concentrated, its specific gravity increases. Excess fluid intake or diseases affecting the ability of the kidneys to concentrate urine can result in low specific gravity readings. A high specific gravity may indicate fluid deficit or dehydration. Steps to measure specific gravity are outlined in Box 18-1 ◆.

Urinary pH. Urinary pH is measured to determine the relative acidity or alkalinity of urine and to assess the client's acid–base status. Quantitative measurement of urine pH is performed in the laboratory, but dipsticks or litmus paper often are used on nursing units or in clinics to obtain less precise pH measurements. Urine normally is slightly acidic, with an average pH of 6 (7 is neutral, less than 7 is acidic, greater than 7 is alkaline).

Glucose. Urine is tested for glucose to screen clients for diabetes mellitus and to assess clients for abnormal glucose tolerance during pregnancy. The amount of glucose in the urine is negligible in all healthy individuals.

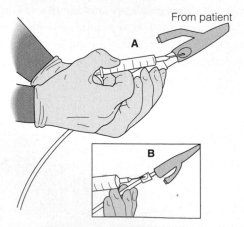

Figure 18-6. ◆ Obtaining a urine specimen from a retention catheter: **A.** From a specific area near the end of the catheter: **B.** From an access port in the tubing.

Figure 18-7. ◆ A urinometer measurement of the specific gravity of the urine is taken at the base of the meniscus.

MEASURING SPECIFIC GRAVITY OF URINE

To Measure with a Urinometer

☑ Wear gloves and pour at least 20 mL of a fresh urine sample into the glass cylinder, or fill the cylinder three-quarters full.

☑ Place the urinometer into the cylinder and give it a gentle spin to prevent it from adhering to the sides of the cylinder.

☑ Hold the urinometer at eye level and read the measurement at the base of the meniscus at the surface of the urine (see Figure 18-7). The depth to which it sinks indicates the specific gravity.

To Measure with a Spectrometer or Refractometer

☑ Be sure to follow the manufacturer's directions.

☑ Don gloves, and place one or two drops of urine on the slide.

☑ Turn on the instrument light, and look into the instrument. The specific gravity will appear on a scope.

☑ Write down the number, then turn off the instrument.

☑ Remove the urine with a damp towel or gauze.

Following the Test

☑ Discard the urine. Clean the equipment with soap and water. Remove gloves.

☑ Document the results of the test on the client's record.

Ketones. *Ketone bodies,* products of the breakdown of fatty acids, normally are not present in the urine but are found in urine of clients with poorly controlled diabetes. Urine ketone testing with reagent tablets or a dipstick also is used to evaluate ketoacidosis in clients who are alcoholic, fasting, starving, or consuming high-protein diets.

Protein. Protein molecules normally are too large to escape from glomerular capillaries into the filtrate. If the glomerular membrane has been damaged, proteins are allowed to escape. Urine testing for the presence of protein generally is done with a reagent strip (dipstick).

Occult Blood. Normal urine is free from blood. When blood is present, it may be clearly visible or not visible (*occult*). Commercial reagent strips are used to test for occult blood in the urine.

Maintaining Normal Urinary Elimination

Most interventions to maintain normal urinary elimination are independent nursing functions. These include promoting adequate fluid intake, maintaining normal voiding habits, and assisting with toileting.

Promoting Fluid Intake. Increasing fluid intake increases urine production, which in turn stimulates the micturition reflex. A normal daily intake averaging 1,500 mL of measurable fluids is adequate for most adult clients.

Many clients have increased fluid requirements, necessitating a higher daily fluid intake. For example, clients who are perspiring excessively (have diaphoresis) or who are experiencing abnormal fluid losses through vomiting, gastric suction, diarrhea, or wound drainage require fluid to replace these losses in addition to their normal daily intake requirements.

Clients who are at risk for urinary tract infection or urinary calculi (stones) should consume 2,000 to 3,000 mL of fluid daily. Dilute urine and frequent urination reduce the risk of urinary tract infection as well as stone formation.

Increased fluid intake may be contraindicated for some clients such as people with kidney failure or heart failure. For these clients, a fluid restriction may be necessary to prevent fluid overload and edema.

Maintaining Normal Voiding Habits. Medical therapies often interfere with a client's normal voiding habits. When a client's urinary elimination pattern is adequate, the nurse helps the client adhere to normal voiding habits as much as possible. Guidelines for assisting clients who are confined to bed to maintain normal voiding habits are listed in Box 18-2 ◆.

Assisting with Toileting. Clients who are weakened by a disease process or are physically impaired require assistance to toilet. The nurse should assist these clients to the bathroom and remain with them if the client is at risk for falling. The bathroom should contain an easily accessible call signal to summon help if needed. Clients also need to be encouraged to use handrails placed near the toilet.

For clients unable to use bathroom facilities, the nurse positions urinary equipment close to the bedside (e.g., urinal, bedpan, commode) and provides the necessary assistance. (See Chapters 13 and 20. 🔗)

Preventing Urinary Tract Infections

The rate of *urinary tract infection (UTI)* in women is about 20 percent yearly compared with a rate of 0.1 percent in men. UTI accounts for 40 percent of all nosocomial infections. Most UTIs are caused by bacteria common to the intestinal environment (e.g., *Escherichia coli*). Women are particularly at risk because of the short urethra and its proximity to the anal and vaginal areas. Nurses provide information and instruction in hygiene and diet to help prevent recurrences of UTI.

Managing Urinary Incontinence

It is important to remember that urinary **incontinence** (inability to control excretion) is not a normal part of aging and often is treatable. Independent nursing interventions for clients with urinary incontinence (UI) include a behavior-oriented

---

BOX 18-2
NURSING CARE CHECKLIST

MAINTAINING NORMAL VOIDING HABITS

Positioning

☑ Assist the client to a normal position for voiding: standing for males; for females, squatting or leaning slightly forward when sitting. These positions enhance movement of urine through the tract by gravity.

☑ If the client is unable to ambulate to the lavatory, use a bedside commode for females and a urinal for males standing at the bedside.

☑ If necessary, encourage the client to push over the pubic area with the hands or to lean forward to increase intra-abdominal pressure and external pressure on the bladder.

Relaxation

☑ Provide privacy for the client. Many people cannot void in the presence of another person.

☑ Allow the client sufficient time to void.

☑ Suggest that the client read or listen to music.

☑ Provide sensory stimuli that may help the client relax.

☑ Pour warm water over the perineum of a female or have the client sit in a warm bath to promote muscle relaxation.

☑ Applying a hot water bottle to the lower abdomen of both men and women may also foster muscle relaxation.

☑ Turn on running water within hearing distance of the client to stimulate the voiding reflex and to mask the sound of voiding for people who find this embarrassing.

☑ Provide ordered analgesics and emotional support to relieve physical and emotional discomfort to decrease muscle tension.

Timing

☑ Assist clients who have the urge to void immediately. Delays only increase the difficulty in starting to void, and the desire to void may pass.

☑ Offer toileting assistance to the client at usual times of voiding, for example, on awakening, before or after meals, and at bedtime.

For Bed-Confined Clients

☑ Warm the bedpan. A cold bedpan may prompt contraction of the perineal muscles and inhibit voiding.

☑ Elevate the head of the client's bed to Fowler's position, place a small pillow or rolled towel at the small of the back to increase physical support and comfort, and have the client flex the hips and knees. This position simulates the normal voiding position as closely as possible.

---

continence training program, prompted voiding, pelvic muscle exercises, positive reinforcement, meticulous skin care, and, for males, application of an external drainage device (condom).

Continence (Bladder) Training. A continence training program requires the involvement of the nurse, the client, and support people. Clients must be alert and physically able to follow a program. The goal of training is to decrease the frequency of UI. A bladder training program may include the following:

◆ Education of the client and support staff.
◆ Bladder training (Box 18-3 ◆), which requires that the client postpone voiding, resist or inhibit the sensation of urgency, and void according to a timetable rather than according to the urge to void.
◆ Delayed voiding provides larger voided volumes and longer intervals between voiding.

Pelvic Muscle Exercises. Pelvic muscle exercises, referred to as Kegel exercises, strengthen pelvic floor muscles in women and can reduce episodes of incontinence. The client can identify perineal muscles by stopping urination midstream or by

tightening the anal sphincter as if to hold a bowel movement. Kegel exercises can be performed anytime, anywhere, sitting or standing—even when voiding.

Maintaining Skin Integrity

Skin that is continually moist becomes *macerated* (softened by soaking). Urine that accumulates on the skin is converted to ammonia, which is very irritating to the skin. Because both skin irritation and maceration predispose the client to skin breakdown and ulceration, the incontinent person requires meticulous skin care. To maintain skin integrity, the nurse washes the client's perineal area with a mild soap and water, rinses it thoroughly, dries it, and provides clean, dry clothing or bed linen. If the skin is irritated, the nurse applies a barrier cream. If it is necessary to pad the client's clothes for protection, the nurse should use products that absorb wetness and leave a dry surface in contact with the skin.

Applying External Urinary Drainage Devices

The application of a condom or external catheter connected to a urinary drainage system is commonly prescribed for inconti-

MediaLink ● Catheter

BOX 18-3
NURSING CARE CHECKLIST

BLADDER TRAINING

☑ Determine the client's voiding pattern and encourage voiding at those times, or establish a regular voiding schedule and help the client to maintain it, whether the client feels the urge or not. The stretching–relaxing sequence of such a schedule tends to increase bladder muscle tone and promote more voluntary control.

☑ Encourage the client to inhibit the urge-to-void sensation when a premature urge to void is experienced.

☑ Instruct the client to practice slow, deep breathing until the urge diminishes or disappears.

☑ When the client finds that voiding can be controlled, the intervals between voiding can be lengthened slightly without loss of continence.

☑ Regulate fluid intake, particularly during evening hours, to help reduce the need to void during the night.

☑ Encourage fluids about half an hour before the voiding time between the hours of 0600 and 1800.

☑ Avoid excessive consumption of citrus juices, carbonated beverages (especially those containing artificial sweeteners), alcohol, and drinks containing caffeine. These irritate the bladder, increasing the risk of incontinence.

☑ Schedule diuretics early in the morning.

☑ Explain to clients that adequate fluid intake is required to ensure adequate urine production to stimulate the micturition reflex.

☑ Apply protector pads to keep the bed linen dry, and provide specially made waterproof underwear to contain the urine and decrease the client's embarrassment.

☑ Assist the client with an exercise program to increase the tone of abdominal and pelvic muscles.

☑ Provide positive reinforcements to encourage continence.

nent males. Use of a condom appliance is preferable to insertion of a retention catheter because the risk of urinary tract infection is minimal.

Methods of applying condoms vary according to how long the condom is worn. Condoms that are worn for a short period are generally applied with elastic tape only. If, however, the condom is to be worn for a longer period (e.g., a few days), additional measures are required to protect the foreskin and to ensure secure attachment. Procedure 18-2 describes how to apply and remove a drainage condom.

Managing Urinary Retention

Interventions that assist the client to maintain a normal voiding pattern, discussed earlier, also apply to urinary retention.

If these actions (described above) are unsuccessful, the physician may order a cholinergic drug such as bethanechol chloride (Urecholine) to stimulate bladder contraction and facilitate voiding. When all measures fail to initiate voiding, urinary catheterization may be necessary to empty the bladder completely. An indwelling Foley catheter may be inserted until the underlying cause is treated. Intermittent straight catheterization (every 3 to 4 hours) may be performed as an alternative because the risk of urinary tract infection is believed by some to be less than with an indwelling catheter.

Urinary Catheterization

Urinary **catheterization** is the introduction of a catheter through the urethra into the urinary bladder. It is usually performed only when absolutely necessary. The urinary structures are normally sterile except at the end of the urethra, the danger exists of introducing microorganisms into the bladder. Once an infection is introduced into the bladder, it can ascend the ureters and eventually involve the kidneys. Thus, strict sterile technique is used for catheterization. Ongoing assessment of clients with retention catheters is a high priority. Box 18-4 ◆ provides guidelines to prevent catheter-associated urinary infections.

Another hazard is trauma, particularly in the male client, whose urethra is longer and more tortuous. It is important to insert a catheter along the normal contour of the urethra. Damage to the urethra can occur if the catheter is forced through strictures or at an incorrect angle.

Catheters are commonly made of rubber or plastics although they may be made from latex or silicone. They are sized by the diameter of the lumen, using the French (Fr) scale: the larger the number, the larger the lumen. Straight catheters are inserted to drain the bladder and then immedi-

BOX 18-4
NURSING CARE CHECKLIST

PREVENTING CATHETER-ASSOCIATED URINARY INFECTIONS

☑ Have an established infection control program.

☑ Catheterize clients only when necessary, by using aseptic technique, sterile equipment, and trained personnel.

☑ Maintain a sterile closed-drainage system.

☑ Do not disconnect the catheter and drainage tubing unless absolutely necessary.

☑ Remove the catheter as soon as possible.

☑ Follow and reinforce good hand-washing technique.

☑ Provide routine perineal hygiene, including cleansing with soap and water after defecation. Prevent contamination of the catheter with feces in the incontinent client.

6.

7.

8.
9.
10.

11.

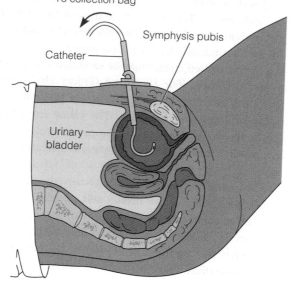

To collection bag

Symphysis pubis

Catheter

Urinary
bladder

Figure 18-14. ◆ Suprapubic catheter in place.

Care of the catheter insertion site involves sterile technique. Dressings around the suprapubic catheter are changed whenever they are soiled with drainage to prevent bacterial growth and reduce the potential for infection. Procedures for cleaning wounds and changing dressings are discussed in Chapter 12. ⚭ Any redness and discharge around the insertion site must be reported.

 EVALUATING

Using the overall goals and desired outcomes identified in the planning stage, the nurse collects data to evaluate such things as skin integrity, risk for infection, and client comfort. The nurse would also collect data about fluid and electrolyte balance.

 DISCHARGE CONSIDERATIONS

UTI can be a recurrent problem for many women. The nurse plays an important role in teaching measures to prevent UTI. Guidelines for nurses to share are listed in Box 18-8 ◆. Although these instructions are especially important for women who have already experienced a UTI, they are useful for anyone.

Nursing Process Case Study:
CLIENT WITH ABDOMINAL INJURY

Mrs. Kennedy, 48, is recovering from an automobile accident in which she sustained blunt trauma to her abdomen. She has

BOX 18-8

TEACHING FOR DISCHARGE

PREVENTING UTIs IN WOMEN
◆ Drink eight 8-ounce glasses of water per day.
◆ Practice frequent voiding (every 2 to 4 hours) to flush bacteria out and prevent organisms from ascending into the bladder. Void immediately after intercourse.
◆ Avoid use of harsh soaps, bubble bath, powder, or sprays in the perineal area.
◆ Avoid tight-fitting pants or other clothing that creates irritation to the urethra and prevents ventilation of the perineal area.
◆ Wear cotton rather than nylon underclothes. Accumulation of perineal moisture facilitates bacterial growth, and cotton enhances ventilation of the perineal area.
◆ Girls and women should always wipe the perineal area from front to back following urination or defecation.
◆ If recurrent UTIs are a problem, take showers rather than baths.
◆ Increase the acidity of urine through regular intake of vitamin C and drinking two to three glasses of cranberry juice daily or take cranberry tablets.

a mild concussion. An indwelling urinary catheter in place until she is able to communicate her need to urinate. Upon entering Mrs. Kennedy's room to collect a urine specimen ordered for culture and sensitivity, you note that Mrs. Kennedy is restless and moaning. Her abdominal dressing is dry and intact and her urinary bag contains about 200 mL of golden-colored urine. Her abdomen is tender and distended. When questioned, Mrs. Kennedy is able to communicate that she is in pain but is unable to communicate the specifics of her pain.

Assessment. VS: T 99.6°F, radial pulse 86, R 24. BP 130/90. WBC is 15,000. Her catheter is patent and urine is clear, amber colored. IV is infusing with D_5W at 75 mL/hr. She has an abdominal incision that is clean and dry, no redness noted.

Diagnosis
◆ Pain
◆ Impaired Skin Integrity
◆ Impaired Urinary Elimination
◆ Anxiety
◆ Impaired Verbal Communication
◆ Risk for Infection

Expected Outcomes
◆ Pain is controlled
◆ Skin integrity effectively managed
◆ Urinary output within normal limits
◆ Client informed about procedures

- Body language assessed for communication
- Wound and catheter maintained without evidence of infection

Planning and Implementation.

- Implement pain control measures
- Monitor and document wound healing
- Maintain and measure urinary output
- Instruct client regarding procedures
- Observe for body language communication
- Monitor for signs and symptoms of infection
- Maintain catheter care

Evaluating. Mrs. Kennedy will remain in the hospital for a week to determine the status of her concussion and results of tests. Her abdominal incision is approximated and healing without signs of infection. She is able to communicate her level of pain on a pain scale. Urinary output is adequate and is a clear straw color. The urinary C&S was positive for organisms and treated with antibiotics. She is ambulating with assistance.

Critical Thinking in the Nursing Process

1. What precautions should be taken when collecting a urine sample from a person with an indwelling urinary catheter and why?
2. What measures can be taken to prevent Mrs. Kennedy from developing a UTI if one is not already present?

Note: The bibliography listings for this and all chapters have been compiled at the back of the book.

PROCEDURE 18-1

Collecting a Urine Specimen for Culture and Sensitivity by Clean Catch

PURPOSE

◆ To determine the presence of microorganisms, the type of organism(s), and the antibiotics to which the organisms are sensitive

EQUIPMENT

◆ Disposable or sterile gloves
◆ Antiseptic towelette, such as povidone–iodine
◆ Sterile cotton balls or 2 × 2 gauze pads
◆ Sterile specimen container
◆ Specimen identification label
◆ Completed laboratory requisition form
◆ Urine receptacle, if the client is not ambulatory
◆ Basin of warm water, soap, washcloth, and towel for the nonambulatory client

INTERVENTIONS

1. Instruct and assist the client appropriately.
   ◆ Inform the client that a urine specimen is required; give the reason, and explain the method to be used to collect it.

2. For an ambulatory client who is able to follow directions, instruct the client how to collect the specimen.
   ◆ Direct or assist the client to the bathroom. Ask the client to wash and dry the genital and perineal area with soap and water. *This removes microorganisms that could contaminate the specimen.*
   ◆ Instruct the client how to clean the urinary meatus with antiseptic towelettes.

FOR FEMALE CLIENTS
   ◆ Use each towelette only once. Clean the perineal area from front to back, and discard the towelette. Use all towelettes provided (usually two or three). *Cleaning from front to back cleans the area of least contamination to the area of greatest contamination.*

FOR MALE CLIENTS
   ◆ If uncircumcised, retract the foreskin slightly to expose the urinary meatus.
   ◆ Using a circular motion, clean the urinary meatus and the distal portion of the penis. Use each towelette only once, then discard. Clean several inches down the shaft of the penis. *This cleans from the area of least contamination to the area of greatest contamination.*

3. For a client who requires assistance, prepare the client and equipment.

◆ Wash the perineal area with soap and water; rinse and dry. Assist the client onto a clean commode or bedpan. If using a bedpan or urinal, position the client as upright as allowed or tolerated.
◆ Open the clean-catch kit, taking care not to contaminate the inside of the specimen container or lid.
◆ Wear clean gloves.
◆ Clean the urinary meatus and perineal area as described in step 2.

4. Collect the specimen from a nonambulatory client or instruct an ambulatory client how to collect it.
   ◆ Instruct the client to start voiding. *Bacteria in the distal urethra and at the urinary meatus are cleared by the first few milliliters of urine expelled.*
   ◆ Place the specimen container into the stream of urine and collect the specimen, taking care not to touch the container to the perineum or penis. Avoid contaminating the interior of the specimen container and the specimen itself.
   ◆ Collect 30 to 60 mL of urine in the container.
   ◆ Cap the container tightly, touching only the outside of the container and the cap (see Figure 18-5).
   ◆ If necessary, clean the outside of the specimen container with disinfectant.
   ◆ Remove gloves if handling another person's urine. Wash hands. *This prevents the spread of infection.*

5. Label the specimen and transport it to the laboratory.
   ◆ Ensure that the specimen label and the laboratory requisition carry the correct information. Attach them

securely to the specimen. *This prevents errors from occurring and ensures good continuity of care.*

- ◆ Arrange for the specimen to be sent to the laboratory immediately. *Bacterial cultures must be started immediately, before any contaminating organisms can grow, multiply, and produce false results.*

6. Document pertinent data.

- ◆ Record collection of the specimen, any pertinent observations of the urine in terms of color, odor, or consistency, and any difficulty in voiding that the client experienced.

◆ SAMPLE DOCUMENTATION

4/12/05	Urine C+S to lab. Urine straw colored,
1200	clear and free from odor. No abnormal
	constituents noted. Client voided freely
	without complaints of difficulty.
	D. Haus LVN

PROCEDURE 18-2
Applying a Condom Catheter

PURPOSES

- ◆ To collect urine and control urinary incontinence
- ◆ To permit the client physical activity without fear of embarrassment because of leaking urine
- ◆ To prevent skin irritation as a result of urine incontinence

EQUIPMENT

- ◆ Leg drainage bag with tubing or urinary drainage bag with tubing
- ◆ Condom sheath
- ◆ Bath blanket
- ◆ Disposable gloves
- ◆ Basin of warm water and soap
- ◆ Washcloth and towel
- ◆ Elastic tape or Velcro strap

INTERVENTIONS

1. Prepare the equipment.

- ◆ Assemble the leg drainage bag or urinary drainage bag for attachment to the condom sheath.
- ◆ Roll the condom outward onto itself to facilitate easier application. *On some models an inner flap will be exposed. This flap is applied around the urinary meatus to prevent the reflux of urine (Figure 18-15 ◆).*

2. Position and drape the client.

- ◆ Position the client in either a supine or a bed-sitting position.
- ◆ Drape the client appropriately with the bath blanket, exposing only the penis. *This provides privacy and comfort.*

3. Inspect and clean the penis.

- ◆ Don gloves.
- ◆ Inspect the penis for skin irritation (contact dermatitis), excoriation, swelling, or discoloration. *The nurse needs to obtain baseline data for use later.*

Figure 18-15. ◆ Before application, roll the condom outward onto itself.

◆ Clean the genital area, and dry it thoroughly. *This minimizes skin irritation and excoriation after the condom is applied.*

4. Apply and secure the condom.
   ◆ Roll the condom smoothly over the penis, leaving 2.5 cm (1 inch) between the end of the penis and the rubber or plastic connecting tube (Figure 18-16 ◆). *This space prevents irritation of the tip of the penis and provides for full drainage of urine.*
   ◆ Secure the condom firmly, but not too tightly, to the penis by wrapping a strip of elastic tape or Velcro around the base of the penis over the condom. *The elastic or Velcro strip should not come in contact with the skin and should hold the condom in place without impeding blood circulation to the penis.*

5. Securely attach the urinary drainage system.
   ◆ Make sure that the tip of the penis is not touching the condom and that the condom is not twisted. *A twisted condom could obstruct the flow of urine.*
   ◆ Attach the urinary drainage system to the condom.
   ◆ Remove gloves.
   ◆ If the client is to remain in bed, attach the urinary drainage bag to the bed frame.
   ◆ If the client is ambulatory, attach the bag to the client's leg (Figure 18-17 ◆). *Attaching the drainage bag to the leg helps control the movement of the tubing and prevents twisting of the thin material of the condom appliance at the tip of the penis.*

Figure 18-16. ◆ Rolling the condom over the penis.

Figure 18-17. ◆ Attaching the urinary drainage bag to the leg.

6. Teach the client about the drainage system.
   ◆ Instruct the client to keep the drainage bag below the level of the condom and to avoid loops or kinks in the tubing.

7. Document pertinent data.
   ◆ Record the application of the condom, the time, and pertinent observations, such as irritated areas on the penis.

8. Inspect the penis 30 minutes following the condom application, and check urine flow.
   ◆ Assess the penis for swelling and discoloration. *These indicate that the condom is too tight.*

9. Change the condom daily, and provide skin care.
   ◆ Remove the elastic or Velcro strip and roll off the condom.
   ◆ Wash the penis with soapy water, rinse, and dry it thoroughly.
   ◆ Assess the foreskin for signs of irritation, swelling, and discoloration.

◆ **SAMPLE DOCUMENTATION**

7/17/04	Condom catheter applied and attached
1430	to gravity drainage. Client tolerated
	procedure well, no complaints of pain.
	Urine clear, straw colored. ———————
	D Haus LVN

PROCEDURE 18-3

Female Urinary Catheterization Using a Straight Catheter

PURPOSES

- To relieve discomfort due to bladder distention or to provide gradual decompression of a distended bladder
- To assess the amount of residual urine if the bladder empties incompletely
- To obtain a urine specimen
- To empty the bladder completely prior to surgery

EQUIPMENT

- Flashlight or lamp
- Mask, if required by agency policy
- Bath blanket or drape
- Soap, a basin of warm water, a washcloth, and a towel
- Disposable gloves

- Bladder ultrasound device (optional)
- A sterile catheterization kit containing:
  Water-soluble lubricant
  Sterile gloves
  Sterile drapes, fenestrated drape (optional) to place over the perineum
  Antiseptic solution
  Cotton balls or gauze squares
  Forceps
  Basin for urine (base of kit can be used)
- Sterile catheter of appropriate size (e.g., for an adult #14 or #16 is often used)
- Specimen container as required
- Bag or receptacle for disposal of the cotton balls

INTERVENTIONS

1. Assess for urinary retention.
   - To palpate the bladder, indent the skin more than 1.3 cm (0.5 in) just above the pubic symphysis by pressing the fingers of one hand on the fingers of the other. *This increases the pressure for palpation.*

2. Prepare the client.
   - Explain the catheterization to the client, and provide privacy. *Exposure of the genitals is embarrassing to most clients. Some people fear that the procedure will be painful; explain that normally a catheterization is painless and that there may be a sensation of pressure.*
   - Assist the client to a supine position, with knees flexed and thighs externally rotated. Pillows can be used to support the knees and to elevate the buttocks. *Raising the client's pelvis gives the nurse a better view of the urinary meatus and reduces the risk of contaminating the catheter.*
   - Drape the client. *This maintains comfort and prevents unnecessary exposure.* Cover the client's chest and abdomen with a bath blanket. Pull the client's gown up over her hips. Cover her legs and feet as for perineal care.
   - Wear disposable gloves. *This prevents transmission of microorganisms.*
   - Wash the perineal–genital area with warm water and soap. *Cleaning reduces the number of microorganisms around the urinary meatus and the possibility of introducing microorganisms with the catheter.*

- Rinse and dry the area well. *Rinsing removes soap that could inhibit the action of the antiseptic if used later.*
- Remove disposable gloves.
- Obtain assistance if the client requires help in maintaining the required position. *The client must remain still throughout the procedure to maintain a clear view of the urinary meatus and prevent contamination of the sterile field.*

3. Prepare the equipment.
   - Adjust the light to view the urinary meatus. It may be necessary to use a flashlight or to place a gooseneck lamp at the foot of the bed.
   - Put on a mask, gown, and cap if required by agency policy.

4. Create a sterile field.
   - At the client's bedside, open a sterile kit and the catheter, if it is packaged separately, and put on the sterile gloves.
   - Drape the client with the sterile drape, being careful to protect its sterility and the sterility of your gloves. Place the drape under the buttocks while keeping the edges cuffed over your gloves. *This prevents contamination of the gloves against the client's buttocks.* If a fenestrated drape is provided, place it over the perineal area, exposing only the labia.
   - Place the sterile kit on the drape between the client's thighs. *This facilitates access to supplies.*
   - Pour the antiseptic solution over the cotton balls, if they are not already prepared and if meatal cleansing with an antiseptic is agency practice (see step 5).

◆ Lubricate the insertion tip of the catheter liberally, and place it in the sterile container ready for use. *Water-soluble lubricant facilitates insertion of the catheter by reducing friction. Lubrication is done at this point because the nurse will subsequently have only one sterile hand available.*

◆ Open the urine specimen container, and keep the top sterile. *This prepares the container for specimen collection.*

5. Clean the meatus with antiseptic (if recommended by agency).

◆ Check agency protocol about cleaning the meatus. *There is controversy regarding the value of meatal cleaning using antiseptics before catheterization.*

◆ Using the nondominant hand, separate the labia minora with your thumb and one finger or another two fingers. Expose the urinary meatus adequately by retracting the tissue of the labia minora in an upward (anterior) direction (Figure 18-18A ◆). Clean first from the meatus downward and then on either side, using a new swab for each stroke (Figure 18-18B). Once the meatus is cleaned, do not allow the labia to close over it. *Keeping the labia apart prevents the risk of contaminating the urinary meatus. Note: Your hand that touches the client becomes unsterile. It remains in position exposing the urinary meatus, while your other hand remains sterile holding the sterile forceps.*

6. Inspect the meatus.

◆ With the urinary meatus exposed (Figure 18-18A), assess any signs, such as excoriation of the tissues surrounding the urinary meatus, swelling of the urinary meatus, or the presence of discharge around the urinary meatus. *This assessment provides baseline data.* If any discharge is present, obtain a culture swab.

7. Insert the catheter until urine flows.

◆ Place the drainage end of the catheter in the urine receptacle. Pick up the insertion end of the catheter with your uncontaminated, sterile, gloved hand, holding it about 5 cm (2 inches) from the insertion tip. *Because the adult female urethra is approximately 1.5 inches long, the catheter is held far enough from the end to allow full insertion into the bladder and to maintain control of the tip of the catheter so it will not accidentally become contaminated.*

◆ Gently insert the catheter into the urinary meatus until urine flows. Insert the catheter in the direction of the urethra. If the catheter meets resistance during insertion, do not force it. *Forceful pressure against the urethra can produce trauma.* Ask the client to take deep breaths. *This helps relax the external sphincter.* If this does not relieve the resistance, discontinue the procedure and report the problem to the nurse in charge. Exercise caution to prevent the catheter tip from becoming contaminated. If it becomes contaminated, discard it.

◆ When the urine flows, transfer your hand from the labia to the catheter to hold it in place. *This prevents its expulsion by a possible bladder contraction.*

Labia majora
Clitoris
Urinary meatus (urethral orifice)
Vagina
Labia minora
Anus

A

B

Figure 18-18. ◆ **A.** To expose the urinary meatus, separate the labia minora and retract the tissue upward. **B.** When cleaning the urinary meatus, move the swab downward.

8. Collect a urine specimen.

◆ Pinch the catheter, and transfer the drainage end of it into the sterile specimen bottle. Usually, 30 mL of urine is sufficient for a specimen. Securely place the top on the specimen container, and set it aside for labeling later.

9. Empty or partially drain the bladder, and then remove the catheter.

◆ For adults experiencing urinary retention, some orders limit the amount of urine drained to 1,000 mL. *Limiting the amount of urine drained has been a controversial issue. Rapid removal of large amounts of urine was once thought to induce engorgement of the pelvic blood vessels and hypovolemic shock. However, retained urine may serve as a reservoir for microorganisms to multiply. Usually agency policy or the physician indicates the amount to be removed and times at which the remaining urine is to be withdrawn. Research findings support the premise that complete drainage of a distended bladder is likely to be more comfortable and certainly seems as safe as threshold clamping.*

◆ Pinch the catheter. *This prevents leakage of urine.* Remove the catheter slowly.

10. Promote client comfort.

◆ Dry the client's perineum with a towel or drape. *Excess lubricant and solution in the area can irritate the skin.*

11. Assess the urine.

◆ Inspect the urine for color, clarity, odor, and the presence of any abnormal constituents, such as blood. Measure the amount of urine.

12. Document the catheterization.

◆ Include assessments before and after the procedure, type and size of catheter inserted, time, characteristics and amount of urine obtained, whether a specimen was sent to the laboratory, and client response to the procedure.

◆ SAMPLE DOCUMENTATION

9/9/05	Urinary straight #14 catheter inserted,
1300	urine spontaneous 300 cc, clear and
	straw colored. Urinalysis and C+S to
	lab. Catheter removed. Client tolerated
	procedure well. ——————————
	D Haus LVN

PROCEDURE 18-4

Male Urinary Catheterization Using a Straight Catheter

PURPOSES

◆ To relieve discomfort due to bladder distention or to provide gradual decompression of a distended bladder

◆ To assess the amount of residual urine if the bladder empties incompletely

◆ To obtain a urine specimen

◆ To empty the bladder completely prior to surgery

EQUIPMENT

◆ See Procedure 18-3. A #16 or #18 catheter is often used for an adult male.

INTERVENTIONS

1. Assess for urinary retention.

◆ Palpate the bladder

2. Prepare the client.

◆ Explain the catheterization, as in Procedure 18-3. Assist the client to a supine position, with the knees slightly flexed and the thighs slightly apart. *This allows greater relaxation of the abdominal and perineal muscles and permits easier insertion of the catheter.*

◆ Drape the client by folding the top bedclothes down so that the penis is exposed and the thighs are covered. Use a bath blanket to cover the client's chest and abdomen.

◆ Wear disposable gloves.

◆ Wash the penis and dry it well.

◆ Remove disposable gloves.

3. Create a sterile field.

◆ Open the sterile tray, and don the sterile gloves.

◆ Place a drape under the penis and a second drape above the penis over the pubic area. If a fenestrated drape is available, place it over the penis and pubic area, exposing only the penis.

◆ Place the sterile kit on the sterile drape over the client's thighs or next to the thigh.

◆ Pour the antiseptic solution over the cotton balls, if they are not already prepared.

mL), and remove the syringe. A special valve prevents backflow of the fluid out of the catheter. Follow agency policy when using a 30-mL balloon. Some agency policies state that only 15 mL of fluid is injected for inflation.

5. Ensure effective balloon inflation.
   ◆ When the balloon is safely inflated, apply slight tension on the catheter until you feel resistance. *Resistance indicates that the catheter balloon is inflated appropriately and that the catheter is well anchored in the bladder.*
   ◆ Then move the catheter slightly back into the bladder. *This keeps the balloon from exerting undue pressure on the neck of the bladder.*

6. Anchor the catheter.
   ◆ Tape the catheter with nonallergenic tape to the inside of a female's thigh or to the thigh or abdomen of a male client (Figures 18-20A and B ◆). Some nurses prefer taping the male catheter to the abdomen whenever there is increased risk of excoriation at the penile–scrotal junction. *Taping restricts the movement of the catheter, thus reducing friction and irritation in the urethra when the client moves. It also prevents skin excoriation at the penile–scrotal junction in the male.*

7. Establish effective drainage.
   ◆ Ensure that the emptying base of the drainage bag is closed.
   ◆ Secure the drainage bag to the bed frame, using the hook or strap provided. Suspend the bag off the floor, but keep it below the level of the client's bladder (Figure 18-18). *Urine flows by gravity from the bladder to the drainage bag. The bag should be off the floor so that the emptying spout does not become grossly contaminated.*
   ◆ Coil the drainage tubing loosely beside the client, so that the remaining tubing runs in a straight line down to the drainage bag. Fasten the vertical tubing to the bedclothes with tape, a tubing clamp, or a safety pin and elastic band (see Figure 18-20). *The drainage tubing should not loop below its entry into the drainage bag, which would impede the flow of urine by gravity.*

8. Document pertinent data.
   ◆ Record the time and date of the catheterization; the type and size of catheter; the reason for catheterization; how much fluid was used to inflate the balloon; assessments before and after the procedure, including amount, color, and clarity of urine obtained; whether a specimen was taken and sent to the laboratory; whether all urine was emptied from the bladder; and the client's response.

A

A

Figure 18-20. ◆ **A.** Tape the catheter to the inside of a female's thigh. **B.** Tape the catheter to the thigh or abdomen of a male client.

◆ **SAMPLE DOCUMENTATION**

12/19/06	Retention catheter 16" inserted, 5cc
1300	balloon inflation. Urine spontaneous with
	300 cc, clear and straw colored.
	Client tolerated procedure well. ———
	Ⓓ Haus LVN

PROCEDURE 18-6

Irrigating a Catheter or Bladder (Closed System)

PURPOSES

◆ To maintain the patency of a urinary catheter and tubing (continuous irrigation)
◆ To free a blockage in a urinary catheter or tubing (intermittent irrigation)

EQUIPMENT

◆ Disposable gloves
◆ Disposable water-resistant sterile towel
◆ Three-way retention catheter in place
◆ Sterile drainage tubing and bag (if not in place)
◆ Sterile antiseptic swabs
◆ Sterile receptacle
◆ Sterile irrigating solution warmed or at room temperature
◆ Infusion tubing
◆ IV pole

INTERVENTIONS

1. Prepare the client.
   ◆ Explain the procedure and its purpose to the client.
   ◆ Provide for privacy and drape the client as needed to allow access to the retention catheter.
   ◆ Wear clean gloves.
     Empty, measure, and record the amount and appearance of urine present in the drainage bag. Discard urine and gloves. *Emptying the drainage bag allows more accurate measurement of urinary output after the irrigation is in place or completed. Assessing the character of the urine provides baseline data for later comparison.*

2. Prepare the equipment.
   ◆ Wash hands.
     Connect the irrigation infusion tubing to the irrigating solution and flush the tubing with solution.
     Connect the irrigation tubing to the input port of the three-way catheter. Connect the drainage bag and tubing to the urinary drainage port if not already in place.

3. Irrigate the bladder.
   a. For continuous irrigation, open the flow clamp on the urinary drainage tubing (if present). *This allows the irrigating solution to flow out of the bladder continuously.*
      ◆ Open the regulating clamp on the irrigating tubing and adjust the flow rate as prescribed by the physician or to 40 to 60 drops per minute if not specified. Assess the drainage for amount, color, and clarity. The amount of drainage should equal the amount of irrigant entering the bladder plus expected urine output.

   b. For intermittent irrigation, determine whether the solution is to remain in the bladder for a specified time.
      ◆ If the solution is to remain in the bladder (a bladder irrigation or instillation), close the flow clamp on the urinary drainage tubing. *Closing the flow clamp allows the solution to be retained in the bladder and in contact with bladder walls.*
      ◆ If the solution is being instilled to irrigate the catheter, open the flow clamp on the urinary drainage tubing. *Irrigating solution flow through the urinary drainage port and tubing, removing mucus shreds or clots.*
      ◆ Open the flow clamp on the irrigating tubing, allowing the specified amount of solution to infuse. Clamp the tubing.
      ◆ After the specified period the solution is to be retained, open the drainage tubing flow clamp and allow the bladder to empty.

4. Assess the client and the urinary output.
   ◆ Assess the client's comfort.
   ◆ Assess the amount, color, and clarity of drainage; note any abnormal constituents such as blood clots, pus, or mucus shreds.
   ◆ To document urine output, empty the drainage bag and measure the contents. Subtract the amount of irrigant instilled from the total volume of drainage to obtain urine output.

5. Document the irrigation.
   ◆ Include all assessments obtained before and after performing the irrigation.

VARIATION: CLOSED IRRIGATION USING A TWO-WAY INDWELLING CATHETER

1. Assemble the equipment, including:
- ♦ Clean disposable gloves
- ♦ Disposable water-resistant towel
- ♦ Sterile irrigating solution
- ♦ Sterile basin
- ♦ Sterile 30- to 50-mL syringe with an 18- or 19-gauge needle
- ♦ Sterile antiseptic swabs

2. Prepare the client (see step 1 of main procedure for catheter irrigation).

3. Prepare the equipment.
- ♦ Wash hands and wear gloves.
- ♦ Place the disposable water-resistant towel under the catheter.
- ♦ For a bladder irrigation or instillation, clamp the drainage tubing distal to the injection port on the tubing or catheter. *Clamping prevents the urine and solution from draining into the drainage bag.* For a catheter irrigation, leave the tubing unclamped.
- ♦ Using aseptic technique, open supplies and pour the irrigating solution into the sterile basin or receptacle. *Aseptic technique is vital to reduce the risk of instilling microorganisms into the urinary tract during the irrigation.*
- ♦ Remove the cap from the needle and draw the prescribed amount of irrigating solution into the syringe, maintaining the sterility of the syringe and solution. Using the antiseptic swab, clean the port on the catheter or drainage tubing through which the solution will be instilled.

4. Irrigate the bladder.
- ♦ Insert the needle into the port.
- ♦ Gently inject the solution into the catheter. In adults, about 30 to 40 mL generally is instilled for catheter irrigations; 100 to 200 mL may be instilled for bladder irrigation or instillation. Smaller amounts are used for children.
- ♦ When the total amount to be instilled has been injected (or for catheter irrigation, when urine is flowing freely), remove the needle from the port and discard the syringe and uncapped needle in an appropriate receptacle (sharps container).
- ♦ After the prescribed dwelling time for a bladder irrigation, remove the clamp from the drainage tubing and allow the urine and irrigating solution to drain into the drainage bag.
- ♦ Assess the drainage for amount, color, and clarity. *The amount of drainage should equal the amount of irrigant entering the bladder plus expected urine output.*

5. Assess the client and the urinary output and document the procedure as previously noted.

♦ SAMPLE DOCUMENTATION

8/8/04	Continuous bladder irrigation maintained.
0700	Occasional clots noted, urine output at
	700 cc this shift. Bladder nondistended
	and no complaints of discomfort. ———
	Ⓓ Haus LVN

Chapter Review

Key Terms by Topics

Use the audio glossary feature of either the CD-ROM or the Companion Website to hear the correct pronunciation of the following key terms.

Structure and function of the urinary system
meatus, micturition, voiding

Factors affecting urinary function
urinary retention, diuretics

Pathologic conditions
calculus, polyuria, diuresis, oliguria, anuria

Nursing care
residual urine, midstream urine, specific gravity, incontinence, catheterization, irrigation, urinary diversion

Key Points

* Urinary elimination depends on normal functioning of the urinary, cardiovascular, and nervous systems. Alterations in function have physical, social, and emotional effects.

* The normal process of urination is stimulated when sufficient urine collects in the bladder to stimulate stretch receptors.

* Alterations in urine production and elimination include polyuria, oliguria, anuria, frequency, nocturia, urgency, dysuria, enuresis, hematuria, incontinence, and retention.

* Assessment of a client's urinary function includes (a) normal voiding patterns, recent changes, past and current problems with urination, and factors influencing the elimination pattern; (b) a physical assessment of the genitourinary system; (c) inspection of the urine for amount, color, clarity, and odor; and, if indicated, (d) testing of urine for specific gravity, pH, and the presence of glucose, ketone bodies, protein, and occult blood.

* Bladder training can often reduce episodes of incontinence.

* Clients with urinary retention are at risk of urinary tract infection. Urinary catheterization is frequently required for clients with urinary retention.

* The most common cause of urinary tract infection is an invasive procedure such as catheterization or cystoscopic examination. Females in particular are prone to ascending urinary tract infections because of their short urethras.

* Nursing interventions include (a) assisting the client to maintain an appropriate fluid intake, (b) assisting the client to maintain normal voiding patterns, (c) monitoring the client's daily fluid intake and output, and (d) maintaining cleanliness of the genital area.

* Care of clients with indwelling catheters is directed toward preventing infection of the urinary tract and encouraging urinary flow through the drainage system.

* When the urinary bladder must be removed, a urinary diversion such as the ileal conduit is formed to allow urine to be eliminated from the body. The client must wear a urine collection device continually over the stoma.

EXPLORE MediaLink

Additional interactive resources for this chapter can be found on the Companion Website at www.prenhall.com/ramont. Click on Chapter 18 and "Begin" to select the activities for this chapter.

For chapter-related NCLEX-style questions and an audio glossary, access the accompanying CD-ROM in this book.

Animations:
* Urinary system dissection
* Renal function
* Catheter
* Furosemide
* Doxazosin

For Further Study

For more about the urinary system, see Figure 10-14.

For more information about cleaning wounds and changing dressings, see Chapter 12.

For more about accurate recording of fluid intake and output, see Chapter 17.

For further discussion of assisting clients who are confined to bed, refer to Chapters 13 and 20.

Critical Thinking Care Map

Caring for a Client with Altered Urinary Elimination

NCLEX-PN Focus Area: Physiological Integrity

Case Study: Mr. Lee Jay is a 54-year-old client being treated for Type 1 diabetes that is out of control. He is incontinent of foul-smelling urine. He complains of thirst and frequent urination. He is 6'3'' and weighs 200 lbs. He states, "I try to maintain my diabetic diet but I'm on a fixed income." Mr. Jay is alert and oriented to person, place, and time. He monitors his glucose about once a week and gives himself insulin injections. He has diminished pedal pulses, and his feet are cool to the touch. The physician has ordered lab tests and an indwelling catheter.

Nursing Diagnosis: Impaired Urinary Elimination

COLLECT DATA

Subjective	Objective
_____	_____
_____	_____
_____	_____
_____	_____
_____	_____
_____	_____
_____	_____

Data Collected
(use those that apply)

- ◆ Diabetes out of control
- ◆ Incontinent
- ◆ Foul-smelling urine
- ◆ Cloudy urine
- ◆ Mucous threads in urine
- ◆ Alert and oriented
- ◆ Weakened
- ◆ Diminished pedal pulses
- ◆ Glucose 440
- ◆ T 99°F
- ◆ BP 140/80
- ◆ Tired
- ◆ Catheter to gravity drainage
- ◆ Thirst
- ◆ Diabetic care compliance

Would you report this data? Yes/No

If yes, to: _____

Nursing Care

_____
_____
_____
_____
_____
_____
_____
_____
_____
_____
_____
_____
_____

Nursing Interventions
(use those that apply)

- ◆ Monitor lab tests.
- ◆ Observe urine for output.
- ◆ Assess urine for abnormal constituents.
- ◆ Assess pedal pulses.
- ◆ Maintain catheter asepsis.
- ◆ Ambulate client TID.
- ◆ Monitor vital signs q4h.
- ◆ Daily weights.
- ◆ Observe stool.

How would you document this? _____
_____
_____
_____
_____

NCLEX-PN Exam Preparation

1. Females are more prone to urinary tract infections (UTIs). This is attributed to the length of the:
   a. Ureters
   b. Urethra
   c. Renal pelvis
   d. Glomeruli

2. The production of abnormally large amounts of urine by the kidneys is known as:
   a. Oliguria
   b. Anuria
   c. Polydipsia
   d. Diuresis

3. The normal adult amount of urine excreted per day is approximately:
   a. 5,000 mL
   b. 3,500 mL
   c. 1,500 mL
   d. 500 mL

4. The purpose of a urine culture is to determine:
   a. Type of microorganisms
   b. Glucose level
   c. Urine concentration
   d. Occult blood

5. The physician has ordered a 24-hour urine specimen. After instructing the client, the nurse will:
   a. Determine the specific gravity
   b. Discard the first void and time the specimen
   c. Test the urine for glucose
   d. Begin timing the 24-hour specimen

6. When obtaining a urine sample from a catheter, the nurse can clamp the catheter for:
   a. 10 minutes
   b. 20 minutes
   c. 30 minutes
   d. 60 minutes

7. The specific gravity of normal urine is approximately:
   a. 1.000 to 1.005
   b. 1.010 to 1.025
   c. 1.025 to 1.030
   d. 1.030 to 1.050

8. Fluid restriction may be initiated for a client with:
   a. Diabetes
   b. Renal calculi
   c. Kidney failure
   d. UTI

9. Which of the following is a measure to prevent UTI recurrence?
   a. Limiting water intake
   b. Encouraging the use of nylon underclothes
   c. Bathing frequently
   d. Drinking cranberry juice, taking vitamin C

10. Your client has returned from surgery with a suprapubic catheter in place. This catheter is introduced through the client's:
    a. Ureter
    b. Kidney
    c. Urethra
    d. Abdomen

Answers for Review Questions, as well as discussion of Case Study and Critical Thinking Care Map questions, appear in Appendix IV.

Chapter 19

Gastrointestinal Elimination

SHARING experiences

"I was taking care of a woman who had surgery for a perforated bowel. She had a colostomy bag. She was having a hard time dealing with her new lifestyle. I spoke with her and tried to comfort and educate her. I taught her how to clean and change the colostomy bag. I also educated her on what foods to avoid and what foods to eat to prevent odor and gas. After I spoke with her, she was instantly relieved. She said, "I guess this isn't so bad. I can do this." She said, "I am so glad you are taking care of me. You have helped me a lot and I appreciate everything you have done. Before you leave today, come and say good-bye. I want to give you a flower to take home with you for all your help." After leaving her room I felt so happy. I was glad that I could help [her] feel more comfortable, first, because of the knowledge I had to educate [her] and, second, because of the compassion I learned going through the VN program. That is when I knew I had made the right decision in choosing this profession. I don't think that in any other profession you would feel as helpful and grateful as I do with nursing.

Renay Jones, LVN Student, North Orange County Regional Occupational Program, Anaheim, CA.

LEARNING outcomes

After completing this chapter, you will be able to:
- Describe the functions of the lower intestinal tract.
- Identify factors that influence fecal elimination and patterns of defecation.
- Distinguish normal from abnormal characteristics and constituents of feces.
- Describe methods used to assess the intestinal tract.
- Differentiate five common fecal elimination problems.
- Describe how to collect stool specimens and test for occult blood.
- Discuss ways to assist toward developing healthy defecation.
- Identify care and management for a ileostomy and colostomy.
- Describe types of enemas and describe the procedure for administering an enema.

MediaLink

www.prenhall.com/ramont

Use the address above to access the free, interactive Companion Website created for this textbook. Get hints, instant feedback, and textbook references to chapter-related NCLEX-style questions. Link to other interesting sites.

Audio Glossary:
Use the Companion Website, or the CD-ROM disk enclosed with your textbook, to hear the pronunciation of key terms in the chapter.

Nurses frequently are involved in assisting clients with elimination problems. These problems can be embarrassing to clients and can cause considerable discomfort.

 # Physiology of Defecation

Elimination of the waste products of digestion from the body is essential to health. The excreted waste products are referred to as **feces** or *stool*.

LARGE INTESTINE

The large intestine extends from the ileocecal (ileocolic) valve, which lies between the small and large intestines, to the anus. The *colon* (large intestine) in the adult is generally about 125 to 150 cm (50 to 60 in) long. It has seven parts: the cecum; ascending, transverse, and descending colons; sigmoid colon; rectum; and anus or external orifice (Figure 19-1 ◆). (See also Figure 10-13. ⊂⊃)

The large intestine is a muscular tube lined with mucous membrane. The muscle fibers are both circular and longitudinal, permitting the intestine to enlarge and contract in both width and length. This expansion and contraction enables **peristalsis,** a wavelike motion that propels intestinal contents forward.

The colon's main functions are the absorption of water and electrolytes, the mucal protection of the intestinal wall, and fecal elimination. The waste products that leave the stomach through the small intestine and then pass through the ileocecal valve are called **chyme.** As much as 1,500 mL of chyme passes into the large intestine daily. Most of it is absorbed in the proximal colon; approximately 100 mL of fluid is excreted in the feces.

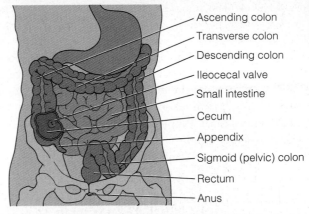

Figure 19-1. ◆ The large intestine and rectum.

- Ascending colon
- Transverse colon
- Descending colon
- Ileocecal valve
- Small intestine
- Cecum
- Appendix
- Sigmoid (pelvic) colon
- Rectum
- Anus

The colon also serves a protective function through mucus secretion. Mucus protects the intestinal wall from bacterial activity and helps hold fecal material together. Products of elimination include flatus and feces. **Flatus** is largely air and the by-products of the digestion of carbohydrates.

RECTUM AND ANAL CANAL

The rectum in the adult is usually 10 to 15 cm (4 to 6 in) long; the most distal portion, 2.5 to 5 cm (1 to 2 in) long, is the anal canal. When the veins in this area become distended, a condition known as hemorrhoids occurs.

The anal canal is bounded by an internal and an external sphincter muscle (Figure 19-2 ◆). The internal sphincter is under involuntary control, and the external sphincter normally is voluntarily controlled.

Defecation or bowel movement is the expulsion of feces from the anus and rectum. The frequency of defecation is highly individual, varying from several times per day to two or three

- Rectum
- Anal-rectal ridge
- Internal anal sphincter
- External anal sphincter
- Anal valve
- Anal canal
- Anal columns

A

- Rectum
- External anal sphincter
- Anal canal

B

Figure 19-2. ◆ The rectum, anal canal, and anal sphincters: **A.** Open; **B.** Closed.

times per week. The amount defecated also varies from person to person. When peristalsis moves the feces into the sigmoid colon and the rectum, the sensory nerves in the rectum are stimulated and the individual becomes aware of the need to defecate.

Expulsion of the feces is assisted by contraction of the abdominal muscles and the diaphragm. This maneuver causes an increase in abdominal pressure, which moves the feces through the anal canal. People who ignore the defecation reflex or who consciously inhibit it may eventually lose sensitivity to the defecation response. Constipation can be the end result.

Feces

Normal feces are made of about 75 percent water and 25 percent solid materials. They are soft but formed. If the feces are propelled very quickly along the large intestine, the expelled feces will be more fluid. If feces move very slowly through the large intestine, feces may be hard and difficult to expel.

Feces are normally brown, chiefly due to the presence of *bilirubin* (a red pigment in bile). Another factor that affects

fecal color is the action of bacteria such as *Escherichia coli* or staphylococci, normally present in the large intestine. The action of microorganisms on the chyme contributes to the odor of feces. Table 19-1 ◆ describes normal and abnormal characteristics of feces.

An adult usually forms 7 to 10 L of flatus (gas) in the large intestine every 24 hours. Air can be swallowed with food and fluids taken by mouth. Other gases are formed through the action of bacteria on the chyme in the large intestine.

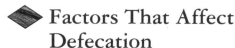

Factors That Affect Defecation

AGE AND DEVELOPMENT

Defecation material and patterns change dramatically from birth to 2½ years. Bowel patterns are established at an early age and are maintained through most of life.

TABLE 19-1	CHARACTERISTICS OF NORMAL AND ABNORMAL FECES		
CHARACTERISTIC	**NORMAL**	**ABNORMAL**	**POSSIBLE CAUSE**
Color	Adult: brown Infant: yellow	Clay or white	Absence of bile pigment (bile obstruction): diagnostic study using barium
		Black or tarry	Drug (e.g., iron); bleeding from upper gastrointestinal tract (e.g., stomach, small intestine); diet high in red meat and dark green vegetables (e.g., spinach)
		Red	Bleeding from lower gastrointestinal tract (e.g., rectum); some foods (e.g., beets)
		Pale	Malabsorption of fats; diet high in milk and milk products and low in meat
		Orange or green	Intestinal infection
Consistency	Formed, soft, semisolid, moist	Hard, dry	Dehydration; decreased intestinal motility resulting from lack of fiber in diet, lack of exercise, emotional upset, laxative abuse
		Diarrhea	Increased intestinal motility (e.g., due to irritation of the colon by bacteria)
Shape	Cylindrical (contour of rectum) about 2.5 cm (1 in) in diameter in adults	Narrow, pencil-shaped, or stringlike stool	Obstructive condition of the rectum
Amount	Varies with diet (about 100–400 g per day)		
Odor	Aromatic: affected by ingested food and person's own bacterial flora	Pungent	Infection, blood
Constituents	Small amounts of undigested roughage, sloughed dead bacteria and epithelial cells, fat, protein, dried constituents of digestive juices (e.g., bile pigments), inorganic matter (calcium, phosphates)	Pus Mucus Parasites Blood Large quantities of fat Foreign objects	Bacterial infection Inflammatory condition Gastrointestinal bleeding Malabsorption Accidental ingestion

DIET

Sufficient bulk (cellulose, fiber) in the diet is necessary to provide fecal volume. **Fiber** is high-residue food that stimulates peristalsis to maintain regularity. Low-residue foods, such as rice, eggs, and lean meats, move more slowly through the intestinal tract. Increasing fluid intake with such foods increases their rate of movement.

Certain foods and irregular eating can result in digestive upsets and, in some instances, the passage of watery stools. Individuals who eat at the same times every day usually have a regularly timed, physiologic response to the food intake and a regular pattern of peristaltic activity in the colon.

Spicy foods can produce diarrhea and flatus in some individuals. Other foods that may influence bowel elimination include the following:

◆ Gas-producing foods, such as cabbage, onions, cauliflower, bananas, and apples
◆ Laxative-producing foods, such as bran, prunes, figs, chocolate, and alcohol
◆ Constipation-producing foods, such as cheese, pasta, eggs, and lean meat

FLUIDS

Daily fluid intake of 2,000 to 3,000 mL is necessary to promote a normal soft, formed stool. When fluid intake is inadequate or output is excessive, the body continues to reabsorb fluid. As a result, the feces becomes hardened and drier than normal. If chyme moves abnormally quickly through the large intestine, however, there is less time for fluid to be absorbed into the blood; as a result, the feces are soft or even watery.

ACTIVITY

Activity stimulates peristalsis, thus facilitating the movement of chyme along the colon. Weak abdominal and pelvic muscles are often ineffective in increasing the intra-abdominal pressure during defecation or in controlling defecation. Weak muscles can result from lack of exercise, immobility, or impaired neurologic functioning. Clients confined to bed are often constipated.

PSYCHOLOGICAL FACTORS

Some people who are anxious or angry experience increased peristaltic activity and subsequent diarrhea. In contrast, people who are depressed may experience slower intestinal motility, resulting in constipation.

DEFECATION HABITS

Hospitalized clients may suppress the urge because of embarrassment about using a bedpan, lack of privacy, or because defecation is too uncomfortable.

MEDICATIONS

Some drugs have side effects that can interfere with normal elimination. Some cause diarrhea; others, such as tranquilizers, morphine, and codeine, cause constipation because they decrease gastrointestinal activity. Iron tablets act more locally on the bowel mucosa to cause constipation.

Some medications are intended to affect elimination directly. **Laxatives/cathartics** are medications that stimulate bowel activity and assist fecal elimination. Other medications soften stool, facilitating defecation. Certain medications, such as dicyclomine hydrochloride (Bentyl), suppress peristaltic activity and sometimes are used to treat diarrhea.

Some medications affect the appearance of the feces. Any drug that causes gastrointestinal bleeding as a side effect (e.g., aspirin products) can cause the stool to be red or black (**tarry**). Iron preparations may cause the stool to be black. Antibiotics may cause a gray-green discoloration because of effects on digestion; and antacids may cause a whitish discoloration or white specks in the stool.

DIAGNOSTIC PROCEDURES

Before certain diagnostic procedures, such as visualization of the sigmoid colon (**sigmoidoscopy**), the client is often restricted from ingesting food or fluid. The client may also be given a cleansing enema prior to the examination.

ANESTHESIA AND SURGERY

General anesthetics cause the normal colon movements to cease or slow down by blocking parasympathetic stimulation. Clients who have regional or spinal anesthesia are less likely to experience this problem.

Surgery that involves direct handling of the intestines can cause intestinal movement to cease temporary. This condition, called **paralytic ileus,** usually lasts 24 to 48 hours. Listening for bowel sounds that reflect intestinal motility is an important nursing assessment following surgery.

PATHOLOGIC CONDITIONS

Spinal cord injuries and head injuries can decrease the sensory stimulation for defecation. Impaired mobility may limit the client's ability to respond to the urge to defecate, resulting in constipation. Poorly functioning anal sphincters may cause the client to experience fecal incontinence.

PAIN

Clients who experience discomfort when defecating often suppress the urge to defecate to avoid the pain. They experience constipation as a result.

 Common Fecal Elimination Problems

Five common problems are related to fecal elimination: constipation, fecal impaction, diarrhea, bowel incontinence, and flatulence.

CONSTIPATION

Constipation is defined as fewer than three bowel movements per week. The client has small, dry, hard stool, or passes no stool for a period of time. Constipation occurs when the movement of feces through the large intestine is slow, allowing time for additional reabsorption of fluid from the large intestine. Constipation is associated with difficult evacuation of stool and increased effort or straining of the voluntary muscles of defecation. It is not associated with a specific number of bowel movements in a set time, because the range of normal varies. Assessment of the person's habits is necessary before a diagnosis of constipation is made. See Box 19-1 ◆ for defining characteristics of constipation.

Constipation can be hazardous to some clients. Straining associated with constipation often is accompanied by holding the breath (**Valsalva maneuver**). This maneuver can present serious problems to people with heart disease, brain injuries, or respiratory disease. Holding the breath increases the intrathoracic and intracranial pressures. To some degree, this pressure can be reduced if the person exhales through the mouth while straining. However, avoiding straining altogether is the best precaution.

FECAL IMPACTION

Fecal **impaction** is a mass or collection of hardened, putty-like feces in the folds of the rectum. Impaction results from prolonged retention and accumulation of fecal material. Fecal impaction is recognized by the passage of liquid fecal seepage and no normal stool. The liquid portion of the feces seeps out around the impacted mass (Figure 19-3 ◆).

The client may experience symptoms that include a frequent but nonproductive urge to defecate, as well as rectal pain. A generalized feeling of illness results. The client becomes anorexic, the abdomen becomes distended, and nausea and vomiting may occur.

The causes of fecal impaction are usually poor defecation habits and constipation. As mentioned, certain medications affect elimination and can contribute to impactions. Substances such as barium used in radiologic examinations of the upper and lower gastrointestinal (GI) tracts can also be a causative factor. After examination of the lower gastrointestinal tract, measures are usually taken to ensure removal of the barium and prevent complications.

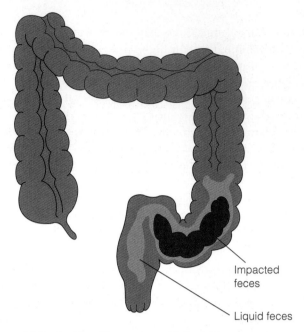

Figure 19-3. ◆ A fecal impaction with liquid feces passing around the impaction.

Impacted feces

Liquid feces

Impaction can be assessed by digital examination of the rectum, during which the hardened mass can often be palpated. Digital examination of the impaction through the rectum should be done gently and carefully, because stimulation of the vagus nerve in the rectal wall can slow the client's heart.

Although fecal impaction can generally be prevented, digital removal of impacted feces is sometimes necessary. When fecal impaction is suspected, the client is often given an oil retention enema, a cleansing enema 2 to 4 hours later, and daily additional cleansing enemas, suppositories, or stool softeners. If these measures fail, manual removal is often necessary.

DIARRHEA

Diarrhea refers to the passage of liquid feces and increased frequency of defecation. Rapid passage of chyme reduces the time available for the large intestine to reabsorb water and electrolytes. The person with diarrhea finds it difficult or impossible to control the urge to defecate. Bowel sounds are increased, and spasmodic cramps occur. Sometimes the client passes blood and excessive mucus; nausea and vomiting may also occur. With persistent diarrhea, irritation of the anal area, perineum, and buttocks generally results. Fatigue, weakness, and dehydration with possible electrolyte imbalance are the results of prolonged diarrhea.

When the cause of diarrhea is irritants in the intestinal tract, diarrhea is thought to be a protective mechanism. However, it can create serious fluid and electrolyte losses in the body (see also Chapter 17). ◯◯ Table 19-2 ◆ lists some of the major causes of diarrhea and the physiologic responses of the body.

BOX 19-1
MANIFESTATIONS OF CONSTIPATION

- ◆ Decreased frequency of defecation
- ◆ Hard, dry, formed stools
- ◆ Straining at stool; painful defecation
- ◆ Reports of rectal fullness, pressure, or incomplete bowel evacuation
- ◆ Abdominal pain, cramps, or distention
- ◆ Use of laxatives
- ◆ Decreased appetite
- ◆ Headache

TABLE 19-2	MAJOR CAUSES OF DIARRHEA
CAUSE	**PHYSIOLOGIC EFFECT**
Psychological stress, (e.g., anxiety)	Increased intestinal motility and mucus secretion
Medications Antibiotics	Inflammation and infection of mucosa due to overgrowth of pathogenic intestinal microorganisms
Iron	Irritation of intestinal mucosa
Cathartics	Irritation of intestinal mucosa
Allergy to food, fluid, drugs	Incomplete digestion of food or fluid
Intolerance of food or fluid	Increased intestinal motility and mucus secretion
Diseases of the colon, e.g.: Malabsorption syndrome	Reduced absorption of fluids
Crohn's disease	Inflammation of the mucosa often leading to ulcer formation
Others Surgical operations	Variable

BOWEL INCONTINENCE

Bowel incontinence, also called fecal incontinence, refers to the loss of voluntary fecal control and gaseous elimination through the anus. Incontinence may occur at specific times, such as after meals, or it may occur irregularly.

Fecal incontinence is generally associated with impaired functioning of the anal sphincter or its nerve supply, such as in some neuromuscular diseases, spinal cord trauma, and tumors of the external anal sphincter muscle.

Fecal incontinence is an emotionally distressing problem that can lead to embarrassment and social isolation. Incontinent feces are acidic and contain digestive enzymes that are highly irritating to skin. Therefore, the area around the anal region should be kept clean and dry and be protected with a moisture barrier ointment.

FLATULENCE

There are three primary causes of flatus: (a) action of bacteria on the chyme in the large intestine, (b) swallowed air, and (c) gas that diffuses from the bloodstream into the intestine.

Flatulence is the presence of excessive *flatus* (or gas) in the intestines. It leads to stretching and inflation of the intestines (intestinal distention). Large amounts of air and other gases can accumulate in the stomach, resulting in gastric distention.

Most gases that are swallowed are expelled through the mouth by **eructation** (belching or burping). Flatulence can occur in the colon, from a variety of causes, such as foods (e.g., cabbage, onions), abdominal surgery, or narcotics. If the gas is propelled by increased colon activity, it may be expelled through the anus. If excessive gas cannot be expelled through the anus, it may be necessary to insert a rectal tube or to provide a return flow enema (also called a Harris Flush) to remove it.

◆ Fecal Diversion Ostomies

An **ostomy** is an opening in the abdominal wall for the elimination of feces or urine. There are many types of ostomies. An **ileostomy** is an opening into the *ileum* (small bowel). A **colostomy** is an opening into the *colon* (large bowel). The purpose of bowel and urinary ostomies is to divert and drain fecal material. Bowel diversion ostomies are often classified according to (a) status (permanent or temporary), (b) location, and (c) the construction of the stoma.

PERMANENCE

Temporary colostomies are generally performed for traumatic injuries or inflammatory conditions of the bowel. They allow the distal diseased portion of the bowel to rest and heal. Permanent colostomies are performed to provide a means of elimination when the rectum or anus is nonfunctional as a result of a birth defect or a disease such as cancer of the bowel. The diseased portion may or may not be removed.

ANATOMIC LOCATION

An ileostomy generally empties from the distal end of the small intestine. An *ascending colostomy* empties from the ascending colon. A *transverse colostomy* empties from the transverse colon. A *descending colostomy* empties from the descending colon. A *sigmoidostomy* empties from the sigmoid colon (Figure 19-4 ◆).

The location of the ostomy affects the character and management of the fecal drainage. The farther along the bowel the ostomy is, the more formed the stool is, because the large bowel reabsorbs water. The frequency of stomal discharge can be controlled better by establishing an ostomy in the large intestine.

OSTOMY MANAGEMENT

Clients with fecal diversions need considerable psychological support, instruction, and physical care. Many agencies contract with enterostomal therapy nurses to assist these clients.

Stoma and Skin Care

Fecal material (**effluent**) from a colostomy or ileostomy is irritating to the peristomal skin. Ileal effluent (products of elimination) is especially irritating because it contains digestive enzymes. The nurse assesses the peristomal skin for irritation each time the appliance is changed. See Box 19-2 ◆ for

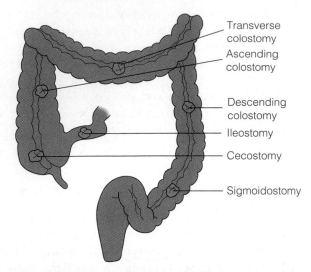

Transverse
colostomy

Ascending
colostomy

Descending
colostomy

Ileostomy

Cecostomy

Sigmoidostomy

Figure 19-4. ◆ The locations of bowel diversion ostomies.

assessing a stoma. Any skin irritation or breakdown needs to be treated immediately.

The skin is kept clean by washing off any excretion and drying the skin thoroughly. An *appliance* (pouch or bag) is then fitted securely to the stoma. Drying the skin before attaching the appliance is crucial, because pouches do not adhere to moist skin, and effluent will leak out. All appliances

---

have three features in common: a pouch to collect the effluent, an outlet at the bottom for easy emptying, and a faceplate. The faceplate is an adhesive ring placed on the client's skin; the pouch attaches to the faceplate.

Odor control is essential to clients' self-esteem. Selecting the appropriate kind of appliance promotes odor control. An intact appliance contains odors. The appliance should be rinsed thoroughly when it is emptied. Deodorizers can be placed in the pouch of the appliance. Oral intake of bismuth subcarbonate can be prescribed by the physician to help control odor.

Disposable ostomy appliances can be used for up to 5 to 7 days. They need to be changed whenever the effluent leaks onto the peristomal skin or when effluent cannot be rinsed completely away. The bag should be monitored for drainage and emptied when it is one-third full. This prevents pulling on the appliance and accidental soiling. If the skin is erythematous (red), eroded, denuded, or ulcerated, it should be changed every 24 to 48 hours to allow appropriate treatment of the skin. If the client complains of pain or discomfort, the area should be carefully inspected. Procedure 19-1 explains how to change a bowel diversion ostomy appliance.

COLLABORATIVE CARE

Diagnostic and Laboratory Studies
Diagnostic studies of the gastrointestinal tract include direct visualization techniques, indirect visualization techniques, and laboratory tests for abnormal constituents.

VISUALIZATION TECHNIQUES. Direct visualization techniques include:

◆ *Anoscopy*—viewing of the anal canal
◆ *Proctoscopy*—viewing of the rectum
◆ *Proctosigmoidoscopy*—viewing of the rectum and sigmoid
◆ *Colonoscopy*—viewing of the large intestine

Indirect visualization of the gastrointestinal tract is achieved by *roentgenography (x-ray films)*. X-rays of the gastrointestinal tract can detect strictures, obstructions, tumors, ulcers, inflammatory disease, or other structural changes such as hiatal hernias. Introduction of a radiopaque substance such as barium enhances visualization of the GI tract. For examination of the upper GI tract or small bowel, the client drinks the barium sulfate ("barium swallow"). For examination of the lower GI tract, the client is given an enema containing the barium, commonly referred to as a "barium enema." These x-rays usually include fluoroscopic examination. That is, the x-ray films are projected onto a screen, which permits continuous observation of the flow of barium. The LPN/LVN prepares the client for the test, maintains NPO status prior to the test if necessary, and follows physician-established protocol.

STOOL SPECIMENS. The nurse is responsible for collecting stool specimens for testing. Before obtaining a specimen, the nurse needs to determine the correct method of obtaining and

---

BOX 19-2
ASSESSING A STOMA

◆ *Stoma color.* The stoma should appear red, similar in color to the mucosal lining of the inner cheek. Very pale or darker-colored stomas with a bluish or purplish hue indicate impaired blood circulation to the area.
◆ *Stoma size and shape.* Most stomas protrude slightly from the abdomen. New stomas normally appear swollen, but swelling generally decreases over 2 or 3 weeks or as long as 6 weeks. Failure of swelling to recede may indicate a problem, such as blockage.
◆ *Slight bleeding.* Initially, the stoma bleeds slightly when the stoma is touched, but other bleeding should be reported.
◆ *Status of peristomal skin.* Any redness and irritation of the peristomal skin—the 5 to 13 cm (2 to 5 in) of skin surrounding the stoma—should be noted.
◆ *Amount and type of feces.* For ileal effluent and feces (effluent from a colostomy), assess amount, color, odor, and consistency. Inspect for abnormalities, such as pus or blood.
◆ *Complaints.* Complaints of a burning sensation under the faceplate may indicate skin breakdown. The presence of abdominal discomfort or distention also needs to be determined.

handling it. In many situations only a single specimen is required. In others, timed specimens are necessary, which require that every stool passed be collected within a designated time period and sent to the laboratory immediately (if ordered).

Nurses need to give clients the following instructions:

◆ Defecate in a clean *bedpan* (receptacle for urine or feces) or bedside commode.
◆ Empty the bladder before specimen collection. If possible, do not contaminate the specimen by urine or menstrual discharge.
◆ Do not place toilet tissue in the bedpan after defecation. Contents of the paper can affect the results.
◆ Notify the nurse as soon as possible after defecation.

NURSING CARE

ASSESSING

The LPN/LVN gathers data by performing a physical examination of the abdomen, rectum, and anus. The nurse inspects the feces and reviews any data obtained from relevant diagnostic tests. Collected data are used in collaboration with the RN when planning care.

Physical examination of the abdomen includes inspection, auscultation, and light palpation (see Chapter 11). 🔗 Auscultation is done before palpation, because palpation can alter peristalsis. Examination of the rectum and anus includes inspection and palpation.

Inspecting the Feces

The client's stool is inspected for color, consistency, shape, amount, odor, and the presence of abnormalities. Table 19-1 provides a summary of normal and abnormal characteristics of stool and possible causes.

DIAGNOSING, PLANNING, and IMPLEMENTING

The LPN/LVN should be aware of appropriate nursing diagnoses related to bowel elimination. Some common NANDA diagnoses for fecal elimination problems are: Constipation, Diarrhea, and Risk for Imbalanced Fluid Volume.

The major goals for clients with fecal elimination problems are to:

◆ Maintain or restore normal bowel elimination pattern
◆ Maintain or regain normal stool consistency
◆ Prevent associated risks such as fluid and electrolyte imbalance, skin breakdown (see Chapter 13), abdominal distention, and pain. 🔗 See Discharge Considerations at the end of the Nursing Care section.

Obtaining Stool Specimens

When obtaining stool samples, the nurse follows these guidelines:

1. Follow medical aseptic technique.
2. Wear disposable gloves to prevent contamination of the hands or of the outside of the specimen container.
3. Use clean tongue blades to transfer the specimen to the container and then dispose of them in the waste container.
4. Collect the amount of stool required. Usually about 2.5 cm (1 inch) of formed stool or 15 to 30 mL of liquid stool is adequate. For some timed specimens, the entire stool passed may need to be sent.
5. Include visible pus, mucus, or blood in sample specimens.
6. For a stool culture, dip a sterile swab into the specimen, preferably where purulent fecal matter is present. Using sterile technique, place the swab in a sterile test tube.
7. Send the specimens to the laboratory immediately (fresh specimens provide the most accurate results). In some instances refrigeration is indicated, because bacteriologic changes take place in stool specimens left at room temperature.

Testing Feces for Occult Blood

Stool is tested for **occult blood** (microscopically visible blood) to detect gastrointestinal bleeding that is not visible to the eye. Bleeding can occur as a result of ulcers, inflammatory disease, or tumors. The test for occult blood (often referred to as the *guaiac test* because it uses blood-sensitive guaiac paper) can be readily performed by the nurse in the clinical area or by the client at home. Refer to Box 19-3 ◆ for client instructions on testing the stool for occult blood.

Certain foods, medications, and vitamin C can produce inaccurate test results. False positive results can occur if the client has recently ingested (a) red meat; (b) raw vegetables or fruits, particularly radishes, turnips, horseradish, and melons; or (c) certain medications that irritate the gastric mucosa and cause bleeding, such as aspirin, iron preparations, and anticoagulants.

Promoting Regular Defecation.

The nurse can help clients in the clinical setting to achieve regular defecation by providing (a) privacy, (b) a regular time for defecation, (c) nutrition and fluids, (d) exercise, and (e) correct positioning.

Privacy. Privacy during defecation is extremely important, but the nurse may need to stay with clients who are too weak to be left alone.

Timing. A client should be encouraged to defecate when the urge to defecate is recognized. Many people have well-established times and routines for defecation that should be part of the client's schedule. Clients should not be hurried but be given adequate time to defecate.

BOX 19-3

TEACHING FOR DISCHARGE

COLLECTING STOOL FOR OCCULT BLOOD TEST

◆ Avoid restricted foods, medications, and vitamin C for the period recommended by the manufacturer and during the test.
◆ Label the specimens with your name, address, age, and date of specimen. Three specimens are collected from consecutive and different bowel movements, to confirm negative results and avoid false-positive results.
◆ Avoid collecting specimens during your menstrual period and for 3 days afterward, or if you have bleeding hemorrhoids or blood in your urine.
◆ Avoid contaminating the specimen with urine or toilet tissue. Empty your bladder before the test. To facilitate specimen collection, transfer the stool to a clean, dry container. Wear disposable gloves.
◆ Use the tongue blade provided to transfer the specimen to the test folder or tape. Only a small amount of stool is required. Take the sample from the center of a formed stool to ensure a uniform sample.
◆ For a Hemoccult test, a thin layer of feces is smeared over the boxes inside the envelope, and a drop of developing solution is applied on the opposite side of the specimen paper. For the Hematest, a thin layer of feces is smeared onto guaiac filter paper, a tablet is placed in the middle of the specimen, and two or three drops of water are added to the tablet.

BOX 19-4

CLIENT TEACHING

MANAGING DIARRHEA

◆ Drink at least 8 glasses of water per day to prevent dehydration.
◆ Avoid alcohol, beverages with caffeine, and excessively cold fluids, which aggravate the problem.
◆ Ingest foods with sodium and potassium. Most foods contain sodium. Potassium is found in dairy products, meats, and many vegetables and fruits, especially tomatoes, potatoes, bananas, peaches, and apricots.
◆ Limit foods containing insoluble fiber, such as whole-wheat and whole-grain breads and cereals, and raw fruits and vegetables.
◆ Increase foods containing soluble fiber, such as oatmeal and skinless fruits and potatoes.
◆ Limit fatty foods (e.g., dairy products and packaged processed meats).
◆ Thoroughly clean and dry the perianal area after passing stool to prevent skin irritation and breakdown. Use soft toilet tissue to clean and dry the area. Apply a moisture-barrier cream or ointment, such as zinc oxide or petrolatum, as needed.
◆ Discontinue medications or foods that cause diarrhea.
◆ When diarrhea has stopped, reestablish normal bowel flora by eating fermented dairy products, such as yogurt or buttermilk.

Nutrition and Fluids. The diet a client needs for regular normal elimination varies, depending on the kind of feces the client currently has, the frequency of defecation, and the types of foods that the client finds assist normal defecation.

◆ For constipation: Increase daily fluid intake, and instruct the client to drink hot liquids and fruit juices, especially prune juice. Include fiber-rich foods in the diet, such as prunes, raw fruit, bran products, and whole-grain cereals and bread.
◆ For diarrhea: Encourage oral intake of fluids and bland food. Eating small amounts of bland foods can be helpful because they are more easily absorbed. Diarrhea can lead to potassium losses. Highly spiced foods and high-fiber foods can aggravate diarrhea. See Box 19-4 ◆ for details about managing diarrhea in the clinical setting and at home.
◆ For flatulence: Limit carbonated beverages, the use of drinking straws, and chewing gum. These increase the ingestion of air. Gas-forming foods, such as cabbage, beans, onions, and cauliflower, should also be avoided.

Exercise. Regular exercise helps clients develop a regular defecation pattern. Weak abdominal and pelvic muscles impede normal defecation. In the clinical setting, encourage ambulatory clients to walk frequently in the room or the hallway.

Positioning. To aid defecation, the best position on a toilet seat for most people seems to be leaning forward. For clients who have difficulty moving themselves to and from the toilet, an elevated toilet seat can be attached to a regular toilet. A bedside commode is often used for the adult client who can get out of bed but is unable to walk to the bathroom. (Figure 19-5 ◆).

Clients restricted to bed may need to use a bedpan. There are two main types of bedpans: the regular high-back pan and the fracture pan (Figure 19-6 ◆). The fracture pan has a low back and is used for clients who cannot raise their buttocks. Nursing guidelines for giving and removing a bedpan are presented in Box 19-5. Female clients use a bedpan for both urine and feces. Male clients use a bedpan for feces and a urinal for urine.

Most male clients are able to use a urinal independently either in bed or when standing at the bedside. The nurse must remain with clients who need support to stand at the bedside. For clients who cannot stand at the bedside, place the urinal between the client's legs with the handle uppermost so that urine will flow into it.

Figure 19-5. ◆ Commode with overlying seat. *Source:* © Elena Dorfman.

Figure 19-6. ◆ Clockwise from the top: The high-back or regular bedpan; male urinal; the slipper or fracture pan. *Source:* © Jenny Thomas.

Teaching about Medications

Antidiarrheal Medications. These medications are usually reserved for treatment of chronic diarrhea (more than 3 to 4 weeks). They slow the motility of the intestine or absorb excess fluid in the intestine.

BOX 19-5
NURSING CARE CHECKLIST

PLACING AND REMOVING A BEDPAN

☑ Provide privacy.

☑ Wear disposable gloves.

☑ If the bedpan is metal, warm it by rinsing it with warm water.

☑ Adjust the bed to a height appropriate to prevent back strain.

☑ Elevate the side rail on the opposite side to prevent the client from falling out of bed.

☑ Ask the client to assist by flexing the knees, resting the weight on the back and heels, and raising the buttocks, or by using a trapeze bar, if present.

☑ Help lift the client as needed by placing one hand under the lower back, resting your elbow on the mattress, and using your forearm as a lever.

☑ Place a regular bedpan so that the client's buttocks rest on the smooth, rounded rim. Place a fracture pan with the flat, low end under the client's buttocks (Figure 19-7 ◆).

☑ For the client who cannot assist, obtain the assistance of another nurse to help lift the client onto the bedpan. Or place the client on his or her side, place the bedpan against the buttocks (Figure 19-8 ◆), and roll the client back onto the bedpan.

☑ To provide a more normal position for the client's lower back, elevate the client's bed to a semi-Fowler's position, if permitted. If elevation is contraindicated,

support the client's back with pillows as needed to prevent hyperextension of the back.

☑ Cover the client with bed linen to maintain comfort and dignity.

☑ Provide toilet tissue, place the call light within reach, lower the bed to the low position, elevate the side rail if indicated, and leave the client alone.

☑ Answer the call bell promptly.

☑ When removing the bedpan, return the bed to the position used when giving the bedpan. Don gloves and hold the bedpan steady to prevent spillage of its contents. Cover the bedpan, and place it on the bedside chair.

☑ If the client needs assistance with cleaning, wipe the client's perineal area with several layers of toilet tissue. If a specimen is to be collected, discard the soiled tissue into a moisture-proof receptacle other than the bedpan. For female clients, clean from the urethra toward the anus to prevent the transfer of rectal microorganisms into the urinary meatus.

☑ Wash the perineal area of dependent clients with soap and water as indicated, and dry the area thoroughly.

☑ For all clients, offer warm water, soap, a washcloth, and a towel to wash the hands.

☑ Assist the client to a comfortable position, empty and clean the bedpan, and return it to the bedside.

☑ Remove and discard your gloves and wash your hands.

☑ Document color, odor, amount, and consistency of urine and feces, and the condition of the perineal area.

Figure 19-7. ◆ Placing a slipper or fracture pan under the buttocks. *Source:* © Elena Dorfman.

Figure 19-8. ◆ Placing a bedpan against a client's buttocks.

Antiflatulent Medications. Antiflatulent agents such as simethicone do not decrease the formation of flatus. They do *coalesce* (pull together) the gas bubbles and facilitate their passage by belching through the mouth or expulsion through the anus.

Cathartics and Laxatives. *Cathartics* are drugs that induce defecation. They can have a strong, purging effect. A *laxative* is mild when compared to a cathartic. It produces frequent soft or liquid stools that are sometimes accompanied by

abdominal cramps. Table 19-3 ◆ describes the different types of laxatives. Some laxatives are given in the form of suppositories. These act in various ways: by softening the feces, by releasing gases such as carbon dioxide to distend the rectum, or by stimulating the nerve endings in the rectal mucosa.

Laxative abuse is believed to be a common problem. Older adults in particular often use laxatives improperly. Continual use of laxatives weakens the bowel's natural responses to fecal distention, and results in chronic constipation.

TABLE 19-3 TYPES OF LAXATIVES

TYPE	ACTION	EXAMPLES	PERTINENT TEACHING INFORMATION
Bulk-forming	Increases the fluid, gaseous, or solid bulk in the intestines	Psyllium hydrophilic mucilloid (Metamucil)	May take 12 or more hours to act. Sufficient fluid must be taken.
Emollient/stool softener	Softens and delays the drying of the feces; permits fat and water to penetrate feces	Docusate sodium (Colace)	Refrigerated oil has less odor. Mixing with fruit juice decreases unpleasant taste.
Wetting agents	Lowers the surface tension of the feces, thus helping water to penetrate the feces	Docusate sodium (Colace)	Slow-acting, may take several days.
Stimulant/irritant	Irritates the intestinal mucosa or stimulates nerve endings in the wall of the intestine, causing rapid propulsion of the contents	Bisacodyl (Dulcolax)	Acts more quickly than bulk-forming agents. Fluid is passed with the feces. May cause cramps. Prolonged use may cause fluid and electrolyte imbalance.
Lubricant	Lubricates the feces in the colon	Mineral oil (Haley's M-O)	Prolonged use inhibits the absorption of some fat-soluble vitamins.
Saline/osmotic	Draws water into the intestine by osmosis, distends bowel, and stimulates peristalsis	Epsom salts, magnesium hydroxide (milk of magnesia), magnesium citrate, sodium phosphate (Fleet enema)	May be rapid acting. Can cause fluid and electrolyte imbalance, particularly in elderly people and children with cardiac and renal disease. Should not be used by elderly clients. Prolonged use inhibits the absorption of some fat-soluble vitamins.

> **clinical ALERT**
>
> Laxatives are contraindicated for client's who have nausea, cramps, fever, vomiting, or undiagnosed abdominal pain.

The client's medication regimen should be examined by the physician and RN to see whether it could be the cause of constipation.

Administering Enemas

An **enema** is a solution introduced into the rectum and large intestine. The purpose of an enema is to distend the intestine and sometimes to irritate the intestinal mucosa, in order to increasing peristalsis and excretion of feces and flatus.

Enemas are classified into three groups: cleansing, retention, and return-flow.

Cleansing Enemas.
Cleansing enemas are intended to remove feces. They are given chiefly to:

◆ Prevent the escape of feces during surgery.
◆ Prepare the intestine for certain diagnostic tests such as x-ray or visualization tests (e.g., colonoscopy).
◆ Remove feces when there is constipation or impaction.
◆ Establish regular bowel function as part of a bowel training program.

Cleansing enemas use a variety of solutions. See Table 19-4 ◆ for commonly used solutions.

Cleansing enemas may also be described as high or low:

1. A *high enema* is given to cleanse as much of the colon as possible.
2. A *low enema* is used to clean the rectum and sigmoid colon only. The client maintains a left lateral position during administration.

The force of flow of the solution is governed by (a) the height of the solution container, (b) size of the tubing, (c) viscosity of the fluid, and (d) resistance of the rectum. The higher the solution container is held above the rectum, the faster the flow and the greater the force (pressure) in the rectum. During most adult enemas, the solution container should be no higher than 30 cm (12 in) above the rectum. During a high cleansing enema, the solution container is usually held 30 to 45 cm (12 to 18 in) above the rectum. This instills the fluid farther to clean the entire bowel.

Retention Enema.
Retention enema introduces oil into the rectum and sigmoid colon. The oil is retained for a relatively long period (e.g., 1 to 3 hours). It acts to soften the feces and to lubricate the rectum and anal canal, thus facilitating passage of the feces.

Return-Flow Enema.
A *return-flow enema* (or *Harris flush*) is used occasionally to expel flatus. Alternating flow of 100 to 200 mL of fluid into and out of the rectum and sigmoid colon stimulates peristalsis. This process is repeated five or six times until the flatus is expelled and abdominal distention is relieved.

Commercially prepared, low-volume, disposable enema kits are commonly used today. The kit includes a flexible bottle of solution with a prelubricated, firm tip. Procedure 19-2 describes how to administer an enema.

Digital Removal of a Fecal Impaction
Digital removal involves breaking up the fecal mass with the finger and removing it in portions.

TABLE 19-4 COMMONLY USED ENEMA SOLUTIONS

SOLUTION	CONSTITUENTS	ACTION	TIME TO TAKE EFFECT	POTENTIAL ADVERSE EFFECTS
Hypertonic	90–120 mL of solution (e.g., sodium phosphate)	Draws water into the colon	5–10 min	Retention of sodium
Hypotonic	500–1,000 mL of tap water	Distends colon, stimulates peristalsis, and softens feces	15–20 min	Fluid and electrolyte imbalance; water intoxication
Isotonic	500–1,000 mL of normal saline (9 mL NaCl to 1,000 mL water)	Distends colon, stimulates peristalsis, and softens feces	15–20 min	Possible sodium retention
Soapsuds	500–1,000 mL (3–5 mL soap to 1,000 mL water)	Irritates mucosa, distends colon	10–15 min	Irritates and may damage mucosa
Oil (mineral, olive, cottonseed)	90–120 mL	Lubricates the feces and the colonic mucosa	30–60 min	

clinical ALERT

Because the bowel mucosa can be injured during the fecal impaction procedure, some agencies limit who can perform digital disimpactions. Rectal stimulation is also contraindicated for some people, because it may result in cardiac arrhythmia.

Manual removal of an impaction can be painful. If facility policy permits, use a well-lubricated, gloved finger and insert the finger into the anal canal as far as you can reach. Loosen and dislodge stool by gently massaging around it. Break up stool by working the finger into the hardened mass, taking care to avoid injury to the mucosa of the rectum. Carefully work stool downward to the end of the rectum and remove it in small pieces. Manual stimulation should be minimal.

Decreasing Flatulence

There are a number of ways to reduce or prevent flatus. They include avoiding gas-producing foods and drinking straws, increasing exercise, moving in bed, and ambulation. Movement stimulates peristalsis, escape of flatus, and reabsorption of gases in the intestinal capillaries. If these measures fail, flatulence may be treated by insertion of a rectal tube.

Bowel Training Programs

For clients who have chronic constipation, frequent impactions, or fecal incontinence, bowel training programs may be helpful. The program is based on factors within the client's control and is designed to help the client establish normal defecation. Such matters as food and fluid intake, exercise, and defecation habits are all considered. Before beginning such a program, clients must understand it and want to be involved.

 EVALUATING

Data are collected to determine whether the client has achieved goals established during the planning phase. Steps toward achieving or maintaining normal bowel elimination patterns and stool consistency are assessed and documented. For clients with ostomies, steps toward self-care are reviewed. If outcomes are not achieved, the nurse should discuss the situation with the RN participating in the client's care.

 DISCHARGE CONSIDERATIONS

The nurse plays an important role in educating clients about bowel elimination. Box 19-6 ◆ provides instructions the nurse can share with clients about maintaining healthy elimination patterns.

To make toileting easier in the home, teach clients and their families to:

◆ Ensure safe and easy access to the toilet. Make sure lighting is appropriate, scatter rugs are removed or securely fastened, and so on.

BOX 19-6

TEACHING FOR DISCHARGE

ESTABLISHING HEALTHY ELIMINATION PATTERNS
◆ Establish a regular exercise regimen.
◆ Include high-fiber foods, such as vegetables, fruits, and whole grains, in the diet.
◆ Maintain fluid intake of 2,000 to 3,000 mL a day.
◆ Do not ignore the urge to defecate.
◆ Allow time to defecate, preferably at the same time each day.
◆ Avoid over-the-counter medications to treat constipation and diarrhea.

◆ Provide instruction as needed about transfer techniques. Suggest ways that garments can be adjusted to make disrobing easier for toileting.
◆ If appropriate, instruct the client to keep a record of time and frequency of stool passage, any associated pain, and color and consistency of the stool.
◆ Provide information about required food and fluid alterations to promote defecation or to manage diarrhea (see Box 19-4).
◆ Discuss problems associated with overuse of laxatives, if appropriate, and the use of alternatives to laxatives, suppositories, and enemas (e.g., Metamucil) (see Table 19-3).
◆ If the client is taking a constipating medication (e.g., narcotic analgesic), discuss the addition of a fiber supplement once a day.
◆ Provide instructions associated with specific elimination problems and treatment, such as constipation, diarrhea, or ostomy care, as discussed above.

Nursing Process Case Study: CLIENT WITH CONSTIPATION

Mrs. Emma Brown is 78-year old widow of 9 months. She lives alone in a low-income housing complex for older people. Her two children live with their families in a city 150 miles away. She has always enjoyed cooking. However, now that she is alone, she does not cook for herself. As a result, she has developed irregular eating patterns and tends to prepare soup-and-toast meals. She gets little exercise and has had bouts of insomnia since her husband's death. For the past month, Mrs. Brown has been having a problem with constipation. She states she has a bowel movement about every 3 to 4 days and her stools are hard and painful to excrete.

Assessment. VS: T 98.6°F, radial pulse 78, R 22. BP 130/84. She complains of anorexia, and her abdomen is bloated. Bowel sounds are diminished.

Diagnosis.

- Constipation
- Risk for Loneliness
- Imbalanced Nutrition: Less Than Body Requirements
- Pain

Expected Outcomes.

- Establish an elimination pattern suitable to lifestyle.
- Examine possible community resources and seek referrals for coping with loneliness.
- Understand fluid importance in stool consistency.
- Participate in planning a routine diet regimen that includes high-fiber foods to decrease constipation.
- Pain associated with bowel movements is controlled.

Planning and Implementation.

- Review bowel pattern and lifestyle.
- Provide resources to client for senior interaction and activity.
- Increase fluids intake and exercise.
- Provide information regarding intestinal physiology.

- Offer a variety of easy to prepare diet menus high in fiber.
- Discuss aids to soften stool.
- Identify pain level associated with bowel movements.

Evaluating. Mrs. Brown has joined a senior center and signed up for an exercise class. She is drinking more fluids. Her diet has more fiber and bran. Mrs. Brown has established a morning routine that provides a relaxing, unhurried time in the bathroom. She heeds the urge to defecate rather than delaying the process. She is preparing a greater variety of foods at scheduled times.

Critical Thinking in the Nursing Process

1. Describe the process of defecation.
2. Teach Mrs. Brown measures and the rationales that will assist her to prevent constipation.

Note: The bibliography listings for this and all chapters have been compiled at the back of the book.

PROCEDURE 19-1

Changing a One-Piece, Drainable Bowel Diversion Ostomy Appliance

PURPOSES

◆ To assess and care for the peristomal skin
◆ To collect effluent for assessment of the amount and type of output
◆ To minimize odors for the client's comfort and self-esteem

EQUIPMENT

◆ Disposable gloves
◆ Electric or safety razor
◆ Bedpan
◆ Solvent (presaturated sponges or liquid)
◆ Moistureproof bag (for disposable pouches)

◆ Cleaning materials, including tissues, warm water, mild soap (optional), washcloth or cotton balls, towel
◆ Tissue or gauze pad
◆ Skin barrier (paste, powder, water, or liquid skin sealant)
◆ Stoma measuring guide
◆ Pen or pencil and scissors
◆ Clean ostomy appliance, with optional belt
◆ Tail closure clamp
◆ Special adhesive, if needed
◆ Stoma guidestrip, if needed
◆ Deodorant (liquid or tablet) for a non-odorproof colostomy bag

INTERVENTIONS

1. Determine the need for an appliance change.
   ◆ Assess the used appliance for leakage of effluent. *Effluent can irritate the peristomal skin.*
   ◆ Ask the client about any discomfort at or around the stoma. *A burning sensation may indicate breakdown beneath the faceplate of the pouch.*
   ◆ Assess the fullness of the pouch. *Pouches need to be emptied when they are one-third to one-half full. The weight of an overly full bag may loosen the faceplate and separate it from the skin, causing the effluent to leak and irritate the peristomal skin.*
   ◆ If there is pouch leakage or discomfort at or around the stoma, change the appliance.

2. Select an appropriate time.
   ◆ Avoid times close to meal or visiting hours. *Ostomy odor and effluent may reduce appetite or embarrass the client.*
   ◆ Avoid times immediately after the administration of any medications that may stimulate bowel evacuation. *It is best to change the pouch when drainage is least likely to occur.*

3. Prepare the client and support people.
   ◆ Explain the procedure to the client and support people. *Changing an ostomy appliance should not cause discomfort, but it may be distasteful to the client. Support persons are often more supportive if properly informed.*
   ◆ Communicate acceptance and support to the client. *It is important to change the appliance competently and quickly.*

   ◆ Provide privacy, preferably in the bathroom, where clients can learn to deal with the ostomy as they would at home.
   ◆ Assist the client to a comfortable sitting or lying position in bed or (preferably) a sitting or standing position in the bathroom. *Lying or standing positions may facilitate smoother pouch application, that is, avoid wrinkles.*
   ◆ Don gloves, and unfasten the belt if the client is wearing one.

4. Shave the peristomal skin of well-established ostomies as needed.
   ◆ Use an electric or safety razor on a regular basis to remove excessive hair. *Hair follicles can become irritated or infected by repeated pulling out of hairs during removal of the appliance and skin barrier.*

5. Empty and remove the ostomy appliance.
   ◆ Empty the contents of the pouch through the bottom opening into a bedpan. *Emptying before removing the pouch prevents spillage of effluent onto the client's skin.*
   ◆ Assess the consistency and the amount of effluent.
   ◆ Peel the bag off slowly while holding the client's skin taut. *Holding the skin taut minimizes client discomfort and prevents abrasion of the skin.*
   ◆ If the appliance is disposable, discard it in a moisture-proof bag.

6. Clean and dry the peristomal skin and stoma.
   ◆ Use toilet tissue to remove excess stool.
   ◆ Use warm water, mild soap (optional), and cotton balls or a washcloth and towel to clean the skin and stoma. Check

agency practice on the use of soap. *Soap is sometimes not advised because it can be irritating to the skin.*

◆ Use a special skin cleanser to remove dried, hard stool. *This emulsifies the stool, making removal less damaging to the skin.*

◆ Dry the area thoroughly by patting with a towel or cotton balls. *Excess rubbing can abrade the skin.*

7. Assess the stoma and peristomal skin.

◆ Inspect the stoma for color, size, shape, and bleeding.

◆ Inspect the peristomal skin for any redness, ulceration, or irritation. *Transient redness after the removal of adhesive is normal.*

◆ Place a piece of tissue or gauze pad over the stoma, and change it as needed. *This absorbs any seepage from the stoma.*

8. Apply paste-type skin barrier if needed.

◆ Fill in abdominal creases or dimples with paste. *This establishes a smooth surface for application of the skin barrier and pouch.*

◆ Allow the paste to dry for 1 to 2 minutes or as recommended by the manufacturer.

9. Prepare and apply the skin barrier (peristomal seal).

FOR A SOLID WAFER OR DISC SKIN BARRIER

◆ Use the guide (Figure 19-9 ◆) to measure the size of the stoma.

◆ On the backing of the skin barrier, trace a circle the same size as the stomal opening.

◆ Cut out the traced stoma pattern to make an opening in the skin barrier. Make the opening no more than 0.3 to 0.4 cm (⅛ to ⅙ in) larger than the stoma. *This minimizes the risk of effluent contacting peristomal skin.*

◆ Remove the backing to expose the sticky adhesive side.

◆ Center the skin barrier over the stoma, and gently press it onto the client's skin, smoothing out any wrinkles or bubbles (Figure 19-10 ◆).

FOR LIQUID SKIN SEALANT

◆ Cover the stoma with a gauze pad. *This prevents contact with the skin sealant.*

Figure 19-9. ◆ A guide for measuring the stoma.

Figure 19-10. ◆ Centering the skin barrier over the stoma.

◆ Either wipe or apply the product evenly around the peristomal skin to form a thin layer of the liquid plastic coating to the same area.

◆ Allow the skin barrier to dry until it no longer feels tacky.

10. Fill in any exposed skin around an irregularly shaped stoma.

◆ Apply paste to any exposed skin areas. Use a non–alcohol-based product if the skin is excoriated. *Alcohol may cause stinging and burning.*
or

◆ Sprinkle peristomal powder on the skin, wipe off the excess, and dab the powder with a slightly moist gauze or an applicator moistened with a liquid skin barrier. *This creates a barrier or seal.*

11. Prepare and apply the clean appliance.

◆ Remove the tissue over the stoma before applying the pouch.

FOR A DISPOSABLE POUCH WITH ADHESIVE SQUARE

◆ If the appliance does not have a precut opening, trace a circle 0.3 to 0.4 cm (⅛ to ⅙ in) larger than the stoma size on the appliance's adhesive square. *The opening is made slightly larger than the stoma to prevent rubbing, cutting, or trauma to the stoma.*

◆ Cut out a circle in the adhesive. Take care not to cut any portion of the pouch.

◆ Peel off the backing from the adhesive seal.

◆ Center the opening of the pouch over the client's stoma, and apply it directly onto the skin barrier (Figure 19-11 ◆).

◆ Gently press the adhesive backing onto the skin and smooth out any wrinkles, working from the stoma outward. *Wrinkles allow seepage of effluent, which can irritate the skin or soil clothing.*

◆ Remove the air from the pouch. *Removing the air helps the pouch lie flat against the abdomen.*

◆ Place a deodorant on the pouch (optional).

Figure 19-11. ◆ Applying the disposable pouch.

◆ Close the pouch by turning up the bottom a few times, fanfolding its end lengthwise, and securing it with a tail closure clamp.

◆ Adjust the teaching plan and nursing care plan as needed. Include on the teaching plan the equipment and procedure used. *Client learning is facilitated by consistent nursing interventions.*

VARIATION: APPLYING THE SKIN BARRIER AND APPLIANCE AS ONE UNIT

◆ If a disc- or wafer-type skin barrier is used, the skin barrier and appliance can be applied as one unit. *Applying the skin barrier and the appliance together not only is quicker but also is thought to reduce the chance of wrinkles. It also is easier for the client to apply without help.*

◆ Prepare the skin barrier by measuring the size of the stoma, tracing a circle on the backing of the skin barrier, and cutting out the traced stoma pattern to make an opening in the skin barrier.

◆ Prepare the appliance by cutting an opening 0.3 to 0.4 cm (⅛ to ⅙ in) larger than the stoma size (if not already present) and peeling off the backing from the adhesive seal.

◆ Center the opening of the pouch over the skin barrier.

◆ Remove the skin barrier backing to expose the sticky adhesive side.

◆ Center the skin barrier and appliance over the stoma, and press it onto the client's skin.

◆ SAMPLE DOCUMENTATION

5/26/05	Ostomy measured, appliance applied.
#1000	Ostomy is brick red in color, no
	bleeding noted. Effluent dark brown,
	watery. Peristomal skin clean and dry.
	Bag secured with ostomy clasp. Client
	tolerated procedure well. ———————
	Ⓓ Haus LVN

PROCEDURE 19-2
Administering an Enema

PURPOSES

◆ To prepare the bowel for a procedure
◆ To relieve constipation

EQUIPMENT

◆ Disposable underpad
◆ Bath blanket
◆ Bedpan or commode

◆ Disposable gloves
◆ Water-soluble lubricant if tubing not prelubricated
◆ Solution container with tubing of correct size and tubing clamp
◆ Correct solution, amount, and temperature (see the accompanying box)
◆ Prepackaged container of enema solution with lubricated tip

INTERVENTIONS

1. Prepare the client.
- Explain the procedure to the client. Indicate that the client may experience a feeling of fullness while the solution is being administered.
- Assist the adult client to a left lateral position, with the right leg as acutely flexed as possible (Figure 19-12 ◆). *This position facilitates the flow of solution by gravity into the sigmoid and descending colon, which are on the left side. Having the right leg acutely flexed provides for adequate exposure of the anus.*
- Place the underpad under the client's buttocks to protect the bed linen, and drape the client with the bath blanket.

2. Prepare the equipment.
- Lubricate about 5 cm (2 in) of the rectal tube (some commercially prepared enema sets already have lubricated nozzles). *Lubrication facilitates insertion through the sphincters and minimizes trauma.*
- Run some solution through the connecting tubing of a large volume enema set and the rectal tube to expel any air in the tubing; then close the clamp. *Air instilled into the rectum, although not harmful, causes unnecessary distention.*

3. Wear gloves, and insert the rectal tube.
- For clients in the left lateral position, lift the upper buttock to ensure good visualization of the anus.
- Insert the tube smoothly and slowly into the rectum, directing it toward the umbilicus (Figure 19-13 ◆). *The angle follows the normal contour of the rectum. Slow insertion prevents spasm of the sphincter.*
- Insert the tube 7 to 10 cm (3 to 4 in) in an adult. *Because the anal canal is about 2.5 to 5 cm (1 to 2 in) long in the adult, insertion to this point places the tip of the tube beyond the anal sphincter into the rectum.*
- If resistance is encountered at the internal sphincter, ask the client to take a deep breath, then run a small amount of solution through the tube to relax the internal anal sphincter.
- Never force tube entry. If resistance persists, withdraw the tube, and report the resistance to the nurse in charge.

Figure 19-13. ◆ Inserting the rectal tube following the direction of the rectum.

4. Slowly administer the enema solution.
- Raise the solution container, and open the clamp to allow fluid flow.
or
Compress a pliable container by hand.
- During most adult low enemas, hold the solution container no higher than 30 cm (12 in) above the rectum. *The higher the solution container is held above the rectum, the faster the flow and the greater the force (pressure) in the rectum.* During a high enema, hold the solution container a little higher (e.g., 45 cm [18 in]). *The fluid must be instilled farther to clean the entire bowel.*
- Administer the fluid slowly. If the client complains of fullness or pain, use the clamp to stop the flow for 30 seconds, and then restart the flow at a slower rate. *Administering the enema slowly and stopping the flow momentarily decrease the likelihood of intestinal spasm and premature ejection of the solution.*
- If you are using a plastic commercial container, roll it up as the fluid is instilled. *This prevents subsequent suctioning of the solution.* See Figure 19-14 ◆.
- After all the solution has been instilled or when the client cannot hold any more and wants to defecate (the

Figure 19-12. ◆ Assuming a left lateral position for an enema. Note the commercially prepared enema.

Figure 19-14. ◆ Rolling up a commercial enema container. *Source:* © Elena Dorfman.

urge to defecate usually indicates that sufficient fluid has been administered), close the clamp, and remove the rectal tube from the anus.

- ◆ Place the rectal tube in a disposable towel as you withdraw it.

5. Encourage the client to retain the enema.

- ◆ Ask the client to remain lying down. *It is easier for the client to retain the enema when lying down than when sitting or standing, because gravity promotes drainage and peristalsis.*
- ◆ Ensure that the client retains the solution for the appropriate amount of time, for example, 5 to 10 minutes for a cleansing enema or at least 30 minutes for a retention enema.

6. Assist the client to defecate.

- ◆ Assist the client to a sitting position on the bedpan, commode, or toilet. *A sitting position facilitates the act of defecation.*
- ◆ Ask the client who is using the toilet not to flush it. *The nurse needs to observe the feces.*
- ◆ If a specimen of feces is required, ask the client to use a bedpan or commode.

7. Record and report relevant data.

- ◆ Record administration of the enema; type of solution; length of time solution was retained; the amount, color, and consistency of the returns; and the relief of flatus and abdominal distention.

VARIATION: ADMINISTERING AN ENEMA TO AN INCONTINENT CLIENT

- ◆ Occasionally, a nurse needs to administer an enema to a client who is unable to control the external sphincter muscle and thus cannot retain the enema solution for

even a few minutes. In that case, the client assumes a supine position with knees flexed on a bedpan. The head of the bed can be elevated slightly, to 30 degrees if necessary for easier breathing, and the client's head and back are supported by pillows. Pressing the buttocks together may help the client to retain the solution. The nurse wears gloves to prevent direct contact with the solution and feces that are expelled over the hand into the bedpan during the administration of the enema.

VARIATION: ADMINISTERING A RETURN-FLOW ENEMA/OR HARRIS FLUSH

- ◆ For a return-flow enema, the solution (100 to 200 mL for an adult) is instilled into the client's rectum and sigmoid colon. Then the solution container is lowered so that the fluid flows back out through the rectal tube into the container. The inflow–outflow process is repeated five or six times (to stimulate peristalsis and the expulsion of flatus), and the solution is replaced several times during the procedure if it becomes thick with feces.

◆ SAMPLE DOCUMENTATION

12/1/05	Cleansing enema given, client tolerated
#0600	750 cc of tap water. Returned soft
	brown stool and water. Client tolerated
	procedure well. D. Haus LVN

Key Terms by Topics

Use the audio glossary feature of either the CD-ROM or the Companion Website to hear the correct pronunciation of the following key terms.

Physiology of defecation
feces, peristalsis, chyme, flatus, defecation,

fiber, laxative, cathartic, tarry, sigmoidoscopy, paralytic ileus

Common fecal elimination problems
constipation, Valsalva maneuver, impaction, diarrhea, flatulence, eructation

Fecal diversion ostomies
ostomy, ileostomy, colostomy, effluent

Nursing care
occult blood, enema

Key Points

◆ The large bowel functions to excrete digestive waste products and help maintain fluid balance.

◆ A regular pattern of fecal elimination with formed, soft stools is essential to health and a sense of well-being. Factors that affect defecation are: developmental level, diet, fluid intake, activity and exercise, psychological factors, regular defecation, medications, diagnostic procedures, anesthesia, and pathologic conditions.

◆ Common fecal elimination problems include constipation, fecal impaction, diarrhea, bowel incontinence, and flatulence.

◆ When inspecting the client's stool, the nurse must observe its color, consistency, shape, amount, odor, and the presence of abnormal constituents.

◆ An adverse effect of constipation is straining during defecation, when the Valsalva maneuver may be used. Cardiac problems may ensue.

◆ An adverse effect of prolonged diarrhea is fluid and electrolyte imbalance.

◆ Digital removal of an impaction should be carried out gently because of vagal nerve stimulation and subsequent depressed cardiac rate. An order is often necessary.

◆ Normal defecation is often facilitated in both well and ill clients by providing privacy, teaching clients to attend to defecation urges promptly, assisting clients to normal sitting positions whenever possible, encouraging appropriate food and fluid intake, and scheduling regular exercise.

◆ Clients who have bowel diversion ostomies require special care, with attention to psychologic adjustment, diet, and stoma and skin care.

EXPLORE MediaLink

Additional interactive resources for this chapter can be found on the Companion Website at www.prenhall.com/ramont. Click on Chapter 19 and "Begin" to select the activities for this chapter.

For chapter-related NCLEX-style questions and an audio glossary, access the accompanying CD-ROM in this book.

Animations:
◆ Digestive system tour ◆ Enema

For Further Study

For detailed information about assessing the abdomen, see Chapter 11.
For more information about maintaining skin integrity, see Chapter 12.
For perineal care, see Chapter 13 and Procedure 13-1.
For further study of fluid balance and nutrition, see Chapter 17.

Critical Thinking Care Map

Caring for a Client with Ulcerative Colitis

NCLEX-PN Focus Area: Physiologic Adaptation

Case Study: Mrs. Dora Davis is a 60-year old client being treated for ulcerative colitis. She was hospitalized for a colectomy; she has a permanent ileostomy. Today marks her third postoperative day. She continues to have pain. When you empty her ileostomy bag, she throws the cover over her head. She is due for discharge in 2 days. The enterostomal nurse has visited and initiated teaching care of the ostomy. Mrs. Davis worries that the bag will break when she gets up. She has confided that she is fearful that her husband will find her unattractive.

Nursing Diagnosis: Deficient Knowledge

COLLECT DATA

Subjective	Objective
_____	_____
_____	_____
_____	_____
_____	_____
_____	_____
_____	_____
_____	_____

Would you report this data? Yes/No

If yes, to: _____

Nursing Care

_____
_____
_____
_____
_____
_____
_____
_____
_____
_____
_____
_____
_____

How would you document this? _____
_____
_____
_____
_____

Data Collected
(use those that apply)

◆ Ileostomy right abdomen
◆ Stoma brick red
◆ Effluent watery, dark brown, flecks of blood
◆ Refuses to look at the ileostomy
◆ Pain
◆ Anxious
◆ Fearful
◆ Peristomal area reddened
◆ Weight 110
◆ Hemoglobin 10
◆ WBC 12,000
◆ Gait steady
◆ UA shows 2+ bacteria
◆ BP 120/86
◆ 99.4°F
◆ Skin turgor slow

Nursing Care
(use all that apply)

◆ Monitor intake and output.
◆ Daily weights.
◆ Increase fluid intake.
◆ Assess stoma.
◆ Inspect peristomal skin.
◆ Monitor lab values.
◆ VS every 4 hours.
◆ Assess skin turgor.
◆ Assess coping mechanisms.
◆ Provide referrals to Ostomy Association.
◆ Include family in teaching.

NCLEX-PN Exam Preparation

TEST-TAKING TIP

Do not spend a long time on one question; go on to the next question. Mark the question and return to it when you have time.

1. When movement of the intestine ceases temporarily after abdominal surgery, it is known as:
   a. Constipation
   b. Volvulus
   c. Ulcerative colitis
   d. Paralytic ileus

2. Using digital removal of a fecal impaction causes rectal stimulation and is contraindicated for:
   a. Renal diseases
   b. Cancer
   c. Cardiac disease
   d. Neurologic disorders

3. Peristalsis is described as:
   a. Gas expulsion from the intestine
   b. Stool formation
   c. Fluid elimination from the intestine
   d. Wavelike contractions of the intestinal muscles

4. Which measure is most often used for the client with a fecal impaction?
   a. Rectal tube
   b. Harris flush
   c. Oil-retention enema
   d. Cathartic

5. Effluent from an ileostomy is irritating to the skin because it contains:
   a. Digestive enzymes
   b. Electrolytes
   c. Bile
   d. Organic salts

6. A stool specimen being tested for blood is called:
   a. C&S test
   b. Guaiac test
   c. Steatorrhea test
   d. Albumin test

7. A common complication of diarrhea is:
   a. Calculus
   b. Potassium loss
   c. Fluid overload
   d. Hypoactive bowel sounds

8. A major side effect of this drug is that it can cause a decrease in gastrointestinal activity leading to constipation:
   a. Colace
   b. Codeine
   c. Catapres
   d. Clonidine

9. A postoperative client is complaining about gas pains. What initial intervention would you suggest?
   a. Bed rest
   b. Drinking with a straw
   c. Ambulation
   d. Lomotil

10. The peristomal site of an ileostomy is reddened and ulcerated. How often would the appliance be changed?
    a. 5 days
    b. Every 4 hours
    c. 24 to 48 hours
    d. Once a week

Answers for Review Questions, as well as discussion of Case Study and Critical Thinking Care Map questions, appear in Appendix IV.

Chapter 20

Activity, Rest, and Sleep

SHARING experiences

I have found that when I took the time to listen, explain, and allow the clients to help to their fullest potential, it ensured a smooth, safe transfer.

Christine Haggard, LVN, Clinical Research Facility, Austin, TX.

LEARNING outcomes

After completing this chapter you will be able to:

- Describe basic elements of normal movement.
- Compare effects of exercise and immobility on body systems.
- Identify and assess factors influencing human mobility including body alignment, activity–exercise patterns, and activity tolerance.
- Use proper body mechanics when positioning, moving, lifting, and ambulating clients.
- Explain the dynamics of sleep.
- Describe variations in sleep patterns throughout the life span.
- Identify factors that affect normal sleep.
- Describe common sleep disorders.
- Describe interventions to promote normal sleep.

MediaLink

www.prenhall.com/ramont

Use the address above to access the free, interactive Companion Website created for this textbook. Get hints, instant feedback, and textbook references to chapter-related NCLEX-style questions. Link to other interesting sites.

Audio Glossary:
Use the Companion Website, or the CD-ROM disk enclosed with your textbook, to hear the pronunciation of key terms in the chapter.

Balanced activity, rest, and sleep are essential to health. Most people equate physical well-being with freedom of mobility. Mobility is vital to independence. Inability to perform routine activities of daily living (ADLs) such as bathing, cooking, shopping, and engaging in recreational sports or work can adversely effect a client's self-esteem and mental health.

Activity

 ## Normal Movement

Body movement is dependent on the integrated and interdependent activity of the musculoskeletal, nervous, and *vestibular* (inner ear) systems. Normal movement involves four bodily aspects: *alignment* (posture), joint mobility, *balance* (stability), and coordination.

ALIGNMENT AND POSTURE

When the body is aligned, organs are properly supported. This allows them to function at their best, while also maintaining balance.

The **line of gravity** is an imaginary vertical line drawn through the body's center of gravity (Figure 20-1 ◆). The **center of gravity** is the point at which all of the body's mass is centered and the base of support (the foundation on which the body rests) achieves balance. In humans, the usual line of gravity is drawn from the top of the head, down between the shoulders, through the trunk slightly anterior to the sacrum, and between the weight-bearing joints (hips, knees) and base of support (feet). In the upright position, the center of gravity occurs in the pelvis approximately midway between the umbilicus and the symphysis pubis. When standing, an adult must center body weight symmetrically along the line of gravity to maintain stability. Greater stability and balance are achieved in the sitting or supine position because a chair or bed provides a wider base of support with a lower center of gravity. When the body is well aligned, there is little strain on the joints, muscles, tendons, or ligaments.

The musculoskeletal system continuously works to maintain erect posture and to offset the constant pull of gravity. The sustained muscle contraction required to maintain the upright position is called **postural tonus.** Posture is one criterion for assessing general health, physical fitness, and beauty. Posture reflects the mood, self-esteem, and personality of an individual.

JOINT MOBILITY

Most skeletal muscles are attached to two bones at the joint. These muscles are defined by the movement they produce and are therefore called flexors, extensors, internal rotators, and so on. Types of synovial joint movement are shown in Table 20-1 ◆.

Flexors are stronger than extensors, so when a person is inactive, joints become pulled into the *flexed* (bent) position. Constant immobility causes muscles to shorten permanently and become fixed in the "flexed" position (see section on immobility below). The **range of motion (ROM)** of a joint is the maximum movement possible for that joint. Range of motion varies by individual and is determined by heredity, age, injury or disease, and level of physical activity. Many mechanisms are responsible for maintaining human balance.

Equilibrium (the sense of balance) depends upon the integration of stimuli from several organs: the muscles and tendons of the head and neck (vestibulospinal input), the eyes (vestibulo-ocular input), and the inner ear. The inner ear or **labyrinth** consists of the cochlea, vestibule, and semicircular canals. The semicircular canals and vestibule govern equilibrium.

Figure 20-1. ◆ Center of gravity and the line of gravity influence standing alignment.

TABLE 20-1	SYNOVIAL JOINT MOVEMENTS AND THEIR ACTIONS			
MOVEMENT	ACTION	MOVEMENT	ACTION
Flexion	Decreasing the angle of the joint (e.g., bending the elbow)	Eversion	Turning the sole of the foot outward by moving the ankle joint
Extension	Increasing the angle of the joint (e.g., straightening the arm at the elbow)	Inversion	Turning the sole of the foot inward by moving the ankle joint
Hyperextension	Further extension or straightening of a joint (e.g., bending the head backward)	Pronation	Moving the bones of the forearm so that the palm of the hand faces downward when held in front of the body
Abduction	Movement of the bone away from the midline of the body	Supination	Moving the bones of the forearm so that the palm of the hand faces upward when held in front of the body
Adduction	Movement of the bone toward the midline of the body	Protraction	Moving a part of the body forward in the same plane parallel to the ground
Rotation	Movement of the bone around its central axis	Retraction	Moving a part of the body backward in the same plane parallel to the ground
Circumduction	Movement of the distal part of the bone in a circle while the proximal end remains fixed		

Factors Affecting Body Alignment and Activity

Numerous factors affect an individual's body alignment, mobility, and daily activity level. These include growth and development, physical health, mental health, nutrition, personal values and attitudes, and other external factors.

GROWTH AND DEVELOPMENT

A person's age and musculoskeletal and nervous system development affect posture, body proportions, body mass, body movements, and reflexes. Refer to Chapter 24 for age-related considerations.

PHYSICAL HEALTH

Mobility is directly affected by any disorder of the musculoskeletal or nervous systems, or by any vestibular (inner ear) disorders. Congenital anomalies, such as hip dysplasia and spina bifida, affect motor function. Musculoskeletal trauma limiting mobility includes strains, sprains, fractures, joint dislocations, amputations, and joint replacement. Nervous system disorders such as cerebral palsy, Parkinson's disease, multiple sclerosis, tumors, infections (e.g., meningitis), and injuries to the spinal cord or brain such as cerebral vascular accidents (strokes) may leave muscles weakened, paralyzed, spastic (with too much muscle tone), or flaccid (without muscle tone). Disorders of the vestibular apparatus, such as ear infection or Ménière's disease, cause **vertigo,** a strong sensation of spinning around in space, which impairs balance.

Illnesses that limit the supply of oxygen to vital organs affect activity tolerance. Examples include chronic obstructive pulmonary disease (COPD), emphysema, anemia, angina, and congestive heart failure (CHF).

MENTAL HEALTH

Mental or *affective* (emotional) disorders affect personal motivation. Anxiety may produce an increase in physical activity. Chronic stress, however, depletes the body's energy reserves, producing fatigue. Slumped posture may indicate lassitude or depression. A depressed client may lack the physical energy required for daily hygiene. Exercise is necessary to mental health. Movement energizes the client and facilitates coping.

NUTRITION

Undernutrition and overnutrition influence body alignment and mobility. Obesity distorts posture and balance, causing strain on muscles and joints. More energy is expended on movement, which produces fatigue.

Effects of Immobility

A sedentary lifestyle or history of inactivity due to injury or illness increases the risk of major disease. The level of risk depends on the duration of inactivity, the client's general health, and sensory awareness. Nurses must understand these risks and encourage client mobility. Early ambulation after illness or surgery is an essential preventive measure.

MUSCULOSKELETAL SYSTEM

Signs of prolonged immobility are most often manifested in the musculoskeletal system. Muscular strength decreases in the absence of physical activity. Common musculoskeletal problems resulting from prolonged immobility include:

◆ *Disuse* **osteoporosis.** Without the stress of weight-bearing activity, bones demineralize. Calcium, which gives bones density and strength, becomes depleted. Despite adequate calcium in the diet, this demineralization process, known as osteoporosis, continues during immobility. Bones become spongy and deformed, and they fracture easily.

◆ *Disuse* **atrophy.** Unused muscles atrophy (decrease in size), losing most of their normal strength and function.

◆ *Contractures.* When muscle fibers are not able to shorten and lengthen for a prolonged time, a contracture (permanent shortening of the muscle) develops. This process involves the tendons, ligaments, and joint capsules causing permanent fixation of the joint—irreversible except by surgical intervention. Joint deformities such as foot drop (Figure 20-2 ◆) and external hip rotation occur when a stronger muscle dominates the opposite muscle.

◆ *Joint pain and stiffness.* Without movement, *collagen* (connective tissue) at the joint becomes **ankylosed** (permanently immobile). In addition, as the bones demineralize, excess calcium may deposit in the joints, contributing to stiffness and pain.

CARDIOVASCULAR SYSTEM

Diminished Cardiac Reserve

Decreased mobility creates an imbalance in the autonomic nervous system, resulting in increased heart rate. During immobility rapid heart rate reduces diastolic pressure, coronary blood flow, and heart capacity available to respond to metabolic demands. Because of this diminished reserve, an immobilized person may experience tachycardia and angina with minimal exertion.

Increased Use of the Valsalva Maneuver

The Valsalva maneuver occurs when forceful exhalation against the closed glottis increases intrathoracic pressure that reduces venous blood return to the heart. This is the kind of breath holding that is done when straining to make a bowel movement or attempting to move up in bed. As the glottis opens and breath is released, blood suddenly surges to the heart. Tachycardia or cardiac arrythmia may result.

Figure 20-2. ◆ Plantar flexion contracture (foot drop).

Orthostatic Hypotension

Orthostatic hypotension (postural hypotension) is common with prolonged bed rest. It is marked by a sudden drop in blood pressure when a client stands and blood pools in the lower extremities. Cerebral perfusion is compromised, creating dizziness or fainting. This sequence is usually accompanied by a sudden and marked increase in heart rate, the body's effort to protect the brain from an inadequate blood supply.

Venous Vasodilation and Stasis

The skeletal muscles of an active person contract with each movement. They compress the blood vessels to pump the blood back to the heart against gravity. Valves in the leg veins, which remain constricted, aid in venous return to the heart by preventing backflow. Atrophied muscles cannot assist in pumping blood back to the heart against gravity. Blood pools in the leg veins, causing vasodilation and engorgement (Figure 20-3 ◆).

Dependent Edema

When venous pressure is great, serum is forced from the blood vessels into the surrounding interstitial space, causing *edema* (swelling). Edema occurs most commonly in the lower body, below the level of the heart. Prolonged bed rest is likely to cause edema at the sacrum. Prolonged sitting generally causes edema in the lower legs.

Thrombophlebitis and Emboli

Venous vasodilation and stasis predispose the client to thrombus (blood clot) formation. Impaired venous return to the heart, blood hypercoagulability, and injury to a vessel wall may result in **thrombophlebitis** (one or more clots loosely attached to an inflamed vessel wall). Thrombi become very

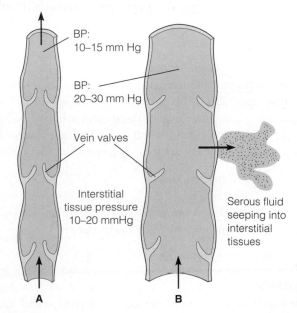

Figure 20-3. ◆ Leg veins: **A,** in a mobile person; **B,** in an immobile person.

dangerous when they break loose. **Emboli** (clots moved from their place of orgin, causing circulatory obstruction elsewhere) may lodge in vessels supplying vital organs. Large pulmonary (lung) emboli may cause **infarction** (death of tissue) and sudden death. Emboli in the coronary or cerebral vessels are equally life threatening.

RESPIRATORY SYSTEM

Decreased Respiratory Movement

In a recumbent, immobile client, ventilation of the lungs is passively altered. The rigid bed presses against the body and curtails chest movement. Abdominal organs push against the diaphragm, further restricting chest movement and lung expansion. An immobile recumbent person rarely sighs, because muscle atrophy affects the respiratory muscles. Without periodic stretching movements, the cartilaginous intercostal joints become fixed in an *expiratory* (sunken chest) position, further restricting the potential for maximum venti-lation. These changes produce shallow respirations and reduced **vital capacity** (the maximum volume of air that can be exhaled after maximum inhalation). Up to 25 to 50 percent of normal vital capacity may be compromised in an immobile, paralyzed client. For more information about oxygenation, see Chapter 16. ☍

Pooling of Respiratory Secretions

Secretions are normally expelled by coughing and posture changes. Inactivity allows respiratory secretions to pool by gravity (Figure 20-4 ◆), interfering with the normal exchange of oxygen and carbon dioxide in the alveoli. Cough may be diminished due to loss of respiratory muscle tone, dehydration (which thickens mucus), or sedatives, which depress the cough reflex. Poor oxygenation and buildup of carbon dioxide in the blood can result in respiratory acidosis, a potentially lethal imbalance of body pH.

Atelectasis

As a result of changes in pulmonary blood flow, bed rest decreases surfactant production. *Surfactant* enables the alveoli to remain open. Decreased surfactant combined with mucus blockage of a bronchiole may cause **atelectasis** (the collapse of a lobe or of an entire lung) distal to the blockage. Immobile, elderly, postoperative clients are at greatest risk of atelectasis.

Hypostatic Pneumonia

Pneumonia (inflammation of the lung) caused by static secre-tions in the alveoli is a common cause of death among weak-ened immobile persons, especially heavy smokers.

METABOLIC SYSTEM

Anorexia

Loss of appetite (*anorexia*) occurs as a result of decreased meta-bolic rate and increased catabolism. Reduced caloric intake is usually a response to decreased energy requirements. Reduced

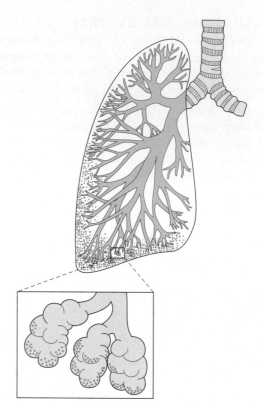

Figure 20-4. ◆ Pooling of secretions in the lungs of an immobile person.

dietary protein intake increases the risk of negative nitrogen balance and malnutrition.

Negative Calcium Balance

Negative calcium balance occurs as a result of calcium loss from bone.

URINARY SYSTEM

Urinary Stasis

Gravity plays an important role in the emptying of the kid-neys and bladder. The client in a supine (back-lying) position must push upward against gravity (Figure 20-5 ◆) to urinate. **Urinary stasis** occurs when urine *stagnates* in (does not move out of) the urinary tract.

Renal Calculi

Negative calcium balance causes increased excretion of cal-cium salts in the urine, which precipitate as crystals or calculi (kidney stones). Prolonged horizontal positioning causes the renal pelvis to become filled with stagnant alkaline urine, cre-ating an ideal environment for calculi formation.

Urinary Retention

Static urine is an excellent medium for bacterial growth. Urinary tract infections (UTIs) are most commonly caused by *Escherichia coli*, the colon bacillus. The normally sterile urinary tract may be contaminated by improper perineal care, an

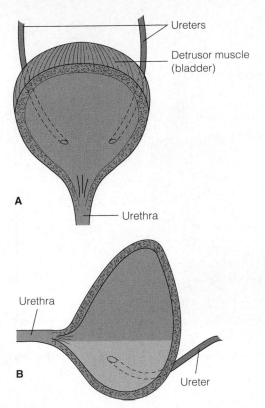

Figure 20-5. ◆ Pooling of urine in the urinary bladder: **A.** The client is in an upright position: **B.** The client is in a back-lying position.

indwelling urinary catheter, or urinary *reflux* (backward flow). See Chapter 18 for conditions related to the urinary tract. ⚭

GASTROINTESTINAL SYSTEM

Decreased peristalsis, colon motility, and strength of the abdominal and perineal muscles used in defecation cause constipation. Disruption of normal bowel habits, caused by the embarrassment or discomfort of using a bedpan, may cause the client to postpone or ignore the urge for elimination. Repeated postponement suppresses the urge and weakens the defecation reflex. A bedfast person may lack the strength required to expel hardened stool. See Chapter 19 for discussion of concerns related to bowel elimination. ⚭

INTEGUMENTARY SYSTEM
Reduced Skin Turgor

Skin can atrophy as a result of prolonged immobility. Shifts in body fluids between fluid compartments can affect the consistency and health of the dermis and subcutaneous tissues, eventually causing a gradual loss in skin *turgor* (elasticity). See Chapter 12 for a full discussion of the skin. ⚭

Skin Breakdown

Normal blood circulation relies on muscle activity. Immobility impedes circulation and diminishes the supply of nutrients. As a result, skin breakdown and formation of pressure ulcers can occur (see Chapter 12).

PSYCHONEUROLOGIC SYSTEM

People who are unable to carry out usual activities related to their roles (e.g., breadwinner, spouse, parent, or athlete) become dependent on others. Loss of independence damages self-esteem, and may in turn provoke exaggerated emotional response. Reactions vary considerably. Some individuals become apathetic or withdrawn; others become angry or aggressive.

COLLABORATIVE CARE

Hospitalized clients with limited mobility due to surgery, trauma, or disease process may need assistive devices in order to regain mobility (Figure 20-6 ◆). In most facilities, selection, fitting, and training in use of these devices is the responsibility of the physical therapy department. It is the LPN's or LVN's responsibility to reinforce the teaching and ensure that the client can use them safely both in the hospital and at home after discharge. See Box 20-1 ◆ for teaching clients to use walking aids.

Mobility Devices

CANES. Three types of canes are used today: the standard straight-legged cane; the tripod or crab cane, which has three feet; and the quad cane, which has four feet and provides the most support.

WALKERS. Walkers are mechanical devices for ambulatory clients who need more support than a cane provides. Walkers come in many shapes and sizes, with devices suited to individual needs. The standard type of walker is made of polished aluminum. It has four legs with rubber tips and plastic hand grips (Figure 20-6B). Many walkers have adjustable legs.

Two- or four-wheeled walkers do not need to be picked up to be moved. However, they are less stable than the standard walkers. Wheeled walkers are used by clients who are too weak or unstable to pick up and move the walker with each step.

CRUTCHES. Crutches may be a temporary need for some people and a permanent one for others. Crutches should enable a person to ambulate independently, so it is important to learn to use them properly. There are several kinds of crutches (Figure 20-6). The most frequently used are the underarm crutch or axillary crutch with hand bars, and the Lofstrand or forearm crutch, which extends to the forearm. The Lofstrand crutch is a single adjustable tube of aluminum to which a curved piece of steel, a rubber-covered hand bar, and a metal forearm cuff are attached. The Canadian or elbow extensor crutch, like the Lofstrand, is made of a single tube of aluminum with lateral attachments, a hand bar, and a cuff for the forearm, but it also has a cuff for the upper arm. This crutch is usually used by clients who require support for weak extensor muscles of the arm (e.g., weak triceps brachii).

A   B   C

Figure 20-6. ◆ Walking aids. **A.** Quad cane. *Source:* © Jenny Thomas. **B.** Standard walker. *Source:* © Elena Dorfman. **C.** Three types of crutches: C1, axillary crutch; C2, Lofstrand crutch; C3, Canadian, or elbow extensor, crutch.

All crutches require suction tips, usually made of rubber, which help to prevent the crutches from slipping on a floor surface. Proper measurement for and fitting of crutches is essential to ensure client safety.

NURSING CARE

The LVN/LPN collects information from the client, from other nurses, and from the client's records. The examination and history are important sources of information about disabilities affecting the client's mobility and activity status, such as contractures, edema, pain in the extremities, or generalized fatigue.

An activity and exercise history is usually part of the comprehensive nursing history form and includes daily activity level, activity tolerance, type and frequency of exercise, and factors affecting mobility. If the client indicates a recent pattern change or difficulties with mobility, a more detailed history is required. This detailed history should include the specific nature of the problem; when it first began and its frequency; its causes, if known; how the problem affects daily living; client coping strategies; and whether these methods have been effective.

 ASSESSING

Body Alignment

Assessment of body alignment includes an inspection of the client while the client stands. To assess alignment the nurse views the client from lateral, anterior, and posterior perspectives.

The "slumped" posture (Figure 20-7 ◆) is the most common problem that occurs when people stand. The neck is flexed far forward, the abdomen protrudes, the pelvis is thrust forward to create *lordosis* (an exaggerated curvature of the lumbar spine), and the knees are markedly hyperextended. Lower back pain and fatigue occur quickly in people with poor posture.

Figure 20-7. ◆ Poor trunk alignment. The arrows indicate the direction in which the pelvis is tilted.

BOX 20-1

TEACHING FOR DISCHARGE

USING WALKING AIDS

Canes
- Hold the cane with the hand on the stronger side of the body to provide maximum support and appropriate body alignment when walking.
- Position the tip of a standard cane (and the nearest tip of other canes) about 15 cm (6 in) to the side and 15 cm (6 in) in front of the near foot, so that the elbow is slightly flexed.

When Maximum Support Is Required
- Move the cane forward about 30 cm (1 ft), or a distance that is comfortable while the body weight is borne by both legs.
- Then move the affected (weak) leg forward to the cane while the weight is borne by the cane and stronger leg.
- Next, move the unaffected (stronger) leg forward ahead of the cane and weak leg while the weight is borne by the cane and weak leg.
- Repeat the steps. This pattern of moving provides at least two points of support on the floor at all times.

As You Become Stronger and Require Less Support
- Move the cane and weak leg forward at the same time, while the weight is borne by the stronger leg.
- Move the stronger leg forward, while the weight is borne by the cane and the weak leg.

Walkers

When Maximum Support Is Required
- Move the walker ahead about 15 cm (6 in) while your body weight is borne by both legs.
- Then move the right foot up to the walker while your body weight is borne by the left leg and both arms.
- Next, move the left foot up to the right foot while your body weight is borne by the right leg and both arms.

If One Leg Is Weaker Than the Other
- Move the walker and the weak leg ahead together about 15 cm (6 in) while your weight is borne by the stronger leg.
- Then move the stronger leg ahead while your weight is borne by the affected leg and both arms.

Crutches
- Follow the plan of exercises developed for you to strengthen your arm muscles before beginning crutch walking.
- Have a health care professional establish the correct length for your crutches and the correct placement of the handpieces. Crutches that are too long force your shoulders upward and make it difficult for you to push your body off the ground. Crutches that are too short will make you hunch over and develop an improper body stance.
- The weight of your body should be borne by the arms rather than the axillae (armpits). Continual pressure on the axillae can injure the radial nerve and eventually cause crutch palsy, a weakness of the muscles of the forearm, wrist, and hand.
- Maintain an erect posture as much as possible to prevent strain on muscles and joints and to maintain balance.
- Each step taken with crutches should be a comfortable distance for you. It is wise to start with a small rather than large step.
- Inspect the crutch tips regularly, and replace them if worn.
- Keep the crutch tips dry and clean to maintain their surface friction. If the tips become wet, dry them well before use.
- Wear a tie shoe with a low heel that grips the floor.

Gait

The characteristic pattern of a person's *gait* (walk) is assessed to determine the client's mobility and risk for injury due to falling. The nurse assesses gait as the client walks into the room or asks the client to walk a distance of 10 feet down a hallway and observes for the following:

- Head is erect, gaze is straight ahead, and vertebral column is upright.
- Heel strikes the ground before the toe.
- Feet are dorsiflexed in the swing phase.
- Arm opposite the swing-through foot moves forward at the same time.
- Gait is smooth, coordinated, and rhythmic, with even weight borne on each foot; it produces minimal body swing from side to side and directs movement straight ahead; and it starts and stops with ease.

The nurse should also note the client's need for a prosthesis or assistive device, such as a cane or walker. For a client who uses assistive aids, the nurse assesses gait without the device and compares the assisted and unassisted gaits.

Appearance and Movement of Joints

Physical examination of the joints involves inspection; palpation; assessment of range of active motion; and, if active motion is not possible, assessment of range of passive motion.

The following joints may be given special attention: neck, shoulder, elbow, wrist, hip, knee, and ankle. Box 20-2 ◆ gives points for the nurse to remember in teaching clients to do active ROM. Assessment of range of motion should not be unduly fatiguing, and the joint movements need to be performed smoothly, slowly, and rhythmically. No joint should be forced. Uneven, jerky movement and forcing can injure the joint and its surrounding muscles and ligaments.

The nurse also assesses the amount of assistance the client requires for the following:

◆ Moving in the bed. In particular, observe for the amount of assistance the client requires for turning:

From a supine position to a lateral position

From a lateral position on one side to a lateral position on the other

From a supine position to a sitting position in bed

◆ Rising from a lying position to a sitting position on the edge of the bed. Healthy people can normally rise without support from the arms.

◆ Rising from a chair to a standing position. Normally this can be done without pushing with the arms.

◆ Range of motion of joints needed to complete transfer movements (see previous section).

◆ Coordination and balance. Determine the client's abilities to hold the body erect, to bear weight and keep balance in a standing position on both legs or only one, to take steps, and to push off from a chair or bed. See Procedure 20-1 for instruction in providing passive range of motion exercises.

Activity Tolerance

By observation, the nurse can predict whether the client has the strength and endurance to participate in activities that require similar expenditures of energy. The most useful measures in predicting activity tolerance are heart rate, strength, and rhythm; respiratory rate, depth, and rhythm; and blood pressure. If the client tolerates an activity well, and if the client's heart rate returns to baseline within 5 minutes after activity, the activity is considered safe. This activity, then, can serve as a standard for predicting the client's tolerance for similar activities.

When collecting data pertaining to the problems of immobility, the nurse uses inspection, palpation, and auscultation; monitors results of laboratory tests; and takes measurements, including body weight, fluid intake, and fluid output.

◆ DIAGNOSING, PLANNING, and IMPLEMENTING

The LVN/LPN in collaboration with the RN develops a nursing care plan using a NANDA list. Examples of NANDA diagnoses that relate to activity are: Activity Intolerance, Impaired Physical Mobility, and Risk for Injury. See Appendix I for a complete NANDA list. ⊂⊃ Positioning, transferring, and ambulating clients are almost always independent nursing functions. The physician usually orders specific body positions only after surgery, anesthesia, or trauma involving the nervous and musculoskeletal systems. All clients should have an activity order written by a physician upon admission.

As part of planning, the nurse is responsible for identifying clients who need assistance with body alignment and determining the degree of assistance required. The nurse must be sensitive to the client's need for independence, yet must provide assistance when warranted.

Most clients require specific knowledge to achieve and maintain proper body mechanics. The nurse is responsible for teaching such skills. For example, a client with a back injury must learn how to get out of bed safely and comfortably; a client with an injured leg needs to know how to transfer from bed to wheelchair safely; and a client with a newly acquired walker needs to learn how to use it safely. Nurses often teach family members or caregivers safe moving, lifting, and transfer techniques in the home setting.

The goals established for clients vary according to the nursing diagnosis and anticipated outcome for each individual. Examples of overall goals for clients with actual or potential problems related to mobility or activity follow:

◆ Increase tolerance for physical activity.

◆ Avoid injury from falling or improper use of body mechanics.

◆ Avoid any complications associated with immobility.

Nursing strategies to maintain or promote body alignment and mobility involve positioning clients appropriately, moving and turning clients in bed, transferring clients, providing ROM exercises, ambulating clients with or without mechanical aids, and preventing the complications of immobility. Whenever positioning, moving, lifting, and ambulat-

---

BOX 20-2
NURSING CARE CHECKLIST

ACTIVE ROM EXERCISES

☑ Perform each ROM exercise as taught to the point of slight resistance, but not beyond, and never to the point of discomfort.

☑ Perform the movements systematically, using the same sequence during each session.

☑ Perform each exercise three times.

☑ Perform each series of exercises twice daily.

For Older Adults

☑ For older adults, it is not essential to achieve full range of motion in all joints. Instead, emphasize achieving a sufficient range of motion to carry out ADLs, such as walking, dressing, combing hair, showering, and preparing a meal.

ing clients, nurses must use proper body mechanics to avoid personal injury. Refer to Chapter 6 for more information related to body mechanics and the nurse.

Positioning Clients

Positioning a client in good body alignment and changing position regularly and systematically are essential aspects of nursing practice. Clients who move easily automatically reposition for comfort. These people generally require minimal assistance from nurses, other than guidance about ways to maintain body alignment and exercise their joints. However, those who are weak, frail, in pain, paralyzed, or unconscious rely on nurses to provide or assist with position changes. For all clients, it is important to assess the skin and provide skin care before and after a position change.

Any position, if unchanged for a prolonged period, becomes detrimental. Frequent changes of position prevent muscle discomfort, pressure damage to superficial nerves and blood vessels, decubiti, and contractures. Position changes maintain muscle tone and stimulate postural reflexes.

When the client is not able to move independently or assist with moving, the preferred method is to have two or more people move or turn the client. Appropriate assistance reduces the risk of muscle strain and body injury to both the client and nurse. See Procedure 20-2 for moving a client in bed.

Sometimes a person who appears well aligned may be experiencing discomfort. To promote the client's proper body alignment, comfort and safety, the nurse should:

- *Make sure the mattress is firm and level* yet yields enough to fill in and support natural body curvatures. Mattress inspection in the home setting is particularly important. A sagging or too soft mattress, or an underfilled water bed may contribute to development of hip flexion contractures or low back strain and pain. A plywood bedboard may be placed beneath a sagging mattress to add support. Some bedboards are hinged to allow the head of the bed to be raised. Bedboards are strongly recommended for clients who are at risk for back problems.
- *Ensure that the bed is clean and dry.* Wrinkled or damp sheets increase the risk of pressure ulcer formation (see Chapter 13 ⊂⊃). Make sure extremities can move freely whenever possible. For example, top sheets need to be loose for the client to move the feet.
- *Place support devices in specified areas* according to the client's position. See Box 20-3 ◆ for commonly used support devices. Use only those devices needed to maintain alignment (such as a trochanter roll, Figure 20-8 ◆) and prevent stress on muscles and joint. If the person is mobile, too many devices limit movement and increase the potential for injury.
- *Avoid placing one body part, particularly one with bony prominences, directly on top of another body part.* Excessive pressure can damage veins and predispose the client to thrombus

> ### BOX 20-3
> ### SUPPORT DEVICES
>
> - *Pillows.* Different sizes are available. Used for support or elevation of a body part (e.g., an arm). Specially designed dense pillows can be used to elevate the upper body.
> - *Mattresses.* There are two types of mattresses: ones that fit on the bed frame (e.g., standard bed mattress) and mattresses that fit on the standard bed mattress (e.g., eggcrate mattress). Mattresses should be evenly supportive. See Chapter 13 for additional information and Table 12-5 for devices that reduce pressure on body parts. ⊂⊃
> - *Bedboards.* The boards are usually made of wood and are placed under the mattress to provide support.
> - *Chair beds.* These beds can be placed into the position of a chair for clients who cannot move from the bed but require a sitting position.
> - *Foot boot.* These are made of a variety of substances. They usually have a firm exterior and padding of foam to protect the skin. They provide support to the feet in a natural position and keep the weight of covers off the toes. Without support, an immobilized client's feet assume a plantar flexion position (foot drop). Prolonged assumption of this position results in permanent contracture of the gastrocnemius muscle and tendon.
> - *Footboard.* A flat panel often made of plastic or wood. It keeps the feet in dorsiflexion to prevent plantar flexion.

Figure 20-8. ◆ Making a trochanter roll: (1) Fold the towel in half lengthwise. (2) Roll the towel tightly, starting at one narrow edge and rolling within approximately 30 cm (1 ft) of the other edge. (3) Invert the roll. Then palpate the greater trochanter of the femur and place the roll with the center at the level of the greater trochanter; place the flat part of towel under the client; then roll the towel snugly against the hip.

Figure 20-10. ◆ Orthopneic position.

Figure 20-12. ◆ Tensing the quadriceps femoris muscles before ambulation.

nausea, tachycardia, and dizziness. If any of these are present, the client should be assisted to the supine position in bed and closely monitored. Box 20-4 ◆ provides client teaching for ways to manage postural hypotension.

◆ EVALUATING

The goals established during the planning phase are evaluated according to specific desired outcomes, also established in that phase. If outcomes are not achieved the nurse, client, and support person if appropriate need to explore the reasons before modifying the care plan.

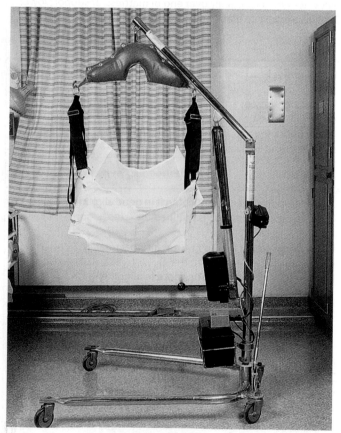

Figure 20-11. ◆ A one-piece seat hydraulic lift. *Source:* © Jenny Thomas.

BOX 20-4

TEACHING FOR DISCHARGE

CONTROLLING POSTURAL HYPOTENSION

◆ Sleep with the head of the bed elevated 8 to 12 inches. This position makes the position change on rising less severe.

◆ Avoid sudden changes in position. Arise from bed in three stages:
   1. Sit up in bed for 1 minute.
   2. Sit on the side of the bed with legs dangling for 1 minute.
   3. Stand with care, holding onto the edge of the bed or another nonmovable object for 1 minute. Gradual changes in position stimulate *renin* (a kidney enzyme that has a role in regulating blood pressure), which prevents a dramatic drop in pressure.

◆ Never bend down all the way to the floor or stand up too quickly after stooping. *Baroreceptors* (sensory nerve endings in the walls of blood vessels) cannot accommodate rapid change.

◆ Postpone activities such as shaving and hair grooming for at least 1 hour after rising. Baroreceptor reflexes are slow to respond after a night of recumbency during sleep.

◆ Wear elastic stockings at night to inhibit venous pooling in the legs.

◆ Be aware that the symptoms of hypotension are most severe at the following times:
   1. 30 to 60 minutes after a heavy meal
   2. 1 to 2 hours after taking an antihypertension medication

◆ Get out of a hot bath very slowly, because high temperatures can lead to venous pooling.

◆ Use a rocking chair to improve circulation in the lower extremities. Even mild leg conditioning can strengthen muscle tone and enhance circulation.

◆ Refrain from any strenuous activity that results in holding the breath and bearing down. This Valsalva maneuver slows the heart rate, leading to subsequent lowering of blood pressure.

Nursing Process Case Study: **CLIENT IN TRACTION**

Kevin Andrews, a 17-year-old high school gymnast, fell from the parallel bars and fractured his left femur. Kevin has been on bed rest in skeletal traction since the accident. He is depressed and bored with the hospital routine of care. Because of painful muscle spasms, he often refuses to be turned or to move voluntarily. His appetite is poor, and he often refuses his hospital meals. He needs encouragement from the nursing staff to cough and deep breathe.

Assessment

◆ Height 175.3 cm (5′ 8″)
◆ Weight 70 kg (154 lbs) on admission
◆ 37° C (98.6° F)
◆ 80 bpm
◆ 16/minute
◆ BP 114/70 mm Hg
◆ Diagnostic Data: chest x-ray negative, urinalysis negative, Hgb 13.3 g/dL, Hct 37%

Diagnosis. The following diagnosis is identified for Kevin: Risk for Disuse Syndrome related to depression and reluctance to move secondary to painful muscle spasms.

Desired Outcomes

◆ Performs activities of daily living within limitation of skeletal traction.
◆ Performs range-of-motion exercises of upper limbs and unaffected lower limb tid.
◆ Uses overhead trapeze q3h to strengthen muscles in upper limbs by day 3.
◆ Traction site remains free of drainage and odor.
◆ Homans' sign remains negative.

Planning and Implementation. The following nursing interventions are implemented for Kevin:

Traction/Immobilization Care

◆ Maintain proper position in bed to enhance traction.
◆ Ensure that the pull of ropes and weights remains along the axis of the fractured bone.

◆ Monitor pin insertion sites.
◆ Perform pin insertion site care.
◆ Monitor circulation, movement, and sensation of affected extremity.
◆ Monitor for complications of immobility.
◆ Administer appropriate skin care at friction points.
◆ Provide trapeze for movement in bed.
◆ Instruct Kevin on the importance of adequate nutrition for bone healing.

Exercise Therapy: Joint Mobility

◆ Determine Kevin's motivation level for maintaining or restoring joint movement.
◆ Explain to Kevin and his family the purpose and plan for joint exercises.
◆ Initiate pain control measures before beginning joint exercise.
◆ Assist Kevin to the optimal body position for each passive or active joint movement.
◆ Encourage active range-of-motion exercises according to a regular schedule.
◆ Collaborate with a physical therapist in developing and executing an exercise program.

Evaluation. Goal partially met. Kevin performs active ROM exercises only once a day and refuses the other two sessions. He uses the overhead trapeze when repositioning frequently throughout the day but is reluctant to bathe and states "Just leave me alone for a while." His appetite has not improved and he eats approximately 40 to 50 percent of each meal. The skin surrounding the pin site remains odorless, dry, and intact. Homans' sign is negative; pulses are strong bilaterally.

Critical Thinking in the Nursing Process

1. What nursing intervention can be done for Kevin to relieve muscle spasms?
2. Kevin is refusing hospital meals. What can you do to improve Kevin's nutritional status needs to promote healing?
3. Describe diversion activities appropriate for a 17-year-old in traction.

Rest and Sleep

Rest and sleep are essential to health. Normal sleep is characterized by minimal physical activity, variable levels of consciousness, changes in the body's physiologic processes, and decreased responsiveness to external stimuli. Some environ-

mental stimuli, such as a smoke detector alarm, will awaken the sleeper, whereas other noises will not. Individuals respond to meaningful stimuli while sleeping and selectively disregard unmeaningful stimuli. Clients often complain that rest and sleep are difficult to achieve in the hospital environment. When deprived of sleep, clients become fatigued, depressed, or irritable. Nurses are responsible for providing an environment conducive to rest and sleep.

 Physiology of Sleep

Sleep is a complex biologic rhythm. When a person's biologic clock coincides with sleep–wake patterns, the person is awake when the physiologic and psychological rhythms are most active and is asleep when the physiologic and psychological rhythms are most inactive. Infants are awake most often in the early morning and the late afternoon. After 4 months of age, infants enter a 24-hour cycle in which they sleep mostly during the night. By the end of the fifth or sixth month, infants' sleep–wake patterns are almost like those of adults.

Two types of sleep have been identified: non–rapid eye movement (NREM or non-REM) sleep and REM (rapid eye movement) sleep.

NREM SLEEP

Most sleep during a night is **NREM sleep.** It is a deep, restful sleep with some decreased physiologic functions. NREM sleep is divided into four stages.

1. Stage I is very light sleep. The person feels drowsy and relaxed. The sleeper can be readily awakened. This stage lasts only a few minutes.
2. Stage II is light sleep during which body processes continue to slow down. The eyes are generally still, the heart and respiratory rates decrease slightly, and body temperature falls. Stage II lasts about 10 to 15 minutes.
3. Stage III occurs when the heart and respiratory rates, as well as other body processes, slow further because of the domination of the parasympathetic nervous system. The sleeper becomes more difficult to arouse.
4. Stage IV signals deep sleep, called delta sleep. The sleeper's heart and respiratory rates are 20 to 30 percent below waking rates. The sleeper is very relaxed, rarely moves, and is difficult to arouse. Stage IV is thought to restore the body physically. During this stage, the eyes usually roll, and some dreaming occurs.

REM SLEEP

REM sleep constitutes about 25 percent of the sleep of a young adult. It usually recurs about every 90 minutes and lasts 5 to 30 minutes. REM sleep is not as restful as NREM sleep. Most dreams take place during REM sleep. Box 20-5 ◆ lists characteristics of sleep.

 Functions of Sleep

Sleep exerts physiologic effects on body systems and restores normal levels of activity and balance within the nervous sys-

---

BOX 20-5
CHARACTERISTICS OF SLEEP

NREM Sleep

◆ Arterial blood pressure falls.
◆ Pulse rate decreases.
◆ Peripheral blood vessels dilate.
◆ Activity of the gastrointestinal tract occasionally increases.
◆ Skeletal muscles relax.
◆ Basal metabolic rate decreases 10 to 30 percent.

REM Sleep

◆ Active dreaming occurs, and dreams are remembered.
◆ The sleeper may be difficult to arouse or may wake spontaneously.
◆ Muscle tone is depressed.
◆ Heart rate and respiratory rate often are irregular.
◆ A few irregular muscle movements occur—in particular, rapid eye movements.
◆ The brain is very active.

Source: Adapted from A. C. Guyton and J. E. Hall, *Textbook of Medical Physiology,* 9th ed. Philadelphia: Saunders, 1996, p. 762–763. Reprinted with permission.

---

tem. The effects of sleep on the body are not fully understood. However, it is known that the activity of the sympathetic nervous system is greater while the person is awake, as are impulses to the body's muscles, which increase muscle tone. During sleep, the activity of the parasympathetic nervous system increases, causing the physiologic changes. Sleep is necessary for protein synthesis and cellular repair.

Research suggests that maintaining a regular sleep–wake rhythm (sleep hygiene) is more important than the actual number of hours slept. Some people, for example, can function well on as little as 5 hours' sleep each night. Reestablishing the sleep–wake cycle (e.g., after the disruption of surgery) is an important aspect of nursing.

 Factors Affecting Sleep

Both the quality and the quantity of sleep are affected by a number of factors. Sleep quality refers to an individual's ability to stay asleep and to get appropriate amounts of REM and NREM sleep. Quantity of sleep is the total time the individual sleeps.

ILLNESS

Illness increases the need for sleep, but disease often disrupts normal sleep rhythms. Respiratory conditions affect sleep. Shortness of breath, nasal congestion, or sinus drainage and coughing disrupt sleep by causing frequent arousal.

People who have gastric or duodenal ulcers may find their sleep disturbed due to pain, the result of increased gastric secretions occurring during REM sleep. Endocrine disorders affect sleep. Hyperthyroidism lengthens presleep time, making it difficult to fall asleep. Hypothyroidism, conversely, decreases Stage IV sleep. Elevated body temperatures can cause some reduction in Stages III and IV NREM sleep and REM sleep.

The need to urinate during the night (*enuresis*) also disrupts sleep. People who awaken at night to urinate sometimes have difficulty getting back to sleep.

ENVIRONMENT

Environment can promote or hinder sleep. Changes in the level of sound, light, and room temperatures adversely affect sleep. Unfamiliar surroundings may contribute to anxiety, which disturbs sleep. Over time, however, most individuals adjust to these changes.

LIFESTYLE

Moderate exercise is conducive to sleep, but excessive exercise can delay sleep. The ability to relax before retiring is an important factor affecting the ability to fall asleep. Shift work affects the quality of rest and sleep. Night shift workers may experience effects of lack of synchronicity between the body's internal clock and waking/working hours. Moving shifts forward (day to evening; evening to night; night to day) can be helpful in preventing fatigue, illness, or work error.

EMOTIONAL STRESS

Anxiety and depression frequently disturb sleep. Anxiety increases the norepinephrine blood levels through stimulation of the sympathetic nervous system.

ALCOHOL AND STIMULANTS

Excessive alcohol intake disrupts REM sleep, although it may hasten the onset of sleep. While making up for lost REM sleep after some of the effects of the alcohol have worn off, people often experience nightmares. Caffeine-containing beverages act as stimulants of the central nervous system, thus interfering with sleep.

SMOKING

Nicotine is a stimulant. Therefore, smokers generally suffer from poor sleep. Smokers have difficulty falling asleep and maintaining sleep. Avoiding tobacco after the evening meal improves sleep.

DIET

Weight change may affect sleep. Weight loss is associated with reduced total sleep time and early awakening. Weight gain is associated with fewer arousals, later awakening, and an increase in total sleep time.

The amino acid L-tryptophan is believed to enhance sleep. Milk and cheese are rich dietary sources of L-tryptophan, which may explain why warm milk helps some people fall asleep.

MOTIVATION

A strong desire to stay awake can counteract fatigue. An individual will find it easier to stay awake when engaged in an interesting activity, whereas boredom invites sleep.

MEDICATIONS

Medications affect the quality of sleep. Sedative–hypnotics (e.g., secobarbital) interfere with Stages III and IV NREM sleep and suppress REM sleep. Beta blockers can cause insomnia and nightmares. Narcotics such as meperidine hydrochloride (Demerol) and morphine and tranquilizers suppress REM sleep and cause frequent awakenings and drowsiness. These drugs may cause some of the following sleep problems: disrupt REM sleep, delay onset of sleep, decrease sleep time, cause nightmares, and increase daytime drowsiness:

◆ Amphetamines
◆ Antidepressants
◆ Beta blockers
◆ Bronchodilators
◆ Caffeine
◆ Decongestants
◆ Narcotics
◆ Steroids

 Common Sleep Disorders

INSOMNIA

Insomnia, the inability to obtain an adequate amount or quality of sleep, is the most common sleep disorder. People suffering from insomnia do not feel refreshed on arising.

Insomnia is most commonly caused by mental overstimulation due to anxiety, but may result from physical discomfort. Clients may become anxious because they think they might not be able to sleep. Drug and alcohol abusers generally suffer from insomnia.

Treatment for insomnia routinely includes a behavior modification plan in which the client learns new habits to foster sleep. The therapeutic value of sleep-inducing drugs is considered debatable since these drugs treat only the symptom and not the root cause of sleeplessness. Furthermore, prolonged usage creates drug dependency.

HYPERSOMNIA

Hypersomnia or excessive daytime sleep (EDS), can result from many diseases. Central nervous system, kidney, liver, or metabolic disorders, such as diabetic acidosis and hypothyroidism, cause sleepiness. Hypersomnia can be linked to mental disorders; depressed persons may use sleep as an escape mechanism.

NARCOLEPSY

Narcolepsy is an underrecognized and poorly understood disorder believed to be genetic or autoimmune. Narcolepsy ◆

sufferers experience regular REM onset sleep attacks lasting from a few seconds to several hours. Nighttime sleep may be fragmented by vivid dreams or nightmares. Central nervous system stimulants such as methylphenidate (Ritalin) or amphetamine may be prescribed to control excessive daytime sleepiness. Tricyclic antidepressants may be given to suppress REM sleep.

SLEEP APNEA

Sleep apnea is the periodic cessation of breathing during sleep. Apnea occurs most often in men over 50 and post-menopausal women. Sufferers may experience up to 600 episodes per night during NREM sleep, each lasting from ten seconds to two minutes. These multiple arousals cause fatigue and EDS.

An apneic episode begins with snoring. Breathing ceases, followed by gasping or snorting as breathing resumes. Breathlessness causes increased carbon dioxide levels in the blood, which trigger awakening.

Treatment is aimed at the cause of the apnea; for example, enlarged tonsils may be removed. The use of a nasal continuous positive airway pressure (CPAP) device at night is often effective.

Sleep apnea profoundly affects a person's work or school performance. In addition, prolonged sleep apnea can cause a sharp rise in blood pressure and may lead to cardiac arrest. Over time, apneic episodes can cause cardiac arrhythmias, pulmonary hypertension, and left-sided heart failure.

PARASOMNIAS

A **parasomnia** is behavior that may interfere with sleep. Examples of this are sleepwalking (*somnambulism*), sleeptalking, bedwetting (*nocturnal enuresis*), nocturnal erection, and teeth grinding and clenching (*bruxism*).

SLEEP DEPRIVATION

Sleep deprivation is the reduction in the amount, quality, or consistency of sleep. This syndrome produces both physiologic and behavioral symptoms whose severity depends on the degree and type of deprivation (i.e., REM or NREM sleep). Combined REM/NREM deprivation increases the severity of symptoms. Table 20-3 ◆ provides types, causes, and manifestations of sleep deprivation.

COLLABORATIVE CARE
Diagnostic Studies

Sleep may be measured objectively in a sleep laboratory by an electroencephalogram (EEG), electromyogram (EMG), and electro-oculogram (EOG) recorded simultaneously. This recording divides sleep into REM and NREM phases. Electrodes are placed on the scalp to record brain waves (EEG), at the outer canthus of each eye to record movement (EOG), and on the chin to record muscle contractions (EMG). Respiratory effort and airflow, ECG, leg movements, and oxygen saturation of arterial blood by pulse oximeter may also be monitored. Pulse oximetry and ECG recordings are of particular significance if sleep apnea is suspected. Video cameras may also be used to record the client's activity (movements, struggling, noisy respirations) during sleep.

TABLE 20-3 TYPES, CAUSES, AND SIGNS OF SLEEP DEPRIVATION

TYPE	CAUSES	CLINICAL SIGNS
REM deprivation	Alcohol, barbiturates, shift work, jet lag, extended ICU hospitalization, morphine, meperidine hydrochloride (Demerol)	Excitability, restlessness, irritability, and increased sensitivity to pain Confusion and suspiciousness Emotional lability
NREM deprivation	All the above plus diazepam (Valium), flurazepam hydrochloride (Dalmane), hypothyroidism, depression, respiratory distress disorders, sleep apnea, and age (common in the elderly)	Withdrawal, apathy, hyporesponsiveness Feeling physically uncomfortable Lack of facial expression Speech deterioration Excessive sleepiness
Both REM and NREM deprivation	As above	Decreased reasoning ability (judgment) and ability to concentrate Inattentiveness Marked fatigue manifested by blurred vision, itchy eyes, nausea, headache Difficulty performing activities of daily living Lack of memory, mental confusion, visual or auditory hallucinations, and illusions

NURSING CARE

ASSESSING

Sleep assessment includes a sleep history including sleep diary, physical examination, and review of diagnostic studies.

A brief general sleep history is obtained for all clients entering a health care facility. This enables the nurse to incorporate the client's needs and preferences in the plan of care.

Sleep Diary

A sleep diary may include all of the following information or selected aspects that pertain to the client's specific problem:

◆ Total number of sleep hours per day
◆ Activities performed 2 to 3 hours before bedtime (type, duration, and time)
◆ Bedtime rituals (e.g., ingestion of food, fluid, or medication, or ADLs like prayer or bathing)
◆ Time of (a) going to bed, (b) trying to fall asleep, (c) falling asleep (approximate), (d) any instances of waking up and duration of these periods, and (e) waking up in the morning
◆ Any worries that the client believes may affect sleep
◆ Factors the client believes have a positive or negative effect on sleep

Physical Examination

Examination includes observation of the client's physical appearance, behavior, and energy level. Evidence of a deviated nasal septum, enlarged neck, obesity and snoring may indicate obstructive sleep apnea. Irritability, restlessness, inattentiveness, slowed speech, yawning, rubbing the eyes, confusion, incoordination, and physical weakness or lethargy also suggest sleep problems.

DIAGNOSING, PLANNING, and IMPLEMENTING

Sleep Deprivation and Sleep Pattern Disturbed are NANDA nursing diagnoses that may be assigned to clients by the RN following assessment. See Appendix I for a complete NANDA list. ⊂⊃ These diagnoses may include further descriptions such as "difficulty falling asleep."

Nursing interventions to enhance clients' sleep primarily involve nonpharmacologic measures. These include teaching sleep hygiene, supporting bedtime rituals; providing a restful environment; and providing comfort measures to promote relaxation and reduce anxiety.

Promoting client sleep during hospitalization is challenging to the nurse, and requires organization, caring, and creativity to control the many external factors affecting sleep. Assistive techniques to promote rest are described in Box 20-6 ◆.

Supporting Bedtime Rituals. Most people have developed presleep routines to help them relax. Altering or eliminating these routines can affect sleep. Common adult bedtime rituals include an evening stroll, listening to music, watching television, taking a bath, and praying. Children's rituals may include a bedtime story, hugging a favorite toy or blanket, and kissing everyone goodnight. Sleep is generally preceded by hygienic routines, such as washing the face and hands (or bathing), brushing the teeth, and voiding.

In institutional settings, nurses can provide similar bedtime rituals. Talking about events like a visit from friends or the weather can help clients relax.

Creating a Restful Environment

To create a restful environment, the nurse needs to ensure safety, reduce sleep interruptions and environmental distractions, and provide room temperature satisfactory to the client. Interventions to reduce environmental distractions, especially noise, were listed in Box 20-6.

Clients must also feel safe in order to rest comfortably. People who are not accustomed to narrow hospital beds may feel more secure with side rails.

Additional safety measures include:

◆ Placing beds in low positions
◆ Using night-lights
◆ Placing call bells within easy reach

Promoting Comfort and Relaxation

Comfort measures are essential to help the client fall asleep and stay asleep, especially when disease interferes with sleep. A concerned, caring attitude, along with the following interventions, can significantly promote client comfort, relaxation, and sleep:

◆ Provide loose-fitting nightwear.
◆ Assist clients with hygienic routines and other bedtime rituals.
◆ Make sure the bed linen is smooth, clean, and dry.
◆ Assist or encourage the client to void before bedtime.
◆ Provide a back massage before sleep (see Procedure 20-5).
◆ Position dependent clients appropriately to aid muscle relaxation.
◆ Provide supportive devices to protect pressure areas.
◆ Schedule medications, especially diuretics, to prevent nocturnal awakenings.
◆ Manage pain by administering analgesics 30 minutes before sleep; change dressings and/or apply warm or cool compresses or splints to painful areas.
◆ Facilitate effective breathing by administering prescribed medications such as bronchodilators before bedtime and position clients appropriately (e.g., semi-Fowler's position).
◆ Encourage slow deep breathing followed by tonic muscle exercises (rhythmic contraction and relaxation) to promote relaxation.

BOX 20-6

TEACHING FOR DISCHARGE

PROMOTING REST AND SLEEP

Sleep Pattern

◆ Establish a regular bedtime and wake-up time for all days of the week to prevent disruptions in your biologic rhythm. Eliminate lengthy naps, or if a daytime nap is necessary, take it at the same time each day and limit the time to 30 minutes, preferably once a day.

◆ Get adequate exercise during the day to reduce stress, but avoid excessive physical exertion 2 hours before bedtime.

◆ Avoid dealing with office work or family problems before bedtime.

◆ Establish a regular routine before sleep such as reading, listening to soft music, taking a warm bath, or doing some other quiet activity you enjoy.

◆ When you are unable to sleep, pursue some relaxing activity until you feel drowsy.

◆ If you have trouble falling asleep, get up and pursue non-strenuous activity until you feel sleepy.

◆ Use the bed mainly for sleep, so that you associate it with sleep.

Environment

◆ Ensure appropriate lighting, temperature, and ventilation.

◆ Keep noise to a minimum; block out extraneous noise as necessary with soft music.

Diet

◆ Avoid heavy meals 3 hours before bedtime.

◆ Avoid alcohol and caffeine-containing foods and beverages (coffee, tea, chocolate) at least 4 hours before bedtime. These act as diuretics, creating the need to void during sleep time.

◆ Decrease fluid intake 2 to 4 hours before sleep if necessary to avoid the need to use the bathroom during sleeping hours.

◆ If a bedtime snack is necessary, consume only light carbohydrates or a milk drink. Heavy or spicy foods can cause gastrointestinal upsets that disturb sleep.

Medications

◆ Use sleeping medications only as a last resort. Take them judiciously (e.g., three times a week). Use over-the-counter medications sparingly because many contain antihistamines that cause daytime drowsiness.

◆ Take analgesics 30 minutes before bedtime to relieve aches and pains.

◆ Consult with your health care provider about adjusting other medications that may cause insomnia.

◆ Encourage the client to share concerns; actively listen and address problems as they arise.

People, especially older adults, are unable to sleep well if they feel cold. Changes in circulation, metabolism, and body tissue density reduce the older person's ability to generate and conserve heat. Interventions to keep elderly clients warm during sleep are listed in Box 20-7 ◆.

Enhancing Sleep with Medications

Sleep medications (most often prescribed on a prn or as-needed basis) include sedative–hypnotics to induce sleep and tranquilizers (benzodiazepines) to decrease anxiety and tension. In institutional settings, the nurse shares responsibility with the client regarding when to administer them. Both nurses and clients must be aware of the actions, effects, and risks of medication prescribed. Medication should be administered only when indicated and once the client has demonstrated understanding of the drug's action and effects. Whenever possible, nonpharmacologic interventions (discussed earlier) are the preferred interventions.

BOX 20-7
NURSING CARE CHECKLIST

HELPING OLDER CLIENTS KEEP WARM IN BED

☑ Before the client goes to bed, warm the bed with hot water bottles or prewarmed bath blankets. Remove the hot water bottle before the client gets into bed to avoid the risk of a burn.

☑ Use 100 percent cotton flannel sheets, if possible, for warmth. Alternatively, apply thermal blankets between the sheet and bedspread.

☑ Encourage the client to wear own clothing, such as flannel nightgown or pajamas, loose-fitting jogging suit, thermal socks, leg warmers, long underwear, sleeping cap (if scalp hair is sparse), sweater, or a favorite quilt or blanket.

EVALUATING

If the desired outcomes are not achieved, the nurse, client, and support people, if appropriate, should explore the reasons. In many facilities, a client care conference may be convened in order to discuss client progress, and analyze collected data. The desired outcome can be continued or revised at that time. If the goal is to be continued, a new timeline will be set.

 DISCHARGE CONSIDERATIONS

Nurses can play a key role in teaching clients how to improve patterns of rest and sleep. This can speed recovery and add to quality of life. Box 20-8 provides discharge teaching about promoting rest and sleep.

Note: The bibliography listings for this and all chapters have been compiled at the back of the book.

BOX 20-8
NURSING CARE CHECKLIST

REDUCING ENVIRONMENTAL DISTRACTIONS IN HOSPITALS

☑ Close window curtains if street lights shine through.
☑ Close curtains between clients in semiprivate and larger rooms.
☑ Reduce or eliminate overhead lighting; provide a night-light at the bedside or in the bathroom.
☑ Close the door of the client's room.
☑ Adhere to agency policy about times to turn off communal televisions or radios.
☑ Lower the ring tone of nearby telephones.
☑ Discontinue use of the paging system after a certain hour (e.g., 2100 hours), or reduce its volume.
☑ Keep required staff conversations at low levels; conduct nursing reports or other discussions in a separate area away from client rooms.
☑ Wear rubber-soled shoes.
☑ Ensure that all cart wheels are well oiled.
☑ Perform only essential nursing tasks during sleeping hours.

PROCEDURE 20-1

Providing Passive Range-of-Motion Exercises

PURPOSE

- ◆ To maintain joint flexibility
- ◆ To provide exercise when the client is unable to accomplish movement actively

EQUIPMENT

- ◆ No special equipment is need except a bed or exercise mat or table.

INTERVENTIONS

1. Perform exercise in an organized format from head to toe. Repeat each movement three times, supporting the joint. *This allows the muscles to stretch and warm.*

2. Observe the client for nonverbal clues of pain. *This can reduce discomfort and prevent further injury.*

3. Neck
   - ◆ Remove pillow.
   - ◆ Flex and extend the neck (Figure 20-13 ◆)
     - ◆ Place palm of one hand under client's head and the other on the chin.
     - ◆ Move head forward from an upright position until the chin rests on the chest.
     - ◆ Move the head back to the resting supine position.
   - ◆ Lateral flexion of neck (Figure 20-14 ◆)
     - ◆ Place heels of the hands on each side of client's cheeks.
     - ◆ Move head laterally toward the right and left shoulders.
   - ◆ Rotation (Figure 20-15 ◆)
     - ◆ Place heels of the hands on client's cheeks.
     - ◆ Turn face as far as possible to the right and left.

4. Shoulder
   - ◆ Flexion/extension (Figure 20-16 ◆).

Figure 20-14. ◆ Right/left lateral flexion.

- ◆ With client's arms at the side, grasp the arm beneath the elbow with one hand and beneath the wrist with the other hand.
- ◆ Raise the arm forward and upward to a position beside the head.
- ◆ Move the arm from a vertical position beside the head forward and down to a resting position at the side of the body.
- ◆ Abduction/adduction (Figure 20-17 ◆)

Figure 20-13. ◆ Head flexion and extension.

Figure 20-15. ◆ Right/left rotation.

Figure 20-16. ◆ Shoulder flexion and extension.

Figure 20-18. ◆ Elbow flexion and extension.

- ◆ Move arm laterally from the resting position at the side to a side position above the head, palm of the hand away from the head.
- ◆ Move the arm laterally from beside the head downward laterally and across the front on the body as far as possible.
- ◆ External/internal rotation
  - ◆ With arm held out to the side at shoulder level and elbow at a right angle and fingers pointing downward, move the arm upward so that the fingers are pointing up and the back of the hand touches the bed or mat.
  - ◆ With arm held out to the side at the level of the shoulder and the elbow bent at a right angle, fingers pointing up, bring the arm forward and down so that the palm touches the mat.
- ◆ Circumduction
  - ◆ Move the arm forward and backward in a full circle.

5. Elbow
- ◆ Flexion/extension (Figure 20-18 ◆)
  - ◆ Bring lower arm forward and upward so that hand is at shoulder level.
  - ◆ Bring lower arm forward and downward, straightening the arm.
- ◆ Rotation for supination/pronation (Figure 20-19 ◆)
  - ◆ Grasp the client's hand with a handshaking motion and turn the palm upward. Make sure only the forearm and not the shoulder moves.
  - ◆ Turn the palm downward, moving only the forearm.

Figure 20-19. ◆ Forearm pronation and supination.

6. Wrist
- ◆ Flexion/extension (Figure 20-20 ◆)
  - ◆ Flex client's arm at the elbow until the forearm is at a right angle to the bed or mat. Support the wrist joint with one hand while manipulating the joint with your other hand.
  - ◆ Bring the fingers of the hand toward the inner aspect of the arm.
  - ◆ Straighten the hand to the same plane as the arm.
- ◆ Hyperflexion
  - ◆ Bend fingers of the hand back as far as possible.
- ◆ Radial flexion (abduction)/ulnar flexion (adduction) (Figure 20-21 ◆)
  - ◆ Bend wrist laterally toward the thumb side.
  - ◆ Bend the wrist laterally toward the fifth finger.

Figure 20-17. ◆ Shoulder abduction and adduction.

Figure 20-20. ◆ Wrist flexion and extension.

Figure 20-21. ◆ Ulnar and radial deviation.

7. Hand and fingers
   ◆ Flexion/extension (Figure 20-22 ◆)
      ◆ Make client's hand into a fist.
      ◆ Straighten the fingers.
   ◆ Hyperextension
      ◆ Gently bend fingers back.
   ◆ Abduction/adduction (Figure 20-23 ◆)
      ◆ Spread fingers of the hand apart.
      ◆ Bring fingers together.
8. Thumb
   ◆ Flexion/extension
      ◆ Move thumb across the palmar surface toward the fifth finger.
      ◆ Move the thumb away from the hand.

Figure 20-22. ◆ Finger flexion and extension.

Figure 20-23. ◆ Finger adduction and abduction.

   ◆ Abduction/adduction
      ◆ Extend the thumb laterally.
      ◆ Move thumb back to the hand.
      ◆ *Note: Can be done when abducting and adducting fingers.*
   ◆ Opposition (Figure 20-24 ◆)
      ◆ Touch thumb to the top of each finger of the same hand.
9. Hip: To exercise hip and leg, place one hand under the client's knee and the other under the ankle.
   ◆ Flexion/extension (Figure 20-25 ◆)
      ◆ Lift the leg and bend the knee, moving the knee up toward the chest as far as possible.
      ◆ Bring leg down, straighten the knee, and lower the leg to the bed.
   ◆ Abduction/adduction (Figure 20-26 ◆)
      ◆ Move the leg to the side away from the client.
      ◆ Move leg back across and in front of the other leg.
      ◆ Slowly raise and lower leg (Figure 20-27 ◆)
   ◆ Circumduction
      ◆ Move the leg in a circle.
   ◆ Internal/external rotation
      ◆ Roll the foot and leg inward.
      ◆ Roll foot and leg outward.
10. Knee
   ◆ Flexion/extension (see Figure 20-25)
      ◆ Bend leg, bringing the heel toward back of thigh. *Note: can be done with hip flexion.*
      ◆ Straighten the leg and return the foot to the bed.

Figure 20-24. ◆ Finger–thumb opposition.

Figure 20-25. ◆ Hip/knee flexion and extension.

Figure 20-26. ◆ Hip abduction and adduction.

11. Ankle
- Extension/flexion (Figure 20-28 ◆)
  - Plantar flexion: move the foot so that the toes are pointed downward.
  - Dorsiflexion: move foot so toes are pointed upward.

12. Foot
- Eversion/inversion
  - Place one hand under the client's ankle and the other over the arch.
  - Turn the whole foot outward.
  - Turn the whole foot inward.

13. Toes
- Flexion/extension (Figure 20-29 ◆)
  - Place one hand over arch.

Figure 20-27. ◆ Straight leg raising.

Figure 20-28. ◆ Ankle dorsiflexion and plantar flexion.

Figure 20-29. ◆ Toe flexion and extension.

- Place the fingers of the other hand over toes and curl downward.
- Place fingers under the toes and bend toes upward.
- Abduction/adduction
  - Spread toes apart.
  - Bring toes together.

◆ SAMPLE DOCUMENTATION

11/3/05	PROM to left lower extremity. Knee
2130	flexion 110 degrees no c/o discomfort.
	Full range on plantar flexion (50
	degrees; 40 degrees yesterday). ———
	D. Smith LPN

PROCEDURE 20-2

Moving a Client in Bed

PURPOSE

◆ To reposition clients who have slid down in bed from the Fowler's position or been pulled down by traction

EQUIPMENT

◆ None needed
◆ Second person may be needed to assist with some clients

INTERVENTIONS

1. Adjust the bed and the client's position.
   ◆ Adjust the head of the bed to a flat position or as low as the client can tolerate. *Moving the client upward against gravity requires more force and can cause back strain.*
   ◆ Raise the bed to the height of your center of gravity.
   ◆ Lock the wheels on the bed and raise the rail on the side of the bed opposite you.
   ◆ Remove all pillows, then place one against the head of the bed. *This pillow protects the client's head from inadvertent injury against the top of the bed during the upward move.*

2. Ask for the client's help in lessening your workload.
   ◆ Ask the client to flex the hips and knees and position the feet so that they can be used effectively for pushing. *Flexing the hips and knees keeps the entire lower leg off the bed surface, preventing friction during movement, and ensures use of the large muscle groups in the client's legs when pushing, thus increasing the force of movement.*
   ◆ Ask the client to:
   a. Grasp the head of the bed with both hands and pull during the move.
   or
   b. Raise the upper part of the body on the elbows and push with the hands and forearms during the move
   or
   c. Grasp the overhead trapeze with both hands and lift and pull during the move. *Client assistance provides additional power to overcome inertia and friction during the move. These actions also keep the client's arms partially off the bed surface, reducing friction during movement, and make use of the large muscle groups of the client's arms to increase the force during movement.*

3. Position yourself appropriately, and move the client.
   ◆ Face the direction of the movement, and then assume a broad stance, with the foot nearest the bed behind the forward foot and weight on the forward foot. Incline your trunk forward from the hips. Flex hips, knees, and ankles.

◆ Place your near arm under the client's thighs (Figure 20-30 ◆). *This supports the heaviest part of the body (the buttocks).* Push down on the mattress with the far arm. *The far arm acts as a lever during the move.*
◆ Tighten your gluteal, abdominal, leg, and arm muscles, and rock from the back leg to the front leg and back again. Then shift your weight to the front leg as the client pushes with the heels and pulls with the arms, so that the client moves toward the head of the bed. *Tightening your muscles helps to prevent strain. Moving the client as you shift your weight adds momentum.*

4. Ensure client comfort.
   ◆ Elevate the head of the bed and provide appropriate support devices for the client's new position.
   ◆ See the sections on positioning clients earlier in this chapter.

Figure 20-30. ◆ Moving a client up in bed.

VARIATION: A CLIENT WHO HAS LIMITED STRENGTH OF THE UPPER EXTREMITIES

◆ Assist the client to flex the hips and knees as in step 2 previously. Place the client's arms across the chest. *This keeps them off the bed surface and minimizes friction during movement.* Ask the client to flex the neck during the move and keep the head off the bed surface.

◆ Position yourself as in step 3, and place one arm under the client's back and shoulders and the other arm under the client's thighs. *This placement of the arms distributes the client's weight and supports the heaviest part of the body (the buttocks).* Shift your weight as in step 3.

VARIATION: TWO NURSES USING A HAND–FOREARM INTERLOCK

Two people are required to move clients who are unable to assist because of their condition or weight. Using the technique described in step 3, with the second staff member on the opposite side of the bed, both of you interlock your forearms under the client's thighs and shoulders and lift the client up in bed.

VARIATION: TWO NURSES USING A TURN SHEET

Two nurses can use a turn sheet to move a client up in bed. *A turn sheet distributes the client's weight more evenly, decreases friction, and exerts a more even force on the client during the move. In addition, it prevents injury of the client's skin, because the friction created between two sheets when one is moved is less than that created by the client's body moving over the sheet.*

◆ Place a drawsheet or a full sheet folded in half under the client, extending from the shoulders to the thighs. Each of you rolls up or fanfolds the turn sheet close to the client's body on either side.

◆ Both of you then grasp the sheet close to the shoulders and buttocks of the client. *This draws the weight closer to the nurses' center of gravity and increases the nurses' balance and stability, permitting a smoother movement.* Then follow the method of moving clients with limited upper extremity strength, described earlier.

TURNING A CLIENT TO A LATERAL OR PRONE POSITION IN BED

Movement to a lateral (side-lying) position may be necessary when placing a bedpan beneath the client, when changing the client's bed linen, or when repositioning the client.

1. Position yourself and the client appropriately before performing the move.

◆ Move the client closer to the side of the bed opposite the side the client will face when turned. *This ensures that the client will be positioned safely in the center of the bed after turning.* Use a pull sheet beneath the client's trunk and thighs to pull the client to the side of the bed. Roll up the sheet as close as possible to the client's body and pull the client to the side of the bed. Adjust the client's head and reposition the legs appropriately.

◆ While standing on the side of the bed nearest the client, place the client's near arm across the chest. Abduct the client's far shoulder slightly from the side of the body. *Pulling the one arm forward facilitates the turning motion. Pulling the other arm away from the body prevents that arm from being caught beneath the client's body during the roll.*

◆ Place the client's near ankle and foot across the far ankle and foot. *This facilitates the turning motion. Making these preparations on the side of the bed closest to the client helps prevent unnecessary reaching.*

◆ Raise the side rail next to the client before going to the other side of the bed. *This ensures that the client, who is close to the edge of the mattress, will not fall.*

◆ Position yourself on the side of the bed toward which the client will turn, directly in line with the client's waistline and as close to the bed as possible.

◆ Incline your trunk forward from the hips. Flex your hips, knees, and ankles. Assume a broad stance with one foot forward and the weight placed on this forward foot.

2. Pull or roll the client to a lateral position.

◆ Place one hand on the client's far hip and the other hand on the client's far shoulder (Figure 20-31 ◆). *This position of the hands supports the client at the two heaviest parts of the body, providing greater control in movement during the roll.*

◆ Tighten your gluteal, abdominal, leg, and arm muscles; rock backward, shifting your weight from the forward to the backward foot; and roll the client onto the side of the body to face you (see Figure 20-31B).

Figure 20-31. ◆ **A, B.** Moving a client to a lateral position.

VARIATION: TURNING THE CLIENT TO A PRONE POSITION

To turn a client to the prone position, follow the preceding steps, with two exceptions:

◆ Instead of abducting the far arm, keep the client's arm alongside the body for the client to roll over. *Keeping the arm alongside the body prevents it from being pinned under the client when the client is rolled.*

◆ Roll the client completely onto the abdomen. It is essential to move the client as close as possible to the edge of the bed before the turn so that the client will be lying on the center of the bed after rolling. Never pull a client across the bed while the client is in the prone position. Doing so can injure a woman's breasts or a man's genitals.

LOGROLLING A CLIENT

Logrolling is a technique used to turn a client whose body must at all times be kept in straight alignment (like a log). *An example is the client with a spinal injury. Considerable care must be taken to prevent additional injury.* This technique requires two nurses or, if the client is large, three nurses. For the client who has a cervical injury, one nurse must maintain the client's head and neck alignment throughout the procedure.

1. Position yourselves and the client appropriately before the move.

◆ Stand on the same side of the bed, and assume a broad stance with one foot ahead of the other.

◆ Place the client's arms across the chest. *Doing so ensures that they will not be injured or become trapped under the body when the body is turned.*

◆ Incline your trunk, and flex your hips, knees, and ankles.

◆ Place your arms under the client as shown in Figure 20-32A ◆ or B, depending on the client's size. *Each staff member then has a major weight area of the client centered between the arms.*

◆ Tighten your gluteal, abdominal, leg, and arm muscles. *This provides support to your back muscles to prevent strain.*

2. Pull the client to the side of the bed.

◆ One nurse counts, "One, two, three, go." Then at the same time, all staff members pull the client to the side of the bed by shifting weight to the back foot. *Moving the client in unison maintains the client's body alignment.*

◆ Elevate the side rail on this side of the bed. *This prevents the client from falling while lying so close to the edge of the bed.*

3. Move to the other side of the bed, and place supportive devices for the client when turned.

◆ Place a pillow where it will support the client's head after the turn. *The pillow prevents lateral flexion of the neck and ensures alignment of the cervical spine.*

◆ Place one or two pillows between the client's legs to support the upper leg when the client is turned. *This pillow prevents adduction of the upper leg and keeps the legs parallel and aligned.*

4. Roll and position the client in proper alignment.

◆ All nurses flex the hips, knees, and ankles and assume a broad stance with one foot forward.

◆ All nurses reach over the client and place hands as shown in Figure 20-33 ◆. *Doing so centers a major weight area of the client between each nurse's arms.*

◆ One nurse counts, "One, two, three, go." Then at the same time, all nurses roll the client to a lateral position.

◆ Place pillows to maintain the client's lateral position. See the discussion of the lateral position.

VARIATION: USING A TURN OR LIFT SHEET

◆ Use a turn sheet to facilitate logrolling. First, stand with another nurse on the same side of the bed. Assume a broad stance with one foot forward, and grasp half of the fanfolded or rolled edge of the turn sheet. On a signal, pull the client toward both of you (Figure 20-34 ◆).

◆ Before turning the client, place pillow supports for the head and legs, as described in step 3 previously. *This helps maintain the client's alignment when turning.* Then go to the other side of the bed (farthest from the client), and assume a stable stance. Reaching over the client, grasp the far edges of the turn sheet, and roll the client toward you (Figure 20-35 ◆). The second nurse (behind the client) helps turn the client and provides pillow supports to ensure good alignment in the lateral position.

Figure 20-32. ◆ Correct arm placement for moving a client to the side of the bed: **A.** Two nurses. **B.** Three nurses.

Figure 20-33. ◆ Correct hand placement for logrolling a client.

Figure 20-34. ◆ Using the turn sheet, the nurses pull the sheet with the client on it to the edge of the bed. *Source: Jenny Thomas.*

MOVING A CLIENT TO A SITTING POSITION ON THE EDGE OF THE BED

The client assumes a sitting position on the edge of the bed before walking, moving to a chair or wheelchair, eating, or performing other activities.

1. Position yourself and the client appropriately before performing the move.
   ◆ Assist the client to a lateral position facing you.

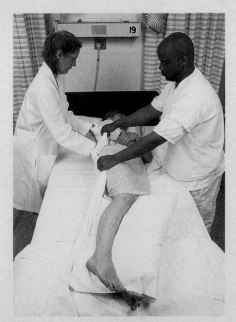

Figure 20-35. ◆ The nurse on the right uses the far edge of the sheet to roll the client toward him; the nurse on the left remains behind the client and assists with turning. *Source: © Jenny Thomas.*

◆ Raise the head of the bed slowly as high as it will go. *This decreases the distance that the client needs to move to sit up on the side of the bed.*
◆ Position the client's feet and lower legs at the edge of the bed. *This enables the client's feet to move easily off the bed during the movement, and the client is aided by gravity into a sitting position.*
◆ Stand beside the client's hips and face the far corner of the bottom of the bed (the angle in which movement will occur). Assume a broad stance, placing the foot nearest the client forward. Incline your trunk forward from the hips. Flex your hips, knees, and ankles (Figure 20-36 ◆).

2. Move the client to a sitting position.
   ◆ Place one arm around the client's shoulders and the other arm beneath both of the client's thighs near the knees (Figure 20-36A). *Supporting the client's shoulders prevents the client from falling backward during the movement. Supporting the client's thighs reduces friction of the thighs against the bed surface during the move and increases the force of the movement.*
   ◆ Tighten your gluteal, abdominal, leg, and arm muscles. *This protects your own muscles from strain.*
   ◆ Lift the client's thighs slightly. *This reduces the friction of the client's thighs and the nurse's arm against the bed surface.*
   ◆ Pivot on the balls of your feet in the desired direction facing the foot of the bed while pulling the client's feet and legs off the bed (Figure 20-36B). *Pivoting prevents twisting of the nurse's spine. The weight of the client's legs swinging downward increases downward movement of the lower body and helps make the client's upper body vertical.*
   ◆ Keep supporting the client until the client is well balanced and comfortable. *This movement may cause some clients to faint.*

Figure 20-36. ◆ **A, B.** Assisting a client to a sitting position on the edge of the bed.

Figure 20-37. ◆ **A, B.** Moving to a sitting position independently.

◆ Assess vital signs (e.g., pulse, respirations, and blood pressure) as indicated by the client's health status.

VARIATION: TEACHING A CLIENT HOW TO SIT ON THE SIDE OF THE BED INDEPENDENTLY

A client who has had recent abdominal surgery or who is weak may have too much abdominal pain or too little strength to sit straight up in bed. This person can be taught to assume a "dangle" position without assistance. Instruct the client to

◆ Roll to the side and lift the far leg over the near leg (Figure 20-37A ◆).
◆ Grasp the mattress edge with the lower arm and push the fist of the upper arm into the mattress (Figure 20-37B).

◆ Push up with the arms as the heels and legs slide over the mattress edge (Figure 20-37B).
◆ Maintain the sitting position by pushing both fists into the mattress behind and to the sides of the buttocks.

◆ SAMPLE DOCUMENTATION

3/16/04	Client attempted dangling position, felt
2:30PM	faint, returned to supine. Reported to
	team leader.
	S. Courant, LVN

PROCEDURE 20-3

Transferring a Client

EQUIPMENT

◆ Transfer (walking) belt

◆ Stretcher (if transferring to stretcher)
◆ Optional: Roller bar or long board (sliding board.

Part A: Transfer Between a Bed and a Chair

INTERVENTIONS

1. Position the equipment appropriately.
  ◆ Lower the bed to its lowest position so that the client's feet will rest flat on the floor. Lock the wheels of the bed. *This helps to prevent risk of fall due to sudden movement.*
  ◆ Place the wheelchair parallel to the bed as close to the bed as possible (Figure 20-38 ◆). Lock the wheels of the wheelchair, and raise the footplate.

2. Prepare and assess the client.
  ◆ Assist the client to a sitting position on the side of the bed. See Procedure 20-2.
  ◆ Assess the client for orthostatic hypotension before moving the client from the bed. *Changes in posture could result in fainting.*
  ◆ Assist the client in putting on a bathrobe and nonskid slippers or shoes. *These provide comfort and safety when walking.*

Figure 20-38. ◆ The wheelchair is placed parallel to the bed as close to the bed as possible. Note that placement of the nurse's feet mirrors that of the client's feet.

◆ Place a transfer belt snugly around the client's waist. Check to be certain that the belt is securely fastened.

3. Give explicit instructions to the client. Ask the client to

◆ Move forward and sit on the edge of the bed. *This brings the client's center of gravity closer to the nurse's.*

◆ Lean forward slightly from the hips. *This brings the client's center of gravity more directly over the base of support and positions the head and trunk in the direction of the movement.*

◆ Place the foot of the stronger leg beneath the edge of the bed and put the other foot forward. *In this way, the client can use the stronger leg muscles to stand and power the movement. A broader base of support makes the client more stable during the transfer.*

◆ Place the client's hands on the bed surface or on your shoulders so that the client can push while standing. *This provides additional force for the movement and reduces the potential for strain on the nurse's back. The client should not grasp the nurse's neck for support. Doing so can injure the nurse.*

4. Position yourself correctly.

◆ Stand directly in front of the client. Incline the trunk forward from the hips. Flex the hips, knees, and ankles. Assume a broad stance, placing one foot forward and one back. Mirror the placement of the client's feet, if possible. *This helps prevent loss of balance during the transfer.*

◆ Encircle the client's waist with your arms, and grasp the transfer belt at the client's back (Figure 20-39 ◆) with thumbs pointing downward. *The belt provides a secure handle for holding onto the client and controlling the movement. Downward placement of the thumbs prevents potential wrist injury as the nurse lifts. By supporting the client in this manner, you keep the client from tilting backward during the transfer.*

◆ Tighten your gluteal, abdominal, leg, and arm muscles.

Figure 20-39. ◆ Using a transfer (walking) belt. *Source:* © Elena Dorfman.

5. Assist the client to stand, and then move together toward the wheelchair.

◆ On the count of three:

  a. Ask the client to push with the back foot, rock to the forward foot, extend (straighten) the joints of the lower extremities, and push or pull up with the hands, while

  b. You push with the forward foot, rock to the back foot, extend the joints of the lower extremities, and pull the client (directly toward your center of gravity) into a standing position.

◆ Support the client in an upright standing position for a few moments. *This allows the nurse and the client to extend the joints and provides the nurse with an opportunity to ensure that the client is all right before moving away from the bed.*

◆ Together, pivot or take a few steps toward the wheelchair.

6. Assist the client to sit.

◆ Ask the client to:

  a. Back up to the wheelchair and place the legs against the seat. *Having the client place the legs against the wheelchair seat minimizes the risk of the client's falling when sitting down.*

  b. Place the foot of the stronger leg slightly behind the other. *This supports body weight during the movement.*

  c. Keep the other foot forward. *This provides a broad base of support.*

  d. Place both hands on the wheelchair arms or on your shoulders. *This increases stability and lessens the strain on the nurse.*

◆ Stand directly in front of the client. Place one foot forward and one back.

◆ Tighten your grasp on the transfer belt, and tighten your gluteal, abdominal, leg, and arm muscles.
◆ On the count of three:
  a. Have the client shift the body weight by rocking to the back foot, lower the body onto the edge of the wheelchair seat by flexing the joints of the legs and arms, and place some body weight on the arms, while
  b. You shift your body weight by stepping back with the forward foot and pivoting toward the chair while lowering the client onto the wheelchair seat.

7. Ensure client safety.
◆ Ask the client to push back into the wheelchair seat. *Sitting well back on the seat provides a broader base of support and greater stability and minimizes the risk of falling from the wheelchair. A wheelchair can topple forward when the client sits on the edge of the seat and leans far forward.*
◆ Lower the footplates, and place the client's feet on them.
◆ Apply a seat belt as required.

VARIATION: ANGLING THE WHEELCHAIR

For clients who have difficulty walking, place the wheelchair at a 45-degree angle to the bed. *This enables the client to pivot into the chair and lessens the amount of body rotation required.*

VARIATION: TRANSFERRING WITHOUT A BELT

◆ For clients who need minimal assistance, place the hands against the sides of the client's chest (not at the axillae) during the transfer (Figure 20-40 ◆). For clients who require more assistance, reach through the client's axillae and place the hands on the client's scapulae during the transfer. Avoid placing hands or pressure on the axillae, especially for clients who have upper extremity paralysis or paresis.
◆ Follow the steps described previously.

VARIATION: TRANSFERRING WITH A BELT AND TWO NURSES

◆ When the client is able to stand, position yourselves on both sides of the client, facing the same direction as the client. Flex your hips, knees, and ankles; grasp the client's transfer belt with the hand closest to the client; and with the other hand support the client's elbows.
◆ Coordinating your efforts, all three of you stand simultaneously, pivot, and move to the wheelchair. Reverse the process to lower the client onto the wheelchair seat.

VARIATION: TRANSFERRING A CLIENT WITH AN INJURED LOWER EXTREMITY

When the client has an injured lower extremity, movement should always occur toward the client's unaffected (strong) side. For example, if the client's right leg is injured and the client is sitting on the edge of the bed preparing to transfer to a wheelchair, position the wheelchair on the client's left side. In this way, the client can use the unaffected leg most effectively and safely.

VARIATION: USING A SLIDING BOARD

Have a client who cannot stand use a sliding board to move without nursing assistance. *This method not only promotes the client's sense of independence but preserves your energy* (Figure 20-41 ◆).

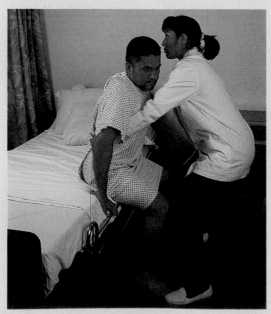

Figure 20-40. ◆ Transferring without a belt. *Source:* © Elena Dorfman.

Figure 20-41. ◆ Using a sliding board. *Source:* © Jenny Thomas.

Part B: Transferring Client Between a Bed and a Stretcher

The stretcher, or gurney, is used to transfer supine clients from one location to another. Whenever the client is capable of accomplishing the transfer from bed to stretcher independently, either by lifting onto it or by rolling onto it, the client should be encouraged to do so. If the client cannot move onto the stretcher independently, at least two nurses are needed to assist with the transfer. More are needed if the client is totally helpless or is heavy.

INTERVENTIONS

1. Adjust the client's bed in preparation for the transfer.
   - Lower the head of the bed until it is flat or as low as the client can tolerate.
   - Raise the bed so that it is slightly higher than the surface of the stretcher. *It is easier for the client to move down an incline.*
   - Ensure that the wheels on the bed are locked.
   - Pull the drawsheet out from both sides of the bed.

2. Move the client to the edge of the bed, and position the stretcher.
   - Roll the drawsheet as close to the client's side as possible.
   - Pull the client to the edge of the bed, and cover the client with a sheet or bath blanket to maintain comfort.
   - Place the stretcher parallel to the bed, next to the client, and lock its wheels.
   - Fill the gap that exists between the bed and the stretcher loosely with the bath blankets (optional).

3. Transfer the client securely to the stretcher.
   - In unison with the other staff members press your body tightly against the stretcher. *This prevents the stretcher from moving.*
   - Roll the pull sheet tightly against the client. *This achieves better control over client movement.*
   - Flex your hips, and pull the client on the pull sheet in unison directly toward you and onto the stretcher. *Pulling downward requires less force than pulling along a flat surface.*
   - Ask the client to flex the neck during the move, if possible, and place arms across the chest. *This prevents injury to these body parts.*

4. Ensure client comfort and safety.
   - Make the client comfortable, unlock the stretcher wheels, and move the stretcher away from the bed.
   - Immediately raise the stretcher side rails and/or fasten the safety straps across the client. *Because the stretcher is high and narrow, the client is in danger of falling unless these safety precautions are taken.*

VARIATION: USING A ROLLER BAR DURING THE TRANSFER

A roller bar is a metal frame covered with longitudinal rollers. Place the bar over the gap between the bed and the stretcher. Using a pull sheet, pull the client onto the roller bar, and roll the client easily onto the stretcher.

VARIATION: USING A LONG BOARD

The long board, which may be referred to as the Smooth Mover or Easyglide, is a lacquered or smooth polyethylene board measuring 45 to 55 cm (18 to 22 in) by 182 cm (72 in) with handholds along its edges. This device may be used by one nurse alone or up to four nurses together. Turn the client to a lateral position away from you, position the board close to the client's back, and roll the client onto the board. Pull the client and board across the bed to the stretcher. Safety belts may be placed over the chest, abdomen, and legs.

VARIATION: USING A THREE-PERSON CARRY (USE CAUTION)

Three people of about equal height stand side-by-side facing the client. Recommendations vary as to which staff member lifts a specific area of the client. Often, the strongest person supports the heaviest part of the client or the tallest person with the longest reach supports the head and shoulders. The stretcher or bed to which the client will be moved is placed at a right angle at the foot of the bed. The wheels of the bed and stretcher are locked. Each person flexes the knees and places the foot nearest to the stretcher slightly forward.

The arms of the lifters are put under the client at the head and shoulders, hips and thighs, and upper and lower legs. The lifters then, on the count of 3, roll the client onto their chests and step back in unison (Figure 20-42 ◆). They then pivot around to the stretcher and lower the client by flexing their knees and hips until their elbows are on the surface of the stretcher. The client is then released on the stretcher surface and is aligned and covered, and the stretcher side rails are raised.

Figure 20-42. ◆ The three carrier lift. *Source:* © Elena Dorfman.

◆ SAMPLE DOCUMENTATION

3/18/04	Found client sitting on edge of bed.
9:30AM	Stated "waiting too long to get help."
	Assisted with transfer to chair. Reminded
	ct. wait for assistance to prevent a fall.
	Son visited ½ hour.
	R. Marino, LVN

PROCEDURE 20-4

Assisting a Client to Walk

PURPOSE

◆ To provide safety for the client who is weak

EQUIPMENT

◆ Walking belt (optional)

INTERVENTIONS

1. Prepare the client for ambulation.

◆ Apply elastic (antiemboli) stockings as required. See Procedure 16-5.

◆ Assist the client to sit on the edge of the bed.

◆ Assess the client carefully for signs and symptoms of orthostatic hypotension (dizziness, light-headedness, pallor, or a sudden increase in heart rate) prior to leaving the bedside.

◆ Ensure that the client is appropriately dressed to walk and wears shoes or slippers with nonskid soles. *Proper attire and footwear prevent chilling and falling.*

◆ Assist the client to stand by the side of the bed until the client feels secure.

◆ Plan the length of the walk with the client, in light of the nursing or physician's orders. Be prepared to shorten the walk according to the person's activity tolerance.

ONE NURSE

2. Ensure client safety while assisting the client to ambulate.

◆ Encourage the client to ambulate independently if the client is able, but walk beside the client.

◆ Remain physically close to the client. *This gives you time to react in case assistance is needed at any point.*

◆ Use a transfer or walking belt if the client is slightly weak and unstable. Make sure the belt is pulled snugly around the client's waist and fastened securely. Grasp the belt at the client's back, and walk behind and slightly to one side of the client (Figure 20-43 ◆).

◆ If it is the client's first time out of bed following surgery, injury, or an extended period of immobility, or if the client is quite weak or unstable, have an assistant follow you and the client with a wheelchair in case it is needed quickly.

◆ If the client is moderately weak and unstable, interlock your forearm with the client's closest forearm, and walk on the client's weaker side. Encourage the client to press the forearm against your hip or waist for stability if desired. In addition, have the client wear a transfer or

Figure 20-43. ◆ Using a transfer (walking) belt to support the client. *Source:* © Elena Dorfman.

walking belt so that you can quickly grab the belt and prevent a fall if the client feels faint.

◆ If the client is very weak and unstable, place your near arm around the client's waist, and with your other arm support the client's near arm at the elbow. Walk on the client's stronger side. Again, have the client wear a transfer or walking belt in case of an emergency.

◆ Encourage the client to assume a normal walking stance and gait as much as possible.

3. Protect the client who begins to fall while ambulating.

◆ If a client begins to experience the signs and symptoms of orthostatic hypotension or extreme weakness, quickly assist the client into a nearby wheelchair or other chair, and help the client to lower the head between the knees. *Lowering the head facilitates blood flow to the brain.*

◆ Stay with the client. *A client who faints while in this position could fall, head first, out of the chair.*

◆ When the weakness subsides, assist the client back to bed.

◆ If a chair is not close by, assist the client to a horizontal position on the floor before fainting occurs (Figure 20-44 ◆). *A vertical position may increase feelings of faintness.*

a. Assume a broad stance with one foot in front of the other. *A broad stance widens the nurse's base of support for stability. Placing one foot behind the other allows the nurse to rock backward and use the femoral muscles when supporting the client's weight and lowering the center of gravity (see step b), thus preventing back strain.*

b. Bring the client backward so that your body supports the person. *Clients who do faint or start to fall and cannot regain their strength or balance usually drop straight downward or pitch slightly forward because of the momentum of ambulating; thus their head, hips, and knees are most vulnerable to injury. Bringing the client's weight backward against the nurse's body allows gradual movement to the floor without injury to the client.*

c. Allow the client to slide down your leg, and lower the person gently to the floor, making sure the client's head does not hit any objects.

TWO NURSES

4. Prepare the client.
   ◆ See step 1 above.

5. Ensure client safety.
   ◆ After the client stands, assume a position with one nurse at either side. Grasp the inferior aspect of the client's upper arm with your nearest hand and the client's lower arm or hand with your other hand (Figure 20-45 ◆). *This provides a secure grip for each nurse.*
   ◆ Optional: Place a walking belt around the client's waist. Each nurse grasps the side handle with the near hand and the lower aspect of the client's upper arm with the other hand.

Figure 20-45. ◆ Two nurses supporting an ambulatory client. *Source:* © Elena Dorfman.

◆ Walk in unison with the client, using a smooth, even gait, at the same speed and with steps the same size as the client's. *This gives the client a greater feeling of security.*

◆ If the client starts to fall and cannot regain strength or balance, each nurse slips an arm under the client's axillae and grasps the client's hands, and together the nurses lower the person gently to the floor or to a nearby chair (Figure 20-46 ◆). *Placing the nurses' arms under the client's axillae evenly balances the client's weight between the two nurses, preventing injury to both the nurses and the client.*

6. Document all relevant information.
   ◆ Document the time of the walk, the distance walked or time taken, and all nursing assessments.

Figure 20-44. ◆ Lowering a fainting client to the floor. *Source:* © Elena Dorfman.

Figure 20-46. ◆ Two nurses lowering a fainting client to the floor. *Source:* © Elena Dorfman.

◆ SAMPLE DOCUMENTATION

9/29/04	Ambulated client from bed to nurse's
1630	station and returned. Client steady, no
	c/o dizziness. "Let's do more tomorrow!"
	E. Ketterer, LPN

PROCEDURE 20-5

Providing a Back Massage

PURPOSES

◆ To relieve muscle tension
◆ To promote physical and mental relaxation
◆ To relieve insomnia

EQUIPMENT

◆ Lotion or oil

INTERVENTIONS

1. Select an appropriate time free of interruptions and distractions.

◆ Provide massage following the bath, before sleeping, and at other times as necessary to achieve relaxation and comfort for the client.

◆ Assist the client to a prone or lateral position in bed. Remove the client's gown, or open the back of the gown.

2. Warm the massage lotion or oil before use. *This prevents the muscles from stiffening when it is used.*

◆ Warm the lotion or oil by pouring and holding it in your hands or placing the container in warm water before applying it to the client's back. *Cold lotion may startle the client and increase discomfort.*

3. Massage the entire back. Two common types of massage strokes are effleurage (stroking the body, pronounced eh-flu-RAJ) and petrissage (kneading or making large quick pinches of the skin, subcutaneous tissue, and muscle, pronounced PET-ri-saj).

◆ Place your hands on either side of the lower spine. Using your palms and fingers, slowly massage using a circular motion and moving upward to the neck, gradually decreasing pressure as you get close to the neck. Use the circular motion over the shoulder blades and then slowly move down the lateral surface of the back (see Figure 20-47 ◆). *Effleurage has a relaxing, sedative effect if slow movement and light pressure are used.*

◆ Repeat this massage pattern for 3 to 4 minutes.

◆ Maintain contact with the skin during the massage.

◆ Use your thumbs to apply friction strokes (strong circular motions).

Figure 20-47. ◆ A back rub pattern.

4. Optional: Petrissage the back and shoulders of the client.
   - ◆ Petrissage first up the vertebral column and then over the entire back. *Petrissage is stimulating, especially if done quickly and with firm pressure.*
   - ◆ Observe the client carefully to ensure that petrissage does not cause pain or discomfort. *If the client grimaces or withdraws from the touch, ease the kneading pressure.*
   - ◆ End the massage with long movements and tell the client you are finishing.

5. Optional: Effleurage and petrissage the upper back and shoulders. *This area often experiences the most tension.*

6. Assist the client to a position of comfort.

7. Document the massage and your observations.

◆ SAMPLE DOCUMENTATION

3/22/05	Client turned left laterally and placed
0800	in Sims' position w/foam wedges. Back
	care including effleurage to lower
	lumbar and sacral area. "Very relaxing."
	Skin intact and pink. ———————
	S. Fontaine, LPN

Chapter Review

Key Terms by Topics

Use the audio glossary feature of either the CD-ROM or the Companion Website to hear the correct pronunciation of the following key terms.

Normal Movement
line of gravity, center of gravity, postural tonus, range of motion (ROM), equilibrium, labyrinth

Factors affecting body alignment and activity
vertigo

Effects of immobility
osteoporosis, atrophy, ankylosed, thrombus, thrombophlebitis, emboli, infarction, vital capacity, atelectasis, urinary stasis

Nursing care
ambulation

Physiology of sleep
NREM sleep, REM sleep

Common sleep disorders
insomnia, hypersomnia, narcolepsy, sleep apnea, parasomnia

Nursing care
effleurage, petrissage

Key Points

- The ability to move freely, easily, and purposefully in the environment is essential for people to meet their basic needs.

- Purposeful coordinated movement relies on the integrated functioning of the musculoskeletal system, the nervous system, and the vestibular apparatus of the inner ear.

- Body alignment and activity are influenced by growth and development, physical health, and prescribed limitations to movement. They are also influenced by mental health, personal values, and attitudes.

- Immobility adversely affects almost every body organ and system. It also can cause psychosocial problems.

- The nurse must (a) prevent the complications of immobility and reduce the severity of any problems resulting from immobility and (b) design exercise programs for clients to promote wellness.

- Positioning a client in good body alignment and changing the position regularly and systematically are essential aspects of nursing practice.

- Safety measures must always be employed when the nurse uses a wheelchair or stretcher to move and transfer clients.

- The nurse should prepare clients for ambulation by helping them become as independent as possible while in bed. Techniques that facilitate normal walking yet provide required physical support are most effective.

- Sleep is a naturally occurring altered state of consciousness in which a person's perceptions of and reactions to the environment are decreased.

- Many factors affect sleep, including illness, age, environment, lifestyle, motivation, emotional stress, diet, smoking, alcohol, and medications.

- Nursing responsibilities to help clients sleep include (a) teaching sleep hygiene, (b) supporting bedtime rituals, (c) creating a restful environment, (d) promoting comfort and relaxation, and (e) administering prescribed medications.

- Nonpharmacologic measures to induce and maintain sleep are always the preferred interventions.

EXPLORE MediaLink

Additional interactive resources for this chapter can be found on the Companion Website at www.prenhall.com/ramont. Click on Chapter 20 and "Begin" to select the activities for this chapter.

For chapter-related NCLEX-style questions and an audio glossary, access the accompanying CD-ROM in this book.

For Further Study

Strategies for preventing strains and sprains in nurses are provided in Chapter 6.

See Figure 11-2 for prone and supine positions.

See Chapter 12 for further discussion of immobility and risk for decubitus ulcer formation.

See Chapter 13 for information on preventing and treating pressure ulcers.

See Chapter 16 for information about oxygenation.

See Chapter 18 for bladder considerations.

See Chapter 19 for more about the effects of immobility on bowel elimination.

See Chapter 24 for age-related considerations in regard to mobility.

Critical Thinking Care Map

Caring for a Client with Sleep Problems

NCLEX-PN Focus Area: Physiological Integrity: Basic Care and Comfort

Case Study: Gillian Marks, 51, states she has a problem falling asleep since her mastectomy 2 months ago. She says fears of prognosis become prominent when she is not active and busy. She has tried reading or watching TV, but neither makes her sleepy or relaxed. She appears agitated and restless. She is receiving her last radiation treatment. A decision has not been made as to the need for chemotherapy.

Nursing Diagnosis: Disturbed Sleep Pattern: Insomnia

COLLECT DATA

Subjective	Objective
_____	_____
_____	_____
_____	_____
_____	_____
_____	_____
_____	_____
_____	_____

Would you report this data? Yes/No

If yes, to: _____

Nursing Care

_____
_____
_____
_____
_____
_____
_____
_____
_____
_____
_____
_____
_____
_____

How would you document this? _____
_____
_____
_____
_____

Data Collected
(use those that apply)

- Weight 126 lbs, 10-lb weight loss since surgery
- BP 128/86
- HR 84 and regular
- RR 16
- WBC 7,000
- H&H 12.8/36
- Skin pale; dark circles around eyes
- Surgical incision clean and healed well
- Radiation site irritated and red

Nursing Interventions
(use those that apply)

- Assess client's sleep patterns and usual bedtime rituals and incorporate these into the plan of care.
- Encourage client to express feelings to others.
- Monitor client's defense mechanisms and supoprt healthy defenses.
- Assess for signs of new onset of depression, depressed mood state, statement of hoplessness, and poor appetite.
- Expect client to meet responsibilities; give positive reinforcement.
- Observe client's medication, diet, and caffeine intake. Look for hidden sources of caffeine.
- Identify causes for and observe client's expression of sorrow.
- Advise client to avoid use of alcohol or hypnotics to induce sleep.
- Assist to resolve ambivalent feelings about illness and management of therapeutic regimen.

NCLEX-PN Exam Preparation

1. The point at which all of the body's mass is centered and the base of support achieves balance is known as the:
   a. Line of gravity
   b. Center of gravity
   c. Line of mobility
   d. Postural tonus

2. Your client has been confined to bed following a musculoskeletal injury. The physician has ordered no weight bearing for an extended period of time. Which of the following conditions would be the biggest concern?
   a. Contractures
   b. Orthostatic hypotension
   c. Osteoporosis
   d. Disuse atrophy

3. Atelectasis, the collapse of a lobe or the entire lung in a bedridden client, is a result of:
   a. Inflammation resulting from static secretions
   b. Reduced vital capacity
   c. Pulmonary emboli
   d. Decreased surfactant and mucus-blocked bronchiole

4. Assistive mobility devices can present a safety hazard for an immobile client. Which of the following statements made by a client would demonstrate the need for additional teaching?
   a. "My crutches are adjusted to the proper length if the pads are touching my underarms."
   b. "It is important to remove throw rugs from around my bed until I am off these crutches."
   c. "I should wear a nonslip sturdy shoe on my unaffected foot."
   d. "The crutches need to have rubber tips to prevent slipping."

5. The position of choice for a client who has difficulty breathing or who is experiencing cardiac problems would be:
   a. Dorsal recumbent
   b. Semi-Fowler's
   c. Orthopneic
   d. Sims'

6. During which stage of NREM (non–rapid eye movement) sleep are body processes dominated by the parasympathetic nervous system?
   a. Stage I
   b. Stage II
   c. Stage III
   d. Stage IV

7. Stage IV sleep is decreased by which of the following conditions?
   a. Hyperthyroidism
   b. Respiratory conditions
   c. Hypothyroidism
   d. Enuresis

8. Treatment for insomnia routinely includes:
   a. Long-term use of sleep-inducing drugs
   b. Behavior modification
   c. Antidepressants
   d. Beta blockers

9. Your client has a history of somnambulism; you understand that to be:
   a. Sleepwalking
   b. Sleep talking
   c. Bedwetting
   d. Teeth grinding

10. A home care client assigned to you suffers from postural hypotension. The RN has recommended that she sit in a rocking chair when out of bed. A family member questions this. Which of the following rationales best explains the suggestion?
    a. Using a rocking chair can strengthen leg muscle tone and enhance circulation.
    b. The rocking motion increases the blood flow to the upper body.
    c. Because she needs help to stand when in the rocking chair, there will be less danger of her falling.
    d. Sitting in the rocking chair will take her mind off her health problems.

Answers for Review Questions, as well as discussion of Case Study and Critical Thinking Care Map questions, appear in Appendix IV.

Medications

SHARING experiences

[Most] clients need more than just a sip of water to take oral medications safely . . . offer water cool enough to taste good to make it easier on them . . . and never, never forget the five "rights"—especially if you're in a hurry!

Valerie A. Gordon-Tate, LPN, LVN, Pediatric Home Care Nurse, Newport News, VA.

LEARNING outcomes

After reading this chapter you will be able to:

- Define selected terms related to the administration of medications.
- Describe legal aspects of administering drugs.
- Identify physiologic factors and individual variables affecting medication action.
- Describe various routes of medication administration.
- Identify essential parts of a medication order.
- Recognize abbreviations commonly used in medication orders.
- List six essential steps to follow when administering medication.
- Describe physiologic variables that alter medication administration and effectiveness.
- Outline steps required to administer oral medications safely.
- Outline steps required for nasogastric and gastrostomy tube medication administration.
- Identify equipment required for parenteral medications.
- Describe LPN/LVN responsibilities in monitoring IV drip rate.
- Describe how to mix selected drugs from vials and ampules.
- Identify sites used for subcutaneous, intramuscular, and intradermal injections.
- Describe essential steps for safely administering parenteral medications by intradermal, subcutaneous, and intramuscular routes.
- Describe essential steps in safely administering topical medications: dermatologic, ophthalmic, otic, nasal, vaginal, respirator inhalation, and rectal preparations.

MediaLink

www.prenhall.com/ramont

Use the address above to access the free, interactive Companion Website created for this textbook. Get hints, instant feedback, and textbook references to chapter-related NCLEX-style questions. Link to other interesting sites.

Audio Glossary:
Use the companion website, or the CD-ROM disk enclosed with your textbook, to hear the pronunciation of key terms in the chapter.

A **medication** is a substance administered for the diagnosis, cure, treatment, relief, or prevention of disease. In the health care context, the words *medication* and *drug* are used interchangeably.

In the United States and Canada, medications are usually dispensed by the order of physicians and dentists. The written direction for the preparation and administration of a drug is called a **prescription.**

A drug may have four different names:

1. The **generic** (family) name, given before a drug becomes official.
2. The *official* name, the name under which it is listed in one of the official publications (e.g., the *United States Pharmacopeia*).
3. The *chemical* name, which describes the drug constituents precisely.
4. The *trademark*, or *brand name*, the name given by the drug manufacturer. Because a drug may be manufactured by several companies, it can have several trade

names. Medications are often available in a variety of forms. Examples are given in Table 21-1 ◆.

Drug Standards

Drugs may have natural (e.g., plant, mineral, and animal) sources, or they may be synthesized in the laboratory. For example, digitalis is plant derived; sodium chloride is a mineral; insulin has animal or human sources, and propoxyphene hydrochloride (the analgesic Darvon) is synthesized in a laboratory.

Drugs vary in strength and activity. Drugs must be pure and of uniform strength if drug dosages are to be predictable in their effect. Therefore, drugs standards have been developed to ensure uniform quality. In the United States, official drugs are those designated by the Federal Food, Drug, and Cosmetic Act. These drugs are officially listed in the *United States Pharmacopeia* (USP) and described according to their source, physical and chemical properties, tests for purity and identity,

TABLE 21-1	TYPES OF DRUG PREPARATIONS		
TYPE	**DESCRIPTION**	**TYPE**	**DESCRIPTION**
Aerosol spray or foam	A liquid, powder, or foam deposited in a thin layer on the skin by air pressure	Ointment (salve, unction)	A semisolid preparation of one or more drugs used for application to the skin and mucous membrane
Aqueous solution	One or more drugs dissolved in water	Paste	A preparation like an ointment, but thicker and stiff, that penetrates the skin less than an ointment
Aqueous suspension	One or more drugs finely divided in a liquid such as water	Pill	One or more drugs mixed with a cohesive material, in oval, round, or flattened shapes
Caplet	A solid form, shaped like a capsule, coated and easily swallowed	Powder	A finely ground drug or drugs; some are used internally, others externally
Capsule	A gelatinous container to hold a drug in powder, liquid, or oil form	Suppository	One or several drugs mixed with a firm base such as gelatin and shaped for insertion into the body (eg, the rectum); the base dissolves gradually at body temperature, releasing the drug
Cream	A nongreasy, semisolid preparation used on the skin		
Elixir	A sweetened and aromatic solution of alcohol used as a vehicle for medicinal agents	Syrup	An aqueous solution of sugar often used to disguise unpleasant-tasting drugs
Extract	A concentrated form of a drug made from vegetables or animals	Tablet	A powdered drug compressed into a hard small disc; some are readily broken along a scored line; others are enteric coated to prevent them from dissolving in the stomach
Gel or jelly	A clear or translucent semisolid that liquefies when applied to the skin		
Liniment	A medication mixed with alcohol, oil, or soapy emollient and applied to the skin		
Lotion	A medication in a liquid suspension applied to the skin	Tincture	An alcoholic or water-and-alcohol solution prepared from drugs derived from plants
Lozenge (troche)	A flat, round, or oval preparation that dissolves and releases a drug when held in the mouth	Transdermal patch	A semipermeable membrane shaped in the form of a disc or patch that contains a drug to be absorbed through the skin over a long period of time

method of storage, assay, category, and normal dosages. In Canada, the *British Pharmacopoeia* is used for the same purpose, although some drugs used in Canada conform to the USP because they are obtained from the United States.

LEGAL ASPECTS OF DRUG ADMINISTRATION

The administration of drugs is controlled by law. See Table 21-2 ◆ for a summary of drug legislation for the United States and Canada.

Nurses must:

1. Know how nursing practice acts in their areas define and limit their functions.
2. Be able to recognize the limits of their own knowledge and skill.

Under the law, nurses are responsible for their own actions whether or not a written order exists. Nurses administer thousands of medications and are responsible for assessing drug effects, including recognizing unfavorable reactions. Since it is impossible to memorize pertinent information about every drug, nurses must rely on references, such as the *Physician's Desk Reference* (PDR) or *Nurse's Drug Guide.* If a physician writes an incorrect order (e.g., Demerol 500 mg instead of Demerol 50 mg), the nurse who administers the incorrect dosage is responsible for the error. Therefore, nurses should question any order that appears unreasonable and refuse to give the medication until the order is clarified.

Another aspect of nursing practice governed by law is the use of controlled substances. In hospitals, controlled substances are kept in a locked drawer, cupboard, medication cart, or computer-controlled dispensing system. Agencies have special forms for recording the use of controlled substances. The information required usually includes the name of the client, drug name, the date and time of administration, the dosage, and the signature of the person who prepared and gave the drug. The name of the physician who ordered the drug may also be part of the record.

Included on this record are the controlled substances wasted during preparation. When a dose or portion of a dose is not used, it must be disposed of according to facility procedure. A second licensed nurse must witness and sign that the drug was wasted and disposed of properly. In most agencies, counts of controlled substances are taken at the end of each shift. The count total should tally with the total at the end of the last shift minus the number used. Discrepancy must be reported immediately.

◆ Effects of Drugs

The **therapeutic effect** of a drug, also referred to as the *desired effect*, is the reason the drug is prescribed. See Table 21-3 ◆ for kinds of therapeutic actions.

A drug **side effect** is an unintended drug action. Unfavorable side effects are called *untoward effects*. Untoward effects may be tolerated for the sake of therapeutic effect. More severe side effects, also called **adverse effects** or *drug reactions*, may justify discontinuing the drug.

Drug toxicity (deleterious effects of a drug on an organism or tissue) results from overdosage, ingestion of a drug intended for external use, and **cumulative effect** (buildup of the drug in the blood because of impaired metab-

TABLE 21-2 IMPORTANT DRUG LEGISLATION FOR UNITED STATES AND CANADA

LEGISLATION	CONTENT
Proprietary or Patent Medicine Act (Can. 1908)	Protects the public against unsafe and ineffective over-the-counter drugs.
Food, Drug, and Cosmetic Act (U.S. 1938)	Implemented by Food and Drug Administration (FDA); requires that labels be accurate and that all drugs be tested for harmful effects.
Durkham-Humphrey Amendment (U.S. 1952)	Clearly differentiates drugs that can be sold only with a prescription, those that can be sold without a prescription, and those that should not be refilled without a new prescription.
Canada Food and Drugs Act (Can. 1953)	Prohibits advertising any food, drug, cosmetic, or device as a cure for certain specified diseases. Sets standards for manufacture, distribution, and sale of all drugs, with the exception of narcotics.
Canadian Narcotic Control Act (Can. 1961)	Allows only authorized people to possess narcotics. Specifies records about narcotics that must be kept.
Kefauver-Harris Amendment (U.S. 1962)	Requires proof of safety and efficacy of a drug for approval.
Comprehensive Drug Abuse Prevention and Control Act (U.S. 1970) (Controlled Substances Act)	Categorizes controlled substances and limits how often a prescription can be filled; established government-funded programs to prevent and treat drug dependence.

TABLE 21-3 THERAPEUTIC ACTIONS OF DRUGS

DRUG TYPE	DESCRIPTION	EXAMPLES
Palliative	Relieves the symptoms of a disease but does not affect the disease itself	Morphine sulfate, aspirin for pain
Curative	Cures a disease or condition	Penicillin for infection
Supportive	Supports body function until other treatments or the body's response can take over	Norepinephrine bitartrate for low blood pressure; aspirin for high body temperature
Substitutive	Replaces body fluids or substances	Thyroxine for hypothyroidism, insulin for diabetes mellitus
Chemotherapeutic	Destroys malignant cells	Busulfan for leukemia
Restorative	Returns the body to health	Vitamin, mineral supplements, B_{12} injections for pernicious anemia

olism or excretion). Some toxic effects become apparent immediately; some are not apparent for weeks or months. Drug toxicity may be avoided by close monitoring of the drug dose and client response.

A **drug allergy** is an immunologic reaction to a drug. When a person is first exposed to a foreign substance (antigen), such as a drug, the body may react by producing antibodies, triggering an allergic reaction. See Table 21-4 ◆ for common mild allergic responses.

TABLE 21-4 COMMON MILD ALLERGIC RESPONSES

SYMPTOM	DESCRIPTION/RATIONALE
Skin rash	Either an intraepidermal vesicle rash or a rash typified by an urticarial wheal or macular eruption; rash is usually generalized over the body
Pruritus	Itching of the skin with or without a rash
Angioedema	Edema due to increased permeability of the blood capillaries
Rhinitis	Excessive watery discharge from the nose
Lacrimal tearing	Excessive tearing
Nausea, vomiting	Stimulation of these centers in the brain
Wheezing and dyspnea	Shortness of breath and wheezing upon inhalation and exhalation due to accumulated fluids and swelling of the respiratory tissues
Diarrhea	Irritation of the mucosa of the large intestine

Drug tolerance occurs when a person requires increases in dosage to maintain the therapeutic effect. Habituating drugs such as opiates, barbiturates, ethyl alchohol, and nicotine produce tolerance. A cumulative effect is the increasing response to repeated doses of a drug, which occurs when the rate of administration exceeds the rate of metabolism or excretion. As a result, the the drug builds up in the client's body unless the dosage is adjusted.

Idiosyncratic effect (unexpected unique bodily response) causes unpredictable abnormal symptoms in clients, including opposite drug actions and over- and underresponse to medications.

A **drug interaction** occurs when the administration of one drug alters the effect of another drug. The effect of each drug may increase (*potentiating or synergistic effect*) or decrease (*inhibiting effect*). Drug interactions may be beneficial or harmful. Foods and other natural substances may interact adversely with a medication. (For example, tetracycline should not be given with milk or milk products because it will decrease the effectiveness of the medication.)

Iatrogenic disease (disease caused unintentionally by medical therapy) can be due to drug administration.

ACTIONS OF DRUGS ON THE BODY

The action of a drug in the body can be described in terms of its half-life. **Half-life** is the time interval required for the body's elimination processes to reduce the concentration of the drug in the body by one half. For example, if a drug's half-life is 8 hours, then the amount of drug in the body is as follows:

Initially: 100%
After 8 hours: 50%
After 16 hours: 25%
After 24 hours: 12.5%
After 32 hours: 6.25%

Because the purpose of most drug therapy is to maintain a constant drug level in the body, repeated doses are required to maintain that level. A person may not respond in the same manner to successive doses. Key terms related to drug actions are listed and described in Box 21-1 ◆.

Absorption

Absorption is the process by which the drug passes into the bloodstream. Unless the drug is administered directly into the bloodstream, absorption is the first step in the movement of the drug through the body. The rate of absorption varies with the route.

FACTORS AFFECTING MEDICATION ACTION

An idiosyncratic effect is unexpected and individual. The drug may have a completely different effect from the normal one or cause unpredictable and unexplained symptoms.

Ethnicity and culture may contribute to differences in responses to medications. It is thought that a toxic reaction may be due to a genetic defect that causes a person to be unable to eliminate a drug or to metabolize a drug too quickly.

Cultural practices can also affect a drug's actions. Herbal remedies may counteract prescribed medications. Age and development may also have an effect on medication. See Box 21-2 ◆ for age-related considerations for medication administration.

Routes of Administration

The route of administration does affect medication action. Pharmaceutical preparations are generally designed for one or two specific routes of administration. Table 21-5 ◆ lists the advantages and disadvantages of various routes of administration. The route of administration should always be indicated when the drug is ordered. When administering a drug, the nurse needs to ensure that the pharmaceutical preparation is appropriate for the route specified.

 Medication Orders

A physician determines the client's medication needs and orders medications. Usually, the order is written, although telephone and verbal orders are acceptable in a number of agencies. Nursing students need to know the agency policies about medication orders. In some hospitals, for example, only licensed nurses are permitted to accept telephone and verbal orders.

Four common medication orders are the stat order, the single order, the standing order, and the prn order.

1. A **stat order** indicates that the medication is to be given immediately and only once.
2. The **single order** or "one-time order" is for medication to be given once at a specified time.
3. The **standing order** may or may not have a termination date. A standing order may be carried out indefinitely (e.g., multiple vitamins daily) until an order is written to cancel it, or it may be carried out for a specified number of days.
4. A **prn order,** "as needed order," permits the nurse to give a medication when, in the nurse's judgment, the client requires it. The nurse must use good judgment about when the medication is needed and when it can be safely administered.

ESSENTIAL PARTS OF A MEDICATION ORDER

The drug order has seven essential parts, as listed in Box 21-3 ◆. Unless it is a standing order, the order should state the number of doses or the number of days the drug is to be administered.

COMMUNICATING A MEDICATION ORDER

A drug order is written on the client's chart by a physician or nurse who receives a telephone or verbal order from a physician. The medication order is then copied by a nurse or clerk to a medication administration record (MAR), often a Kardex. Increasingly, nurses are provided with daily computer-generated MARs. This method saves time and reduces errors caused by hand copying of the physician's order.

Medication administration records (Figure 21-1 ◆) vary in form, but all include the client's name, room, and bed number; drug name and dose; and times and method of administration. In some agencies, the date the order was prescribed and the date the order expires are also included.

The nurse should always question the physician about any order that is *ambiguous* (unclear or difficult to read), *unusual* (e.g., an abnormally high dosage of a medication), or contraindicated by the client's condition. When the LPN/LVN judges that a physician-ordered medication is inappropriate, the following actions are required:

1. Discuss the order with the RN and/or the nursing supervisor.

> ## BOX 21-1
> ## KEY TERMS RELATED TO DRUG ACTION
>
> ◆ **Onset of action**: The time after administration when the body initially responds to the drug
> ◆ **Peak plasma level**: The highest plasma level achieved by a single dose when the elimination rate of a drug equals the absorption rate
> ◆ **Drug half-life** (elimination half-life): The time required for the elimination process to reduce the concentration of the drug to one half what it was at initial administration
> ◆ **Plateau**: A maintained concentration of a drug in the plasma during a series of scheduled doses
> ◆ **Absorption**: The process by which a drug passes into the bloodstream

(Text continues on p. 507)

TABLE 21-5 ROUTES OF ADMINISTRATION

ROUTE	ADVANTAGES	DISADVANTAGES
Oral	Most convenient Usually least expensive Safe, does not break skin barrier Administration usually does not cause stress	Inappropriate for clients with nausea or vomiting Drug may have unpleasant taste or odor Inappropriate when gastrointestinal tract has reduced motility Inappropriate if client cannot swallow or is unconscious Cannot be used before certain diagnostic tests or surgical procedures Drug may discolor teeth, harm tooth enamel Drug may irritate gastric mucosa Drug can be aspirated by seriously ill clients
Sublingual	Same as for oral, *plus* Drug can be administered for local effect Drug is rapidly absorbed into the bloodstream More potent than oral route because drug directly enters the blood and bypasses the liver	If swallowed, drug may be inactivated by gastric juice Drug must remain under tongue until dissolved and absorbed
Buccal	Same as for sublingual	Same as for sublingual
Rectal	Can be used when drug has objectionable taste or odor Drug released at slow, steady rate	Dose absorbed is unpredictable
Vaginal	Provides local therapeutic effect	Limited use
Topical	Provides a local effect Few side effects	May be messy and may soil clothes Drug can enter body through abrasions and cause systemic effects
Transdermal	Prolonged systemic effect Few side effects Avoids gastrointestinal absorption problems	Leaves residue on the skin that may soil clothes
Subcutaneous	Onset of drug action faster than oral	Must involve sterile technique because breaks skin barrier More expensive than oral Can administer only small volume Slower than intramuscular administration Some drugs can irritate tissues and cause pain Can be anxiety producing
Intramuscular	Pain from irritating drugs is minimized Can administer larger volume than subcutaneous Drug is rapidly absorbed	Breaks skin barrier Can be anxiety producing
Intradermal	Absorption is slow (this is an advantage in testing for allergies)	Amount of drug administered must be small Breaks skin barrier
Intravenous	Rapid effect	Limited to highly soluble drugs Drug distribution inhibited by poor circulation
Inhalation	Introduces drug throughout respiratory tract Rapid localized relief Drug can be administered to unconscious client	Drug intended for localized effect can have systemic effect Of use only for the respiratory system

☐ Seton Medical Center 100 Spurway Ave • Daly City ☐ Seton Medical Center Coastside 100 Marine Blvd • Moss Beach	**MEDICATION ADMINISTRATION RECORD**		**PAGE 1 OF 1** 5 0507-02

VERIFIED BY: _____ **DATE:** _____

DIAGNOSIS: *#ALOC

                 *#PNEUMONIA

ALLERGIES: NO KNOWN DRUG ALLERGIES

PRN#:

MRN#:   **AGE:**

ADM: 08-04-01   **SEX:**

DOB: **HT:**

DR.   **HT:**

GENERATED: 08-07-01   07:32am

FOR PERIOD: 08-07-01   08:00

THROUGH: 08-08-01   07:59

START	STOP	MEDICATION/I.V./IVPB/IRRIGATION	0800-1559	1600-2359	0000-0759
08-06 17	09-05 16	FERROUS SULFATE 300MG=5ML TWICE A DAY PO (FESO4)□□□□□□ (973539)	09	17	
08-06 17	09-05 16	DOCUSATE SODIUM 100MG=1UDCUP TWICE A DAY PO (COLACE) 100MG/30ML UD□□ □□ (973532) HOLD FOR LOOSE STOOL	09	17	
08-05 09	09-04 08	ASCORBIC ACID 500MG=1TAB TWICE A DAY PO (VITAMIN C) 500MG TAB□□□□ (972096)	09	17	
08-05 09	09-04 08	LEVOTHYROXINE 0.05MG=1TABDAILY PO (SYNTHROID) 0.05MG TAB□□□□ (972095)	09		
08-05 09	09-04 08	ASPIRIN 325MG=1 TAB DAILY PO (ASPIRIN) 325MG TAB□□□□□ (972094) *W/FOOD TO AVOID GI UPSET	09		
08-04 23	08-14 22	CEFUROXIME ADDV. 1.500GM=1VIAL EVERY 8 HOUS IV (KEFUROX) 1.5GM ADDV□□□□□ (971776) *ATTACH TO D5W 50ML ADDV BAG *ACTIVATE BEFORE UNFUSION* * INFUSE OVER 30 MINS*	14	22	06

─────── **PRN ORDERS** ───────

START	STOP	MEDICATION/I.V./IVPB/IRRIGATION	0800-1559	1600-2359	0000-0759
08-04 23	09-03 22	ACETAMINOPHEN 650MG=1SUPP EVERY 4 HOURS AS NEEDED PR (TYLENOL) 650MG SUPP□□□□□ (971779)			

INITIALS	SIGNATURE	SHIFT	INITIALS	SIGNATURE	SHIFT	INITIALS	SIGNATURE	SHIFT

SITE CODES: A. Right Upper Outer Gluteus   C. Right Outer Aspect Arm   E. Right Ventrogluteal   G. Abdomen   J. Left Thigh
             B. Left Upper Outer Quadrant Gluteus   D. Left Outer Aspect Arm   F. Left Ventrogluteal   H. Right Thigh

Figure 21-1. ◆ Medication administration record. *Source:* Courtesy of Seton Medical Center, Daly City, CA. Reprinted with permission.

BOX 21-2 AGE-RELATED CONSIDERATIONS FOR MEDICATION ADMINISTRATION

Infants and Children

◆ Knowledge of human growth and development is essential for the nurse. Oral medications for children are usually prepared in sweetened liquid form to make them more palatable. Never disguise with a necessary food (like formula, milk, or juice), because the child may refuse that food in the future. Parents may provide suggestions.

◆ Infants usually require small dosages because of their body size and the immaturity of their organs, especially the liver and kidneys. They often do not have all the enzymes required for drug metabolism and therefore may require different medications than adults. In adolescence or adulthood, allergic reactions may occur to drugs formerly tolerated.

◆ Children tend to fear any unfamiliar procedures, especially those in which needles are used. The nurse must acknowledge that the child will experience pain; denying this fact only fosters distrust. After an injection, the nurse (or parent) should cuddle and speak softly to the infant and/or give a toy to dispel the child's association of the nurse with pain.

Variation: Giving Oral Medications to Infants and Children

◆ Select an appropriate vehicle to measure and administer the medication, for example, plastic disposable cup, plastic syringe without needle, or tuberculin syringe. Whenever possible, give children a choice about use of a spoon, dropper, or syringe.

◆ Dilute the oral medication, if indicated, with a small amount of water. Many oral medications are readily swallowed if they are diluted with a small amount of water. If large quantities of water are used, the child may refuse to drink the entire amount and receive only a portion of the medication.

◆ Unless contraindicated, crush medications that are not supplied in liquid form and mix them with substances available on most pediatric units, such as honey, flavored syrup, jam, or a fruit puree. *Note:* When selecting a substance to mix with a medication, avoid *essential* food items such as milk, cereal, and orange juice. If these foods are used, the child may refuse them in the future.

◆ Disguise disagreeable-tasting medications with sweet-tasting substances mentioned previously. However, present any altered medication to the child honestly and not as a food or treat.

◆ To prevent nausea, pour a carbonated beverage over finely crushed ice and give it before or immediately after the medication is administered.

◆ To prevent aspiration and choking, position infants in a semireclining position, and administer the medication slowly in divided doses by spoon or a plastic syringe.

◆ If using a spoon, retrieve and refeed medication that is thrust outward by the infant's tongue.

◆ If using a syringe, place it along the side of the infant's tongue. This position prevents gagging and expulsion of the medication.

◆ A child's parents or guardians may be able to provide valuable information on how best to give the child medications. However, a nurse may need to partially restrain a child who refuses to cooperate or consistently resists despite explanation, encouragement, and attempts to determine the reason for the behavior.
  a. Place the child in your lap with the right arm behind you.
  b. Grasp the child's left hand firmly with your left hand.
  c. Secure the head between your arm and body.

◆ Follow all medication with a drink of water, juice, a soft drink, or a Popsicle or frozen juice bar. This removes any unpleasant aftertaste.

◆ For children who take sweetened medications on a long-term basis, follow the medication administration with oral hygiene. These children are at high risk for dental caries.

◆ For a young child, use a doll to demonstrate the procedure. This facilitates cooperation and decreases anxiety.

◆ For a young child or infant, enlist assistance to immobilize the arms and head. The parent may hold the infant or young child. This prevents accidental injury during medication administration.

Adults

◆ Maternal health considerations: During pregnancy, women must be very careful about taking medications. Most drugs are contraindicated because of the possible adverse effects on the fetus.

◆ Older adult physiologic changes that affect responses to medications:
  ◆ Decreased gastric mobility and decreased gastric acid production and blood flow can impair drug absorption.
  ◆ Increased adipose tissue and decreased total body fluid proportionate to the body mass can increase the possibility of drug toxicity.
  ◆ Decreased number of protein-binding sites and changes in the blood–brain barrier. The latter permits fat-soluble drugs to move readily to the brain, often resulting in dizziness and confusion. This is particularly evident with beta blockers.
  ◆ Impaired circulation delays the action of medications given intramuscularly or subcutaneously. Digitalis, which is frequently taken by older people, can accumulate to toxic levels and be lethal.

◆ Older adults usually require smaller dosages of drugs, especially CNS depressants. Then reactions to medications, particularly sedatives, are unpredictable and often bizarre. Reactions to sedatives include irritability, confusion, disorientation, restlessness, and incontinence. Nurses therefore need to observe clients carefully for untoward reactions.

◆ Because memory and visual acuity may be impaired, the nurse needs to develop simple, realistic plans for clients to follow at home. For example, clients are more likely to remember to take medications if they are scheduled to be taken with meals or at bedtime. If they are likely to forget whether they have taken their medications, a special container for medications can be employed. An empty container indicates that the person has already taken the pills. If the person has poor visual acuity, the nurse or a family member can be write out the plan in block letters large enough to be read.

◆ Older adult psychosocial problems (related to physiologic changes, past experiences, and established attitudes toward medications):
   ◆ Taking several different medications daily. The possibility of error increases with the number of medications taken.

◆ The greater number of medications also compounds the problem of drug interactions. A general rule to follow is to take as few medications as possible.

◆ Attitudes of older people toward medical care and medications vary. Older people tend to believe in the wisdom of the physician more readily than younger people. Some older people are bewildered by the prescription of several medications and may passively accept their medications and "cheek" them, spitting out tablets or capsules after the nurse leaves the room. For this reason, the nurse is advised to stay with clients until they have swallowed the medications. Others may be suspicious of medications and actively refuse them.

◆ Older people are mature adults capable of reasoning. Therefore, the nurse needs to explain the reasons for and the effects of medications. This education can prevent clients from continuing to take a medication long after there is a need for it or discontinuing a drug too quickly. For example, clients should know that diuretics will cause them to urinate more frequently and may reduce ankle edema. Instructions about medications need to be given to all clients. These instructions should include when to take the drugs, what effects to expect, and when to consult a physician.

---

2. Contact the physician and discuss the rationale for believing the medication or dosage to be inappropriate.

3. Document in notes the following: time the physician was notified, by whom, information conveyed to the physician, and the physician's response (using the physician's words, if possible).

4. If the physician cannot be reached, document all attempts to contact the physician and the reason for withholding the medication.

5. If someone else gives the medication, document data about the client's condition before and after the medication.

6. If an incident report is indicated, clearly document factual information.

BOX 21-3
ESSENTIAL PARTS OF A DRUG ORDER

◆ Full name of the client
◆ Date and time the order is written
◆ Name of the drug to be administered
◆ Dosage of the drug
◆ Route of administration
◆ Frequency of administration
◆ Signature of the person writing the order

 ## Systems of Measurement

Three systems of measurement are used for the administration of medication: the metric system, the apothecaries' system, and the household system.

METRIC SYSTEM

The **metric system** is a decimal system based on units of 10. Units can be multiplied or divided by 10 to form secondary units. Multiples are calculated by moving the decimal point to the right, and division by moving the decimal point to the left.

Basic units of measurement are the meter, the liter, and the gram. Prefixes (from Latin) indicate subdivision of the basic unit: deci (1/10 or 0.1), centi (1/100 or 0.01), and milli (1/1,000 or 0.001). Multiples of the basic unit (from Greek) are deka (10), hecto (100), and kilo (1000). See Figure 21-2 ◆ for examples. In nursing practice, the kilogram (kg) is the

Volume   **Weight**

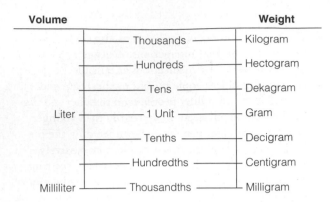

Thousands ——— Kilogram
Hundreds ——— Hectogram
Tens ——— Dekagram
Liter ——— 1 Unit ——— Gram
Tenths ——— Decigram
Hundredths ——— Centigram
Milliliter ——— Thousandths ——— Milligram

Figure 21-2. ◆ Basic metric measurements of volume and weight.

TABLE 21-6	APPROXIMATE EQUIVALENTS: METRIC, APOTHECARIES', AND HOUSEHOLD SYSTEMS		
METRIC	**APOTHECARIES'**	**HOUSEHOLD**	
Volume			
1 mL	15 minims (min or m)	15 drops (gtt) 1 tablespoon (Tbsp)	
5 mL	7.5 min	1 measuring teaspoon	
7.5 mL	112.5 min	1 household teaspoon	
15 mL	4 fluid drams (f)	1 tablespoon	
30 mL	1 fluid ounce (f)	1 fluid ounce	
500 mL	1 pint (pt)	1 pint	
1,000 mL	1 quart (qt)	1 quart	
4,000 mL	1 gallon (gal)	1 gallon	
Weight			
1 mg (milligram)	1/60 grain	—	
60 mg	1 grain	—	
1 g (gram)	15 grains	—	
4 g	1 dram	—	
30 g	1 ounce	—	
500 g	1.1 pound (lb)	—	
1,000 g (1 kg [kilogram])	2.2 lb	—	

only multiple of the gram used, and the milligram (mg) and microgram (mcg or µg) are subdivisions. Fractional parts of the liter are usually expressed in milliliters (mL).

APOTHECARIES' SYSTEM

The **apothecaries' system** predates the metric system. The basic unit of weight in the apothecaries' system is the grain (gr), likened to a grain of wheat, and the basic unit of volume is the minim, a volume of water equal in weight to a grain of wheat. The word *minim* means "the least." Other units of weight are the dram, the ounce, and the pound. The units of volume are the fluid dram, the fluid ounce, the pint, the quart, and the gallon.

Quantities in the apothecaries' system are often expressed by lowercase Roman numerals (ii, iv, ix, etc.), particularly when the unit of measure is abbreviated. The Roman numeral follows the unit of measure.

HOUSEHOLD SYSTEM

Household system measures may be used when more accurate systems of measure are not required. Included in household measures are drops, teaspoons, tablespoons, cups, and glasses. Although pints and quarts are often found in the home, they are defined as apothecaries' measures. See Table 21-6 ◆ for measurement equivalents of metric, apothecary, and household system.

> **clinical ALERT**
>
> A household teaspoon may hold 7.5 mL. This caution should be included in discharge instructions. It is advisable to use a medication cup or spoon with mL markings, to prevent overdose of a drug.

CONVERTING UNITS OF WEIGHT AND MEASURE

Sometimes drugs are dispensed from the pharmacy in grams when the order specifies milligrams, or they are dispensed in milligrams though ordered in grains. For example, a physician orders morphine gr 1/4. The medication is available only in milligrams. The nurse knows that 1 mg equals 1/60 gr or 60

mg equals 1 grain. To convert the ordered dose to milligrams, the nurse calculates as follows:

$$\text{If } 60 \text{ mg} = 1 \text{ gr}$$
$$\text{Then } x \text{ mg} = 1/4 \text{ gr } (0.25 \text{ gr})$$
$$x = \frac{(60 \times 0.25)}{1}$$
$$x = 15 \text{ mg}$$

Converting Weights within the Metric System

It is quite simple to find equivalent units of weight within the metric system, because the system is based on units of 10. Only three metric units of weight are used for drug dosages: the gram (g), milligram (mg), and microgram (mcg or µg); 1,000 mg or 1,000,000 mcg equals 1 g. Equivalents are computed by dividing or multiplying. For example, to change milligrams to grams, the nurse divides the number of milligrams by 1,000. The simplest way to divide by 1,000 is to move the decimal point three places to the left:

$$500 \text{ mg} = ? \text{ g}$$

Move the decimal point three places to the left:

$$\text{Answer} = 0.5 \text{ g}$$

Conversely, to convert grams to milligrams, multiply the number of grams by 1,000, or move the decimal point three places to the right:

$$0.006 \text{ g} = ? \text{ mg}$$

Move the decimal point three places to the right:

$$\text{Answer} = 6 \text{ mg}$$

Converting Weights and Measures Between Systems

When preparing client medications, a nurse may need to convert weights or volumes from one system to another.

The units of weight most commonly used in nursing practice are the gram, milligram, and kilogram; and the grain and the pound. Household units of weight are generally not applicable (see Table 21-6). Learning these equivalents helps the nurse make weight conversions easily.

CALCULATING DOSAGES

Several formulas can be used to calculate drug dosages. One formula uses ratios:

$$\frac{\text{Dose on hand}}{\text{Quantity on hand}} = \frac{\text{Desired dose}}{\text{Quantity desired } (n)}$$

For example, erythromycin 500 mg is ordered. It is supplied in a liquid form containing 250 mg in 5 mL. To calculate the dosage, the nurse uses the formula

$$\frac{\text{Dose on hand (250 mg)}}{\text{Quantity on hand (5 mL)}} = \frac{\text{Desired dose (500 mg)}}{\text{Quantity desired } (n)}$$

Then the nurse cross-multiplies:

$$250 \times n = 5 \times 500$$
$$250 \times n = 2{,}500$$
$$n = \frac{2{,}500}{250}$$
$$n = 10 \text{ mL}$$

Therefore, the dose ordered is 10 mL. The nurse can also use the following formula to calculate dosages:

$$\frac{\text{Desired dose}}{\text{Dose on hand}} \times \text{Quantity on hand}$$

For example, heparin is often distributed in large vials in prepared dilutions of 10,000 units per mL. If the order calls for 5,000 units, the nurse can use the formula above to calculate:

$$n = \frac{5{,}000}{10{,}000} \times 1 \text{ mL}$$
$$n = 1/2 \text{ mL} = 0.5 \text{ mL}$$

Therefore, the nurse injects 0.5 mL for a 5,000-unit dose.

Dosages for Children

Although dosage is stated in the medication order, nurses must understand something about the safe dosage for children. Unlike adult dosages, children's dosages are not always standard. Body size significantly affects dosage.

Figure 21-3. ◆ Nomogram with estimated body surface area. A straight line is drawn between the child's height (on the left) and the child's weight (on the right). The point at which the line intersects the surface area column is the estimated body surface area.

BODY SURFACE AREA. Body surface area is determined by using a **nomogram** and the child's height and weight. This is considered to be the most accurate method of calculating a child's dose. Standard nomograms give a child's body surface area according to weight and height (Figure 21-3 ◆). The formula is the ratio of the child's body surface area to the surface area of an average adult (1.7 square meters, or 1.7 m²), multiplied by the normal adult dose of the drug:

$$\text{Child's dose} = \frac{\text{Surface area of child (m}^2)}{1.7 \text{ m}^2} \times \text{Normal adult dose}$$

For example, a child who weighs 10 kg and is 50 cm tall has a body surface area of 0.4 m². Therefore, the child's dose of tetracycline corresponding to an adult dose of 250 mg would be as follows:

$$\text{Child's dose} = \frac{0.4 \text{ m}^2}{1.7 \text{ m}^2} \times 250 \text{ mg}$$
$$= 0.23 \times 250 = 58.82 \text{ mg}$$

Equipment

SYRINGES

To administer parenteral medications, nurses use injectable equipment: **Syringes** have three parts: the *tip*, which connects with the needle; the *barrel*, or fluid chamber, on which the scales are printed; and the *plunger*, which fits inside the barrel (Figure 21-4 ◆).

To handle a syringe aseptically, the nurse may touch the outside of the barrel and the plunger handle. The nurse must avoid letting any unsterile object contact the tip or inside of the barrel, the shaft of the plunger, or the shaft or tip of the needle.

Syringes differ in size, shape, and material. The three most commonly used types are the standard hypodermic syringe, the insulin syringe, and the tuberculin syringe (Figure 21-5 ◆). Hypodermic syringes come in 2-, 2.5-, and 3-mL sizes. They usually have two scales marked on them: the minim and the milliliter. The milliliter scale is the one normally used; the minim scale is used for very small dosages.

Insulin syringes are similar to hypodermic syringes, but they have a specially calibrated scale for use with U-100 insulin. In North America all insulin syringes are calibrated this way. Most insulin syringes are disposable and have a nonremovable needle. Low-dose insulin syringes are also available. The correct choice of syringe is based on the insulin dose. The tuberculin syringe is a narrow-barrel syringe, calibrated in tenths and hundredths of a milliliter (up to 1 mL) on one scale and in sixteenths of a minim (up to 1 minim) on the other scale. Originally designed to administer tuberculin, this syringe is useful for administering other drugs, particularly when a small, precise measurement is necessary (e.g., pediatric doses).

Other syringes are manufactured in several sizes such as 5, 10, 20, and 50 mL. Most syringes used today are made of plastic and are individually packaged for sterility in a paper

Figure 21-5. ◆ Three kinds of syringes: **A.** Hypodermic syringe marked in tenths (0.1) of milliliters and in minims: **B.** Insulin syringe marked in 100 units; **C.** Tuberculin syringe marked in tenths and hundredths (0.01) of cubic millimeters and in minims.

wrapper or a rigid plastic container (Figure 21-6 ◆). The syringe and needle may be packaged together or separately.

Injectable medications are frequently supplied in disposable, prefilled unit-dose systems such as (a) ready-to-use syringes or (b) prefilled sterile cartridges and needles that require the attachment of a reusable holder (injection system) before use (Figure 21-7 ◆). Examples of the latter system are the Tubex and Carpuject injection systems. The manufacturers provide specific directions for use. Because most prefilled cartridges are overfilled, excess medication must be ejected before the injection to ensure the right dosage.

NEEDLES

Needles are made of stainless steel, and most are disposable. A needle has three parts: the **hub,** which fits onto the syringe; the **cannula,** or shaft, which is attached to the hub; and the **bevel,** which is the slanted part of the tip (Figure 21-8 ◆).

Figure 21-4. ◆ The three parts of a syringe.

Figure 21-6. ◆ Disposable plastic syringes and needles: top, with syringe and needle exposed; middle, with plastic cup over the needle; bottom, with plastic case over the needle and syringe. *Source:* © Elena Dorfman.

C

Figure 21-7. ◆ **A.** Syringe and prefilled sterile cartridge with needle. **B.** Assembling the device. **C.** The cartridge slides into the syringe barrel, turns, and locks at the needle end. The plunger then screws into the cartridge end. *Source:* © Elena Dorfman.

Needles have variable characteristics:

1. *Slant or length of the bevel.* Bevel length varies. Long-bevel needles are sharpest. They are best for subcutaneous and intramuscular injections because they cause the least discomfort.

2. *Length of the shaft.* The shaft length of commonly used needles varies 1.25 to 5 cm from (1/2 to 2 inches). The appropriate needle length is chosen according to the client's muscle development, the client's weight, and the type of injection.

Figure 21-8. ◆ The parts of a needle.

3. *Gauge (or diameter) of the shaft.* The gauge varies from 18 to 28. The larger the gauge number, the smaller the diameter of the shaft. Smaller gauges produce less tissue trauma, but larger gauges are necessary for viscous medications, such as penicillin.

Additional equipment is need for intravenous administration.

◆ Routes of Administration

ORAL MEDICATIONS

The oral route is the most common medication route. So long as a client can swallow effectively and retain the drug in the stomach, this is the route of choice. Procedure 21-1 describes how to give oral medications. Oral medications are contraindicated when a client is vomiting, has gastric or intestinal suction, is unconscious, or has swallowing difficulty, such as after a stroke. Such clients in the hospital are usually on orders for "nothing by mouth" (**NPO**).

There are two variations on the oral medication route, sublingual and buccal. In **sublingual** administration the drug is placed under the tongue (Figure 21-9 ◆). The drug is absorbed into the blood vessels on the underside of the tongue. Nitroglycerin is one example of a drug commonly given in this manner.

Figure 21-9. ◆ Sublingual administration of a tablet.

Figure 21-10. ◆ Buccal administration of a tablet.

Buccal means pertaining to the cheek. In buccal administration the tablet is held in the mouth next to the mucous membranes of the cheek until it dissolves (Figure 21-10 ◆). The medication acts locally on the mucous membrane or systemically when the drug is swallowed with saliva.

NASOGASTRIC AND GASTROSTOMY MEDICATIONS

For the client who is getting nothing by mouth (NPO) and has a nasogastric (NG) or gastrostomy (G) tube in place, medication may be administered via the tube. See also Procedures 17-2 and 17-3. ⊕

PARENTERAL MEDICATIONS

LPNs and LVNs give **parenteral** (injectable) medications. The routes are **intradermal** (ID or into the dermis or skin), **subcutaneous** (SC or SQ, below the skin), **intramuscular** (IM or into the muscle), and, in some states, **intravenous** (IV or into the vein). Figure 21-11 ◆ illustrates the different angles of these injections and different ways of holding the syringe to administer them. Administration of medications via the parenteral route is discussed in the Nursing Care section of this chapter.

Because parenteral medications are absorbed rapidly and are irretrievable once injected, the nurse must prepare and administer them carefully and accurately. Administering parenteral drugs requires the same nursing knowledge as for oral and topical drugs. However, because injections are invasive procedures, aseptic technique must be used to minimize the risk of infection.

MediaLink ● **Animation: Injections**

Figure 21-11. ◆ Angles of needle insertion for four types of injection.

TOPICAL MEDICATIONS

Topical medications are those that are applied locally to the skin or to mucous membranes in areas such as the eye, external ear canal, nose, vagina, and rectum. Traditionally, topical application to the skin was limited to medications intended to produce a local effect at the administration site. However, several medications (e.g., nitroglycerin and estrogen) have been "packaged" in special transdermal delivery systems that gradually release a predictable amount of active substance into the bloodstream for as long as a week.

NURSING CARE

 ASSESSING

When LPNs/LVNs are assigned the responsibility of administering medication, they must review the client's chart, including the medication history and nursing notes for assessment data, and discuss any concerns with the RN or physician.

 DIAGNOSING, PLANNING, and IMPLEMENTING

Providing Safety in Medication Administration

When administering any drug, regardless of the route of administration, the nurse must follow certain procedures. For a description of these procedures, see Table 21-7 ◆. Box 21-4 ◆ lists the five "rights" and the three "checks" for accurate drug administration. The nurse who prepares the medication must also administer it to the client. Medications must never be left unattended on the medication cart or at the client's bedside.

Observing Client's Response to the Drug

The kinds of behavior that reflect the action or lack of action of a drug and its untoward effects (both minor and major) are as variable as the purposes of the drugs themselves. For example, the effectiveness of a sedative–hypnotic may be directly observed by how well the client sleeps. The effectiveness of an antispasmodic must be based on the client's report of pain relief. It is essential to chart the client's drug response, but written notes are only one facet of communication needed for

TABLE 21-7	RULES FOR MEDICATION ADMINISTRATION
THE NURSE MUST ALWAYS	**DESCRIPTION**
Identify the client	In hospitals, most clients wear some sort of identification (ID), such as a wristband with name and hospital ID number. Before giving the client any drug, check the ID band against the medication administration record (MAR). As a double check, ask the client to state his name.
Inform the client	If the client is unfamiliar with the medication, the nurse should explain the intended action as well as any side effects or adverse effects that might occur.
Administer the drug	Read medication orders and records carefully; check both the client and drug name against the names on the drug packaging. If the client's medication is kept in a medication cart or computerized dispensary, check against this also.
Provide adjunctive interventions as indicated	Clients may need physical assistance, such as positioning for an injection. They may need teaching about measures to enhance drug effectiveness, such as changes in diet and fluid intake. Clients may express fear of medication. The LVN/LPN can allay fear through active listening and by offering factual information and emotional support.
Record the drug administered	The facts recorded in the chart, in ink or by computer printout, are name of the drug, dosage, method of administration, specific relevant data such as pulse rate (taken in most settings prior to the administration of digitalis), and any other pertinent information. The record should also include the exact time of administration and the signature of the nurse providing the medication. Many medication records are designed flowchart style so that the nurse signs once on the page and initials each medication administered. Any prn or stat medications, as well as the client's response to the drug, are recorded separately and should be documented in the nursing/progress notes. Nurses must be aware of all the medications a client is taking, and be alert for interactions.
Evaluate the client's response to the drug	In all nursing activities, nurses need to be aware of the medications that a client is taking and record their effectiveness as assessed by the client and the nurse on the client's chart. The nurse may also report the client's response to the RN or the physician.

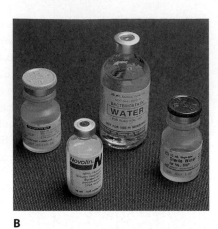

A   B

Figure 21-12. ◆ **A.** Ampules. **B.** Vials.

continuity of care. The LVN/LPN should also verbally report the client's response to the team leader or physician.

Administering Oral Medications

The nurse provides oral medications and water or other liquid as appropriate for the client. The nurse remains with the client while the client swallows the medicine and assists if necessary. (*Note:* The nurse should be aware that some clients "pouch" medications in the cheek instead of swallowing them.)

Sublingual and buccal medications are placed under the tongue or between the cheek and the gum. They are not swallowed but allowed to dissolve in the mouth.

Administering Nasogastric and Gastrostomy Medications

Clients may be NPO because of illness, surgery, or another procedure. Medication may then be administered via nasogastric or gastrostomy tube. Guidelines for administering medications by NG or G tubes are shown in Box 21-5 ◆.

Assisting with IV Medication Administration

LPN/LVNs, once are licensed and certified in IV therapy, may be responsible for starting and hanging IVs. Until then, the LPN/LVN is responsible for assessing the site and removing the delivery system, once an order has been given to discontinue. Box 21-6 ◆ provides instructions for discontinuing an intravenous injection. See also Procedure 17-4. ⚭

Preparing Injectable Medications

Injectable medications can be prepared by withdrawing the medication from an ampule or vial into a sterile syringe, using prefilled syringes, or via needleless injection system.

Ampules and Vials. Ampules and vials (Figure 21-12 ◆) are frequently used to package sterile parenteral medications. An **ampule** is a clear glass container with a distinctive shape usually designed to hold a single dose of a drug. Ampule capacity ranges from 1 mL to 10 mL or more. Most ampules have colored score markings for opening. Refer to Procedure 21-2 for steps in preparing medications from ampules and vials.

A **vial** is a small glass bottle with a sealed rubber cap. Vials come in different sizes, from single to multidose and have a metal or plastic cap that protects the rubber seal.

Mixing Medications in One Syringe. Frequently, clients need more than one drug injected at the same time. To spare the client the experience of being injected twice, two drugs (if compatible) can be mixed together in one syringe (see Procedure 21-2 for how to mix medications in one syringe).

Preventing Needle-Stick Injuries

One of the most potentially hazardous procedures that health care personnel face is using and disposing of needles and sharps.

clinical **ALERT**

Needle-stick injuries present a major risk for infection with hepatitis B virus, human immunodeficiency virus (HIV), and many other pathogens. Standards have been set by the Occupational Safety and Health Administration (OSHA) to prevent such injuries.

To prevent needle-stick injury, the nurse must follow these guidelines carefully and consistently:

◆ Always use the designated puncture-proof disposal container provided (Figure 21-13 ◆). Never throw sharps in wastebaskets. Never leave them unattended in public or client care areas.
◆ Handle all sharps with care, including any items that can cut or puncture skin, such as needles, surgical blades, lancets, razors, broken glass (including capillary pipettes and open ampules), exposed dental wires, reusable items (e.g., large-bore needles, hooks, rasps, drill points), or ANY SHARP INSTRUMENT!
◆ Never bend or break needles before disposal.
◆ Never recap used needles except under specified circumstances (e.g., when transporting a syringe to the laboratory for an arterial blood gas or blood culture).

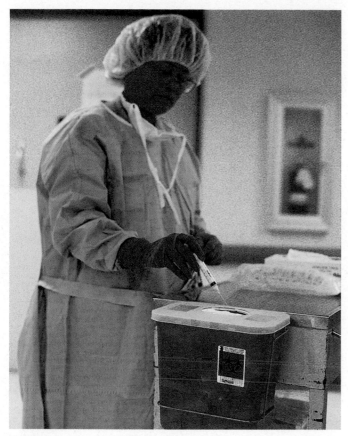

Figure 21-13. ◆ Disposal container for contaminated needles and other sharps. *Source:* © Elena Dorfman.

◆ If you must recap a needle, use the one-handed "scoop" method. Set the needle cap and syringe horizontally on a flat surface. Insert the needle into the cap, using one hand (Figure 21-14 ◆). Use your other hand to pick up the cap; tighten it to the needle hub.

If an accidental needle-stick injury occurs, follow specific steps outlined by the agency. A summary of these steps is provided in Box 21-7 ◆. Safety syringes are now available to protect health care workers.

Administering Intradermal Injections

An intradermal injection is the administration of a drug into the dermal layer of the skin just beneath the epidermis (see

Figure 21-14. ◆ Recapping a used needle using the scoop method. *Source:* © Elena Dorfman.

BOX 21-5
NURSING CARE CHECKLIST

ADMINISTERING MEDICATIONS BY NASOGASTRIC OR GASTROSTOMY TUBE

☑ Always check with the pharmacist to see if the client's medications come in liquid form, because liquids are less likely to cause tube obstruction.

☑ If not available, determine if the drug may be safely crushed. Enteric-coated, sustained-action, buccal, and sublingual medications should never be crushed.

☑ Dissolve crushed tablets in warm water. Cold liquids may congeal or cause client discomfort.

☑ Read medication labels carefully before opening a capsule.

☑ Open capsules and mix the contents with water only with the pharmacist's advice.

☑ Do not administer whole or undissolved medications.

☑ If the tube is connected to suction, disconnect the suction and keep the tube clamped for 20 to 30 minutes after giving the medication to enhance absorption.

☑ Always check and confirm NGT placement before administering medications by checking gastric pH or by auscultating air.

☑ Flush the tube with at least 15 to 30 mL (5 to 10 mL for children) of water before administering medications.

☑ If you are giving several medications, administer each one separately and flush with at least 5 mL (3 mL for children) of water between each.

☑ When you have finished administering all medications, flush with another 15 to 30 mL of water to clear the tube.

Sources: Data from Lehmann, S., & Barber, J. (1991, November). Giving medication by feeding tube: How to avoid problems. *Nursing 91*, p. 61; and Petrosino, B. M., Christian, B. J., Wolfe, J., et al. (1989, December). Implications of selected problems with nasoenteral tube feeding. *Critical Care Quarterly, 12,* 1.

Figure 21-11). Intradermal injections generally use only a small amount of liquid, such as 0.1 mL. This method of administration is frequently indicated for allergy and tuberculin tests and for vaccinations. Common sites for intradermal injections are the inner lower arm, the upper chest, and the back beneath the scapulae (Figure 21-15 ◆). Typically, the left arm is used for tuberculin tests and the right arm is used for all other tests.

The equipment normally used is a 1-mL syringe calibrated into hundredths of a milliliter. The needle is short and fine. After the site is cleaned, the skin is held tautly, and the syringe is held at about a 15-degree angle to the skin, with the bevel of the needle upward. The needle is then inserted through the epidermis

Figure 21-15. ◆ Body sites commonly used for intradermal injections.

Epidermis
Dermis
Subcutaneous tissue

Figure 21-16. ◆ For an intradermal injection: **A,** the needle enters the skin at a 15 degree angle; and **B,** the medication forms a bleb under the epidermis.

into the dermis, and the fluid is injected. The drug produces a small bleb just under the skin (Figure 21-16 ◆). The needle is then withdrawn quickly, and the site is very lightly wiped with

an antiseptic swab. The area is not massaged because the medication may disperse into the tissue or out through the needle insertion site. Intradermal injections are absorbed slowly through blood capillaries in the area.

Administering Subcutaneous Injections

Many kinds of drugs (such as insulin and heparin) are administered *subcutaneously* (just beneath the skin). Common sites for subcutaneous injections are the outer aspect of the upper arms and the anterior aspect of the thighs. These areas are convenient and normally have good blood circulation. Other areas that can be used are the abdomen, the scapular areas of the upper back, and the upper ventrogluteal and dorsogluteal areas (Figure 21-17 ◆). Only small doses (0.5 to 1 mL) of medication are usually injected via the subcutaneous route. Refer to Procedure 21-3 for instructions about subcutaneous injections.

BOX 21-6
NURSING CARE CHECKLIST

DISCONTINUING INTRAVENOUS DEVICE

- ☑ Check physician's order.
- ☑ Gather appropriate equipment.
- ☑ Identify the client and explain the procedure.
- ☑ Wash hands and don gloves.
- ☑ Stabilize needle or catheter while removing tape.
- ☑ Remove needle or catheter carefully and smoothly, keeping it almost flush with skin.
- ☑ Do not press down on top of needle point while it is in the vein.
- ☑ Quickly press sterile pad over venipuncture site, and hold firmly until bleeding stops.
- ☑ Hold pressure for several minutes if client's drug therapy prolongs bleeding.
- ☑ Apply clean pad and tape in place.
- ☑ Elevate arm to reduce venous pressure and help facilitate clot formation.
- ☑ Observe venipuncture site for redness, swelling, or hematoma.
- ☑ Dispose of equipment.
- ☑ Wash hands.
- ☑ Check site again in 15 minutes.
- ☑ Record volume infused on intake and output (I&O) sheet.
- ☑ Document.

BOX 21-7
WHAT TO DO IF NEEDLESTICK OCCURS

If you experience a needle-stick or sharp injury or were exposed to blood or other body fluids of a client during the course of your work, immediately follow these steps or those prescribed by the facility:

- ◆ Wash needlesticks and cuts with soap and water.
- ◆ Flush splashes to nose, mouth, or skin with clean water.
- ◆ Irrigate eyes with clean water, saline, or sterile irrigants.
- ◆ Report the incident to your supervisor.
- ◆ Immediately seek medical treatment.

Source: Recommendations courtesy of the National Institute for Occupational Health and Safety.

Figure 21-17. ◆ Body sites commonly used for subcutaneous injections.

Administering Intramuscular Injections

Injections into muscle tissue (IM injections) are absorbed more quickly than subcutaneous injections because of the greater blood supply to the body muscles. Muscles can also take a larger volume of fluid without discomfort than subcutaneous tissues can, although the amount varies somewhat, depending on muscle size, muscle condition, and the site used. An adult with well-developed muscles can usually safely tolerate up to 4 mL of medication in the gluteus medius and gluteus maximus muscles.

A major consideration in the administration of intramuscular injections is the selection of a safe site located away from large blood vessels, nerves, and bone. Several body sites can be used for IM injections (Figure 21-18 ◆). See Procedure 21-3B for administering IM injections.

Ventrogluteal Site. The ventrogluteal site is in the gluteus medius muscle, which lies over the gluteus minimus. The ventrogluteal site is the preferred site for IM injections because the area (a) contains no large nerves or blood vessels; (b) provides the greatest thickness of gluteal muscle consisting of both the gluteus medius and gluteus minimus; (c) is sealed off by bone; and (d) contains consistently less fat than the buttock area, thus eliminating the need to determine the depth of subcutaneous fat.

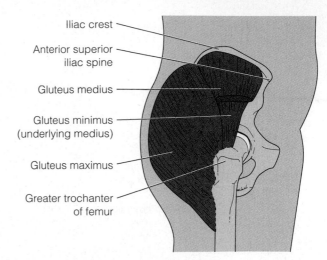

Figure 21-18. ◆ Lateral view of the right buttock showing the three gluteal muscles used for intramuscular injections.

The client position for the injection can be a supine, prone, or side-lying position. To establish the exact site, the nurse places the heel of the hand on the client's greater trochanter, with the fingers pointing toward the client's head. The right hand is used for the left hip, and the left hand for the right hip. With the index finger on the client's anterior superior iliac spine, the nurse stretches the middle finger dorsally, palpating the crest of the ilium and then pressing below it. The triangle formed by the index finger, the third finger, and the crest of the ileum is the injection site (Figure 21-19 ◆).

Vastus Lateralis Site. The vastus lateralis muscle is usually thick and well developed in both adults and children. It is recommended as the site of choice for IM injections for infants. Because there are no major blood vessels or nerves in the area, it is desirable for infants whose gluteal muscles are poorly developed. It is located on the anterior lateral aspect of the thigh (Figure 21-20 ◆). The middle third of the muscle is

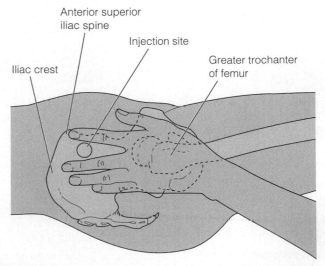

Figure 21-19. ◆ The ventrogluteal site for an intramuscular injection.

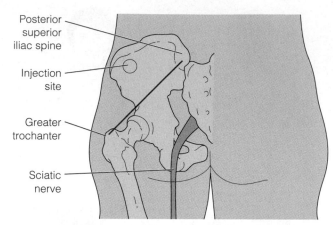

Figure 21-21. ◆ The dorsogluteal site for an intramuscular injection.

Figure 21-20. ◆ **A.** The vastus lateralis muscle of the upper thigh, used for intramuscular injections. **B.** The vastus lateralis site of the right thigh, used for an intramuscular injection.

suggested as the site. This is established by dividing the area between the greater trochanter of the femur and the lateral femoral condyle into thirds and selecting the middle third (Figure 21-20B). The client can assume a back-lying or a sitting position for an injection into this site.

Dorsogluteal Site. The dorsogluteal site is composed of the thick gluteal muscles of the buttocks (Figure 21-21 ◆). The dorsogluteal site can be used for adults and for children with

well-developed gluteal muscles. Because these muscles are developed by walking, this site should not be used for children under 3 years unless the child has been walking for at least 1 year. The nurse must choose the injection site carefully to avoid striking the sciatic nerve, major blood vessels, or bone.

The nurse palpates the posterior superior iliac spine, then draws an imaginary line to the greater trochanter of the femur. This line is lateral to and parallel to the sciatic nerve. The injection site is lateral and superior to this line. Palpating the ilium and the trochanter is important. Visual calculations alone can result in an injection that is too low and that injures other structures.

The client needs to assume a prone position with the toes pointed inward, or a side-lying position with the upper knee flexed and in front of the lower leg. These positions promote muscle relaxation and minimize discomfort from the injection.

Deltoid Site. The deltoid muscle is found on the lateral aspect of the upper arm. It is not used often for IM injections, because it is a relatively small muscle and is very close to the radial nerve and radial artery. It is sometimes considered for use in adults because of rapid absorption from the deltoid area, but no more than 1 mL of solution can be administered. This site is recommended for the administration of hepatitis B vaccine in adults.

To locate the densest part of the muscle, the nurse palpates the lower edge of the acromion and the midpoint on the lateral aspect of the arm that is in line with the axilla. A triangle within these boundaries indicates the deltoid muscle about 5 cm (2 in) below the acromion process (Figure 21-22 ◆). Another method of establishing the deltoid site is to place four fingers across the deltoid muscle, with the first finger on the acromion process. The site is three fingerbreadths below the acromion process (see Figure 21-22B).

Procedure 21-3B describes how to administer an IM injection using the Z-track technique. This technique is recommended for IM injections. Vistaril (hydroxyzine hydrochloride solution) is an example of a medication that requires Z-track injection.

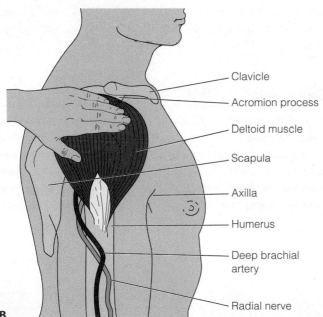

Figure 21-22. ◆ **A.** The deltoid muscle of the upper arm, used for intramuscular injections. **B.** A method of establishing the deltoid muscle site for an intramuscular injection.

Although it is common practice to add 0.2 cc of air following the drawing up of medication, research has shown that use of an air bubble in the syringe is unnecessary with modern disposable syringes and can be potentially dangerous, causing overdoses (Beyea & Nicoll, 1996, pp. 34–35). Syringes are now calibrated to deliver correct dosages without the use of an air bubble.

Administering Topical Applications

Skin Applications. Topical skin or dermatologic preparations include ointments, pastes, creams, lotions, powders, sprays, and patches. See Table 21-1 earlier in this chapter. Before applying a dermatologic preparation, thoroughly clean the area with mild soap and water and pat it dry. Medication absorption is affected by the buildup of skin secretions and previous topical medication. Human skin harbors microorganisms, so nurses should wear gloves when administering skin applications and always use surgical asepsis when an open wound is present.

Ophthalmic Instillations. Preparations for the eye (**ophthalmics**) come as liquids or ointments. Procedure 21-4 illustrates how to administer ophthalmic medications.

Otic Instillations. Medical aseptic technique is used to instill **otics** (ear preparations) unless the tympanic membrane is damaged, in which case sterile technique is required. The position of the external auditory canal varies with age. In the child under 3 years of age, it is directed upward. In the adult, the external auditory canal is an S-shaped structure about 2.5 cm (1 in) long.

Procedure 21-5 explains how to administer otic instillations.

Nasal Instillations. Nasal instillations (nose drops and sprays) usually are instilled for their *astringent* effect (to shrink swollen mucous membranes), to loosen secretions and facilitate drainage, or to treat infections of the nasal cavity or sinuses. Nasal decongestants are the most common nasal instillations. Many of these products are available without a prescription. Clients need to be taught to use these agents with caution. Chronic use of nasal decongestants may lead to a *rebound effect*, an increase in nasal congestion after the decongestant action has ended. If excess decongestant solution is swallowed, serious systemic effects may also develop, especially in children. Saline drops are safer as a decongestant for children.

Usually, clients self-administer sprays. In the supine position with the head tilted back, the client holds the tip of the container just inside the nares and inhales as the spray enters the nasal passages. For clients who use nasal sprays repeatedly, the nares need to be assessed for irritation. In children, nasal sprays are given with the head in an upright position to prevent excess spray from being swallowed.

The client should also be instructed to (a) breathe through the mouth to prevent aspiration of medication into the trachea and bronchi, (b) remain in a back-lying position for at least 1 minute so that the solution will come into contact with all of the nasal surface and (c) avoid blowing the nose for several minutes.

Vaginal Instillations. Vaginal medications, or instillations are inserted as creams, jellies, foams, or suppositories to treat infection or to relieve vaginal discomfort, such as itching, dryness, or pain. See Procedure 21-6 for administering vaginal instillations.

Rectal Instillations. Insertion of medications into the rectum in the form of suppositories is a frequent practice. Rectal administration is a convenient and safe method of giving certain medications.

When rectal medication is to be given for constipation, the nurse should check the chart for the last bowel movement (b.m.) recorded if there is no b.m. recorded, then a digital exam should be done before giving suppository. To insert a rectal suppository:

◆ Assist the client to a left lateral position, with the upper leg flexed.
◆ Fold back the top bedclothes to expose the buttocks.
◆ Don a glove on the hand used to insert the suppository.
◆ Unwrap the suppository and lubricate the smooth rounded end, or see manufacturer's instructions. The rounded end is usually inserted first, and lubricant reduces irritation of the mucosa.
◆ Lubricate the gloved index finger.
◆ Encourage the client to relax by breathing through the mouth.
◆ Insert the suppository gently into the anal canal, rounded end first (or according to manufacturer's instructions), along the rectal wall using the gloved index finger (Figure 21-23 ◆). For an adult, insert the suppository beyond the internal sphincter (i.e., 10 cm [4 in]); for a child or infant, insert it 5 cm (2 in) or less.
◆ Avoid embedding the suppository in feces.
◆ Press the client's buttocks together for a few minutes.
◆ Ask the client to remain in the left lateral or supine position for at least 5 minutes to help retain the suppository. The suppository should be retained for at least 30 to 40 minutes or according to manufacturer's instructions.

Medication is occasionally given by enema. An example of this would be Kayexalate (sodium polystyrene sulfonate) to treat hyperkalemia (excessive potassium).

Respiratory Inhalation Drugs. Medications administered by inhalation, such as bronchodilators, are frequently prescribed for clients with chronic respiratory disease such as asthma, emphysema, or bronchitis. Medications by inhalation are often administered by a respiratory technologist via *nebulizer* (a machine that aerosolizes liquid as a fine mist delivered by mouthpiece or facial mask). See Chapter 16 for more information. ☞ A *metered-dose inhaler* (MDI) is a handheld nebulizer (HHN) that can be used by clients to self-administer measured doses of an aerosol medication. To ensure correct delivery of the prescribed medication, nurses need to instruct clients on correct MDI use. To release medication through the mouthpiece, the client compresses the canister by hand while inhaling, and medication is released (Figure 21-24 ◆). An extender or spacer may be attached to the mouthpiece to facilitate medication absorption for better results. *Spacers* are holding chambers into which the medication is fired and from which the client inhales, so that the dose is not lost by exhalation. Box 21-8 ◆ provides instructions for clients about using a metered-dose inhaler (MDI). Newer, breath-activated MDIs are being produced in which inhalation triggers the release of a premeasured dose of medication.

Irrigations An irrigation (or *lavage*) is the washing out of a body cavity by a stream of water or other fluid, which may contain medication. Guidelines for administering eye and ear irrigations are shown in Box 21-9 ◆.

◆ EVALUATING

After administering medication, the nurse observes the client to determine the effectiveness of the medication. The nurse also monitors the client for possible adverse effects and reports these to the team leader and physician. The nurse must promptly document administration of medications to provide client safety and prevent accidental overdose of medications.

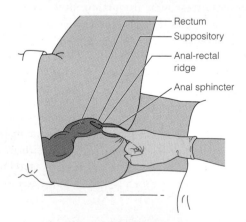

Rectum
Suppository
Anal-rectal ridge
Anal sphincter

Figure 21-23. ◆ Inserting a rectal suppository beyond the internal sphincter and along the rectal wall.

Figure 21-24. ◆ The inhaler positioned away from the open mouth. *Source:* © Jenny Thomas.

BOX 21-8

CLIENT TEACHING

USING A METERED-DOSE INHALER

- Make sure the canister is firmly and fully inserted into the inhaler.
- Remove the mouthpiece cap and, holding the inhaler upright, shake the inhaler for 3 to 5 seconds to mix the medication evenly.
- Tilt the head back slightly.
- Hold the canister upside down.
  a. Hold the MDI 1 to 2 cm (0.5 to 1 in) from the open mouth (Figure 21-24 ◆).
  b. Put the mouthpiece far enough into the mouth so that it extends beyond the teeth. Close the lips tightly around the mouthpiece. An MDI with a spacer or extender is always placed in the mouth.

Administering the Medication

- Inhale and exhale for several breaths, inhaling slowly and deeply through the nose.
- Then inhale slowly and deeply through the mouth while at the same time pressing down once on the medication canister. Continue to inhale for 2 to 3 seconds.
- Hold your breath for 5 to 10 seconds or longer, if possible.
- Remove the inhaler from or away from the mouth.
- Exhale slowly through pursed lips.

- If another puff is prescribed, wait for 1 to 3 minutes before the next inhalation. Remember to reshake the inhaler.
- After the inhalation is completed, rinse mouth with tap water and blow the nose to remove any remaining medication and reduce irritation and risk of infection.
- Clean the MDI mouthpiece after each use. Use mild soap and water, rinse it, and let it air dry before replacing it on the device.
- Disinfect the mouthpiece weekly by soaking it for 20 minutes in 1 pint of water and 2 ounces of vinegar.
- Store the canister at room temperature. Avoid extremes of temperature.
- Follow the physician's orders about frequency of use.
- Report adverse reactions such as restlessness, palpitations, nervousness, or rash to your physician.

Sources: Data from Weixler, D. (1994, July). Correcting metered dose inhaler misuse. *Nursing 94, 24,* 62–64; and Borkgren, M., & Gronkiewicz, C. (1995, January). Update your asthma care from hospital to home. *American Journal of Nursing, 95*(1), 28.

Nursing Process Case Study: CLIENT WITH AN EMERGENCY APPENDECTOMY

Kevin Ketron is a 20-year-old client who just returned to the nursing unit from surgery after undergoing an emergency appendectomy.

Assessment. Client is awake and complaining of mild incisional pain. Dressing is dry and intact. Intravenous infusion of lactated Ringer's solution running at 125 mL/hr. Following surgery he received Kefzol (a cephalosporin antibiotic) 1 g intravenously q4h until he was able to tolerate fluids. He now has been placed on oral Suprax (cefixime) 200 mg twice daily until discharged and for 1 week after returning home. He also has an order for morphine sulfate 10 mg to be given q3h intramuscularly as necessary for pain.

Diagnosis. The following diagnoses are identified for Kevin:

- Deficient Fluid Volume related to fluid restriction; nausea and vomiting
- Ineffective Health Maintenance related to deficient knowledge regarding self-care following appendectomy

- Pain, Acute related to surgial incision
- Risk for Infection related to surgical incision

Expected Outcomes

- Maintain normal blood presure, pulse, and body temperature.
- Follow mutually agreed upon health care maintenance plan.
- Use pain rating scale to identify current level of pain intensity and determine a comfort level.
- Remain free from symptoms of infection.

Planning and Implementation

- Monitor vital signs q4h; observe for decreased pulse volume and increase in body temperature.
- Provide fresh water and oral fluids preferred by the client; provide prescribed diet and snacks.
- Ensure that follow-up appointment is scheduled before discharge.
- Provide detailed instruction for self-care, medications, and wound care; evaluate understanding of discharge instructions.
- Tell client to report location, intensity (using pain scale), and quality when experiencing pain.

ADMINISTERING EYE AND EAR IRRIGATION

☑ Assess the site and surrounding structures for exudate, erythema, swelling, discharge, or other lesions before the irrigation. Determine the client's chief complaints (burning, pain, itching, etc.).

☑ Assemble required equipment: irrigating solution; appropriate irrigating syringe; receptacle to receive irrigation returns (e.g., kidney-shaped basin); moisture-proof drape; and cotton swabs as needed.

☑ Position the client appropriately in a sitting or lying position with the head tilted toward the affected eye or ear.

☑ Place the fluid-receiving receptacle below the affected area and a moisture-resistant pad beneath the receptacle.

☑ Put on disposable gloves.

☑ Clean the eyelids or ear meatus before the irrigation as necessary, using moistened cotton swabs.

Administering the Irrigation

Eye Irrigation

☑ Expose the lower conjunctival sac by separating the lids with the thumb and forefinger to prevent reflex blinking. Or, to irrigate in stages, first hold the lower lid down, then hold the upper lid up. Exert pressure on the bony prominences of the cheekbone and beneath the eyebrow when holding the eyelids to minimize the possibility of pressing the eyeball and causing discomfort.

☑ Fill and hold the eye irrigator about 2.5 cm (1 in) above the eye to ensure an even, safe pressure of the solution.

☑ Irrigate the eye, directing the solution on the lower conjunctival sac and from the inner canthus to the outer canthus. Directing the solution in this way prevents possible injury to the cornea and prevents fluid and contaminants from flowing down the nasolacrimal duct.

☑ Irrigate until the solution leaving the eye is clear (no discharge is present) or until all the solution has been used.

☑ Dry around the eye with cotton balls.

Ear Irrigation

☑ Straighten the ear canal.

☑ Insert a rubber-tipped syringe into the auditory meatus, and direct the solution gently upward against the top of the canal. The solution is instilled gently because strong pressure from the fluid can cause discomfort and damage the tympanic membrane.

☑ Dry the outside of the ear with absorbent cotton balls. Place a cotton fluff in the auditory meatus to absorb the excess fluid.

☑ Assist the client to a side-lying position on the affected side. Lying with the affected side down helps drain the excess fluid by gravity.

For All Irrigations

☑ Assess the client for any discomfort and the appearance and odor of the fluid returns.

☑ Document all relevant information, including all nursing assessments and interventions relative to the procedure; the type, concentration, amount, and temperature of the solution used; the appearance of the returns; and the presence of any discomfort.

◆ Describe adverse effects of unrelieved pain.

◆ Discuss client's fear of undertreated pain, overdose, and addiction.

◆ When opioids are administered, assess pain intensity, sedation, and respiratory status.

◆ Use proper hand-washing techniques before and after giving care to client.

◆ Follow Standard Precautions and wear gloves during any contact with blood and body fluids.

◆ Perform dressing changes using sterile technique.

◆ Ensure client's appropriate hygienic care with hand washing; bathing; and hair, nails, and perineal care performed by the nurse or client.

Evaluation. Vital signs on second postoperative day are 98.8/76/18, BP 128/78. He is taking a clear liquid diet, tolerated well with no complaints of nausea or vomiting.

Discharge planning was initiated. The client will check with his roommate on ability to drive him to his follow-up appointment. Mr. Ketron was able to identify signs and symptoms of infection and describe when a physician should be notified. He understands the need to request pain medication while pain is still manageable. His pain is being maintained at a 2 to 3 level with prn M/S q4h. The incision site is clean and dry with no drainage. Edges are well approximated, staples removed and steri-strips applied. Client has taken a shower.

Critical Thinking in the Nursing Process

1. It is always possible that a person receiving antibiotic drugs may experience side effects or an allergic reaction to the drug. How does an allergic reaction differ from a drug side effect?

2. Mr. Ketron is complaining of pain, and you have prepared his IM injection of morphine. How will you select the best site to give the morphine injection?

3. Mr. Ketron has been placed on oral antibiotics now that he is able to tolerate food and oral fluids. What difference, if any, does it make if this drug is given before or after meals?

Note: The Bibliography listings for this and all chapters have been compiled at the back of the book.

Administering Oral Medications

PURPOSE

◆ To provide a medication that has systemic effects or local effects on the gastrointestinal tract or both (see specific drug action)

EQUIPMENT

◆ Medication tray or cart
◆ Disposable medication cups: small paper or plastic cups for tablets and capsules, waxed or plastic calibrated medication cups for liquids
◆ Medication administration record (MAR) or computer printout
◆ Pill crusher
   or
◆ Syringe of appropriate size for child's mouth and medication amount
◆ Straws to administer medications that may discolor the teeth or to facilitate the ingestion of liquid medication for certain clients

INTERVENTIONS

1. Verify the client's ability to take medication orally.
   ◆ Determine whether the client can swallow well, is NPO, nauseated or vomiting, has gastric suction, or has diminished or absent bowel sounds.

2. Verify the order for accuracy.
   ◆ Check the accuracy of the MAR or of the printout with the physician's written order. *It should contain the following information: (a) client's name, (b) drug name and dosage, (c) time for administration, and (d) route of administration.*
   ◆ Check the expiration date.
   ◆ Report any discrepancies in the order to the nurse in charge or the physician, as agency policy dictates.

3. Obtain appropriate medication.
   ◆ Read the MAR and take the appropriate medication from the shelf, drawer, or refrigerator. The medication may be dispensed from the bottle, box, or unit-dose package.
   ◆ Compare the label of the medication container or unit-dose package against the order on the MAR. If these are not identical, recheck the client's chart. If there is still a discrepancy, check with the nurse in charge or the pharmacist. *These checks are essential in providing the correct medication.*

4. Prepare the medication.
   ◆ Prepare the correct amount of medication for the required dose, using aseptic technique.
   ◆ While preparing the medication, recheck the MAR with each prepared drug and container. *This second check reduces the chance of error.*

TABLETS OR CAPSULES

   ◆ Pour the required number into the bottle cap, and then transfer the medication to the disposable cup without touching the tablets (Figure 21-25 ◆). Usually, all tablets or capsules to be given to the client are placed in the same cup.
   ◆ Keep narcotics and medications that require specific assessments, such as pulse measurements, respiratory rate or depth, or blood pressure, separate from the

Figure 21-25. ◆ Pouring a tablet into the container cap.

Figure 21-26. ◆ A cutting device can be used to divide tablets. *Source:* © Elena Dorfman.

others. *This enables the nurse to withhold the medication if indicated.*

◆ Break scored tablets as needed to obtain the correct dosage. Use a file or cutting device if necessary (Figure 21-26 ◆). Discard unused tablet pieces according to agency policy.

◆ If the client has difficulty swallowing, crush the tablets to a fine powder with a pill crusher or between two medication cups or spoons. Mix the powder with a small amount of soft food (e.g., custard, applesauce). *Note:* Check with pharmacy before crushing tablets. *Sustained-action, enteric-coated, buccal, or sublingual tablets should not be crushed.*

◆ Place packaged unit-dose capsules or tablets (Figure 21-27A ◆) directly into the medicine cup. Do not remove the wrapper until at the bedside. *The wrapper keeps the medication clean and facilitates identification.*

A

B

Figure 21-27. ◆ Unit-dose packages: **A,** tablets; **B,** liquid medications. *Source:* © Elena Dorfman.

LIQUID MEDICATION

◆ Thoroughly mix the medication before pouring. Discard any mixed medication changed in appearance. *Changes in appearance may indicate contamination or expiration of the medication.*

◆ Remove the cap and place it upside down on the countertop. *This helps to avoid contaminating its inside.*

◆ Hold the bottle so the label is next to your palm, and pour the medication away from the label (Figure 21-28 ◆). *This prevents the label from becoming soiled and illegible as a result of spilled liquids.*

◆ Hold the medication cup at eye level and fill it to the desired level, using the bottom of the meniscus (crescent-shaped upper surface of a column of liquid) to align with container scale (Figure 21-29 ◆). *This method ensures accuracy of measurement.*

◆ Before capping the bottle, wipe the lip with a paper towel. *This prevents the cap from sticking.*

◆ When giving small amounts of liquids (e.g., less than 5 mL), prepare the medication in a sterile syringe without the needle.

◆ Keep unit-dose liquids in their package and open them at the bedside.

ORAL NARCOTICS

◆ If an agency uses a manual recording system for controlled substances, check the narcotic record for the previous drug count and compare it with the supply available. *Some medication, including narcotics, are kept in plastic containers that are sectioned and numbered. This allows the drugs to be controlled securely.*

Figure 21-28. ◆ Pouring a liquid medication from a bottle.

Base of meniscus

Figure 21-29. ◆ The bottom of the meniscus is the measuring guide.

◆ Remove the next available tablet and drop it in the medicine cup.

◆ After removing a tablet, record the necessary information on the appropriate narcotic control record and sign it. *Note: Computer-controlled dispensing systems allow access only to the selected drug and automatically record its use.*

ALL MEDICATIONS

◆ Place the prepared medication and MAR together on the tray or cart.

◆ Return the bottle, box, or envelope to its storage place and recheck the label on the container. *This third check further reduces the risk of error.*

◆ Avoid leaving prepared medications unattended. *This precaution prevents potential mishandling errors.*

5. Administer the medication at the correct time.

◆ Identify the client by comparing the name and hospital number on the medication record or list with the name and number on the client's identification bracelet and by asking the client's name. *Accurate identification is essential to prevent error.*

◆ Explain the purpose of the medication and how it will help, using language that the client can understand. Include relevant information about effects; for example, tell the client receiving a diuretic to expect an increase in urine. *Information facilitates acceptance of and compliance with the therapy.*

◆ Assist the client to a sitting position or, if not possible, to a side-lying position. *These positions facilitate swallowing and prevent aspiration.*

◆ Take the required assessment measures, such as pulse and respiratory rates or blood pressure. Take the apical pulse rate before administering digitalis preparations. Take blood pressure before giving hypotensive drugs. Take the respiratory rate prior to administering narcotics. *Narcotics depress the respiratory center.* If any of the findings are above or below the predetermined parameters, consult the physician before administering the medication.

◆ Give the client sufficient water or preferred juice to swallow the medication. Before using juice, check for any food and medication incompatibilities. *Fluids ease swallowing and facilitate absorption from the gastrointestinal tract.* Liquid medications other than antacids or cough preparations are generally diluted with 15 mL (0.5 oz) of water to facilitate absorption.

◆ If the client is unable to hold the pill cup, use the pill cup to introduce the medication into the client's mouth, and give only one tablet or capsule at a time. *Putting the cup to the client's mouth maintains the cleanliness of the nurse's hands. Giving one medication at a time eases swallowing.*

◆ If an older child or adult has difficulty swallowing, ask the client to place the medication on the back of the tongue before taking the water. *Stimulation of the back of the tongue produces the swallowing reflex.*

◆ If the medication has an objectionable taste, ask the client to suck a few ice chips beforehand, or give the medication with juice, applesauce, or bread if there are no contraindications. *The cold will desensitize the taste buds, and juices or bread can mask the taste of the medication.*

◆ If the client says that the medication you are about to give is different from what the client has been receiving, do not give the medication without checking the original order. *Most clients are familiar with the appearance of medications taken previously. Unfamiliar medications may signal a possible error.*

◆ Stay with the client until all medications have been swallowed. *The nurse must see the client swallow the medication before the drug administration can be recorded.* A physician's order or agency policy is required for medications left at the bedside.

6. Document each medication given.

◆ Record the medication given, dosage, time, any complaints or assessments of the client, and your signature.

◆ If medication was refused or omitted, record this fact on the appropriate record; document the reason, when possible, and the nurse's actions according to agency policy. *Recording the fact and the reason communicates the greatest amount of information, so that the charge nurse or physician can follow up.*

7. Dispose of all supplies appropriately.

◆ Return the medication records to the appropriate file for the next administration time.

◆ Replenish stock (e.g., medication cups) and return cart to medicine room.

◆ Discard used disposable supplies.

8. Evaluate the effects of the medication.

◆ Return to the client when the medication is expected to take effect (usually 30 minutes). *This allows you to evaluate the effects of the medication on the client.*

◆ SAMPLE DOCUMENTATION

10/25/05	Digoxin 1mg held. AP 54. Will reassess
0900	in 1 hour. Other vs within normal limits.
	No c/o chest pain or dyspnea. ————
	M. Wirthwood LVN

PROCEDURE 21-2

Preparing Medications

EQUIPMENT

◆ MAR or computer printout
◆ Ampule of sterile medication, or two vials of medication, or one vial and one ampule, or two ampules, or one vial or ampule and one cartridge
◆ File (if ampule is not scored) and small gauze square, or ampule opener

◆ Antiseptic swabs
◆ Sterile needle and syringe
◆ Filter needle (optional) (now mandated by JCAHO for use with ampule)
◆ Additional sterile subcutaneous or intramuscular needle (optional)
◆ Sterile water or normal saline, if drug is in powdered form

Part A: Ampules

INTERVENTIONS

1. Check the medication order, including drug administration. *This ensures accuracy.*
   ◆ Check the label on the ampule carefully against the MAR or client's chart to make sure that the correct medication is being prepared.
   ◆ Follow the three checks for administering medications. Read the label on the medication (a) before it is taken off the shelf, (b) before withdrawing the medication, and (c) after placing it back on the shelf.

2. Prepare the medication ampule for drug withdrawal.
   ◆ Flick the upper stem of the ampule several times with a fingernail or, holding the upper stem of the ampule, make a large circle with the arm extended. *This will bring all the medication down to the main portion of the ampule.*
   ◆ Partially file the neck of the ampule, if necessary, to start a clean break.
   ◆ Place a piece of sterile gauze between your thumb and the ampule neck or around the ampule neck, and break off the top by bending it toward you (Figure 21-30 ◆). *The sterile gauze protects the fingers from the broken glass and any glass fragments will spray away from the nurse.*
   or
   Place the antiseptic wipe packet over the top of the ampule before breaking off the top. *This method ensures that all the glass fragments fall into the packet and reduces the risk of cuts.*
   ◆ Dispose of the top of the ampule in the sharps container.

3. Withdraw the medication.
   ◆ Place the ampule on a flat surface.
   ◆ Obtain a filter needle to withdraw the medication.

Figure 21-30. ◆ Breaking the neck of an ampule. *Source:* © Jenny Thomas.

Disconnect the existing needle with cap on; attach the filter needle to the syringe. *Filter needles prevent glass particles from being drawn up with the medication.*
◆ Remove the cap from the filter needle and insert the needle into the center of the ampule. Do not touch the rim of the ampule with the needle to keep it sterile. Withdraw the required dosage.
◆ If necessary, tilt the ampule slightly to access all the medication(Figure 21-31 ◆).

Figure 21-31. ◆ Withdrawing a medication from an ampule. *Source:* © Jenny Thomas Photography.

◆ If a filter needle was used to withdraw the medication, replace it with a regular needle; tighten the cap at the hub before injecting the client.

◆ If a filter needle was not used, recap the needle using a safety device. *This prevents needle-stick injury.*

Part B: Preparing Medications from Vials

INTERVENTIONS

1. Check the medication order, including drug administration, to ensure accuracy.

◆ Check the label on the vial carefully against the MAR or client's chart to make sure that the correct medication is being prepared.

◆ Follow the three checks for administering medications. Read the label on the medication (a) before it is taken off the shelf, (b) before withdrawing the medication, and (c) after placing it back on the shelf.

2. Prepare the medication vial for drug withdrawal.

◆ Mix the solution, if necessary, by rotating the vial between the palms of the hands, not by shaking. *Some vials contain aqueous suspensions, which settle when they stand. In some instances shaking is contraindicated because it may cause the mixture to foam.*

◆ Remove the protective metal cap, and clean the rubber cap of a previously opened vial with an antiseptic wipe by rubbing in a circular motion. *The antiseptic cleans the cap of dust or grease and reduces the number of microorganisms.*

3. Withdraw the medication.

◆ Attach a filter needle as agency practice dictates to draw up premixed liquid medications from multidose vials. *The filter prevents any solid particles from being drawn up through the needle.*

◆ Ensure that the needle is firmly attached to the syringe.

◆ Remove the cap from the needle; then draw up into the syringe the amount of air equal to the volume of the medication to be withdrawn.

◆ Carefully insert the needle into the upright vial through the center of the rubber cap, maintaining the sterility of the needle.

◆ Inject the air into the vial, keeping the bevel of the needle above the surface of the medication (Figure 21-32 ◆). *The air will allow the medication to be drawn out easily because negative pressure will not be created inside the vial. The bevel is kept above the medication to avoid creating bubbles in the medication.*

◆ Withdraw the prescribed amount of medication using either of the following methods:

a. Hold the vial down (i.e., with the base lower than the top); move the needle tip so that it is below the fluid level; and withdraw the medication (Figure 21-33 ◆). Avoid drawing up the last drops of the vial. *Proponents of this method say that keeping the vial in the upright*

Figure 21-32. ◆ Injecting air into a vial. *Source:* © Jenny Thomas.

A

B

Figure 21-33. ◆ **A.** Withdrawing a medication from a vial that is held with the base down. **B.** Withdrawing a medication from an inverted vial. *Source:* © Elena Dorfman.

position while withdrawing the medication allows particulate matter to precipitate out of the solution. Leaving the last few drops reduces the chance of withdrawing foreign particles.

or

b. Invert the vial; ensure the needle tip is below the fluid level; and gradually withdraw the medication (Figure 21-33B). *Keeping the tip of the needle below the fluid level prevents air from being drawn into the syringe.*

◆ Hold the syringe and vial at eye level to determine that the correct dosage of drug is drawn into the syringe. Eject air remaining at the top of the syringe into the vial.

◆ When the correct volume of medication is obtained, withdraw the needle from the vial, and replace the cap over the needle, thus maintaining its sterility.

◆ If necessary, tap the syringe barrel to dislodge any air bubbles present in the syringe. *The tapping motion will cause the air bubbles to rise to the top of the syringe where they can be ejected out of the syringe.*

◆ Replace the filter needle, if used, with a regular needle and cover of the correct gauge and length before injecting the client.

VARIATION: PREPARING AND USING MULTIDOSE VIALS

◆ Read the manufacturer's directions.

◆ Withdraw an equivalent amount of air from the vial before adding the solvent, unless otherwise indicated by the directions.

◆ Add the amount of sterile water or saline indicated in the directions.

◆ If a multidose vial is reconstituted, label the vial with the date and time it was prepared, the amount of drug contained in each milliliter of solution, and your initials. *Time is an important factor to consider in the expiration of these medications.*

◆ Once the medication reconstituted, store it in a refrigerator or as recommended by the manufacturer.

Part C: Mixing Medications Using One Syringe

INTERVENTIONS

1. Check the medication order for accuracy.

◆ Check the label on the ampule or vial carefully against the MAR or client's chart. *This makes sure that the correct medication is being prepared.*

◆ Follow the three checks for administering medications. Read the label on the medication (a) before it is taken off the shelf, (b) before withdrawing the medication, and (c) after placing it back on the shelf.

◆ Before preparing and combining the medications, ensure that the total volume of the injection is appropriate for the injection site.

2. Prepare the medication ampule or vial for drug withdrawal.

◆ See Part A of this procedure for an ampule.

◆ Inspect the appearance of the medication for clarity. *Some medications are always cloudy. Preparations that have changed in appearance should be discarded.*

◆ If using insulin, thoroughly mix the solution in each vial prior to administration. Rotate the vials between the palms of the hands and invert the vials. *Mixing ensures an adequate concentration and thus an accurate dose. Shaking insulin vials can make the medication frothy, making precise measurement difficult.*

◆ Clean the tops of the vials with antiseptic swabs.

3. Withdraw the medications.

MIXING MEDICATIONS FROM TWO VIALS

◆ Withdraw a volume of air equal to the volume of medications to be withdrawn from vials A and B.

◆ Inject a volume of air equal to the volume of medication to be withdrawn into vial A.

◆ Withdraw the needle from vial A and inject the remaining air into vial B.

◆ Withdraw the required amount of medication from vial B. The same needle is used to inject air into and withdraw medication from the second vial. *It must not be contaminated with the medication in vial A.*

◆ Using a newly attached sterile needle, withdraw the required amount of medication from vial A. If using a syringe with a fused needle, withdraw the medication from vial A. The syringe now contains a mixture of medications from vials A and B. *With this method, neither vial is contaminated by microorganisms or by medication from the other vial.*

◆ See also the Variation later in this procedure.

MIXING MEDICATIONS FROM ONE VIAL AND ONE AMPULE

◆ First prepare and withdraw the medication from the vial. Ampules do not require the addition of air prior to withdrawal of the drug.

◆ Then withdraw the required amount of medication from the ampule.

MIXING MEDICATIONS FROM ONE CARTRIDGE AND ONE VIAL OR AMPULE

◆ First ensure that the correct dose of the medication is in the cartridge. Discard any excess medication and air.

◆ Draw up the required medication from a vial or ampule into the cartridge. Note that when withdrawing medication from a vial, an equal amount of air must first be injected into the vial.

◆ If the total volume to be injected exceeds the capacity of the cartridge, use a syringe with sufficient capacity to withdraw the desired amount of medication from the vial or ampule, and transfer the required amount from the cartridge to the syringe.

VARIATION: MIXING INSULINS

The following is an example of mixing 10 units of regular insulin and 30 units of NPH insulin, which contains protamine.

Figure 21-34. ◆ Mixing two types of insulin together.

◆ Inject 30 units of air into the NPH vial and withdraw the needle. (There should be no insulin in the needle.) The needle should not touch the insulin (Figure 21-34 ◆, step 1).

◆ Inject 10 units of air into the regular insulin vial and immediately withdraw 10 units of regular insulin (Figure 21-34, steps 2 and 3).

◆ Reinsert the needle into the NPH insulin vial and withdraw 30 units of NPH insulin (Figure 21-34, step 4). (The air was previously injected into the vial.)
By using this method, you avoid adding NPH insulin to the regular insulin.

◆ SAMPLE DOCUMENTATION

6/7/05		
Focus		
pain	0200	D—c/o incisional pain 7/10.
		Incision free of drainage and
		redness. Edges well approximated.
		A—Vistaril 50 mg, Demerol 75 mg IM
		R—pain 2/10 resting comfortably
		_____ A. Johnson LVN

PROCEDURE 21-3
Administering Injections

PURPOSE

◆ To provide a medication the client requires (see specific drug action)

◆ For subcutaneous: To allow slower absorption of a medication compared with either the intramuscular or intravenous route

EQUIPMENT

◆ Client's MAR or computer printout
◆ Sterile medication (usually provided in an ampule or vial)
◆ Syringe and needle of a size appropriate for the amount of solution to be administered
◆ Antiseptic swabs
◆ Dry sterile gauze for opening an ampule (optional)
◆ Disposable gloves

Part A: Intramuscular

INTERVENTIONS

1. Check the medication order for accuracy.
   - ◆ See Procedure 21-1, step 1.

2. Prepare the medication from the vial or ampule.
   - ◆ See Procedure 21-2 (ampule or vial).
   - ◆ Whenever feasible, change the needle on the syringe before the injection. *Because the outside of a new needle is free of medication, it does not irritate subcutaneous tissues as it passes into the muscle.*
   - ◆ Invert the syringe needle uppermost and expel all excess air.

3. Identify the client, and assist the client to a comfortable position.
   - ◆ Check the client's arm band, and ask the client to tell you his or her name. *This verifies identity.*
   - ◆ Assist the client to a supine, lateral, prone, or sitting position, depending on the chosen site. If the target muscle is the gluteus medius (ventrogluteal site), have the client in the supine position flex the knee(s); in the lateral position, flex the upper leg; and in the prone position, "toe in." *Appropriate positioning promotes relaxation of the target muscle.*
   - ◆ Obtain assistance to immobilize an infant or young child. The parent may hold the infant or young child. *This prevents accidental injury during the procedure.*

4. Select, locate, and clean the site.
   - ◆ Wash hands.
   - ◆ Select a site free of skin lesions, tenderness, swelling, hardness, or localized inflammation and one that has not been used frequently.
   - ◆ If injections are to be frequent, alternate sites. If necessary, discuss with the prescribing physician an alternative method of providing the medication.
   - ◆ Determine whether the size of the muscle is appropriate to the amount of medication to be injected. *An average adult's deltoid muscle can usually absorb 0.5 mL of medication, although some authorities believe 1 mL can be absorbed by a well-*

developed deltoid muscle. The gluteus medius muscle can often absorb 1 to 4 mL, although 4 mL may be very painful.
   - ◆ Locate the exact site for the injection. (See the discussion of sites earlier in this chapter.)
   - ◆ Don gloves.
   - ◆ Clean the site with an antiseptic swab. Using a circular motion, start at the center and move outward about 5 cm (2 in).
   - ◆ Transfer and hold the swab between the third and fourth fingers of your nondominant hand in readiness for needle withdrawal, or position the swab on the client's skin above the intended site. Allow skin to dry prior to injecting medication.

5. Prepare the syringe for injection.
   - ◆ Remove the needle cover without contaminating the needle.
   - ◆ Confirm that the medication and the dose are both correct.
   - ◆ If using a prefilled unit-dose medication, be careful to avoid dripping medication on the needle prior to injection. If this does occur, wipe the medication off the needle with a sterile gauze. *Medication left on the needle can cause pain when it is tracked through the subcutaneous tissue.*

6. Inject the medication using a Z-track technique.
   - ◆ Use the nondominant hand to pull the skin laterally and downward approximately 2.5 cm (1 inch) at the site (Figure 21-35 ◆). Under some circumstances, such as for an emaciated client or an infant, the muscle may be pinched. *Pulling the skin and subcutaneous tissue or pinching the muscle makes it firmer and facilitates needle insertion.*
   - ◆ Holding the syringe between the thumb and forefinger (as if holding a pencil), pierce the skin quickly at a 90-degree angle (Figure 21-36 ◆), and insert the needle into the muscle. *Using a quick motion lessens the client's discomfort.*
   - ◆ Aspirate by holding the barrel of the syringe steady with your nondominant hand and by pulling back on the plunger with your dominant hand. If blood appears in the syringe, withdraw the needle, discard the syringe, and

Figure 21-35. ◆ Inserting an intramuscular needle at a 90-degree angle using the Z-track method: **A,** skin pulled to the side; **B,** skin released. *Note:* When the skin returns to its normal position after the needle is withdrawn, a seal is formed over the intramuscular site. This prevents seepage of the medication into the subcutaneous tissues and subsequent discomfort.

Figure 21-36. ◆ Administering an intramuscular injection into the ventrogluteal site. *Source:* © Jenny Thomas.

prepare a new injection. *This step determines whether the needle has been inserted into a blood vessel.*

◆ If blood does not appear, inject the medication steadily and slowly, holding the syringe steady. *Injecting medication slowly permits it to disperse into the muscle tissue, thus decreasing*

the client's discomfort. Holding the syringe steady minimizes discomfort.

7. Withdraw the needle.
  ◆ Withdraw the needle slowly and steadily. *This minimizes tissue injury.*
  ◆ Apply gentle pressure at the site with a dry sponge. Do not massage the site. *Massaging the site can result in tissue irritation.*
  ◆ If bleeding occurs, apply pressure with a dry sterile gauze until it stops.

8. Discard the uncapped needle and attached syringe into the proper receptacle.
  ◆ Remove gloves. Wash hands.

9. Document all relevant information.
  ◆ Include the time of administration, drug name, dose, route, and the client's reactions.

10. Assess effectiveness of the medication at the time it is expected to act.

Part B: Subcutaneous Injection

INTERVENTIONS

1. Check the medication order for accuracy.
  ◆ See Procedure 21-1, step 1.

2. Prepare the medication from the vial or ampule.
  ◆ See Procedure 21-2 (ampule or vial).

3. Identify the client, and assist the client to a comfortable position.
  ◆ Check the client's arm band and ask the client's name.
  ◆ Assist the client to a position in which the arm, leg, or abdomen can be relaxed, depending on the site to be used. *A relaxed position of the site minimizes discomfort.*
  ◆ Obtain assistance in holding an uncooperative client or small child. *This prevents injury due to sudden movement after needle insertion.*

4. Select and clean the site.
  ◆ Select a site free of tenderness, hardness, swelling, scarring, itching, burning, or localized inflammation. Select a site that has not been used frequently. *These conditions could hinder the absorption of the medication and also increase the likelihood of injury and discomfort at the injection site.*
  ◆ Don gloves.
  ◆ Cleanse the skin with antiseptic per agency protocol. Swab the center of the site in a widening circle to about 5 cm (2 in). Let the skin dry completely. *The mechanical action of swabbing removes skin secretions, which contain microorganisms.*
  ◆ Hold the swab between the third and fourth fingers of the nondominant hand, or position the swab on the client's skin above the intended site. *This keeps the swab accessible when the needle is withdrawn.*

5. Prepare the syringe for injection.

  ◆ Remove the needle cap while waiting for the antiseptic to dry. Pull the cap straight off to avoid contaminating the needle by the outside edge of the cap. *The needle will become contaminated if it touches anything but the inside of the cap, which is sterile.*
  ◆ Confirm that the medication and the dosage are both correct. *This prevents medication error.*

6. Inject the medication.
  ◆ Grasp the syringe in your dominant hand by holding it between your thumb and fingers. With palm facing to the side or upward for a 45-degree-angle insertion, or with the palm downward for a 90-degree-angle insertion, prepare to inject (Figure 21-37 ◆; see also Figure 21-11).

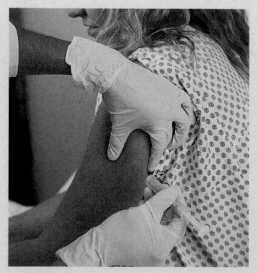

Figure 21-37. ◆ Administering a subcutaneous injection into pinched tissue. *Source:* © Elena Dorfman.

◆ Using the nondominant hand, pinch or spread the skin at the site, and insert the needle using the dominant hand and a firm steady push. *The nondominant hand can be used to immobilize the extremity of an infant or a young child as the needle is inserted.* Recommendations vary about whether to pinch or spread the skin and at what angle to administer subcutaneous injections. The most important consideration is the depth of the subcutaneous tissue in the area to be injected. *If the client has more than 1/2 inch of adipose tissue in the injection site, it would be safe to administer the injection at a 90-degree angle with the skin spread. If the client is thin or lean and lacks adipose tissue, the subcutaneous injection should be given with the skin pinched and at a 45- to 60-degree angle.*

◆ When the needle is inserted, move your nondominant hand to the end of the plunger. Some nurses find it easier to move the nondominant hand to the barrel of the syringe and the dominant hand to the end of the plunger. If the nondominant hand is holding the extremity of an infant or small child, use the dominant hand to aspirate and inject the medication.

◆ Aspirate by pulling back on the plunger. If blood appears, withdraw the needle, discard the syringe, document the occurrence and prepare a new injection. If no blood appears, inject the medication. *Subcutaneous medications can be very dangerous if injected directly into the bloodstream since these drugs require slow absorption.* See variation for administering a heparin injection.

◆ Inject the medication by holding the syringe steady and depressing the plunger with a slow, even pressure. *Holding the syringe steady and injecting the medication at an even pressure minimizes discomfort for the client.*

7. Remove the needle.

◆ Remove slowly and smoothly, pulling along the line of insertion while depressing the skin with your nondominant hand. *Depressing the skin places countertraction on it and minimizes the client's discomfort when the needle is withdrawn.*

◆ If bleeding occurs, apply pressure to the site with dry sterile gauze until it stops. *Bleeding rarely occurs after subcutaneous injection.*

8. Dispose of supplies appropriately.

◆ Discard the uncapped needle and attached syringe into designated receptacles. *Proper disposal protects the nurse and others from injury and contamination. The CDC recommends not capping the needle before disposal to reduce the risk of needlestick injuries.*

◆ Remove gloves. Wash hands.

9. Document all relevant information.

◆ Document the medication given, dosage, time, route, any assessments, and add your signature.

◆ Many agencies prefer that medication administration be recorded on the medication record. *The nurse's notes are used when prn medications are given or when there is a special problem.*

10. Assess the effectiveness of the medication at the time it is expected to act.

VARIATION: ADMINISTERING A HEPARIN INJECTION

The subcutaneous administration of heparin requires special precautions because of the drug's anticoagulant properties.

◆ Select a site on the abdomen away from the umbilicus and above the level of the iliac crests. *Some agencies support the practice of subcutaneous injection of heparin in the thighs or arms as alternate sites to the abdomen.*

◆ Use a 3/8-inch, 25- or 26-gauge needle, and insert it at a 90-degree angle. If a client is very lean or wasted, use a needle longer than 3/8 inch, and insert it at a 45-degree angle. The arms or thighs may be used as alternate sites.

◆ Do not aspirate when giving heparin by subcutaneous injection. *Aspiration can possibly damage the surrounding tissue and cause bleeding as well as bruising.*

◆ Do not massage the site after the injection. *Massaging could cause bleeding and ecchymoses and hasten drug absorption.*

◆ Alternate the sites of subsequent injections.

◆ SAMPLE DOCUMENTATION

1/30/05	Pen VK 500,000 u IM rt. thigh.
2:30 PM	Client tolerated well.
	P. Bullock, LPN

Administering Ophthalmic Instillations

PURPOSES

◆ To provide an eye medication the client requires (e.g., an antibiotic) to treat an infection or for other reasons (see specific drug action)

EQUIPMENT

◆ Disposable gloves
◆ Sterile absorbent sponges soaked in sterile normal saline
◆ Medication
◆ Dry sterile absorbent sponges
◆ Sterile eye dressing (pad) as needed and paper eye tape to secure it

INTERVENTIONS

1. Check the medication order and the medication.
   ◆ Check the physician's order for the preparation, strength, and number of drops. Also confirm the prescribed frequency of the instillation and which eye is to be treated. Abbreviations are frequently used to identify the eye: OD (right eye), OS (left eye), OU (both eyes).
   ◆ Check the expiration date and ensure that the medication is clearly labeled.

2. Prepare the client.
   ◆ Check the client's identification band, and ask the client's name.
   ◆ Explain the technique to the client or to the parents of an infant or child. *The administration of an ophthalmic medication is not usually painful. Ointments are often soothing to the eye, but some liquid preparations may sting initially.*
   ◆ Assist the client to a comfortable position, either sitting or lying.

3. Clean the eyelid and the eyelashes.
   ◆ Don sterile gloves.
   ◆ Use sterile cotton balls moistened with sterile irrigating solution or sterile normal saline, and wipe from the inner canthus to the outer canthus. *If not removed, material on the eyelid and lashes can be washed into the eye. Cleaning toward the outer canthus prevents contamination of the other eye and the lacrimal duct.*

4. Administer the eye medication.
   ◆ Check the ophthalmic preparation for the name, strength, and number of drops if a liquid is used. Draw the correct number of drops into the shaft of the dropper if a dropper is used. If ointment is used, discard the first bead. *Checking medication data is essential to prevent a medication error. The first bead of ointment from a tube is considered to be contaminated.*

   ◆ Instruct the client to look up to the ceiling. Give the client a dry sterile absorbent sponge. *The person is less likely to blink if looking up. While the client looks up, the cornea is partially protected by the top eyelid.* A sponge is needed to press on the nasolacrimal duct after a liquid instillation or to wipe excess ointment from the eyelashes after an ointment is instilled.

   ◆ Expose the lower conjunctival sac by placing the thumb or fingers of your nondominant hand on the client's cheekbone just below the eye and gently drawing down the skin on the cheek. If the tissues are edematous, handle the tissues carefully to avoid damaging them. *Placing the fingers on the cheekbone minimizes the possibility of touching the cornea, avoids putting any pressure on the eyeball, and prevents the person from blinking or squinting.*

   ◆ Approach the eye from the side and instill the correct number of drops onto the outer third of the lower conjunctival sac. Hold the dropper 1 to 2 cm (0.4 to 0.8 in) above the sac (Figure 21-38 ◆). *The client is less likely to blink if a side approach is used. When instilled into the conjunctival sac, drops will not harm the cornea as they might if dropped directly on it.* The dropper must not touch the sac or the cornea.
   or
   ◆ Holding the tube above the lower conjunctival sac, squeeze 2 cm (0.8 in) of ointment from the tube into the lower conjunctival sac from the inner canthus outward (Figure 21-39 ◆).

   ◆ Instruct the client to close the eyelids but not to squeeze them shut. Closing the eye spreads the medication over the eyeball. *Squeezing can injure the eye and push out the medication.*

Figure 21-38. ◆ Instilling an eyedrop into the lower conjunctival sac. *Source:* © Elena Dorfman.

- For liquid medications, press firmly or have the client press firmly on the nasolacrimal duct for at least 30 seconds (Figure 21-40 ◆). Check agency practice. *Pressing on the nasolacrimal duct prevents the medication from running out of the eye and down the duct.*

5. Clean the eyelids as needed. Wipe the eyelids gently from the inner to the outer canthus to collect excess medication.

Figure 21-39. ◆ Instilling an eye ointment into the lower conjunctival sac. *Source:* © Jenny Thomas.

Figure 21-40. ◆ Pressing on the nasolacrimal duct. *Source:* © Jenny Thomas.

6. Apply an eye pad if needed, and secure it with paper eye tape.
7. Assess the client's response.
   - Assess responses immediately after the instillation and again after the medication should have acted.
8. Document all relevant information.
   - Record nursing assessments and interventions. Include the name of the drug, the strength, the number of drops if a liquid, the time, and the response of the client.

◆ SAMPLE DOCUMENTATION

03/24/06	Presented at ER following work-related
1930	injury. Experienced severed pain in rt.
	eye while using grinding wheel.
	Fluorescein NA 2 gtts instilled OD.
	Seen by Dr. Wilson .5 mm sliver metal
	sliver removed. Eye irrigated with 25 cc
	NSS. Eye patch applied. ————
	R. Nelson, LPN

PROCEDURE 21-5

Administering Otic Instillations

PURPOSES

◆ To soften earwax so that it can be readily removed at a later time
◆ To provide local therapy to reduce inflammation, destroy infective organisms in the external ear canal, or both
◆ To relieve pain

EQUIPMENT

◆ Disposable gloves (optional)
◆ Cotton-tipped applicator
◆ Correct medication bottle with a dropper
◆ Flexible rubber tip (optional) for the end of the dropper, which prevents injury from sudden motion, for example, by a child or disoriented client
◆ Cotton fluff

INTERVENTIONS

1. Check the medication order.
   ◆ Check the physician's order for the kind of medication; the time, amount, and dosage; and which ear is to be treated.

2. Prepare the client.
   ◆ Check the client's identification band, and ask the client's name.
   ◆ Obtain assistance to immobilize an infant or young child. *This prevents accidental injury due to sudden movement during the procedure.*
   ◆ Assist the client to a side-lying position with the ear being treated uppermost.

3. Clean the pinna of the ear and the meatus of the ear canal.
   ◆ Don gloves if infection is suspected.
   ◆ Use cotton-tipped applicators and solution to wipe the pinna and auditory meatus. Remove any discharge before the instillation so that it won't be washed into the ear canal.

4. Administer the ear medication.
   ◆ Warm the medication container in your hand, or place it in warm water for a short time. *This promotes client comfort.*
   ◆ Partially fill the ear dropper with medication.
   ◆ Straighten the auditory canal. For an infant, gently pull the pinna down and back (Figure 21-41 ◆). For an adult or a child older than 3 years of age, pull the pinna upward and backward. *The auditory canal is straightened so that the solution can flow the entire length of the canal.*
   ◆ Instill the correct number of drops along the side of the ear canal (Figure 21-42 ◆).

Normal position

Figure 21-41. ◆ Straightening the ear canal of a child by pulling the pinna down and back.

◆ Press gently but firmly a few times on the tragus of the ear. Pressing on the tragus assists the flow of medication into the ear canal.
◆ Ask the client to remain in the side-lying position for about 5 minutes. This prevents the drops from escaping and allows the medication to reach all sides of the canal cavity.

Figure 21-42. ◆ Instilling ear drops.

◆ Insert a small piece of cotton fluff loosely at the meatus of the auditory canal for 15 to 20 minutes. Do not press it into the canal. *The cotton helps retain the medication when the client is up. If pressed tightly into the canal, the cotton would interfere with the action of the drug and the outward movement of normal secretions.*

5. Assess the client's response.
   ◆ Assess the character and amount of discharge, appearance of the canal, discomfort, and so on, immediately after the instillation and again when the medication is expected to act. Inspect the cotton ball for any drainage.

6. Document all relevant information.
   ◆ Document all nursing assessments and interventions relative to the procedure.

◆ Include the time, the dose, and any complaints of pain. *Many agencies use flowsheets; others may require that a notation be made on the nurse's notes.*

◆ **SAMPLE DOCUMENTATION**

12/02/05	Impacted cerumen x2 weeks. Deborex
0930	gtts ii each ear daily x 5 days.
	Prepared for ear irrigation. 100 cc
	warm H_2O via Asepto syringe.
	Otoscopic exam revealed clear ear
	canal. Tolerated procedure well. ———
	O. Pearson, LVN

PROCEDURE 21-6

Administering Vaginal Instillations

PURPOSES

◆ To treat or prevent infection
◆ To reduce inflammation
◆ To relieve vaginal discomfort

EQUIPMENT

◆ Drape
◆ Correct vaginal suppository or cream
◆ Applicator for vaginal cream
◆ Disposable gloves
◆ Lubricant for a suppository
◆ Disposable towel
◆ Clean perineal pad

INTERVENTIONS

1. Check the medication order and identify the client.
   ◆ Carefully check the physician's order for the specific medication ordered, its dosage, and the time of administration.
   ◆ Check the client's identification band, and ask the client's name.

2. Prepare the client.
   ◆ Explain to the client that a vaginal instillation is normally a painless procedure, and in fact may bring relief from itching and burning if an infection is present. *Many people feel embarrassed about this procedure,*

and some may prefer to perform the procedure themselves if instruction is provided.
   ◆ Provide privacy, and ask the client to void. *If the bladder is empty, the client will have less discomfort during the treatment, and the possibility of injuring the vaginal lining is decreased.*

3. Position and drape the client appropriately.
   ◆ Assist the client to a back-lying position with the knees flexed and the hips rotated laterally.
   ◆ Drape the client appropriately so that only the perineal area is exposed.

4. Prepare the equipment.

◆ Unwrap the suppository, and put it on the opened wrapper.

or

Fill the applicator with the prescribed cream, jelly, or foam. Directions are provided with the manufacturer's applicator.

5. Assess and clean the perineal area.
   ◆ Don gloves. *Gloves prevent contamination of the nurse's hands from vaginal and perineal microorganisms.*
   ◆ Inspect the vaginal orifice; note any redness, edema, odor, or discharge from the vagina; and ask about any vaginal discomfort.
   ◆ Provide perineal care to remove microorganisms. *This decreases the chance of moving microorganisms into the vagina.*

6. Administer the vaginal suppository, cream, foam, or jelly.
   ◆ Lubricate the rounded (smooth) end of the suppository, which is inserted first. *Lubrication facilitates insertion.*
   ◆ Lubricate your gloved index finger.
   ◆ Expose the vaginal orifice by separating the labia with your nondominant hand.
   ◆ Insert the suppository about 8 to 10 cm (3 to 4 in) along the posterior wall of the vagina, or as far as it will go (Figure 21-43 ◆). The posterior wall of the vagina is about 2.5 cm (1 in) longer than the anterior wall because the cervix protrudes into the uppermost portion of the anterior wall. The anterior wall is usually about 6 to 7.5 cm (2.5 to 3 in).
   ◆ Withdraw the finger, and remove the gloves, turning them inside out. Discard appropriately. *Turning the gloves inside out prevents the spread of microorganisms.*
   ◆ Ask the client to remain lying in the supine position for 5 to 10 minutes following insertion. The hips may also be elevated on a pillow. *This position allows the medication to flow into the posterior fornix after it has melted.*

Figure 21-44. ◆ Using an applicator to instill a vaginal cream.

VAGINAL CREAM, JELLY, OR FOAM

   ◆ Gently insert the applicator about 5 cm (2 in).
   ◆ Slowly push the plunger until the applicator is empty (Figure 21-44 ◆).
   ◆ Remove the applicator and place it on the towel. *The applicator is put on the towel to prevent the spread of microorganisms.*
   ◆ Discard the applicator if disposable or clean it according to the manufacturer's directions.
   ◆ Remove the gloves, turning them inside out. Discard appropriately.
   ◆ Ask the client to remain lying in the supine position for 5 to 10 minutes following the insertion.

7. Ensure client comfort.
   ◆ Dry the perineum with tissues as required.
   ◆ Apply a clean perineal pad and a T-binder if there is excessive drainage.

8. Document all relevant information.
   ◆ Record the instillation and assessments as for other medications and instillations.

9. Assess and document the client's response.

◆ SAMPLE DOCUMENTATION

05/21/05	C/O of vaginal itching, white cheese-like
1900	discharge and burning on urination.
	Completed 10-day course of ABT.
	Terconazole via applicator
	intravaginally.
	T. Mallesen, LPN

Figure 21-43. ◆ Instilling a vaginal suppository.

Chapter Review

Key Terms by Topics

Use the audio glossary feature of either the CD-ROM or the Companion Website to hear the correct pronunciation of the following key terms.

Introduction
medication, prescription, generic

Effects of drugs
therapeutic effect, side effect, adverse effect, drug toxicity, cumulative effect, drug

allergy, drug tolerance, idiosyncratic effect, drug interaction, iatrogenic disease, half-life, absorption

Medication orders
stat order, single order, standing order, prn order

Systems of measurement
metric system, apothecaries' system, household system, nomogram

Equipment
syringes, hub, cannula, bevel

Routes of administration
NPO, sublingual, buccal, parenteral, intradermal, subcutaneous, intramuscular, intravenous

Nursing care
ampule, vial, ophthalmics, otics

Key Points

◆ Nursing practice acts define limits on the nurse's responsibilities regarding medications.

◆ Medications have several names. Nurses need to know the generic and trade names of a medication and be aware of both its therapeutic and side effects.

◆ Adverse effects of medications include drug toxicity, drug allergy, drug tolerance, idiosyncratic effect, and drug interactions.

◆ Various routes are used to administer medications: oral, sublingual, buccal, parenteral, topical, or via a nasogastric or gastrostomy tube.

◆ Medication orders must include the client name, date and time the order is written, name of the medication, dosage, route, frequency of administration, and signature of the person writing the order. Nurses must question any unclear orders before implementing the order.

◆ Three systems of measurement are used: the metric system, the apothecaries' system, and the household system. Weights and measures may need to be converted by the nurse within these three systems.

◆ When administering medications the nurse observes the five rights to ensure accurate administration. When preparing medications, the nurse checks the medication container label against the medication card form or printout three times.

◆ The nurse who prepares the medication administers it and must never leave a prepared medication unattended.

◆ The nurse always identifies the client appropriately before administering a medication and stays with the client until the medication is taken.

◆ Medications, once given, are documented as soon as possible after administration.

◆ When mixing insulins in the same syringe, air should be injected into the cloudy (intermediate- or long-acting) insulin vial first, followed by air into the clear (short-acting) vial. The short-acting (clear) insulin should be drawn up first, followed by the cloudy

(intermediate- or long-acting). There should never be contamination of the short-acting insulin.

◆ Proper site selection is essential for an intramuscular injection to prevent tissue, bone, and nerve damage. The nurse should always palpate anatomic landmarks when selecting a site.

◆ Clients receiving a series of injections should have the injection sites rotated.

◆ After use, needles should not be recapped but must be placed in puncture-resistant containers.

EXPLORE MediaLink

Additional interactive resources for this chapter can be found on the Companion Website at www.prenhall.com/ramont.
Click on Chapter 21 and "Begin" to select the activities for this chapter.

For chapter-related NCLEX-style questions, and an audio glossary, access the accompanying CD-ROM in this book.
Animations: Diuretics

For Further Study

For more details on respiratory therapy, see Chapter 16, "Oxygenation."

For further information about inserting a nasogastric tube, see Procedure 17-2.

For information about administering tube feedings, see Procedure 17-3.

For information about discontinuing an intravenous device, see Procedure 17-4.

Critical Thinking Care Map

Caring for a Client with IDDM (Insulin-Dependent Diabetes Mellitus)

NCLEX-PN Focus Area: Health Promotion and Maintenance

Case Study: Marissa Gonsalves is a 27-year-old elementary schoolteacher newly diagnosed with Type 1 diabetes mellitus. She also attends school at night with plans to complete her master's degree in the spring. She lives with three roommates who have shared a house since their college days. She expresses concern over her diagnosis. "It will be hard to follow the diet at home. I don't eat on a regular schedule on my school nights and my roommates are big snackers."

Nursing Diagnosis: Ineffective Management of Therapeutic Regimen

COLLECT DATA

Subjective	Objective
_____	_____
_____	_____
_____	_____
_____	_____
_____	_____
_____	_____

Would you report this data? Yes/No

If yes, to: _____

Nursing Care

_____
_____
_____
_____
_____
_____
_____
_____
_____
_____
_____
_____

How would you document this? _____
_____
_____
_____
_____

Data Collected

- Weight 156 lbs
- Fasting blood sugar 164 mg/mL
- Urine shows presence of ketones
- VS: 99/132/28, BP 100/54
- Complains of excessive thirst and frequent urination
- States "I have been so tired, but it is probably because I am working and going to school"
- Started on insulin injection and blood glucose monitoring; client hesitant to perform monitoring and injections herself
- 1,800-cal ADA diet

Nursing Interventions
(use those that apply)

- Review daily actions that are not therapeutic.
- Provide information about the therapeutic regimen in various formats (video, brochures, written instructions).
- Pay meticulous attention to foot care.
- Monitor skin condition at least once a day, determine whether client is experiencing loss of sensation.
- Assess client's locus of control related to her health.
- Deliberate with the client on changes that are possible to meet therapeutic goals.
- Observe and report signs of infection such as redness, warmth, discharge, and increased body temperature.
- Demonstrate and allow client to perform monitoring amd self-injection under supervision.

NCLEX-PN Exam Preparation

1. Demerol 50 mg has been ordered for your client. On checking the narcotic cabinet, you find a Demerol 75-mg prefilled syringe on hand. Which of the following is the appropriate action?
   a. Inform your client that he will have to wait until the pharmacy brings the correct dose of medication.
   b. Call the physician and request a different order.
   c. Waste 25 mg of Demerol in front of a licensed witness.
   d. Give your client an injection of 50 mg and dispose of the syringe with the remainder in the sharps container.

2. The physician has written an order that is illegible. It appears to be to 5 mg of Ativan. The order in fact was 0.5 mg. Who is responsible for the error?
   a. The nurse who administers the incorrect dosage is responsible for the error.
   b. The physician who wrote the illegible order is responsible.
   c. The unit secretary who transcribed the order is responsible.
   d. The charge nurse who verified the order is responsible.

3. The reason the drug is prescribed is known as the:
   a. Side effect
   b. Untoward effect
   c. Therapeutic effect
   d. Adverse effects

4. Your client is experiencing unpredictable abnormal symptoms including opposite drug action. You know this to be a(n):
   a. Drug tolerance
   b. Idiosyncratic effect
   c. Iatrogenic disease
   d. Drug interaction

5. The physician has ordered Valium 5 mg "Stat" for agitation. You understand the order to mean:
   a. The drug is to be given as needed.
   b. The medication is to be given immediately and only once.
   c. The order may be carried out indefinitely until an order is written to cancel it.
   d. The drug is to be given according to the facility policy.

6. A preop order is given for atropine 1/300 gr. On hand you have a multidose vial containing 1 mg/mL. What volume of the drug would you give?
   a. 1/3 mL
   b. 0.2 mL
   c. 1 mL
   d. 2 mL

7. You are providing discharge instructions for a mother of a 2-year-old. The physician has written a prescription for 1 teaspoon amoxicillin q6h × 10 days. Which of the following statements would assure that the mother understands the instructions?
   a. "I will used his favorite spoon to measure his medication."
   b. "I will disguise the medicine in his milk to be sure he will take it."
   c. "I will give him the medication with meals and his last dose before he goes to bed.
   d. "I will need to use a medicine cup to measure the correct dose."

8. You are preparing a subcutaneous injection of heparin for your client. You will be giving 4,000 U. On hand you have 5,000 U/mL. Which of the following is the best syringe to use?
   a. An insulin syringe because it is calibrated in units with a 5/8-Inch needle
   b. A tuberculin syringe because it is calibrated in tenths (0.1)
   c. A 2-cc syringe with a 22-gauge 2.5-cm (1-inch) needle
   d. A 3-cc syringe with a 23-gauge 3-cm (1.5-inch) needle

9. The primary reason why nurses should wear gloves when administering topical medications is:
   a. Human skin harbors microorganisms.
   b. Topical medication can cause skin irritation on the nurse.
   c. Topical medications on the nurse's hands can be transferred to another client.
   d. Skin preprations must be applied using sterile technique.

10. The dorsogluteal site should not be used for infants because:
    a. It is difficult to restrain a child in the proper position to use this site.
    b. This muscle is developed by walking so it should not be used until the child has been walking for 1 year.
    c. Medication is absorbed slowly from this location.
    d. The area is very vascular so there is a tendency for extensive bruising.

Answers for Review Questions, as well as discussion of Case Study and Critical Thinking Care Map questions, appear in Appendix IV.

Chapter 22

Perioperative Nursing

SHARING experiences

"*I always wanted to be a doctor, but that was out of my reach. I became an EMT about the same time my brother-in-law became an RN. After watching him and listening to him, I decided this was the field for me.*"

Darrin Rodriguez, LPN student, Practical Nursing Program, Idaho State University, Pocatello, ID.

LEARNING outcomes

After completing this chapter, you will be able to:

- Describe the phases of the perioperative period.
- Discuss various types of surgery according to degree of urgency, degree of risk, and purpose.
- Identify nursing responsibilities in planning perioperative nursing care.
- Describe essential preoperative teaching, including pain control, moving, leg exercises, and coughing and deep-breathing exercises.
- Describe essential aspects of preparing a client for surgery, including skin preparation.
- Identify potential postoperative complications and describe nursing interventions to prevent them.
- Describe appropriate wound care for a postoperative client.

MediaLink

 www.prenhall.com/ramont

Use the address above to access the free, interactive Companion Website created for this textbook. Get hints, instant feedback, and textbook references to chapter-related NCLEX-style questions. Link to other interestIng sites.

Audio Glossary:
Use the Companion Website, or the CD-ROM disk enclosed with your textbook, to hear the pronunciation of key terms in the chapter.

Surgery is a unique experience of a planned physical alteration encompassing three phases: preoperative, intraoperative, and postoperative. The *preoperative phase* occurs prior to surgery; the *intraoperative phase* occurs during surgery; and the *postoperative phase* occurs following surgery. These three phases are together referred to as the **perioperative period.** The LPN's/LVN's responsibilities are usually confined to client care in the postoperative period, although preoperative preparation is within the scope of the vocational/practical nurse.

Surgical procedures are commonly grouped in one of three ways:

1. *Purpose.* Surgical procedures may be categorized according to their purpose; see Box 22-1 ◆.
2. *Degree of urgency.* Surgery is classified by its urgency and necessity to preserve the client's life, body part, or body function. **Emergency surgery** is performed immediately to preserve function or the life of the client. **Elective surgery** is performed when a condition is not immediately life threatening or to improve the client's life.
3. *Degree of risk.* Surgery is also classified as major or minor according to the degree of risk to the client. *Major surgery* involves a high degree of risk. In contrast, *minor surgery* normally involves little risk, produces few complications, and is often performed on an outpatient basis as "day surgery." The degree of risk involved in a surgical procedure is affected by the client's age, general health, nutritional status, use of medications, and mental status. See Box 22-2 ◆ for health problems that increase surgical risk.

BOX 22-1
PURPOSE OF SURGICAL PROCEDURES

Diagnostic Confirms or establishes a diagnosis (e.g., biopsy of a mass in a breast)

Palliative Relieves or reduces pain or symptoms of a disease; does not cure (e.g., resection of nerve roots)

Ablative Removes a diseased body part (e.g., removal of a gallbladder [cholecystectomy])

Reconstructive Restores function or appearance that has been lost or reduced (e.g., breast implant)

Transplant Replaces malfunctioning structures (e.g., hip replacement)

 Preoperative Phase

PREOPERATIVE CONSENT

Prior to any surgical procedure, clients must sign a consent form, which is generally supplied by the agency. This requirement protects clients from having any surgical procedure they do not want or do not understand. It also protects the hospital and the health personnel from a claim by the client or family that permission was not granted. The consent form becomes a part of the client's record and goes to the operating room with the client.

SCREENING TESTS

The physician orders preoperative diagnostic tests or screening tests and examinations to determine abnormalities.

BOX 22-2 RISK FACTORS FOR CLIENTS NEEDING SURGERY

◆ Malnutrition can lead to delayed wound healing, infection, and reduced energy. Protein and vitamins are needed for wound healing; vitamin K is essential for blood clotting.

◆ Obesity leads to hypertension, impaired cardiac function, and impaired respiratory ventilation. Obese clients are also more likely to have delayed wound healing and wound infection because adipose tissue impedes blood circulation and its delivery of nutrients, antibodies, and enzymes required for wound healing.

◆ Cardiac conditions such as angina pectoris, recent myocardial infarction, hypertension, and congestive heart failure weaken the heart. Well-controlled cardiac problems generally pose minimal operative risk.

◆ Blood coagulation disorders may lead to severe bleeding, hemorrhage, and subsequent shock.

◆ Upper respiratory tract infections or chronic obstructive lung diseases such as emphysema adversely affect pulmonary function, especially when exacerbated by the effects of general anesthesia. They also predispose the client to postoperative lung infections.

◆ Renal disease or insufficiency impairs regulation of the body's fluids and electrolytes and excretion of drugs and other toxins.

◆ Diabetes mellitus predisposes the client to wound infection and delayed healing.

◆ Liver disease (e.g., cirrhosis) impairs the liver's abilities to detoxify medications used during surgery, produce the prothrombin necessary for blood clotting, and metabolize nutrients essential for healing.

◆ Uncontrolled neurologic disease such as epilepsy may result in seizures during surgery or recovery.

◆ Aspirin increases blood coagulation time and risk of hemorrhage; it needs to be discontinued several days prior to surgery.

TABLE 22-1 ROUTINE PREOPERATIVE SCREENING TESTS	
TEST	**RATIONALE**
Complete blood count (CBC)	RBCs, hemoglobin (Hgb), and hematocrit (Hct) are important to the oxygen-carrying capacity of the blood; WBCs are an indicator of immune function
Blood grouping and cross-matching	Determined in case blood transfusion is required during or after surgery
Serum electrolytes (Na^+, K^+, Ca^{2+}, Mg^{2+}, Cl^-, HCO_3^-)	To evaluate fluid and electrolyte status
Fasting blood glucose	High levels may indicate undiagnosed diabetes mellitus
Blood urea nitrogen (BUN) and creatinine	To evaluate renal function
ALT, AST, LDH, and bilirubin	To evaluate liver function
Serum albumin and total protein	To evaluate nutritional status
Urinalysis	To determine urine composition and possible abnormal components (e.g., protein or glucose) or infection
Chest x-ray	To evaluate respiratory status and heart size
Electrocardiogram (ECG)	To identify preexisting cardiac problems or disease

Abnormalities may warrant treatment prior to surgery. See Table 22-1 ◆ for routine preoperative screening tests.

NURSING CARE

ASSESSING

Preoperative assessment includes collecting and reviewing specific client data to determine the client's needs both pre- and postoperatively. Physical, psychological, and social needs are determined during assessment.

Preoperatively, the nurse performs a brief but complete physical assessment, paying particular attention to systems that could affect the client's response to anesthesia or surgery. Respiratory and cardiovascular assessments provide baseline data for evaluating the client's postoperative status. They also may alert care providers to a problem (e.g., a respiratory infection or irregular pulse rate) that may affect the client's response to surgery and anesthesia.

DIAGNOSING, PLANNING, and IMPLEMENTING

A number of NANDA nursing diagnoses may be appropriate for the preoperative client. The LPN/LVN will help implement many of the interventions. Some common nursing diagnoses for perioperative clients are: Anxiety and Deficient Knowledge.

Planning should involve the client and support people. The length of the preoperative period affects preoperative care and planning. When the client is admitted several days before surgery, a nursing care plan and teaching plan can be developed. Goals for preoperative clients are to be physically, mentally, and emotionally prepared for surgery.

Preoperative Teaching

Preoperative teaching is a vital part of nursing care. Studies have shown that preoperative teaching reduces clients' anxiety and postoperative complications. It also increases their satisfaction with the surgical experience. Good preoperative teaching aids the client's return to work and other activities of daily living.

Preoperative instructions for all clients are summarized in Box 22-3 ◆. Procedure 22-1 provides guidelines for teaching clients about moving, leg exercises, deep breathing, and coughing.

Providing Physical Preparation

Preoperative physical preparation includes the following areas: nutrition and fluids, elimination, hygiene, medications, rest, care of valuables and prostheses, special orders, and surgical skin preparation. In many agencies a preoperative checklist is used on the day of surgery. The nurse checks the agency's forms and follows appropriate recording procedures. Two things are essential:

1. All pertinent records (laboratory records, x-ray films, consents) must be assembled and completed so that operating and recovery room personnel can refer to them.

BOX 22-3

CLIENT TEACHING

PREOPERATIVE INSTRUCTIONS

Preoperative Regimen

◆ Explain the need for preoperative tests (e.g., laboratory, x-ray, ECG).
◆ Discuss bowel preparation, if required.
◆ Discuss skin preparation, including operative area and preoperative bath or shower.
◆ Discuss preoperative medications, if ordered.
◆ Explain individual therapies ordered by the physician, such as intravenous therapy, the insertion of a urinary catheter or nasogastric tube, use of a spirometer, or antiemboli stockings.
◆ Discuss the visit by the anesthetist.
◆ Explain the need to restrict food and oral fluids at least 8 hours before surgery.
◆ Provide a general timetable for perioperative events, including the time of surgery.
◆ Discuss the need to remove jewelry, makeup, and all prostheses (e.g., eyeglasses, hearing aids, complete or partial dentures, wig) immediately before surgery.
◆ Inform client about the preoperative holding area, and give the location of the waiting room for support people.
◆ Teach deep-breathing and coughing exercises, leg exercises, ways to turn and move (see Procedure 22-1), and splinting techniques.

2. All physical preparation must be completed to ensure client safety.

Nutrition and Fluids. Adequate hydration and nutrition promote healing. Nurses need to record any signs of malnutrition or fluid imbalance.

Many preoperative clients are listed as NPO (nothing by mouth). Because anesthetics depress gastrointestinal functioning and create a danger that the client may vomit and aspirate vomitus during administration of a general anesthetic, the client usually fasts at least 6 to 8 hours before surgery. Some recent research, however, no longer supports preoperative fasting (Winslow & Crenshaw, 2002). Facility policy should be followed.

Elimination. Enemas before surgery are no longer routine, but cleansing enemas may be ordered if bowel surgery is planned. After surgery involving the intestines, peristalsis often doesn't return for 24 to 48 hours.

Prior to surgery, a retention catheter may be ordered to ensure that the bladder remains empty. This helps prevent inadvertent injury to the bladder, particularly during pelvic surgery. If the client does not have a catheter, it is important to empty the bladder prior to receiving preoperative medications.

Hygiene. In some settings, clients are asked to bathe or shower the evening or morning of surgery (or both). The purpose of hygienic measures is to reduce the risk of wound infection. The bath includes a shampoo whenever possible.

In most agencies, skin preparation is carried out during the intraoperative phase. The purpose of surgical skin prep is to reduce the risk of postoperative infection.

The client's nails should be trimmed and free of polish. All cosmetics should be removed so that the nail beds, skin, and lips are visible for assessing circulation during and after surgery.

Surgical caps may be worn the day of surgery by clients in some hospitals. The surgical caps contain the client's hair and trap microorganisms on the hair and scalp.

Immediately before surgery, the nurse removes, or asks the client to remove, all hair pins and clips. Clips could cause pressure or accidental damage to the scalp when the client is unconscious. The client also removes personal clothing and puts on an operating room gown.

Valuables. Valuables such as jewelry and money should be sent home with support people. If this is impossible, they are labeled and placed in safekeeping (see discussion in Chapter 8 and Figure 8-2). ⊖⊃ If a client wishes not to remove a wedding band, the nurse can tape it in place. However, wedding bands must be removed if there is danger of the fingers swelling after surgery. Situations requiring removal of rings are cast application to an arm and mastectomy with removal of the lymph nodes, because they may cause edema of the arm and hand.

Prostheses. All **prostheses** (artificial body parts, such as partial or complete dentures, contact lenses, artificial eyes, and artificial limbs), as well as eyeglasses, wigs, and false eyelashes, must be removed before surgery.

Medications. Preoperative medications may be given on the hospital unit or after the client goes to the operating room. Commonly used preoperative medications include:

◆ Sedatives and tranquilizers, such as secobarbital and diazepam (Valium) to reduce anxiety and ease anesthetic induction
◆ Narcotic analgesics, such as morphine and meperidine (Demerol) to provide client sedation and reduce the required amount of anesthetic
◆ Anticholinergics, such as atropine, scopolamine, and glycopyrrolate (Robinul) to reduce oral and pulmonary secretions and prevent laryngospasm
◆ Histamine-receptor antihistamines, such as cimetidine (Tagamet) and ranitidine (Zantac) to reduce gastric fluid volume and gastric acidity
◆ Neuroleptanalgesic agents, such as Innovar to induce general calmness and sleepiness

Preoperative medications, which will be given at a scheduled time or "on call," that is, when the operating room notifies the nurse to give the medication.

Vital Signs. The nurse assesses and records physical measurements or vital signs for baseline data. Abnormal findings, such as elevated blood pressure or elevated temperature, must be reported.

Antiemboli Stockings. **Antiemboli stockings** are firm elastic hose that compress the veins of the legs and facilitate the return of venous blood to the heart. They are intended to prevent the formation of blood clots in the legs and edema of the legs and feet. These stockings are frequently applied both preoperatively and postoperatively. See Procedure 22-2 for steps in applying antiemboli stockings.

Sequential Compression Devices. Clients who are undergoing surgery may benefit from a **sequential compression device (SCD)** to promote venous return from the legs. SCDs inflate and deflate plastic sleeves wrapped around the legs to promote venous flow. See Procedure 16-5 for steps in applying a sequential compression device.

 EVALUATING

The nurse evaluates specific desired outcomes. For example, the nurse would check whether vital signs are stable, the client understands and is ready for the upcoming surgery, and the client has learned how to do postoperative exercises.

 Intraoperative Phase

RNs work intraoperatively as members of the surgical team, advocating for the client, maintaining safety, and continually assessing the needs of the client and the team. An LPN/LVN can also work in this specialized area with additional training.

TYPES OF ANESTHESIA

Anesthesia, the alteration in the level of sensation and consciousness, is classified as *general* (comprehensive) or *regional* (specific). **Conscious sedation,** in which a client is conscious and has an increased pain threshold during surgery, is a minimal form of anesthesia. Anesthetic agents usually are administered by an anesthesiologist or nurse-anesthetist. See Box 22-4 ◆ for a detailed explanation of the types of anesthesia.

 Postoperative Phase

Nursing during the postoperative phase is especially important for the client's recovery. Anesthesia impairs the ability of clients to respond to environmental stimuli and to help themselves, although the degree of consciousness of clients will vary. Moreover, surgery itself traumatizes the body by disrupting protective mechanisms and homeostasis.

BOX 22-4
TYPES OF ANESTHESIA

General anesthesia is the loss of all sensation and consciousness.

◆ Protective reflexes such as cough and gag reflexes are lost.
◆ Blocks awareness centers in the brain so that amnesia (loss of memory), analgesia (insensibility to pain), hypnosis (artificial sleep), and relaxation (rendering a part of the body less tense) occur.
◆ Administered by intravenous infusion or by inhalation of gases through a mask or an endotracheal tube.

Regional anesthesia is the temporary interruption of the transmission of nerve impulses to and from a specific area or region of the body.

◆ *Topical* (surface) *anesthesia* is applied directly to the skin and mucous membranes, open skin surfaces, wounds, and burns.
◆ *Local anesthesia* (infiltration) is injected into a specific area and is used for minor surgical procedures such as suturing a small wound or performing a biopsy. *Nerve block* is a technique in which the anesthetic agent is injected into and around a nerve or small nerve group that supplies sensation to a small area of the body.
◆ *Spinal anesthesia* is injected, by way of a lumbar puncture, into the subarachnoid space surrounding the spinal cord. Spinal anesthesia is often categorized as a low, mid, or high spinal.
◆ *Epidural* (peridural) anesthesia is an injection of an anesthetic agent into the epidural space, the area inside the spinal column but outside the dura mater.

Conscious sedation produces minimal depression of the level of consciousness

◆ Used alone or in conjunction with regional anesthesia for diagnostic tests and surgical procedures.
◆ Ability to consciously maintain a patent airway and respond verbally and physically retained.
◆ Increases the client's pain threshold.
◆ Induces a degree of amnesia but allows for prompt reversal of its effects.
◆ Rapid return to normal activities of daily living.

IMMEDIATE POSTANESTHETIC PHASE

In the recovery room (postanesthesia care room or PACU), the unconscious client is usually cared for by an RN. After the client has stablized, he or she will be transferred to a nursing unit where an LPN/LVN may be assigned to continue postoperative care.

PREPARING FOR ONGOING CARE OF THE POSTOPERATIVE CLIENT

While the client is in the operating room, the client's bed and room are prepared for the postoperative phase. The nurse must obtain and set up any special equipment, such as an intravenous pole, suction, oxygen equipment, and orthopedic appliances (e.g., traction). If these are not requested on the client's record, the nurse should consult with the perioperative nurse or surgeon.

NURSING CARE

ASSESSING

As soon as the client returns to the nursing unit, the RN conducts an initial assessment. The sequence of these activities varies with the situation. The surgeon's postoperative orders will be consulted to learn the following:

◆ Food and fluids permitted by mouth
◆ Intravenous solutions and intravenous medications
◆ Position in bed
◆ Medications ordered (e.g., analgesics, antibiotics)
◆ Laboratory tests
◆ Intake and output, which in some agencies are monitored for all postoperative clients
◆ Activity permitted, including ambulation

The nurse also checks the PACU record for the following data:

◆ Operation performed
◆ Presence and location of any drains
◆ Anesthetic used
◆ Postoperative diagnosis
◆ Estimated blood loss
◆ Medications administered in the recovery room

Assessments are usually made every 15 minutes until vital signs stabilize, every hour for the next 4 hours, then every 4 hours for the next 2 days. *Note:* Assessments *must* be made as often as the client's condition requires. The nurse performs the assessments described below.

Level of Consciousness

Assess orientation to time, place, and person. Most clients are fully conscious but drowsy when returned to their unit. Assess reaction to verbal stimuli and ability to move extremities.

Vital Signs

Take the client's vital signs (pulse, respiration, blood pressure, and oxygen saturation level) every 15 minutes until stable or in accordance with agency protocol. Compare initial findings with postanesthesia care unit (PACU) data. In addition, assess the client's lung sounds and assess for signs of common circu-

latory problems, such as postoperative hypotension, hemorrhage, or shock. (See Procedures in Chapter 16 for more about oxygenation.) Potential postoperative problems with related manifestations and preventive measures are listed in Table 22-2 ◆.

Skin Color and Temperature

Skin color and temperature, particularly that of the lips and nail beds, are indicators of **tissue perfusion** (passage of blood through the vessels). Pale, cyanotic, cool, and moist skin may indicate circulatory problems.

Comfort

Assess at the times the client's vital signs are obtained and as needed between vital sign measurements. Assess the location and intensity of the pain. Do not assume that reported pain is incisional. Other causes may include muscle strains, flatus, and angina. Ask the client to rate pain on a scale of 0 to 10, with 0 being no pain and 10 the worst pain imaginable. Evaluate the client for objective indicators of pain: pallor, perspiration, muscle tension, and reluctance to cough, move, or ambulate. Determine when and what analgesics were last administered, and assess the client for any side effects of medication such as nausea and vomiting. (See Chapter 15 for in-depth discussion of pain.)

Fluid Balance

Assess the type and amount of intravenous fluids, flow rate, and infusion site. LPN/LVN responsibilities related to IV therapy are defined in the scope of practice in each individual state. Monitor the client's fluid intake and output. In addition to watching for shock, assess the client for signs of circulatory overload, and monitor serum electrolytes.

Dressing and Bedclothes

Inspect the client's dressings and bedclothes underneath the client. Excessive bloody drainage on dressings or on bedclothes, often appearing underneath the client, can indicate hemorrhage. Record amount of drainage on dressings by describing the diameter of the stains or by noting the number and type of dressings saturated with drainage.

Drains and Tubes

Determine color, consistency, and amount of drainage from all tubes and drains. All tubes should be *patent* (open), and tubes and suction equipment should be functioning. Drainage bags must be hanging properly. See Chapter 12 for more information about wound care.

Document the client's time of arrival and all assessments. Many agencies have progress flow records for this purpose. Alter the frequency, parameters, and priorities to meet the individual needs of the client.

(Text continues on p. 550.)

TABLE 22-2 **POTENTIAL POSTOPERATIVE PROBLEMS**

PROBLEM/DESCRIPTION	CAUSE	CLINICAL SIGNS	PREVENTIVE INTERVENTIONS
Respiratory Pneumonia—inflammation of the alveoli	Infection, toxins, or irritants causing inflammatory process	Elevated temperature, cough, expectoration of blood-tinged or purulent sputum, dyspnea, chest pain	Deep-breathing exercises and coughing, moving in bed, early ambulation
Infectious pneumonia—may be limited to one or more lobes (*lobar*) or occur as scattered patches throughout the lungs (*bronchial*); also can involve interstitial tissues of lungs	Common organisms include *Streptococcus pneumoniae*, *Haemophilus influenzae*, and *Staphylococcus aureus*		
Hypostatic pneumonia	Immobility and impaired ventilation result in atelectasis and promote growth of pathogens		
Aspiration pneumonia—inflammatory process caused by irritation of lung tissue by aspirated material, particularly hydrochloric acid (HCl) from the stomach	Aspiration of gastric contents, food, or other substances; often related to loss of gag reflex		
Atelectasis—a condition in which alveoli collapse and are not ventilated	Mucous plugs blocking bronchial passageways, inadequate lung expansion, analgesics, immobility	Dyspnea, tachypnea, tachycardia; diaphoresis, anxiety; pleural pain, decreased chest wall movement; dull or absent breath sounds; decreased oxygen saturation (SaO_2)	Deep-breathing exercises and coughing, moving in bed, early ambulation
Pulmonary embolism—blood clot that has moved to the lungs and blocks a pulmonary artery, thus obstructing blood flow to a portion of the lung	Stasis of venous blood from immobility, venous injury from fractures or during surgery, use of oral contraceptives high in estrogen, preexisting coagulation or circulatory disorder	Sudden chest pain, shortness of breath, cyanosis, shock (tachycardia, low blood pressure)	Turning, ambulation, antiemboli stockings, sequential compression devices (SCDs)
Circulatory Hypovolemia—inadequate circulating blood volume	Fluid deficit, hemorrhage	Tachycardia, decreased urine output, decreased blood pressure	Early detection of signs; fluid and/or blood replacement
Hemorrhage—internal or external bleeding	Disruption of sutures, insecure ligation of blood vessels	Overt bleeding (dressings saturated with bright blood; bright, free-flowing blood in drains or chest tubes), increased pain, increasing abdominal girth, swelling or bruising around incision	Early detection of signs

(continued)

TABLE 22-2	POTENTIAL POSTOPERATIVE PROBLEMS (*continued*)		
PROBLEM/DESCRIPTION	**CAUSE**	**CLINICAL SIGNS**	**PREVENTIVE INTERVENTIONS**
Hypovolemic shock—inadequate tissue perfusion resulting from markedly reduced circulating blood volume	Severe hypovolemia from fluid deficit or hemorrhage	Rapid weak pulse, dyspnea, tachypnea; restlessness and anxiety; urine output less than 30 mL/hr; decreased blood pressure; cool, clammy skin, thirst, pallor	Maintain blood volume through adequate fluid replacement, prevent hemorrhage; early detection of signs
Thrombophlebitis—inflammation of the veins, usually of the legs and associated with a blood clot	Slowed venous blood flow due to immobility or prolonged sitting; trauma to vein, resulting in inflammation and increased blood coagulability	Aching, cramping pain; affected area is swollen, red, and hot to touch; vein feels hard; discomfort in calf when foot is dorsiflexed or when client walks (Homans' sign)	Early ambulation, leg exercises, antiemboli stockings, SCDs, adequate fluid intake
Thrombus—Blood clot attached to wall of vein or artery (most commonly the leg veins)	As for thrombophlebitis for venous thrombi; disruption or inflammation of arterial wall for arterial thrombi	*Venous:* same as thrombophlebitis *Arterial:* pain and pallor of affected extremity; decreased or absent peripheral pulses	*Venous:* same as thrombophlebitis *Arterial:* maintaining prescribed position; early detection of signs
Embolus—foreign body or clot that has moved from its site of formation to another area of the body (e.g., lungs, heart, or brain)	Venous or arterial thrombus; broken intravenous catheter, fat, or amniotic fluid	In venous system, usually becomes a pulmonary embolus (see pulmonary embolism); signs of arterial emboli may depend on the location	As for thrombophlebitis or thrombus; careful maintenance of IV catheters
Urinary Urinary retention—inability to empty the bladder, with excessive accumulation of urine in the bladder	Depressed bladder muscle tone from narcotics and anesthetics; handling of tissues during surgery on adjacent organs (rectum, vagina)	Fluid intake larger than output; inability to void or frequent voiding of small amounts, bladder distention, suprapubic discomfort, restlessness	Monitoring of fluid intake and output, interventions to facilitate voiding, urinary catheterization as needed
Urinary tract infection (UTI)—Inflammation of the bladder, ureters, or urethra	Immobilization and limited fluid intake, instrumentation of the urinary tract	Burning sensation when voiding, urgency, cloudy urine, lower abdominal pain	Adequate fluid intake, early ambulation, aseptic straight catheterization only as necessary, good perineal hygiene
Gastrointestinal Nausea and vomiting	Pain, abdominal distention, ingesting food or fluids before return of peristalsis, certain medications, anxiety	Complaints of feeling sick to the stomach, retching or gagging	IV fluids until peristalsis returns; then clear fluids, full fluids, and regular diet; antiemetic drugs if ordered; analgesics for pain
Constipation—Infrequent or no stool passage for abnormal length of time (e.g., within 48 hours after solid diet started)	Lack of dietary roughage, analgesics (decreased intestinal motility), immobility	Absence of stool elimination, abdominal distention, and discomfort	Adequate fluid intake, high-fiber diet, early ambulation
Tympanites—retention of gases within the intestines	Slowed motility of the intestines due to handling of the bowel during surgery and the effects of anesthesia	Obvious abdominal distention, abdominal discomfort (gas pains), absence of bowel sounds	Early ambulation; avoid using a straw, provide ice chips or water at room temperature

(*continued*)

TABLE 22-2 POTENTIAL POSTOPERATIVE PROBLEMS (*continued*)

PROBLEM/DESCRIPTION	CAUSE	CLINICAL SIGNS	PREVENTIVE INTERVENTIONS
Paralytic ileus—intestinal obstruction characterized by lack of peristaltic activity	Handling the bowel during surgery, anesthesia, electrolyte imbalance, wound infection	Abdominal pain and distention; constipation; absent bowel sounds; vomiting	IV fluids until peristalsis returns; gradual reintroduction of oral feeding; early ambulation
Wound Wound infection—inflammation and infection of incision or drain site	Poor aseptic technique; laboratory analysis of wound swab identifies causative microorganism	Purulent exudate, redness, tenderness, elevated body temperature, wound odor	Keeping wound clean and dry, surgical aseptic technique when changing dressings
Wound dehiscence—separation of a suture line before the incision heals	Malnutrition (emaciation, obesity), poor circulation, excessive strain on suture line	Increased incision drainage, tissues underlying skin become visible along parts of the incision	Adequate nutrition, appropriate incisional support and avoidance of strain
Wound evisceration—Extrusion of internal organs and tissues through the incision	Same as for wound dehiscence	Opening of incision and visible protrusion of organs	Same as for wound dehiscence
Psychological Postoperative depression—mental disorder characterized by altered mood	Weakness, surprise nature of emergency surgery, news of malignancy, severely altered body image, or other personal matter; may be a physiologic response to some surgeries	Anorexia, tearfulness, loss of ambition, withdrawal, rejection of others, feelings of dejection, sleep disturbances (insomnia, excessive sleeping)	Adequate rest, physical activity, opportunity to express anger and other negative feelings

MediaLink ● Morphine

◆ DIAGNOSING, PLANNING and IMPLEMENTING

Surgery can involve many body systems both directly and indirectly and is a complex experience for the client. So, nursing diagnoses focus on a wide variety of actual, potential, and collaborative problems. See Appendix I for list of NANDA diagnoses for the postoperative client. ⊖⊃ Some of the most common nursing diagnoses for postoperative clients are Impaired Skin Integrity and Risk for Infection. Potential problems that may be experienced by the postoperative client are summarized in Table 22-2.

Postoperative care planning and discharge planning begin in the preoperative phase when preoperative teaching is implemented.

Some major client outcomes after surgery include maintaining comfort, healing, achieving wellness, and avoiding complications of surgery.

Pain Management

Pain is usually greatest 12 to 36 hours after surgery, decreasing after the second or third postoperative day. (See Chapter 15 for a more in-depth discussion of pain and pain management. ⊖⊃) During the initial postoperative period, the physician may prescribe one of the following:

1. Patient-controlled analgesia (PCA) (self-administration of opioid medication by programmed infusion pump).
2. Continuous analgesic administration through an intravenous or epidural catheter. PRN parenteral or oral analgesics should be administered on a routine basis (every 2 to 6 hours, depending on the drug, route, and dose) for the first 24 to 36 hours. When routine analgesic administration is no longer necessary, the prescribed analgesic is generally given before scheduled activities and rest periods. Clients need to be reminded that analgesics are most effective when taken on a regular basis or before pain becomes severe. An anti-inflammatory agent is often administered in conjunction with a narcotic analgesic to enhance pain relief.

Nurses can provide nonpharmacologic measures in addition to prescribed analgesia. These include ensuring that the client is warm and providing back rubs, position changes, diversional activities, and adjunctive measures such as use of imagery.

Positioning

Position the client as ordered. Clients who have had spinal anesthetics usually lie flat for 8 to 12 hours. An unconscious or semiconscious client is placed on a side with the head slightly elevated, if possible, or in a position that allows fluids to drain from the mouth. Unless contraindicated, elevation of affected extremities (e.g., following foot surgery) with the distal extremity higher than the heart promotes venous drainage and reduces swelling.

Deep-Breathing and Coughing Exercises

Deep-breathing exercises help remove mucus, which can form and remain in the lungs due to the effects of general anesthetic and analgesics. (These drugs depress the action of both the cilia of the mucous membranes lining the respiratory tract and the respiratory center in the brain.) Deep breathing increases lung expansion and prevents the accumulation of secretions. It helps prevent pneumonia and **atelectasis** (collapse of the alveoli), which may result from stagnation of fluid in the lungs (see Procedure 22-1).

An incentive spirometer is often ordered for the postoperative client to encourage deep breathing. This device measures the flow of air inhaled through a mouthpiece. See Chapter 16 for information about how to use an incentive spirometer. 🔗 The client is instructed to breathe in through the mouthpiece until a certain level is achieved (usually measured by a ball within an enclosed chamber). Inhalation and ventilation are enhanced using the incentive spirometer.

Deep breathing frequently initiates the coughing reflex. Voluntary coughing in conjunction with deep breathing helps the client move and expel respiratory tract secretions (see Procedure 22-1).

Encourage the client to do deep-breathing and coughing exercises hourly, or at least every 2 hours, during waking hours for the first few days. Assist the client to a sitting position in bed or on the side of the bed. The client can splint the incision with a pillow when coughing, or the nurse can splint the incision for the client to reduce discomfort.

Leg Exercises

Encourage the client to do leg exercises taught in the preoperative period every 1 to 2 hours during waking hours. Muscle contractions compress the veins, preventing the stasis of blood in the veins, a cause of thrombus formation and subsequent thrombophlebitis and emboli. Contractions also promote arterial blood flow (see Procedure 22-1).

Moving and Ambulation

Encourage the client to turn from side to side at least every 2 hours. This allows alternate lungs to expand fully (the uppermost lung will have full expansion). Clients who practice turning before surgery usually find it easier to do after surgery. Avoid placing pillows or rolls under the client's knees because pressure on the popliteal blood vessels can reduce blood circulation to and from the lower extremities.

The client should ambulate as soon as possible after surgery in accordance with the surgeon's orders. Generally, clients begin ambulation the evening of the day of surgery or the first day after surgery, unless contraindicated. Early ambulation prevents respiratory, circulatory, urinary, and gastroin-

testinal complications. It also prevents general muscle weakness. Schedule ambulation for periods after the client has taken an analgesic or when the client is comfortable. Ambulation should be gradual, starting with the client sitting on the bed and dangling the feet over the side.

A client who cannot ambulate is periodically assisted to a sitting position in bed, if allowed, and turned frequently. The sitting position permits the greatest lung expansion.

Hydration

Intravenous infusions replace body fluids lost either before or during surgery. When oral intake is permitted, initially offer only small sips of water. Large amounts of water can induce vomiting because of the affects of anesthetics and narcotic analgesics on stomach motility. The client who cannot take fluids by mouth may be allowed by the surgeon's orders to suck ice chips. Provide mouth care and place a mouthwash at the client's bedside. Postoperative clients often complain of thirst and a dry, sticky mouth. These discomforts are a result of the preoperative fasting period, preoperative medications (such as atropine), and loss of body fluid.

Measure the client's fluid intake and output for at least 2 days or until fluid balance is stable without an intravenous infusion. Ensuring adequate fluid balance is important. Sufficient fluids keep the respiratory mucus membranes and secretions moist, thus facilitating the expectoration of mucus during coughing. Also, an adequate fluid balance is important to maintain renal and cardiovascular function.

Diet

The surgeon orders the client's postoperative diet. Depending on the extent of surgery and the organs involved, the client may be allowed nothing by mouth (NPO) for several days or may be able to resume oral intake when nausea is no longer present. When "diet as tolerated" is ordered, offer clear liquids first. If the client tolerates these with no nausea, the diet can often progress to full liquids and then to a regular diet, provided gastrointestinal functioning is normal. Assess the return of peristalsis by auscultating the abdomen (see Chapter 11). 🔗 Gurgling and rumbling sounds indicate peristalsis. Bowel sounds should be carefully assessed every 4 to 6 hours. Oral fluids and food are usually started after the return of peristalsis. Very weak clients will need assistance to eat.

Observe the client's tolerance of the food and fluids ingested. Note and report the passage of flatus or abdominal distention.

Urinary Elimination

Provide measures that promote urinary elimination. For example, help male clients stand at the bedside, or female clients to a bedside commode if allowed. Ensure that fluid intake is adequate. Report to the surgeon if a client does not void within 8 hours following surgery, unless another time frame is specified.

Generally, I&O records (see Figure 17-5) are kept for at least 2 days or until the client reestablishes fluid balance without an IV or catheter in place. ⟳

Suction

Some clients return from surgery with a gastric or intestinal tube in place and orders to connect the tube to suction. For more information about gastrointestinal tubes, see Chapter 17. ⟳ The suction ordered can be continuous or intermittent. Intermittent suction is applied when a single-lumen gastric tube is used to reduce the risk of damaging the mucous membrane near the distal port of the tube. Continuous suction may be applied if a double-lumen tube is in place. Fluids and electrolytes must be replaced intravenously when gastric suction or continuous drainage is ordered. Nasogastric tubes may be irrigated if the lumen becomes clogged. They are generally irrigated before and after tube feedings or the instillation of medications. Nasogastric irrigation may require a physician's order, particularly following gastrointestinal surgery. Procedure 22-3 describes the management of gastrointestinal suction. See also Procedure 17-3. ⟳

Suction may also be applied to other drainage tubes such as chest tubes or a wound drain. The type and amount of suction is ordered by the physician. A suction regulator with a drainage receptacle connects to a wall outlet that provides negative pressure. Check the receptacle frequently to prevent excess drainage from interfering with the suction apparatus. Empty or change the receptacle according to agency policy. Portable electric suction units or pumps (e.g., the Gomco pump) may be used in the home or when wall suction is not available.

Wound Care

Most clients return from surgery with a sutured wound covered by a dressing, although in some cases the wound may be left unsutured. Dressings are inspected regularly to ensure that they are clean, dry, and intact. Excessive drainage may indicate hemorrhage, infection, or an open wound.

See Chapter 12 for information about wound drainage, cleaning wounds, wound irrigation, hot and cold applications, and supporting and immobilizing wounds. ⟳

When dressings are changed, the nurse assesses the wound for appearance, size, drainage, swelling, pain, and the status of a drain or tubes. Details about these assessments are outlined in Box 22-5 ◆.

Not all surgical dressings require changing. Sometimes surgeons in the operating room apply a dressing that remains in place until the sutures are removed, and no further dressings are required. In many situations, however, surgical dressings are changed regularly to prevent the growth of microorganisms.

In some instances, a client may have a Penrose drain inserted directly into the incision. In this situation, the main surgical incision is considered cleaner than the surgical stab

---

BOX 22-5
NURSING CARE CHECKLIST

ASSESSING SURGICAL WOUNDS

☑ *Appearance.* Inspect color of wound and surrounding area and approximation of wound edges.

☑ *Size.* Note size and location of dehiscence (partial or total rupturing of a sutured wound), if present. If internal organs are visible (evisceration), notify physician immediately!

☑ *Drainage.* Observe location, color, consistency, odor, and degree of saturation of dressings. Note number of gauzes saturated or diameter of drainage on gauze.

☑ *Swelling.* Observe the amount of swelling; minimal to moderate swelling is normal in early stages of wound healing.

☑ *Pain.* Expect severe to moderate postoperative pain for 3 to 5 days; persistent severe pain or sudden onset of severe pain may indicate internal hemorrhaging or infection.

☑ *Drains or tubes.* Inspect drain security and placement, amount and character of drainage, and functioning of collecting apparatus, if present.

---

wound made for the drain insertion, because there is usually considerable drainage. The main incision is therefore cleaned first.

clinical ALERT

Materials that were used to clean a stab wound are never used again to clean the main incision. The main incision must be kept free of the microorganisms around the stab wound.

Cleaning a wound and applying a sterile dressing are detailed in Procedure 22-4.

Wound Drains and Suction. Surgical drains, such as a Penrose drain, are inserted to permit the drainage of excess serosanguineous fluid and purulent material and to promote healing of underlying tissues. These drains may be inserted and sutured through the incision line, but they are most commonly inserted through stab wounds a few centimeters away from the incision line so that the incision itself may be kept dry. Without a drain, some wounds would heal on the surface and trap the discharge inside, and an abscess might form.

A **closed wound drainage system** consists of a drain connected to either an electric suction or a portable drainage suction, such as a Hemovac (Figure 22-1 ◆) or Jackson-Pratt. The closed system reduces the possible entry of microorganisms into the wound through the drain. The drainage tubes are sutured in place and connected to a reservoir. These portable wound suctions also provide for accurate

Figure 22-1. ◆ Closed wound drainage system (Hemovac).

measurement of the drainage. Generally, the suction is discontinued from 3 to 5 days postoperatively or when the drainage is minimal. Nurses are responsible for maintaining the wound suction, which hastens the healing process by draining excess exudate that might otherwise interfere with the formation of granulation tissue.

When emptying the container, the nurse should wear gloves and avoid touching the drainage port.

Sutures. **Sutures** are threads used to sew body tissues together. Sutures used to attach tissues beneath the skin are often made of an absorbable material that disappears in several days. Skin sutures, by contrast, are made of a variety of nonabsorbable materials. Silver wire clips or staples are also available. Usually, skin sutures are removed 7 to 10 days after surgery.

The physician orders the removal of sutures. In some agencies, only physicians remove sutures; in others, registered nurses and nursing students with appropriate supervision may do so. The LPN/LVN should review the LPN/LVN scope of practice regarding suture and staple removal. Many states permit the removal of these on well-approximated, uncomplicated surgical wounds. (For review of wound healing, see Chapter 12. ⊗)

Sterile technique and special suture scissors are used in suture removal. The scissors have a short, curved cutting tip that readily slides under the suture (Figure 22-2). Wire clips or staples are removed with a special instrument that squeezes the center of the clip to remove it from the skin (Figure 22-2B). Nursing care guidelines for removing sutures are provided in Box 22-6 .

◆ EVALUATING

Using the goals developed during the planning stage, the nurse collects data to evaluate whether the identified goals and desired outcomes have been achieved. The nurse collects data about client comfort, healing, restoring wellness, and preventing risks associated with surgery.

◆ DISCHARGE CONSIDERATIONS

The nurse reviews the client's self-care abilities, such as the ability to manage hygiene and other self-care, to perform wound care as needed, to manage tubes and stomas, and to manage prescribed medications. The nurse teaches about required supplies (dressings, hypoallergenic tape, etc.) or assistive devices (cane, raised toilet seat, grab bars in the shower). The client must know what occurrences might indicate a complication, and when to call the nurse or physician. Referrals and support systems should all be reviewed before discharge.

Nursing Process Case Study:
A POSTSURGICAL CLIENT

Mr. Teng is a 77-year-old client with a history of chronic obstructive pulmonary disease. Currently, his respiratory condition is being controlled with medications, and he is free of infection. He has just been transferred to the PACU following a hernia repair performed under spinal anesthesia.

A   **B**

Figure 22-2. ◆ **A.** Suture scissors. **B.** Removing surgical clips.

BOX 22-6
NURSING CARE CHECKLIST

REMOVING SKIN SUTURES

☑ Before removing skin sutures, verify the orders for suture removal and whether a dressing is to be applied following the suture removal.

☑ Inform the client that suture removal may produce slight discomfort, such as a pulling or stinging sensation, but should not be painful.

☑ Remove dressings and clean the incision in accordance with agency protocol

☑ Put on sterile gloves.

Plain Interrupted Sutures

☑ Grasp the suture at the knot with a pair of forceps.

☑ Place the curved tip of the suture scissors under the suture as close to the skin as possible, either on the side opposite the knot (Figure 22-3 ◆) or directly under the knot. Cut the suture. *Sutures are cut as close to the skin as possible on one side of the visible part because the suture material that is visible to the eye is in contact with resident bacteria of the skin and must not be pulled beneath*

the skin during removal. Suture material that is beneath the skin is considered free from bacteria.

☑ With the forceps, pull the suture out in one piece. Inspect the suture carefully to make sure that all suture material is removed. *Suture material left beneath the skin acts as a foreign body and causes inflammation.*

☑ Discard the suture onto a piece of sterile gauze or into a moistureproof bag. Be careful not to contaminate the forceps tips.

☑ Remove alternate sutures so that remaining sutures keep the skin edges in close approximation and prevent dehiscence. If no dehiscence occurs, remove the remaining sutures. If dehiscence does occur, do not remove the remaining sutures and report the dehiscence to the nurse in charge.

☑ If steri-strips are ordered by the physician, apply them to the wound after removing the sutures or clips. Reapply a dressing, if indicated.

☑ Instruct the client about follow-up wound care, such as contacting the physician if wound discharge appears.

Figure 22-3. ◆ Removing a plain interrupted skin suture.

Assessment. His BP is 132/88, P 84, R 28, and tympanic temperature 97.8° F. He is awake and stable.

Diagnosis. Ineffective Breathing Pattern.

Expected Outcomes.

◆ Performs deep breathing, coughing and incentive spirometry as instructed
◆ Normal auscultated breath sounds
◆ Adequate respiratory excusion (depth)

Planning and Implementation.

◆ Monitor respiratory rate, depth and ease of respiration

◆ Monitor client's oxygen saturation and blood gases
◆ Encourage client to take deep breaths at prescribed intervals and do controlled coughing
◆ Assist client to sit on side of bed and splint abdomen with pillow while coughing
◆ Teach client to use incentive spiromter

Evaluation. Client demonstrates ability to use incentive spirometer, cough, and deep breathe, q2h while awake. Splints abdomen while coughing to decrease discomfort. Lungs clear, no signs and symptoms of respiratory infection.

Critical Thinking in the Nursing Process

1. What factors place Mr. Teng at increased risk for the development of complications during and after surgery?
2. Speculate about why Mr. Teng's surgeon and anesthesiologist decided to perform Mr. Teng's surgery under regional anesthesia as opposed to general anesthesia?
3. What postoperative precautions are especially important to Mr. Teng in view of his chronic lung condition?

Note: The bibliography listings for this and all chapters have been compiled at the back of the book.

PROCEDURE 22-1

Teaching Moving, Leg Exercises, Deep Breathing, and Coughing

PURPOSES

◆ To maintain blood circulation
◆ To stimulate respiratory function and lung aeration, preventing atelactasis and pneumonia
◆ To decrease stasis of gas in the intestines
◆ To facilitate early ambulation
◆ To stimulate blood circulation, thereby preventing thrombophlebitis and thrombus formation

EQUIPMENT

◆ Pillow

INTERVENTIONS

1. Show the client ways to turn in bed and to get out of bed.
   ◆ Instruct a client who will have a right abdominal incision or a right-sided chest incision to turn to the left side of the bed and sit up as follows:
   a. Flex the knees.
   b. Splint the wound by holding the left arm and hand or a small pillow against the incision. *This minimizes pressure against the incision and reduces pain.*
   c. Turn to the left while pushing with the right foot and grasping a partial side rail on the left side of the bed with the right hand. *This puts least pressure on the side with the incision.*
   d. Come to a sitting position on the side of the bed by using the right arm and hand to push down against the mattress and swinging the feet over the edge of the bed.
   ◆ Teach a client with left abdominal or left-sided chest incision to perform the same procedure but splint with the right arm and turn to the right.
   ◆ For clients with orthopedic surgery (e.g., hip surgery), use special aids, such as a trapeze, to assist with movement.
2. Teach the client the following three leg exercises.
   ◆ Alternate dorsiflexion and plantar flexion of the feet (see Figure 22-4 ◆). This exercise is sometimes referred to as calf pumping, because it alternately contracts and relaxes the calf muscles, including the gastrocnemius muscles (see also Figures 20-12 and 20-28). ⊂⊃
   ◆ Flex and extend the knees, and press the backs of the knees into the bed while dorsiflexing the feet. Instruct clients who cannot raise their legs to do isometric exercises that contract and relax the muscles.

Figure 22-4. ◆ Flexing and extending the knees.

◆ Raise and lower the legs alternately from the surface of the bed. Flex the knee of the stable leg and extend the knee of the moving leg (see Figure 22-5 ◆). This exercise contracts and relaxes the quadriceps muscles.

Figure 22-5. ◆ Raising and lowering the legs.

3. Demonstrate deep-breathing (diaphragmatic) exercises as follows.

- ◆ Place your hands palms down on the border of your rib cage, and inhale slowly and evenly through the nose until the greatest chest expansion is achieved (Figure 22-6 ◆).
- ◆ Hold your breath for 2 to 3 seconds.
- ◆ Then exhale slowly through the mouth.
- ◆ Continue exhalation until maximum chest contraction has been achieved.

4. Help the client perform deep-breathing exercises.

- ◆ Ask the client to assume a sitting position.
- ◆ Place the palms of your hands on the border of the client's rib cage to assess respiratory depth.
- ◆ Ask the client to perform deep breathing, as described in step 3.

5. Instruct the client to cough voluntarily after a few deep inhalations.

- ◆ Ask the client to inhale deeply, hold the breath for a few seconds, and then cough once or twice.
- ◆ Ensure that the client coughs deeply and does not just clear the throat.

6. Demonstrate ways to splint the abdomen when coughing, if the incision will be painful when the client coughs.

- ◆ Show the client how to support the incision by placing the palms of the hands on either side of the incision site or directly over the incision site, holding the palm of one hand over the other. *Coughing uses the abdominal and*

Figure 22-6. ◆ Demonstrating deep breathing. *Source:* © Elena Dorfman.

Figure 22-7. ◆ Splinting an incision with a pillow while coughing. *Source:* © Elena Dorfman.

other accessory respiratory muscles. Splinting the incision may reduce pain while coughing if the incision is near any of these muscles.

- ◆ Show the client how to splint the abdomen with clasped hands and a firmly rolled pillow held against the client's abdomen (Figure 22-7 ◆).

7. Inform the client about the expected frequency of these exercises. *This prepares the client mentally to perform them in the recovery period.*

- ◆ Instruct the client to start the exercises as soon after surgery as possible. This promotes good oxygenation.
- ◆ Encourage clients with abdominal or chest surgery to carry out deep breathing and coughing at least every 2 hours, taking a minimum of five breaths at each session. Note, however, that the number of breaths and frequency of deep breathing varies with the client's condition. *People who are susceptible to pulmonary problems may need deep-breathing exercises every hour. People with chronic respiratory disease may need special breathing exercises (e.g., pursed-lip breathing), abdominal breathing, exercises using various kinds of incentive spirometers).* See Chapter 16. ∞

8. Document the teaching and all assessments.

◆ **SAMPLE DOCUMENTATION**

12/13/05	Client coughing and deep breathing
1430	q 2 hours. Splinting abdomen while
	coughing. Lungs clear. ————
	T. Thompson, LPN

PROCEDURE 22-2

Applying Antiemboli Stockings

PURPOSES

- ◆ To facilitate venous return from the lower extremities
- ◆ To prevent venous stasis and venous thrombosis
- ◆ To reduce peripheral edema

EQUIPMENT

- ◆ Tape measure
- ◆ Clean antiemboli stockings of appropriate size and of the type ordered
- ◆ Talcum powder

INTERVENTIONS

1. Take measurements as needed to obtain the appropriate size stockings.
   - ◆ Measure the length of both legs from the heel to the gluteal fold (for thigh-length stockings) or from the heel to the popliteal space (for knee-length stockings).
   - ◆ Measure the circumference of each calf and each thigh at the widest point.
   - ◆ Compare the measurements to the size chart to obtain stockings of correct size. Obtain two sizes if there is a significant difference. *Stockings that are too large for the client do not place adequate pressure on the legs to facilitate venous return and may bunch, increasing the risk of pressure and skin irritation. Stockings that are too small may impede blood flow to the feet and cause discomfort.*

2. Select an appropriate time to apply the stockings.
   - ◆ Apply stockings in the morning, if possible, before the client arises. *In sitting and standing positions, the veins can become distended so that edema occurs; the stockings should be applied before this happens.*

   - ◆ Assist the client who has been ambulating to lie down and elevate the legs for 15 to 30 minutes before applying the stockings. *This facilitates venous return and reduces swelling.*

3. Prepare the client.
   - ◆ Assist the client to a lying position in bed.
   - ◆ Wash and dry the legs as needed.
   - ◆ Dust the ankles with talcum powder. *This eases application.*

4. Apply the stockings.
   - ◆ Reach inside the stocking from the top, and grasping the heel, turn the upper portion of the stocking inside out over the foot portion. *Firm elastic stockings are easier to fit over the foot and calf when inverted in this manner rather than bunching the stocking up.*
   - ◆ Ask the client to point the toes, and position the stocking on the client's foot, taking care to place the toe and heel portions of the stocking appropriately (Figure 22-8 ◆). *Pointing the toes makes application easier.*
   - ◆ Grasp the upper edge of the stocking and gently pull the stocking over the leg, turning it right side out in the process (Figure 22-8B).

A   **B**

Figure 22-8. ◆ **A.** Applying the inverted stocking over the toes. **B.** Pulling the stocking snugly over the leg. *Source:* © Elena Dorfman.

clinical ALERT

If you are having trouble adjusting stockings over a client's foot, this technique may help. Place the foot in a small plastic bag. (A clean bedside trash bag works well.) Adjust the stocking over the bag-covered foot and up the leg. Once the stocking has been adjusted, pull the plastic bag out through the open toe of the stocking. The elastic stocking will be smooth and wrinkle free without discomfort to the client.

◆ Inspect the client's leg and stocking, smoothing any folds or creases. Ensure that the stocking is not rolled down or bunched at the top or ankle. *Folds and creases can cause skin irritation under the stocking; bunching of the stocking can further impair venous return.*

◆ Remove the hose for 30 minutes every 8 hours, inspecting the legs and skin while the hose are off. *This allows early detection of problems.*

◆ Soiled hose may be laundered by hand with warm water and mild soap. Hang to dry.

5. Document the procedure.

◆ Record the procedure, your assessment data, and when the stockings are removed and reapplied.

◆ **SAMPLE DOCUMENTATION**

4/30/05	antiemboli stockings removed for
0900	bathing. Bilateral pedal pulses strong
	and regular. Skin warm, dry and
	pink. No evidence of edema. Homan's
	sign negative. Stockings replaced,
	client ambulated from bed to chair. ⸺
	K. Turner, LVN

PROCEDURE 22-3

Managing Gastrointestinal Suction

PURPOSES

◆ To relieve abdominal distention
◆ To maintain gastric decompression after surgery
◆ To remove blood and secretions from the gastrointestinal tract
◆ To relieve discomfort (e.g., when a client has a bowel obstruction)
◆ To maintain the patency of the nasogastric tube

EQUIPMENT

◆ Gastrointestinal tube in place in the client
◆ Basin
◆ 50-mL syringe with an adapter
◆ Stethoscope
◆ Suction device for either continuous or intermittent suction
◆ Connector and connecting tubing
◆ Disposable gloves
◆ Graduated container as required to measure gastric drainage
◆ Cotton-tipped applicators
◆ Ointment or lubricant
◆ Disposable irrigating set containing a sterile 50-mL syringe, moisture-resistant pad, basin, and graduated container
◆ Sterile normal saline (500 mL) or the ordered solution

INTERVENTIONS

INITIATING SUCTION

1. Position the client appropriately.

◆ Assist the client to a semi-Fowler's position if it is not contraindicated. *In semi-Fowler's position the tube is not as likely to lie against the wall of the stomach and will therefore suction most efficiently. Semi-Fowler's position also prevents reflux of gastric contents, which could lead to aspiration.*

2. Confirm that the tube is in the stomach.

◆ Aspirate stomach contents and check their acidity using a pH test strip.

◆ Insert air into the tube with the syringe and listen with a stethoscope over the stomach (just below the xiphoid process) for a swish of air.

◆ Use other methods in accordance with agency protocol.

3. Set and check the suction.

◆ Connect the appropriate suction regulator to the wall suction outlet and the collection device to the regulator. Intermittent suction regulators generally are used with single-lumen tubes and apply suction for a set interval (15 to 60 seconds), followed by an interval of no suction. Intermittent suction is set at 80 to 100 mm Hg or as ordered by the physician. Check the suction level by occluding the drainage tube and observing the regulator dial during a suction cycle. Continuous suction regulators are used with double-lumen (e.g., Salem sump) nasogastric tubes. Set continuous suction as ordered by the physician, or at 60 to 120 mm Hg.

◆ If using a portable suction machine, turn on the machine and regulate the suction as above. The Gomco pump has two settings: low intermittent for single-lumen tubes, and high for double-lumen tubes.

◆ Test for proper suctioning by holding the open end of the suction tube to the ear and listening for a sucking noise or by occluding the end of the tube with a thumb.

4. Establish gastric suction.

◆ Connect the gastrointestinal tube to the tubing from the suction by using the connector.

◆ If a Salem sump tube is in place, connect the larger lumen to the suction equipment. This double-lumen tube has a smaller tube running inside the primary suction tube. *The smaller tube provides a continuous flow of atmospheric air through the drainage tube at its distal end and prevents excessive suction force on the gastric mucosa at the drainage outlets. Damage to the gastric mucosa is thus avoided.*

◆ Always keep the air vent tube of a Salem sump tube open and above the level of the stomach when suction is applied. *Closing the vent would stop the sump action and cause mucosal damage. Keeping the end of the air vent tube higher than the stomach prevents reflux of gastric contents into the air lumen of the tube.*

◆ After suction is applied, watch the tubing for a few minutes until the gastric contents appear to be running through the tubing into the receptacle. A Salem sump tube makes a soft, hissing sound when it is functioning correctly.

◆ If the suction is not working properly, check that all connections are tight and that the tubing is not kinked.

◆ Coil and pin the tubing on the bed so that it does not loop below the suction bottle. *If the tubing falls below the suction bottle, the suction may be obstructed because of the pressure required to push the fluid against gravity.*

5. Assess the drainage.

◆ Observe the amount, color, odor, and consistency of the drainage. *Normal gastric drainage has a mucoid consistency and is either colorless or yellow-green because of the presence of bile. A coffee-grounds color and consistency may indicate bleeding.*

◆ Test the gastric drainage for pH and blood (by using Hematest) when indicated. *A person who has had gastrointestinal surgery can be expected to have some blood in the drainage.*

MAINTAINING SUCTION

6. Assess the client and the suction system regularly.

◆ Assess the client every 30 minutes until the system is running effectively and then every 2 hours, or as the client's health indicates, to ensure that the suction is functioning properly. *If the client complains of fullness, nausea, or epigastric pain or if the flow of gastric secretions is absent in the tubing or in the collection bottle, ineffective suctioning or blockage of the nasogastric tube is likely.*

◆ Inspect the suction system for patency of the system (eg, kinks or blockages in the tubing) and tightness of the connections. *Loose connections can permit air to enter and thus decrease the effectiveness of the suction by decreasing the negative pressure.*

7. Relieve blockages if present.

◆ Don gloves.

◆ Check the suction equipment. To do this, disconnect the nasogastric tube from the suction over a collecting basin (to collect gastric drainage), and then, with the suction on, place the end of the suction tubing in a basin of water. *If water is drawn into the drainage bottle, the suction equipment is functioning properly, but the nasogastric tube is either blocked or positioned incorrectly.*

◆ Reposition the client (e.g., to the other side) if permitted. *This may facilitate drainage.*

◆ Rotate the nasogastric tube, and reposition it. This step is contraindicated for clients with gastric surgery. *Moving the tube may interfere with gastric sutures.*

◆ Irrigate the nasogastric tube as agency protocol states or on the order of the physician. See steps 11 to 13.

8. Prevent reflux into the vent lumen of a Salem sump tube. *Reflux of gastric contents into the vent lumen may occur when stomach pressure exceeds atmospheric pressure. In this situation, gastric contents follow the path of least resistance and flow out the vent lumen rather than the drainage lumen.* To prevent reflux:

◆ Place the vent tubing higher than the client's stomach.

◆ Keep the drainage collection container below the level of the client's stomach and do not allow it to become overfull. *A collection device placed above the level of fluid in the stomach or that is too full may interfere with drainage, allowing reflux of gastric contents into the air lumen.*

◆ Keep the drainage lumen free of particulate matter that may obstruct the lumen. See steps 11 to 13 for irrigating a nasogastric tube.

9. Ensure client comfort.
   ◆ Clean the client's nostrils as needed, using the cotton-tipped applicators and water. Apply a water-soluble lubricant or ointment.
   ◆ Provide mouth care every 2 to 4 hours and as needed. *Some postoperative clients are permitted to suck ice chips or a moist cloth to maintain the moisture of the oral mucous membranes.*

10. Empty the drainage receptacle according to agency policy or physician's order.
    ◆ Clamp the nasogastric tube, and turn off the suction.
    ◆ Don gloves.
    ◆ If the receptacle is graduated, determine the amount of drainage.
    ◆ Disconnect the receptacle.
    ◆ If the receptacle is not graduated, empty the contents into a graduated container and measure.
    ◆ Inspect the drainage carefully for color, consistency, and presence of substances (e.g., blood clots).
    ◆ Discard and replace a full receptacle or rinse the receptacle with warm water and reattach it to the suction. Check agency policy.
    ◆ Turn on the suction and unclamp the nasogastric tube.
    ◆ Observe the system for several minutes to make sure function is reestablished.
    ◆ Go to step 14.

IRRIGATING A GASTROINTESTINAL TUBE

11. Prepare the client and the equipment.
    ◆ Place the moisture-resistant pad under the end of the gastrointestinal tube.
    ◆ Turn off the suction.
    ◆ Don gloves.
    ◆ Disconnect the gastrointestinal tube from the connector.
    ◆ Determine that the tube is in the stomach. See step 2 above and Chapter 17. ⊂⊃ *This ensures that the irrigating solution enters the client's stomach.*

12. Irrigate the tube.
    ◆ Draw up the ordered volume of irrigating solution in the syringe; 30 mL of solution per instillation is usual, but up to 60 mL may be given per instillation if ordered.
    ◆ Attach the syringe to the nasogastric tube, and slowly inject the solution.
    ◆ Gently aspirate the solution. *Forceful withdrawal could damage the gastric mucosa.*

◆ If you encounter difficulty in withdrawing the solution, inject 20 mL of air and aspirate again, and/or reposition the client or the nasogastric tube. *Air and repositioning may move the end of the tube away from the stomach wall.* If aspirating difficulty continues, reattach the tube in intermittent low suction, and notify the nurse in charge or physician.
◆ Repeat the preceding steps until the ordered amount of solution is used.
◆ *Note:* A Salem sump tube can also be irrigated through the vent lumen without interrupting suction. However, only small quantities of irrigant can be injected through this lumen compared to the drainage lumen.
◆ After irrigating a Salem sump tube, inject 10 to 20 mL of air into the vent lumen while applying suction to the drainage lumen. *This tests the patency of the vent and ensures sump functioning.*

13. Reestablish suction.
    ◆ Reconnect the nasogastric tube to suction.
    ◆ If a Salem sump tube is used, inject the air vent lumen with 10 mL of air after reconnecting the tube to suction.
    ◆ Observe the system for several minutes to make sure it is functioning.

14. Document all relevant information.
    ◆ Record the time suction was started. Also record the pressure established, the color and consistency of the drainage, and nursing assessments.
    ◆ During maintenance, record assessments, supportive nursing measures, and data about the suction system.
    ◆ When irrigating the tube, record verification of tube placement; the time of the irrigation; the amount and type of irrigating solution used; the amount, color and consistency of the returns; the patency of the system following the irrigation; and nursing assessments. *Remember the saying, "If it isn't documented, it wasn't done."*

◆ SAMPLE DOCUMENTATION

8-26-04	Abdominal distention decreased;
7:30 AM	bowel sounds present in all 4 quadrants;
	450 cc of dark coffee ground gastric
	drainage; oral mucous pink and moist.
	D. Wilson, LPN

PROCEDURE 22-4

Cleaning a Sutured Wound and Applying a Sterile Dressing

PURPOSES

◆ To promote wound healing by primary intention
◆ To prevent infection
◆ To assess the healing process
◆ To protect the wound from mechanical trauma

EQUIPMENT

◆ Bath blanket (if necessary)
◆ Moisture-proof bag
◆ Mask (optional)
◆ Acetone or another solution (if necessary to loosen adhesive)
◆ Disposable gloves

◆ Sterile gloves
◆ Sterile dressing set; if none is available, gather the following sterile items from a central supply cart:
  ◆ Drape or towel
  ◆ Gauze squares
  ◆ Container for the cleaning solution
  ◆ Cleaning solution (e.g., normal saline)
  ◆ Two pairs of forceps (thumb or artery)
  ◆ Gauze dressings and surgipads
  ◆ Applicators or tongue blades to apply ointments
  ◆ Additional supplies required for the particular dressing (e.g., extra gauze dressings and ointment, if ordered)
  ◆ Tape, tie tapes, or binder

INTERVENTIONS

1. Prepare the client and assemble the equipment.
   ◆ Acquire assistance for changing a dressing on a restless or confused adult. *The person might move and contaminate the sterile field or the wound.*
   ◆ Assist the client to a comfortable position in which the wound can be readily exposed. Expose only the wound area, using a bath blanket to cover the client, if necessary. *Unnecessary exposure is physically and psychologically distressing to most people.*
   ◆ Make a cuff on the moistureproof bag for disposal of the soiled dressings, and place the bag within reach. It can be taped to the bedclothes or bedside table. *Making a cuff helps keep the outside of the bag free from contamination by the soiled dressings and prevents subsequent contamination of the nurse's hands or of sterile instrument tips when discarding dressing or sponges. Placement of the bag within reach prevents the nurse from reaching across the sterile field and the wound and potentially contaminating these areas.*
   ◆ Put on a face mask, if required. *Some agencies require that a mask be worn for surgical dressing changes to prevent contamination of the wound by droplet spray from the nurse's respiratory tract.*

2. Remove binders and tape.
   ◆ Remove binders, if used, and place them aside. Untie tie tapes, if used.
   ◆ If adhesive tape was used, remove it by holding down the skin and pulling the tape gently but firmly toward the wound. *Pressing down on the skin provides*

   countertraction against the pulling motion. Tape is pulled toward the incision to prevent strain on the sutures or wound.
   ◆ Use a solvent to loosen tape, if required. *Moistening the tape with acetone or a similar solvent lessens the discomfort of removal, particularly from hairy surfaces.*

3. Remove and dispose of soiled dressings appropriately.
   ◆ Put on clean disposable gloves, and remove the outer abdominal dressing or surgipad.
   ◆ Lift the outer dressing so that the underside is away from the client's face. *The appearance and odor of the drainage may be upsetting to the client.*
   ◆ Place the soiled dressing in the moistureproof bag without touching the outside of the bag. *Contamination of the outside of the bag is avoided to prevent the spread of microorganisms to the nurse and others.*
   ◆ Remove the under dressings, taking care not to dislodge any drains. If the gauze sticks to the drain, support the drain with one hand and remove the gauze with the other.
   ◆ Assess the location, type (color, consistency), and odor of wound drainage, and the number of gauzes saturated or the diameter of drainage collected on the dressings.
   ◆ Discard the soiled dressings in the bag as before.
   ◆ Remove gloves, dispose of them in the moisture-proof bag, and wash hands.

4. Set up the sterile supplies.
   ◆ Open the sterile dressing set, using surgical aseptic technique.
   ◆ Place the sterile drape beside the wound.

◆ Open the sterile cleaning solution, and pour it over the gauze sponges in the plastic container.
◆ Put on sterile gloves.

5. Clean the wound, if indicated.
   ◆ Clean the wound, using your gloved hands or forceps and gauze swabs moistened with cleaning solution.
   ◆ If using forceps, keep the forceps tips lower than the handles at all times. *This prevents their contamination by fluid traveling up to the handle and nurse's wrist and back to the tips.*
   ◆ Use the cleaning methods illustrated and described in Figure 22-9 ◆ or one recommended by agency protocol.
   ◆ Use a separate swab for each stroke, and discard each swab after use. *This prevents the introduction of microorganisms to other wound areas.*
   ◆ If a drain is present, clean it next, taking care to avoid reaching across the cleaned incision. Clean the skin around the drain site by swabbing in half or full circles from around the drain site outward, using separate swabs for each wipe (Figure 22-9C). *This ensures that clean areas are not contaminated.*
   ◆ Support and hold the drain erect while cleaning around it. Clean as many times as necessary to remove the drainage.
   ◆ Dry the surrounding skin with dry gauze swabs as required. Do not dry the incision or wound itself. *Moisture facilitates wound healing.*

6. Apply dressings to the drain site and the incision.
   ◆ Place a precut 4 × 4 gauze snugly around the drain (Figure 22-10 ◆), or open a 4 × 4 gauze to 4 × 8, fold it lengthwise to 2 × 8, and place the 2 × 8 around the drain so that the ends overlap. *This dressing absorbs the drainage and helps prevent it from excoriating the skin. Using precut gauze or folding it as described, instead of cutting the gauze, prevents any threads from coming loose and getting into the wound, where they could cause inflammation and provide a site for infection.*

Figure 22-10. ◆ Precut gauze in place around a drain.

   ◆ Apply the sterile dressings one at a time over the drain and the incision. Place the bulk of the dressings over the drain area and below the drain, depending on the client's usual position. *Layers of dressings are placed for best absorption of drainage, which flows by gravity.*
   ◆ Apply the final surgipad, remove gloves, and dispose of them. Secure the dressing with tape or ties.

7. Document the procedure and all nursing assessments.

◆ **SAMPLE DOCUMENTATION**

2/18/05	Incision clean and dry, edges pink, well
1430	approximated, sutures in place. Moderate
	ammount of serous sanguinous drainage on
	dressing, no evidence of inflammation or odor.
	Incisional pain 4/10. Incision cleaned with
	nss. Covered with sterile dressing and secured.
	B. Harvey, LVN

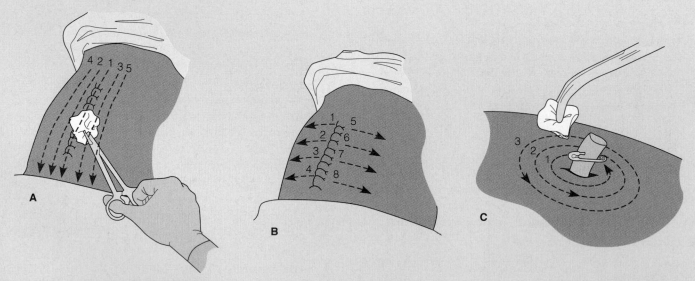

Figure 22-9. ◆ Methods of cleaning surgical wounds: **A.** Cleaning the wound from top to bottom, starting at the center. **B.** Cleaning a wound outward from the incision. **C.** Cleaning around a drain site. For all methods, a clean sterile swab is used for each stroke.

Chapter Review

Key Terms by Topics

Use the audio glossary feature of either the CD-ROM or the Companion Website to hear the correct pronunciation of the following key terms.

Introduction
surgery, perioperative period, diagnostic, palliative, ablative, reconstructive, transplant, emergency surgery, elective surgery

Preoperative phase
prostheses, antiemboli stockings, sequential compression device (SCD)

Intraoperative nursing care
anesthesia, conscious sedation

Postoperative Nursing Care
closed wound drainage system, sutures

Key Points

◆ Surgery is a unique experience that creates stress and necessitates physical and psychological changes. Factors such as age, general health, nutritional status, medication use, and mental status affect a client's risk during surgery.

◆ Clients must agree to surgery and sign an informed consent.

◆ Preoperative teaching should include moving, leg exercises, and coughing and deep-breathing exercises. Good postoperative teaching helps prevent postoperative complications.

◆ Physical preparation includes the following areas: nutrition and fluids, elimination, hygiene, rest, medications, care of valuables and prostheses, special orders, and surgical skin preparation.

◆ A preoperative checklist provides a guide to and documentation of a client's preparation before surgery.

◆ Initial and ongoing assessment of the postoperative client includes level of consciousness, vital signs, oxygen saturation, skin color and temperature, comfort, fluid balance, dressings, drains, and tubes.

◆ The overall goals of nursing care during the postoperative period are to promote comfort and healing, restore the highest possible level of wellness, and prevent associated risks such as infection or respiratory and cardiovascular complications.

◆ Surgical aseptic technique (sterile technique) is used when changing dressings on surgical wounds to promote healing and reduce the risk of infection. Sutures, wire clips, or staples are generally removed 7 to 10 days after surgery.

EXPLORE MediaLink

Additional interactive resources for this chapter can be found on the Companion Website at www.prenhall.com/ramont. Click on Chapter 22 and "Begin" to select the activities for this chapter.

For chapter-related NCLEX-style questions and an audio glossary, access the accompanying CD-ROM in this book.

Animation:
◆ Integumentary repair
◆ Lidocaine
◆ Morphine

For Further Study

For handling of client valuables prior to surgery, see discussion in Chapter 8 and Figure 8-2.

For information about assessing the return of peristalsis by auscultating the abdomen, see Chapter 11.

See Chapter 12 for in-depth discussion of stages of wound healing, information about wound drainage, cleaning wounds, wound irrigation, hot and cold applications, and supporting and immobilizing wounds.

For a more in-depth discussion of pain and pain management, see Chapter 15.

For client instructions on using the incentive spirometer, see Chapter 16.

For more information on use of sequential compression devices, see Chapter 16 and Procedure 16-5.

For more information about gastrointestinal tubes, see Chapter 17 and Procedure 17-3. For an illustration of an intake and output record, see Figure 17-5.

For illustration of leg exercises, see also Figures 20-12 and 20-28.

Critical Thinking Care Map

Caring for a Client with an Amputated Arm

NCLEX-PN Focus Area: Psychosocial Integrity: Coping and Adaptation

Case Study: Tim Broughton is a 22-year-old college student. Six days ago, he was involved in a motorcycle accident. After every attempt to save his right arm, amputation below the shoulder was performed 2 days ago.

Nursing Diagnosis: Disturbed Body Image

COLLECT DATA

Subjective	Objective

Would you report this data? Yes/No

If yes, to: _____

Nursing Care

_____
_____
_____
_____
_____
_____
_____
_____
_____
_____
_____
_____
_____

How would you document this? _____
_____
_____
_____
_____

Data Collected
(use those that apply)

- Vital signs stable
- Complains of pain
- Refuses to respond to nurse's questions about pain level
- Will not look at limb during dressing change
- "I wish I had died in the accident; life will never be the same."
- Dressing dry and intact
- Wound healing without signs of infection

Nursing Interventions
(use those that apply)

- Contact physician for social worker or psychologist referral
- Acknowledge denial, anger, or depression as normal.
- Teach the importance of range-of-motion exercises.
- Ask client to describe past experiences with pain and effectiveness of methods used to manage pain.
- Encourage client to make own decisions, participate in plan of care, and accept both inadequacies and strengths.
- Obtain assistive devices needed for activity.
- Allow client gradual exposure to body change.
- Help client to accept help from others.
- Teach family appropriate care of surgical site.

NCLEX-PN Exam Preparation

TEST-TAKING TIP

Remember the order of priority of AIRWAY, BREATHING and CIRCULATION!

1. Preoperative teaching is a vital part of nursing care. Good preoperative teaching:
   a. Shortens the length of hospitalization
   b. Facilitates the client's return to work and other activities of daily living
   c. Reduces postoperative pain
   d. Increases anxiety in the client

2. You are preparing clients for surgery. Several clients request that they be allowed to wear their wedding ring. Of the following, which client must remove the ring, rather than having it secured with tape?
   a. A 65-year-old male scheduled for a TURP (transurethral prostatectomy)
   b. A 31-year-old female having a repeat c-section
   c. A 72-year-old female having a total hip replacement
   d. A 49-year-old female scheduled for a left modified radical mastectomy

3. Postoperative assessments are usually made every 15 minutes until vital signs stabilize. Of the following, which client would require qh vital signs?
   a. Stable vital signs on the day of discharge
   b. Stable vital signs 3 hours postop
   c. Client with hypotension and depressed respirations 2 hours postop
   d. Temperature of 99.8° F second day postop

4. A client returns to the unit following surgery in which spinal anesthesia was administered. You need to give instructions to the nursing assistant about positioning the client. Of the following positions, which is the most appropriate for this client?
   a. Reverse Trendelenburg
   b. On his or her left side with head slightly elevated
   c. Flat for 8 to 12 hours
   d. Semi-Fowler's

5. You are teaching deep breathing and coughing to your client who is having surgery later today. Which of the following statements indicates the need for further teaching?
   a. "I will lie prone and flat while coughing to control pain."
   b. "I will hold a pillow against my abdomen during coughing."
   c. "After taking a deep breath, I will cough forcefully."
   d. "I will take a deep breath through my nose prior to coughing."

6. A postoperative client is complaining of pain. Of the following, which is the most accurate way to assess the severity of pain?
   a. Assess the client's vital signs.
   b. Ask the client if the pain is mild, moderate, or severe.
   c. Observe physiologic signs such as grimace or sweating.
   d. Ask the client to rate the pain using a scale of 0–10.

7. One day following surgery your client is to begin to ambulate. He asks, "Why can't I just stay in bed until I feel better?" Of the following, which would be the best response?
   a. "Your doctor has written an order for you to walk, and I must follow the doctor's orders."
   b. "If you walk to the chair, it will be easier to change the bed while you are up."
   c. "Walking is one of the best ways to prevent respiratory and circulatory complications."
   d. "You will never feel better if you just lie in bed."

8. You are preparing your client for surgery. Of the following assessment information, what needs to be reported to the physician immediately?
   a. Vital signs 98.8–84–20 BP 132/80
   b. The client reports he took his pills with sips of water before coming to the hospital.
   c. The client tells you he doesn't understand what they are going to do, and he is not sure he wants to go through with the surgery.
   d. The client is allergic to morphine sulfate.

9. Reflux of gastric contents into the vent lumen may occur when stomach pressure exceeds atmospheric pressure. In order to prevent this, you would:
   a. Clamp the vent tube and turn up the suction.
   b. Place the vent tubing higher than the client's stomach.
   c. Place the vent tube lower than the stomach.
   d. Irrigate the tube via the vent.

10. You are removing staples for an abdominal surgical incision. The wound opens and a portion of the intestine protrudes from the opening. You know this occurrence to be:
    a. Secondary intention
    b. Dehiscence
    c. Evisceration
    d. Granulation

Chapter 23

Client Teaching

SHARING experiences

"The first time I realized I wanted to be a nurse was when I was younger and I looked at my mom talking to the mother of a sick child. This mother was so concerned, and she seemed to put all her trust in my mother. And I want that. I want people to trust me to take care of them."

Briseida Ramirez, LVN Student, North Orange County Regional Occupational Program, Anaheim, CA.

LEARNING outcomes

After completing this chapter, you will be able to:
- Discuss the three main concepts of learning theory.
- Describe the three domains of learning.
- Identify factors that influence learning throughout life.
- Contrast the nursing process and teaching process.
- Identify the LVN's/LPN's role in client teaching.
- Describe essential aspects of a teaching plan.
- Identify effective teaching strategies.
- Discuss the challenges of teaching clients of different cultures.
- Identify methods to evaluate learning.
- Demonstrate effective documentation of teaching–learning activities.

MediaLink

www.prenhall.com/ramont

Use the address above to access the free, interactive Companion Website created for this textbook. Get hints, instant feedback, and textbook references to chapter-related NCLEX-style questions. Link to other interesting sites.

Audio Glossary:
Use the Companion Website, or the CD-ROM disk enclosed with your textbook, to hear the pronunciation of key terms in the chapter.

Client education is a major nursing responsibility—both legally and professionally. Legislation regarding nursing defines client teaching as an independent nursing function. In 1992, the American Hospital Association passed the Patients' Bill of Rights mandating client education as a right of all clients.

Learning

Client education is an integrated and multifaceted teaching–learning process in which the nurse and client work together to change unhealthy client behaviors. Client education is dynamic. Each participant communicates information, emotions, perceptions, and attitudes to the other. Areas for client education include health promotion, protection, and maintenance (Box 23-1 ◆).

Learning is a lifelong process of acquiring knowledge or skills that cannot be solely accounted for by human growth. This process is demonstrated by changes in behavior (see Box 23-2 ◆). Each client has unique learning needs regarding intellectual knowledge, skills, or behaviors.

An important aspect of learning is an individual's desire to learn and to act on the learning. In health care, **compliance** is the extent to which a person's behavior coincides with medical or health advice. Compliance is best demonstrated when the client embraces learning and then follows through with appropriate and expected behaviors. For example, a newly diagnosed client with diabetes would show compliance by willingly studying the special diet and then planning meals accordingly.

BOX 23-2
ATTRIBUTES OF LEARNING

Learning is:

- An experience that occurs inside the learner
- The discovery of the personal meaning and relevance of ideas
- A consequence of experience
- A collaborative and cooperative process
- An evolutionary process
- A process that is both intellectual and emotional

Nurses can use the following concepts about learners as a guide for teaching adult clients:

- As people mature, they move from dependence to independence. See Chapter 24. ◈
- An adult's previous experiences can be used as a resource for learning.
- An adult's readiness to learn is often related to a developmental task or social role.
- People are more oriented to learning when the material is useful immediately, not sometime in the future.

LEARNING THEORIES

The three main theories of human learning are behaviorism, cognitivism, and humanism.

BOX 23-1 AREAS FOR CLIENT EDUCATION

Promotion of Health

- Increasing a person's level of wellness
- Growth and development topics
- Fertility control
- Hygiene
- Nutrition
- Exercise
- Stress management
- Lifestyle modification
- Resources within the community

Prevention of Illness/Injury

- Health screening (e.g., blood glucose levels, blood pressure, blood cholesterol, Pap test, mammograms, vision, hearing, routine physical examinations)
- Reducing health risk factors (e.g., lowering cholesterol level)
- Specific protective health measures (e.g., immunizations, use of condoms, use of sunscreen, use of medication, umbilical cord care)

- First aid
- Safety (e.g., using seat belts, helmets, walkers)

Restoration of Health

- Information about tests, diagnosis, treatment, medications
- Self-care skills or skills needed to care for family member
- Resources within health care setting and community

Adapting to Altered Health and Function

- Adaptations in lifestyle
- Problem-solving skills
- Adaptation to changing health status
- Strategies to deal with current problems (e.g., home IV skills, medications, diet, activity limits, prostheses)
- Strategies to deal with future problems (e.g., fear of pain with terminal cancer, future surgeries, or treatments)
- Information about treatments and likely outcomes
- Referrals to other health care facilities or services
- Facilitation of strong self-image
- Grief and bereavement counseling

Behaviorism

Behaviorism is the belief that environment influences behavior, which is the essential factor determining human action. Edward Thorndike, who pioneered the twentieth-century behaviorist movement, asserted that learning should be based on the learner's behavior. B. F. Skinner introduced the importance of positive reinforcement to encourage a person to repeat desired action. Bandura claimed that most learning comes from observation and instruction rather than personal trial and error; so, most people imitate or model observed behavior. Imitation and modeling of healthy behaviors are key goals of client teaching.

Cognitivism

Cognitivism defines learning largely as a complex thinking process. The learner constantly structures and processes information from many sources. Cognitivists emphasize the importance of individual perception and motivation, as well as the teacher–learner relationship and environment. Developmental readiness and individual readiness (called client *motivation*) are other key factors.

J. Piaget and B. Bloom are important cognitive theorists. Bloom (1956) identified three *domains* (or areas) of learning: cognitive, affective, and psychomotor. The **cognitive domain** includes knowing, comprehending, and applying. The **affective domain** includes feelings, emotions, interests, attitudes, and appreciations. The **psychomotor domain** includes motor skills (such as giving an injection). Nurses should address each domain in client teaching. For example, a three-point teaching on colostomy care would include the following:

1. Demonstration of irrigation technique (*psychomotor* domain)
2. Discussion of safe fluid volume for irrigation (*cognitive* domain)
3. Discussion of the client's change in body image (*affective* domain)

Humanism

Humanism (humanistic learning theory) focuses on both cognitive and affective qualities of the learner. Leading humanists include Abraham Maslow and Carl Rogers. According to humanistic theory, each individual is a unique composite of biologic, psychologic, social, cultural, and spiritual factors. Learning focuses on self-development, achieving full potential, and learning what the person needs (what is relevant). Autonomy and self-determination are most important. Learning is self-motivated, self-initiated, and self-evaluated. So, the learner is an active participant in every phase of the teaching process.

APPLYING LEARNING THEORIES

Each mode of teaching has benefits and drawbacks. Behaviorism is useful but may be hard to apply to complex learning sit-

uations. It also may limit the learner's role in the teaching process. Cognitivism recognizes complex and multiple learning domains. However, it may not address external factors that are beyond the nurse's control. Humanism addresses the client's first interest (him- or herself), but this may inhibit the teacher's role in the process. See Table 23-1 ◆ for nursing applications of each mode of teaching.

FACTORS THAT FACILITATE LEARNING

Motivation

Motivation to learn is the desire to do so. It greatly influences how quickly and how much a person learns. Motivation is generally greatest when the client recognizes a need and believes he or she can meet it by learning. It is not enough for the need to be identified and verbalized by the nurse. The need must be experienced by the client. Often, the nurse's primary task in teaching is to help the client (or significant others) to recognize the need. For example, smokers with heart

TABLE 23-1	APPLICATION OF LEARNING THEORY
NURSING THEORY	**NURSING ACTIONS**
Behaviorism	• Encourage learner problem solving through trial and error. • Encourage repetitive practice and redemonstration. • Praise the learner and provide positive feedback. • Provide role models of desired behavior
Cognitivism	• Assess the learner's developmental capacity and readiness to learn. • Adapt teaching strategies accordingly. • Recognize the role of personality in selecting teaching methods to target different learning styles. • Recognize the role of perception in learning by using multisensory teaching methods. • Provide an environment conducive to learning. • Encourage a positive teacher–learner relationship.
Humanism	• Encourage self-directed and active learning by serving as a facilitator, resource, or mentor for the learner. • Encourage learners to establish and evaluate goals. • Expose the learner to relevant new information and ask appropriate questions to encourage fact seeking.

disease need to understand the effects of nicotine before they recognize the need to quit.

Readiness

Readiness to learn is the demonstration of behaviors or cues that reflect the learner's motivation to learn at a specific time. Readiness reflects not only desire or willingness but ability to learn at a given time. The nurse's role in teaching is to identify and develop client readiness. For example, a client may want to learn ostomy care, but postoperative pain or a change in body image may inhibit him. The nurse can provide pain medication and emotional support to enhance readiness.

Active Involvement

Active involvement in the learning process makes learning faster and more meaningful (Figure 23-1 ◆). It also improves **retention** (holding, keeping; in the case of learning, retention means active remembering). *Active learning* promotes critical thinking and strengthens problem-solving ability. *Passive learning* (listening to lectures or watching television, for example) is much less effective. For example, clients who are actively learning about their therapeutic diets may be more able to apply the principles being taught to their cultural food preferences and their usual eating habits.

Relevance

Relevance is importance or applicability. The knowledge or skill to be learned must be personally relevant to the learner. The client can learn more easily if he can connect the new knowledge to what he already possesses. For example, a morbidly obese patient may be more motivated to lose weight if he remembers having more energy when he weighed less. The

Figure 23-1. ◆ Learning is facilitated when the client is interested and actively involved.

nurse should emphasize and validate the relevance of learning throughout the teaching process.

Feedback

Feedback is shared information that relates a person's performance to the desired goal. Feedback must accompany the practice of psychomotor skills; it must be meaningful to help the person learn those skills. Praise, redirection, constructive criticism, and advice are ways of providing *positive feedback*. *Negative feedback,* such as ridicule, anger, or sarcasm, inhibits learning. Such feedback is viewed as a type of punishment and may cause clients to avoid the teacher.

Nonjudgmental Support

People learn best when they believe they are accepted and will not be judged. Clients who expect to be judged (especially as "poor" students) will not learn as well as those who feel respected and accepted. Once learners have succeeded in accomplishing a task or understanding an idea, they gain self-confidence in their ability to learn. Self-confidence increases motivation and reduces anxiety and fear of failure.

Simple to Complex

Material that is logically organized and proceeds from the simple to the complex is easiest to learn. Such organization enables the learner to comprehend and assimilate knowledge to promote new understanding. Simple and complex are relative terms, however. What is simple for one client may be complex for another.

Repetition

Repetitive practice of key facts and skills aids retention of newly introduced concepts. When combined with positive feedback from the nurse, repetition improves skill performance and the client's ability to apply this knowledge to other settings.

Timing

People retain concepts best when the time between initial learning and active use is short. As time between learning and practicing increases, retention decreases.

For example, if an asthmatic is prescribed an inhaler for PRN use and effectively demonstrates "practice" use one time, this does not mean that he or she may remember how to use it three weeks later during an episode.

Environment

Environmental factors affect learning. The optimal learning environment promotes physical and psychological comfort (see Chapter 20). ⊂⊃ It is well lit (including glare-free lighting), well ventilated, neither too hot nor too cold, and with a minimum of noise and other distractions. Privacy is essential to some kinds of learning, such as when discussing confidential issues or demonstrating techniques like perineal or ostomy care. Anxious or shy clients, however, may prefer to have a support person present. To ensure privacy, nurses should teach when visitors or other interruptions are unlikely.

FACTORS THAT INHIBIT LEARNING

Many internal and external factors can create barriers to the learning process (Table 23-2 ◆).

Emotions

Emotions such as fear, anxiety, anger, and depression can impede learning. Clients experiencing intense emotions are preoccupied and unable to concentrate on incoming messages. Fear and anxiety may be minimized by providing factual information to counteract uncertainty or irrational thoughts. Severely depressed clients may require psychiatric and/or drug therapy to increase motivation and participation in the teaching process.

Physiologic Events

Learning can be inhibited by physiologic events such as a critical illness, pain, or sensory deficits.

clinical ALERT

The nurse must identify and reduce physiologic barriers to learning before teaching. When a client cannot concentrate and apply energy to learning, the learning itself becomes impaired.

Cultural Barriers

Cultural barriers to learning include language and values. Foreign language is a common barrier. Western medicine may conflict with clients' native healing beliefs and cultural practices. For example, a client who comes from a culture that does not value slimness may have difficulty learning about a reducing diet. To be effective, the nurse should directly address such conflict. Support persons such as translators should be involved whenever there is a language barrier.

TABLE 23-2 BARRIERS TO LEARNING

BARRIER	EXPLANATION	NURSING IMPLICATIONS
Acute illness	Client requires all resources and energy to cope with illness.	Defer teaching until client is less ill.
Pain	Pain decreases ability to concentrate.	Deal with pain before teaching.
Prognosis	Client can be preoccupied with illness and unable to concentrate on new information.	Defer teaching to a better time.
Biorhythms	Mental and physical performances have a circadian (daily) rhythm.	Adapt time of teaching to suit client.
Emotion (e.g., anxiety, denial, depression, grief)	Emotions require energy and distract from learning.	Deal with emotions and possible misinformation first.
Language	Client may not be fluent in the nurse's language.	Obtain services of an interpreter or nurse with appropriate language skills.
Age Older adults Children	Vision, hearing, and motor control can be impaired in older adults. Children have a shorter attention span.	Consider sensory and motor deficits in teaching plan. Plan shorter and more active learning episodes.
Culture/Religion	There may be cultural or religious restrictions on certain types of knowledge, for example, birth control information.	Assess the client's cultural/religious needs when planning learning activities.
Physical disability	Visual, hearing, sensory, or motor impairments may interfere with a client's ability to learn.	Plan teaching activities appropriate to learner's physical abilities. For example, provide audio learning tools for visually impaired or reading-disabled clients.
Mental disability	Impaired cognitive ability may affect the client's capacity for learning.	Assess client's capacity for learning, and plan teaching activities to complement the client's ability while planning more complex learning for the client's caregivers.

Psychomotor Ability

It is important that the LPN/LVN be aware of a client's psychomotor skills when collaborating with the RN to develop a teaching plan or in cooperation with other disciplines such as Physical Therapy. The following physical abilities are important for learning psychomotor skills:

1. *Muscle strength.* For example, an elderly client who cannot rise from a chair because of insufficient leg and muscle strength cannot be expected to learn to lift herself out of a bathtub.

2. *Motor coordination. Gross motor coordination* (coordination of large muscle groups) is necessary for walking. For example, a client who has advanced amyotrophic lateral sclerosis (ALS) involving the lower limbs will probably be unable to use a walker. Likewise, fine motor coordination is needed when doing precise motions such as eating with a fork.

3. *Energy.* Learning psychomotor skills requires increased energy. The elderly and infirm often have limited energy resources, so practice sessions should be scheduled when the client's energy level is at its peak.

4. *Sensory acuity.* People depend on sight for most learning (e.g., walking with crutches, changing a dressing, drawing a medication into a syringe). Visually impaired clients often need assistance to carry out such tasks.

◆ Teaching

Teaching is a system of activities intended to produce specific learning. Individualized teaching emphasizes reducing health risks and taking specific action to increase the client's level of personal wellness (see Box 23-1).

The teaching process and the nursing process are much alike. Table 23-3 ◆ compares the two processes.

TEACHING CLIENTS AND THEIR FAMILIES

Nurses teach clients and their families in varied environments such as the home, a hospital, assisted living, or a long-term

Figure 23-2. ◆ Teaching activities may need to include hands-on client participation. *Source:* © Elena Dorfman.

care facility. Clients may be instructed in groups or in one-on-one sessions (Figure 23-2 ◆.) For example, a nurse may teach about diabetic foot care to several clients at once, or the nurse may teach privately about wound care while changing a client's dressing. Nurses are often responsible for teaching clients' spouses and other caregivers.

Despite time constraints caused by short hospital stays, nurses are expected to provide education that will ensure the client's safe transition from one level of care to another. Nurses must make appropriate plans for follow-up education in the client's home. Discharge plans must include documentation of all teaching before discharge, and the learning goals yet to be achieved. See Chapters 8 and 9 for more information about discharge and documentation. ∞

TEACHING IN THE COMMUNITY

Nurses often participate in community health education programs. Teaching may be voluntary, such as for the Red Cross, or it may be compensated employment, such as for a government

STEP	TEACHING PROCESS	NURSING PROCESS
1	Collect data; analyze client's learning strengths and deficits.	Collect data; analyze client's strengths and deficits.
2	Make educational diagnoses.	Make nursing diagnoses.
3	Prepare teaching plan: • Write learning objectives. • Select content and time frame. • Select teaching strategies.	Plan nursing goals/desired outcomes, and select interventions.
4	Implement teaching plan.	Implement nursing strategies.
5	Evaluate client learning based on achievement of learning objectives.	Evaluate client outcomes based on achievement of goal criteria.

TABLE 23-3 COMPARISON OF THE TEACHING PROCESS AND THE NURSING PROCESS

agency. Community teaching may be to large groups with a common interest in some aspect of health, such as nutrition, cardiopulmonary resuscitation (CPR), or bicycle and swimming safety. Community education programs can also be for small groups or individual learners, such as childbirth classes.

TEACHING HEALTH PERSONNEL

Nurses are responsible for supporting and maintaining the profession by teaching each other. In many facilities, nurses are required to present staff development sessions to colleagues. Experienced LPNs or LVNs may function as preceptors for new graduate LPNs/LVNs or for newly employed LPNs/LVNs. LPN/LVNs reinforce teaching begun by the clinical nurse specialist and other members of the health care team. In some settings the LPN/LVN is responsible for all client teaching.

NURSING CARE

◆ ASSESSING

Comprehensive assessment of learning needs incorporates data from the nursing history, physical assessment, and the client's support system. LPN/LVN observations are vital to the success of the overall assessment. Data collection should include information regarding all aspects of learning, including readiness, motivation, reading ability, and comprehension level. The nurse also comes to know the common learning needs that groups of people with similar health problems have. The LPN/LVN must be constantly aware of changes in the client's health status and report these observations as learning needs and health status change.

Several elements in the nursing history provide clues to learning needs:

◆ Age (and developmental status) dictate the choice of appropriate teaching strategies and health teaching content.

◆ Clients' perceptions of their current health problems and concerns may indicate knowledge deficits.

◆ A client's health beliefs and practices are always important to consider. Nurses must recognize that sometimes a client's health beliefs may interfere with healthful changes, and that it will not be possible to change that individual's core beliefs. Clients who do make changes usually believe they are personally at risk; they believe that the risk is serious; and they believe that changes in lifestyle will help to prevent the undesired outcome.

◆ The client's cultural group may have beliefs and practices related to diet, health, illness, and lifestyle. It is important to know how a client's practices and values affect their learning needs and their willingness to learn. Although clients may understand the health care information being taught, they may avoid it in the home where folk medical practices prevail. It is important to know whether any advice or treatments given by the doctor conflict with their values or beliefs. If they seek the advice of traditional healers, or use herbs or folk treatments, it is important to verify whether their medical doctor knows about these. For additional information, see Chapter 26, as well as the section on transcultural teaching later in this chapter. ⟨∞⟩

◆ Economic factors can affect a client's learning. For example, elderly clients with diabetes may not have enough money to buy a large supply of sterile insulin syringes. The concern about cost may make it hard for them to focus on learning to administer the insulin.

◆ Learning styles vary. Some people are *visual learners* and learn best by watching or reading text. *Auditory learners* learn best by verbal explanations. Many learn best through touch and feel (*haptic learners*), such as by manipulating equipment to discover how it works. Some learn best in groups. For others, thinking about a skill and its logic promotes learning. The nurse should ask clients how they prefer to learn and have learned best in the past. The nurse can also discover a client's learning style by varying activies and techniques when teaching.

◆ In the client's support system, there may be others who can assist the client's learning. Family members or close friends may help reinforce health teaching to maintain lifestyle changes at home.

The physical examination provides useful clues to the client's learning needs, such as mental status, energy level, and nutritional status. The exam provides data about the client's physical capacity (such as vision, hearing, and muscle strength) to learn and perform self-care. This information is vital in developing the teaching plan.

Readiness to Learn

A client who is ready to learn may seek information by asking questions and requesting reading materials. The client who is not yet ready is unlikely to demonstrate these behaviors and may even engage in avoidance behavior. For example, the nurse may ask, "When would you like me to show you how to inject insulin?" and the client might respond, "Oh, my wife will take care of everything."

The nurse assesses for the following:

◆ *Physical readiness.* Is the client in pain, fatigued, or immobile? If so, the client may not be ready.

◆ *Emotional readiness.* Is the client motivated toward self-care? Clients who are anxious, depressed, or grieving over their health status are not ready.

◆ *Cognitive readiness.* What is the client's level of consciousness? Is disease (such as stroke) affecting the client's cognition? Are drugs affecting the client's judgment or concentration? If so, the client may not yet be ready to learn.

Nurses can promote learning readiness by providing physical and emotional support during the critical stage of recovery. As the client stabilizes physically and emotionally, the nurse can provide opportunities to learn.

MOTIVATION

As discussed earlier, motivation is usually greatest when the client is ready, the learning need is recognized, and the information being offered is meaningful (relevant) to the client.

Nurses can increase a client's motivation by:

- Relating the learning to something the client values
- Creating a welcoming, nonthreatening learning environment in which the client is likely to succeed
- Encouraging autonomy and independence
- Demonstrating a positive attitude about the client's ability to learn
- Offering positive reinforcement and emotional support during the learning process

Reading Level

The nurse should not assume that a client's reading level is equal to the level of formal education achieved. Nurses should ask clients about their reading proficiency. However, clients with literacy problems may be reluctant to discuss the issue. Reading materials for clients with low literacy should be at the eighth grade level (or lower).

 DIAGNOSING, PLANNING, and IMPLEMENTING

There are three basic NANDA-approved nursing diagnoses that directly relate to the learning process: Deficient Knowledge, Health-Seeking Behavior, and Noncompliance. These diagnoses are used when a client's learning needs are the primary concern.

Whenever the diagnostic label Deficient Knowledge is used, either the client is seeking health information or the nurse has identified a learning need. An example of this would be: *Deficient Knowledge: Low-Calorie Diet* related to inexperience with newly ordered therapy.

When the diagnostic label Health Seeking Behavior is used, the client is seeking health-related information. This diagnosis is especially appropriate for clients attending community health education programs. A sample NANDA label would be: *Health Seeking Behavior: Exercise and Activity* related to desire to improve health behaviors and decrease risk of heart disease.

Whenever the diagnostic label Noncompliance is used, factors are present that prevent the person from following advice given by health professionals.

clinical ALERT

The diagnosis Noncompliance must be used with caution, because failure to follow health care advice is not always the result of an unwilling attitude.

Noncompliance, as a nursing diagnosis, is associated with the desire to comply, but the inability to do so because of intervening factors (Carpenito, 1997, p.575). Intervening factors include communication barriers and financial limitations. A sample diagnosis is: *Noncompliance: Hygienic Colostomy Care* related to insufficient funds to purchase necessary supplies.

A teaching plan is developed, using information collected during the nursing history and physical assessment, as well as observations from the LPN/LVN. Involving the client in this process is essential. Involved clients are more motivated and are more likely to achieve learning goals.

Determining Teaching Priorities

In the initial planning phase, the client and nurse collaborate to prioritize learning needs. For example, a client with heart disease may not be ready to learn about other lifestyle changes until she satisfies her need to learn how "to make food taste good without adding salt." Nurses can also use theoretical frameworks, such as Maslow's hierarchy of needs (see Figure 4-4), to establish priorities. ⛓

Setting Learning Objectives

Learning objectives are equivalent to desired outcomes for other nursing diagnoses. They are written in the same way. Like client outcomes, learning objectives would do the following:

1. State the client (learner) behavior or performance, not nurse behavior. For example, "Will identify personal risk factors for heart disease" (*client behavior*), not "Teach the client about cardiac risk factors" (*nurse behavior*).
2. Reflect an observable, measurable activity. The performance may be visible (e.g., walking) or invisible (e.g., adding a column of figures). The performance of an objective might be written: "Selects low-fat foods from a menu" (observable), not "understands low-fat diet" (unobservable). Verbs used for learning objectives would include such things as "defines, describes, identifies, selects," and so on. Outcomes would avoid words like "knows, understands, believes, and appreciates." They are neither observable nor measurable.
3. Use modifiers as required to clarify what, where, when, or how the behavior will be performed. For example, "Irrigates colostomy independently as taught" tells how the client does the task.
4. Specify the time by which learning should have occurred. For example, "The client will state three things that affect blood sugar level by end of second class on diabetes."

Learning objectives can reflect the learner's command of simple to complex concepts. For example, the learning objective "The client will list cardiac risk factors" simply requires the learner to identify all cardiac risk factors. In contrast, the learning objective "The client will list *personal* cardiac risk factors" requires that the learner learn how general cardiac risk factors apply to his or her own behaviors.

Choosing Content

The content of teaching is determined by learning objectives. For instance, "Identify appropriate sites for insulin injection" means the nurse must include content about the body sites suitable for insulin injections. Nurses can select among many sources of information including books, nursing journals, and other nurses and physicians. Whatever sources the nurse chooses, content should be:

◆ Accurate
◆ Current
◆ Based on learning goals (outcomes)
◆ Adjusted for the learner's age, culture, and ability
◆ Consistent with information the nurse is teaching
◆ Selected with consideration of how much time and what resources are available for teaching

Selecting Teaching Strategies

The method of teaching that the nurse chooses should be suited to the individual, to the material to be learned, and to the teacher (Figure 23-3 ◆). For example, the person who cannot read needs to have material presented in other ways. The best strategy for teaching how to give an injection is not lecturing but demonstration. Teachers who lead group sessions should be poised, confident, and skilled at group facilitation. People who are visually oriented should be taught with visual aids. See Table 23-4 ◆ for selected teaching strategies.

Ordering Learning Experiences

To conserve nursing resources, some health agencies have developed their own teaching guides. These guides feature standardized content and teaching methods that all staff nurses are expected to use when teaching. Standardized teaching plans are convenient. These guides ensure consistent content for the learner, and they reduce the confusion that might occur when

Figure 23-3. ◆ Teaching materials and strategies should be suited to the client's age and learning abilities.

more than one teacher is involved. Consistency of content is key, whether the nurse develops an original teaching plan or uses a standardized format. For example, when teaching multistep procedures (like ostomy care) the nurse should repeat the steps in the same sequence, without altering the order. If possible, the nurse should use the same brands and types of equipment the client will be using at home. Instructions for the nurse in client teaching are provided in Box 23-3 ◆.

The nurse needs to be flexible in implementing any teaching plan because the plan may need revising. The client may tire sooner than anticipated or be faced with too much information too quickly.

clinical ALERT

Report
The LPV/LVN should report any changes in the client's physical or psychosocial condition that might require alteration in the teaching plan.

The client's needs may change. External factors may intervene. For example, the nurse and the client may have planned for the client to self-irrigate his colostomy at 10 A.M., but when the time comes, he wants more information before actually doing it himself. In this case, the nurse would discuss the desired information, provide written information, and defer teaching until the next day. The LPN/LVN would collaborate with the team leader and document accordingly. (See Table 23-2 for barriers to learning.)

Implementing Client Education

When structuring client teaching sessions, the nurse should keep the following eight principles in mind:

1. **The optimal time for each session depends largely on the learner.** Whenever possible, ask the client for help to choose the best time, for example, when they feel most rested or when no other activities are scheduled.
2. **The pace of teaching affects learning.** A very rapid pace may confuse or frustrate the learner. When the pace is too slow, the client may become bored and distracted. (Loss of interest may also indicate that the client is fatigued.)
3. **Position and location affect learning.** Most people associate their bed with rest and sleep, not with learning. A client who is shown a videotape while in bed is more likely to become drowsy during instruction than a client who is sitting in a bedside chair.
4. **Teaching aids foster learning and attentiveness.** When selecting teaching aids, the nurse should choose identical products (such as ostomy pouches) to those the client will be using. When planning audiovisual presentations, the nurse should ensure that all equipment is functioning well before starting the session. Teaching aids should be appropriate to the client's developmental level (see Figure 23-3). For example, some anatomical models may contain tiny plastic parts that pose a choking hazard to young children.

TABLE 23-4	SELECTED TEACHING STRATEGIES	
STRATEGY	MAJOR TYPE OF LEARNING	CHARACTERISTICS
Explanation or description (e.g., lecture)	Cognitive	Teacher controls content and pace. Learner is passive; therefore retains less information than when actively participating. Feedback is determined by teacher. May be given to individual or group.
One-to-one discussion	Affective, cognitive	Encourages participation by learner. Permits reinforcement and repetition at learner's level. Permits introduction of sensitive subjects.
Answering questions	Cognitive	Teacher controls most of content and pace. Teacher must understand question and what it means to learner. Learner may need to overcome cultural perception that asking questions is impolite and may embarrass the teacher. Can be used with individuals and groups. Teacher should confirm personal responses by asking the learner, "Does that answer your question?"
Demonstration	Psychomotor	Often used with explanation. Can be used with individuals, small or large groups. Does not permit use of equipment by learners; learner is passive.
Discovery	Cognitive, affective	Teacher guides problem-solving situation. Learner is active participant; retention of information is high.
Group discussions	Affective, cognitive	Group members assist and learn from each other. Teacher needs to keep the discussion focused and prevent monopolization by one or two learners.
Practice	Psychomotor	Allows repetition and immediate feedback. Permits hands-on experience.
Printed and audiovisual materials	Cognitive	Forms include books, pamphlets, films, programmed instruction, and computer learning. Learners can proceed at their own speed. Nurse can act as resource person, need not be present during learning. Potentially ineffective if reading level is too high. Teacher needs to select language that meets learner needs if English is a second language.
Role-playing	Affective, cognitive	Permits expression of attitudes, values, and emotions. Can assist in development of communication skills. Involves active participation by learner. Teacher must create supportive, safe environment for learners to minimize anxiety.
Modeling	Affective, psychomotor	Nurse sets example by attitude, psychomotor skill.
Computer-assisted learning programs	All types of learning	Learner is active. Learner controls pace. Provides immediate reinforcement and review. Use with individuals or groups.

Box 23-4 ◆ lists teaching tools that are specifically useful for children.

5. **Learning is more effective through self-directed activity.** The nurse can encourage independent learning by enabling the client to explore alternative sources of information. If the client chooses, the nurse may provide a list of related health topics to research.

6. **Repetition reinforces learning.** Summarizing content, rephrasing (using other words), and approaching the material from another point of view are ways of repeating and clarifying content. For instance, after discussing the kinds of foods that can be included in a diet, the nurse describes the foods again, but in the context of the three meals eaten during one day.

BOX 23-3
NURSING CARE CHECKLIST

GENERAL TEACHING AND CLIENT TEACHING

General Teaching Guidelines

☑ **All teaching should be individualized.** If certain activities do not assist the learner, the nurse should make adaptations. For example, explanation alone may not be able to teach a client to handle a syringe. Actually handling the syringe may be more effective.

☑ **When the learner is involved in planning, the desire to learn is increased.**

☑ **Rapport between teacher and learner is essential.** The nurse should take time to establish rapport before teaching.

☑ **Teaching should build upon the client's existing knowledge base.** For example, a person who already knows how to cook can use this knowledge when learning to prepare food for a special diet.

☑ **Communication must be clear, concise, and mutually understood.** For example, a client may understand the terms "damp" and "wet" to have very different meanings. So, when the nurse says, "Don't get the abdominal incision wet," the client may immediately understand that he may not shower or bathe, but may think that wiping the incision with a damp wash cloth is allowed. The nurse should explain that no water or moisture should touch the incision.

☑ **Teaching that involves a number of the learner's senses often enhances learning.** For example, when teaching about changing a surgical dressing, the nurse can tell the client about the procedure (hearing), show how to change the dressing (sight), and show how to manipulate the equipment (touch).

☑ **Goal-setting (determining learning objectives and outcomes) must be appropriate to the client's lifestyle and resources.** For example, it would be unreasonable to expect a woman to soak in a tub of hot water four times a day if she did not have a bathtub or hot running water.

Client Teaching Guidelines

☑ **Discover the client's knowledge or skill level.** Ask questions or have the client complete a written form, such as a pretest.

☑ **Identify fear, anxiety, or other barriers to learning. Address the source of anxieties before beginning to teach.** For example, a client's spouse may be reluctant to learn tracheostomy care due to fear of suffocating the client during suctioning.

☑ **Begin with relevant information in an area of client readiness.** For example, an adolescent may want to know how he may continue to play football before he can learn how to administer insulin to himself.

☑ **Teach the basics first.** Make sure the client demonstrates understanding of a procedure before you teach variations or give information on special circumstances or "trouble-shooting." For example, when teaching a client to insert a retention catheter, explain the basic procedure in its entirety before discussing what to do if the catheter fails to drain properly.

☑ **Plan to review.** Schedule time to clarify content and to answer any questions the learner(s) may have.

---

7. **Organize the material; connect new information to what the client has already learned.** For example, "You understand how urine flows down a catheter from the bladder. Now I will show you how to push fluid up the catheter to rinse the bladder."

8. **Always use simple language.** If possible, eliminate medical jargon. Even common terms like urine and feces may be unfamiliar to clients. Avoid common abbreviations such as RR (recovery room) or CAD (coronary artery disease).

Teaching Strategies. Nurses can choose from a number of special teaching strategies. Any strategy the nurse selects must be appropriate for the learner and the learning goals.

Client Contracting. A learning contract with a client specifies certain objectives and when they are to be met. Here is an example of a self-contract:

I, Amy Martin, will jog for 20 minutes three times per week for a period of 2 weeks and will then buy myself six yellow roses.

Amy Martin
July 30, 2006

The contract, drawn up and signed by the client and the nurse, should specify learning objectives, responsibilities of the client and the nurse, and the methods of follow-up and evaluation. The learning contract allows for freedom, mutual respect, and mutual responsibility. Contracts may be revised when the client chooses to set new goals.

Group Teaching. Group instruction is economical, and it provides members with an opportunity to share and learn from others. A small group allows for discussion in which everyone can participate. A large group often requires a lecture

POPULATION FOCUS

TEACHING TOOLS FOR CHILDREN

◆ **Visits**. Visiting the hospital and treatment rooms; seeing people dressed in uniforms, scrub suits, protective gear.

◆ **Dress-up**. Touching and dressing up in the clothing they will see and wear.

◆ **Coloring books**. Using coloring books to prepare for treatments, surgery, or hospitalization; shows what rooms, people, and equipment will look like.

◆ **Storybooks**. Storybooks describe how the child will feel, what will be done, and what the place will look like. Parents can read these stories to children several times before the experience. Younger children like this repetition.

◆ **Dolls**. Practicing procedures on dolls or teddy bears that they will later experience; gives a sense of mastery of the situation. Custom dolls are often available for inserting tubes and giving injections, for example.

◆ **Puppet play**. Puppets can be used in role-play situations to provide information and show the child what the experience will be like; they help the child express emotions.

◆ **Health fairs**. Health fairs can educate children about their bodies and ways to stay healthy. Fairs can focus on high-risk problems children face, such as accident prevention, poison control, and other topics identified in the community as a concern.

technique or use of films, videos, slides, or role-playing by teachers. All members involved in group instruction should have a common need (e.g., prenatal health or preoperative instruction). It is also important to consider sociocultural factors when forming a group (see Chapter 26). ⮔

Computer-Assisted Instruction (CAI). Computer-assisted instruction is constantly advancing. Now, computers can be used to teach:

◆ Complex problem-solving skills
◆ Application of information
◆ Psychomotor skills

"Virtual reality" programs and video clips can allow the client to "see" how the heart pumps blood or how nerves send messages to the brain. Learning is becoming increasingly visual.

Discovery/Problem Solving. In using the discovery/problem-solving technique, the nurse presents some initial information and then asks the learners a question or presents a situation related to the information. The learner applies the new information to the situation and decides what to do. Learners can work alone or in groups. This technique is well suited to family learning. The teacher guides the learners through the

thinking process to reach the best solution or the best action to take in the situation. For example, the nurse-educator might present information on diabetes and glucose management. Then the nurse might ask the learners how they think their insulin and diet should be adjusted if their morning glucose was too low. In this way, clients learn what critical components they need to consider to reach the best solution to the problem.

Behavior Modification. Behaviorists believe that (a) human behaviors are learned and can be selectively strengthened, weakened, eliminated, or replaced and (b) a person's behavior is under conscious control. **Behavior modification** is a system of positive reinforcement in which desirable behavior is regarded and undesirable behavior is ignored. For example, clients trying to quit smoking are not criticized when they smoke, but they are praised or rewarded when they go without a cigarette for a certain period of time. The effectiveness of a behavior modification plan may be increased by including a client contract. The contract outlines the behavior modification plan and lists specific rewards.

Transcultural Teaching. When nurse and client come from different ethnic or cultural backgrounds, natural communication barriers may exist. These barriers include language, differing concepts of time, or cultural beliefs and practices that may influence compliance with client teaching and health care. See Chapter 26 for more information on culturally competent nursing. ⮔ Guidelines for teaching clients from other ethnic or cultural groups are listed in Box 23-5 ◆.

The nurse should treat the client's cultural healing beliefs with respect and try to identify whether they are in agreement or in conflict with what is being taught. The nurse can then focus on the ones in agreement to promote the integration of new learning with familiar health practices. The client will need an explanation of why certain folk healing practices are harmful, and how the recommended health practices will improve health.

◆ EVALUATING

Evaluating Learning

Evaluation is both an ongoing and a final process in which the client, the LPN/LVN in collaboration with the RN, and often the support people determine what has been learned. Learning is measured against the learning goals that were selected in the planning phase. For example, the objective "Selects foods that are low in carbohydrates" can be evaluated by asking the client to name such foods or to select low-carbohydrate foods from a list.

The best method for evaluating depends on the type of learning (cognitive, psychomotor, or affective). For cognitive learning, the client demonstrates the acquired knowledge. The client might:

◆ Select the solution to a problem using the new knowledge
◆ Take written tests

BOX 23-5

POPULATION FOCUS

TRANSCULTURAL TEACHING GUIDELINES

◆ **Enlist the aid of a translator when necessary.**

◆ **Obtain foreign language teaching materials.** The translator can assist by reading the materials to the nurse and can assist the nurse with adaptations of the material.

◆ **Use visual aids.** Many pictures, charts, and diagrams have universal meaning. Videos can allow the client to observe a skill or procedure, despite a language barrier. Audiovisual materials in which English is spoken slowly and clearly can benefit a client who may be learning English.

◆ **Use clear, simple language.** Avoid long sentences and big words. Use concrete rather than abstract terms. Avoid medical jargon.

◆ **Avoid slang or colloquialisms.** The client may think you mean these literally.

◆ **Present only one idea at a time.**

◆ **Phrase questions positively.** For example, it is much better to say, "Do you understand how far you may bend your hip after surgery?" is a much better question than to say, "You don't know how far you may bend your hip, do you?"

◆ **Validate verbal communication in writing.** This is especially important if understanding the client's speech is a problem. For example, during an assessment, write down numbers or phrases and have the client read them to verify accuracy.

◆ **Use humor very cautiously.** Meaning can change in the translation process.

◆ **Specifically invite the client to ask questions or request help.** In some cultures, expressing a need is not appropriate. Expressing confusion or asking to be shown something again may be considered rude. Some clients may feel that asking questions or stating a lack of understanding may cause the nurse to "lose face."

◆ **Confirm nonverbal cues.** A client who nods, uses eye contact, or smiles may not really understand what is being taught. In some cultures these signals are merely indicators of respect.

◆ **Identify cultural gender issues.** When explaining procedures or functioning related to personal areas of the body, it may be appropriate to have a nurse of the same sex do the teaching. Because of modesty concerns, and cultural taboos about male–female interaction, it is wise to have a female nurse teach a female client about personal care, birth control, sexually transmitted diseases, and other potentially sensitive areas. If a translator is

needed during explanation of procedures or teaching, the translator should also be female.

◆ **Include the family in planning and teaching.** This promotes trust and mutual respect. Identify the authoritative family member and incorporate that person into the planning and teaching to promote compliance and support of health teaching. In some cultures, the male head of household is the critical family member to include in health teaching; in other cultures, it is the eldest female member.

◆ **Consider the client's time orientation**. The client may be oriented to the past, present, future, or a combination of these. Cultures with a predominant orientation to the present include the Mexican American, Navajo Native American, Appalachian, Eskimo, and Filipino American cultures. Preventing future problems may be less significant for these clients, so teaching prevention may be difficult. For example, teaching a client why and when to take medications may be more difficult if the client is oriented to the present. In such instances, the nurse can emphasize preventing short-term problems. Schedules tend to be very flexible in present-oriented societies. Failure to keep clinic appointments or to arrive on time is common in clients who have a present-time orientation. The nurse can help by arranging transportation and by accommodating these clients when they do come rather than rescheduling an appointment that they probably will not keep. Teaching clients to take medications at bedtime or with a meal does not necessarily mean that these activities will occur at the same time each day. For this reason, the nurse should assess the client's daily routine before teaching the client to pair a treatment or medication with a daily event. When teaching a client when to take medication, the nurse should determine whether a clock or watch is available to the client and whether the client can tell time.

◆ **Identify cultural health practices and beliefs**. Noncompliance with health teaching may be related to conflict with folk medicine beliefs. Noncompliance may also be related to lack of understanding or fatalism, a belief system in which life events are held to be predestined or fixed in advance and the individual is powerless to change them. To encourage compliance, the nurse may need to involve the client in learning about the causes and preventability of certain disorders.

◆ Respond to oral questioning (e.g., restate information or give correct responses to questions)

◆ Self-report and self-monitor during follow-up phone calls, home visits, or computer-assisted instruction

For psychomotor skills, evaluation is best done by observing how well the client carries out a procedure such as changing a dressing.

Affective learning is more difficult to evaluate. The nurse may listen to the client's responses to questions, note how the client speaks about relevant subjects, and observe the client's behavior that expresses feelings and values. For example, have parents learned to value health enough to have their children immunized?

Following evaluation, teaching may have to be modified or repeated. Follow-up teaching in the home or by phone may be needed.

Behavior change does not always take place immediately. Often, individuals accept change intellectually first and then change their behavior only periodically (for example, a person who knows that she must lose weight may diet and exercise off and on).

If the new behavior is to replace the old behavior, it must emerge gradually; otherwise, the old behavior may prevail. The nurse can support behavior change by anticipating client vacillation and by providing encouragement.

Evaluating Teaching

It is important for nurses to evaluate their own teaching and the content of the teaching program, just as they evaluate the effectiveness of nursing interventions for other nursing diagnoses. Evaluation should include all aspects of teaching, including timing, teaching strategies, content quality, and so on. The nurse may find, for example, that the client was excited about understanding how to control her diabetes and was motivated to learn more.

Both the client and the nurse should evaluate the learning experience. The client should be asked for detailed feedback. Feedback questionnaires and videotapes of the learning sessions can be helpful.

The nurse should not feel ineffective as a teacher if the client forgets some of what is taught. Forgetting is normal and should be anticipated. Having the client write down information, repeating it during teaching, giving handouts on the information, and having the client be active in the learning process all promote retention.

Documenting

Documentation of the teaching process is essential. Charting provides a legal record that the teaching occurred, and it communicates the teaching to other health professionals. If teaching is not documented, legally it did not occur.

Responses to teaching should always be documented. What did the client or support person say or do to indicate that learning occurred? Has the client demonstrated mastery of a skill or the acquisition of knowledge? Such documented responses provide evidence of learning. Many agencies have multiple-copy client teaching forms that include the medical and nursing diagnoses, the treatment plan, and the client education (see Figure 8-4). 🔗 After the teaching session is completed, the client and the nurse sign the form and a copy of the form is given to the client to reinforce content and provide a record of the teaching. A second copy of the completed and signed form is placed in the client's chart.

Key aspects of the teaching process to be documented in the client record include:

- Diagnosed learning needs
- Learning objectives
- Topics taught
- Client outcomes
- Need for additional teaching
- Resources provided

The nurse's written teaching plan should include:

- Actual information and skills taught
- Teaching strategies used
- Time framework and content for each class
- Teaching outcomes and methods of evaluation

Nursing Process Case Study:
CLIENT WITH LACERATION

Kevin Brewer is a 24-year-old male college student admitted to the ER with a 7-cm (2.5-in) laceration on the left lower anterior leg, which occurred during a hockey game. The laceration was cleaned, sutured, and bandaged. The client was given an appointment to return to the health clinic in 10 days for suture removal. Client states that he lives in the college dormitory and is able to care for the wound if given instructions. Client states he is able to read and understand English.

Assessment. Mr. Brewer complains of a pain level of 5 related to the laceration to his left leg. Stated pain at a level of 1, 35 minutes after administration of prn pain medication. Client is able to ambulate with a slow, steady gait. His roommate is on his way to the ER to drive the client home.

Diagnosis. The current nursing diagnosis for Mr. Brewer is: Deficient Knowledge related to wound care.

Expected Outcomes. The expected outcomes specify that Mr. Brewer will:

- Be able to describe signs and symptoms of wound infection
- Respond to questions regarding wound care and perform return demonstration of wound cleansing and bandaging
- Identify equipment needed for wound care
- Describe appropriate action if complications arise
- Identify date, time, and location of follow-up appointment for suture removal

Planning and Implementation. The following nursing interventions are planned and implemented:

- Instruct client on what to look for regarding signs and symptoms of wound infection and appropriate action to take if complications arise.
- Demonstrate wound cleansing and bandaging, and allow time for a return demonstration by the client.

◆ Lay out equipment needed for wound care in front of client and encourage client to handle and become familiar with equipment.

◆ Provide written instructions for all implementations to client.

◆ Provide an appointment card for client with details for date, time, and location of suture removal appointment.

Evaluation. After teaching session, Mr. Brewer was able to fulfill all expected outcomes without difficulty.

Critical Thinking in the Nursing Process

1. Why is it necessary for Mr. Brewer to be able to identify the signs and symptoms of wound infection?
2. Why is it important for Mr. Brewer to be able to give a return demonstration of wound care?
3. Why should Mr. Brewer be allowed to handle the equipment needed for wound care?

Note: The bibliography listings for this and all chapters have been compiled at the back of the book)

Chapter Review

🔊))) Key Terms by Topics

Use the audio glossary feature of either the CD-ROM or the Companion Website to hear the correct pronunciation of the following key terms.

Learning
client education, learning, compliance, behaviorism, cognitivism, cognitive domain, affective domain, psychomotor domain, humanism, motivation, readiness, retention, relevance, feedback

Teaching
teaching, behavior modification

Key Points

* Teaching clients and families about their health needs is a major role of the nurse.

* Learning is represented by a change in behavior.

* Three main theories of learning are behaviorism, cognitivism, and humanism.

* There are three learning domains: cognitive, affective, and psychomotor.

* Factors to facilitate learning include: motivation, readiness, active involvement, relevance, feedback, nonjudgmental support, repetition, timing, environment, and progression from simple to complex concepts.

* Factors such as emotions, certain physiologic events, psychomotor deficits, and cultural barriers may impede learning.

* Learning objectives guide the content of the teaching plan and are written in terms of client or learner behavior.

* Teaching strategies should be suited to the client, the material to be learned, and the teacher. They should be adjusted to the client's developmental level and health status.

* Teaching methods and materials must be adapted for clients who are illiterate, elderly, or from different cultural backgrounds.

* Documentation of client teaching is essential to communicate the teaching to other health professionals and to provide a record for legal and accreditation purposes.

EXPLORE MediaLink

Additional interactive resources for this chapter can be found on the Companion Website at www.prenhall.com/ramont. Click on Chapter 23 and "Begin" to select the activities for this chapter.

For chapter-related NCLEX-Style questions and an audio glossary, access the accompanying CD-ROM in this book.

Animations:
* Video: dry powdered inhaler
* Video: metered dose inhaler
* Video: peak flow meter

🔗 For Further Study

For Maslow's hierarchy of needs, see Figure 4-4.

For more information on documentation of client teaching, see Chapter 8 and Figure 8-4.

For documentation methods and guidelines, see Chapter 9.

For environmental considerations, see Chapter 20.

Further steps to improve culturally competent nursing are discussed in Chapter 26.

For growth and developmental issues as they affect clients, see Chapter 24.

Critical Care Thinking Map

Caring for a Client with Deficient Knowledge

NCLEX-PN Focus Area: Physiological Integrity

Case Study: Mrs. Yorty, 59, is an African-American bank vice president who is heavily relied on by her boss and coworkers. Three days ago she was admitted to the hospital with complaints of shortness of breath and mild chest pain. A diagnostic evaluation indicates that she has significant coronary artery disease but has not yet suffered a heart attack. Her physician indicated that Mrs. Yorty will need to make significant lifestyle changes to reduce her heart attack risk. Mrs. Yorty states that she rests a lot after work so she doesn't overwork her heart.

Nursing Diagnosis: Deficient Knowledge

COLLECT DATA

Subjective	Objective

Would you report this data? Yes/No

If yes, to: _____

Nursing Care

_____
_____
_____
_____
_____
_____
_____
_____
_____
_____
_____

How would you document this? _____
_____
_____
_____
_____

Data Collected

(use those that apply)

- Weight 180 lbs
- Height 5'1"
- Blood pressure 140/100
- Pulse 80
- Temperature 98.5
- Blood oxygen level 98%
- Lung sounds clear bilaterally
- Complains of shortness of breath on mild exertion
- Complains of occasional mild chest pain
- States she rests a lot after work so she doesn't overwork her heart
- States she has smoked 1 pack of cigarettes a day for 25 years

Nursing Interventions

(use those that apply)

- Encourage client to make dietary changes. Stress importance of cutting back on fat, especially saturated fats which may help reduce cholesterol
- Encourage client to eat a well-balanced diet with at least five servings of fruits and vegetables a day.
- Obtain a physician's order for the client to meet with the hospital dietitian.
- Explain to client that physical activity can reduce her risk of heart attack. However, her doctor will prescribe how much activity she may do based on the severity of her coronary artery disease.
- Explain to client that smoking is a major risk factor and that by quitting she can significantly cut her risk of a heart attack.
- Instruct client that she will die of a heart attack if she doesn't stop smoking.

NCLEX-PN Exam Preparation

1. The health educator asks you to use Bandura's modeling theory to teach an infant care class for teenage parents. Which of the following methods would be most appropriate?

   a. Lecture, video, and handouts
   b. Demonstration, return demonstration
   c. Rewarding the participants for a good job
   d. Reading material and paper and pencil tests

2. Information about tests, diagnosis, treatment, and medications would be covered in which area of client teaching?

   a. Promotion of Health
   b. Prevention of Illness/Injury
   c. Restoration of Health
   d. Adapting to Altered Health and Function

3. Your client is scheduled for her first meeting with the physical therapist for mobility training following TKR. When you administer pain medication prior to the session, the client's family asks why. Your best response is:

   a. "The next dose is due during the time physical therapy is scheduled. I don't want to interrupt them."
   b. "The medication will take effect, so she will be able to rest following therapy."
   c. "Your mother wants medication, so I need to give it to her."
   d. "Pain decreases ability to concentrate, so the pain needs to be controlled before teaching begins."

4. You have just told your outpatient surgical client not to get the incision wet until after his follow-up visit. Which statement demonstrates a need for more instruction?

   a. "I will not take a shower until I see the doctor."
   b. "I will only wipe the area with a damp wash cloth daily."
   c. "I will be careful not to get the area wet while washing."
   d. "The dressing should be kept clean and dry until I see the doctor."

5. You have been teaching your client self administration of insulin. The first two times, she prepared the injection correctly. This morning she states, "I can't do it. How will I be able to take care of myself at home?" Of the following, which is the most appropriate nursing diagnosis?

   a. Powerlessness related to a perceived lack of control.
   b. Deficient Knowledge related to disease process.
   c. Ineffective Therapeutic Regimen Management related to difficulty in modifying personal habits.
   d. Risk for Injury related to deficient sensory perception

6. An elderly Vietnamese client does not maintain eye contact during discharge instructions. The nurse should interpret this behavior to mean that:

   a. She does not understand the instructions.
   b. She is not interested in what is being said.
   c. She may feel eye contact is a sign of disrespect.
   d. She prefers that the instructions be given by the physician.

7. You are assigned to teach a group of 4- and 5-year-olds about the Food Pyramid. Using your understanding of appropriate client teaching, which method would you select for this group?

   a. Lecture and printed handouts
   b. Plastic foods to be placed appropriately on the pyramid
   c. The "Hungry Caterpillar" story, plus a puppet and colorful pyramid and foods
   d. Cooking class using food from each group

8. An elderly man with dementia lives with family who work full time. You are assigned to do a safety assessment of the client to ascertain if he can be alone during the daytime. Which statement demonstrates an understanding of your report by the family?

   a. "We will tell him not to cook while we're out."
   b. "There is a list of emergency numbers by the phone."
   c. "We will be looking into a senior day care center where Dad can stay during our work hours."
   d. "Dad has always been so independent, I can't bear to see him this way."

9. Feedback is necessary for successful learning to take place. Feedback can be positive or negative. Negative feedback:

   a. is viewed as punishment and may cause clients to avoid the teacher.
   b. is a way of getting the client's attention and works well in some instances.
   c. can be used if presented in a joking manner.
   d. is a form of behavioral modification.

10. An elderly client is being discharged from the hospital. The client is alert, but she has a mild hearing loss. Her husband has cataracts. The daughter is parking the car. You wish to complete discharge so you can take your scheduled lunch. What is the most appropriate procedure for administering discharge instructions?

    a. Begin the instruction, since the client is alert.
    b. Wait for the daughter, so they all can be instructed at the same time.
    c. Write out the instructions for the daughter.
    d. Since the husband's hearing is intact and the client is able to read, provide an explanation accompanied with written Instructions.

Answers for Review Questions, as well as discussion of Case Study and Critical Care Thinking Map questions, appear in Appendix IV.

You are a newly graduated LPN assigned to a medical–surgical unit. You have been assigned to three clients.

Mr. Ramos is a 58-year-old male who was admitted for a prostatectomy (TURP) this morning. He is predominantly Spanish speaking, though he knows a few words of English and understands a little if he is spoken to slowly. He has returned from surgery. Initially, he was sedated but begins to be more alert. He appears agitated and is yelling loudly at his roommate, who puts on his call light to summon the nurse. The roommate states, "Mr. Ramos is trying to climb out of bed and he is frightening me."

Mr. Drew is a 53-year-old male who was admitted directly from his physician's office with chest pain. His BP is 168/90 with tachycardia (heart rate 102). He is diaphoretic and is complaining of nausea.

Mr. Melezack is a 64-year-old male who had a colon resection 3 days ago. His NG tube has been clamped and he has been started on clear liquids. It was reported that he tolerated them well. The doctor has ordered that the tube can be removed if there is no nausea or vomiting.

TIME MANAGEMENT

You have received report. Using your knowledge of the three clients' diagnoses and present needs, prioritize your care for the shift.

CRITICAL THINKING

Mr. Drew's lab work has come back. You observe that his CPK values are within normal limits and that his chest pain is relieved with sublingual nitroglycerin spray. He will be discharged in the morning, and you are to begin his discharge planning. In your teaching plan, state what activities would decrease the chance of recurrent angina and the risk factors that need to be controlled to decrease effects of heart disease.

COMPASSIONATE CARING

Mr. Ramos is frightening his roommate and trying to climb out of bed. He has an IV line and a three-way catheter, which is draining dark red urine with clots. Outline the steps you would take to protect Mr. Ramos from himself and to relieve the concerns of the roommate.

COMMUNICATION AND TEAM BUILDING

The client care assistant reports to you that Mr. Melezack is complaining of abdominal pain. He has vomited and asks to see you right away. After you go to his room to assess his present status, you will need to document and report your findings to the appropriate individuals. Write a medical record entry, using the focus charting method. State what information needs to be reported and to whom.

UNIT

IV

Promoting Psychosocial Health

Chapter 24 ▸ Life Span Development

Chapter 25 ▸ Client Communication

Chapter 26 ▸ Delivering Culturally Competent Care

Chapter 27 ▸ Sensory Perception

Chapter 28 ▸ Self-Concept

Chapter 29 ▸ Sexuality

Chapter 30 ▸ Stress and Coping

Chapter 31 ▸ Loss, Grieving, and Death

Chapter 24

Life Span Development

SHARING experiences

"While in clinicals for my LPN, I [worked at] a hospital that had a psych unit on the eighth floor. I was assigned to care for an elderly woman, who was post CVA [stroke], on the sixth floor Med/Surg unit. She kept saying, "A man is walking outside my window!" I brought this to the attention of the staff RN, who chuckled and informed me that [this was] a delusional "after effect" of the CVA. After I had tried without success to convince the woman that we were six floors up and that she did not have a man outside her window, I went to the window and opened the curtain. I looked and then went to the staff RN and told her that I [had not had] a CVA but I did see a man outside the window. It took 10 minutes to convince her to look for herself. As it turned out, a male client from the psych ward had opened a window and climbed down as far as the sixth floor ledge [before] he became stuck! . . . That was the day I learned one of the most valuable lessons in nursing. No matter what clients may be telling you, never assume that they are "delusional." When in doubt, check it out."

Mark S. Reef, LPN, BSN, RN, Howard Community Hospital, Kokomo, IN.

LEARNING outcomes

After completing this chapter, you will be able to:
- Differentiate growth from development.
- List factors that influence growth and development.
- Describe significant characteristics and nursing implications of stages of growth and development from infancy through old age.
- Trace stages of psychosocial development according to Erikson.
- Explain Piaget's phases of cognitive development.
- Describe moral development according to Kohlberg.
- Describe spiritual development according to Fowler.
- Describe usual physical development through the life span.
- Identify characteristic tasks of different stages of development.
- Identify selected health problems associated with young, middle-aged and older adults.
- Identify health assessment and health promotion activities from birth through older adult.
- List examples of health-promotion topics from young adulthood through old adulthood.

MediaLink

www.prenhall.com/ramon

Use the address above to access the free, interactive Companion Website created for this textbook. Get hints, instant feedback, and textbook references to chapter-related NCLEX-style questions. Link to other interesting sites.

Audio Glossary:
Use the Companion Website, or the CD-ROM disk enclosed with your textbook, to hear the pronunciation of key terms in the chapter.

Often used interchangeably, the terms *growth* and *development* have different meanings. **Growth** refers to physical change and increase in size. Indicators of growth include height, weight, bone size, and dentition. While the pattern of physiologic growth is similar for all people, growth rates vary during different stages of growth and development. For example, the growth rate is rapid during the prenatal, neonatal, infancy, and adolescent stages, but slows during childhood, and is minimal during adulthood.

Development is an increase in the complexity of function and skill progression. It refers to the person's capacity and skill to adapt to the environment. Development is the behavioral aspect of growth which includes the ability to walk, to talk, and to run.

◆ Processes of Growth and Development

Growth and development take place in an organized way, although it does not progress at the same rate with all individuals.

- *Cephalocaudally*—from the head down or literally from head (cephalo) to tail (caudal) (e.g., the infant gains head control before control of extremities)
- *Proximal to distal*—from the midline of the body to the extremities (e.g., the infant rolls over before grasp is perfected)
- *General to specific* (e.g., walking is learned before running or skipping)

Growth and development are independent, interrelated processes. For example, an infant's muscles, bones, and nervous system must grow to a certain point before the infant can sit up or walk. Growth generally takes place during the first 20 years of life; development continues after that. Principles of growth and development are described in Box 24-1 ◆.

The factors that influence growth and development are genetic and environmental. The genetic inheritance of an individual is established at conception. It remains unchanged throughout life and determines such characteristics as sex, physical stature, and race. Environmental factors include family, religion, climate, culture, school, community, and nutrition. For example, poorly nourished children are more likely to have infections than are well-fed children and may not attain their full height potential.

RELATIONSHIP BETWEEN GROWTH AND DEVELOPMENT

The rate of a person's growth and development is highly individual. However, the sequence of growth and development is predictable. Stages of growth usually correspond to certain developmental changes, as shown in Table 24-1 ◆.

Growth and development are commonly thought of as having five major components:

- **Physiologic** (relating to physical processes in the human body)
- **Psychosocial** (pertaining to the relationship between oneself and others)
- **Cognitive** (having to do with awareness of and interaction between oneself and the environment)
- **Moral** (relating to judgments of right or wrong

BOX 24-1 PRINCIPLES OF GROWTH AND DEVELOPMENT

- Growth and development are continuous, orderly, sequential processes influenced by maturational, environmental, and genetic factors.
- All humans follow the same pattern of growth and development.
- The sequence of each stage is predictable, although the time of onset, the length of the stage, and the effects of each stage vary with the person.
- Learning can either help or hinder the maturational process, depending on what is learned.
- Each developmental stage has its own characteristics.
- Growth and development occur in a cephalocaudal direction. They start at the head and move to the trunk, legs, and feet. This pattern is particularly obvious at birth, when the head of the infant is disproportionately large.
- Growth and development occur from the center of the body outward. For example, infants can roll over before they can grasp an object with the thumb and second finger.
- Development proceeds from simple to complex, or from single acts to integrated acts. To drink and swallow from

a cup, for example, the child must first learn eye–hand coordination, grasping, hand–mouth coordination, controlled tipping of the cup, and then mouth, lip, and tongue movements to drink and swallow.
- Development becomes increasingly differentiated. Differentiated development begins with a generalized response and progresses to a skilled specific response. For example, an infant's initial response to a stimulus involves the total body; a 5-year-old child can respond more specifically with laughter or fear.
- Certain stages of growth and development are more critical than others. It is known that the first 10 to 12 weeks after conception are critical. The incidence of congenital anomalies as a result of exposure to certain viruses, chemicals, or drugs is greater during this stage than others.
- The pace of growth and development is uneven. Asynchronous development is demonstrated by rapid growth of the head during infancy and of the extremities at puberty.

TABLE 24-1	STAGES OF GROWTH AND DEVELOPMENT		
STAGE	**AGE**	**SIGNIFICANT CHARACTERISTICS**	**NURSING IMPLICATIONS**
Neonatal	Birth–28 days	Behavior is largely reflexive and develops to more purposeful behavior.	Assist parents to identify and meet unmet needs.
Infancy	1 month–1 year	Physical growth is rapid.	Control the infant's environment so that physical and psychologic needs are met.
Toddlerhood	1–3 years	Motor development permits increased physical autonomy. Psychosocial skills increase.	Safety and risk-taking strategies must be balanced to permit growth.
Preschool	3–6 years	The preschooler's world is expanding. New experiences and the preschooler's social role are tried during play. Physical growth is slower.	Provide opportunities for play and social activity.
School age	6–12 years	Stage includes the preadolescent period (10 to 12 years). Peer group increasingly influences behavior. Physical, cognitive, and social development increases, and communication skills improve.	Allow time and energy for the school-age child to pursue hobbies and school activities. Recognize and support child's achievement.
Adolescence	12–20 years	Self-concept changes with biologic development. Values are tested. Physical growth accelerates. Stress increases, especially in face of conflicts.	Assist adolescents to develop coping behaviors. Help adolescents develop strategies for resolving conflicts.
Young adulthood	20–40 years	A personal lifestyle develops. Person establishes a relationship with a significant other and a commitment to something.	Accept adult's chosen lifestyle and assist with necessary adjustments relating to health. Recognize the person's commitments. Support change as necessary for health.
Middle adulthood	40–65 years	Lifestyle changes due to other changes; for example, children leave home, occupational goals change.	Assist clients to plan for anticipated changes in life, to recognize the risk factors related to health, and to focus on strengths rather than weaknesses.
Older adulthood Young-old	65–74 years	Adaptation to retirement and changing physical abilities is often necessary. Chronic illness may develop.	Assist clients to keep physically and socially active and to maintain peer group interactions.
Middle-old	75–84 years	Adaptation to decline in speed of movement, reaction time, and sensory abilities and increasing dependence on others may be necessary.	Assist clients to cope with loss (e.g., hearing, eyesight, death of loved one). Provide necessary safety measures.
Old-old	85 and over	Increasing physical problems may develop.	Assist clients with self-care as required, and with maintaining as much independence as possible.

◆ **spiritual** (pertaining to relationship with God or a Higher Power).

A knowledge of growth and development is essential for nurses if they are to identify developmental needs and problems and participate in health assessment and promotion. Growth and development encompass the prenatal period and the life span: from the neonate to older adult including the physical, psychosocial, cognitive, moral, and spiritual aspects of each life stage.

 Conception and Prenatal Development

Prenatal or intrauterine development lasts approximately 38 to 40 weeks. Traditionally, pregnancy has been divided into three periods, called *trimesters*, each of which lasts about 3 months. Each trimester includes certain landmarks for developmental changes in the mother and the fetus. There are two phases of intrauterine life: embryonic and fetal.

The *embryonic phase* is the period during which the fertilized ovum develops into an organism with most of the features of the human. This period takes place during the first trimester of pregnancy. During the first 3 weeks:

1. The embryo is implanted.
2. Tissues differentiate into three layers. From these layers all of the body's complex organs and systems are formed.
3. Placental function starts. Its functions are to exchange nutrients and gases between the embryo or fetus and the mother.
4. The fetal membranes differentiate.

The fetal phase of development is characterized by a period of rapid growth in the size of the fetus. Both genetic and environmental factors affect its growth.

At the end of the second trimester, the fetus resembles a small baby. The skin appears wrinkled, red, and transparent. A protective covering (called *vernix caseosa*) begins to develop over the skin. This is a white cheeselike substance that adheres to the skin. *Lanugo*, a fine downy hair, also covers the body. At about 5 months, the mother first perceives movement by the fetus, and the first fetal heartbeat may be heard.

At the end of the third trimester the fetus has developed to approximately 20 inches and 7.0 to 7.5 pounds. The lanugo has disappeared, and the skin is a more normal color and appears less wrinkled. The last 2 months in utero are largely devoted to accumulating weight.

◆ Neonates and Infants (Birth to 1 Year)

Babies are considered neonates from birth to the end of 1 month. Infants are babies from 1 month of age to 1 year.

PHYSICAL DEVELOPMENT

An infant's basic task is survival, which requires breathing, sleeping, sucking, eating, swallowing, digesting, and eliminating. Infants undergo significant physiologic change in these areas: weight, length, head growth, vision, and motor development.

Weight

Just after birth, most infants lose 5 to 10 percent of their birth weight because of fluid loss. This weight loss is normal, and infants usually regain that weight in about 1 week. Usual weight gain is 5 to 7 ounces weekly for 6 months. By 5 months of age infants usually reach twice their birth weight, and by age 12 months, three times their birth weight.

Length

The average length of a newborn is about 20 inches. Two recumbent lengths are measured (Figure 24-1 ◆): the crown-to-rump length (the sitting length), which is approximately the same as the head circumference, and the head-to-heel length (from the top of the head to the base of the heels). By

Figure 24-1. ◆ Measuring an infant head to heel, from the top of the head to the base of the heels. *Source:* © Elena Dorfman.

12 months, the infant's length increases by approximately one half of the birth length.

Head and Chest Circumference

Assessment of head circumference is of particular importance in infants and children to determine the growth rate of the skull and the brain. An infant's head should be measured at every visit to the physician or nurse until the child is 2 years old (Figure 24-2 ◆).

Normal head circumference (*normocephaly*) is often related to chest circumference. The chest circumference of the newborn is usually less than the head circumference. As the infant grows, the chest circumference becomes larger than the head circumference.

Head Molding

The heads of most newborn babies are misshapen because of the molding of the head that occurs during vaginal deliveries. Molding of the head is made possible by **fontanelles** (unossified membranous gaps) in the bone structure of the skull and by overriding of the sutures (junction lines of the skull bones). Within a week, a newborn's head usually regains its symmetry. The posterior fontanelle closes from 4 to 8 weeks after birth.

Figure 24-2. ◆ An infant's head circumference is measured around the skull, above the eyebrows. *Source:* © Elena Dorfman.

MediaLink Growth Chart Birth—36 months

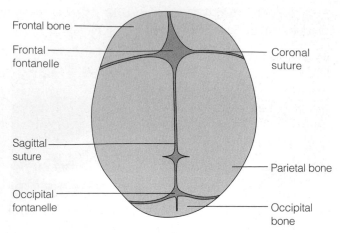

Figure 24-3. ◆ The bones of the skull, showing the fontanelles and the suture lines.

The larger anterior fontanelle, which is diamond-shaped, closes between 9 and 18 months (Figure 24-3 ◆).

Sensory Abilities

VISION. The newborn can follow large moving objects and blinks in response to bright light.

- The newborn eyes cannot focus on close objects.
- At 4 months, the infant can recognize familiar objects and follow moving ones.
- At 6 months, the infant can perceive colors.
- At 9 months, most can recognize facial characteristics and often smile in response to a familiar face.
- At 12 months, depth perception has developed.

HEARING

- Newborns with intact hearing will react with a startle to a loud noise. Newborn hearing screenings are now mandated prior to hospital discharge, in many locals. Computerized equipment makes this possible. Within a few days they can tell the difference between their mother's voice and that of another woman.
- At 5 months of age, the infant will pause while sucking in order to listen to the mother's voice.
- A 9-month-old infant is able to locate the source of sounds and recognizes familiar ones.
- At 1 year, the infant listens to sounds, begins to distinguish words, and responds to simple commands.

SMELL AND TASTE. The senses of smell and taste are functional shortly after birth. Newborns prefer sweet tastes and tend to decrease their sucking in response to liquids with a salty content. They are able to recognize the smell of their mother's milk and respond to this smell by turning toward the mother.

TOUCH. The sense of touch is well developed at birth. Skin-to-skin touching is important for an infant's development.

The infant responds positively to the warmth, love, and security it perceives when touched, held, and cuddled. The newborn is also sensitive to temperature extremes and pain; however, babies react diffusely and cannot isolate the discomfort.

REFLEXES. The **reflexes** of the newborn are unconscious, involuntary responses. They are neither learned nor consciously carried out; rather, they are nervous system responses to a number of stimuli. Box 24-2 ◆ describes infant reflexes.

Motor Abilities

Motor development is the development of the baby's abilities to move and to control the body (Figure 24-4 ◆). See Table 24-2 ◆ for examples of motor and social development in infants.

BOX 24-2
INFANT REFLEXES

- *Sucking reflex:* A feeding reflex that occurs when the infant's lips are touched. The reflex persists throughout infancy.
- *Rooting reflex:* A feeding reflex elicited by touching the baby's cheek, causing the baby's head to turn to the side that was touched. This reflex usually disappears after 4 months.
- *Moro reflex:* Often assessed to estimate the maturity of the central nervous system. A loud noise, a sudden change in position, or an abrupt jarring of the crib elicits this reflex. The infant reacts by extending both arms and legs outward with the fingers spread, then suddenly retracting the limbs. Often, the infant cries at the same time. This reflex disappears after 4 months.
- *Palmar grasp reflex:* Occurs when a small object is placed against the palm of the hand, causing the fingers to curl around it. This reflex disappears after 3 months.
- *Plantar reflex:* Similar to the palmar grasp reflex; an object placed just beneath the toes causes them to curl around it. This reflex disappears after 8 months.
- *Tonic neck reflex (TNR) or fencing reflex:* A postural reflex. When a baby who is lying on its back turns its head to the right side, for example, the left side of the body shows a flexing of the left arm and the left leg. This reflex disappears after 4 months.
- *Stepping reflex (walking or dancing reflex):* Can be elicited by holding the baby upright so that the feet touch a flat surface. The legs then move up and down as if the baby were walking. This reflex usually disappears at about 2 months.
- *Babinski reflex:* When the sole of the foot is stroked, the big toe rises and the other toes fan out. A newborn baby has a positive Babinski. After age 1, the infant exhibits a negative Babinski; that is, the toes curl downward. A positive Babinski after age 1 indicates brain damage.

Figure 24-4. ♦ An infant sits without support at 6 months of age.

PSYCHOSOCIAL DEVELOPMENT

Erikson described eight stages of development in humans (Table 24-3 ♦). According to Erikson, the central crisis at this stage is trust versus mistrust. Infants depend on the primary caregivers for all their physiologic and psychological needs. The newborn reacts socially to caregivers by paying attention to the face or voice and by cuddling when held. It is able to interact with the environment by responding to various stimuli such as touch and sound.

COGNITIVE DEVELOPMENT

According to Piaget, **cognitive development** is a result of interaction between an individual and the environment. Piaget identified stages and significant behaviors for different age groups (Table 24-4 ♦). Infants' initial period of cognitive development was named the sensorimotor phase.

MORAL DEVELOPMENT

Infants associate right and wrong with pleasure and pain. What gives them pleasure is right, since they are too young to reason otherwise. In later months and years, children can tell easily and quickly by changes in parental facial expressions and voice tones that their behavior is either approved or disapproved.

HEALTH ASSESSMENT AND PROMOTION

Nursing care of infants involves some specific tests. General care of infants and children in discussed under Nursing Care later in this chapter.

Apgar Scoring

Newborn babies can be assessed immediately by the Apgar scoring system. This provides a numeric indicator of the baby's physiologic capacities to adapt to extrauterine life. Apgar scoring is usually carried out 60 seconds after birth and is repeated in 5 minutes. Those with very low scores require special resuscitative measures and care. Apgar scoring is listed in Table 24-5 ♦.

During ongoing assessments, the nurse examines and observes the infant, taking into account variations that occur with developmental age and activity. Health promotion guidelines for infants, toddlers, and preschoolers are shown in Table 24-6 ♦.

Developmental Screening Tests

Development can be assessed by observing the infant's behavior and by using standardized tests such as the Denver Developmental Screening Test (DDST). The DDST is used to screen children from birth to 6 years of age. The test is intended to estimate the abilities of a child compared to those of an average group of children of the same age and ethnic group.

TABLE 24-2	EXAMPLES OF MOTOR AND SOCIAL DEVELOPMENT IN INFANCY	
AGE	MOTOR DEVELOPMENT	SOCIAL DEVELOPMENT
Newborn	Turns head from side to side when in a prone position Grasps by reflex when object is placed in palm of hand	Displays displeasure by crying and satisfaction by soft vocalizations Attends to adult face and voice by eye contact and quieting
6 months	Lifts chest and shoulders off table when prone, bearing weight on hands Manipulates small objects	Starts to imitate sounds Vocalizes one-syllable sounds:"ma ma,""da da"
9 months	Creeps and crawls Beginner pincer grasp with thumb and forefinger	Complies with simple verbal commands Displays fear of being left alone (e.g., going to bed) Waves "bye-bye"
12 months	Walks alone with help Uses spoon to feed self	Clings to mother in unfamiliar situations Demonstrates emotions such as anger and affection

TABLE 24-3	ERIKSON'S EIGHT STAGES OF DEVELOPMENT				
STAGE	AGE	CENTRAL TASK	INDICATORS OF POSITIVE RESOLUTION	INDICATORS OF NEGATIVE RESOLUTION
Infancy	Birth–18 months	Trust versus mistrust	Learning to trust others	Mistrust, withdrawal, estrangement
Early childhood	18 months– 3 years	Autonomy versus shame and doubt	Self-control without loss of self-esteem Ability to cooperate and to express oneself	Compulsive self-restraint or compliance Willfulness and defiance
Late childhood	3–5 years	Initiative versus guilt	Learning the degree to which assertiveness and purpose influence the environment Beginning ability to evaluate one's own behavior	Lack of self-confidence Pessimism, fear of wrongdoing Overcontrol and overrestriction of own activity
School age	6–12 years	Industry versus inferiority	Beginning to create, develop, and manipulate Developing sense of competence and perseverance	Loss of hope, sense of being mediocre Withdrawal from school and peers
Adolescence	12–20 years	Identity versus role confusion	Coherent sense of self Plans to actualize one's abilities	Feelings of confusion, indecisiveness, and possible antisocial behavior
Young adulthood	18–25 years	Intimacy versus isolation	Intimate relationship with another person Commitment to work and relationships	Impersonal relationships Avoidance of relationship, career, or lifestyle commitments
Adulthood	25–65 years	Generativity versus stagnation	Creativity, productivity, concern for others	Self-indulgence, self-concern, lack of interests and commitments
Maturity	65 years to death	Integrity versus despair	Acceptance of worth and uniqueness of one's own life Acceptance of death	Sense of loss, contempt for others

Source: From Childhood and society, 2nd., (pp. 247–274), by E. Erikson, 1963, New York: W. W. Norton. Copyright 1950, © 1963 by W. W. Norton & Company, Inc., renewed © 1978, 1991 by Erik H. Erikson. Reprinted by permission.

 ## Toddlers (1 to 3 Years)

Toddlers develop from having no voluntary control to being able to walk and speak. They also learn to control their bladder and bowels, and they acquire all kinds of information about their environment.

PHYSICAL DEVELOPMENT

Toddlers are usually chubby, with relatively short legs and a large head (Figure 24-5 ◆). The face appears small when compared to the skull. Toddlers have a pronounced lumbar lordosis and a protruding abdomen. The abdominal muscles develop gradually with growth, and the abdomen flattens.

Weight

Two-year-olds can be expected to weigh approximately four times their birth weight. The weight gain is about 5 lbs

Figure 24-5. ◆ The toddler appears chubby with relatively short legs and a large head. *Source:* © Michael Newman.

TABLE 24-4 PIAGET'S PHASES OF COGNITIVE DEVELOPMENT		
PHASES AND STAGES	AGE	SIGNIFICANT BEHAVIOR
Sensorimotor phase	Birth–2 years	
Stage 1 Use of reflexes	Birth–1 month	Most action is reflexive.
Stage 2 Primary circular reaction	1–4 months	Perception of events is centered on the body. Objects are extension of self.
Stage 3 Secondary circular reaction	4–8 months	Acknowledges the external environment. Actively makes changes in the environment.
Stage 4 Coordination of secondary schemata	8–12 months	Can distinguish a goal from a means of attaining it.
Stage 5 Tertiary circular reaction	12–18 months	Tries and discovers new goals and ways to attain goals. Rituals are important.
Stage 6 Inventions of new means	18–24 months	Interprets the environment by mental image. Uses make-believe and pretend play.
Preconceptual phase	2–4 years	Uses an egocentric approach to accommodate the demands of an environment. Everything is significant and relates to "me." Explores the environment. Language development is rapid. Associates words with objects.
Intuitive thought phase	4–7 years	Egocentric thinking diminishes. Thinks of one idea at a time. Includes others in the environment. Words express thoughts.
Concrete operations phase	7–11 years	Solves concrete problems. Begins to understand relationships such as size. Understands right and left. Cognizant of viewpoints.
Formal operations phase	11–15 years	Uses rational thinking. Reasoning is deductive and futuristic.

Source: From *The origin of intelligence in children,* by J. Piaget, 1966, International Universities Press, Inc., Copyright © 1966. Adapted with permission.

between 1 year and 2 years and about 2 to 5 lbs between 2 and 3 years.

Height
A toddler's height can be measured as height or length. Height is measured while the toddler stands, and length is measured while the toddler is in a recumbent position. Between ages 1 and 2 years, the average growth in height is 4 to 5 inches, and between 2 and 3 years it slows to 2½ to 3½ inches.

Head Circumference
The head circumference of the toddler increases about 1 inch on average. By 24 months, the head is 80 percent of the average adult size and the brain is 70 percent of its adult size.

Sensory Abilities
Visual acuity is fairly well established at 1 year; average estimates of acuity for the toddler are 20/70 at 18 months and 20/40 at 2 years of age. Accommodation to near and far objects is fairly well developed by 18 months and continues to mature with age. Hearing in the 3-year-old is at adult levels. The taste buds of the toddler are sensitive to the natural flavors of food, and the 3-year-old prefers familiar odors and tastes. Touch is a very important sense, and a distressed toddler is often soothed by tactile sensations.

Motor Abilities
Fine muscle coordination and gross motor skills improve during toddlerhood.

At 18 months, the child can:

TABLE 24-5	APGAR SCORING SYSTEM TO ASSESS THE NEWBORN		
	SCORE		
SIGN	0	1	2
1. Heart rate	Absent	Slow (below 100 per minute)	Above 100 per minute
2. Respirations	Absent	Slow, irregular	Regular rate, crying
3. Muscle tone	Flaccid	Some flexion of extremities	Active movements
4. Reflex irritability	None	Grimace	Cries
5. Color	Body pale or cyanotic	Body pink (for African-American babies, pink mucous membranes), extremities blue	Body completely pink, pink mucous membranes in African-American babies

◆ Pick up small beads and place them in a receptacle
◆ Hold a spoon and a cup
◆ Walk upstairs with assistance
◆ Crawl down the stairs

   At 2 years, toddlers can:

◆ Hold a spoon and put it into the mouth correctly
◆ Run(with steady gait)
◆ Balance on one foot
◆ Ride a tricycle

   By 3 years most children are toilet trained, with occasional night time accidents or when playing.

PSYCHOSOCIAL DEVELOPMENT

Toddlers begin to develop their sense of autonomy by asserting themselves with the frequent use of the word *no*. Parents need to have a great deal of patience coupled with an understanding of the importance of this developmental milestone. See Table 24-3 of the Erikson's stage for toddlers.

   Although toddlers like to explore the environment, they always need to have a significant person nearby. During the toddler stage, receptive and expressive language skills are developing quickly. Children can understand words and follow directions long before they can actually form them into sentences. By 1 year of age, toddlers can recognize their own names.

COGNITIVE DEVELOPMENT

According to Piaget, the toddler completes the fifth and sixth stages of the sensorimotor phase and starts the preconceptual phase at about 2 years of age (see Table 24-4).

MORAL DEVELOPMENT

Kohlberg established six stages of **moral development** (Table 24-7 ◆). According to Kohlberg, the first level of moral development is the preconventional when children respond to punishment and reward. During the second year of life, chil-dren begin to know that some activities elicit affection and approval.

SPIRITUAL DEVELOPMENT

Fowler theorized six stages of **spiritual development** (Table 24-8 ◆). According to Fowler, the toddler's stage of spiritual development is undifferentiated. Toddlers may be aware of some religious practices, but they are primarily involved in learning knowledge and emotional reactions rather than establishing spiritual beliefs. A toddler may repeat short prayers at bedtime, conforming to a ritual, because praise and affection result.

HEALTH ASSESSMENT AND PROMOTION

Assessment activities for the toddler are similar to those for the infant in terms of measuring weight, length (height), and vital signs. Promoting health and wellness includes such areas as accident prevention, toilet training, and good dental hygiene. See Table 24-6 for Health promotion guidelines. See also the Nursing Care section below.

 # Preschoolers (4 and 5 Years)

During the preschool period physical growth slows, but control of the body and coordination increase greatly.

PHYSICAL DEVELOPMENT

By the time children are 4 or 5 years old, they appear taller and thinner than toddlers. The preschooler's brain reaches almost its adult size by 5 years. The extremities of the body grow more quickly than the body trunk, making the child's body appear somewhat out of proportion.

Weight, Height, and Sensory Abilities

Weight gain in preschool children is generally slow. By 5 years they have added only another 7 to 12 lbs to their 3-year-

TABLE 24-6 HEALTH PROMOTION GUIDELINES FOR INFANTS, TODDLERS, AND PRESCHOOLERS

GUIDELINES	INFANTS	TODDLERS	PRESCHOOLERS
Health Examinations	At 2 weeks and at 2, 4, 6, and 12 months	At 15 and 18 months and then as recommended by the physician Dental visit starting at age 3 Hearing tests by 18 months or earlier	Every 1 to 2 years
Protective Measures	Immunizations: diphtheria–pertussis–tetanus (DPT), oral poliovirus vaccine (OPV), measles–mumps–rubella (MMR), *Haemophilus influenzae* type B, and hepatitis B and varicella vaccines as recommended (see Chapter 30) Fluoride supplements if there is inadequate water fluoridation (less than 0.7 parts per million [ppm]) Screening for tuberculosis Screening for phenylketonuria (PKU) Prompt attention for illnesses Appropriate skin hygiene and clothing	Immunizations: continuing DPT, OPV series, measles–mumps–rubella (MMR), *Haemophilus influenzae* type B, and hepatitis B vaccines as recommended Screenings for tuberculosis and lead poisoning Fluoride supplements if there is inadequate water fluoridation (less than 0.7 ppm)	Immunizations: continuing DPT, OPV series, measles–mumps–rubella (MMR) vaccine; other immunizations as recommended (see Chapter 30) Screening for tuberculosis Vision and hearing screening Regular dental screenings and fluoride treatment
Safety	Importance of supervision Car seat, crib, playpen, bath, and home environment safety measures Feeding measures (e.g., avoid propping bottle) Providing toys with no small parts or sharp edges	Importance of supervision and teaching child to obey commands Home environment safety measures (e.g., lock medicine cabinet) Outdoor safety measures (e.g., close supervision near water) Appropriate toys	Educating child about simple safety rules (e.g., crossing the street) Teaching child to play safely (e.g., bicycle and playground safety) Educating to prevent poisoning
Nutrition	Breast-feeding and bottle-feeding techniques Formula preparation Feeding schedule Introduction of solid foods Need for iron supplements at 4–6 months	Importance of nutritious meals and snacks Teaching simple mealtime manners Dental care	Importance of nutritious meals and snacks
Elimination	Characteristics and frequency of stool and urine elimination Diarrhea and its effects	Toilet training techniques	Teaching proper hygiene (e.g., washing hands after using bathroom)
Rest/Sleep	Usual sleep and rest patterns	Dealing with sleep disturbances	Dealing with sleep disturbances (e.g., nightmares)
Sensory Stimulation/Play	Touch: holding, cuddling, rocking Vision: colorful, moving toys Hearing: soothing voice tones, music, singing Play: toys appropriate for development	Providing adequate space and a variety of activities Toys that allow "acting on" behaviors and provide motor and sensory stimulation	Providing times for group play activities Teaching child simple games that require cooperation and interaction Providing toys and dress-ups for role-playing

TABLE 24-7 KOHLBERG'S STAGES OF MORAL DEVELOPMENT

LEVEL AND STAGE	DEFINITION	EXAMPLE
Level I Preconventional Stage 1: Punishment and obedience orientation Stage 2: Instrumental-relativist orientation	The activity is wrong if one is punished, and the activity is right if one is not punished. Action is taken to satisfy one's needs	A nurse follows a physician's order so as not to be fired. A client in hospital agrees to stay in bed if the nurse will buy the client a newspaper.
Level II Conventional Stage 3: Interpersonal concordance (good boy, nice girl) Stage 4: Law and order orientation	Action is taken to please another and gain approval. Right behavior is obeying the law and following the rules.	A nurse gives elderly clients in hospital sedatives at bedtime because the night nurse wants all clients to sleep at night. A nurse does not permit a worried client to phone home because hospital rules stipulate no phone calls after 9:00 PM.
Level III Postconventional Stage 5: Social contract, legalistic orientation Stage 6: Universal-ethical principals	Standard of behavior is based on adhering to laws that protect the welfare and rights of others. Personal values and opinions are recognized, and violating the rights of others is avoided. Universal moral principles are internalized. Person respects other humans and believes that relationships are based on mutual trust.	A nurse arranges for an East Indian client to have privacy for prayer each evening. A nurse become an advocate for a hospitalized client by reporting to the nursing supervisor a conversation in which a physician threatened to withhold assistance unless the client agreed to surgery.

Source: Adapted from R. Duska and M. Whelan, *Moral Development: A Guide to Piaget and Kohlberg.* Copyright 1975 by The Missionary Society of St. Paul the Apostle in the State of New York. Used by permission of Paulist Press.

TABLE 24-8 FOWLER'S STAGES OF SPIRITUAL DEVELOPMENT

STAGE	AGE	DESCRIPTION
0. Undifferentiated	0–3 years	Infant unable to formulate concepts about self or the environment
1. Intuitive–projective	4–6 years	A combination of images and beliefs given by trusted others, mixed with the child's own experience and imagination
2. Mythic–literal	7–12 years	Private world of fantasy and wonder; symbols refer to something specific; dramatic stories and myths used to communicate spiritual meanings
3. Synthetic–conventional	Adolescent or adult	World and ultimate environment structured by the expectations and judgments of others; interpersonal focus
4. Individuating–reflexive	After 18 years	Constructing one's own explicit system; high degree of self-consciousness
5. Paradoxical–consolidative	After 30 years	Awareness of truth from a variety of viewpoints
6. Universalizing	Maybe never	Becoming an incarnation of the principles of love and justice

Source: Data from J. Fowler and S. Keen, *Life maps: Conversations in the journey of faith* (Waco, TX: Word Books, 1985) and A. Hollander, *How to help your child have a spiritual life: A parents' guide to inner development* (New York: A & W Publishers, 1980).

old weight. Preschool children grow about 2.0 to 2.5 inches each year.

VISION. Preschool children are generally *hyperopic* (far-sighted), that is, unable to focus on near objects. By the end of the preschool years, visual ability has improved to approximately 20/30.

HEARING AND TASTE. The hearing of the preschool child has reached optimal levels, and the ability to listen (attending to and comprehending what is said) has matured since the toddler age. As for the sense of taste, preschoolers show their preferences by asking for something "yummy," and may refuse something they consider "yucky."

Motor Abilities

By 5 years of age, children are able to wash their hands and face and brush their teeth. They are self-conscious about exposing their bodies and go to the bathroom without telling others. Typically, preschool children run with increasing skill each year. By 5 years of age, they run skillfully and can jump three steps. Preschoolers can balance on their toes and dress themselves without assistance.

PSYCHOSOCIAL DEVELOPMENT

Erikson writes that the major developmental crisis of the preschooler is initiative versus guilt (see Table 24-3). Parents can enhance the self-concept of the preschooler by providing opportunities for new achievements where the child can learn, repeat, and master.

The self-concept of the preschooler is also based on gender identification. Preschoolers are aware of the two sexes and identify with the correct one. They may mimic the parent's behavior, attitudes, and appearance (Figure 24-6 ◆).

Preschool children gradually emerge as social beings. At the age of 3 or 4, they learn to play with a small number of their peers. They gradually learn to play with more people as they grow older. Preschoolers also learn about their feelings; they know the words *cry, sad,* and *laugh,* and the feelings related to them. They also begin to learn how to control their feelings and behavior. The preschooler uses the same types of coping mechanisms in response to stress as the toddler does, although protest behavior (kicking, screaming) is less likely to occur in the older preschooler.

COGNITIVE, MORAL, AND SPIRITUAL DEVELOPMENT

The preschooler's cognitive development, according to Piaget, is the phase of intuitive thought (see Table 24-4). Reading skills also start to develop at this age.

Preschoolers are capable of prosocial behavior, that is, any action that a person takes to benefit someone else. The term prosocial is synonymous with kind and connotes sharing, helping, protecting, giving aid, befriending, showing affection, and giving encouragement. Moral behavior to a preschooler may mean taking turns at play or sharing. It is

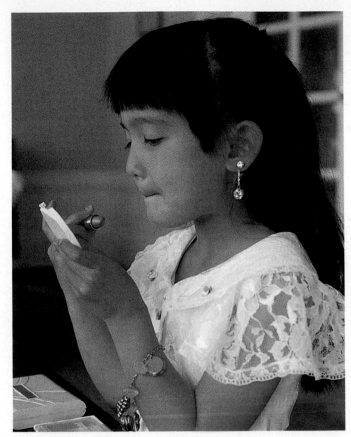

Figure 24-6. ◆ Preschoolers often identify with the parent of the same sex and like to mimic behavior. *Source:* © Elena Dorfman.

important for parents to answer preschoolers' "why" questions and discuss values with them (see Table 24-7).

Many preschoolers enroll in Sunday school or faith-oriented classes. The preschooler usually enjoys the social interaction of these classes (see Table 24-8). Faith at this stage is primarily a result of the teaching of significant others, such as parents and teachers.

HEALTH ASSESSMENT AND PROMOTION

During assessment, the preschooler can often participate in answering questions with assistance from parents or caregivers. Health promotion guidelines for the preschooler are shown in Table 24-6. Further information on nursing care is provided below.

◆ School-Age Children (6 to 12 Years)

The school-age period starts when children are about 6 years of age, when the deciduous teeth are shed. This period includes the preadolescent *(prepuberty)* period. It ends at about 12 years, with the onset of puberty. **Puberty** is the age when the reproductive organs become functional and secondary sex characteristics develop. See Chapter 29 for further discussion of sexuality and sexual development. ⊘⊙ In general, the period from 6 to 12 years is one of rapid and dramatic change.

PHYSICAL DEVELOPMENT

Weight, Height, and Sensory Abilities

The school-age child gains weight rapidly and thus appears less thin than previously. At 6 years boys tend to weigh about 2 lbs more than girls. The weight gain of school children from 6 to 12 years of age averages 7 lbs per year, but the major weight gains occur from age 10 to 12 for boys and from 9 to 12 for girls.

At 6 years both boys and girls are about the same height. Before puberty, children of both sexes have a growth spurt, girls between 10 and 12 years and boys between 12 and 14 years. Thus, girls may well be taller than boys at 12 years, but boys are usually stronger.

VISION. The depth and distance perception of children 6 to 8 years of age is accurate. By age 6 children have full binocular vision. The eye muscles are well developed and coordinated, and both eyes can focus on one object at the same time. 20/20 vision is usually well established between 9 and 11 years of age.

HEARING AND TOUCH. Auditory perception is fully developed in school-age children, who are able to identify fine differences in voices, both in sound and in pitch. At this stage, children also have a well-developed sense of touch and are able to locate points of heat and cold on all body surfaces. They are also able to identify an unseen object, such as a pencil or a book, simply by touch. This ability is called *stereognosis*.

Prepubertal Changes

Little change takes place in the reproductive and endocrine systems until the prepuberty period. During prepuberty, at about ages 9 to 13, endocrine functions slowly increase. This change in endocrine function can result in increased perspiration and more active sebaceous glands.

Motor Abilities

During the middle years (6 to 10), children perfect their muscular skills and coordination. By 9 years most children are becoming skilled in games of interest, such as football or baseball. These skills are often associated with school, and many of them are learned there. By 9 years most children have sufficient fine motor control for such activities as building models or sewing.

PSYCHOSOCIAL DEVELOPMENT

At this time children begin to create and develop a sense of competence and perseverance. School-age children are motivated by activities that provide a sense of worth. They concentrate on mastering skills that will help them function in the adult world (Figure 24-7 ◆; see also Table 24-3).

Figure 24-7. ◆ Expanding cognitive skills enable school-age children to interact cooperatively in activities of an increasingly complex nature, as shown by the children playing this board game. *Source:* © Jane Wattenburg.

As they grow older, schoolchildren learn to play with more children at one time. Usually, the 6- or 7-year-old is a member of a peer group. This group can be a greater influence than the family in teaching attitudes.

The schoolchild's self-concept continues to mature. Children recognize similarities and differences between themselves and others. School-age children compare themselves with others and obtain feedback from teachers and peers.

COGNITIVE, MORAL, AND SPIRITUAL DEVELOPMENT

According to Piaget, the ages 7 to 11 years mark the phase of concrete operations (see Table 24-4). During this stage the child changes from egocentric interactions to cooperative interactions.

Some school-age children are at Kohlberg's stage 1 of the preconventional level (punishment and obedience); that is, they act to avoid being punished. Some school-age children, however, are at stage 2 (instrumental-relativist orientation). These children do things to benefit themselves. Fairness (everyone getting a fair share or chance) becomes important (see Table 24-7).

According to Fowler, the school-age child is at stage 2 in spiritual development, the mythic–literal stage. Children learn to distinguish fantasy from fact. Spiritual facts are those beliefs that are accepted by a religious group. Parents and the minister, rabbi, or priest help the child distinguish fact from fantasy. These people still influence the child more than peers in spiritual matters. (see Table 24-8).

School-age children may ask many questions about God and religion in these years and will generally believe that God is good and always present to help. Just before puberty, children become aware that their prayers are not always answered and become disappointed.

HEALTH ASSESSMENT AND PROMOTION

During the assessment interview the nurse responds to questions from the parent or other caregiver, gives appropriate feedback, and lends encouragement and support. Promoting health and wellness includes dental hygiene and regular dental examinations, safety measures to prevent accidents, promoting physical fitness, supporting autonomy and self-esteem, and hygiene measures to prevent infections. See Table 24-9 ◆ for health promotion guidelines for school-age children and adolescents.

 ## Adolescents (12 to 18 years)

Adolescence is the period during which the person becomes physically and psychologically mature and acquires a personal identity. At the end of this critical period in development, the person is ready to enter adulthood and assume its responsibilities. Puberty is the first stage of adolescence in which sexual organs begin to grow and mature.

PHYSICAL DEVELOPMENT

Height, Weight, and Structure

During puberty, growth is markedly accelerated compared to the slow, steady growth of the child. This period, marked by sudden and dramatic physical changes, is referred to as the adolescent growth spurt. In boys, the growth spurt usually begins between ages 12 and 16; in girls, it begins earlier, usually between ages 10 and 14. Because the growth spurt begins earlier in girls, many girls surpass boys in height at this time.

Physical growth continues throughout adolescence. Growth is fastest for boys at about 14 years, and the maximum height is often reached at about 18 or 19 years. Some men add another 1 or 2 cm to their height during their 20s as the vertebral column gradually continues to grow. During the period

TABLE 24-9	HEALTH PROMOTION GUIDELINES FOR SCHOOL-AGE CHILDREN AND ADOLESCENTS	
GUIDELINES	SCHOOL-AGE CHILDREN	ADOLESCENTS
Health Examinations	Annual physical examination or as recommended	As recommended by the physician
Protective Measures	Immunizations as recommended Screening for tuberculosis Periodic vision, speech, and hearing screenings Regular dental screenings and fluoride treatment Providing accurate information about sexual issues (e.g., reproduction, AIDS)	Immunizations as recommended, such as adult tetanus–diphtheria (Td) vaccine and hepatitis B vaccine Screening for tuberculosis Periodic vision and hearing screenings Regular dental assessments Obtaining and providing accurate information about sexual issues
Safety	Using proper equipment when participating in sports and other physical activities (e.g., helmets, pads) Encouraging child to take responsibility for own safety (e.g., participating in bicycle and water safety courses)	Adolescent's taking responsibility for using motor vehicles safely (e.g., completing a driver's education course, wearing seat belt and helmet) Making certain that proper precautions are taken during all athletic activities (e.g., medical supervision, proper equipment) Parents' keeping lines of communication open and being alert to signs of substance abuse and emotional disturbances in the adolescent
Nutrition, Elimination, Exercise	Importance of child not skipping meals and eating a balanced diet Experiences with food that may lead to obesity Utilizing positive approaches for elimination problems (e.g., enuresis)	Importance of healthy snacks and appropriate patterns of food intake and exercise Factors that may lead to nutritional problems (e.g., obesity, anorexia nervosa, bulimia) Balancing sedentary activities with regular exercise
Play and Social Interactions	Providing opportunities for a variety of organized group activities Accepting realistic expectations of child's abilities Acting as role models in acceptance of other persons who may be different Providing a home environment that limits TV viewing and video games and encourages completion of homework	Encouraging adolescent to establish relationships that promote discussion of feelings, concerns, and fears Parents' encouraging adolescent peer group activities that promote appropriate moral and spiritual values Parents' acting as role models for appropriate social interactions Parents' providing a comfortable home environment for appropriate adolescent peer group activities

of 10 to 18 years of age, the average American male doubles his weight and grows about 16 inches.

Growth is noted first in the musculoskeletal system. This growth follows a sequential pattern: The head, hands, and feet are the first to grow to adult status. Next, the extremities reach their adult size. Because the extremities grow before the trunk, the adolescent looks leggy, awkward, and uncoordinated. After the trunk grows to full size, the shoulders, chest, and hips grow. Skull and facial bones also change proportions: The forehead becomes more prominent, and the jawbones develop.

Glandular Changes

The eccrine and apocrine glands increase their secretions and become fully functional during puberty.

Sexual Characteristics

During puberty, both primary and secondary sex characteristics develop. Primary sexual characteristics relate to the organs necessary for reproduction, such as the testes, penis, vagina, and uterus. Secondary sexual characteristics differentiate the male from the female but do not relate directly to reproduction. See discussion in Chapter 29. ⬭

The first noticeable sign that puberty has begun in males is the appearance of pubic hair. Sexual maturity is achieved by age 18.

Often, the first noticeable sign of puberty in females is the appearance of the breast bud, although the appearance of hair along the labia may precede this. The milestone of female puberty is the *menarche* (beginning of menstrual cycles), which occurs about 2 years after the breast bud appears. At first, menstrual periods are scanty and irregular and may occur without ovulation. Ovulation is usually established 1 to 2 years after menarche. Female internal reproductive organs reach adult size about age 18 to 20.

PSYCHOSOCIAL DEVELOPMENT

The psychosocial task of the adolescent is the establishment of identity. The danger of this stage is role confusion (see Table 24-3). Because of the adolescent's dramatic body changes, the development of a stable identity is difficult. Adolescents who are accepted, loved, and valued by family and peers generally tend to gain confidence and feel good about themselves. Adolescents who have difficulty forming relationships or who are perceived by peers as too different and not included in adolescent cliques may develop less favorable self-images and have low self-esteem.

Adolescents still need guidance from their parents, although they appear to neither want it nor need it. However, adolescents need to know that their parents care about them and that their parents still want to help them. Restrictions and guidance need to be presented in a manner that makes adolescents feel loved. They need consistency in guidance and fewer restrictions than previously. They should have the independence they can handle yet know that their parents will assist them when they need help.

During adolescence, peer groups assume great importance (Figure 24-8 ◆).

COGNITIVE DEVELOPMENT

Cognitive abilities mature during adolescence. Between the ages of 11 and 15, the adolescent begins formal operations stage of cognitive development (see Table 24-4). The adolescent becomes more informed about the world and environment. Adolescents use new information to solve everyday problems and can communicate with adults on most subjects.

MORAL DEVELOPMENT

According to Kohlberg, the young adolescent is usually at the conventional level of moral development. Most still accept the Golden Rule and want to abide by social order and existing laws. Adolescents examine their values, standards, and morals. They may discard the values they have adopted from parents in favor of values they consider more suitable. See Kohlberg's stages of moral development in Table 24-7.

SPIRITUAL DEVELOPMENT

According to Fowler, the adolescent or young adult reaches the synthetic–conventional stage of spiritual development (see Table 24-8). The adolescent may reconcile the differences in one of the following ways:

◆ Deciding any differences are wrong
◆ Compartmentalizing the differences (For example, a friend may not be able to go to dances on Friday evenings because of religious observances, but the friend can share activities on other days.)
◆ Obtaining advice from a significant other, such as a parent or a minister

Often, the adolescent believes that various religious beliefs and practices have more similarities than differences.

Figure 24-8. ◆ Adolescent peer group relationships enhance a sense of belonging, self-esteem, and self-identity. *Source:* © Elena Dorfman.

HEALTH ASSESSMENT AND PROMOTION

Adolescents are usually self-directed in meeting their health needs. Because of maturation changes, however, they need teaching and guidance in a number of health care areas.

Promoting health and wellness includes screening for tobacco, alcohol, and drug use and for sexual practices, and checking blood pressure, height, and weight. See Table 24-9 for health promotion guidelines for adolescents.

 ## Young Adults (20 to 40 Years)

Legally, a person in the United States can vote at 18 years. Another criterion of adulthood is financial independence, which is also highly variable. Some adults are financially dependent on their families for many years during prolonged education.

Adulthood may also be indicated by moving away from home and establishing one's own living arrangements. Many adults under 30 continue to live with parents due to high housing costs and unemployment rates, as well as social issues such as high divorce rates, single parenting, and the problems resulting from substance abuse. Some young people who are employed full time receive only minimum wage and are unable to earn enough money to be totally self-supporting.

Young adults are typically busy people who face many challenges. They are expected to assume new roles at work, in the home, and in the community, and to develop interests, values, and attitudes related to these roles.

PHYSICAL DEVELOPMENT

People in their early 20s are in their prime years physically. The musculoskeletal system is well developed and coordinated. This is the period when athletic endeavors reach their peak.

Although physical changes are minimal during this stage, weight and muscle mass may change as a result of diet and exercise. In addition, extensive physical and psychosocial changes occur in pregnant and lactating women. These changes are discussed in maternal/child textbooks.

PSYCHOSOCIAL DEVELOPMENT

In contrast to the minimal physical changes, psychosocial development and stresses of the young adult are great. (See Chapter 30.) Young adults face a number of new experiences and changes in lifestyle as they progress toward maturity.

Remaining single is becoming the lifestyle of more and more young adults. Many people choose to remain single, perhaps to pursue an education and then to have the freedom to pursue their chosen vocation. Some unmarried individuals choose to live with another person of the opposite or same sex and share living arrangements and certain expenses. Some unmarried people are gay or lesbian and live with or are involved with a partner to whom they are committed.

The multiple roles of adulthood (citizen, worker, taxpayer, homeowner, wife/husband, daughter/son, brother/sister, parent, friend, etc.) may also create stress as a result of role conflict (Figure 24-9 ◆). See Table 24-3 for Erikson's stage for young adults.

COGNITIVE, MORAL, AND SPIRITUAL DEVELOPMENT

Cognitive structures were completed during the formal operations period, from roughly 11 to 15 years (see Table 24-4).

Young adults who have mastered the previous stages of Kohlberg's theory of moral development now enter the post-conventional level (see Table 24-7). At this time, the person is able to separate self from the expectations and rules of others and to define morality in terms of personal principles.

According to Fowler, the individual enters the individuating–reflective period sometime after 18 years of age (see Table 24-8).

HEALTH ASSESSMENT AND PROMOTION

Young adults are usually interested in meeting their health needs. However, because of the many stresses and changes that occur throughout this 20-year period, the nurse needs to offer teaching and guidance in several health care areas. The nurse may wish to discuss some or all of the health promotion topics outlined for adults in Table 24-10 ◆.

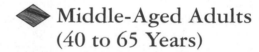 ## Middle-Aged Adults (40 to 65 Years)

The middle years, from 40 to 65, have been called the years of stability and consolidation. For most people, it is a time when children have grown and moved away or are moving away from home. Thus, partners generally have more time for and with each other and time to pursue interests they may have deferred for years.

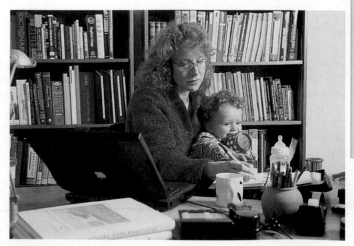

Figure 24-9. ◆ Many young women combine active careers with motherhood. *Source:* © Elena Dorfman.

TABLE 24-10 HEALTH PROMOTION GUIDELINES FOR YOUNG ADULTS, MIDDLE-AGED ADULTS, AND OLDER ADULTS

GUIDELINES	YOUNG ADULTS	MIDDLE-AGED ADULT	OLDER ADULTS
Health Tests and Screenings	Routine physical examination (every 1–3 years for females; every 5 years for males) Immunizations as recommended, such as tetanus–diphtheria (Td) boosters Regular dental assessments (e.g., annually) Periodic vision and hearing screenings Breast self-examination monthly, 1 week after onset of period Professional breast examination every 1–3 years Papanicolaou smear annually or at onset of sexual activity Testicular self-examination every month Screening for cardiovascular disease (e.g., cholesterol test every 5 years if results are normal; blood pressure to detect hypertension; baseline electrocardiogram at age 35 for males) Tuberculosis skin test every 2 years	Routine physical examination (annually for females; every 2–3 years or as directed by physician for males) Immunizations as recommended, such as a tetanus booster every 10 years and influenza and pneumococcal vaccinations Regular dental assessments (e.g., yearly) Tonometry for signs of glaucoma and other eye disease every 2–3 years or annually if indicated Breast self-examination as for young adults and first day of every month after menopause Testicular self-examination monthly Screenings for cardiovascular disease (e.g., blood pressure measurement; electrocardiogram and cholesterol test as directed by the physician) Screenings for colorectal, breast, cervical, uterine, and prostate cancer Screening for tuberculosis every 2 years	As for middle-aged adults
Safety	Motor vehicle safety reinforcement (e.g., using designated drivers when drinking, maintaining brakes and tires) Sun protection measures Workplace safety measures Water safety reinforcement (e.g., no diving in shallow water)	Motor vehicle safety reinforcement, especially when driving at night Workplace safety measures Home safety measures: keeping hallways and stairways lighted and uncluttered, using smoke detectors, using nonskid mats and hand rails in the bathrooms	Home safety measures to prevent falls, fire, burns, scalds, and electrocution Motor vehicle safety reinforcement, especially when driving at night Precautions to prevent pedestrian accidents
Nutrition/ Exercise and Elimination	Importance of adequate iron intake in diet Nutritional and exercise factors that may lead to cardiovascular disease (e.g., obesity, cholesterol and fat intake, lack of vigorous exercise)	Importance of adequate protein, calcium, and vitamin D in diet Nutritional and exercise factors that may lead to cardiovascular disease (e.g., obesity, cholesterol and fat intake, lack of vigorous exercise) An exercise program that emphasizes skill and coordination	Importance of a well-balanced diet with fewer calories to accommodate lower metabolic rate and decreased physical activity Importance of sufficient amounts of vitamin D and calcium to prevent osteoporosis Nutritional and exercise factors that may lead to cardiovascular disease (e.g., obesity, cholesterol and fat intake, lack of exercise) A regular program of moderate exercise to maintain joint mobility, muscle tone, and bone calcification Importance of adequate roughage in the diet, adequate exercise, and at least six 8-ounce glasses of fluid daily to prevent constipation

(continues)

TABLE 24-10	HEALTH PROMOTION GUIDELINES FOR YOUNG ADULTS, MIDDLE-AGED ADULTS, AND OLDER ADULTS (*continued*)		
GUIDELINES	**YOUNG ADULTS**	**MIDDLE-AGED ADULT**	**OLDER ADULTS**
Social Interactions	Encouraging personal relationships that promote discussion of feelings, concerns, and fears Setting short- and long-term goals for work and career choices	The possibility of a midlife crisis: Encourage discussion of feelings, concerns, and fears Providing time to expand and review previous interests Retirement planning (financial and possible diversional activities), with partner if appropriate	Encouraging intellectual and recreational pursuits Encouraging personal relationships that promote discussion of feelings, concerns, and fears Availability of social community centers and programs for seniors

PHYSICAL DEVELOPMENT

A number of changes take place during the middle years. At 40, most adults can function as effectively as they did in their 20s. However, during ages 40 to 65 many physical changes take place. Normal changes of aging, which become more pronounced among older adults, are described in Table 24-11 ◆.

PSYCHOSOCIAL DEVELOPMENT

Before the mid-1900s, the developmental tasks of middle-aged adults received little attention. Havighurst outlined seven tasks for this age group (Table 24-12 ◆). Erikson views the developmental choice of the middle-aged adult as generativity versus stagnation (see Table 24-3). *Generativity* is defined as the concern for establishing and guiding the next generation. In other words, the concern about providing for the welfare of humankind is equal to the concern of providing for self.

The middle-aged person looks older and feels older. Although people of these ages are reaching their prime, they begin to recognize that time is at a premium and that life is finite. Youthfulness and physical strength can no longer be taken for granted.

Some researchers suggest that it is not the events themselves that make midlife a crisis, but an individual's response to these life events. Internal and external resources include physical health, family income, the social support system, intelligence, and personality. Thus, the crisis or transitions of midlife are not just within the individual but rather between the individual and the individual's world.

COGNITIVE, MORAL, AND SPIRITUAL DEVELOPMENT

The middle-aged adult's cognitive and intellectual abilities change very little. Cognitive processes include reaction time, memory, perception, learning, problem solving, and creativity. Learning continues and can be enhanced by increased motivation at this time in life.

Middle-aged adults are able to carry out all the strategies described in Piaget's phase of formal operations (see Table 24-4).

According to Kohlberg, the adult can move beyond the conventional level to the postconventional level (see Table 24-7).

Not all adults progress through Fowler's stages to the fifth, called the paradoxical–consolidative stage. At this stage, the individual can view "truth" from a number of viewpoints (see Table 24-8). In middle age, people tend to be less dogmatic about religious beliefs. People in this age group often rely on spiritual beliefs to help them deal with illness, death, and tragedy.

HEALTH ASSESSMENT AND PROMOTION

Guidelines for health promotion for the middle-aged adult are shown in Table 24-10. Further discussion of nursing care is provided in the Nursing Care section on page 608.

◆ Older Adults (Over 65 Years)

In 2000, the number of Americans age 65 and older was about 14 percent of the population. By the year 2030, that percentage is projected to increase to more than 18 percent of the population. The group of older individuals who are 85 years and older is rapidly increasing. Census projections estimate that the population over 85 will almost triple by the year 2020 (U.S. Bureau of the Census, 2000).

Various systems are used to categorize the aging population. *Frail elderly*, a term used to described the extremely aged, is more likely to be used to describe the elderly individual who has significant physiologic and functional impairment, whatever the age.

PHYSICAL CHANGES

As the person ages, a number of physical changes occur; some are visible, some are not. Table 24-11 summarizes normal physical changes associated with aging.

PSYCHOSOCIAL DEVELOPMENT

According to Erikson, the developmental task at this time is ego integrity versus despair (see Table 24-3). People who attain ego integrity view life with a sense of wholeness and

TABLE 24-11	NORMAL PHYSICAL CHANGES ASSOCIATED WITH AGING
PHYSICAL CHANGES	**RATIONALE**
Integumentary	
Increased skin dryness	Decrease in sebaceous gland activity and tissue fluid
Increased skin pallor	Decreased vascularity
Increased skin fragility	Reduced thickness and vascularity of the dermis; loss of subcutaneous fat
Progressive wrinkling and sagging of the skin	Loss of skin elasticity, increased dryness, and decreased subcutaneous fat
Brown "age spots" (lentigo senilus) on exposed body parts (e.g., face, hands, arms)	Clustering of melanocytes (pigment-producing cells)
Decreased perspiration	Reduced number and function of sweat glands
Thinning and graying of scalp, pubic, and axillary hair	Progressive loss of pigment cells from the hair bulbs
Slower nail growth and increased thickening with ridges	Increased calcium deposition
Neuromuscular	
Decreased speed and power of skeletal muscle contractions	Decrease in muscle fibers
Slowed reaction time	Diminished conduction speed of nerve fibers and decreased muscle tone
Loss of height (stature)	Atrophy of intervertebral discs
Osteoporosis	Bone demineralization
Joint stiffness	Deterioration of joint cartilage
Impaired balance	Decreased muscle reaction time and coordination
Sensory/perceptual	
Loss of visual acuity	Degeneration leading to lens opacity (cataracts), thickening, and inelasticity **(presbyopia)**
Increased sensitivity to glare and decreased ability to adjust to darkness	Changes in the ciliary muscles; rigid pupil sphincter; decrease in pupil size
Partial or complete glossy white circle around the periphery of the cornea (arcus senilis)	Fatty deposits
Progressive loss of hearing (presbycusis)	Changes in the structures and nerve tissues in the inner ear; thickening of the eardrum
Decreased sense of taste, especially the sweet sensations at the tip of the tongue	Decreased number of taste buds in the tongue because of tongue atrophy
Decreased sense of smell	Atrophy of the olfactory bulb at the base of the brain (responsible for smell perception)
Increased threshold for sensations of pain, touch, and temperature	Possible nerve conduction and neuron changes
Pulmonary	
Decreased ability to expel foreign or accumulated matter	Decreased elasticity and ciliary activity
Decreased lung expansion; less effective exhalation; reduced vital capacity; and increased residual volume	Weakened thoracic muscles; calcification of costal cartilage, making the rib cage more rigid; dilation from inelasticity of alveoli
Difficult, short, heavy, rapid breathing (dyspnea) following exertion or intense exercise	Diminished delivery and diffusion of oxygen to the tissues to repay the normal oxygen debt because of changes in both respiratory and vascular tissues
Cardiovascular	
Reduced cardiac output and stroke volume, particularly during increased activity or unusual demands; may result in shortness of breath on exertion and pooling of blood in the extremities	Increased rigidity and thickness of heart valves (hence decreased filling/emptying abilities); decreased contractile strength
Reduced elasticity and increased rigidity of arteries	Increased calcium deposits in the muscular layer
Increase in diastolic and systolic blood pressure	Inelasticity of systemic arteries and increased peripheral resistance
Orthostatic hypertension	Reduced sensitivity of the blood pressure–regulating baroreceptors

TABLE 24-11	**NORMAL PHYSICAL CHANGES ASSOCIATED WITH AGING**

PHYSICAL CHANGES	RATIONALE
Gastrointestinal	
Delayed swallowing time	Alterations in the swallowing mechanism
Increased tendency for indigestion	Gradual decrease in digestive enzymes, reduction in gastric pH, and slower absorption rate
Increased tendency for constipation	Decreased muscle tone of the intestines; decreased peristalsis
Urinary	
Reduced filtering ability of the kidney and impaired renal function	Decreased number of functioning nephrons (basic functional units of the kidney) and arteriosclerotic changes in blood flow
Less effective concentration of urine	Decreased tubular function
Urinary urgency and urinary frequency	Enlarged prostate gland in men; weakened muscles supporting the bladder or weakness of the urinary sphincter in women
Tendency for a nocturnal frequency and retention of residual urine	Decreased bladder capacity and tone
Genitals	
Prostate enlargement (benign) in men	Exact mechanism is unclear; possible endocrine changes
Multiple changes in women (shrinkage and atrophy of the vulva, cervix, uterus, fallopian tubes, and ovaries; reduction in secretions; and changes in vaginal flora)	Diminished secretion of female hormones and more alkaline vaginal pH

derive satisfaction from past accomplishments. They view death as an acceptable completion of life. By contrast, people who despair often believe they have made poor choices during life and wish they could live life over. For other viewpoints on developmental tasks of the older adult, see Box 24-3 ◆.

Retirement

Today, a majority of the people over 65 are unemployed. However, many who are healthy continue to work on a full- or part-time basis. Work offers these people a better income, a sense of self-worth, and the chance to continue long-established routines. Some need to work for economic reasons.

Retirement can be a time when projects or recreational activities deferred for a long time can be pursued (Figure 24-

10 ◆). The lifestyle of later years is to a large degree formulated in youth. People who attempt suddenly to refocus and enrich their lives at retirement usually have difficulty. The later years can foster a sense of integrity and continuity, or they can be years of despair.

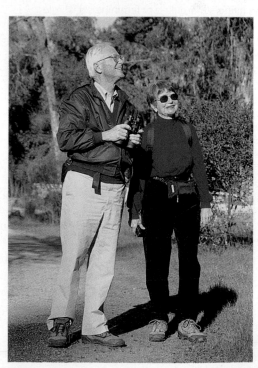

Figure 24-10. ◆ Middle-aged adults have time to pursue interests that may have been put aside for child care. *Source:* © Elena Dorfman.

BOX 24-3	

POPULATION FOCUS

DEVELOPMENTAL TASKS OF THE OLDER ADULT
- Adjusting to decreasing physical strength and health; safeguarding mental health
- Adjusting to retirement and reduced income; establishing a comfortable routine
- Adjusting to the death of a spouse
- Establishing an explicit affiliation with one's age group; keeping involved
- Meeting social and civic obligations
- Establishing satisfactory living arrangements
- Maintaining marital and family relations

TABLE 24-12 HAVIGHURST'S AGE PERIODS AND DEVELOPMENTAL TASKS

Infancy and Early Childhood
1. Learning to walk
2. Learning to take solid foods
3. Learning to talk
4. Learning to control the elimination of body wastes
5. Learning sex differences and sexual modesty
6. Achieving psychologic stability
7. Forming simple concepts of social and physical reality
8. Learning to relate emotionally to parents, siblings, and other people
9. Learning to distinguish right from wrong and developing a conscience

Middle Childhood
1. Learning physical skills necessary for ordinary games
2. Building wholesome attitudes toward oneself as a growing organism
3. Learning to get along with age-mates
4. Learning an appropriate masculine or feminine social role
5. Developing fundamental skills in reading, writing, and calculating
6. Developing concepts necessary for everyday living
7. Developing conscience, morality, and a scale of values
8. Achieving personal independence
9. Developing attitudes toward social groups and institutions

Adolescence
1. Achieving new and more mature relations with age-mates of both sexes
2. Achieving a masculine or feminine social role
3. Accepting one's physique and using the body effectively
4. Achieving emotional independence from parents and other adults
5. Achieving assurance of economic independence
6. Selecting and preparing for an occupation
7. Preparing for marriage and family life

8. Developing intellectual skills and concepts necessary for civic competence
9. Desiring and achieving socially responsible behavior
10. Acquiring a set of values and an ethical system as a guide to behavior

Early Adulthood
1. Selecting a mate
2. Learning to live with a partner
3. Starting a family
4. Rearing children
5. Managing a home
6. Getting started in an occupation
7. Taking on civic responsibility
8. Finding a congenial social group

Middle Age
1. Achieving adult civic and social responsibility
2. Establishing and maintaining an economic standard of living
3. Assisting teenage children to become responsible and happy adults
4. Developing adult leisure-time activities
5. Relating oneself to one's spouse as a person
6. Accepting and adjusting to the physiologic changes of middle age
7. Adjusting to aging parents

Later Maturity
1. Adjusting to decreasing physical strength and health
2. Adjusting to retirement and reduced income
3. Adjusting to death of a spouse
4. Establishing an explicit affiliation with one's age group
5. Meeting social and civil obligations
6. Establishing satisfactory physical living arrangements

Source: From Robert J. Havighurst, *Developmental tasks and education, 3e.* Published by Allyn and Bacon, Boston, MA. Copyright © 1972 by Pearson Education

Economic Changes

The financial needs of elderly people vary considerably. Food and medical costs alone are often a financial burden. Adequate financial resources enable the older person to remain independent.

Problems with income are often related to low retirement benefits, lack of pension plans for many workers, and the increased length of the retirement years. Nurses should be aware of the costs of health care. For example, the nurse or the client can request the physician to order lower-priced medications.

Relocation

During late adulthood, many people experience relocation. A variety of factors may lead to this decision. The home may be too large or too expensive, maintainance may become burden-

some or impossible. Decreased mobility may require living on one floor with more accessible bathroom facilities.

Leaving the family home and the neighbors and friends of several decades may be a difficult decision. Relocation for some is voluntary. The person may be seeking a more moderate climate with better recreational facilities geared to a more leisurely lifestyle. Adjustment will be much easier for the elderly person making a voluntary move.

Some elderly people must relocate to assistend living or long-term care facilities. The decision to enter a nursing home is frequently made when elderly people can no longer care for themselves, often because of problems of mobility and memory impairment. An increasing number of nursing home residents are in the very old age group (85 years and over), and most are women.

Maintaining Independence and Self-Esteem

Most elderly people thrive on independence (Figure 24-11). It is important to them to be able to look after themselves even if they have to struggle to do so. Although it may be difficult for younger family members to watch an older person completing tasks in a slow, determined way, aging people need this sense of accomplishment. To maintain the elderly adult's sense of self-respect, nurses and family members need to encourage them to do as much as possible for themselves, provided that safety is maintained. Nurses need to acknowledge the elderly client's ability to think, reason, and make decisions. Most elderly people are willing to listen to suggestions and advice, but they do not want to be ordered around. The nurse can support a decision by an elderly client even if eventually the decision is reversed because of failing health.

Facing Death

Well-adjusted aging couples usually thrive on companionship. Many couples rely increasingly on their mates for this company. When a mate dies, the remaining partner inevitably experiences feelings of loss, emptiness, and loneliness. These emotions are associated with **grieving,** the process of reacting to loss. Many are capable and manage to live alone. However, reliance on younger family members increases as age advances and ill health occurs. More women than men face bereavement and solitude because women usually live longer. Older people are often reminded of the brevity of life by the death of friends. Independence established prior to loss of a mate makes this adjustment period easier. A person who has some meaningful friendships, economic security, ongoing interests in the community, or private hobbies and a peaceful philosophy of life copes more easily with bereavement. Successful relationships with children and grandchildren are also of inestimable value. See Chapter 31 for a discussion about facing death. ⚭

COGNITIVE DEVELOPMENT

Piaget's phases of cognitive development end with the formal operations phase. Intellectual capacity includes perception, cognitive agility, memory, and learning.

Perception, or the ability to interpret the environment, depends on the acuteness of the senses. If the aging person's senses are impaired, the ability to perceive the environment and react appropriately is diminished. Changes in the nervous system may also affect perceptual capacity.

Changes in the cognitive structures occur as a person ages. It is believed that there is progressive loss of neurons. In addition, blood flow to the brain decreases, the meninges appear to thicken, and brain metabolism slows. In older adults, changes in cognitive abilities are more often a difference in speed than in ability. Overall, the older adult maintains intelligence, problem solving, judgment, creativity, and other well-practiced cognitive skills. Intellectual loss generally reflects a disease process. Most older adults do not experience cognitive impairments.

Memory is also a component of intellectual capacity. In older adults, retrieval of information from long-term memory can be slower, especially if the information is not frequently used. Most age-related differences occur in short-term memory. Older adults tend to forget the recent past. This forgetfulness can be improved by the use of memory aids, making notes or lists, and placing objects in consistent locations.

It is suggested that the older person remains mentally active to maintain cognitive ability at the highest possible level. Lifelong mental activity, particularly verbal activity, helps the older person retain a high level of cognitive function and may help maintain long-term memory. Cognitive impair-

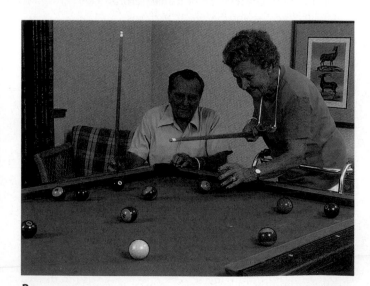

A   B

Figure 24-11. ◆ **A.** Many elderly people find creative outlets during retirement. **B.** Retirement provides time for enjoying hobbies.
*Source for **A**:* © Elena Dorfman/AWL.

ment that interferes with normal life is not considered part of normal aging. A decline in intellectual abilities that interferes with social or occupational functions should always be regarded as abnormal. Family members should be advised to seek prompt medical evaluation.

MORAL DEVELOPMENT

According to Kohlberg, moral development is completed in the early adult years. Most old people stay at Kohlberg's conventional level of moral development (see Table 24-7). The value and belief patterns that are important to older adults. Cultural background, life experiences, gender, religion, and socioeconomic status all influence one's values. The nurse must identify and consider the specific values of the older client when nursing care is planned.

SPIRITUAL DEVELOPMENT

Often, the older person's knowledge becomes wisdom, an inner resource for dealing with both positive and negative life experiences. Many older people have strong religious convictions and continue to attend religious meetings or services. Involvement in religion often helps the older adult to resolve issues related to the meaning of life, to adversity, or to good fortune. The "old-old" person who cannot attend formal services often continues religious participation in a more private manner. According to Fowler, some people enter the sixth stage of spiritual development, universalizing (see Table 24-8).

HEALTH ASSESSMENT AND PROMOTION

Assessment activities may include questions about the following:

◆ Usual dietary pattern
◆ Any problems with bowel or urinary elimination
◆ Activity/exercise and sleep/rest patterns
◆ Family and social activities and interests
◆ Any problems with reading, writing, or problem solving
◆ Adjustment to retirement or loss of partner

Health care professionals must also be alert for:

◆ Symptoms of depression
◆ Risk factors for suicide
◆ Signs of abnormal bereavement
◆ Changes in cognitive function
◆ Medications that increase risk of falls
◆ Signs of physical abuse or neglect
◆ Skin lesions (malignant and peripheral)
◆ Tooth decay, gingivitis, loose teeth

Older persons are usually concerned about their health and are interested in information and behavioral strategies directed toward improving it. The nurse may wish to discuss some or all of the health promotion topics outlined in Table 24-10.

NURSING CARE

ASSESSING

Data for assessment should always take into consideration the normal growth and developmental level of the client. For example, normal assessment information for an infant would include head circumference as well as height and weight. Normal assessment data for a 14-year-old girl would include presence and frequency of menstrual cycles.

DIAGNOSING, PLANNING, and IMPLEMENTING

Nursing diagnoses for clients with developmentally related concerns might include: Risk for Impaired Parenting, Relocation Stress Syndrome, and Situational Low Self-Esteem.

Planning at all levels of nursing care should incorporate an understanding of the client's age, developmental level, and any particular issues that might affect the client's progress toward wellness.

Awareness of a client's developmental level is especially important in implementing nursing care. A young child will usually respond better if a parent or safe adult is present for nursing care. An adolescent may prefer to have the parent leave the room during physical examination (especially a parent of the opposite sex). An older adult with age-related hearing impairment would benefit from having a family member or caregiver present to listen to discharge instructions.

Sensitivity to developmental issues is a great aid to nurses both in listening and in providing teaching. (See also Chapter 23. ⊙)

EVALUATING

The nurse collects data to determine whether outcomes have been met. If goals have not been achieved, the nurse can consider the need to adapt interventions to address developmental needs more closely.

Nursing Process Case Study:
CARING FOR A CLIENT WITH INVOLUTIONAL DEPRESSION

Sandra Peterson is a 48-year-old woman experiencing perimenopause. She feels that she is "losing her mind." She constantly forgets things and her mood is unpredictable. She often becomes irritable for no apparent reason and shortly thereafter is depressed and feels guilty for being hypercritical of her family and also herself. She has a tendency to overdramatize events. According to her family, she "always has to be right." In addition, Sandra accidentally burns herself every time she uses the oven, because she refuses to recognize the limitations of her aging body. Her arms have burn scars that are obviously months old. However, this time, she has sustained a severe burn. Sandra lives with her husband, but the close family frequently interacts, although she reports, "My kids continually make excuses not to attend family gatherings."

Assessment.

- C/o persistent physical symptoms that do not respond to treatment: headaches, digestive disorders, chronic pain.
- Weight 135, height 62'', increase of 7 lbs over the last month
- VS: 97.2–76–18 BP 110/78, c/o palpitations
- Lab test
- H&H 12.8, 33
- T_3, T_4 within normal
- Serum calcium low

Nursing Diagnosis.
The following nursing diagnoses have been identified for Mrs. Peterson:

- Chronic Low Self-Esteem related to repeated unmet expectations
- Disturbed Energy Field related to disharmony
- Self-Mutilation related to inability to express tension verbally

Expected Outcomes.

- Verbalizes increased self-acceptance through use of positive self statements
- States feeling of relaxation
- States appropriate ways to cope with increased psychological or physiological tension

Planning and Implementation.

- Demonstrate and promote effective communication techniques.
- Encourage realistic and achievable goal setting; recognize the value of attempts and accomplishment.
- Assist client with evaluating the impact of family on feelings of self-worth.
- Adminster therapeutic touch to induce relaxation.
- Validate the client's feelings and concerns related to sense of disharmony or energy disturbance.
- Provide medical treatment for injuries. Use careful aseptic technique when caring for burns.
- Assess for signs of depression, anxiety and impulsivity.
- Establish trust.

Evaluation.
On recheck, the client reports participating in yoga class 3x per week for relaxation. Reports that she has had no injuries this week. No digestive problems or headaches this week. Family reports she seems less stressed.

Critical Thinking in the Nursing Process

1. What might be some of the reasons for Sandra's burns?
2. According to Erikson's Developmental Stages, Sandra is in the generativity vs. stagnation stage. Her behavior demonstrates negative resolution (self-indulgence, self-concern, and lack of interest and commitments). What recommendations could you make as a nurse that would help produce positive resolution?
3. Sandra's family is very concerned about her injuries and behavior. What can they do to help her through this difficult time?

Note: The bibliography listings for this and all chapters have been compiled at the back of the book.

Chapter Review

Key Terms by Topics

Use the audio glossary feature of either the CD-ROM or the Companion Website to hear the correct pronunciation of the following key terms.

Introduction
growth, development, physiologic, psychosocial, cognitive, moral, spiritual

Neonates and Infants
fontanelles, motor development, reflexes, cognitive development

Toddlers
moral development, spiritual development

School-Age Children
puberty

Older adults
grieving

Key Points

* Growth and development are influenced by both genetics and environment. Development begins at conception and continues into old age.

* Growth and development have 5 major components: physiologic, psychosocial, cognitive, moral, and spiritual.

* Developmental theories provide information to help the health care professional understand what is taking place.

* Health assessment and promotion activites by the nurse assist the client to meet developmental milestones.

* As the population grows older, growth and development needs of the elderly will impact health care to a greater extent.

 EXPLORE **MediaLink**

Additional interactive resources for this chapter can be found on the Companion Website at www.prenhall.com/ramont. Click on Chapter 24 and "Begin" to select the activities for this chapter.

For chapter-related NCLEX-style questions and an audio glossary, access the accompanying CD-ROM in this book.

Animations:

* Heart
* Head and neck
* Abdomen
* Upper extremity
* Lower extremity
* Head and face
* Thorax and abdomen
* Pelvis and abdomen
* Lower leg

* Atlas and axis
* Clavicle and scapula
* Humerus
* Hand
* Hip
* Femur
* Tibia and fibula
* Foot
* L dopa

For Further Study

For more about teaching clients, see Chapter 23.
For information related to self-concept, see Chapter 28.
For more about sexual development and function, see Chapter 29.
For discussion about the effects of stress, See Chapter 30
For information about grief and dying, see Chapter 31.

Critical Thinking Care Map

Caring for a Client with Risk for Injury

NCLEX-PN Focus Area: Safety

Case Study: Todd Underwood, a 2-year-old, is brought into the clinic by his mother, Kelly. He has been brought in for a recheck following an ear infection. When you enter the exam room to take his vital sign, you observe Kelly frantically chasing Todd around the room. He is climbing on the furniture, opening all the cupboards, and pulling the paper off the exam table. Kelly states, "I'm worn out from chasing him and worried about his safety. Over the weekend he got into the medicine cabinet and was able to open several bottles. He also has learned how to unlock the patio door, which leads to the backyard jacuzzi."

Todd lives with his parents. A 12-year-old half-sister visits on alternate weekends.

Nursing Diagnosis: Risk for Injury/Trauma

COLLECT DATA

Subjective	Objective
_____	_____
_____	_____
_____	_____
_____	_____
_____	_____
_____	_____

Would you report this data? Yes/No

If yes, to: _____

Nursing Care

_____
_____
_____
_____
_____
_____
_____
_____
_____
_____
_____
_____

How would you document this? _____
_____
_____
_____
_____

Data Collected
(use those that apply)

- 2-year-old male child
- Lives with parents
- Half-sister, child of father's previous marriage, visits alternate weekends
- Both parents work outside the home
- Is cared for by maternal grandmother during the week
- VS: T 98.8°F (tympanic), 80–18
- Weight 29 lbs
- Height 34 inches
- Amoxicillin 500 mg (10-day course completed 2 days ago)
- Diet: Appetite fair. Grandmother has trouble getting him to sit down for meals, usually resorts to finger food. Takes a bottle at night.

Nursing Interventions
(use those that apply)

- Teach caregiver the need for close supervision of young children.
- Provide poison control number to mother.
- Instruct parent to keep syrup of ipecac in home first aid kit.
- Assist parents in devising a plan to child proof home.
- Inform parents of available CPR and first aid training in the community.
- Advise parent to eliminate all sweets from the child's diet.
- Explain individual differences in child temperaments and compare and contrast with the reality of parent expectations.
- Discuss sound disciplinary techniques (e.g., time out).
- Initiate referrals to parent education opportunities and stress management training.
- Observe for cause of family problem.
- Help caregiver find personal time to meet own needs and learn stress management.

NCLEX-PN Exam Preparation

1. You are assessing a 2-month-old infant. The mother tells you that he has been lifting his head and looking around but cannot roll over. She is expressing concerns about the baby's development. Your best response would be:

   a. "Don't worry, he will roll over at about 4 months."
   b. "Development is very individualized, but it does progress in an orderly manner. Once he develops head and chest control, you should expect rolling over to follow."
   c. "Babies who sleep on their backs don't try to roll over as soon."
   d. "Heavier babies are slower to roll over."

2. You are caring for a client who has undergone total hip replacement surgery. The physician is now recommending that the client be transferred to a long-term care facility for rehabilitation. The client states, "I would rather die than go there. My life is over. I will never be able to care for myself again." You understand that the client is in which stage of development according to Erikson's theory?

   a. Autonomy vs. shame and doubt
   b. Generativity vs. stagnation
   c. Integrity vs. despair
   d. Intimacy vs. isolation

3. A 10-year-old boy wishes to build a stand to sell lemonade on the front lawn. His mother, by encouraging his effort and desire to work, helps him achieve the development of Erikson's task of:

   a. Autonomy
   b. Industry
   c. Identity
   d. Ego integrity

4. You are assigned to measure and weigh a 5-month-old infant who has been brought into the clinic. The infant's birth weight was 7 lbs 2 oz. Using your knowledge of normal growth patterns, you would expect the weight today to be approximately:

   a. 10 lbs 11 oz
   b. 12 lbs
   c. 14 lbs 4 oz
   d. 21 lbs 6 oz

5. The extremities of the body grow more quickly than the body trunk, making the child's body appear somewhat out of proportion. This statement describes which period of development?

   a. Infant
   b. Toddler

   c. Preschooler
   d. School age

6. You have been assigned to care for a elderly client who is scheduled for surgery in the morning. The client is anxious, cannot sleep, and wishes to phone a family member. Because the hospital rules stipulate no phone calls after 9 P.M., you do not allow the call. Your actions demonstrate which stage of moral development according to Kohlberg?

   a. Stage 1: Punishment and obedience orientation
   b. Stage 3: Interpersonal concordance
   c. Stage 4: Law and order orientation
   d. Stage 6: Universal–ethical principles

7. An adult who relies on spiritual beliefs to help him or her deal with illness, death, or tragedy is progressing to which stage of spiritual development according to Fowler?

   a. Intuitive–projective
   b. Mythical–literal
   c. Synthetic–conventional
   d. Paradoxical–consolidative

8. Establishing satisfactory physical living arrangements is a developmental task according to:

   a. Erikson
   b. Fowler
   c. Kohlberg
   d. Havighurst

9. According to Erikson, if an individual expresses a sense of loss and contempt for others, it is an indication of unmet developmental needs during which of the following stages?

   a. Trust vs. mistrust
   b. Initiative vs. guilt
   c. Identity vs. role confusion
   d. Integrity vs. despair

10. You have been studying life span development. While visiting your elderly but healthy neighbor, a family member has some questions concerning aging. Which of the following statements is correct?

    a. "Most older adults have periods of confusion."
    b. "Older adults are likely to become senile."
    c. "Older adults have slower reaction time."
    d. "Older adults need more calories to maintain weight."

Answers for Review Questions, as well as discussion of Case Study and Critical Thinking Care Map questions, appear in Appendix IV.

Client Communication

Chapter
25

SHARING experiences

66 *Dealing with clients in the hospital setting can present challenges, especially for male nursing students. I have found that if I'm proficient in my skills, professional in my attitude, and compassionate in my care, I can meet the needs of my assigned clients—male or female, ambula-* *tory or bedridden, young or old. I may not choose to spend my career working with some types of clients who have been assigned to me as a student, but I will have learned something from each of them.* 99

Mohammad Naz, LVN student, North Orange County Regional Occupational Program, Anaheim, CA.

LEARNING outcomes

After completing this chapter, you will be able to:
- Describe essential aspects of communication and the communication process.
- Differentiate between verbal and nonverbal communication.
- Describe factors influencing the communication process.
- Explain techniques the nurse can use to help the client express thoughts, feelings, and concerns.
- Describe barriers to the development of therapeutic relationships.
- Discuss questions and approaches to use when interviewing clients.
- Identify factors that influence interviews with clients.

MediaLink

www.prenhall.com/ramont

Use the address above to access the free, interactive Companion Website created for this textbook. Get hints, instant feedback, and textbook references to chapter-related NCLEX-style questions. Link to other interesting sites.

Audio Glossary:
Use the Companion Website, or the CD-ROM disk enclosed with your textbook, to hear the pronunciations of key terms in the chapter.

Communication is a critical skill for nurses. It is the primary means by which nurse–client relationship occurs. It is the process by which humans meet their survival needs, build relationships, and experience joy. In nursing, communication is used to gather information, to teach and persuade, and to express caring and comfort.

The term **communication** has various meanings, depending on the context in which it is used. To some, communication is the exchange of information or thoughts between two or more people. This kind of communication uses talking and listening or writing and reading. Painting, dancing, and storytelling are other methods of communication. In addition, gestures and body actions convey thoughts to others, sometimes "speaking louder than words."

The intent of any communication is to obtain a response. Communication has two main purposes: to influence others, and to obtain information. *Helpful communication* encourages a sharing of information, thoughts, or feelings between two or more people. *Unhelpful communication* hinders or blocks the transfer of information and feelings. Communication techniques that help or hinder effective communication are discussed later in this chapter. See Tables 25-1 ◆ and 25-2 ◆.

◆ Factors Influencing Communication

Many factors, such as developmental stages, personal space, and environment, influence the communication process in a therapeutic setting. In addition, the roles and relationship of the speaker and the listener affect communication between them.

DEVELOPMENT

Language, psychosocial development, and intellectual development move through stages across the life span. Knowledge of a client's developmental stage allows the nurse to modify the message to reach the listener. This is particularly true in a client teaching situation.

From an early age, females and males communicate differently. Girls tend to use language to seek confirmation, minimize differences, and establish intimacy. Boys use language to establish independence and negotiate status within a group. These differences can continue into adulthood, so the same communication may be interpreted differently by a man and a woman. Many studies have found that men and women communicate differently in both content and process of communication. There is evidence to suggest that more effective communication occurs when the care provider and the client are of the same gender.

Because each person has unique personality traits, values, and life experiences, each perceives and interprets messages and experiences differently. It is important for the nurse

to be aware of a client's values and to validate or correct perceptions to avoid creating barriers in the nurse–client relationship. (**Validation** is a form of feedback that provides confirmation that both parties have the same basic understanding of the message and the feedback.)

PERSONAL SPACE

Personal space is the distance people prefer in interactions with others. When someone who wants to communicate steps too close, the receiver automatically steps back a pace or two. It is a natural protective instinct for people to maintain a certain amount of space immediately around them. The amount of personal space varies with individuals and cultures. When providing nursing care, the nurse may need to invade a client's personal space. It is important to be aware of this and to warn the client when this will occur.

Territoriality is a concept of the space and things that an individual considers as belonging to the self. For example, clients in a hospital often consider their territory as bounded by the curtains around the bed unit. If a visitor or nurse removes a chair to use at another bed, the client may feel upset or somewhat threatened. Nurses should obtain permission from clients to remove, rearrange, or borrow objects in their hospital area.

ROLES AND RELATIONSHIPS

Roles and relationships affect the communication process. Roles vary when communication occurs. Choices of words and tone of voice are different, depending on the roles of the communicators. Nursing student and instructor, client and physician, and parent and child are examples of such roles. The specific relationship between communicators is also significant. The nurse who meets with a client for the first time needs to establish a relationship with that client.

ENVIRONMENT

Communication occurs best in a comfortable, private environment. Nurses should be careful to provide both comfort and privacy. Environmental distractions, such as loud noises or people walking into the room, can impair and distort communication.

GROUP COMMUNICATION

A **group** is two or more people who have shared needs and goals, who take each other into account in their actions, and who thus are held together and set apart from others because of their interactions.

Examples of groups are families, peer groups, work groups, and religious groups. Communication within a group depends on each member of the group and their *motivations* (the reasons for their participation in the group.)

Self-help groups are formed of individuals who share a similar health, social, or daily living problem. The belief is that people who have experienced such a problem understand it better than those who have not had the experience. Examples of

TABLE 25-1	THERAPEUTIC COMMUNICATION TECHNIQUES	
TECHNIQUE	**DESCRIPTION**	**EXAMPLES**
Using silence	Accepting pauses or silences that may extend for several seconds or minutes without interjecting any verbal response.	Sitting quietly (or walking with the client) and waiting attentively until the client is able to put thoughts and feelings into words.
Providing general leads	Using statements or questions that (a) encourage the client to verbalize; (b) choose a topic of conversation; and (c) facilitate continued verbalization.	"Perhaps you would like to talk about…." "Would it help to discuss your feelings?" "Where would you like to begin?" "And then what?" "I follow what you are saying."
Being specific and tentative	Making statements that are specific rather than general, and tentative rather than absolute.	"You scratched my arm." (specific statement) "You are as clumsy as an ox." (general statement) "You seem unconcerned about Mary." (tentative statement) "You don't give a damn about Mary and you never will." (absolute statement)
Using open-ended questions	Asking broad questions that lead or invite the client to explore (elaborate, clarify, describe, compare, or illustrate) thoughts or feelings. Open-ended questions specify only the topic to be discussed and invite answers that are longer than one or two words.	"I'd like to hear more about that." "Tell me about…." "How have you been feeling lately?" "What brought you to the hospital?" "What is your opinion?" "You said you were frightened yesterday. How do you feel now?"
Using touch	Providing appropriate forms of touch to reinforce caring feelings. Because tactile contacts vary considerably among individuals, families, and cultures, the nurse must be sensitive to the differences in attitudes and practices of clients and self.	Putting an arm over the client's shoulder. Placing your hand over the client's hand.
Restating or paraphrasing	Actively listening for the client's basic message and then repeating those thoughts and/or feelings in similar words. This conveys that the nurse has listened and understood the client's basic message and also offers clients a clearer idea of what they have said.	*Client*: "I couldn't manage to eat any dinner last night—not even the dessert." *Nurse*: "You had difficulty eating yesterday." *Client*: "Yes, I was very upset after my family left." *Client*: "I have trouble talking to strangers." *Nurse*: "You find it difficult talking to people you do not know?"
Seeking clarification	A method of making the client's broad overall meaning of the message more understandable. It is used when paraphrasing is difficult or when the communication is rambling or garbled. To clarify the message, the nurse can restate the basic message or confess confusion and ask the client to repeat or restate the message. Nurses can also clarify their own message with statements.	"I'm puzzled." "I'm not sure I understand that. "Would you please say that again" "Would you tell me more?" "I meant this rather than that." "I guess I didn't make that clear—I'll go over it again."
Perception checking or seeking consensual validation	A method similar to clarifying that verifies the meaning of *specific words* rather than the overall meaning of a message.	*Client*: "My husband *never* gives me any presents." *Nurse*: "You mean he has *never* given you a present for your birthday or Christmas?" *Client*: "Well—not *never*. He does get me something for my birthday and Christmas, but he never thinks of giving me anything at any other time."

(continues)

TABLE 25-1	THERAPEUTIC COMMUNICATION TECHNIQUES *(continued)*	
TECHNIQUE	**DESCRIPTION**	**EXAMPLES**
Offering self	Suggesting one's presence, interest, or wish to understand the client without making any demands or attaching conditions that the client must comply with to receive the nurse's attention.	"I'll stay with you until your daughter arrives." "We can sit here quietly for a while; we don't need to talk unless you would like to." "I'll help you to dress to go home."
Giving information	Providing, in a simple and direct manner, specific factual information the client may or may not request. When information is not known, the nurse states this and indicates who has it or when the nurse will obtain it.	"Your surgery is scheduled for 11 AM tomorrow." "You will feel a pulling sensation when the tube is removed from your abdomen." "I do not know the answer to that, but I will find out from Mrs. King, the nurse in charge."
Acknowledging	Giving recognition, in a nonjudgmental way, of a change in behavior, an effort the client has made, or a contribution to a communication. Acknowledgment may be with or without understanding, verbal or nonverbal.	"You trimmed your beard and mustache and washed your hair." "I notice you keep squinting your eyes. Are you having difficulty seeing?" "You walked twice as far today with your walker."
Clarifying time or sequence	Helping the client clarify an event, situation, or happening in relationship to time.	*Client:* "I vomited this morning." *Nurse:* "Was that after breakfast?" *Client:* "I feel that I have been asleep for weeks." *Nurse:* "You had your operation Monday, and today is Tuesday."
Presenting reality	Helping the client to differentiate the real from the unreal.	"That telephone ring came from the program on television." "That's not a dead mouse in the corner; it is a discarded washcloth." "Your magazine is here in the drawer. It has not been stolen."
Focusing	Helping the client expand on and develop a topic of importance. It is important for the nurse to wait until the client finishes stating the main concerns before attempting to focus. The focus may be an idea or a feeling; however, the nurse often emphasizes a feeling to help the client recognize an emotion disguised behind words.	*Client:* "My wife says she will look after me, but I don't think she can, what with the children to take care of, and they're always after her about something—clothes, homework, what's for dinner that night." *Nurse:* "You are worried about how well she can manage."
Reflecting	Directing ideas, feelings, questions, or content back to clients to enable them to explore their own ideas and feelings about a situation.	*Client:* "What can I do?" *Nurse:* "What do you think would be helpful?" *Client:* "Do you think I should tell my husband?" *Nurse:* "You seem unsure about telling your husband."
Summarizing and planning	Stating the main points of a discussion to clarify the relevant points discussed. This technique is useful at the end of an interview or to review a health teaching session. It often acts as an introduction to future care planning."	"During the past half hour we have talked about...." "Tomorrow afternoon we may explore this further." "In a few days I'll review what you have learned about the actions and effects of your insulin."

self-help groups include Alcoholics Anonymous (the first of this type), and groups for those who have experienced stillbirth, divorce, drug abuse, cancer, mental illness, or diabetes.

Nurses may spend time together outside of work to help relieve work-related stress. Nurses who understand work stress can help encourage and support others. They can share the joys of success and the frustration of failure.

 ## Modes of Communication

Communication is generally carried out in two different modes: verbal and nonverbal. *Verbal communication* uses the spoken or written word. *Nonverbal communication* uses other forms, such as gestures, facial expressions, and touch. Although both kinds of communication occur at the same time, as much as 80

TABLE 25-2	BARRIERS TO COMMUNICATION	
TECHNIQUE	**DESCRIPTION**	**EXAMPLES**
Stereotyping	Offering generalized and oversimplified beliefs about groups of people that are based on experiences too limited to be valid. These responses categorize clients and negate their uniqueness as individuals.	"Two-year-olds are brats." "Women are complainers." "Men don't cry." "Most people don't have any pain after this type of surgery."
Agreeing and disagreeing	Akin to judgmental responses, agreeing and disagreeing imply that the client is either right or wrong and that the nurse is in a position to judge this. These responses deter clients from thinking through their position and may cause a client to become defensive.	*Client*: "I don't think Dr. Broad is a very good doctor. He doesn't seem interested in his patients." *Nurse*: "Dr. Broad is head of the Department of Surgery and is an excellent surgeon."
Being defensive	Attempting to protect a person or health care services from negative comments. These responses prevent the client from expressing true concerns. The nurse is saying, "You have no right to complain." Defensive responses protect the nurse from admitting weaknesses in the health care services, including personal weaknesses.	*Client*: "Those night nurses must just sit around and talk all night. They didn't answer my light for over an hour." *Nurse*: "I'll have you know we literally run around on nights. You're not the only client, you know."
Challenging	Giving a response that makes clients prove their statement or point of view. These responses indicate that the nurse is failing to consider the client's feelings, making the client feel it necessary to defend a position.	*Client*: "I felt nauseated after that red pill." *Nurse*: "Surely you don't think I gave you the wrong pill?" *Client*: "I feel as if I am dying." *Nurse*: "How can you feel that way when your pulse is 60?" *Client*: "I believe my husband doesn't love me." *Nurse*: "You can't say that; why, he visits you every day."
Probing	Asking for information chiefly out of curiosity rather than with the intent to assist the client. These responses are considered prying and violate the client's privacy. Asking "why" is often probing and places the client in a defensive position.	*Client*: "I was speeding along the street and didn't see the stop sign." *Nurse*: "Why were you speeding?" *Client*: "I didn't ask the doctor when he was here." *Nurse*: "Why didn't you?"
Testing	Asking questions that make the client admit to something. These responses permit the client only limited answers and often meet the nurse's need rather than the client's.	"Who do you think you are?" (forces people to admit their status is only that of client) "Do you think I am not busy?" (forces the client to admit that the nurse really is busy)
Rejecting	Refusing to discuss certain topics with the client. These responses often make clients feel that the nurse is rejecting not only their communication but also the clients themselves.	"I don't want to discuss that. Let's talk about ..." "Let's discuss other areas of interest to you rather than the two problems you keep mentioning." "I can't talk now. I'm on my way for coffee break."
Changing topics and subjects	Directing the communication into areas of self-interest rather than considering the client's concerns is often a self-protective response to a topic that causes anxiety. These responses imply that what the nurse considers important will be discussed and that clients should not discuss certain topics.	*Client*: "I'm separated from my wife. Do you think I should have sexual relations with another woman?" *Nurse*: "I see that you're 36 and that you like gardening. This sunshine is good for my roses. I have a beautiful rose garden."
Unwarranted reassurance	Using clichés or comforting statements of advice as a means to reassure the client. These responses block the fears, feelings, and other thoughts of the client.	"You'll feel better soon." "I'm sure everything will turn out all right." "Don't worry."

(continues)

TABLE 25-2	BARRIERS TO COMMUNICATION *(continued)*	
TECHNIQUE	DESCRIPTION	EXAMPLES
Passing judgment	Giving opinions and approving or disapproving responses, moralizing, or implying one's own values. These responses imply that the client must think as the nurse thinks, fostering client dependence.	"That's good (bad)." "You shouldn't do that." "That's not good enough." "What you did was wrong (right)."
Giving common advice	Telling the client what to do. These responses deny the client's right to be an equal partner. Note that giving *expert* rather than common advice is therapeutic.	*Client*: "Should I move from my home to a nursing home?" *Nurse*: "If I were you, I'd go to a nursing home, where you'll get your meals cooked for you."

to 90 percent of what is actually communicated is nonverbal. Learning about nonverbal communication is very important for nurses so that they can develop effective communication patterns and relationships with clients.

VERBAL COMMUNICATION

Verbal communication is largely conscious. People choose the words they use. Their choices are often guided by their culture, socioeconomic background, age, and education. As a result, countless possibilities exist for the way ideas are exchanged.

NONVERBAL COMMUNICATION

Nonverbal communication is sometimes called *body language*. It includes gestures, body movements, touch, and physical appearance (Figure 25-1 ◆). Nonverbal behavior is controlled less consciously than verbal behavior. Because of this, nonverbal communication often tells others more about what a person is feeling than what is actually said. Nonverbal communication either reinforces or contradicts what is said verbally. If a nurse says to a client, "I'd be happy to sit here and talk to you

for a while," yet glances nervously at a watch every few seconds, the actions contradict the verbal message. The client is more likely to believe the nonverbal behavior, which says, "I am very busy and need to leave."

Observing and interpreting the client's nonverbal behavior is an essential skill for nurses to develop. To observe nonverbal behavior efficiently, the nurse must make a systematic assessment of the person's overall physical appearance, posture, gait, facial expressions, and gestures. The nurse should always exercise caution in interpreting, and always confirm any observation with the client.

Nonverbal communication varies widely among cultures. Even behaviors such as smiling and handshaking can mean different things in different cultures.

Personal appearance, clothing, and adornments can say a lot about a person. Clothing may convey social and financial status, culture, religion, group association, and self-concept. Jewelry may be worn as a decoration or as a protection against harm. When the symbolic meaning of an object is unfamiliar, the nurse should ask about its significance.

How a person dresses is often an indicator of how the person feels. When a person known for immaculate grooming becomes sloppy in appearance, the nurse may suspect a physical illness or a loss of self-esteem.

The ways people walk and carry themselves are often reliable indicators of self-concept, current mood, and health. The posture of people when they are sitting or lying can also indicate feelings or mood. The nurse can validate the interpretation of the behavior by saying, for example, "You look like it really hurts you to move. I'm wondering how your pain is and if you might need something to make you more comfortable?"

No part of the body is as expressive as the face. Facial expressions can convey surprise, fear, anger, disgust, happiness, and sadness. When the message is not clear, it is important to get feedback to be sure what the person intends.

Nurses need to be aware of their own facial expressions and what they are communicating to others. Clients are quick to notice the nurse's expression, particularly when they feel unsure or uncomfortable. It is impossible to control all facial

Figure 25-1. ◆ Appropriate forms of touch can communicate caring.

expression. However, in some circumstances the nurse must learn to control expressions like fear or disgust.

Eye contact is another essential element of facial communication. In many cultures, mutual eye contact means you recognize the other person and are willing to maintain communication.

Gestures

Hand and body gestures may emphasize and clarify the spoken word. They may occur without words to indicate a particular feeling or to give a sign. Some gestures, however, may have different meanings, depending on one's culture. For example, the American gesture meaning "shoo" or "go away" means "come here" or "come back" in some Asian cultures.

For people with special communication problems, such as the deaf, the hands are invaluable in communication. Many deaf people learn sign language. Ill persons who are unable to reply verbally can similarly devise a communication system using the hands. (See also Chapter 27. ⬡)

 ## Therapeutic Communication

Therapeutic communication is client-centered, goal-directed, and time-limited communication. Nurses use therapeutic communication to determine client concerns, problems, and feelings. It is important for the nurse to know how to help clients explore their own feelings and how to avoid shutting down communication by saying the wrong thing.

THERAPEUTIC TECHNIQUES

Nurses can use a variety of responses to a client's comments to help them explore or expand on the client's thoughts and feelings. This is important if the nurse is to help the client achieve goals and overcome obstacles. Table 25-1 ◆ earlier in the chapter lists therapeutic communication techniques with examples. See also Chapter 23. ⬡

As you talk with clients, you will find you are most comfortable using certain techniques such as offering self, using touch, and providing general leads (Figure 25-2 ◆).

Figure 25-2. ◆ The nurse's facial expression and touch communicate warmth and caring. *Source:* © Elena Dorfman.

However, it is good to try new techniques periodically, especially if the techniques you usually use do not seem to be working.

Communication techniques should be comfortable for you, so that the conversation flows and is not stilted. Be careful not to overuse any one technique, as it may seem to the client that you are being insincere or uncaring. Overuse of silence or reflecting, for example, may slow down communication.

BARRIERS TO COMMUNICATION

Have you ever had a conversation with someone who responded in a way that made you feel it was useless to keep talking to them? Chances are good that you experienced a barrier to communication. Everyone uses communication barriers from time to time, but nurses need to be especially careful to avoid them when speaking with clients. Communication barriers are described in Table 25-2 ◆. It is very important to recognize when a barrier to communication has been used. You may respond to a client and then realize that you have used a barrier. When this happens, it is perfectly acceptable to say, "Let me say that differently" or "I'm sorry, that did not come out the way I meant it." If you realize later that you have used a barrier and shut down communication with a client, you can speak with the client again. You can tell the client that you would like to talk about the subject again and that you did not mean to be abrupt earlier. See Table 25-2 earlier in the chapter for examples of barriers to communication.

PRINCIPLES OF COMMUNICATION FOR THE CLINICAL SETTING

Effective communication in the clinical setting can be accomplished using the following communication principles:

◆ Use therapeutic communication techniques to communicate with clients.
◆ Think before you speak. Communicating with a client is different than speaking with a friend or another student. Share only what is appropriate, and always remember ethical principles and confidentiality.
◆ Be quiet and gentle in your communication. Do not communicate in any way that could increase the stress or discomfort of clients, families, or staff.
◆ Ask appropriate questions. Questions are asked to obtain information needed to care for clients, not to satisfy your curiosity. You should not make it a habit to read charts or look up information on the computer on clients to whom you are not assigned. When information is needed for educational purposes, the client's name and personal information must be removed. Client records should not be copied and removed from the hospital by a student.
◆ Keep information confidential. Do not talk about clients or their families in inappropriate places. Avoid discussing clients in the elevator, cafeteria, or anywhere visitors can overhear. See Chapter 32 for guidelines on Health

Insurance Portability and Accountability Act of 1996 (HIPPA), effective 4/14/03. ⊂⊃

◆ Be respectful in your communication. Speak to physicians, nursing assistants, instructors, and visitors with equal respect.

◆ Find out what you don't know. Don't pretend that you know something if you don't. This could inadvertently harm a client. Do not expect your instructor to give you all the answers. Instead, take responsibility for your own learning.

◆ Give a clear concise report. Shift report is an important form of communication (see Chapter 9). ⊂⊃

ATTENTIVE LISTENING

Attentive listening or **active listening** involves listening for key themes in communication with clients. The nurse should not interrupt the speaker, should take time to think about the message, and should ask questions to clarify or obtain additional information if needed. Attentive behaviors are a type of nonverbal communication. The nurse should lean slightly toward the client and have direct eye contact with the client. (Clients may have personal or cultural reasons for not returning eye contact. In these cases, the nurse would still make sure to make eye contact often.) The nurse should use open and expansive gestures as well as nonverbal cues such as nodding and smiling.

Attentive listening is a highly developed skill, but it can be learned with practice. A nurse can convey attentiveness in various ways. Common responses are nodding the head, uttering "uh huh" or "mmm," repeating the words that the client has used, or saying "I see what you mean." Each nurse has characteristic ways of responding, and the nurse must take care not to sound insincere or phony.

◆ Interviewing

An interview is a planned communication or a conversation with a purpose, for example, to get or give information. Interviewing is used in most phases of the nursing process, and is especially important when obtaining the nursing health history.

There are two approaches to interviewing: directive and nondirective. The *directive interview* is structured and is used to discover specific information. The nurse explains the purpose of the interview and asks closed questions (see the next section) that call for specific data. The client gives responses without discussion. Directive interviews are used to gather and to give information when time is limited, such as in an emergency situation.

A *nondirective interview* allows the client to control the situation. *Rapport,* an understanding between two or more people, is built in this type of interview. The nurse encourages communication by asking open-ended questions (see the next section) and by providing empathetic responses.

A combination of directive and nondirective approaches is usually appropriate during the information-gathering inter-

view. The nurse begins by asking open-ended questions to determine areas of concern for the client. If, for example, a client expresses worry about surgery, the nurse pauses to explore the client's worry and to provide support. Simply to note the worry, without dealing with it, can leave the impression that the nurse does not care about the client's concerns or dismisses them as unimportant. As the interview evolves, the nurse may use closed questions to obtain more specific data and to complete the nursing health history. See the nursing care checklist in Box 25-1 ◆ for guidelines for wording verbal communication.

KINDS OF INTERVIEW QUESTIONS

Questions are classified as closed or open ended, and as neutral or leading. **Closed-ended questions,** used in the directive interview, generally require only "yes" or "no" or short factual answers giving specific information. Thus, the amount of information gained is generally limited. Closed questions often begin with "when," "where," "who," "what," "do (did, does)," "is (are, was)" and sometimes "how." Examples of closed questions are "What medication did you take?", "Are you having pain now? Show me where it is.", "How old are you?", and "When did you fall?" The highly stressed person and the person who has difficulty communicating will find closed-ended questions easier to answer than open-ended questions.

Open-ended questions, used in the nondirective interview, invite clients to discover and explore their thoughts or feelings. They allow clients the freedom to talk about what they wish. An open-ended question specifies only the broad topic to be discussed and invites answers longer than one or two words. The open-ended question is useful at the beginning of an interview or to change topics and to elicit attitudes.

The type of question a nurse chooses depends on the situation. For example, the nurse asks closed-ended questions in an emergency when information must be obtained quickly. Nurses often find it necessary to use a combination of closed- and open-ended questions throughout an interview to obtain needed information. A comparison of open- and closed-ended questions appears in Box 25-2 ◆.

A *neutral question* is a question the client can answer without direction or pressure from the nurse. Examples are: "How do you feel about that?" and "Why do you think you had the operation?" A *leading question,* by contrast, directs the client's answer. The phrasing of the question suggests what answer is expected. Examples are: "You're stressed about surgery tomorrow, aren't you?" and "You will take your medicine, won't you?" The leading question gives the client less opportunity to decide whether the answer is true or not. Leading questions create problems if the client gives inaccurate responses in order to please the nurse. This can result in inaccurate data.

PLANNING THE INTERVIEW AND SETTING

Before beginning an interview, the nurse reviews available information. Certain factors are crucial in planning interviews:

BOX 25-1
NURSING CARE CHECKLIST

GUIDELINES FOR WORDING VERBAL COMMUNICATION

☑ Pay attention to your tone of voice, manner, and pace of speech. They can change the feeling and impact of the message. Your intonation can express enthusiasm, sadness, anger, or amusement. Your pace of speech may indicate interest, anxiety, boredom, or fear.

☑ Use simple terms and give complete information. Complex technical terms become natural to nurses, but laypeople often misunderstand them. Instead of saying to a client, "The nurses will be catheterizing you tomorrow for a urine analysis," it may be more understandable to say, "Tomorrow we need to get a sample of your urine, so we will collect it by putting a small tube into your bladder." Speak clearly and briefly. A message that is direct and simple will be more effective. *Clarity* is saying precisely what you mean, and *brevity* is using the fewest words necessary. The result is a message that is simple and clear.

☑ Use consistency in verbal and nonverbal communication. The nurse's behavior must match the words spoken. When the nurse tells the client, "I am interested in hearing what you have to say," the nonverbal behavior would include the nurse facing the client, making eye contact, and leaning forward.

☑ Keep communication relevant and well timed. The timing of any message needs to be appropriate to ensure that words are heard. Messages should address the person's interests and concerns, and be given when the client can hear and understand them. Nurses need to be aware of both relevance and timing when communicating with clients.

☑ Avoid asking several questions at once or asking questions without waiting for an answer. For example, a nurse might enter a client's room and say in one breath, "Good morning. How are you this morning? Did you sleep well last night? Your husband is coming to see you before your surgery, isn't he?" The client no doubt would wonder which question to answer first.

☑ Be adaptable when communicating. Spoken messages should be adapted to behavioral cues from the client. What the nurse says and how it is said must show sensitivity. For example, a nurse who is usually friendly and jovial may notice that a client seems very withdrawn and distressed. The nurse should modify his or her tone of speech with this client, and share observations about the client's expression and mood.

☑ Be *credible* (believable). Credibility may be the most important requirement for effective communication. Nurses foster credibility by being consistent, dependable, and honest. They should be knowledgeable about what is being discussed and have accurate information. Nurses should convey confidence and certainty in what they are saying. If they don't know the answer, they should say so. "I don't know the answer to that, but I will find someone who does."

☑ Use humor, but use it with care. Humor can be a positive and powerful tool in the nurse–client relationship. Humor can help clients adjust to difficult and painful situations by providing a different perspective and promoting a sense of well-being. The physical act of laughter can be both an emotional and physical release that reduces tension. Healthful humor must be distinguished from harmful humor. Healthful humor elicits laughter; it is appropriate to the situation and protects a person's dignity. Harmful humor ridicules other people by laughing at them. Humor is also harmful if used to avoid resolving problems.

1. *Time.* Nurses need to schedule interviews with hospitalized clients for a time when the client is comfortable and when interruptions are unlikely. Nurses should schedule interviews with home care clients at a time selected by the client. In all instances, the client should be comfortable and unhurried.

2. *Place.* The place for an interview should be comfortable, well lit, private, and quiet. Most people are uncomfortable about answering personal questions or expressing strong feelings in the sight or hearing of others.

3. *Seating arrangements.* When a client is in bed, the nurse can sit at a 45-degree angle to the bed. This position is less formal than sitting behind a table or standing at the foot of the bed. During an initial admission interview, a client may feel less confronted if there is an overbed table between the client and the nurse. Sitting on a client's bed may make the client uncomfortable.

4. *Distance.* People feel uncomfortable when talking to someone who is too close or too far away. Most people feel comfortable at a distance of 3 to 4 feet during an interview. Some clients require more or less personal space, depending on their cultural and personal needs. Variables in the personal space people require are illustrated in Box 25-3 ◆.

Height also affects communication. When a nurse is standing and looking down at a client, the client may feel intimidated.

BOX 25-2 COMPARISON OF OPEN- AND CLOSED-ENDED QUESTIONS

Open-ended questions are questions or statements that require more than a yes or no or other short response (usually begin with "what" or "how").

"How have you been feeling lately?"
"What brought you to the hospital?"
"How did you feel in that situation?"
"Would you describe more about how your relate to your child?"
"What would you like to talk about today?"

Closed-ended questions are questions that can be answered by yes or no or other single word answers.

"Are you feeling okay?"
"Do you know why you have been admitted?"
"Did that situation caused you to feel depressed or upset?"
"Do you have a good relationship with your children?"
"Would you like to talk about what is bothering you today?"

STAGES OF AN INTERVIEW

An interview has three major stages: the opening or introduction, the body or development, and the closing.

The Opening

The opening can be the most important part of the interview because what is said and done at that time sets the tone for the remainder of the interview. The purposes of the opening are to establish rapport and orient the interviewee.

Establishing rapport is a process of creating goodwill and trust. It can begin with a greeting ("Good morning, Mr. Johnson") or a self-introduction ("Good morning. I'm Becky James, a nursing student") accompanied by nonverbal gestures such as a smile, a handshake, and a friendly manner. A brief amount of small talk about the person, the weather, sports, and families is appropriate to develop rapport, but too much superficial talk can cause anxiety. The nurse then orients the client by explaining the purpose and nature of the interview, what information is needed, how long it will take, and what is expected of the client. The nurse usually states that the client has the right not to provide data and tells the client how the information will be used.

The following is an example of an interview introduction:

STEP 1: ESTABLISH RAPPORT

Nurse: Hello Ms. Goodwin. I'm Sharon Fellows and I will be assisting with your care today. I am a nursing student at the technical center.

BOX 25-3

POPULATION FOCUS

PERSONAL SPACE VARIABLES BY CULTURE OR ETHNIC GROUP

◆ African: Close personal space; touching acceptable within families and extended families.
◆ Chinese: distant personal space; direct eye contact avoided and touch by strangers not acceptable.
◆ Eastern Indian: direct eye contact shows lack of respect; handshake permissible only between males.
◆ European-American, Canadian, and British: Personal space at least 18 inches between individuals during conversation.
◆ Filipino: Touching is permissible; if eye contact is established, it must be maintained.
◆ Germans: Space is sacred; even furniture placement maintains distance.
◆ Iraqi: Touch and embracing are the acceptable greeting.
◆ Israeli: Demonstrative touch.
◆ Japanese: Touch not encouraged; handshake acceptable; distant personal space; eye contact is considered disrespectful.
◆ Mexican: Close personal space; touch is acceptable even with those of same sex.
◆ Native American: Periods of silence during communication shows respect; close personal space—no boundaries; limited eye contact.
◆ Saudi: Hand holding between men is acceptable; men may only touch females within the family.

Client: It's nice to meet you. My sister-in-law teaches at the technical center. Do you know Dorothy Goodwin?

Nurse: No, I don't believe I have met her. What does she teach?

Client: Something in computers. I don't actually understand it! Will you be bringing me my medicine today?

STEP 2: ORIENTATION

Nurse: Yes, that will be part of my responsibilities. I also need to ask you a few questions about your health and illness. Do you need any pain medicine or other medicines before we talk for about 10 minutes?

Client: No, I am fine. Just wondered if you would be doing the medicines today.

Nurse: I will. Don't hesitate to ask for anything you need.

Client: What do you need to know?

Nurse: I need to ask you about what you might need after you leave the hospital. If you don't want to discuss something I bring up, just let me know. I will be making notes so we can arrange for you to have follow-up doctor visits and nursing care if you need it.

Client: I probably will. My husband cannot do much because he is nearly blind and has a heart condition. My daughter will be coming to stay for a few days, though.

The Body

In the body of the interview, the client communicates what he or she thinks, feels, knows, and perceives in response to questions from the nurse. The nurse can make the transition from the opening stage to this stage by asking an open-ended question that is related to the stated purpose such as, "What brought you to the hospital today?"

The nurse must use communication techniques that make both parties feel comfortable and serve the purpose of the interview (Figure 25-3 ◆). See communication techniques in Table 25-1 ◆. Brief guidelines for communicating during an interview are outlined in Box 25-4 ◆.

The Closing

The nurse usually terminates the interview when the needed information has been obtained. In some cases, however, a client terminates it. For example, the client may decide not to give any more information or be unable to offer more information because of fatigue. The closing is important in maintaining rapport. The following techniques are commonly used to close an interview:

1. Signal that the interview is coming to an end by offering to answer questions: "Do you have any questions?" "I would be glad to answer any questions you have." Be sure to allow time for the person to answer, or the offer will be regarded as insincere.

2. Declare completion of the purpose or task by saying "Well, that's about all I need to know for now" or "Well, those are all the questions I have for now." Preceding a

Figure 25-3. ◆ The nurse conveys attentive listening through a posture of involvement.

> ### BOX 25-4
> ### NURSING CARE CHECKLIST
>
> ## COMMUNICATION DURING AN INTERVIEW
>
> ☑ Listen attentively, using all your senses, and speak slowly and clearly.
> ☑ Use language the client understands, and clarify points that are not understood.
> ☑ Plan questions to follow a logical sequence.
> ☑ Ask only one question at a time. Double questions limit the client to one choice and may confuse both the nurse and the client.
> ☑ Allow the client the opportunity to look at things the way they appear to him or her and not the way they appear to the nurse or someone else.
> ☑ Do not impose your own values on the client.
> ☑ Avoid using personal examples, such as saying, "If I were you. . ."
> ☑ Nonverbally convey respect, concern, interest, and acceptance (see Figure 25-3 ◆).
> ☑ Use and accept silence to help the client search for more thoughts or to organize them.
> ☑ Use eye contact and be calm, unhurried, and sympathetic.

remark with the word "well" generally signals that the end of the interaction is near.

3. State appreciation or satisfaction about what was accomplished: "I really enjoyed meeting you, and I think we accomplished a great deal." "Those are all the questions I have. Thank you for your time and help." "The questions you have answered will be helpful in planning your nursing care."

NURSING CARE

 ## ASSESSING

Good nursing requires an understanding of the many factors involved in communicating. A client may state that she is "all set" for the next day's gallbladder surgery. However, the nurse may observe that the client has a fearful expression and is trembling. If the nurse focuses only on the client's verbal communication, he or she is unlikely to provide good care or an accurate documentation.

The nurse collects assessment data through closed- or open-ended questions, depending on the task at hand and the time available. When collecting data for a shift change, the nurse might focus on vital signs, status of IVs, and so on.

When giving a client a sponge bath before sleep, the nurse might ask open-ended questions that would give the client the opportunity to reminisce and think of pleasant events.

DIAGNOSING, PLANNING, and IMPLEMENTING

Certain nursing diagnoses that may affect communication with a client are Anxiety, Coping, Denial, Hopelessness, and Disturbed Sensory Perception. Be prepared to address the client's feelings, and to adapt the pace and style of your communication.

The following interventions are useful in interviewing clients:

◆ Before beginning an interview, know what information to collect. This ensures that the exchange with the client is smooth and efficient. It also frees you to observe the client more during the interaction.

◆ Schedule interviews at a time that is as convenient as possible for the client, and when interruptions are not likely to occur. Allow home care clients to select a time. This allows the interview to be relaxed and unhurried. Scheduling a time without interruptions is helpful because most people are uncomfortable about answering personal questions or expressing strong feelings in the sight or hearing of others.

◆ If possible, sit at a 45-degree angle to the bed or chair where the client is, and about 3 or 4 feet from the client. Sitting too close to, or standing over, the client can make the client feel threatened. Sitting far away may suggest lack of interest.

◆ Open the interview with a friendly greeting and introduce yourself. If appropriate, start with some general conversation. Then explain why you are there. This approach expresses respect for the client and builds rapport. The client can be more relaxed about the interview once its purpose is stated.

◆ Ask an open-ended question that is related to the stated purpose, is easy to answer, and does not embarrass or place stress on the person. This helps make the transition into the main part of the interview.

◆ Throughout the interview, use good communication techniques. If you feel you have put up a block to communication, apologize and restate the question in a better way. Pay attention to both verbal and nonverbal messages from the client.

◆ When the necessary information has been obtained, ask if the client has any questions. If the client decides to stop the interview, state what you have accomplished and, if needed, say what follow-up will be required. Suggest a follow-up time. If all questions have been answered, the open-ended question signals that the interview is ending. If a client is too tired or refuses to give any more information, the restatement will help them to know what has been accomplished and what more they will be asked to do at another time.

◆ Thank clients for their time and express hope for a positive outcome. This again expresses your respect and concern for them.

EVALUATING

In evaluating professional communications with clients, the nurse first looks at the client's verbal and nonverbal expressions of comfort. Does the client seem relaxed, or does he appear flushed and tense? Does the client express satisfaction at understanding better, or does he appear anxious and confused?

The nurse also mentally reviews the interaction to determine the success of the communication process. What communication techniques were effective in the situation? Which were not effective? Did any blocks to communication arise? Was a way found to move past them? If not, can the nurse think of a possible way past the block now that the interaction is over? Has the nurse experienced any similar communications that might provide insights?

Nursing Process Case Study: CLIENT AFFECTED BY NURSE COMMUNICATION BARRIERS

Mr. Levowitz is currently in the recovery room after surgery to remove prostate cancer that had spread to his abdomen. His wife comes into the room crying. The LPN asks her what is wrong. Mrs. Levowitz continues to sob and is unable to answer. The nurse gets chairs for herself and Mrs. Levowitz and urges her to sit down. She says, "Come on now. The news can't be that bad, can it?" Mrs Levowitz responds that the doctor has said the cancer is so bad, there is nothing they can do. The LPN then says, "I am so very sorry. That must be difficult news to hear." Mrs. Levowitz cries a bit longer, then says she doesn't know how she can live without him. The nurse tells her, "You should wait and see how the chemotherapy and radiation treatments go before you think about living without him. Things may still turn out all right." Mrs. Levowitz grasps at that hope and says, "Oh, do you really think those treatments could help him? That he doesn't really have cancer that bad?" The LPN says, "It's been known to happen. I really have to go see some other clients now. Everything will be okay for you. It will turn out just fine."

Assessment. The client and his wife live alone in a small cottage several miles outside the city. Mrs. Levowitz does not drive and has always been a stay-at-home wife. She also expresses concerns about caring for him at home and getting him to his treatment appointments. Mr. Levowitz is very controlled and sits quietly, not joining in the conversation with the LPN and his wife.

Diagnosis. The nursing diagnoses for Mr. Levowitz (and significant others) include the following:

* Caregiver Role Strain related to need for significant home care
* Compromised Family Coping related to inadequate resources available
* Anticipatory Grieving related to potential loss of significant others
* Ineffective Role Performance related to change in physical capacity to resume prior role

Expected Outcomes

* Caregiver identifies resources available to help in giving care.
* Identifies need for and seeks outside support.
* Plans for future one day at a time.
* Accepts physical limitation regarding role responsibility and considers ways to change lifestyle to accomplish goals associated with role performance.

Planning and Implementation

* Monitor caregiver for psychological distress and signs of depression.
* Assess health of the caregiver at intervals, especially if she has a chronic illness in addition to caregiver role.
* Help caregiver identify ways to equitably distribute workload among family.
* Assist in finding transportation for treatment and family visits.
* Refer family to appropriate resources for assistance as indicated.

* Involve client and family in planning care as much as possible.
* Use therapeutic communication with open-ended questions such as "What are your fears and thoughts?"
* Actively listen to client's/family's expression of grief. Do not interrupt, do not tell own story, and do not offer meaningless platitudes such as, "It will be better this way."
* Refer to family counseling as needed for adjustment of role change.
* Identify way to compensate for physical disabilities.

Evaluation. Mr. Levowitz spoke with social worker; arrangements were made for them to move temporarily to an assisted living arrangement during treament; Mr. Levowitz expressed that "I will keep an open mind, maybe we will consider moving permanently to the assisted living apartment." Both client and wife expressed a desire to discuss the future once a therapeutic communication dialogue was started. Mr. Levowitz expressed an understanding of his physical limitation, but stated, "They can't get rid of me that easily. I am going to fight this as long as my wife is by my side."

Critical Thinking in the Nursing Process

1. What communication techniques did the LPN use?
2. What barriers to communication did the nurse create?
3. What non-verbal communication did the nurse employ?
4. How might the nurse correct the barriers she used with Mrs. Levowitz?

Note: The bibliography listings for this and all chapters have been compiled at the back of the book.

Chapter Review

Key Terms by Topics

Use the audio glossary feature of either the CD-ROM or the Companion Website to hear the correct pronunciation of the following key terms.

Introduction
communication, reflecting

Factors influencing communication
validation, group

Therapeutic communication
therapeutic communication, active listening

Interviewing
closed-ended questions, open-ended questions

Key Points

* Communication is a critical nursing skill used to gather information, to teach and persuade, and to express caring and comfort.

* Communication is a two-way process that involves the sender of the message and the receiver of the message. Messages are both verbal and nonverbal.

* The effectiveness of verbal communication depends on many factors, including pace and intonation, simplicity, clarity and brevity, timing, relevance, adaptability, and credibility.

* Nonverbal communication includes personal appearance, posture and gait, facial expressions, and gestures. It often reveals more about a person's thoughts and feelings than words do. The "receiver" is more likely to believe a nonverbal message than a verbal one.

* When communication is effective, verbal and nonverbal expressions are consistent.

* When assessing verbal and nonverbal behaviors, nurses need to consider cultural influences. A single nonverbal expression can indicate a variety of feelings, and one word can have several meanings.

* Many techniques facilitate therapeutic communication: attentive listening; paraphrasing; clarifying; using open questions and statements; focusing; being specific; using touch and silence; clarifying reality, time, or sequence; providing general leads; and summarizing.

* To communicate well, the nurse must be seen as trustworthy. Offering unvalidated reassurance, stating approval or disapproval, giving common (not expert) advice, stereotyping, and being defensive are all things that destroy trust.

EXPLORE MediaLink

Additional interactive resources for this chapter can be found on the Companion Website at www.prenhall.com/ramont. Click on Chapter 25 and "Begin" to select the activities for this chapter.

For chapter-related NCLEX-style questions and an audio glossary, access the accompanying CD-ROM in this book.

∞ For Further Study

For further information about giving end of shift reports, see Chapter 9.

For more discussion of communication as it relates to teaching and learning, see Chapter 23.

See Chapter 27 for more information about dealing with clients with sensory impairments.

See Chapter 32 for information about Health Insurance Portability accountability act.

Critical Thinking Care Map

Caring for a Client with Anorexia

NCLEX-PN Focus Area: Coping and Adaptation

Case Study: Erlene, age 18, has been diagnosed with anorexia. She expresses that she feels she is fat, although she admits to losing 15 pounds in the last 2 months. She is planning to leave home to go to college in about 3 months. She has come for her college physical. Her mother accompanies her and insists on being in the room during the exam. She attempts to answer all questions directed to Erlene.

Nursing Diagnosis: Ineffective Family Therapeutic Regimen Management

COLLECT DATA

Subjective	Objective
_____	_____
_____	_____
_____	_____
_____	_____
_____	_____
_____	_____

Would you report this data? Yes/No

If yes, to: _____

Nursing Care

_____
_____
_____
_____
_____
_____
_____
_____
_____
_____
_____
_____
_____

How would you document this? _____
_____
_____
_____
_____

Data Collected
(use those that apply)

- Height 5' 9"
- Weight 98 pounds (down from 117 two months ago).
- LMP 3 months ago.
- VS: T 96.8/ P 100/ R 18; BP 90/66
- Exercises 2 hours per day in addition to cheerleading practice
- Mother states she is a straight A student and very popular: "We are so proud of Erlene. She has a full scholarship to my college. She is going to be an attorney just like her father."
- Erlene is asked what she eats on a normal day. Mother replies, "She is so busy she just grabs breakfast on the run. I am sure she eats lunch at school; she says she isn't hungry at dinnertime."
- When Erlene is sent to restroom to collect a urine sample, her mother states, "She hasn't had a period in 3 months. Do you think she could be pregnant?"
- Takes no prescription medications; does admit to taking laxatives for "constipation"

Nursing interventions
(use those that apply)

- Review with family members the congruence and incongruence of family behaviors and health related goal.
- Help family to mobilize social support.
- Identify barriers that cause impaired social interaction.
- Encourage client to use "I" statements and to accept responsibility for and consequences of actions.
- Review client's currrent medication.
- Collaborate with other consultants regarding strategies for working with families.
- Facilitate modeling and role-playing for family regarding healthy ways to communicate and interact.
- Establish open and trusting relationship with the family.
- Provide sufficient knowledge to support family decisions regarding therapeutic regimens.
- Assess client's level of anxiety and physical reaction to anxiety.
- Review symptoms of specific disorder and work with family toward developing a greater awareness of symptoms.
- Model age and cognitively appropriate caregiver skills by communicating with the client at an appropriate cognitive level.

NCLEX-PN Exam Preparation

1. When a nursing student sits on a client's bed while conducting an admission interview, he or she is disregarding the client's need for:
   a. Confidentiality
   b. Personal space
   c. Eye contact
   d. Acceptance

2. Questions that begin with "when," "where," "who," "what," "do (did, does)," "is (are, was)" and sometimes "how" can be described as:
   a. Leading questions
   b. Open-ended questions
   c. Close-ended questions
   d. Attentive questions

3. The opening can be the most important part of the interview because:
   a. It sets the tone for the remainder of the interview, establishes rapport, and orients the interviewee.
   b. It states appreciation or satisfaction about accomplishments.
   c. The client communicates what he or she thinks, feels, knows, and perceives in response to questions from the nurse.
   d. The nurse can make the transition by asking an open-ended question that is related to the stated purpose.

4. When the nurse makes a systematic assessment of the person's overall physical appearance, posture, gait, facial expressions, and gestures he or she is:
   a. Communicating nonverbally
   b. Observing or interpreting nonverbal behavior
   c. Contradicting what the client is saying verbally
   d. Making unfounded judgment about the client

5. You are attempting to establish a therapeutic relationship with a client. Which of the following statements would support this attempt?
   a. "I have at least 30 minutes I can spend with you, until it is time for your family session."
   b. "I understand how frustrated you must be that you will have to remain in the hospital over the holidays. I had surgery one year ago at Thanksgiving. It was really depressing."
   c. "I am sure your surgery will be fine; you have a very good doctor."
   d. "If I were you, I would get another opinion before I agreed to surgery."

6. The communication between you and your client has been going quite well, when you inadvertently used a communication barrier. Your best reaction would be to:
   a. Change the subject and continue talking with the client.
   b. Stop and make a statement such as "I'm sorry, that didn't come out the way I meant it."
   c. Ignore your mistake. The client probably didn't notice.
   d. End the session, and leave the room as quickly as possible.

7. Active or attentive listening can best be described as:
   a. Interrupting the client to clarify information being given
   b. Leaning forward slightly, making eye contact, and giving nonverbal clues while listening
   c. Making notes so that you don't miss what the client is saying
   d. Frequently looking at your watch or out the window, so that the client will realize that he has a time limit

8. "You are stressed about your surgery tomorrow, aren't you?" is an example of a(n):
   a. Neutral question
   b. Open-ended question
   c. Leading question
   d. Directed interview question

9. The portion of the interview in which the client communicates what he or she thinks, feels, knows, and perceives is known as
   a. Establishing rapport
   b. Orientation
   c. The opening
   d. The body

10. You have completed the interview with your client. Which of the following statements or actions would best signal the client that the interview is coming to an end?
    a. Glance at your watch, close the chart, and stand.
    b. "Well, I really enjoyed meeting with you, I think we have accomplished a great deal."
    c. "I have other clients I need to see. I will stop back later on."
    d. "Time really flew. I have all the information I need."

Answers for Review Questions, as well as discussion of Case Study and Critical Thinking Care Map questions, appear in Appendix IV.

Delivering Culturally Competent Care

Chapter
26

SHARING experiences

I work as the only nurse on night shift to care for sixty-two people on an Alzheimer's unit. We have several Latino clients. Most of them don't speak English, but I haven't really had any problem with this. When they're in pain, you can figure it out. Some know enough to say, *"mucho pain," but [when dealing] with Alzheimer's, it's just common sense to look for the nonverbal [cues].*

Rose Syass, LPN, The Manor Retirement Center, Las Vegas, NV.

LEARNING outcomes

After completing this chapter, you will be able to:
- Describe the concept of culture.
- Differentiate concepts of cultural awareness, cultural sensitivity, and cultural competence.
- Identify factors related to communication with culturally diverse clients and colleagues.
- Identify health views of culturally diverse clients: magico-religious, biomedical, and holistic.
- Describe ways to overcome cultural barriers to health care.
- Assess clients from a cultural perspective and plan culturally competent client care.

Cultural competence in nursing is provision of safe and effective health care regardless of population or setting. It is more than recognition by the health care community that clients come from varied backgrounds and that this diversity affects the individual's health beliefs. Culturally competent care begins with the nurse's self-understanding.

Culture is defined as "the learned, shared, and transmitted values, beliefs, norms, and life way practices of a particular group that guide thinking, decisions, and actions in patterned ways." The experience of culture is universal and varies within each group. Box 26-1 ◆ describes some characteristics of culture. A **subculture** is a smaller group sharing a specific characteristic (such as age, gender, ethnic origin, or occupation) within the larger cultural group. For example, student nurses belong to both the "student" and "medical" subcultures.

Nurses and clients may share the same dominant culture (such as North American culture), but they may not share the same health beliefs.

Nurses need to be aware that although individuals from the same groups share common beliefs, values, and experiences, subcultures create diversity. **Diversity** refers to the "fact or state of being different." Differentiating factors such as age, gender, sexual orientation, ethnicity, race, religion, educational or socioeconomic status, and dwelling area (rural vs. urban) may influence clients' health beliefs and expectations.

BOX 26-1
CHARACTERISTICS OF CULTURE

◆ *Culture is learned.* It is neither instinctual nor innate. Learning occurs through life experiences beginning with birth.

◆ *Culture is taught.* Verbal and nonverbal communication from family and peers transmits culture. All animals can learn, but only humans pass along culture.

◆ *Culture is social.* It originates and develops through the interactions of people: families, groups, and communities.

◆ *Culture is dynamic.* Customs, beliefs, and practices change as people adapt to changes in environment. For example, the cultural family norm of the multigenerational household may change when education or employment requires children to leave home or illness forces elderly grandparents to reside in an extended care facility.

◆ *Culture exists on many levels.* It is most easily recognized at the material level. For example, art, tools, and clothes reveal aspects of culture. Abstract concepts such as values, beliefs, and traditions may be more difficult to discover.

◆ *Culture is satisfying.* Gratification strengthens habits and beliefs. Cultural habits persist only as long as they satisfy human needs.

The terms *culture, diversity, ethnicity,* and *race* are often used interchangeably, but they are not synonymous. **Ethnicity** has been defined as "a consciousness of belonging to a group that is differentiated from others by symbolic markers (culture, biology, territory). This experience is rooted in the bonds of a shared past." Religion and geographic background are common factors that help define ethnicity.

Race is the classification of people according to shared biologic characteristics, genetic markers, or features such as skin color, hair texture, and blood type. Different ethnic groups can belong to the same race, as many subcultures are found within an ethnic group. Culture should never be confused with race or ethnicity.

Understanding clients' varying cultural beliefs and needs is essential to nursing practice. A nurse with cultural competence possesses the knowledge, skill, and ability to provide safe and effective health care regardless of population or setting. It was once thought that by hiring a culturally diverse staff, a health care institution would automatically be able to meet the needs of a diverse client population. However, staff diversity does not guarantee cultural sensitivity. The aim of culturally competent care, as outlined in the second goal of the *Healthy People 2010* document, is the elimination of health disparities (U.S. Dept of Health & Human Services, 2000).

A broad range exists in the distribution of health care services delivered in America. For example, members of certain racial, ethnic and socioeconomic groups experience more limited access to health care. Although a diverse population may be one of our nation's greatest assets, it presents our greatest challenge: to provide affordable, comprehensive, and culturally competent, community-based care to all members of our society.

◆ Concepts Related to Culture

Cultural patterns are learned. Therefore, it is important to understand that members of a particular group may not share identical cultural experiences.

Two important terms identify the differences and similarities among peoples of different cultures. **Culture-universals** are the commonalities of values, norms of behavior, and life patterns among different cultures. **Culture-specifics** are those values, beliefs, and patterns of behavior that tend to be unique to a designated culture rather than shared with members of other cultures. For example, most cultures have ceremonies to celebrate the passage from childhood to adulthood; this practice is a culture-universal. However, different cultural groups celebrate this important life event in very different ways (Figure 26-1 ◆). In Latin or Hispanic cultures, the "quince" or "quinceañero" party, which celebrates a girl's 15th birthday, signifies that the young girl has now become a woman. In the Jewish tradition, the bar mitzvah (for boys) and the bat mitzvah (for girls) are celebrations of the passage to adulthood.

Figure 26-1. ◆ Celebrations of the passage to adulthood. Celebrations like the Jewish Bar Mitzvah mark the official beginning of adulthood. *Source:* © Elena Dorfman.

 ## Culture and Health Care

The cultural beliefs and practices regarding health and illness of North America's many different ethnic and cultural groups are important considerations when planning nursing care. Madeleine Leininger pioneered transcultural nursing in 1970. She observed caring in different cultures and subcultures of the world. Leininger analyzed these varying health and illness values, beliefs, and practices to establish a system of providing culturally competent nursing care. Box 26-2 ◆ describes the differences between health status, health beliefs, and health behaviors.

Every culture has two coexisting health care systems: professional and indigenous. A **professional** system is highly structured and maintained by individuals who have completed formal studies. The **indigenous** system consists of traditional folk medicine. **Folk medicine** is defined as those health beliefs and practices that derive from cultural traditions rather than from modern medicine's scientific base. An indigenous system exists long before a professional system develops in a culture. Professionals may devalue an indigenous system, considering it unscientific, "primitive," or even "quackery." Leininger emphasizes that the goal of health care professionals should be to creatively integrate the best of both systems for the benefit of the people served. See Chapter 3 for description of Leininger's nursing theory. ⊖⊃

HEALTH BELIEFS AND PRACTICES

Sociocultural forces such as politics, economics, religion and the predominant health care system can influence the client's health status, beliefs, and health behavior (see Box 26-2). In

---

BOX 26-2 DIFFERENTIATING HEALTH STATUS, BELIEFS, AND BEHAVIORS

- **Health status**—State of health of an individual at a given time. A report of health status may include anxiety, depression, or acute illness and thus describe the individual's problem in general. Health status can also describe such specifics as pulse rate and body temperature.
- **Health beliefs**—Concepts about health that an individual believes true. Such beliefs may or may not be founded on fact. Some of these are influenced by culture, such as the "hot–cold" system of some Hispanic Americans. In this system, health is viewed as a balance of hot and cold qualities within a person. Citrus fruits and some fowl are considered cold foods, and meats and bread are hot foods. In this context hot and cold do not denote temperature or spiciness but innate qualities of the food. For example, a fever is said to be caused by an excess of hot foods. Another example of a culturally related health belief is the belief that health and illness are closely associated with the amount and quality of blood in the body. For example, some Southerners say that "high blood," meaning too much blood in the body, causes headaches and dizziness.
- **Health behaviors**—The actions people take to understand their health state, maintain an optimal state of health, prevent illness and injury, and reach their maximum physical and mental potential. Behaviors such as eating wisely, exercising, paying attention to signs of illness, following treatment advice, avoiding known health hazards such as smoking, taking time for rest and relaxation, and managing one's time effectively are all examples. Health behavior is intended to prevent illness or disease or to provide for early detection of disease. Nurses preparing a plan of care with an individual need to consider the person's health beliefs before they suggest a change in health behaviors.

1999, Margaret Andrews and Joyceen Boyle described three views of health beliefs:

- **Magico-religious.** Health and illness are controlled by supernatural forces. Clients may believe that illness is a form of punishment, brought on by opposing God's will or by magic worked against them. Healing may also be be viewed as dependent on "God's will." Strongly held beliefs can produce real physical illness. These illnesses may require "alternative" treatments such as prayer, rituals, or placebo.
- Scientific or biomedical. Illness is caused by microorganisms or the breakdown of the human body. Clients with biomedical health beliefs generally expect medications, treatments, or surgery to cure disease.

◆ Holistic. Health is maintained when opposing forces of nature are in balance or harmony. All elements of nature are assigned characteristics such as gender, light, temperature, and force. The Chinese concept of "yin and yang" and the "hot–cold" theory of illness in Hispanic cultures are examples of holistic belief systems. For example, when a Chinese client has a "yin" disease (such as cancer) he or she may want to consume foods with opposite "yang" properties (masculine, bright, hot, dry and strong) (Giger & Davidhizar, 1999, p. 69). The term *holistic* is commonly used by nurses to mean treating (and considering) the whole person, not just the medical diagnosis the person might have.

Most clients have mixed health beliefs and practices, combining elements of folk medicine with professional care. Because folk healing is more culturally based, it may be more comfortable and less frightening to the client. Furthermore, clients with limited incomes or limited access to professional care may turn to folk healing. For example, many people continue to use chicken soup as a remedy for colds and "flu." Nurses should remember that treatments once considered to be folk medicine (like acupuncture and massage) are now employed in the delivery of professional health care.

CULTURAL PATTERNS

Cultural groups respond to the environment and each other in patterned ways that reflect their values and beliefs. Responses to social organization, communication, space, time, nutrition, and biologic events (pain, life, death) vary by group.

Social Patterns

The family is the basic unit of society. Cultural values can determine intrafamily communication, norm for family size, and roles for each member. In some families, the man is considered the provider and decision maker. The woman may need to consult her husband prior to making decisions regarding medical treatment for herself or her children. Other families are matriarchal—that is, the mother or grandmother is considered the family leader and decision maker.

The value placed on children and the elderly within a society is culturally derived. In some cultures, children are not physically disciplined, but allowed to interact with their environment while the caregivers provide subtle direction to prevent harm. In many societies, the elderly are highly respected as founts of the culture's wisdom. Responsibility for elder care is influenced by culture. In many cultures, aged parents who cannot live independently live with their adult children.

Sex-role behavior is determined by culture. Some cultures have a prevailing concept of *machismo*, or male superiority. The positive aspects of machismo require that the adult male provide for and protect his family, including extended family members. The woman is expected to maintain the home and raise the children.

Sex-role behaviors can change dramatically, however. In many homes, women and men both work outside the home and both share in household responsibilities (Figure 26-2 ◆).

Cultural values may also dictate the extent of the family's involvement in the client's care. In some cultures, many family members—even entire clans—may want to visit and participate in the client's care. The nurse should evaluate the positive benefits of family participation in the client's care and modify visiting policies as appropriate. The number of individuals wishing to participate in the client's care may depend on the degree of impact the illness has on the family. For example, a single adult child may belong to a culture that discourages placing a severely disabled parent in a nursing home. Therefore, many extended family members may become involved in providing at-home care for the client. Box 26-3 ◆ lists factors that determine the impact of illness on the family.

Naming systems differ according to culture. For example, in Japan and Vietnam the family (surname) comes first and the given name second. Other titles may be used to delineate gender, child, or adult status. In traditional Japanese culture, adults address each other by their surname followed by "san," meaning Mr., Mrs., or Miss. An example is "Maurakami san." Children are referred to by their first names followed by "kun" for boys and "chan" for girls. In the southern United States, it is customary to combine a title with a first name (such as "Miss Lillian") to connote respect for elder status.

Sikhs and Hindus traditionally have three names. Hindus have a personal name, a complimentary name, then a

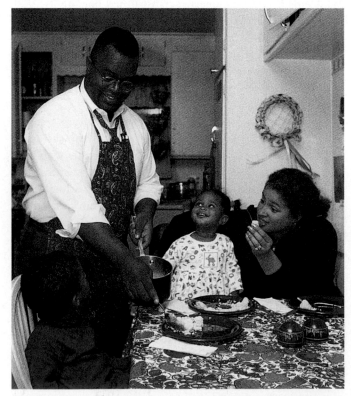

Figure 26-2. ◆ Role patterns within traditional families are changing.

BOX 26-3 FACTORS DETERMINING THE IMPACT OF ILLNESS ON THE FAMILY

- The nature of the illness, which can range from minor to life threatening
- The duration of the illness, which ranges from short term to long term
- The residual effects of the illness, including none to permanent disability
- The meaning of the illness to the family and its significance to family systems
- The financial impact of the illness, which is influenced by factors such as insurance and ability of the ill member to return to work
- The effect of the illness on future family functioning (e.g., previous patterns may be restored or new patterns may be established)

family name. Complimentary name should not be confused with an ordinary middle name. A complimentary name is given as an honor, such as in the case of "Mahatma" (Great Soul), which was bestowed on Mohandas K. Gandhi. Sikhs have a personal name, then the title Singh for men and Kaur for women, then the family name. Names by marriage also vary. In the Hispanic culture a woman who marries retains her father's name and also takes her husband's, such as "Gonzales y Herrera" or "Zeta-Jones."

Communication

Communication and culture are closely interconnected. Communicating effectively with clients is essential in providing culturally competent nursing care.

The most obvious cultural difference is in verbal communication: language, intonation, rhythm, speed, pronunciation, and silence. In North America, the dominant language is English. However, American English differs from "Queen's English" as spoken in Great Britain and other countries of the world. Immigrants who speak English can still encounter language difficulty because English words may have different meanings or pronunciations based on local culture. For example, in the United States, a "boot" is a kind of shoe, whereas in England the word "boot" can also refer to the trunk of car.

Spanish is the second most commonly spoken language in the United States. It is the primary language in many regions of the world, including Spain, South and Central America, Mexico, the Caribbean, and the Philippines. Like English, Spanish consists of many dialects. Therefore, people from different Latino cultures may communicate in Spanish, yet not completely understand each other.

For clients who have limited knowledge of English, the nurse should avoid slang, euphemisms, medical jargon, and abbreviations. Adding gestures or pictures to verbal communication can increase a client's understanding. The nurse

should speak slowly and at normal volume to convey respect. Loud speech may be considered offensive.

When a language barrier exists, a translator may be necessary. Guidelines for using an interpreter are shown in Box 26-4 ◆. Interpreters must be able to provide accurate and unbiased translation. Some schools and health care institutions do not permit student nurses to translate discussions on consent for procedures because the student's lack of knowledge about the procedure may lead the student to provide inaccurate information. Students should determine an institution's policy before agreeing to translate.

Cultural values influence the subject matter and progression of verbal communication. In some cultures, it is believed that social courtesies should be exchanged before business or personal topics are introduced. The sharing of family information or intimate personal details with outsiders—even health care professionals—may be considered taboo. Although nurses may feel pressured to communicate quickly, a client may be offended if the nurse immediately asks personal questions. Discussing general topics first can convey that the nurse is courteous and concerned for the client. This enables the nurse to develop rapport with the client before progression to a more personal discussion.

Culture also determines who may participate in conversations. For example, in some cultures, all discussions regard-

BOX 26-4
NURSING CARE CHECKLIST

USING AN INTERPRETER

- ☑ Avoid asking a member of the client's family, especially a child or spouse, to act as interpreter. The client, not wishing to worry family members, may not provide complete or accurate information.
- ☑ Be aware of gender and age differences. It is preferable to use an interpreter of the same sex as the client to avoid embarrassment and faulty translation of sexual matters.
- ☑ Avoid an interpreter who is politically or socially incompatible with the client. For example, a Bosnian Serb may not be the best interpreter for a Muslim, even if he speaks the language.
- ☑ Address the questions to the client, not to the interpreter.
- ☑ Ask the interpreter to translate as closely as possible the words used by the nurse.
- ☑ Speak slowly and distinctly. Do not use metaphors, for example, "Does it swell like a grapefruit?" or "Is the pain stabbing like a knife?"
- ☑ Observe the facial expressions and body language that the client assumes when listening and talking to the interpreter.

ing health care must include the family decision maker, such as the spouse, grandparent, or eldest son. Some societies have taboos regarding conversations between persons of the opposite sex and/or between married and single persons.

Nonverbal communication includes silence, touch, eye movement, facial expressions, and body posture. Some cultures are quite comfortable with long periods of silence, whereas others consider it appropriate to speak before the other has finished talking. Many people value silence and view it as essential to understanding another's needs, or to preserve privacy. Some cultures view silence as a sign of respect. Others use silence to convey passive agreement.

Culture dictates which forms of touch are appropriate. In some societies, touch is expected as a social courtesy. In American culture, for example, the firm handshake is a recognized form of greeting that conveys character and strength. In some European cultures, greetings may include a kiss on one or both cheeks with the handshake. In other societies, however, touch is considered magical (and dangerous) because of the belief that the soul can leave the body on physical contact. Therefore, casual touching is forbidden. In many cultures, for example, a kiss is not an appropriate public greeting between persons of the opposite sex—even those who are family members. However, a kiss on the cheek is acceptable as a greeting between members of the same sex. Nurses should observe client–family interactions for cues to an appropriate degree of touch. The nurse should also observe the client's responses to ordinary touch necessary to provide care. For example, note the client's reaction to the physical examination or bath.

Facial expressions can also vary among cultures. Expressions can convey a meaning opposite to what is felt or understood. For example, a smile may not indicate understanding or agreement. Instead, smiling may be a simple demonstration of respect, or an attempt to please the nurse.

Eye movement during communication has cultural foundations. In Western cultures, direct eye contact is valued and regarded as a sign of attentiveness. It conveys self-confidence, openness, interest, listening, and honesty. Lack of eye contact may be interpreted as secretiveness, shyness, guilt, lack of interest, or even as a sign of mental illness. In contrast, other cultures may view direct eye contact as impolite or an invasion of privacy. The nurse should not misinterpret the character of a client who avoids eye contact.

Body posture and gesture are learned aspects of culture. Across cultures, finger pointing, the "V" sign with index and middle fingers, and the "thumbs up" sign have different meanings. For example, the "V" hand signal means "victory" in some cultures, but is an offensive gesture in others.

Space Orientation

Space is a relative concept that includes the individual, the body, the surrounding environment, and objects within that environment. The relationship between the individual's own body and objects and persons within space is learned and influ-

enced by culture. For example, in nomadic societies, space is not owned. Area is occupied temporarily until the tribe moves on. In Western societies, people tend to be more territorial, as reflected in phrases such as "Get out of my space." The nurse must be aware of the client's response to movement toward the client. A client may withdraw if the nurse is perceived as being too close. The nurse will need to explain the need for close contact, then obtain permission to continue.

Clients in long-term care facilities, or those who are hospitalized for an extended time, may want to personalize their space. These individuals may want to control where objects are placed on a bedside cabinet or overbed table. Nurses must be responsive to clients' needs to exert some control over the environment. When there are no medical contraindications, clients should be encouraged to wear their own clothing or have objects of personal significance. Wearing cultural dress and having personal cultural objects in one's environment promotes individuality, enhances cultural identity, and builds self-esteem.

Time Orientation

Time orientation refers to an individual's focus on the past, the present, or the future. Most cultures combine all three orientations, but one tends to dominate. The American focus on time tends to be directed to the future, with emphasis on linear or "clock" time and schedules. European-Americans often plan ahead—for the coming week, for vacation, for retirement. The culture of nursing and health care values time. Appointments are scheduled and treatments prescribed with time parameters (often according to the clock). Medication orders generally include how often medicine is to be taken and when (e.g., digoxin, 0.25 mg once daily, at 10:00 A.M.). This kind of scheduling works well for future-oriented clients.

In contrast, when caring for clients who are oriented to the present it is important to avoid fixed schedules. Instead, the nurse may offer a time range for treatments and activities. For example, instead of instructing the client to take digoxin every day at 10:00 A.M., the nurse may tell the client to take it every day in the morning, or after rising from bed.

Nutrition

Most cultures have staple foods, that is, foods that are plentiful or readily accessible in the environment. For example, the staple food for Asians is rice and for Eastern Europeans is wheat.

Even clients who have lived in the United States or Canada for several generations often continue to eat the foods of their cultural homeland.

The ways foods are prepared and served are cultural practices. For example, in the United States, a traditional food served on the Thanksgiving holiday is stuffed turkey. However, in different regions of the country the stuffing recipe varies. In the South, stuffing is usually made from cornbread, whereas in New England, it often has seasoned wheatbread and chestnuts. Preparation of daily staple foods may vary by subculture. For example, some Asians enjoy steamed rice; others prefer boiled rice.

Food-related cultural practices include infant feeding and weaning behaviors. Preferences for breast or bottle feeding and when to introduce solid foods vary by culture.

Religious practice associated with specific cultures affects diet. Religions have rules regarding what, how, and when foods may be consumed. Orthodox Judaism and Islam prohibit the ingestion of pork products. Orthodox Jews observe kosher customs, eating only those foods inspected and prepared according to dietary laws. For example, the eating of milk and meat products at the same meal is forbidden. Observant Buddhists, Hindus, and Sikhs are strict vegetarians. Some Christian denominations (such as Seventh Day Adventists) prohibit meat, caffeine, and alchohol consumption. Christians, Jews, and Muslims may participate in religious fasts. For example, observant Roman Catholics abstain from meat on Ash Wednesday and Good Friday. Orthodox Jews fast on Yom Kippur (Day of Atonement). Muslims fast during the month of Ramadan. (In all three religions, people may be excused from these fasts because of ill health.)

Religious fasting is sometimes a hidden aspect that adversely affects the client's care. For example, during Ramadan, Muslims go without food or water from sunrise to sunset. Doing so increases the risk of kidney problems or *syncope* (heatstroke) in some geographic areas. Fasting could also mean that the client would refuse medication during these hours. Individuals who do not eat pork due to religious dietary restriction may also not accept drugs developed from pork derivative, such as insulin. A diabetic client with these beliefs should use human insulin.

Pain

Beliefs regarding and responses to pain vary among ethnic and racial groups. Response to pain must be understood in relation to the client's perception of pain and its impact on the family. In some cultures, pain is considered "divine retribution." The individual is expected to accept pain without complaint to atone for sins. In other cultures, self-infliction of pain is a sign of mourning or grief. Pain infliction is an integral aspect of some cultures' ritual rites of passage; tolerance of pain signifies strength and endurance. In some cultures, pain tolerance is associated with masculinity. Boys are taught to "take it like a man" and "big boys don't cry." In other cultures, men may express pain to receive attention and sympathy.

If a client does not complain, do not assume the client is pain free. Nurses must remain aware that cultural beliefs may prohibit clients from reporting discomfort. Facial grimaces, infrequent talking, muscle tension, and vital sign changes may indicate pain. The nurse is responsible for observing such changes and offering pain relief to the client as appropriate.

Pain treatment varies by culture. In European-American cultures, medication is typically sought for pain relief. In other cultures, heat, cold, relaxation, or other techniques are used.

Death

Most cultures believe in an "afterlife," wherein a component of human existence (which some call the "soul") continues following the death of the body. Many cultures believe the soul is judged by merit. Some believe it goes to a place of eternal comfort or torment (such as the Judeo-Christian concept of Heaven and Hell). Others (such as Buddhists and Hindus) believe the soul is reincarnated. Death may be less threatening to individuals who believe they have behaved well in life because they expect a reward—eternal joy or another happier life on Earth. Unnatural or untimely deaths may be considered divine punishments.

Cultural beliefs about prolonging life (including artificial life support), organ donation, autopsy, preparation of the body, and cremation are closely allied to religion. Prolonging life is generally encouraged. However, some religions discourage the practice, either as a rule or in certain circumstances. Christian Scientists, for example, are unlikely to use medical means to prolong life. Jews generally oppose prolonging life after irreversible brain damage. In hopeless illness, Buddhists may permit euthanasia. Some religions prohibit the removal of body parts and dictate that all body parts be given appropriate burial.

Organ donation is prohibited by Jehovah's Witnesses and Muslims, whereas Buddhists in America consider it an act of mercy and encourage it. Autopsy and cremation may be prohibited, opposed, or discouraged by Orthodox Jews, Eastern Orthodox Christians, Muslims, and Jehovah's Witnesses. Hindus, in contrast, prefer cremation. The casting of human ashes on sacred rivers is a Hindu death ritual.

Nurses must be knowledgeable about clients' death-related rituals. For example, dying Roman Catholic and Eastern Orthodox Christians may receive the Sacraments of the Anointing of the Sick and Eucharist (Holy Communion). Hindus may engage in bedside chanting. Rituals may include special procedures for washing, dressing, positioning, and shrouding the dead. The nurse must ensure that any ritual items present in the health care agency (such as medals or prayer beads) are given to the family or to the funeral home. See Chapter 31 for additional information concerning death and dying.

◆ Culturally Sensitive Care

Kittler and Sucher (1990) suggest a four-step process to improve cultural sensitivity:

1. **Know your own cultural heritage.** For example, do you value stoic behavior in relation to pain? Are the rights of the individual valued over and above the rights of the family? Only by knowing your own culture (values, practices, and beliefs) can you be ready to learn about another's. Awareness of biases can enables the nurse to modify personal behavior that may compromise care. When unable to do so, another nurse should be asked to take over the client's care.

2. **Understand the client's culture as described by the client.** Avoid assuming that all people of the same ethnic background share the same culture. When the nurse understands the client's culture as it affects that individual, mutual respect is more likely to develop.

3. **Understand adaptations the client has made to live in a North American culture.** Identify the client's unique preferences in health practices, diet, hygiene, and so on.

4. **Form a nursing care plan with the client that incorporates his or her culture.** In this way, cultural values, practices, and beliefs can be incorporated with care and judgment.

BARRIERS TO CULTURAL SENSITIVITY

Ethnocentrism, stereotyping, prejudice, and discrimination are common barriers to cultural sensitivity, and therefore to competent care.

Ethnocentrism refers to the view that the beliefs and values of one's own culture are superior to those of other cultures. Ethnocentrism occurs in health care when professional caregivers believe that the only valid health care beliefs and practices are their own. Nurses who take a transcultural view, however, value their own beliefs and practices while respecting the beliefs and practices of others. **Stereotyping** is assuming that all members of a culture or ethnic group are alike. For example, a nurse may assume that all Italians express pain verbally or that all Chinese like rice. Stereotyping may be either positive or negative and is frequently an outcome of racism or discrimination. Nurses must identify clients' unique beliefs, needs, and values to avoid stereotyping.

Prejudice is a strongly held opinion about some topic or group of people. Such opinion may be based on experience, fear, or misinformation. Positive prejudice often stems from ethnocentrism.

Discrimination is defined as "the differential treatment of individuals or groups based on categories such as race, ethnicity, gender, social class, or exceptionality." For example, a nurse takes a child who is waiting in an emergency department ahead of another child. The child taken ahead appears clean, is neatly dressed, and is smiling; the other child appears dirty, is wearing worn clothes, and is angry. Racism is the belief that race is the primary determinant of human traits and capacities and that racial differences result in an inherent superiority of a particular race. It is related to ethnocentrism and is a common cause of discrimination.

It is important for nurses to be culturally sensitive and to convey this sensitivity to clients, support people, and other health care personnel (Box 26-5 ◆).

All phases of the nursing process are affected by the client's and the nurse's cultural values, beliefs, and behaviors. As the client's culture and the nurse's culture come together in the nurse–client relationship, a unique cultural environment is created that can improve or impair the client's outcome. Self-awareness of personal biases can enable nurses to develop modifying

BOX 26-5
NURSING CARE CHECKLIST

CONVEYING CULTURAL SENSITIVITY

☑ **Always ask clients how they wish to be addressed.** Use surnames (e.g., Mrs. Aylia, Dr. Rush) unless invited to do otherwise. Ask the client the term they prefer to use when referring to ethnic origin or sexual orientation. Terms can vary and may be influenced by the client's age or gender.

☑ **Provide a formal introduction.** Upon meeting a client for the first time, state your name and title (e.g., Maria Fernandez, LPN). Explain your role in the client's care. Introductions are the best times to learn proper pronunciation of the client's names.

☑ **Inquire about the client's personal health and general health beliefs.** Determine if the client's beliefs are congruent with the dominant health care culture. If not, establish whether the incongruency will have a negative impact on the client's health.

☑ **Never make assumptions.** Avoid stereotypes and always ask about anything you don't understand.

☑ **Respect clients' values, beliefs, and practices.** If you don't agree with them, and this conflict is causing distress, request that another nurse be assigned to care for the client.

☑ **Demonstrate respect for clients' support persons.** In some cultures, health care decisions are made by family members. Some clients choose significant others outside the family to make these decisions for them.

☑ **Be authentic.** Remain true to your own values, but be honest about conflict or knowledge you may lack regarding the client's culture.

☑ **Demonstrate sincere effort to obtain client trust.** Understand, however, that trust may develop slowly or not at all.

behaviors or (if they are unable to do so) to remove themselves from situations where care may be compromised. The nurse must also consider the cultural values of the health care setting because those too may influence the client's outcome.

NURSING CARE

 ASSESSING

The cultural assessment is a cornerstone of culturally competent care. Prior to an interview, the nurse determines the client's language and proficiency in English. A goal of the cultural assessment is to understand and differentiate the client's health status, health beliefs, and health behaviors (see Box 26-2).

To obtain assessment data, the nurse uses broad statements and open-ended questions that encourage clients to express themselves fully (Andrews & Boyle, 1999). See Box 26-6 ◆ for examples of questions.

The nurse can learn about the client's communication patterns and orientation to space by observing nonverbal behavior. It is unnecessary to complete a total cultural assessment for every client. Instead, nurses need to collect enough basic cultural data to identify patterns of behavior that may either facilitate or interfere with a nursing strategy or treatment plan.

 ## DIAGNOSING, PLANNING, and IMPLEMENTING

Developing a culturally sensitive care plan involves accommodating the client's viewpoint and negotiating with the client.

Negotiation is a collaborative process. It acknowledges that the nurse–client relationship is *reciprocal* (works in both

directions) and that differences of opinion exist between the nurse and client regarding health, illness, and treatment. Successful negotiation requires expert communication skills, such as responding empathetically, validating information, and effectively summarizing content. Negotiation is necessary when cultural treatment practices conflict, or when cultural practices are considered harmful to the client's well-being. The nurse must determine precisely how the client is managing the illness, what practices could be harmful, and which practices can be safely combined with Western medicine. For example, mixing antihypertensive medication or replacing insulin therapy with herbs may be potentially dangerous. In situations where harm may occur, the nurse needs to inform the client about possible outcomes.

When a client chooses to follow only cultural practices and refuses all prescribed medical or nursing interventions, nursing goals for the client must be modified.

 ## EVALUATING

Transcultural nursing care is challenging. Creativity, knowledge, and flexibility are required to discover the meaning of clients' behaviors and to modify nursing interventions to make them culturally acceptable. Nurses should actively learn from each transcultural nursing situation they encounter to improve the delivery of culture-specific care to future clients. Box 26-7 ◆ offers suggestions for providing culturally competent nursing care.

 ## DISCHARGE CONSIDERATIONS

Nurses identify community resources that are available to assist clients of different cultures. The hospital social worker or discharge planner are a good resource for community resources. The client's church or a community center can also

---

BOX 26-6 EXAMPLES OF OPEN-ENDED QUESTIONS FOR A CULTURAL ASSESSMENT

Cultural Affiliation
I am interested in learning about your cultural heritage. Can you tell me about where you came from and how long you have lived in this country?

Beliefs About Current Illness
What do you call your problem? Why did it start when it did? What does your sickness do to your body? What are the chief problems your sickness has caused for you personally, for your family, and at work?

Health Care Practices
What kinds of things do you do to maintain health? For example, what types of food do you eat to maintain health? Do you eat different foods when you are sick?

Illness Beliefs and Care Practices
What kind of things do you do to treat illness? Do you use traditional healers (curandero or herbalist, minister, monk, priest, spiritualist, or shaman)?
What special remedies are generally used for the illness you have? What remedies are you currently using (e.g., herbal remedies, potions, massage, wearing of talismans, copper bracelets, or charms)?

Family Life and Support System
I would like to learn about your family. Is there someone in your family who usually makes health care decisions? Who will be able to help you during and after treatment? Do you need help to contact these people?

BOX 26-7 NURSING CARE CHECKLIST

PROVIDING CULTURALLY COMPETENT CARE TO FAMILIES

- ☑ Learn the rituals, customs, and practices of the major cultural groups with whom you come into contact. Learn to appreciate the richness of diversity as an asset rather than a hindrance in your practice.
- ☑ Identify your own personal biases, attitudes, prejudices, and stereotypes.
- ☑ Include cultural assessment of the client and family as part of overall assessment.
- ☑ Recognize that it is the client's (or family's) right to make their own health care choices.
- ☑ Convey respect and cooperate with traditional helpers and caregivers.

provide resources, especially if the client and his or her family are not acclimated to the community as a whole.

Nursing Process Case Study: PROVIDING CULTURALLY SENSITIVE CARE

Rachel was born to a Jewish couple and is Jewish by race and religion. Her father died when she was 10 years old and her mother remarried 3 years later. Rachel was legally adopted by her Italian stepfather, who was a devout Catholic. Although the family participated in Catholic-Italian traditions, Rachel's mother taught her many Jewish traditions as well, so that her heritage would be preserved. Rachel is now 58 years old, practices traditions from both her Jewish and Italian upbringing, and is dying of cancer. "I have been thinking about dying. Although I haven't been very religious as an adult, I think I would like to speak to a rabbi." You are the nurse caring for Rachel during her final days.

Assessment.

- States that only living relative is 86-year-old stepfather
- 58-year-old female, weight 97 lbs.
- NPO; complains of nausea and vomiting
- Stage 1 pressure sore on coccyx
- VS: T 100.6° F (38.1° C), P 86, R 18, BP 140/70
- IV for hydration and PCA for pain management

Diagnosis. The following nursing diagnoses are developed for Rachel:

- Risk for Spiritual Distress
- Risk for Loneliness
- Powerlessness

Expected Outcomes. The expected outcomes for the plan of care are that Rachel will:

- State acceptance of suggestions to enhance spirituality
- Demonstrate positive use of time alone when socialization is not possible

- State feelings of powerlessness and other feelings related to powerlessness (e.g., anger, sadness, hopelessness)

Planning and Implementation. The following nursing interventions are implemented for Rachel:

- Perform spiritual assessment to determine whether client's usual means of spirituality are useful during physical distress.
- Encourage client to use usual means of spirituality to face challenges with psychosocial problems.
- Validate feelings regarding loss.
- Encourage client to pray or offer to pray with client.
- Assess for the influence of cultural beliefs on ability to cope with spiritual distress.
- Assess for the influence of cultural beliefs, norms, and values on the client's feelings of powerlessness.
- Promote a sense of ethnic attachment.
- Validate the client's feelings regarding isolation and loneliness.

Evaluation. Client met with rabbi and also with the hospital's Catholic chaplain. Expresses concern for elderly stepfather's ability to cope if her funeral follows Jewish custom. Stepfather visited; they discussed her spiritual issues. Stepfather agreed to a Jewish service, but asked for Rachel's permission to hold a Memorial Mass following her burial. Rachel expressed a peaceful feeling and experienced a restful night's sleep.

Critical Thinking in the Nursing Process

1. How may Rachel's mixed cultural background pose a dilemma for you as her nurse or her family?
2. How may Rachel's culture affect her approach to death and the care of her body following her death?
3. How would you document this?

Note: The bibliography listings for this and all chapters have been compiled at the back of the book.

Chapter Review

Key Terms by Topics

Use the audio glossary feature of either the CD-ROM or the Companion Website to hear the correct pronunciation of the following key terms.

Introduction
cultural competence, culture, subculture, diversity, ethnicity, race

Concepts related to culture
culture-universals, culture-specifics

Culture and health care
health status, health beliefs, health behaviors, professional, indigenous, folk medicine, magico-religious

Culturally sensitive care
ethnocentrism, stereotyping, prejudice, discrimination

Key Points

◆ An individual's ethnic and cultural background can influence beliefs, values, and practices.

◆ Personal characteristics modify an individual's cultural values, beliefs, and practices.

◆ Cultures have varying patterns of human response to social organization, space, time, nutrition, and biologic events (birth, pain and death).

◆ When assessing a client, the nurse considers the client's cultural values, beliefs, and practices related to health and health care.

◆ Culturally competent care begins with the nurse's own cultural self-awareness.

◆ Negotiation is a vital skill required in transcultural nursing.

EXPLORE MediaLink

Additional interactive resources for this chapter can be found on the Companion Website at www.prenhall.com/ramont. Click on Chapter 26 and "Begin" to select the activities for this chapter.

For chapter-related NCLEX-style questions and an audio glossary, access the accompanying CD-ROM in this book.

∞ For Further Study

For a description of Leininger's nursing theory, see Chapter 3.

For additional information concerning death and dying, see Chapter 31.

Critical Thinking Care Map
Caring for a Child Receiving Home Remedies
NCLEX-PN Focus Area: Psychosocial Integrity

Case Study: One-year-old Oahn Tran, a Vietnamese girl, was brought in by her father because of wheezing and a persistent cough. While checking her vital signs, you notice bright red circular dermabrasions, about the size of the opening of a shot glass. She has them all over her back, legs, and arms. You ask the father what the sores are from and he replies, "Her grandmother, who lives with us, performs Giac on her. In our culture, in order to draw out a bad force within the child, we place small, heated glasses on the skin, which forms suction. It leaves those marks." The sight of these sores still concerns you and you think of reporting it as abuse.

Nursing Diagnosis: Risk for Caregiver Role Strain

COLLECT DATA

Subjective	Objective

Would you report this data? Yes/No

If yes, to: _____

Nursing Care

How would you document this? _____

Data Collected
(use those that apply)

- One-year-old child with stuffy nose and cough
- URI of 3 days' duration
- Fever 102.2° F (39° C)
- Respirations 28 and shallow, nasal flaring, and retraction
- Chest x-ray nonspecific inflammation
- Viral culture of nasal swab reveals RSV (respiratory syncytial virus)
- Admitted to hospital and placed in isolation

Nursing Interventions
(use those that apply)

- Maintain a patent airway at all times.
- Negotiate with family regarding aspects of health behavior that will need to be modified.
- Assess for the influences of cultural beliefs, norms, values, and expectations on the family experience of care giving.
- Negotiate with parent regarding the aspects of caregiving that can be modified and still honor cultural beliefs.
- Encourage family support groups or other service providers.
- Encourage critical thinking to consider strategies for changes in behavior.
- Assess for the influence of cultural beliefs, norms, and values on the client's and families perception of risk for injury.
- Acknowledge racial/ethnic differences at the onset of care.
- Auscultate breath sounds q2h.
- Monitor respiratory patterns, including rate, depth, and effort.
- Position client to optimize respirations.

NCLEX-PN Exam Preparation

1. The nurse should consider which of the following when working with a client of a different ethnic group?
   a. Culture-universals
   b. Culture-specifics
   c. Cultural stereotypes
   d. Subcultures

2. Race is defined by which of the following characteristics?
   a. Culture and territory
   b. Biological characteristics and genetic markers
   c. Common social and cultural heritage
   d. Transmitted values and beliefs

3. A client who seeks care from an herbalist prior to seeking care from a physician is said to have used:
   a. An indigenous health care system
   b. A professional health care system
   c. An ineffective mode of treatment
   d. Cultural "quackery"

4. A Caucasian nurse who was born and raised in the American culture and views Western medicine as the only option can be said to be:
   a. Prejudiced
   b. Culturally sensitive
   c. Ethnocentric
   d. Culturally competent

5. When a nurse makes a statement based on ethnic stereotyping ("Italians have no pain tolerence"), the nurse has assumed that:
   a. All members of an ethnic group are alike.
   b. All members of a cultural group have the same health beliefs.
   c. Commonalities occur among cultures.
   d. Individuals of specific groups respond to medical treatment differently.

6. Your assigned client has just been informed that she has advanced breast cancer. Chemotherapy has been recommended. Her response is, "I won't have chemotherapy. If it is God's will, I will get better without treatment." Her health beliefs can be described as:
   a. Scientific
   b. Biomedical
   c. Holistic
   d. Magico-religious

7. A young Asian mother brings in her 3-year-old for follow-up after recurrent ear infections. The physician suggests surgery to place ear tubes. The mother becomes agitated when pushed to schedule surgery. With your knowledge of cultural responses you determine that:
   a. She doesn't understand why the procedure must be done.
   b. It is important to consider who has the authority to make health care decisions in the family.
   c. She is concerned that her health insurance may not pay for the procedure.
   d. An interpreter should be provided when consent for surgery is being obtained.

8. You are assigned to work with the lactation specialist. A Hispanic mother who had expressed a desire to breast-feed is giving her baby a bottle. She states, "I don't have any milk yet. I will breast feed when I get home." From her statement you would conclude the following:
   a. She does not understand the importance of colostrum to provide immunity for the baby.
   b. She not understand the concept of supply and demand for milk production.
   c. Some cultural groups are extremely modest and are not comfortable breast-feeding unless in private.
   d. She really doesn't plan to breast-feed. She just feels pressured by the staff to agree to it.

9. A Jewish rabbi in traction refuses your help to eat roast beef, vegetables, roll, butter, and a carton of milk. Which of the following statements would be appropriate?
   a. "It is very important that you have protein and calcium in order for your body to heal."
   b. "If you don't like the meal they have sent I can see what else is available."
   c. "I know it is difficult to be dependent. Once you are out of traction you will be able to do it on your own."
   d. "Do you follow kosher dietary laws? I will have the dietitian speak with you about your special needs."

10. A non–English-speaking client arrives on the medical unit. No interpreter is available. To expedite admission, the nurse asks the family to interpret for the client. Based on your knowledge of culturally competent care, which of the following would explain why insufficient health information was received?
    a. The family members do not understand the medical questions asked.
    b. The client does not wish family members to know about her problem.
    c. The client is reluctant to answer personal questions.
    d. The client feels the nurse will not try to understand her problem because of the language barrier.

Answers for Review Questions, as well as discussion of Case Study and Critical Thinking Care Map Questions, appear in Appendix IV.

Chapter 27

Sensory Perception

SHARING experiences

"Nursing, to me, is the single best way I can give back to the community. Using our hands for the benefit of others is what makes us human—especially when it involves basic needs mixed with compassion."

Valarie Gray, LPN student, Practical Nursing Program, Idaho State University, Pocatello, ID.

LEARNING outcomes

After completing this chapter, you will be able to:
- Describe factors influencing the sensory experience.
- Discuss factors that place a client at risk for sensory disturbances.
- Describe essential components in assessing a client's sensory–perceptual function.
- Identify clinical signs and symptoms of sensory overload and deprivation.
- List and describe methods of preventing sesory overload and deprivation
- Discuss nursing interventions for managing acute sensory deficits.
- Describe factors that affect the amount and quality of sensory stimulation.
- Explain the key points related to diagnosis, planning, and implementing care.
- Identify strategies to promote and maintain orientation to person, place, time, and situation for confused and unconscious clients.
- Discuss the process of evaluation to determine if goals and outcomes have been achieved.

MediaLink

 www.prenhall.com/ramont

Use the address above to access the free, interactive Companion Website created for this textbook. Get hints, instant feedback, and textbook references to chapter-related NCLEX-style questions. Link to other interesting sites.

Audio Glossary:
Use the Companion Website, or the CD-ROM disk enclosed with your textbook, to hear the pronunciation of key terms in the chapter.

An individual's senses are essential for growth, development, and survival. Sensory stimuli give meaning to events in the environment. Any alteration in people's sensory functions can affect their ability to function within the environment. For example, many clients have impaired sensory functions that put them at risk in the health care setting. Nurses can help them find ways to function safely in this often confusing environment.

Components of the Sensory Process

For an individual to be aware of the surroundings, four aspects of the sensory process must be present:

- *Stimulus*—An agent or act that stimulates a nerve receptor.
- *Receptor*—A nerve cell acts as a receptor by converting the stimulus to a nerve impulse. Most receptors are specific, that is, sensitive to only one type of stimulus, such as visual, auditory, or touch.
- *Impulse conduction*—The impulse travels along nerve pathways to the spinal cord or directly to the brain. For example, auditory impulses travel to the organ of Corti in the inner ear. From there the impulses travel along the eighth cranial nerve to the temporal lobe of the brain.
- *Perception*—Perception, or awareness and interpretation of stimuli, takes place in the brain, where specialized brain cells interpret the nature and the quality of the sensory stimuli. The level of consciousness affects the perception of the stimuli.

SENSORY RECEPTION AND PERCEPTION

The sensory process, therefore, involves two major components: reception and perception. **Sensory reception** is the process of receiving stimuli or data. These stimuli are either external or internal. External stimuli are *visual* (sight), *auditory* (hearing), **olfactory** (smell), *tactile* (touch), and **gustatory** (taste). Gustatory stimuli can be internal as well. Other types of internal stimuli are kinesthetic or visceral. **Kinesthetic** refers to awareness of the position and movement of body parts. For example, a person walking is aware of which leg is forward. **Visceral** refers to organs that may produce stimuli that make a person aware of them (e.g., a full stomach). Regardless of the type of stimuli received, **sensory perception** involves the conscious organization and translation of the data or stimuli into meaningful information.

Arousal Mechanism

For the person to receive and interpret stimuli, the brain must be alert. The brain has the capacity to adapt to sensory stimuli. For example, a person living in a city may not notice traffic noise that someone from a rural area would find loud and disturbing. Not all sensory stimuli are acted on; some are stored by the memory to be used at a later date.

Cognition (cerebral functioning) involves such processes as conscious thought, reality orientation, problem solving, judgment, and comprehension.

Awareness is the ability to perceive environmental stimuli and body reactions and to respond appropriately through thought and action. The normal, alert person can assimilate many kinds of information at one time. There are several states of awareness, as shown in Table 27-1 ◆.

Sensory Alterations

People become accustomed to certain sensory stimuli. When these change markedly, the individual may experience discomfort. For example, when clients enter a hospital they usually experience stimuli that are different in quantity and quality from those they experience at home. These changes may cause clients to become confused and disoriented (see Table 27-1).

Nurses are aware of behaviors that result from changes in stimuli. Hospitals and other institutions pay more attention now to color, sound, privacy, and social interaction for clients, so that the stimuli more resemble those in the home environment. Changes in stimuli can result in alterations from sensory deprivation, sensory overload, and sensory deficits.

SENSORY DEPRIVATION

Sensory deprivation is generally thought of as a decrease in or lack of meaningful stimuli. Because of this reduced stimulation, a person becomes more acutely aware of the remaining stimuli and often perceives these in a distorted manner. Thus, the person often experiences alterations in perception, cogni-

TABLE 27-1	STATES OF AWARENESS
STATE	**DESCRIPTION**
Full consciousness	Alert; oriented to time, place, person; understands verbal and written words
Disoriented	Not oriented to time, place, or person
Confused	Reduced awareness, easily bewildered; poor memory, misinterprets stimuli; impaired judgment
Somnolent	Extreme drowsiness but will respond to stimuli
Semicomatose	Can be aroused by extreme or repeated stimuli
Coma[a]	Will not respond to verbal stimuli

[a]See Glasgow Coma Scale, Table 11-2.

tion, and emotion. Box 27-1 ◆ describes clinical signs of sensory deprivation.

SENSORY OVERLOAD

Sensory overload generally occurs when a person is unable to process or manage the amount or intensity of sensory stimuli. Three factors contribute to sensory overload:

* Increased quantity or quality of internal stimuli, such as pain, dyspnea, anxiety
* Increased quantity or quality of external stimuli, such as a noisy health care setting, intrusive diagnostic studies, contacts with many strangers
* Inability to disregard stimuli selectively, perhaps as a result of nervous system disturbances or medications that stimulate the arousal mechanism

Sensory overload can prevent the brain from ignoring or responding to specific stimuli. The person usually feels overwhelmed and does not feel in control. It is important for nurses to remember that the sights and sounds that are familiar to them often represent overload to clients. People who have sensory overload may appear fatigued. They often cannot internalize new information and experience cognitive overload as a result of everything that is happening to them. Such factors as pain, lack of sleep, and worry can also contribute to sensory overload. See Box 27-1 for common manifestations of sensory overload.

SENSORY DEFICITS

A **sensory deficit** is impaired reception, perception, or both, of one or more of the senses. Blindness and deafness are sensory deficits. When only one sense is affected, other senses may become more acute to compensate for the loss. However, sudden loss of eyesight can result in disorientation.

When there is a gradual loss of sensory function, individuals often develop behaviors to compensate for the loss. Sometimes these behaviors are unconscious. For example, a person with gradual hearing loss in the right ear may unconsciously turn the left ear toward a speaker. When the loss is sudden, however, compensatory behavior often takes days or weeks to develop.

Some neurologic diseases cause changes in the kinesthetic sense and tactile perceptions. Diseases of the inner ear, for example, can cause loss of kinesthetic sense.

Clients with sensory deficits are at risk of both sensory deprivation and sensory overload. Persons with visual problems may be unable to read, watch television, or recognize nurses by sight. An unfamiliar environment can add to their confusion. Blind people often have highly structured home environments, and the diversity and unfamiliarity of the hospital environment can create sensory overload. At the same time, impaired vision often results in an inability to move around readily or socialize with others.

SENSORY AIDS

Many sensory aids are available for clients who have visual and hearing deficits, as listed in Box 27-2 ◆. Sensory aids can be used in the health care setting as well as in the home. In all situations, the assistance of support people needs to be enlisted whenever possible to help the client deal with the deficit. See also Chapter 13. ᴳᴰ

Factors Affecting Sensory Function

A number of factors affect the amount and quality of sensory stimulation, including a person's developmental stage, culture, level of stress, medications and illness, and lifestyle.

DEVELOPMENTAL STAGE

As children grow, they learn that certain sensations provide cues for behavior they have already learned. For example, parents model stopping and looking both ways before crossing a street. Children learn that stopping on a curb is associated with this safety behavior. Adults have many learned responses to sensory cues. Therefore, the sudden loss or impairment of any sense has a profound effect on both the child and adult.

CULTURE

An individual's culture often determines the amount of stimulation that a person considers usual or "normal." For example, a child raised in a large, active Latino family may be accustomed to more stimulation than an only child raised in a European American family. A sudden change in cultural surroundings experienced by immigrants or visitors to a new

---

BOX 27-1 MANIFESTATIONS OF SENSORY DEPRIVATION AND SENSORY OVERLOAD

Sensory Deprivation

* Excessive yawning, drowsiness, sleeping
* Decreased attention span, difficulty concentrating, decreased problem solving
* Impaired memory
* Periodic disorientation, general confusion, or nocturnal confusion
* Preoccupation with somatic complaints, such as palpitations
* Hallucinations or delusions
* Crying, annoyance over small matters, depression
* Apathy, emotional lability

Sensory Overload

* Complaints of fatigue, sleeplessness
* Irritability, anxiety, restlessness
* Periodic or general disorientation
* Reduced problem-solving ability and task performance
* Increased muscle tension

BOX 27-2 SENSORY AIDS FOR VISUAL AND HEARING DEFICITS

Visual

- ◆ Eyeglasses of the correct prescription, clean and in good repair
- ◆ Adequate room lighting, including night lights
- ◆ Sunglasses or shades on windows to reduce glare
- ◆ Bright, contrasting colors in the environment
- ◆ Magnifying glass
- ◆ Phone dialer with large numbers
- ◆ Clock and wristwatch with large numbers
- ◆ Color code or texture code on stoves, washer, medicine containers, and so on
- ◆ Colored or raised rims on dishes
- ◆ Reading material with large print
- ◆ Braille or recorded books
- ◆ Seeing-eye dog

Hearing

- ◆ Hearing aid in good order
- ◆ Lip reading
- ◆ Sign language
- ◆ Amplified telephones
- ◆ Telecommunication device for the deaf (TDD)
- ◆ Amplified telephone ringers and doorbells
- ◆ Flashing alarm clocks
- ◆ Flashing smoke detectors

country, especially where there are differences in language, dress, and cultural behaviors, may also result in sensory overload or cultural shock.

It is important that nurses be sensitive to what stimulation is culturally acceptable to a client. For example, in some cultures touch is comforting; in others it is considered intrusive or offensive.

STRESS

During times of increased stress, people may find their senses already overloaded and thus seek to decrease sensory stimulation. For example, a client dealing with physical illness, pain, hospitalization, and diagnostic tests may wish to have only close support people visit. In addition, the client may need the nurse's help to decrease unnecessary stimuli (e.g., noise) as much as possible. See also Chapter 8. ⊂⊃

MEDICATIONS AND ILLNESS

Certain medications can alter an individual's awareness of environmental stimuli. Narcotics and sedatives, for example, can decrease awareness of stimuli. Some antidepressants can alter perceptions of stimuli.

Certain diseases, such as atherosclerosis, restrict blood flow to the receptor organs and the brain, thereby decreasing awareness and slowing responses. Uncontrolled diabetes mel-

litus can impair vision. Some central nervous system diseases cause varying degrees of paralysis and sensory loss.

LIFESTYLE AND PERSONALITY

Lifestyle influences the quality and quantity of stimulation to which an individual is accustomed. A client who is employed in a large company may be accustomed to many diverse stimuli. A client who is self-employed and works in the home is exposed to fewer, less diverse stimuli. Personality differences also affect an individual's comfort regarding the quantity and quality of stimuli. While some people delight in constantly changing stimuli and excitement, others prefer a more structured life with few changes.

◆ The Confused Client

Confusion can occur in clients of all ages, but it is most commonly seen in older people. The causes of confusion can be physiologic or situational. The most common causes of confusion are:

- ◆ Drug effects, such as potentiating effects of multiple drug use and drug intoxication
- ◆ Physiologic disturbances, such as hypoxia, dehydration, metabolic or fluid imbalances, neurologic disorders, infectious processes, and nutritional deficiencies
- ◆ Abrupt loss of a significant person or persons
- ◆ Multiple losses in a short time span
- ◆ A move to a radically different environment

Clients who are confused often know something is wrong and want help. Box 27-3 ◆ describes nursing interventions to help orient the confused person to time, place, person, and situation.

NURSING CARE

◆ ASSESSING

During the course of a head-to-toe assessment, the LPN/LVN has the opportunity to gather information on the client's level of sensory–perceptual functioning. The examination should reveal whether the senses are impaired. It is helpful to collect information about the client's specific visual and hearing abilities; perception of heat, cold, light, touch, and pain in the limbs; and awareness of the position of the body parts. This information is useful as the LPN/LVN collaborates with the RN on planning and implementation.

It may be necessary to perform additional sensory tests. These tests may be performed by the LPN/LVN, the RN, or a specialist (e.g., audiologist or speech therapist). Specific sensory tests include:

MediaLink ◆ Cross-Section of the Ear

MediaLink ◆ Ear Abnormalities

PROMOTING ORIENTATION TO TIME, PLACE, PERSON, AND SITUATION

☑ Wear a readable name tag.

☑ Address the person by name and introduce yourself frequently: "Good morning, Mr. Richards. I am Betty Brown. I will be your nurse today."

☑ Identify time and place as indicated: "Today is December 5, and it is 8:00 in the morning."

☑ Ask the client, "Where are you?" and orient the client to place (e.g., nursing home) if indicated.

☑ Place a calendar and clock in the client's room. Mark holidays with ribbons, pins, or other means.

☑ Speak clearly and calmly to the client, allowing time for your words to be processed and for the client to give a response.

☑ Provide frequent face-to-face contact.

☑ Provide clear, concise explanations of each treatment procedure or task.

☑ Reinforce reality by interpreting unfamiliar sounds, sights, and smells. Correct any misconceptions of events or situations.

☑ Schedule activities (e.g., meals, bath, activity and rest periods, treatments) at the same time each day to provide a sense of security. If possible, assign the same caregivers.

☑ Keep familiar items in the client's environment (e.g., photographs), and keep the environment uncluttered. A disorganized, cluttered environment increases confusion.

☑ Encourage the client to wear familiar or personal clothing and to arrange personal hygiene articles in order of use as needed.

☑ Encourage participation in familiar activities or hobbies to emphasize the client's strengths rather than problems.

☑ Tell the client when you are leaving and when you will return.

◆ Visual acuity test (using a Snellen chart or other reading material such as a newspaper) and visual fields test (see Chapter 11, Procedure 11-1) ⊕

◆ Hearing acuity test (such as whisper test, Weber test, Rinne tuning fork test) and observation of client in conversation with others

◆ Olfactory test, by identifying specific aromas

◆ Gustatory test, by identifying three tastes such as lemon, salt, and sugar

◆ Tactile test, by testing light touch, sharp and dull sensation, two-point discrimination, hot and cold sensation, vibration sense, position sense, and **stereognosis** (the

ability to recognize objects by touching or manipulating them).

The LPN/LVN should also determine whether sensory adaptive devices that the client uses (eyeglasses, hearing aids) function properly. Special care should be taken to protect eyeglasses and hearing aids from breakage or loss. A client whose glasses or hearing aids are lost or damaged will be unable to participate fully in his or her care and recovery.

Clients at risk for sensory–perceptual alterations need to be identified to ensure that preventive measures can be initiated. Box 27-4 ◆ identifies clients who are at risk for sensory deprivation or sensory overload.

Client Environment

The LVN/LPN must continuously be aware of quantity, quality, and type of stimuli produced in the environment. The client's environment may produce insufficient stimuli, placing the client at risk for sensory deprivation. It may contain too many stimuli, placing the client at risk for sensory overload (Figure 27-1 ◆). Nonstimulating environments include those that severely restrict physical activity and limit social contact with family and friends. Because appropriate or meaningful stimuli decrease the incidence of sensory deprivation, the nurse must consider the client's health care environment for the presence of the following stimuli:

◆ Radio or other auditory device (e.g., cassette player), television

◆ Clock or calendar

◆ Reading material (or toys for children)

◆ Number and compatibility of roommates

◆ Number of visitors

Social Support Network

The degree of isolation a person feels is significantly influenced by the quality and quantity of support from family members and friends. It is important for the nurse to ask

Figure 27-1. ◆ A client in an intensive care unit (ICU) may experience sensory overload.

BOX 27-4

POPULATION FOCUS

CLIENTS AT RISK FOR SENSORY DEPRIVATION OR SENSORY OVERLOAD

Sensory Deprivation

- Clients confined in a nonstimulating or monotonous environment in the home or health care agency
- Clients who have impaired vision or hearing
- Clients with mobility restrictions such as quadriplegia with bed rest, traction apparatus, paraplegia
- Clients who are unable to process stimuli (e.g., clients who have brain damage or who are taking medications that affect the central nervous system)
- Clients with a communicable disease (e.g., AIDS)
- Clients who have emotional disorders (e.g., depression) and withdraw within themselves
- Clients who have limited social contact with family and friends (e.g., clients from a different culture)

Sensory Overload

- Clients who have pain or discomfort
- Clients who are acutely ill and have been admitted to an acute care facility
- Clients who are being closely monitored in an ICU (see Figure 27-1) and have intrusive tubes such as IVs, catheters, or nasogastric or endotracheal tubes
- Clients who have decreased cognitive ability (e.g., head injury)

(a) whether the client lives alone, (b) who visits and when, and (c) whether any signs indicate social deprivation. Social deprivation might be evidenced by withdrawal from contact with others to avoid embarrassment or dependence on others, negative self-image, reports of lack of meaningful communication with others, and absence of opportunities to discuss fears or concerns that facilitate coping mechanisms.

DIAGNOSING, PLANNING, and IMPLEMENTING

The LPN/LVN should become familiar with diagnostic labels for sensory–perceptual problems. This will be useful in preparing to collaborate with the RN.

Examples of nursing diagnoses for which sensory–perceptual alterations is the etiology include:

- Risk for Injury related to sensory–perceptual alterations, such as decreased depth perception or decreased sense of smell
- Impaired Home Maintenance Management related to sensory–perceptual alterations (declining visual abilities)
- Risk for Impaired Skin Integrity related to sensory–perceptual alterations (reduced tactile sensation)

- Impaired Verbal Communication related to sensory–perceptual alterations, such as altered level of consciousness or sensory overload
- Self Care Deficit: Bathing/Hygiene related to sensory–perceptual alterations, such as diminished kinesthetic sense
- Social Isolation related to sensory–perceptual alterations, such as impaired hearing

Client outcomes for sensory–perceptual alterations are to:

- Maintain the function of existing senses.
- Develop an effective communication mechanism.
- Prevent injury.
- Prevent sensory overload or deprivation.
- Reduce social isolation.
- Perform activities of daily living independently and safely.

Examples of nursing interventions for clients with sensory–perceptual alterations are:

- Increase, reduce, or eliminate environmental stimuli to achieve appropriate sensory input.
- Identify and implement appropriate safety precautions.
- Ensure access to and use of assistive devices such as eyeglasses and hearing aids.
- Promote the use of existing senses.
- Provide methods for meaningful communication through touch, writing implements, or other methods as indicated.
- Encourage social interaction with family, friends, and other components of the client's social support network.
- Provide information about social services, community resources, occupational therapy, and other appropriate resources as indicated.

Nurses can assist clients with sensory alterations by promoting healthy sensory function, by adjusting environmental stimuli, and by helping clients to manage acute sensory deficits.

Promoting Healthy Sensory Function

Early screening to detect problems in the visual and hearing functions is essential. For example, children with chronic ear infections and people who live or work in an environment where there is a high noise level should receive routine auditory testing. Women who are considering pregnancy should be advised of the importance of testing for syphilis and rubella, which can cause hearing impairments in newborns. Periodic vision screening of all newborns and children is recommended to detect congenital blindness, strabismus, and refractive errors. Newborn hearing screenings are now possible. Many states are mandating this testing. Hospital nurseries can perform the test with relative ease and in a timely manner. The screening provides valuable information and guidelines for further testing.

Healthy sensory function can be promoted with environmental stimuli that provide appropriate and varied sensory input. As many senses as possible should be stimulated. Colors, sounds, textures, smells, and changes in body position can provide various sensations. Nurses can teach parents to stimulate infants and children, and family members to stimulate an elderly person. Social activities often help stimulate the mind and the senses.

Nurses should teach clients general health measures and ways of preventing sensory loss, such as getting regular eye examinations and controlling chronic diseases like diabetes. Box 27-5 ◆ provides client teaching to prevent sensory impairment.

Preventing Sensory Deprivation

For clients who are at risk for sensory deprivation, nurses can increase environmental stimuli in a number of ways. For example, newspapers, books, and television can stimulate the visual and auditory senses. Providing objects that are pleasant to touch, such as a pet to stroke, can provide tactile and inter-

active stimulation. Clocks that differentiate night from day by color can help orient a client to time. The sense of smell can be stimulated by the presence of fresh flowers or plants (Figure 27-2 ◆).

Arrangements should also be made for people to visit and talk with the client regularly. Many church and community groups provide visitors to "shut-ins," that is, people who are confined to their homes or who reside in nursing homes. Box 27-6 ◆ provides measures to prevent sensory deprivation.

Preventing Sensory Overload

For clients who are at risk of overstimulation, nurses should reduce the number and type of environmental stimuli. The nurse can counteract sensory overload by blocking stimuli and by helping the client organize the stimuli and alter responses to the stimuli.

Dark glasses can partially block light rays, and a window shade or drape can reduce visual stimulation. Earplugs reduce auditory stimuli, as do soft background music and earphones. The odor from a draining wound can be minimized by keeping the dressing dry and clean and by applying a liquid deodorant on a gauze near the wound.

Another method of blocking stimuli is to provide rest intervals free of interruptions. Sometimes the number of visitors and the length of visits must be restricted. Also, if the nurse carries out several nursing measures together, the client can have a scheduled quiet period before the next activity.

By explaining sounds in the environment, when clients understand their meaning, stimuli are frequently less confusing and more easily ignored. People can also learn to alter their responses to the stimuli. Clients can employ relaxation techniques to reduce anxiety and stress despite continual sensory stimulation. Box 27-6 also gives nursing measures to prevent sensory overload.

BOX 27-5

CLIENT TEACHING

PREVENTING SENSORY IMPAIRMENTS

◆ Have regular health examinations.
◆ Have regular eye examinations as recommended by the physician or pediatrician to screen for eye problems. For clients ages 40 and over, a medical eye examination is generally recommended every 3 to 5 years, or every 1 to 2 years if there is a family history of glaucoma.
◆ Seek early medical attention (a) if signs suggesting visual impairment arise (e.g., failure to react to light, or reduced eye contact from an infant), (b) if the child complains of an earache or has an ear infection, and (c) for persistent eye redness, discharge or increased tearing, growths on or near the eye, pupil asymmetry or other irregularity, or any pain or discomfort.
◆ Obtain regular immunizations of children against diseases capable of causing hearing loss (e.g., rubella, mumps, and measles).
◆ Avoid giving infants and toddlers toys with long pointed handles and keep pointed instruments (e.g., scissors and screwdrivers) out of reach. Supervise preschoolers when they use scissors.
◆ Make sure that toddlers do not walk or run with a pointed object in hand. Teach preschoolers to walk carefully when carrying such objects as sticks or scissors.
◆ Teach school-age children and adolescents the proper use of sports equipment (e.g., hockey sticks) and power tools.
◆ Wear protective eye goggles when using power tools, riding motorcycles, spraying chemicals, and so on.
◆ Wear ear protectors when working in an environment with high noise levels or brief loud impulse noises (e.g., blasting).
◆ Wear dark glasses to avoid damage from ultraviolet rays and never look directly into the sun.

Figure 27-2. ◆ Activities can be planned to combine social contact and stimulation of different senses.

BOX 27-6
NURSING CARE CHECKLIST

PREVENTING SENSORY DEPRIVATION AND SENSORY OVERLOAD

Preventing Sensory Deprivation

☑ Encourage the client to use eyeglasses and hearing aids.

☑ Address the client by name and touch the client while speaking if this is not culturally offensive.

☑ Communicate frequently with the client, and maintain meaningful interactions (e.g., discuss current events).

☑ Provide a telephone, radio and/or TV, clock, and calendar.

☑ Provide murals, pictures, sculptures, and wall hangings. Many libraries and museums will lend artwork free of charge, or a local school may provide art projects developed by their students.

☑ Have family and friends bring freshly cut flowers and plants.

☑ Consider having a resident keep a pet such as fish, a cat, or a bird, or make arrangements for pets to visit on a regular basis.

☑ Include different textured objects to feel such as a sheepskin pillow, silk scarf, soft blanket, or other inanimate object.

☑ Increase tactile stimulation through physical care measures such as back massages, hair care, and foot soaks.

☑ Encourage social interaction through activity groups or visits by family and friends.

☑ Encourage the use of crossword puzzles or games to stimulate mental function.

☑ Encourage environment changes such as a walk through a mall, or for an immobilized client, sitting near a window or at a place on the nursing unit where the client can watch local traffic.

☑ Encourage the use of self-stimulation techniques such as singing, humming, whistling, or reciting.

Preventing Sensory Overload

☑ Minimize unnecessary light, noise, and distraction. Provide dark glasses and earplugs as needed.

☑ Control pain as indicated.

☑ Introduce yourself by name and address the client by name.

☑ Provide orienting cues, such as clocks, calendars, equipment, and furniture in the room.

☑ Provide a private room.

☑ Limit visitors.

☑ Plan care to allow for uninterrupted periods for rest or sleep.

☑ Schedule a routine of care so the client knows when and what to expect (post the schedule for the client wherever possible).

☑ Speak in a low tone of voice and in an unhurried manner.

☑ Provide new information gradually to enable the client to process the meaning. When providing information, ask the client to repeat it so that there are no misunderstandings.

☑ Describe any tests and procedures to the client beforehand.

☑ Reduce noxious odors. Empty a commode or bedpan immediately after use; keep wounds clean and covered; use a room deodorizer when indicated; and provide good ventilation.

☑ Take time to discuss the client's problems and to correct misinterpretations.

☑ Assist the client with stress-reducing techniques.

Promoting the Use of Other Senses

When assisting clients who have a sensory deficit, the nurse needs to encourage the use of sensory aids to support residual sensory function, promote the use of other senses, communicate effectively, and ensure client safety.

When one sense is lost, the nurse can teach the client to use other senses to supplement the loss. The type of stimulation needs to be adapted to the client's specific deficit. For example, for the visually impaired client, stimulation of hearing, taste, smell, and touch can be encouraged. A radio, audiotapes of music or books, or clocks that chime can be used for

auditory stimulation. Diets that include a variety of flavors, temperatures, and textures can be planned to stimulate the taste buds. Fresh flowers, fragrances, brewing coffee, and baking can stimulate the sense of smell. Measures such as providing a massage, hair brushing, different textures in clothing and upholstery fabrics, and pets can be used to stimulate touch receptors.

Communicating Effectively

Communication with clients who have sensory deficits should convey respect, enhance the person's self-esteem, and ensure the exchange of correct information. A person with a hearing impairment has to concentrate more than other people and therefore tires more readily. Fatigue compounded by an illness can further reduce the person's ability to hear. A person with a visual impairment is unable to observe nonverbal cues during communication and relies largely on the spoken word and tone of voice. Guidelines for communicating with people who are visually or hearing impaired are listed in Box 27-7 ◆.

Ensuring Client Safety

Nurses must implement safety precautions in health care settings for clients with sensory deficits and teach them special precautions to ensure their safety at home.

Impaired Vision. For clients with visual impairments nurses need to do the following in a health care setting:

◆ Orient the client to the arrangement of room furnishings and maintain an uncluttered environment.

◆ Keep pathways clear and do not rearrange furniture without re-orienting the client. Ensure that housekeeping personnel are informed about this.

◆ Organize self-care articles within the client's reach and orient the client to their location.

◆ Keep the call light within easy reach and place the bed in the lowest position.

◆ Assist with ambulation by standing to the client's side, walking about 1 foot ahead, and allowing the person to grasp your arm. Confirm whether the client prefers grasping your arm with the dominant or nondominant hand.

Impaired Hearing. Clients with impaired hearing need to have call lights answered in person, since they may be unable to respond to voice on the intercom.

The Unconscious Client. The person who is unconscious and unable to respond to the spoken word nevertheless can often hear what is spoken. It is therefore important that nurses talk to the client as though they were understood, using a normal tone of voice and speaking before touching the client. Nurses should also try to keep the environmental noises at a minimum so that the client can focus on words. The following are some additional measures nurses can take in caring for the unconscious client:

BOX 27-7
NURSING CARE CHECKLIST

COMMUNICATING WITH CLIENTS WITH VISUAL OR HEARING DEFICITS

Visual Deficit

☑ Always announce your presence when entering the client's room and identify yourself by name.

☑ Stay in the client's field of vision if the client has a partial vision loss.

☑ Speak in a warm and pleasant tone of voice. Some people tend to speak louder than necessary when talking to a blind person.

☑ Always explain what you are about to do before touching the person.

☑ Explain the sounds in the environment.

☑ Indicate when the conversation has ended and when you are leaving the room.

Hearing Deficit

☑ Before initiating conversation, convey your presence by moving to a position where you can be seen or by gently touching the person.

☑ Decrease background noises (e.g., radio) before speaking.

☑ Talk at a moderate rate and in a normal tone of voice. Shouting does not make your voice more distinct and in some instances makes understanding more difficult.

☑ Address the person directly. Do not turn away in the middle of a remark or story. Make sure the person can see your face easily and that it is well lighted.

☑ Avoid talking when you have something in your mouth, such as chewing gum. Avoid covering your mouth with your hand.

☑ Keep your voice at about the same volume throughout each sentence, without dropping the voice at the end of each sentence.

☑ Always speak as clearly and accurately as possible. Articulate consonants with particular care.

☑ Do not "overarticulate"; mouthing or overdoing articulation is just as troublesome as mumbling. Pantomime or write ideas, or use sign language or finger spelling as appropriate.

☑ Use longer phrases, which tend to be easier to understand than short ones. For example, "Will you get me a drink of water?" presents much less difficulty than "Will you get me a drink?" Word choice is important: "Fifteen cents" and "fifty cents" may be confused, but "half a dollar" is clear.

☑ Pronounce every name with care. Make a reference to the name for easier understanding, for example, "Joan, the girl from the office" or "Sears, the big downtown store."

☑ Change to a new subject at a slower rate, making sure that the person follows the change to the new subject. A key word or two at the beginning of a new topic is a good indicator.

◆ Orient the unconscious client to self, time, and place.
◆ Listen carefully to the support person's concerns. Often, they simply want to express them.
◆ Maintain the same schedule each day. *Routine gives the client a sense of security*.
◆ Touch and stroke the unconscious client.
◆ To the support persons, explain what is happening, and encourage them to talk to and touch the client as though the client were conscious. *This auditory and tactile stimulation supports the client and may restore some degree of consciousness*.
◆ Always address the client by name, and explain beforehand the care to be provided. Unconscious clients require bathing, skin care, turning, feeding, and assistance with elimination needs.

EVALUATING

Using the measurable desired outcomes developed during the planning stage, the nurse collects data needed to judge whether client goals and outcomes have been achieved. Such data might include:

◆ Client's use of assistive devices (e.g., hearing aid, large-print reading materials) to support sensory functioning
◆ Client's participation in social activities to reduce social isolation
◆ Client's verbalizing that closed curtains helped him rest better in the afternoon

If outcomes are not achieved, the nurse and client, and support caregivers if appropriate, need to explore the reasons before modifying the care plan.

DISCHARGE CONSIDERATIONS

To provide for continuity of care, the nurse must consider the client's needs for assistance in the home or residential treatment setting. Some clients with severe alterations in sensory–perceptual functioning may be discharged to an assisted living facility that provides the specific support the client requires. Discharge planning incorporates a reassessment of the client's abilities for self-care, the availability and skills of support people, financial resources, and the need for referrals and home health services. Box 27-8 ◆ outlines areas to assess before discharge in regard to sensory–perceptual alterations. A major aspect of discharge planning involves the instructional needs of the client and family.

Nursing Process Case Study: CLIENT IN ICU

Mrs. Dodd is a 51-year-old client who is being cared for in the critical care unit following an automobile accident in which she suffered extensive traumatic injuries. Mrs. Dodd is con-

---

> ### BOX 27-8
> ### ASSESSING FOR DISCHARGE
>
> #### SENSORY–PERCEPTUAL ALTERATIONS
>
> ◆ *Self-care abilities:* Ability to care for self while adapting to sensory impairment
> ◆ *Safety:* Physical safety of client's environment including lighting, noise, access, lack of clutter or obstructions, use of stairs, assistive devices with respect to sensory impairment, such as flashing fire alarms or telephones for hearing impaired
> ◆ *Level of knowledge:* Assistive devices available; ways to maximize use of other senses; local, regional, or national organizations that may provide education, training, support, or other assistance, such as the National Braille Association, Guide Dogs for the Blind, the National Association of the Deaf

nected to several monitoring devices, has an intubation tube and ventilator to assist her with respirations, and is receiving various pain and other medications.

Assessment BP 150/90, P 60, R 14 (on mechanical ventilator), PCO_2 40 mm Hg. ET tube in place. Responds to verbal commands and tactile stimuli. Burr holes to evacuate epidural hematoma. Stable pelvic fracture. No evidence of internal bleeding or shock. Around the clock IV pain control.

Diagnosis Disturbed Sensory Perception related to excessive environmental stimuli.

Expected Outcomes

◆ Demonstrates relaxed body movements and facial expression
◆ Will respond to caregiver with eye blinks

Planning and Implementation

◆ Identify name and purpose when approaching client bedside.
◆ Orient to time, place, person, and surroundings.
◆ Pay attention to client's emotional needs.
◆ Minimize unnecessary light, noise, and distraction.
◆ Monitor pain control.
◆ Plan care to allow for uninterrupted periods of rest.
◆ Describe any test and procedure or activity prior to initiating.
◆ Provide client with alternate form of communication.

Evaluation Mrs. Dodd appears less anxious today as evidenced by relaxed facial expression. She is provided with 2 hours of uninterrupted rest q shift. She is responding to yes and no questions with eye blinks and is beginning to make her needs known.

Critical Thinking in the Nursing Process

1. Identify factors that place Mrs. Dodd at risk for the development of sensory deprivation or overload.
2. How can you intervene to help Mrs. Dodd during this stressful event?

3. How might care of a client in the home setting differ from the care of a client such as Mrs. Dodd who is receiving care in the critical care unit?

Note: The bibliography listings for this and all chapters have been compiled at the back of the book.

Chapter Review

🔊 Key Terms by Topics

Use the audio glossary feature of either the CD-ROM or the Companion Website to hear the correct pronunciation of the following key terms.

Components of the Sensory Process
stimulus, receptor, sensory reception, olfac-

tory, gustatory, kinesthetic, visceral, sensory perception

Sensory alterations
sensory deprivation, sensory overload, sensory deficit

Nursing care
stereognosis

Key Points

* Sensory deprivation occurs when a person receives decreased sensory input or monotonous or meaningless sensory input.

* Sensory overload occurs when a person experiences excessive sensory input and is unable to process or manage the stimuli. The person feels overwhelmed and not in control.

* Clients at risk for sensory deprivation include those who are homebound or institutionalized, those on bed rest or isolation precautions, or those with sensory deficits.

* Clients at risk for sensory overload include those in pain, those in intensive care units, or those with intrusive and uncomfortable monitoring or treatment equipment.

* Nurses and support caregivers need to devise and implement effective communication mechanisms for clients who have visual and hearing impairments.

* Confused clients and unconscious clients need care that is directed to promoting their orientation to time, place, person, and situation.

🌐 EXPLORE MediaLink

Additional interactive resources for this chapter can be found on the Companion Website at www.prenhall.com/ramont. Click on Chapter 27 and "Begin" to select the activities for this chapter.

For chapter-related NCLEX-style questions and an audio glossary, access the accompanying CD-ROM in this book.

Animations:
* Ear abnormalities
* Middle ear dynamics
* Fluoxetine
* Pilocarpine

🔗 For Further Study

For further discussion of orienting clients, see Chapter 8.
For information about assessing sensory function, see Chapter 11.
For more about care of hearing aids, see Chapter 13.

Critical Thinking Care Map

Caring for the Client with Sensory–Perceptual Alteration

NCLEX-PN Focus Area: Physiological Adaptation

Case Study: Julia Hagstrom is an 80-year-old widow who has recently become a resident of an extended care facility. Just prior to her admission she underwent surgery for the removal of cataracts and also experienced difficulty with hearing. Her children were concerned about her physical safety and lack of socialization and urged her to enter a nursing home. Mrs. Hagstrom had cared for herself independently for 15 years in her own home. Three days after admission the nurse finds the client somewhat confused and disoriented to person, place, and time. She appears restless, withdrawn, and her syntax is sometimes inappropriate. She states "I'm afraid of all of these strange creatures in this orphanage."

Nursing Diagnosis: Disturbed Sensory Perception

COLLECT DATA

Subjective	Objective
_____	_____
_____	_____
_____	_____
_____	_____
_____	_____
_____	_____

Would you report this data? Yes/No

If yes, to: _____

Nursing Care

_____
_____
_____
_____
_____
_____
_____
_____
_____
_____
_____
_____

How would you document this? _____
_____
_____
_____
_____

Data Collected

(use those that apply)

- Height: 63"
- Weight: 122 lbs.
- VS: T 98.6°F, P 72, R 18, BP 128/74
- Rinne test: negative
- Diagnostic data (chest x-ray, CBC, and urinalysis) all negative

Nursing Interventions

(use those that apply)

- Provide a consistent physical environment and a daily routine.
- Consider environmental and human factors that may limit dressing/grooming ability.
- Observe for cause of inability to feed self independently.
- Provide caregiver who is familiar to Mrs. Hagstrom.
- Provide low-stimulation environment for Mrs. Hagstrom because disorientation may be increased by overstimulation.
- Encourage independent decision making by reviewing options and their possible consequences with client.
- Provide for adequate rest, sleep, and daytime naps.
- Assess family and living environment for social dynamics.
- Facilitate use of hearing aids, as appropriate.
- Obtain Mrs. Hagstrom's attention through touch.

NCLEX-PN Exam Preparation

TEST-TAKING TIP

Identify the issue of the question. The issue is the specific subject content that the question is asking about. The issue of the question can include: a drug, a side effect or toxic effect of the drug, a procedure, a complication, or a specific nursing action.

1. Stimulus, receptor, impulse conduction, and perception must be present for an individual to be aware of the surroundings. The stimulus can be described as:
   a. A nerve cell that converts the agent to an impulse
   b. An agent that acts on a nerve receptor
   c. An impulse that travels along nerve pathways to the spinal cord or directly to the brain
   d. An interpretation that takes place in the brain

2. Your primary nurse instructs you to complete an assessment of awareness on a "somnolent" client. You understand that to mean that the client:
   a. Is not oriented to time, place, or person
   b. Has reduced awareness and impaired judgment
   c. Has extreme drowsiness, but will respond to stimuli
   d. Can be aroused by extreme or repeated stimuli

3. Several foreign-born nursing assistants are speaking to each other in their native language while feeding residents in the dayroom. Of the following, which is the most appropriate statement you as the nurse should make when discussing the problem?
   a. The facility has an all English rule. Anyone not complying will be placed on a 2-day suspension.
   b. Family members are complaining about the non-English conversation going on in front of residents.
   c. Since many of the residents are confused, they won't understand what you are discussing, so you should speak in English.
   d. Conversing in a foreign language can cause sensory deprivation for the residents. Please speak English and include them in the conversation.

4. Your client comes to the nurse's station several times each day to ask what time the activities start. Which is the most appropriate action to help the client be more independent?
   a. Tell him to check the activity board at the end of the hall.
   b. Tell him you will come to get him at the appropriate time.
   c. Place a clock and an activity schedule in his room.
   d. Page clients on the overhead system when it is time to come to the dayroom.

5. When caring for an unconscious client, the nurse should keep environmental noise to a minimum and speak to the client during care because:
   a. It will be reassuring for the family when they visit.
   b. Clients often hear what is being said even though they cannot respond.
   c. It will prevent sensory deprivation.
   d. It will help the time pass more quickly.

6. Safety issues for the visually impaired are particularly important during ambulation. Which is the appropriate method for assisting a visually impaired individual?
   a. Walk about 1 foot ahead, and allow the person to grasp your arm.
   b. Grasp the client's arm with your dominant hand and walk in front of the client.
   c. Provide the client with a white cane and begin mobility training.
   d. Instruct client that a family member will need to accompany him when he walks.

7. You are caring for a recently widowed elderly client in her home. She is showing signs of confusion. Of the following, which is the likely cause?
   a. Head injury related to trauma
   b. Abrupt loss of a significant person
   c. Discomfort with her environment or caregiver
   d. An undiagnosed medical problem

8. You are working in a long term care facility. Many of the clients have visual and hearing deficits. When discussing ways to meet their sensory needs, which is the highest priority?
   a. Ensuring a safe environment and preventing sensory deprivation
   b. Including the clients in monthly outings
   c. Calling family to suggest that they visit at least weekly
   d. Including the clients in group meetings so they can talk about their deficits

9. Clients age 40 and over, with a family history of glaucoma, should have a medical eye examination:
   a. Every 1 to 2 years
   b. Every 3 to 5 years
   c. Whenever symptoms occur
   d. When recommended by their optometrist

10. One of the clients in a skilled nursing facility is attempting to climb out of bed. She is insisting that she must see her husband right now. Of the following statements, which is the most appropriate one to make to a confused client?
    a. "I just spoke with your husband; he is fine; now go to sleep."
    b. "Stay in bed, or we will have to restrain you."
    c. "This is the hospital. I am your nurse. Let me sit with you while you fall back to sleep."
    d. "You are disturbing all the other residents. You must be quiet or I will have to give you some medication."

Chapter 28

Self-Concept

SHARING experiences

"I am owned,
Not by people or possessions.
For people change and possessions flee.
I believe in a calling much higher
Than the human eye can see.
I am owned by a belief, a promise,
That I will joyfully and willing help,
Even though I may be weary or misunderstood.

So I may reflect peace to the aged, that they
May savor their wisdom.
Bring delight to the young,
For this world, these ways,
They shall inherit.
Life will present many paradoxes.
This is my duty, my promise, because I am
A peacemaker, a friend, a healer, a nurse."

Kelly C. Goetz, LVN, Fullerton, CA.

LEARNING outcomes

After completing this chapter, you will be able to:

- Identify four personal and social dimensions of self-concept.
- Explain Erikson's theory of the effects of psychosocial crises on self-concept and self-esteem.
- Describe the four components of self-concept.
- Identify common stressors affecting self-concept and coping strategies.
- Describe nursing actions designed to achieve identified goals for clients with altered self-concept.
- Describe ways to enhance the self-esteem of older adults.

MediaLink

www.prenhall.com/ramont

Use the address above to access the free, interactive Companion Website created for this textbook. Get hints, instant feedback, and textbook references to chapter-related NCLEX-style questions. Link to other interesting sites.

Audio Glossary:
Use the Companion Website, or the CD-ROM disk enclosed with your textbook, to hear the pronunciation of key terms in the chapter.

A positive self-concept is essential to a person's mental and physical health. Individuals with a positive self-concept are better able to develop and maintain interpersonal relationships and resist psychological and physical illness. Nurses have a responsibility not only to identify people with a negative self-concept, but also to identify the possible causes in order to help people develop a more positive view of themselves.

A nurse's own self-concept is also important. Nurses who feel positive about themselves are better able to help clients meet their needs.

Self-concept is a complex idea that influences:

◆ How one thinks, talks, and acts
◆ How one sees and treats another person
◆ Choices one makes
◆ Ability to give and receive love
◆ Ability to take action and to change things

Self-concept is a view of oneself from several angles. These include:

◆ *Self-knowledge:* The knowledge that one has about oneself, including insights into one's abilities, nature, and limitations
◆ *Self-expectation:* What one expects of oneself; may be a realistic or unrealistic expectation
◆ *Social self:* How a person is perceived by others and society
◆ *Social evaluation:* The appraisal of oneself in relationship to others, events, or situations

Formation of Self-Concept

A person is not born with a self-concept; rather, it develops as a result of social interactions with others. According to Erik Erikson, a social theorist, people face certain developmental tasks associated with eight psychosocial stages of life. The success with which a person copes with these developmental crises largely determines the development of self-concept. Inability to cope results in self-concept problems at the time, and often, later in life. See Table 28-1 ◆ for behaviors indicating successful and unsuccessful resolution of these developmental crises.

There are three broad steps in the development of one's self-concept:

1. The infant learns that the physical self is separate and different from the environment.
2. The child internalizes others' attitudes toward self.
3. The child and adult internalize the standards of society.

Each person's self-concept is like a collage. At the center of the collage are the beliefs and images that are most vital to the person's identity. They constitute core self-concept. For example: "I am competent/incompetent"; "I am male/female." Images and beliefs that are less important to the person are on the periphery. For example: "I am left-/right-handed"; "I am athletic/unathletic."

People are thought to base their self-concept on how they perceive and evaluate themselves in these areas:

◆ Vocational performance
◆ Intellectual functioning
◆ Personal appearance and physical attractiveness
◆ Sexual attractiveness and performance
◆ Being liked by others
◆ Ability to cope with and resolve problems
◆ Independence

Components of Self-Concept

There are four components of self-concept: body image, role performance, personal identity, and self-esteem.

BODY IMAGE

The image of physical self, or **body image,** is how a person perceives the size, appearance, and functioning of the body and its parts. A person's body image develops partly from others' attitudes and responses to that person's body and partly from the individual's own exploration of the body. As the parents or caregivers respond to the child with smiles, holding, and touching, and also as the child explores its own body sensations during breast-feeding, thumb sucking, and the bath, body image develops (Figure 28-1 ◆). Cultural and societal values also influence a person's body image.

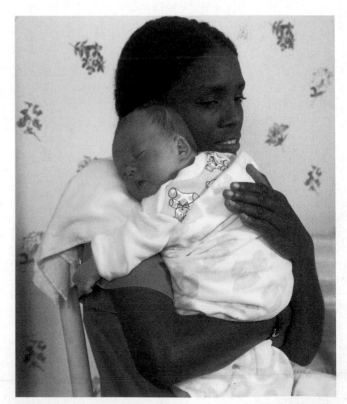

Figure 28-1. ◆ Children's attitude toward themselves is learned in part by the ways they are held and touched as infants.

TABLE 28-1	EXAMPLES OF BEHAVIORS ASSOCIATED WITH ERIKSON'S STAGES OF PSYCHOSOCIAL DEVELOPMENT	
STAGE: DEVELOPMENTAL CRISIS	BEHAVIORS INDICATING POSITIVE RESOLUTION	BEHAVIORS INDICATING NEGATIVE RESOLUTION
Infancy: Trust vs. mistrust	Requesting assistance and expecting to receive it Expressing belief of another person Sharing time, opinions, and experiences	Restricting conversation to superficialities Refusing to provide a person with information Being unable to accept assistance
Toddlerhood: Autonomy vs. shame and doubt	Accepting the rules of a group but also expressing disagreement when it is felt Expressing one's own opinion Easily accepting deferment of a wish fulfillment	Failing to express needs Not expressing one's own opinion when opposed Overconcern about being clean
Early childhood: Initiative vs. guilt	Starting projects eagerly Expressing curiosity about many things Demonstrating original thought	Imitating others rather than developing independent ideas Apologizing and being very embarrassed over small mistakes Verbalizing fear about starting a new project
Early school years: Industry vs. inferiority	Completing a task once it has been started Working well with others Using time effectively	Not completing tasks started Not assisting with the work of others Not organizing work
Adolescence: Identity vs. role confusion	Asserting independence Planning realistically for future roles Establishing close interpersonal relationships	Failing to assume responsibility for directing one's own behavior Accepting the values of others without question Failing to set goals in life
Early adulthood: Intimacy vs. isolation	Establishing a close, intense relationship with another person Accepting sexual behavior as desirable Making a commitment to that relationship, even in times of stress and sacrifice	Remaining alone Avoiding close interpersonal relationships
Middle-aged adults: Generativity vs. stagnation	Being willing to share with another person Guiding others Establishing a priority of needs, recognizing both self and others	Talking about oneself instead of listening to others Showing concern for oneself in spite of needs of others Being unable to accept interdependence
Older adults: Integrity vs. despair	Using past experience to assist others Maintaining productivity in some areas Accepting limitations	Crying and being apathetic Not accepting changes Demanding unnecessary assistance and attention from others

Body image encompasses the functioning of the body and its parts. It also includes body prostheses, such as artificial limbs, dentures, and hairpieces, as well as devices required for functioning, such as wheelchairs, canes, and eyeglasses. Past as well as present perceptions are part of one's body image.

The various information and entertainment media have played a part over the years in how individuals view themselves and others. If a person's body image closely resembles one's body ideal, the individual is more likely to think positively about the physical and nonphysical components of the self.

A person with a healthy body image will normally show concern for both health and appearance. This person will seek help if ill and will include health-promoting practices in daily activities. A person who has an unhealthy body image is likely to be overly concerned about minor illness and to neglect activities like sleep and a healthy diet that are important to health.

The person with body image disturbance may ignore a body part that is significantly changed by illness or trauma (see also Chapter 22). ⊂⊃ Some individuals may also express feelings of helplessness, hopelessness, powerlessness, and vulnerability, and may exhibit self-destructive behavior such as over- or undereating or suicide attempts.

ROLE PERFORMANCE

A **role** is a set of expectations about how the person occupying one position behaves toward a person occupying another position. Role **performance** relates what a person does in a particular role to the behaviors expected of that role. Each person usually has several roles, such as husband, parent, brother, son, employee, friend. Some roles are assumed for only limited periods, such as client, student, and ill person. People need to know who they are in relation to others and what society expects for the positions they hold. To relate or interact appropriately with others, people also need to know the role positions that others occupy. Failure to master a role creates frustration and feelings of inadequacy, often lowering self-esteem.

PERSONAL IDENTITY

A person's **personal identity** is the conscious sense of individuality and uniqueness that is continually evolving throughout life. People often view their identity in terms of name, sex, age, race, ethnic origin or culture, occupation or roles, talents, and other situational characteristics (e.g., marital status and education).

Personal identity also includes a person's beliefs and values, personality, and character.

SELF-ESTEEM

Self-esteem is one's judgment of one's own worth, that is, how that person's standards and performances compare to others and also to one's ideal self. If a person's self-concept does not match with the ideal self, then low self-esteem results. Parents can encourage self-esteem

◆ *History of success and failure.* People who have a history of failures come to see themselves as a failure, whereas people with a history of successes will have a more positive self-concept, making more successes likely.
◆ *Illness.* Illness and trauma can also affect the self-concept. People respond to illness and aging in a variety of ways: acceptance, denial, withdrawal, and depression are common reactions.

NURSING CARE

 ASSESSING

Before conducting a psychosocial assessment, the nurse must establish trust and a working relationship with the client. In Neeb's *Fundamentals of Mental Health Nursing* (2001), the following guidelines are suggested for nurse–client interviewing:

◆ *Be honest.* Tell the client the purpose of the interview.
◆ *Be assertive.* If the interview is mandatory (intake, preoperative), the client must understand that it is required. Arrange a mutually accepted time to conduct the interview so the client will be prepared.
◆ *Be sensitive.* Sometimes the questions are very difficult or embarrassing for the client to answer. Assure the client that you understand his or her feelings and that information shared by the client is part of his or her medical record
◆ *Use empathy.* Let the client know that you are interested in what is being said and that you are there to be helpful.
◆ *Use open-ended questions.* Personalize the questions as much as possible. Use this time to discuss and clarify as much information as you can to avoid having to repeat parts of the interview later.

This assessment can be used in either the acute care or home care environment. It is the nurse's responsibility to use therapeutic communication and to remain sensitive to the effect that cultural influences will have on the client's behaviors and needs. It is also important that the nurse identify any stressors that may affect aspects of the self-concept. See Box 28-1 ◆ for examples of stressors that may place a client at risk for problems with self-concept.

When stressors are identified, the nurse should also identify the client's coping style and determine whether this style is effective by asking the client such questions as:

◆ When you have a problem or face a stressful situation, how do you usually deal with it?
◆ Do these methods work?

Personal Identity

When assessing self-concept, the information the nurse first needs is about the client's personal identity. This involves who

Factors Affecting Self-Concept

Major factors that affect a person's self-concept are:

◆ *Development.* As an individual develops, the factors that affect the self-concept change. For example, whereas an infant requires a supportive, caring environment, a child requires freedom to explore and learn.
◆ *Family and culture.* A young child's values are largely influenced by the family and culture. Later on, peers influence the child and thereby affect the sense of self. When the child is confronted by differing expectations from family, culture, and peers, the child's sense of self is often confused.
◆ *Stressors.* Stressors can strengthen the self-concept as an individual copes successfully with problems. On the other hand, stressors can cause maladaptive responses including substance abuse, withdrawal, and anxiety.
◆ *Resources.* Internal resources such as confidence and values can affect the self-concept. External resources such as a support network, sufficient finances, and organizations can also influence self-concept. Generally the greater the number of resources a person has and uses, the more positive the effect on the self-concept.

BOX 28-1
STRESSORS AFFECTING SELF-CONCEPT

Identity Stressors
- Change in physical appearance (e.g., facial wrinkles)
- Declining physical, mental, or sensory abilities
- Inability to achieve goals
- Relationship concerns
- Sexuality concerns
- Unrealistic ideal self
- Membership in a minority group
- Cultural dissonance

Body Image Stressors
- Loss of body parts (e.g., amputation, mastectomy, hysterectomy)
- Loss of body functions (e.g., from heart disease, renal disease, spinal cord injury, cerebrovascular accident, neuromuscular disease, arthritis, declining mental or sensory abilities)
- Disfigurement (e.g., through pregnancy, severe burns, facial blemishes, colostomy, ileostomy, tracheostomy, laryngectomy)

Self-Esteem Stressors
- Lack of positive feedback from significant others
- Repeated failures
- Unrealistic expectations
- Inability to cope with life stressors
- Abusive relationship
- Loss of financial security

Role Stressors
- Loss of parent, spouse, child, or close friend
- Change or loss of job
- Retirement
- Divorce or separation
- Illness
- Hospitalization
- Ambiguous role expectations
- Conflicting role expectations
- Inability to meet role expectations

BOX 28-2 ASSESSING CLIENTS: PERSONAL IDENTITY, BODY IMAGE, AND ROLE RELATIONSHIPS

PERSONAL IDENTITY
- How would you describe yourself as a person?
- What do you like about yourself?
- How do others describe you as a person?
- What are your personal strengths, talents, and abilities?
- What would you change about yourself if you could?
- Does it bother you a lot if someone doesn't like you?
- Is it hard for you to say no when you want to say no?

BODY IMAGE
- Is there any part of your body you would like to change?
- Are you comfortable discussing your surgery?
- How do you feel about your appearance?
- What changes in your body do you expect after surgery?
- How have significant others in your life reacted to changes in your body?

FAMILY RELATIONSHIPS
- Tell me about your family.
- What is your home like?
- Is there anyone you are especially close to or distant from in your family?
- What are your relationships like with your other relatives?
- What are your responsibilities in the family, and is there anything you would like to change?
- How well do you feel you accomplish what is expected of you?
- Do you see yourself as being treated equally in your family?
- Are you proud of your family members?
- Do you feel your family members are proud of you?
- Tell me how you spend your time each day.

WORK ROLES AND SOCIAL ROLES
- Do you like your work?
- How do you get along at work?
- What about your work would you like to change if you could?
- How do you spend your free time?
- Are you involved in any community groups?
- Are you most comfortable alone, with one other person, or in a group?
- Who is most important to you?
- Whom do you seek out for help?

the client believes he or she is. See Box 28-2 ◆ for examples of assessment questions to ask.

Body Image
If there are indications of a body image disturbance, the nurse should assess the client carefully for possible functional or physical problems. See Box 28-2 for examples of questions to ask about body image.

Self-Esteem
A nurse can ask the following questions to determine a client's self-esteem:

- Are you satisfied with your life?
- How do you feel about yourself?
- Are you accomplishing what you want?
- What goals in life are important to you?

Some behaviors that might reflect low self-esteem are listed in Box 28-3 ◆. Be sure to determine the client's cultural background first, in order not to misinterpret specific cultural behaviors as indications of low self-esteem (see Chapter 26).

Role Relationships

The nurse assesses the client's satisfactions and dissatisfactions associated with role responsibilities and relationships. Family roles are especially important to people. Relationships can be supportive and promote growth. At the opposite extreme, however, relationships can be highly stressful, especially when violence and abuse are present. To obtain information related to the client's family relationships and satisfaction or dissatisfaction with work roles and social roles, the nurse might ask some of the questions shown in Box 28-2. Questions need to be individualized according to each client's age and situation.

◆ DIAGNOSING, PLANNING, and IMPLEMENTING

The NANDA nursing diagnostic labels will be used by the RN. Common nursing diagnoses for this area are Disturbed Body Image, Ineffective Role Performance, and Chronic Low Self-Esteem. The LVN/LPN's role may be to collaborate with the client, the RN, or other caregivers. A list of NANDA diagnoses can be found in Appendix A. ∞

The LVN/LPN who has little experience in intervening with clients with altered self-concept may wish to consult with a clinical specialist or a more experienced nurse to develop effective plans. The nurse and client set goals to enhance the client's self-concept.

The goals established vary according to the diagnoses and defining characteristics related to each individual. Examples of overall goals are:

BOX 28-3 MANIFESTATIONS OF LOW SELF-ESTEEM

- ◆ Avoids eye contact
- ◆ Stoops in posture and moves slowly
- ◆ Is poorly groomed and has an unkempt appearance
- ◆ Is hesitant or halting in speech
- ◆ Is overly critical of self (e.g., "I'm no good," "I'm ugly," or "People don't like me.")
- ◆ May be overly critical of others
- ◆ Is unable to accept positive remarks about self
- ◆ Encourages reprimands from others, to punish self
- ◆ Apologizes frequently
- ◆ Verbalizes feelings of hopelessness, helplessness, and powerlessness, such as "I really don't care what happens," "I'll do whatever anyone wants," or "Whatever is destined will happen."

- ◆ Develop a realistic and positive perception of body appearance and function.
- ◆ Increase feelings of self-worth.
- ◆ Perform new roles responsibly and capably.

Nurses must always establish a therapeutic relationship, in order to assist clients to evaluate themselves and make behavioral changes.

Identifying Areas of Strength

Healthy people often perceive their problems and weaknesses more clearly than they perceive their assets and strengths. When a client has difficulty identifying personality strengths and assets, the nurse needs to provide the client with a set of guidelines or a framework. Box 28-4 ◆ provides a framework for identifying personality strengths.

Nurses can employ the following specific strategies to help clients identify personal strengths:

BOX 28-4 FRAMEWORK FOR IDENTIFYING PERSONALITY STRENGTHS

Note past, present, and anticipated future participation in any of the following:

- ◆ Hobbies and crafts
- ◆ Expressive arts such as writing, painting, sketching, or music appreciation
- ◆ Sports and outdoor activities, including spectator sports
- ◆ Education, training, and related areas (including self-education)
- ◆ Work, vocation, job, or position

In addition, determine which of these might apply:

- ◆ Sense of humor and the ability to laugh at oneself and take kidding
- ◆ Health status including healthy aspects of body function and good health maintenance practices
- ◆ Special aptitudes such as sales or mechanical ability; a "green thumb"; ability to recognize and enjoy beauty; ability to solve problems; a liking for adventure or pioneering; having stick-to-itiveness, perseverance, and the drive or will needed to get things done
- ◆ Relationship strengths, including the ability to make people feel comfortable, the capacity to enjoy being with people, being aware of people's needs and feelings, being able to listen
- ◆ Emotional strengths including the capacity to give and receive warmth, affection, and love; the ability to "take" anger and to feel and express a wide range of emotions; the capacity for empathy
- ◆ Spiritual strengths such as religious faith or love of God, membership and participation in church and related activities

◆ Stress positive thinking rather than self-negation.
◆ Notice and verbally reinforce client strengths.
◆ Encourage the setting of attainable goals.
◆ Acknowledge goals that have been attained.
◆ Provide honest, positive feedback.

Maintaining a Sense of Self

Sometimes people who are ill not only are unaware of their strengths but also are separated from a sense of self. Nurses can use these techniques to help clients maintain a sense of self:

◆ Communicate worth by looks and touch (e.g., eye contact, a smile, a touch on the hand or shoulder).
◆ Respect the client's privacy and sensitivities.
◆ Provide a simple explanation before starting a procedure.
◆ Listen attentively to the client's concerns.
◆ Recognize the client's individuality by addressing the client by name.
◆ Accept the client's responses.

Assisting Clients with Altered Self-Concept

Nurses assisting clients who have an altered self-concept must establish a therapeutic relationship. To do this the nurse must possess self-awareness and effective communication skills (see Chapters 23 and 25). ⊂⊃ The following nursing interventions may help clients analyze the problem and change self-concept:

◆ Encourage clients to appraise the situation and express their feelings.
◆ Encourage clients to ask questions.
◆ Provide accurate information.
◆ Become aware of distortions, inappropriate or unrealistic standards, and faulty labels in clients' speech.
◆ Explore the client's positive qualities and strengths.
◆ Encourage clients to express positive self-evaluation more than negative self-evaluation.
◆ Avoid criticism.
◆ Teach clients to substitute negative self-talk ("I can't walk to the store anymore") with positive self-talk ("I can walk half a block each morning"). Negative self-talk reinforces a negative self-concept.

Assisting Clients with Disturbed Body Image

Surgery (ostomies, amputations, mastectomies) can have a profound effect on people's body image and self-concept. Treatments for illness, such as chemotherapy, can also radically alter a person's physical appearance (Figure 28-2 ◆). Clients with conditions like anorexia nervosa or bulimia carry a distorted self-image. To assist all these clients, the nurse establishes a therapeutic nursing relationship, practices good communication skills, and provides nursing care as described above.

Many facilities use critical pathways for clients following surgery. These pathways outline expected outcomes on a

Figure 28-2. ◆ One of the most common threats to body image at any age is hair loss induced by chemotherapy. Use of hats or wigs can sometimes improve self-concept.

day to day basis. For an example of a Critical Pathway for a client following a total mastectomy, see Appendix V. ⊂⊃

Enhancing Self-Esteem

People who have relatively high self-esteem appear to be adjusted, happy, and competent. Box 28-5 ◆ describes age-related considerations for enhancing self-esteem in children.

BOX 28-5

POPULATION FOCUS

WAYS TO ENHANCE SELF-ESTEEM IN CHILDREN

Basic Attitudes
◆ Security and trust
◆ Identity
◆ Belonging
◆ Purpose
◆ Personal competence

Key Ingredients
◆ Love and acceptance
◆ Firmness
◆ Consistency
◆ Establishment of expectations

Ways to Meet Child's Needs
◆ Take time to be with child.
◆ Physical contact conveys caring better than words.
◆ Provide reasonable rules that can serve as guidelines for new situations.
◆ Give positive feedback.
◆ Convey faith and confidence in the child's ability to achieve goals.

EVALUATING

The nurse, client, and significant others need to understand that to change beliefs, feelings, and behaviors affecting self-esteem requires time and ongoing effort. Unlike many physical problems (e.g., wounds) where healing can be observed quickly, improving one's self-concept can be a continuing concern and is not so easily evaluated. New crises can cause clients to doubt themselves and revert to former feelings of inadequacy. People learn slowly from each new situation and gradually gain new strategies for feeling satisfied with themselves.

Nursing Process Case Study: CLIENT WITH SELF-CONCEPT ISSUES

You are working in the community clinic. You have been assigned to do an admission workup on walk-in clients. You enter the exam room and encounter a 21-year-old young man with long hair, wearing foundation and mascara, and who is dressed somewhat effeminately. The name on his chart is Brian Breshear, yet when you address him by that name, he flinches and hardly looks up. In response to your question of what brings him in today, he softly replies, "I don't think I am supposed to be in this body. I want to learn about a sex change operation."

Assessment Male client, height 5'6", weight 134 lb; speaks with almost inaudible voice; responds only to direct questions. Vital signs are within normal limits T 98.6, P 78, R 20, BP 122/76. Client appears anxious; wringing hands and avoiding eye contact.

Diagnosis The following nursing diagnoses have been developed for Brian:

- Anxiety related to Disturbed Body Image
- Ineffective Role Performance/Disturbed Personal Identity
- Risk for Compromised Family Coping

Expected Outcomes The expected outcomes for the plan of care are that Brian will:

- Relate an increase in psychological and physiologic comfort.
- Verbalize and demonstrate increased feelings of self-concept.
- Verbalize the need for assistance with situation.
- Relate community resources available.

Planning and Implementation The following nursing interventions are implemented for Brian:

- Be direct and nonjudgmental.
- Encourage him to express his feelings, especially about the way he feels, thinks, or views himself.
- Provide reliable information, and reinforce information already given.
- Provide for opportunity to share with others going through the same experience.
- Establish a trusting nurse–client relationship.
- Provide information on psychological and physiological counseling and referrals.
- Assess level of anxiety.
- Provide reassurance and comfort.
- Encourage realistic appraisal of the situation: dispel guilt and myths.
- If indicated, ask family members to consider the situation from Brian's perspective.

Evaluation Brian related at his next medical visit that he had attended a counseling appointment with family members. They were able to share their feelings and concerns. His parents indicated that they will be supportive of any decision he makes. He will continue to participate in individual counseling sessions as well as attending a group. He has decided not to seek a surgical consult until a complete medical workup has been done and he has had the opportunity to work through some issues with the counselor and his family.

Critical Thinking in the Nursing Process

1. It is extremely important that the nurse establish a nonjudgmental, supportive therapeutic relationship with Brian. What are some of the communication techniques that you could use to establish this relationship?
2. Brian's father calls the clinic very upset, because the counselor wishes to see the family along with Brian. You have answered the phone. What is the most appropriate response to give to the father?
3. Brian has decided to place any plans for surgury on hold for now. How can you support him in this decision and later if he decides to go ahead with a sex change operation?

Note: The bibliography listings for this and all chapters have been compiled at the back of the book.

Chapter Review

Key Terms by Topics

Use the audio glossary feature of either the CD-ROM or the Companion Website to hear the correct pronunciation of the following key terms.

Introduction
Self-concept

Components of self-concept
body image, role, performance, personal identity, self-esteem

Key Points

* A positive self-concept is essential to a person's physical and psychological well-being.
* A person's self-perception can differ from the person's perception of how others see the person and from the ideal self (how the person would like to be).
* Components of self-concept include body image, role performance, personal identity, and self-esteem.
* Because a positive self-concept is basic to health, one of the nurse's major responsibilities is to assist clients whose self-concept is disturbed to develop a more positive and realistic image of themselves.
* A trusting client–nurse relationship is essential for the effective assessment of a client's self-concept, for providing help and support, and for motivating client behavior change.

EXPLORE MediaLink

Additional interactive resources for this chapter can be found on the Companion Website at www.prenhall.com/ramont. Click on Chapter 28 and "Begin" to select the activities for this chapter.

For chapter-related NCLEX-style questions and an audio glossary, access the accompanying CD-ROM in this book.

Animations:
* Gender identity
* Gender identity: early memories
* Gender identity: self-esteem
* Fluoxetine

For Further Study

For more about surgery and client self-concept, see Chapter 22.
For in-depth discussion of client teaching, see Chapter 23.
For more information about client communication, see Chapter 25.
For further study of cultural awareness and culturally competent nursing, see Chapter 26.

Critical Thinking Care Map

Caring for a Client with an Amputation

NCLEX-PN Focus Area: Safety

Case Study: Craig is a 20-year-old male college student who was involved in an automobile accident 3 days ago, suffering a traumatic amputation of his left lower leg. Craig's mother has remained with him since the accident and is very supportive. His father is grief stricken and having difficulty dealing with Craig's condition, because Craig was captain of his college basketball team and had hopes of becoming a professional basketball player. Craig's condition is stable and he is being placed into a rehabilitation program immediately. Soon, he will be fitted for a leg prosthesis. Usually an outgoing individual, Craig is somber and untalkative. He does not look at his leg when dressings are being changed and he refuses to discuss his rehabilitation program.

Nursing Diagnosis: Situational Low Self-Esteem

COLLECT DATA

Subjective
_____
_____
_____
_____
_____
_____
_____

Objective
_____
_____
_____
_____
_____
_____
_____

Would you report this data? Yes/No

If yes, to: _____

Nursing Care

_____
_____
_____
_____
_____
_____
_____
_____
_____
_____
_____
_____
_____
_____

How would you document this? _____
_____
_____
_____

Data Collected
(use all that apply)

- Somber and untalkative
- 20-year-old male student
- Refuses to discuss rehabilitation
- Automobile accident 3 days ago
- Father is grief stricken and having difficulty dealing with Craig's condition because traumatic amputation of his left lower leg
- Condition is stable
- Mother at bedside
- Captain of his college basketball team, shared aspirations of becoming a professional basketball player
- To be fitted for a leg prosthesis
- Usually an outgoing individual
- Does not look at his leg when dressings are being changed
- Rehabilitation program to begin immediately
- Mother very supportive

Nursing Interventions
(use those that apply)

- Actively listen to, demonstrate respect for, and accept the client.
- Encourage client to get up and use crutches within 2 days.
- Assess for intergenerational family problems that can overwhelm coping abilities.
- Assess client for anger and identify previous outlets for anger.
- Have client list strengths.
- Encourage client to reminisce about basketball.
- Accept client's own pace in working through grief and crisis situation.
- Assess the strengths and deficiencies of the family system.
- Talk to family about the importance of sharing feelings and ways to do so.
- Note other stressors in the family.
- Assess for unhealthy coping mechanisms such as substance abuse.
- Provide information about support groups.
- Assess client's support system.

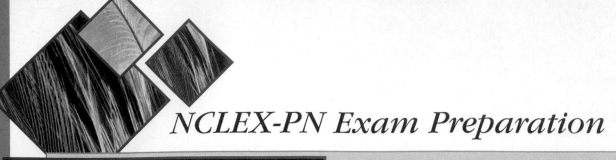

NCLEX-PN Exam Preparation

1. The knowledge that one has about oneself, including insight into one's abilities and limitations, is known as:
   a. Self-expectation
   b. Self-knowledge
   c. Social self
   d. Social evaluation

2. Individuals face certain developmental tasks associated with eight psychosocial stages of development. The success with which a person copes with these developmental crises largely determines the development of self-concept. Psychosocial development was outlined by:
   a. Sigmund Freud
   b. Lawrence Kohlberg
   c. Erik Erikson
   d. Aaron Beck

3. There are three broad steps in the development of one's self-concept: learning that the physical self is separate from the environment, internalizing others' attitudes toward self, and:
   a. Overcoming the pressures of society
   b. Overcoming separation anxiety
   c. Internalizing personality development
   d. Internalizing the standards of society

4. An adolescent female with anorexia nervosa has lost over 25% of her normal weight. When she looks in the mirror, she expresses the feeling that she is "fat." Of the following nursing diagnoses, which is appropriate for dealing with self-concept issues?
   a. Risk for Powerlessness
   b. Disturbed Body Image
   c. Imbalanced Nutrition, Less Than Body Requirements
   d. Ineffective Family Therapeutic Regimen Management

5. People who are ill may be unaware of their strengths and also are separated from a sense of self. Nurses can use many techniques to help clients maintain a sense of self. Which of the following is the best way to communicate worth by looks and touch?
   a. Refrain from making eye contact so as not to embarrass the client.
   b. Make no physical contact with client unless necessary for care.
   c. Encourage client to look at surgical site to promote self-acceptance.
   d. Make eye contact and touch client lightly on hand or shoulder when providing comfort.

6. Negative self-talk reinforces a negative self-concept. Of the following statements, which would represent negative-self talk by a client?
   a. "I am worried that I may have limitations when I am discharged."
   b. "I can't mow my lawn anymore."
   c. "Even though I may not be able to mow the lawn, I can still enjoy my flower garden."
   d. "I will be glad to be in my own home even though I will need to have someone stay with me."

7. The nurse can best demonstrate empathy by which of the following statements.
   a. "I know exactly how you feel."
   b. "I am sure you are very devastated by your diagnosis. I know I would be."
   c. "Dealing with serious illness can be very difficult. We can talk if you like, or I would be happy to just sit here with you quietly."
   d. "Although things look pretty bad today, they will get better as time goes on."

8. During the course of a psychosocial interview a nurse asks the client, "What goals in life are important to you?" The question is asked to determine:
   a. The client's self-esteem
   b. The client understanding of the care plan
   c. If the client has a disturbed body image
   d. The client's ability to cope with family roles

9. Nurses should establish a therapeutic relationship. The purpose of this is to:
   a. Provide client health teaching
   b. Assist clients to evaluate themselves and make behavioral changes
   c. Be able to carry out the needed assessments and care
   d. Provide a safe enviroment for the hospitalized client

10. During the assessment interview the nurse wishes to gather information about the client's family role. Of the following questions, which would provide the best access to information?
    a. "Are you married, and how many children do you have?"
    b. "Are you worried about your family while you are hospitalized?"
    c. "Tell me about how you family is adjusting to your illness."
    d. "Would you like to tell me about your family?"

Sexuality

Chapter

29

SHARING experiences

"In my thirty years of experience as a nurse in Geriatrics, I have found that attempting to take away the elderly's way of expressing their sexuality can be detrimental to their mental as well as their physical well-being. Growing old doesn't mean losing our sexuality. Much strength can be found in companionship."

Sandy Groff, LPN, D.O.N., Colonial Hall Assisted Living, Willow Street, PA.

LEARNING outcomes

After completing this chapter, you will be able to:
- Define key terms related to sexuality.
- Describe sexual development and concerns across the life span.
- Identify factors influencing sexuality throughout the life span.
- Discuss essential aspects of the sexual response cycle.
- Describe physiologic changes in sexuality in males and females throughout the life span.
- Identify the forms of male and female sexual dysfunction.
- List the elements of a focused interview about sexual concerns.
- Recognize health-promotion teaching related to reproductive issues.

MediaLink

www.prenhall.com/ramont

Use the address above to access the free, interactive Companion Website created for this textbook. Get hints, instant feedback, and textbook references to chapter-related NCLEX-style questions. Link to other interesting sites.

Audio Glossary:
Use the Companion Website, or the CD-ROM disk enclosed with your textbook, to hear the pronunciation of key terms in the chapter.

Sexuality is important to each person's identity throughout the life span. Each person has the capacity to function as a sexual being. The client's sexuality needs to be considered when they enter the health care system. The nurse must understand the normal sexual response and focus on the holistic nature of care to effectively support the sexual health of their clients during the life cycle.

Sex Versus Sexuality

Sexuality is influenced by the biologic, psychological, sociologic, cultural, and spiritual aspects of being. The words *sex* and *sexuality* are used interchangeably, and often incorrectly, to define different aspects of sexual being. **Sex** is the term most commonly used to denote biologic male or female status, but it is also used to describe specific sexual behavior, such as sexual intercourse. According to Masters, Johnson, and Kolodny (1995, p. 3), "The word **sexuality** generally has a broader meaning since it refers to all aspects of being sexual. Sexuality means a dimension of personality instead of referring to a person's capacity for erotic response alone."

Sexuality is subject to lifelong dynamic change. Normal developmental alterations and health status may necessitate adaptations in sexual expressions, but individuals continue to express sexuality in a variety of ways. To recognize if the client is sexually healthy the nurse must explore the biologic, psychological, and sociocultural dimensions of sexuality.

Pediatric and Adolescent Considerations

From birth, infants are assigned the gender of male or female, and by 3 years of age they begin to develop a gender identity. Preschoolers become increasingly aware of their own and others' body parts. During the school-age years, gender-role behavior is learned. See Table 29-1 ◆ for sexual development throughout the life span.

Parents need to be the primary educators of children at an early age. However, peers, teachers, media, and toys also teach about sexual issues. Parents need to learn how to answer questions and what information to provide for their children starting in the preschool years. Formal structured comprehensive sex education programs are available through the Sex Information and Education Council of the U.S. in New York. The programs are for age kindergarten through grade 12 (Leifer, 1999).

Although there is an increasing awareness today of sexuality and sexual functioning, some people still hold myths and misconceptions about sexuality. Many of these are handed down in families and cultures. Table 29-2 ◆ lists some common sexual myths and misconceptions.

PUBERTY

During **puberty** in early adolescence (12 to 13 years), primary and secondary sex characteristics develop, and children need information about body changes. For boys, the testes and scrotum increase in size, the skin over the scrotum becomes darker, pubic hair grows, and axillary sweating begins. Development of the genitals to adult size takes about 5 to 6 years. For girls, the pelvis and hips broaden, the breast tissues develop, pubic hair grows, axillary sweating begins, vaginal secretions become milky and change from an alkaline to an acid pH, and vaginal flora changes.

Girls need to be taught about **menstruation** (monthly uterine bleeding) and related self-care. Teenagers have irregular menstruation initially, which may lead to embarrassment because of stained clothing. They can be taught to watch for signs of approaching menstruation, such as tender breasts, water retention, or the appearance of skin eruptions or pimples. Parents and nurses should advise teenage girls to wash their hands thoroughly before inserting a tampon, to change tampons frequently, to alternate them with sanitary pads, and to use pads at night. These measures help to decrease risk of infection. Thorough cleaning of the genital area and wiping from front to back will also help to prevent infection and odors.

Dysmenorrhea (painful menstruation) is common among adolescent females and causes much short-term absenteeism. Cramping, lower abdominal pain radiating to the back and upper thighs, nausea, vomiting, diarrhea, and headaches result from powerful uterine contractions that cause pain.

SEXUAL ABUSE

All children need to be taught information about sexual abuse, including what it is and what to report to a responsible adult. **Sexual abuse** is any involvement of a child in an act designed to provide sexual gratification to an adult (Clark, 2003). Of the estimated 1 million children abused each year approximately 11% involve sexual abuse (Clark, 2003). This abuse cannot always be seen (Ball & Bindler, 1999). The child may have feelings of guilt, shame, anger, hostility, and low self-esteem that can lead to a self-destructive life and possibly suicide. Factors that increase the risk of sexual abuse are listed in Box 29-1 ◆.

Children who have been victims of sexual abuse may display some or all of these symptoms: pain, itching, bruising,

MediaLink ● Video: Sexual Abuse

BOX 29-1

POPULATION FOCUS

CHILDREN AT RISK FOR SEXUAL ABUSE
- ◆ Natural father is absent.
- ◆ Child is female.
- ◆ Mother is employed outside the home.
- ◆ Relationship with the parent is poor; conflict exists.
- ◆ Parent is substance abuser or socially isolated.

TABLE 29-1	SEXUAL DEVELOPMENT THROUGH THE LIFE SPAN	
STAGE	**CHARACTERISTICS**	**NURSING INTERVENTIONS AND TEACHING GUIDELINES**
Infancy Birth to 18 months	Given gender assignment of male or female. Differentiates self from others gradually. External genitals are sensitive to touch. Male infants have penile erections; females, vaginal lubrication. Dress and toys are gender oriented.	Self-manipulation of the genitals is normal. Caregivers need to recognize these behaviors as common in children.
Toddler 1–3 years	Continues to develop gender identity. Able to identify own gender.	Body exploration and genital fondling is normal. Use correct names for body parts. Children from single-parent homes should have contact with adults of both sexes.
Preschooler 4–5 years	Becomes increasingly aware of self. Explores own and playmates' body parts. Learns correct names for body parts. Learns to control feelings and behavior. Focuses love on parent of the opposite sex.	Answer questions about "where babies come from" honestly and simply. Parental overreaction to exploration of genitals and masturbation can lead to feelings that sex is "bad."
School Age 6–12 years	Has strong identification with parent of same sex. Tends to have friends of the same sex. Has increasing awareness of self. Continues self-stimulating behavior. Learns the role and concepts of own gender as part of the total self-concept. At about 8 or 9 years becomes concerned about specific sex roles and often approaches parents with explicit concerns about sexuality and reproduction.	Provide parents and children with opportunities to express their concerns and ask questions regarding sex. Answer all questions with factual data and perhaps follow up with appropriate books and other material. Advise parents to discuss basic information about sexual intercourse, menstruation, and reproduction with children at about 10 years of age. If helpful, give children reading material and then discuss it with them.
Adolescence 12–18 or 20 years	Primary and secondary sex characteristics develop. Menarche takes place. Develops relationships with the opposite sex. Masturbation is common. May participate in sexual activity.	Adolescents require information about body changes. Peer groups have great importance at this time and assist in forming sexual roles. Dating helps adolescents prepare for adult roles. Parents influence values and beliefs regarding behavior. Teenagers require information about contraceptive measures and precautions to take in regard to sexually transmitted diseases (STDs).
Young Adulthood 20–40 years	Sexual activity is common. Many prefer cohabitation instead of marriage; however, many marry and start families by age 30. Establishes own lifestyle and values. Many couples share financial obligations and household tasks.	Young adults often require information about measures to prevent unwanted pregnancies (i.e., abstinence or contraceptive devices). Require information to prevent STDs. Regular communication is required to understand partner's sexual needs and to work through problems and stresses.

(continues)

	TABLE 29-1	SEXUAL DEVELOPMENT THROUGH THE LIFE SPAN *(continued)*	

STAGE	CHARACTERISTICS	NURSING INTERVENTIONS AND TEACHING GUIDELINES
Middle Adulthood 40–65 years	Men and women experience decreased hormone production. The menopause occurs in women, usually anywhere between 40 and 55 years. The climacteric occurs gradually in men. Quality rather than the number of sexual experiences becomes important. Divorce is common. Individuals establish independent moral and ethical standards.	Women and men may need help adjusting to new roles. People may require counseling to help them reevaluate and direct their energies. Encourage couples to look at the positive aspects of this time of life.
Late Adulthood 65 years and over	Interest in sexual activity may continue. Sexual activity becomes less frequent. Women's vaginal secretions diminish, and breasts atrophy. Men produce fewer sperm and need more time to achieve an erection and to ejaculate.	Elderly people can continue sexual activity. Couples may require counseling about adapting their affection and sexual needs to physical limitations.

bleeding of genitals; stains or blood in underwear; withdrawn or aggressive behavior; or unusual sexual behavior. Whenever a child exhibits any of these manifestations, it is important to rule out other causes, such as infection, improper genital hygiene practices, or pinworm infestation. The nurse must identify how she feels regarding this subject to be able to deal with the parents and victims of child abuse. Nursing management includes further prevention of injury, providing support-

ive care, reinforcing the importance of follow-up, and reporting suspected abuse.

clinical ALERT

All states have child abuse laws that require professionals, including nurses, to report suspected child abuse (Ball & Bindler, 1999).

	TABLE 29-2	COMMON SEXUAL MISCONCEPTIONS

MISCONCEPTION	FACT
Nearly all men over 70 years old are impotent.	Sexual desire and ability decrease very little after middle age.
Masturbation causes mental instability.	Masturbation is not the cause of any mental imbalance or abnormality.
Sexual activity weakens a person.	There is no evidence that sexual activity weakens a person.
Women who have experienced orgasm are more likely to become pregnant.	Conceiving is not related to orgasm.
A large penis provides greater sexual satisfaction to women than a small penis.	Sexual satisfaction results from the entire experience of sex; size of penis is not the determining factor.
Alcohol is a sexual stimulant.	Alcohol is a relaxant and central nervous system depressant. Chronic alcoholism is associated with impotence.
Intercourse during menstruation is dangerous.	There is no physiologic basis for abstinence during menses.
The face-to-face coital position is the only moral and proper one.	Various positions offer pleasure and can be acceptable.

All adolescents want to know about sex but are often uneasy about discussing these concerns with their parents. Nurses, the schools, and the family need to provide accurate information. During the nursing assessment, teenagers should be asked directly what they know about sex, contraception, and reproduction. Sometimes a teenager's information is based on popular myths, not on fact. The nurse should discuss factual information about sex, sexual actions and their consequences; the individual's right to decide how to express oneself sexually; and the responsibilities that go with sexual activity.

Adolescents should be taught about **rape** (intercourse in which one person is an unwilling or unconsenting party). They should also be taught about date rape. **Date rape** occurs when a person manipulates a social interaction in order to have nonconsensual intercourse. Date rape often involves substances such as alcohol or other central nervous system (CNS) depressants, which cause the victim to fall asleep before the rape takes place. It is important to teach that rape is a violent act that should be reported, and that the victim is not to blame for being raped.

CULTURE AND SEXUALITY

Sexuality is structured and regulated by the individual's culture (see Chapter 26). 🔗 Culture influences the sexual nature of dress, rules about marriage, expectations of role behavior and social responsibilities, and specific sex practices. Societal attitudes vary widely. Attitudes about childhood sexual play, premarital sex, and homosexuality may be restrictive or permissive. Some cultures have specific sex practices. For example, puberty rites of adolescent males in native African and Australian cultures include **circumcision** (removal of the foreskin of the penis). Circumcision is also practiced on many male infants, especially among Jews. Female body beautification is carried out in some cultures to make the body more decorative. This involves forming *keloids* (scars) from above the chest to the groin on girls of 4 to 5 years of age. Female circumcision or female genital mutilation (FGM) is still practiced in some parts of Africa today. It involves either excision of the clitoris, the labia minora, and the labia majora, or closure of the vagina **(infibulation).** The reasons for sexual mutilation vary. Infibulation may be done to guarantee the bride's virginity. Excision of the clitoris is intended to reduce sexual desire and vulnerability to temptation. In 1980, the World Health Organization and the United Nations Children's Fund (UNICEF) unanimously recommended that all forms of female circumcision be abolished. In 1996, the U.S. Congress passed legislation making practicing FGM on girls under 18 a federal criminal offense (Brady, 1998).

STD PREVENTION

Both males and females experience increased sexual motivation *(libido)* during puberty and adolescence as a result of hormonal and body changes. Certain drugs also increase libido.

Responsible sexual behavior involves the prevention of sexually transmitted diseases and the prevention of unwanted pregnancy.

Sexually transmitted diseases (STDs) are diseases transmitted by sexual activity. STDs are the most common bacterial infections among adolescents. They need education about these diseases, preventive measures, and early treatment. Table 29-3 ◆ lists the common types and symptoms of STDs for which teenagers should seek medical care. The nurse should also inform the teenager about the various methods of birth control: pills, diaphragms, intrauterine devices (IUDs), the rhythm method, and condoms, to prevent an unplanned pregnancy. These are discussed later in this chapter.

The prevention of STDs is an essential part of sexual health teaching. Increases in these diseases are due to two factors: changing sexual mores that permit increased sexual activity, and an increase in the number of sexual partners. Because the term *sexually transmitted disease* raises feelings of guilt, shame, and fear, people frequently do not seek medical help as early as they should. In fact, many STDs can be treated quickly and effectively. Others may have serious consequences if they are not treated early. For example, a woman who develops pelvic inflammatory disease (PID) may have damage to the reproductive structures and may become sterile.

Some infections (*Trichomonas* and *Candida*) can also be acquired nonsexually. *Trichomonas* can survive on bed linen, clothing, and towels, so it can be transmitted without direct sexual contact. *Candida* is a yeast, which usually lives harmlessly in the body but can multiply to cause an infection. It is not something that is transferred from one partner to another through sexual contact.

Cervical cancer, though not a sexually transmitted disease, is more of a risk for women with multiple sexual partners, with human papillomavirus, or with genital herpes (Nettina, 2001).

There is still no long-term effective treatment for human immunodeficiency virus (HIV), which leads to acquired immune deficiency syndrome (AIDS). Anxiety about AIDS transmission has caused many individuals to alter their sexual behavior. Condoms made of latex or polyurethane can help reduce the likelihood of STDs, but even these sometimes allow transmission of disease. Up to 6% of condoms break or fall off during intercourse. Although the use of condoms has been described as "safe sex," the only truly safe sex is sex within a monogamous relationship or abstinence from sex. Methods for preventing the transmission of STDs are described in Box 29-2 ◆.

PREVENTION OF UNWANTED PREGNANCIES

Prevention of unwanted pregnancies should be addressed not only with adolescents but also with couples who are planning

TABLE 29-3 TYPES AND MANIFESTATIONS OF STDS

DISEASE	MALE	FEMALE
Gonorrhea	Painful urination; urethritis with watery white discharge, which may become purulent.	May be asymptomatic; or vaginal discharge, pain, and urinary frequency may be present.
Syphilis	Chancre, usually on glans penis, which is painless and heals in 4–6 weeks; secondary symptoms—skin eruptions, low-grade fever, inflammation of lymph glands—in 6 weeks to 6 months after chancre heals.	Chancre on cervix or other genital areas, which heals in 4–6 weeks; symptoms same as for male.
Genital warts (condyloma acuminatum)	Single lesions or clusters of lesions growing beneath or on the foreskin, at external meatus, or on the glans penis. On dry skin areas, lesions are hard and yellow-gray. On moist areas, lesions are pink or red and soft with a cauliflower like appearance.	Lesions appear at the bottom part of the vaginal opening, on the perineum, the vaginal lips, inner walls of the vagina, and the cervix.
Herpes genitalis (herpes simplex of the genitals)	Primary herpes involves the presence of painful sores or large, discrete vesicles that last for weeks; vesicles rupture. Recurrent herpes is itchy rather than painful; it lasts for a few hours to 10 days.	Same as for males.
Chlamydial urethritis	Urinary frequency; watery, mucoid urethral discharge.	Commonly a carrier; vaginal discharge, dysuria, urinary frequency.
Trichomoniasis	Slight itching; moisture on top of penis; slight, early morning urethral discharge. Many males are asymptomatic.	Itching and redness of vulva and skin inside thighs; copious watery, frothy vaginal discharge.
Candidiasis	Itching, irritation, discharge, plaque of cheesy material under foreskin.	Red and excoriated vulva; intense itching of vaginal and vulvar tissues; thick, white, cheesy or curdlike discharge.
Acquired immune deficiency syndrome (AIDS)	Symptoms can appear anytime from several months to several years after acquiring the virus. The person has reduced immunity to other diseases. Symptoms include any of the following for which there is no other explanation: persistent heavy night sweats; extreme fatigue; severe weight loss; enlarged lymph glands in neck, axillae, or groin; persistent diarrhea; skin rashes; blurred vision or chronic headache; harsh, dry cough; thick gray-white coating on tongue or throat.	

the time of their first birth and want to space children and limit family size. Nurses need to be familiar with various contraceptive methods and their advantages, disadvantages, contraindications, effectiveness, safety, and cost. Contraceptive methods are outlined in Box 29-3 ◆. It is important to teach that some methods (such as coitus interruptus) are far less effective than others, and that sometimes a combination of methods can be used.

SCREENING FOR CANCER

Monthly breast self-examination (BSE) for females (Figure 29-1 ◆) and monthly testicular self-examination (TSE) for males (Figure 29-2 ◆) should be started in adolescence. Early detection of cancer results in a greater chance of cure and less complex treatment. Clients need to be assured that most lumps discovered are not cancerous. However, it is essential that all lumps or abnormalities be checked by a physician for accurate diagnosis. All nursing history assessments of clients need to

include the client's understanding and practice of BSE or TSE. Self-examination involves both inspection and palpation procedures and should be conducted once a month.

For BSE, a regular time is best, such as 1 week following menstruation, when breast tenderness and fullness caused by

Figure 29-1. ◆ Using a circular pattern to palpate the right breast.

Figure 29-2. ◆ Rolling the testicle between the thumb and fingers.

fluid retention have subsided. Women who examine themselves regularly become familiar with the shape and texture of their breasts.

The best time for TSE is after a warm bath or shower when the scrotal sac is relaxed. Men should also be taught to inspect and palpate their breasts, because they have some glandular tissue beneath each nipple, a potential site for malignancy. For specific techniques of self-examination, see Boxes 29-4 ◆ and 29-5 ◆. Clients should also be informed about the American Cancer Society's cancer screening guidelines for asymptomatic people. ACS recommendations include: breast examination by a health care provider every 3 years from age 20 to 39 and yearly thereafter, screening mammogram every year from age 40, annual Pap test beginning at age 18, yearly rectal exam with blood test for prostate-specific antigen (PSA) for men over age 50, yearly stool exam for colon cancer, and yearly testicular exam beginning at age 15 (Nettina, 2001). See also Chapter 11. ∞

BOX 29-2

CLIENT TEACHING

PREVENTING TRANSMISSION OF STDS
- ◆ Have one sexual partner.
- ◆ Use condoms in nonmonogamous and homosexual relationships or other relationships that have the potential for STD transmission.
- ◆ Talk openly with sexual partners about how to have "safe sex" and be honest about any history of an STD.
- ◆ Abstain from sexual activity with a partner known to have or suspected of having an STD.
- ◆ Report to a health care facility for examination whenever in doubt about possible exposure or when signs of an STD are evident.
- ◆ When an STD is diagnosed, notify all partners and encourage them to seek treatment.
- ◆ Avoid unnecessary transfusions of blood or blood products. Use *autologous transfusions* (donation of own blood before surgery) for elective surgery whenever possible.

BOX 29-3
METHODS OF CONTRACEPTION

- ◆ Abstinence
- ◆ Coitus interruptus (withdrawal of the penis before ejaculation)
- ◆ Fertility awareness (identification of the days of the month when conception could take place and abstaining during that time)
- ◆ Mechanical barriers: vaginal diaphragm, cervical cap, condom
- ◆ Chemical barriers: insertion of spermicidal foams, creams, jellies, or suppositories into the vagina before intercourse
- ◆ Intrauterine devices (IUDs)
- ◆ Hormonal barriers: oral contraceptives (birth control pills), subdermal implants of synthetic progestin
- ◆ Surgical sterilization: tubal ligation and vasectomy
- ◆ Abortion

Maternal and Infant Considerations

Sexual development of the infant was outlined in Table 29-1 ◆. Sexuality begins before birth. Sex determination can be made by the 11th to the 14th week of gestation (Nettina, 2001). When an infant is born, gender is assigned. In rare cases of **hermaphroditism,** the infant has both testicular and ovarian tissue, and it may be difficult to determine gender (Mosby's Medical, Nursing, and Allied Health Dictionary, 2001). This can be very upsetting and may have a profound impact on both parents and child. Chromosomal studies and other diagnostic tests may need to be completed to determine the proper gender (Novak & Broom, 1999).

PREGNANCY AND POSTPARTUM

Pregnancy may enhance sexuality for a woman and her partner, or it may decrease desire, depending on the individual. Body image, a central part of the sense of self, changes constantly during pregnancy and can affect one's sexuality. Pregnancy can affect sexual desire if it is associated with physical discomfort, fear of injury to the fetus, or perceived loss of attractiveness. Alternate positions for intercourse may need to be used. Monthly BSE should continue throughout pregnancy.

Safety can sometimes be an issue in pregnancy. Intercourse may worsen situations with repeated miscarriage, uterine abnormalities, premature labor, premature rupture of membranes, vaginal bleeding, or abdominal pain (Sherwen, Scoloven, & Weingarten, 1999).

Following delivery, libido is often reduced for about 4 weeks due to decreased vaginal lubrication, thinner vaginal walls, pain or fear of pain after an episiotomy, and a slower

BOX 29-4

CLIENT TEACHING

BREAST SELF-EXAMINATION

Inspection Before a Mirror

Look for any change in size or shape; lumps or thickenings; any rashes or other skin irritations; dimpled or puckered skin; any discharge or change in the nipples (e.g., position or asymmetry). Inspect the breasts in all of the following positions:

◆ Stand and face the mirror with your arm relaxed at your sides or hands resting on the hips; then turn to the right and the left for a side view (look for any flattening in the side view).

◆ Bend forward from the waist with arms raised over the head.

◆ Stand straight with the arms raised over the head and move the arms slowly up and down at the sides. (Look for free movement of the breasts over the chest wall.)

◆ Press your hands firmly together at chin level while the elbows are raised to shoulder level.

Palpation: Lying Position

◆ Place a pillow under your right shoulder and place the right hand behind your head. This position distributes breast tissue more evenly on the chest.

◆ Use the finger pads (tips) of the three middle fingers (held together) on your left hand to feel for lumps.

◆ Press the breast tissue against the chest wall firmly enough to know how your breast feels. A ridge of firm tissue in the lower curve of each breast is normal.

◆ Use small circular motions all the way around the rim of your breast (see Figure 29-1) starting and ending at the same place (e.g., the 12 o'clock position). Then move your fingers in toward the nipple about 2 cm and feel all the way around again. Repeat this action as many times as necessary until the entire breast is covered.

◆ Bring your arm down to your side and feel under your armpit, where breast tissue is also located.

◆ Repeat the exam on your left breast, using the finger pads of your right hand.

Palpation: Standing or Sitting

◆ Repeat the examination of both breasts while upright with one arm behind your head. This position makes it easier to check the area where a large percentage of breast cancers are found, the upper outer part of the breast and toward the armpit.

◆ Report any changes to your health care provider promptly.

◆ **Optional:** Do the upright BSE in the shower. Soapy hands glide more easily over wet skin.

---

response to stimulation. Postpartum clients should be cautioned about safe sexual activities. Sexual activity should be avoided until the episiotomy is healed and *lochia* (vaginal discharge after birth) has stopped, to prevent infection and trauma (Leifer, 1999).

Contraception should also be addressed before the client leaves the hospital. The nurse should reinforce the fact that ovulation and pregnancy can occur before the 6-week checkup, even if the client is breast-feeding.

Once an infant arrives, there is less time and energy for intimacy and privacy. Sexuality often becomes secondary to needs of the family. This may take a toll on the relationship.

INFERTILITY

Infertility (inability to conceive a child) is a growing problem in the United States. About 15% of couples are unable to achieve pregnancy (Leifer, 1999). Couples sometimes pursue their careers and wait until later in adulthood to have children. These individuals can have psychological reactions to infertility, including guilt, isolation, depression, and stress on the relationship. Much time, patience, and money may be invested in dealing with infertility. Cultural and religion can also have a great impact.

Infertility resulting from tubal ligation or vasectomy may enhance or interfere with sexual performance and pleasure, depending on how it is seen by the individuals involved.

 Adult Health Considerations

Sexuality and sexual identity are important to the adult client. A major part of a person's self-identity develops through experience during the young and middle adult years. Sexual identity consists of biological sex, gender identity, and sexual orientation. Traditional family and cultural values influence gender identity. Traditional adult male roles included being the breadwinner, heterosexual lover, and father, and expressing feelings in a controlled fashion. Women were expected to express their emotions more freely, to be more gentle and sensitive, and to be more concerned than men with clothing and appearance. However, many people now challenge these stereotypes. Men are freer now to be sensitive, and women are capably functioning as competitive and assertive executives and world leaders. Gender identity also includes one's comfort with his or her biological sex. Occasionally, a person has the genitalia, secondary sex characteristics, and hormonal influence of one gender but truly identifies with the other gender.

BOX 29-5

CLIENT TEACHING

TESTICULAR SELF-EXAMINATION

◆ Choose one day of each month (e.g., the first or last day of each month) to examine yourself.

◆ Examine yourself when you are taking a warm shower or bath.

◆ Place the index and middle fingers under the testicles and the thumbs on top.

◆ Roll each testicle between the thumb and fingers of each hand, feeling for lumps, thickening, or a hardening in consistency (see Figure 29-2). The testes should feel smooth.

◆ Palpate the *epididymis,* a cordlike structure on the top and back of the testicle. The epididymis feels soft and not as smooth as a testicle.

◆ Locate the spermatic cord, or *vas deferens*, which extends upward from the scrotum toward the base of the penis. It should feel firm and smooth.

◆ Using a mirror, inspect your testicles for swelling, any enlargement, or lumps in the skin of the testicle. Report any lumps or other changes to your health care provider promptly.

SEXUAL ORIENTATION

Sexual orientation is the preference of a person for one sex or the other. Types of sexual orientation are listed in Box 29-6 ◆. The determiners of sexual orientation are unknown. It is believed that homosexual identity often begins in childhood and may even have a genetic basis. Estimates of the percentage of the population with a homosexual orientation vary from 2 or 3 percent to at least 10 percent. Because these individuals grow up acutely aware of the discrimination they face in North America, many do not disclose their sexual orientation, and accurate figures have not been established. See also Chapter 28. ⊂⊃

BOX 29-6
TYPES OF SEXUAL ORIENTATION

◆ *Heterosexual:* A person who is sexually attracted to persons of the opposite gender

◆ *Bisexual:* A person who is sexually attracted to persons of both sexes

◆ *Homosexual:* A person who is sexually attracted to persons of same gender

◆ *Transsexual:* A person who is of a certain biological gender but who has feelings of the opposite sex

◆ *Transvestite:* A person who desires to wear clothes or take on the role of the opposite sex

It is important for the nurse to understand characteristics of sexual development through the life span, in order to be able to determine variations. Young adults develop a value system and learn to respect the values of others. Cohabitation may be chosen instead of marriage. Sexual activity is common and may include experimentation with various sexual expressions.

NORMAL SEXUAL RESPONSE

Young adult men and women are often concerned about normal sexual response, both for themselves and their partners. Many problems arise in relationships because of basic differences in the male and female sexual response patterns. Couples need to communicate their needs to one another early in their courtship so that a successful intimate relationship can develop and grow. Young adults should also be aware that because sexual needs and responses may change, each partner should listen and respond to the needs of the other.

There are many methods of sexual stimulation. Manual or oral stimulation of the genital area can be used as a prelude to genital **intercourse** (the sexual union of two persons, most commonly by penetration of the penis into the vagina).

The most common form of sexual activity with the adult is heterosexual genital intercourse, also known as **coitus** or *copulation*. A variety of positions are used in sexual intercourse. The choice of intercourse positions and activities depends on physical comfort and beliefs, values, and attitudes about different practices.

During sexual arousal, two primary physiologic changes occur: *vasocongestion* (congestion of the blood vessels in the genital area) and *myotonia* (increased muscle tension). One model of physiologic response identifies four phases of physiologic changes: excitement, plateau, orgasm, and resolution (Masters & Johnson, 1966, p. 4). Table 29-4 ◆ summarizes the physiologic changes associated with each of the phases of the sexual response cycle in both males and females. It is important for the nurse to understand the normal sexual response, and to remember that many variations in this cycle also are considered normal.

clinical ALERT

The use of condoms during anal sex is particularly important. Because anorectal tissue is not self-lubricating, a lubricant must be used on the condom. Also, since normal bacterial flora from the bowel can produce infections in other parts of the body, the used condom should be removed and another applied before inserting the penis into other body orifices.

Anal intercourse is a key risk factor in the spread of HIV due to rectal trauma, which gives the virus immediate access to the bloodstream. Although diverse sexual activity is more widely accepted today, it is necessary to note that in many jurisdictions, anal intercourse has been legally defined as sodomy, an offense punishable by law.

TABLE 29-4	PHYSIOLOGIC CHANGES IN THE SEXUAL RESPONSE CYCLE		
PHASE OF THE SEXUAL RESPONSE CYCLE	SIGNS PRESENT IN BOTH SEXES	SIGNS PRESENT IN MALES ONLY	SIGNS PRESENT IN FEMALES ONLY
Excitement	Increased muscle tension Moderate increase in heart rate, respirations, and blood pressure Sex flush (less prevalent in men than in women; present in 75% of women) Nipple erection (60% of men and most women)	Penile erection Tensing, thickening, and elevation of the scrotum Partial elevation and increase in size of testicles	Enlargement of the clitoral glans Vaginal lubrication Widening and lengthening of vaginal barrel Separation and flattening of the labia majora Reddening of the labia minora and vaginal wall Breast tumescence (enlargement) and enlarged areolae
Plateau	Increased voluntary and involuntary myotonia Abdominal, intercostal, anal, and facial muscle contraction Accelerated heart rate and respiratory rate, and increased blood pressure Sex flush (appearance in some men late in the phase; spread over the entire body in women)	Increase in penile circumference at the coronal ridge (base of the prepuce), and deepening of color 50% increase in testicular size, and elevation close to the perineum Appearance of a few drops of mucoid secretions from the bulbourethral glands at tip of penis; may contain sperm	Retraction of the clitoris under the hood Appearance of the orgasmic platform (increase in the size of the outer one third of the vagina and the labia minora) Slight increase in the width and depth of the inner two thirds of the vagina Further reddening of the labia minora Appearance of a few drops of mucoid secretion from the Bartholin's glands to lubricate inner labia Further increase in breast size and areolar enlargement
Orgasmic	Involuntary spasms of muscle groups throughout the body Diminished sensory awareness Involuntary contractions of the anal sphincter Peak heart rate (110–180 bpm), respiratory rate (40/min or greater), and blood pressure (systolic 30–80 mm Hg and diastolic 20–50 mm Hg above normal)	Rhythmic, expulsive contractions of the penis at 0.8-sec intervals Emission of seminal fluid into the prostatic urethra from contraction of the vas deferens and accessory organs (stage 1 of the expulsive process) Closing of the internal bladder sphincter just before ejaculation to prevent retrograde ejaculation into bladder Orgasm may occur without ejaculation Ejaculation of semen through the penile urethra and expulsion from the urethral meatus. The force of ejaculation varies from man to man and at different times but diminishes after the first two to three contractions (stage 2 of the expulsive process)	Approximately 5–12 contractions in the orgasmic platform at 0.8-sec intervals Contraction of the muscles of the pelvic floor and the uterine muscles Varied pattern of orgasms, including minor surges and contractions, multiple orgasms, or a single intense orgasm similar to that of the male

(continues)

TABLE 29-4	PHYSIOLOGIC CHANGES IN THE SEXUAL RESPONSE CYCLE (*continued*)		
PHASE OF THE SEXUAL RESPONSE CYCLE	SIGNS PRESENT IN BOTH SEXES	SIGNS PRESENT IN MALES ONLY	SIGNS PRESENT IN FEMALES ONLY
Resolution	Reversal of vasocongestion in 10–30 min; disappearance of all signs of myotonia within 5 min Genitals and breasts return to their preexcitement states Sex flush disappears in reverse order of appearance Heart rate, respiratory rate, and blood pressure return to normal Other reactions include sleepiness, relaxation, and emotional outbursts such as crying or laughing	A **refractory period** during which the body will not respond to sexual stimulation; varies, depending on age and other factors, from a few moments to hours or days	

Condoms are used for contraception as well as for preventing STDs. Contraception was discussed in the Maternal–Infant Consideration section.

Some alternative forms of sexual expression for the adult may be illegal or harmful to others. These include *voyeurism* (seeking sexual arousal by observing the body of another); *sadomasochistic bondage* (heterosexual or homosexual activities that involve inflicting pain or experiencing pain during sexual stimulation); and *pedophilia* (sexual acts with children).

Some clients may act out sexually or be sexually aggressive toward other clients or the nurse. Their behaviors may infringe on the rights of others or be harmful to others. Nurses need to respond to this behavior as unacceptable. However, they also need to recognize it as a possible expression of a sexual concern or problem that the client may be experiencing (Box 29-7 ◆).

Some clients experience **sexual dysfunction** (undesired, altered sexual function). The ability to engage in genital intercourse is of great importance to most people. Many people experience transient problems with their ability to respond to sexual stimulation or to maintain the response. A smaller percentage of people experience long-standing problems. Many factors may interfere with sexual response including physical dysfunction, stress, illness, overwork, religion. Sexual dysfunction can be further divided into male and female dysfunction.

Three male types of dysfunction are erectile dysfunction, premature ejaculation, and retarded ejaculation. **Erectile dysfunction,** more commonly referred to as **impotence,** is the inability to achieve or maintain an erection sufficient for sexual satisfaction for oneself or one's partner and can occur at any age. Erectile dysfunction can be caused by physiologic or psychological factors. Physiologic factors include (a) neurologic disorders created by spinal cord injuries, injury to the genitals or perineal nerves, extensive surgery such as abdominal–perineal bowel resections, radical perineal prostatectomy, diabetes mellitus, multiple sclerosis, and Parkinson's disease; and (b) prolonged use of drugs, such as alcohol, sedatives, heroin, antidepressants, antipsychotics (phenothiazines), and antihypertensives; (c) traumatic early sexual experiences (e.g., rejection); and (d) boredom associated with the specific partner. Some of these disorders can particularly come into play with the busy lifestyle of the young adult. With the long workdays and activities in families, satisfying sexuality can be difficult.

In the female, the four dysfunctions are orgasmic dysfunction, vaginismus, dyspareunia, and vulvodynia. **Orgasmic dysfunction** is the inability of a woman to achieve orgasm. Orgasmic dysfunction can be caused by drugs, alcohol, aging, and anatomic abnormalities of the genitals. However, most cases have psychological causes, including hostility between partners, fear or guilt about enjoying the sexual act, and concern about performance. Therapy usually involves helping both partners to establish new attitudes about sex. Pelvic muscle exercises (Kegel exercises) can also increase the woman's capacity to achieve orgasm by increasing the strength of the pubococcygeal muscle.

There are many medications that can have effects on sexuality in the adult. These include many prescription medications and social drugs that can affect sexual desire and response. Table 29-5 ◆ lists various medications that affect sexual function (Clayton & Stock, 2001). Early traumatic sexual experiences or boredom with a sexual partner can also depress sexual responsiveness.

The nurse can assist the client in identifying any sexual dysfunction by performing a thorough assessment. Assessment guidelines for sexual dysfunction are discussed in the Nursing Care section.

TABLE 29-5	DRUGS AFFECTING SEXUAL FUNCTION

Antihypertensive

Thiazide diuretics
Beta blockers
Alpha-adrenergic blockers
Sympatholytics
Spironolactone

Central Nervous System Depressants

Phenothiazides
Monoamine oxidase inhibitors
Serotonin reuptake inhibitors

Cardiovascular

Digoxin
Clofibrate
Gemfibrozil

Miscellaneous Agents

Substances of abuse (alcohol, cocaine, marijuana, nicotine)
Alkylating agents
Anabolic steroids
Estrogens
Corticosteriods
Cimetidine
5-alpha-reductase inhibitors

Geriatric Health Considerations

As the client enters the older adult stage, the reproductive system slows down. The climacteric in the male is not as dramatic as in the female; changes are more gradual. Most experts say there is not a true climacteric in the male, but that the decline in male sexual desire is related to the decline in physical strength and aging of all the body tissues (Porth, 2002). Although testosterone levels decline with age, the ability to remain fertile may extend into old age.

FACTORS AFFECTING SEXUAL RESPONSE

Sexuality may be far more broadly defined by older adults. Their definition may include such things as touching, hugging, romantic gestures (e.g., giving or receiving roses), comfort, warmth, dressing up, joy, spirituality, and beauty. Interest in sexual activity is not lost as men age. However, more time is needed to achieve an erection and to ejaculate. More direct genital stimulation is required to achieve an erection. The volume of ejaculated fluid decreases. The intensity of contractions with orgasm may decrease. The refractory period after orgasm is longer.

Older women remain capable of multiple orgasms and may, in fact, experience an increase in sexual desire after the menopause. However, vaginal lubrication and elasticity

BOX 29-7 NURSING STRATEGIES FOR INAPPROPRIATE SEXUAL BEHAVIOR

- ◆ Identify the behavior you expect: "Please call me by my name, not 'honey,' " or, "I expect you to keep yourself covered when I am in the room. If you are feeling hot or something is uncomfortable, let me know, and I will try to make you more comfortable."
- ◆ Set firm limits: Take the client's hand and move it away, use direct eye contact, and say, "Don't do that!"
- ◆ Communicate that the behavior is not acceptable by saying, for example, "I really do not like the things you are saying," or, "I see you are not dressed. I will be back in 10 minutes and will help you with breakfast when you have your clothes on."
- ◆ Tell the client how the behavior makes you feel: "When you act like that toward me, I don't want to come into your room. It embarrasses me and makes it hard for me to give you the kind of nursing care you need."
- ◆ Try to refocus clients from the inappropriate behavior to their real concerns and fears. Sometimes people talk like that when they are concerned about the sexual part of their life and how their illness will affect them. Offer to discuss sexuality concerns: "All morning you have been making very personal sexual comments about yourself. Are there things that you have questions about or would like to talk about?"
- ◆ Clarify the consequences of continued inappropriate behavior (avoidance, withdrawal of services, no chance to help resolve underlying concerns of client).
- ◆ Report the incident to your nursing instructor, charge nurse, or clinical nurse specialist. Discuss the incident, your feelings, and possible interventions.
- ◆ If you feel you are not being successful in getting the client to change behavior, ask your supervisor to assign another nurse to the client.

decrease with menopause and decreased estrogen levels, and phases of the sexual response cycle may take longer to occur. There is a possibility of pain during sexual activity and intercourse **(dyspareunia)** related to vaginal dryness or chronic health conditions like diabetes or arthritis. Lack of privacy may be a concern for older adults who live with family or in a rehabilitation or nursing home facility.

Personal values can influence sexuality in the older adult. Cultural and religious guidelines define acceptable behavior, forbidden behavior, and the consequences of breaking sexual rules. For example, many groups hold virginity before marriage to be the rule, and view forms of sexual expression other than male–female intercourse as wrong and unnatural.

Many personal values conflict with the more flexible values of society that have developed over the last few decades, including premarital sex and homosexuality. These conflicts create marked anxiety and potential sexual dysfunction in some individuals.

Among adults one person may view a sexual behavior as bizarre, perverted, or wrong while another may feel that it is completely natural and right. Examples include masturbation, oral or anal intercourse, and cross-dressing. Many people accept sexual expression of various forms if it is performed by consenting adults, is practiced in privacy, and is not harmful. Couples need to explore and communicate about various types of sexual expression to prevent domination of sexual decision making by one member of the couple.

Heart disease, diabetes, degenerative joint disease, STDs, cerebrovascular accident (CVA), and disorders that cause mental deterioration may interfere with the sexuality of the older adult. Heart disease frequently influences sexual expression. Older adults are at risk for myocardial infarction and are often anxious about their sexuality and sexual activity. Concerns about the effect of sexual activity on the heart may cause people to restrict or avoid intercourse. Education by health professionals can alleviate client fears following heart surgery or hospitalization for alterations in heart function. Clients can be taught to resume sexual activity based on reactions to exercise. They can be told to avoid sexual intercourse after large meals or consumption of alcoholic beverages. They can be taught safe positions to assume, as well as signs of distress.

Many men with long-term diabetes mellitus develop erectile dysfunction. Women who have diabetes may experience orgasmic dysfunction, difficulty experiencing arousal, loss of vaginal lubrication, and painful intercourse related to *Monilia* infection of the vagina.

Any surgical procedure has the potential to alter a person's body image, especially when the surgery involves mutilating, removing, or altering parts of the body. Examples include amputation of a leg, radical neck surgery, excision of large portions of the lower jaw, and ostomies. The impact is even greater when the surgery alters or removes body parts linked directly with sexual functioning. Such surgery includes mastectomy, hysterectomy, and vaginal excision in women; and **orchiectomy** (removal of the testicles) and penectomy in men. Feelings of ugliness and loss of masculinity or femininity are common after these surgeries. These surgeries are more common among older adults.

Many people also have concerns about their reactions to a partner's surgical procedure. Having discussions with both individuals to provide facts can be very helpful. For example, many men delay seeking medical advice and treatment because they fear that prostatectomy will cause impotence. However, surgical approaches for prostatectomy do not result in impotence. *Retrograde ejaculation* (ejaculation of seminal fluid into the bladder) sometimes results; this affects fertility. In most instances, however, the man may resume sexual activity in 6 to 8 weeks. Ejaculate will be decreased or absent and the urine is often cloudy.

Joint disease may indirectly affect sexual function because of pain, stiffness, loss of joint motion, and fatigue. Such symptoms influence sexual motivation as well as sexual positioning and methods. Chronic pain often decreases sexual motivation. Altered positions for coitus may be necessary, and alternative ways to express sexual stimulation and warmth may need to be emphasized.

STDs can be transmitted by the older adult population. These include gonorrhea, chlamydia, syphilis, genital herpes, trichomoniasis, HIV or AIDS, and genital warts. Frequently, older adults lack knowledge in this area, thinking they are exempt from STDs. The presence of an STD is often unknown when transmission occurs.

Another problem that can occur with the older adult population is altered mental status. Because mind and thought are both involved in sexual functioning, any impairment of the mind may affect sexual expression. For example, depression lowers libido and can affect both the depressed and the nondepressed partner. Some clients with mental disorders or brain injury may behave in an inappropriate sexual manner, such as touching their genitals, removing their clothing, or seeking frequent sexual activity. Clients with Alzheimer's disease may not remember any previous sexual contact with their partners.

Most geriatric clients take many prescription medications, which have side effects that can affect sexual functioning. Older adults may need medications to enhance sexual motivation. With the introduction of drugs like Viagra, there is increasing awareness of alternatives for those with these problems, including possible use of Viagra for women (Napoli, 1999).

NURSING CARE

 ## ASSESSING

When assessing a client for sexual concerns, the nurse should be aware of the person's developmental level. It is important to speak in clear, understandable terms to clients of any age, and to use the proper names for body parts and sexual activities. The nurse may need to ask specifically about any concerns or problems related to sexuality.

The nurse can assist the client in identifying any sexual dysfunction by performing a thorough assessment. An example of assessment guidelines is provided in Box 29-8 ◆.

 ## DIAGNOSING, PLANNING, and IMPLEMENTING

Nursing diagnoses that might be seen in clients with sexual health issues are: Sexual Dysfunction, Ineffective Sexuality Patterns, Deficient Knowledge (contraceptive methods), Rape-Trauma Syndrome, or Interrupted Family Processes.

BOX 29-8 ASSESSING CLIENTS: SEXUAL HEALTH HISTORY

Women

◆ When did your menstrual periods first begin, and when did you have your last menstrual period?

◆ What is the usual length of your period in days and usual amount of bleeding?

◆ Do you have any concerns about the amount or regularity of your menstrual flow?

◆ If periods are irregular, problematic, or have stopped: Have you been evaluated for this change or done anything yourself to deal with it?

◆ Are you having any burning with urination, any vaginal itching or discharge, midcycle spotting, pain with intercourse, or any other problems?

◆ Have you ever been pregnant? (Explore number and outcome of pregnancies, including miscarriages and induced abortions.)

◆ How often do you do breast self-examination?

◆ Is there a history of breast or ovarian cancer in your family?

◆ When did you have your last Pap test and mammogram?

Men

◆ Are you having any difficulty with initiating urination, urinary frequency, or frequent urination at night?

◆ Are you having any itching or discharge from your penis?

◆ How often do you do testicular self-examination?

◆ Is there a history of testicular cancer in your family?

Men and Women

◆ Are you currently sexually active?

◆ What do you do to protect yourself from infection when you are sexually active?

◆ Have you ever had a sexually transmitted disease?

◆ Has any disease, injury, surgery, medication, or other situation affected your sexual health and happiness or your feelings about yourself as a woman or man?

◆ Do you have any questions about your sexual health or functioning, or is there anything else we have discussed that you would like clarified or explained?

Outcomes for clients with concerns about sexuality might include:

◆ Client seeks consultation with urologist about enlarged prostate.

◆ Client verbalizes the need to discuss dyspareunia with spouse and to use lubricants during intercourse.

◆ Client plans visit to gynecologist to obtain Pap smear and to learn about possible insertion of IUD.

◆ Client states that rape was not her fault.

◆ Mother states that she will nap when the baby naps for the next 4 weeks.

Nurses can best assist clients to deal with problems related to sexuality if they first resolve some of their own feelings about the issue. Using the proper anatomic terms can help with this. Stating the facts clearly and simply is also important. Because views of sexuality are closely tied to one's culture, nurses should take time to clarify their own views on sexuality, and to identify values they hold about sex and sexual relationships. There are many ethical issues related to sexuality, including:

◆ Contraception
◆ Abortion
◆ Sexual preference
◆ Types of sexual activity

 clinical **ALERT**

No matter what the nurse's upbringing and value system, it is important to approach the client with the client's needs in mind.

Education and emotional support are two important aspects of nursing care related to sexuality and reproductive concerns. The nurse can teach the importance of communicating with a spouse or sexual partner, and of adapting to physical changes as a normal part of life. In clients with multiple sexual partners, the nurse should provide guidelines for safer sex (see Box 29-2).

◆ EVALUATING

The nurse reviews client outcomes related to specific sexual concerns. Both physical and emotional aspects of the client's concern are reassessed. The nurse may request referrals for specialized care.

Nursing Process Case Study: CLIENT WITH INEFFECTIVE SEXUALITY PATTERNS

Jeffery Stevens is a 55-year-old carpet installer who is hospitalized with a myocardial infarction. He has been moved from the cardiac care unit (CCU) to the medical floor. He has had several episodes of chest pain relieved by medication. He has repeatedly made inappropriate sexual comments and gestures to the nursing staff.

Assessment Mary Jennings, Mr. Stevens's night shift nurse, reported to the night charge nurse that Mr. Stevens stated, "Why don't you crawl up in here with me to keep me warm?" She states Mr. Stevens also stated, "A little heart attack can't keep me down." He stated, "My wife will be too afraid after what happened the other night when I came into the hospital to ever have sex again."

Ms. Jennings notes on the nurse's notes that Mr. Stevens had chest pain at 2200 relieved by Nitroglycerin gr 1/150 × 1 sublingual and that shortness of breath was also noted at this time. He has had no arrhythmias on the telemetry since moving to the floor. His BP was 134/82, P 64, R 22.

Diagnosis The current nursing diagnoses for Mr. Stevens are as follows:

◆ Ineffective Sexuality Patterns related to altered self-concept
◆ Deficient Knowledge related to absence of sexual teaching
◆ Ineffective Sexuality Pattern related to fear of chest pain

Expected Outcomes The expected outcomes specify that Mr. Stevens will:

◆ Identify factors contributing to altered self-concept
◆ Gain knowledge about sexual activity following a myocardial infarction
◆ Experience decreased pain with sexual activity

Planning and Implementation The following nursing interventions are planned and implemented:

◆ Question to identify or clarify reasons for sexual comments and actions.
◆ Consistently refocus inappropriate sexual comments and actions to client's underlying fears and concerns.
◆ Allow expression of concern about sexual functioning or identity.
◆ Acquire information on usual sexual pattern and expectations.
◆ Identify limitations on sexual activity caused by myocardial infarction with cardiac rehabilitation team.
◆ Explain appropriate modifications in sexual practices in response to these limitations, including engaging in sexual activity after rest. Usually early in the morning is best after a period of 4 to 8 weeks (when physician advises).

◆ Instruct client to terminate sexual activity if chest pain or dyspnea occurs.
◆ Teach client to take nitroglycerin as prescribed by the physician before sexual activity if angina occurs during sexual activity.
◆ Advise client to avoid intercourse 1 to 2 hours after a heavy meal or after alcohol consumption.
◆ Instruct client to avoid sexual activity when stressed.

Evaluation By the end of the shift Ms. Jennings was able to determine that Mr. Stevens normally had sexual activity two to three times a week with his wife and that they were engaging in sexual activity when he experienced his myocardial infarction. Mr. Stevens had stated he and his wife had been married for 27 years and he was afraid he would not be able to maintain the previous sexual relationship they had experienced. He also stated the chest pain he was continuing to have made him worry he would never be able to have sexual activity again without pain. Ms. Jennings was also able to give Mr. Stevens information on sexual activity following a myocardial infarction included in his cardiac rehabilitation notebook provided for him to take with him on discharge.

Critical Thinking in the Nursing Process

1. Why was Mr. Stevens making inappropriate sexual comments and gestures?
2. What other information would have been helpful in this situation?
3. Who else should be including in teaching Mr. Stevens about sexual activity during the cardiac rehabilitation process?

Note: The bibliography listings for this and all chapters have been compiled at the back of the book.

Chapter Review

Key Terms by Topics

Use the audio glossary feature of either the CD-ROM or the Companion Website to hear the correct pronunciation of the following key terms.

Sex versus sexuality
sex, sexuality

Pediatric and adolescent considerations
puberty, menstruation, dysmenorrhea, sexual abuse, rape, date rape, circumcision, infibulation, sexually transmitted disease (STD)

Maternal and infant considerations
hermaphroditism, infertility

Adult health considerations
sexual orientation, intercourse, coitus, sexual dysfunction, erectile dysfunction, impotence, orgasmic dysfunction

Geriatric health considerations
dyspareunia, orchiectomy

Key Points

- Sexuality is important to all ages throughout the life span. It is not just gender or the sex act, but a whole dimension of personality.

- Puberty is a key time in the development of sexuality. Children need to be educated about the changes in their bodies and about the reproductive process. Parents should be primary educators in this area, but many times children learn about sexual matters from their peers.

- Different cultures view sexuality and sexual activities differently. It is important to recognize one's own values about sexuality and to respect the client's values when giving client care. The focus should always be on client needs.

- Suspected sexual abuse must always be reported. Victims of abuse should be reminded that they are not to blame for being abused.

- The adult's sexuality evolves through sexual experiences. A person's sexual identity consists of biological sex, gender identity, and sexual orientation.

- Inappropriate comments or actions by a client may signal a concern the client wishes to discuss. However, it is important to address the inappropriate actions immediately and state appropriate expectations clearly.

- Older adults continue to function sexually despite physical changes. They learn to adapt sexual activity to physical limitations.

EXPLORE MediaLink

Additional interactive resources for this chapter can be found on the Companion Website at www.prenhall.com/ramont. Click on Chapter 29 and "Begin" to select the activities for this chapter.

For chapter-related NCLEX-style questions and an audio glossary, access the accompanying CD-ROM in this book.

Animation:
- oogenesis
- spermatogenesis
- physical abuse
- oogenesis and spermatogenesis
- leaving abuse behind
- sexual abuse

For Further Study

For more information about physical assessment, see Chapter 11.
For additional information about cultural values, see Chapter 26.
For further study about client self-concept, see Chapter 28.

Critical Thinking Care Map

Caring for a Client with Altered Sexuality

NCLEX-PN Focus Area: Psychosocial Integrity

Case Study: Nancy Johnson is a 43-year-old who had a mastectomy 4 days ago for cancer of the breast. She states "I'll never be the same" as the LVN makes her morning rounds. She also states her husband has been very attentive assisting her but that he deserves more.

Nursing Diagnosis: Ineffective Sexuality Pattern

COLLECT DATA

Subjective	Objective
_____	_____
_____	_____
_____	_____
_____	_____
_____	_____
_____	_____

Would you report this data? Yes/No

If yes, to: _____

Nursing Care

_____
_____
_____
_____
_____
_____
_____
_____
_____
_____
_____
_____
_____
_____

How would you document this? _____
_____
_____
_____
_____
_____

Data Collected

(use those that apply)

- Client works as an administrative assistant in a large law firm.
- States she will never be the same
- Medicated with Vicodin 2 tablets at 0800 and 1200
- States husband deserves more
- Reach for Recovery visited on the first and second postop days.
- Looks down when speaking
- Holds robe tightly around chest
- Dressing on left breast clean/dry/intact
- Husband noted to be at bedside since returned from surgery and has not left the hospital
- Stayed in bed with face covered all morning
- Jackson–Pratt drain in place × 2
- Refused to ambulate in the hall
- Looked through mail brought to room by volunteer
- Ate 10% of breakfast and lunch

Nursing Interventions

(use those that apply)

- Encourage client to express feelings about the way she feels about sexuality related to loss of the breast.
- Discuss the usual feelings of clients who are postoperative mastectomy and ways to cope.
- Discuss with client importance of Reach for Recovery follow-up.
- Instruct in the importance of communication with husband to work through feelings toward acceptance.
- Discuss available support groups in the community and obtain necessary contacts for follow-up (American Cancer Society).
- Encourage client to discuss sexuality issues with the primary health care provider.

NCLEX-PN Exam Preparation

1. The school nurse has been working with a group of adolescents helping them to identify myths and common misconceptions about sexuality. If the school nurse's teaching has been effective, which of the following statements will the students identify as a myth or common misconception about sexuality?

   a. Masturbation is harmless.
   b. Conceiving is unrelated to orgasm.
   c. Sexual desire decreases little after middle age.
   d. Alcohol is a sexual stimulant.

2. During a bath procedure, a client asks the nurse which sexual position is the correct position during sexual intercourse. The best answer by the nurse would be which of the following answers?

   a. "The position that offers the most pleasure and is acceptable to both partners."
   b. "A position in which both partners are able to see the face of the other partner."
   c. "It is improper for you to ask this question and we need to focus on your bath."
   d. "A variety of positions with frequent change of position is accepted as correct."

3. A parent informs the nurse that his son who is in early adolescence has had an increase in the size of the testes and scrotum, with the skin over the scrotum becoming darker. The nurse recognizes these signs as most likely being related to which of the following causes?

   a. Testicular cancer
   b. Normal growth and development
   c. Excessive masturbation
   d. Late phase of testicular herniation

4. While working with a child, the nurse finds the child has symptoms associated with sexual abuse of a child. The nurse most needs to do which of the following things?

   a. Ask the child if she has been sexually abused.
   b. Confront the parent(s) or caregivers about having sexually abused the child.
   c. Report suspected child sexual abuse to the state agency dealing with child abuse.
   d. Discuss the findings with other health care professionals.

5. Anyone in the United States who does an infibulation on a child under age 18 is considered by the courts to be doing which of the following things?

   a. Practicing procedures acceptable in some cultures
   b. Practicing medicine without a license to do so
   c. Committing a federal criminal offense
   d. Committing a misdemeanor

6. In educating teenagers about sexually transmitted diseases, the nurse will explain that a person is more at risk of cervical cancer if she has which of the following problems or diagnoses?

   a. Human papillomavirus
   b. Trichomoniasis
   c. Herpes-zoster virus
   d. Candidiasis

7. When teaching clients about prevention of unwanted pregnancies, the nurse will point to which of the following methods of contraception as most ineffective?

   a. Diaphram
   b. Coitus interruptus
   c. Birth control pills
   d. Intrauterine devices

8. A parent asks the nurse when gender determination can be made in the developing fetus. The nurse will explain that gender determination can be made by which of the following weeks of gestation?

   a. 3 to 6 weeks
   b. Around 7 weeks
   c. Around 9 weeks
   d. 11 to 14 weeks

9. When working with a female client who has orgasmic dysfunction, the nurse will explore a number of possible causes with the client, but will keep in mind that the majority of cases of orgasmic dysfunction have which of the following underlying causes?

   a. Alcohol or other drugs
   b. Aging
   c. Psychological causes
   d. Anatomic abnormalities

10. The nurse working with an older client who has had heart surgery or has been hospitalized for alterations in heart function will most likely need to teach the client to avoid which of the following things?

    a. Having orgasm with sexual intercourse
    b. Sexual intercourse after large meals or drinking alcohol
    c. Having sexual intercourse more than once a month
    d. Sexual intercourse just before going to sleep

Answers for Review Questions, as well as discussion of Case Study and Critical Thinking Care Map questions, appear in Appendix IV.

Stress and Coping

SHARING experiences

I just wished I had entered nursing sooner. Because of "life getting in the way," it was later in my life that I became an LVN. Nursing had been my lifelong dream. I was not disap- *pointed, because it has been the most rewarding experience. I have met some of the most amazing and inspiring people doing a job I love. It doesn't get much better than that.*

Marilyn Runnells, LVN, North Orange County Regional Occupational Program, Anaheim, CA.

LEARNING outcomes

After completing this chapter, you will be able to:

- Explain three models of stress.
- Discuss physiologic indicators of stress.
- Differentiate four levels of anxiety.
- Identify behaviors related to specific defense mechanisms.
- Discuss types of coping and coping strategies.
- Describe interventions to help clients minimize and manage stress.
- Describe warning signs of job-related stress or burnout for the nurse.

MediaLink

www.prenhall.com/ramont

Use the address above to access the free, interactive Companion Website created for this textbook. Get hints, instant feedback, and textbook references to chapter-related NCLEX-style questions. Link to other interesting sites.

Audio Glossary:
Use the Companion Website, or the CD-ROM disk enclosed with your textbook, to hear the pronunciations of key terms in the chapter.

Stress is a universal phenomenon. All people experience it. It can be described as tension between two opposing forces. Not all stress is harmful. Limited stress can raise energy levels, which may be an asset when faced with certain tasks, such as a test. Excessive stress may cause physical illness and/or psychological distress.

◆ ![diamond] **Concepts of Stress**

Stress is a condition that requires a response. It has many consequences:

◆ *Physiologic*—can threaten a person's physiologic homeostasis
◆ *Emotional*—can produce negative or unconstructive feelings about the self
◆ *Intellectual*—can influence a person's perceptual and problem-solving abilities
◆ *Social*—can alter a person's relationship with others
◆ *Spiritual*—can challenge one's beliefs and values

Figure 30-1 ◆ illustrates the physical consequences of prolonged or excessive stress.

An individual is considered to be mentally healthy if he or she is able to love (form relationships), work, and cope simulta-

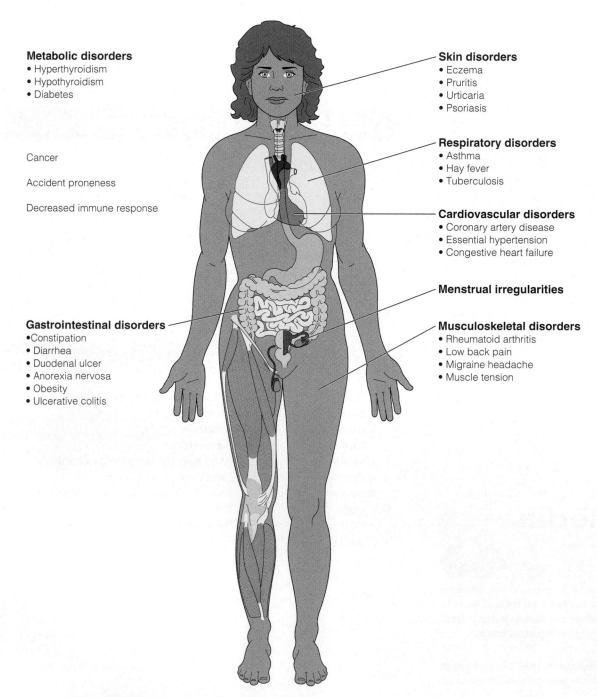

Metabolic disorders
• Hyperthyroidism
• Hypothyroidism
• Diabetes

Cancer

Accident proneness

Decreased immune response

Gastrointestinal disorders
•Constipation
• Diarrhea
• Duodenal ulcer
• Anorexia nervosa
• Obesity
• Ulcerative colitis

Skin disorders
• Eczema
• Pruritis
• Urticaria
• Psoriasis

Respiratory disorders
• Asthma
• Hay fever
• Tuberculosis

Cardiovascular disorders
• Coronary artery disease
• Essential hypertension
• Congestive heart failure

Menstrual irregularities

Musculoskeletal disorders
• Rheumatoid arthritis
• Low back pain
• Migraine headache
• Muscle tension

Figure 30-1. ◆ Many physical disorders can be caused or aggravated by stress.

neously. Coping with stress then becomes an important factor in maintaining mental homeostasis or emotional balance.

SOURCES OF STRESS

Sources of stress can be broadly classified as either internal or external **stressors.** They may also be developmental or situational stressors, or both. Internal stressors originate within a person. Examples are receiving a diagnosis of cancer or experiencing feelings of depression. External stressors originate outside the individual. Examples are moving to another city, experiencing a death in the family, or feeling pressure from peers. Developmental stressors occur at predictable times throughout an individual's life. Within each developmental stage, certain tasks must be achieved to prevent or reduce stress. Examples of these tasks are shown in Table 30-1 ◆. Situational stressors are unpredictable and may occur at any time during life. Situational stress may be positive or negative. Examples of this type of stress include:

TABLE 30-1	SELECTED STRESSORS ASSOCIATED WITH DEVELOPMENTAL STAGES
DEVELOPMENTAL STAGE	**STRESSORS**
Child	Resolving conflict between independence and dependence Beginning school Establishing peer relationships and adjustments Coping with peer competition
Adolescent	Accepting changing physique Developing relationships involving sexual attraction Achieving independence Choosing a career
Young adult	Getting married Leaving home Managing a home Getting started in an occupation Continuing one's education Rearing children
Middle adult	Accepting physical changes of aging Maintaining social status and standard of living Helping teenage children to become independent Adjusting to aging parents
Older adult	Accepting decreasing physical abilities and health Accepting changes in residence Adjusting to retirement and reduced income Adjusting to death of spouse and friends

- ◆ Death of a family member
- ◆ Marriage or divorce
- ◆ Birth of a child
- ◆ New job
- ◆ Illness

MODELS OF STRESS

The three main models for explaining the effects of stress are stimulus based, response based, and transaction based. Nurses use knowledge of these models to help clients practice healthy coping responses and change unhealthy, unproductive responses.

Stimulus-Based Model

In the stimulus-based model, stress is defined as a life event, or a set of circumstances, that arouses physiological and/or psychological reactions that may increase the individual's vulnerability to illness. Holmes and Rahe (1967) assigned a numerical value to 43 life changes or events. The scale of stressful life events is used to document a person's relatively recent experiences, such as divorce, pregnancy, and retirement. In this view, both positive and negative events are considered stressful.

Research has shown that people who have a high level of stress are often more prone to illness. They also have a lowered ability to cope with an illness and subsequent stress. Similar scales have since been developed, but all such scales require caution because the degree of stress an event presents can be highly individual.

Response-Based Model

Stress may also be considered as a response to illness. Hans Selye, a recognized authority in the field of stress, observed, "Whether a man suffers from severe blood loss, an infection or advanced cancer; he loses his appetite, strength, and ambition; usually he also loses weight and even his facial expression betrays his illness. I felt that the syndrome of 'Just being sick,' which is essentially the same no matter what disease we have, could be analyzed and expressed scientifically" (Selye, 1976, p. 12).

Selye realized that changes in the body occurred in the presence of stress, and this became the basis of his identification of the *general adaptation syndrome (GAS)*. He proposed three stages in this syndrome (1976, p. 38): alarm reaction, resistance, and exhaustion. Refer to Figure 30-2 ◆ for an illustration of these stages. Selye's General Adaptation Syndrome depicts a range of physiologic responses to stressors in the body as a whole.

Transaction-Based Model

The transactional view was developed by Richard Lazarus in 1965. It focuses on individual differences in response to stress, rather than to events or reactions. The transactional view attempts to answer the following: Which factors lead some persons, and not others, to respond effectively to stressful

Figure 30-2. ◆ A stress syndrome, termed the general adaptation syndrome (GAS) by Hans Selye, evolves in three stages. Stages 1 and 2 (the alarm reaction and the stage of resistance) are continuously repeated throughout a lifetime cycle. If resistance cannot be sustained, Stage 3 (the stage of exhaustion) occurs, causing altered psychological and physiologic functioning.

events? Why are some persons more sensitive and vulnerable to stressful events? And why are some persons able to adapt over longer periods than others to stressful events?

The Lazarus Transactional Stress theory includes cognitive, affective, and adaptive (coping) responses. This theory states that the person and the environment are inseparable; each affects and is affected by the other. Stress refers to "any event in which environmental demands, internal demands, or both, tax or exceed the adaptive resources of an individual, social system, or tissue system" (Monat & Lazarus, 1991, p. 3). The individual responds to perceived environmental changes by adaptive (coping) responses. See the Coping section later in this chapter.

INDICATORS OF STRESS

Indicators of an individual's stress may be physiological, psychological, or cognitive.

Physiologic Indicators

Responses to stress vary depending on the individual's perception of events. The physiologic signs and symptoms of stress

result from the activation of the sympathetic and neuroendocrine systems of the body. The autonomic nervous system reacts to a percieved threat by releasing large amounts of epinephrine (adrenaline) and cortisone into the body. The person is then ready for "fight or flight." **Fight or flight** can be described as a generalized response to an emergency situation. This includes internal stimulation of the sympathetic nervous system and the adrenal glands. The heart and respiratory rates, blood pressure, and blood flow to the muscles are increased. This response prepares the body to either flee or fight (Thomas, 2001). Box 30-1 ◆ describes the physiological indicators of stress.

Psychologic Indicators

Psychological responses to stress include such reactions as anxiety, fear, anger, and depression.

ANXIETY. A common reaction to stress is anxiety. **Anxiety** can be described as a state of mental uneasiness, apprehension, dread, or foreboding. It can also be a feeling of helplessness related to an unidentified threat to self or significant relationships. Anxiety can be experienced at the conscious, subconscious, or unconscious levels. It differs from fear in four ways:

1. The source of anxiety may not be identifiable; the source of fear is identifiable.
2. Anxiety is related to the future, that is, to an anticipated event. Fear is related to the present.
3. Anxiety is vague, whereas fear is definite.

BOX 30-1
MANIFESTATIONS OF STRESS

- ◆ Pupils dilate to increase visual perception when serious threats to the body arise.
- ◆ Sweat production (diaphoresis) increases to control elevated body heat due to increased metabolism.
- ◆ The heart rate increases, which leads to an increased pulse rate to transport nutrients and by-products of metabolism more efficiently.
- ◆ Skin is pallid because of constriction of peripheral blood vessels, an effect of norepinephrine.
- ◆ The rate and depth of respirations increase because of dilation of the bronchioles, promoting hyperventilation.
- ◆ Urinary output decreases.
- ◆ The mouth may be dry.
- ◆ Peristalsis of the intestines decreases, resulting in possible constipation and flatus.
- ◆ For serious threats, mental alertness improves.
- ◆ Muscle tension increases to prepare for rapid motor activity or defense.
- ◆ Blood sugar increases because of release of glucocorticoids and gluconeogenesis.

4. Anxiety is the result of psychological or emotional conflict; fear is the result of a physical or psychological reality.

All people experience anxiety to some degree most of the time. Mild or moderate anxiety helps people accomplish developmental tasks and meet goals. In this sense, anxiety is an effective coping strategy. For example, mild anxiety motivates students to study. Excessive anxiety, however, often has destructive effects. The overly anxious student may be unable to sleep or to eat, and may do poorly on a test as a result.

Anxiety may be manifested on four levels:

1. Mild anxiety produces a slight arousal state that enhances perception, learning, and productive abilities. Most healthy people experience mild anxiety, perhaps as a feeling of mild restlessness that prompts a person to seek information and ask questions.
2. Moderate anxiety increases the arousal state to a point where the person expresses feelings of tension, nervousness, or concern. Perceptual abilities are narrowed. Attention is focused on a particular aspect of a situation.
3. Severe anxiety consumes most of the person's energies and requires intervention. The person, unable to focus on what is really happening, focuses on only one specific detail of the situation causing the anxiety.

4. Panic is an overpowering, frightening level of anxiety that causes the person to lose control. It is experienced less frequently than other levels of anxiety. A panicked person may distort events as a result of altered perception.

Table 30-2 ◆ lists indicators of different levels of anxiety.

FEAR. **Fear** is an emotion or feeling of apprehension aroused by impending danger, pain, or other perceived threat. People may fear something that has already occurred, a current threat, or something they believe will happen. The fear may or may not be based in reality. For example, beginning nursing students may fear their first experience in a client care setting. They may be worried that clients will not want to be cared for by students or that they might inadvertently harm the clients. The nursing students' feelings of fear are real and will probably elicit a stress response. However, the instructor arranges the students' first client assignment so that the students' feared outcomes are unlikely to occur.

ANGER. **Anger** is an emotional state that includes feelings of animosity or strong displeasure. Many people feel guilty when they feel anger because they have been taught that to feel angry is wrong. When anger is expressed in a nonalienating

TABLE 30-2	INDICATORS OF LEVELS OF ANXIETY			
LEVEL OF ANXIETY				
CATEGORY	**MILD**	**MODERATE**	**SEVERE**	**PANIC**
Verbalization changes	Increased questioning	Voice tremors and pitch changes	Communication difficult to understand	Communication may not be understandable
Motor activity changes	Mild restlessness Sleeplessness	Tremors, facial twitches, and shakiness Increased muscle tension	Increased motor activity, inability to relax Fearful facial expression	Increased motor activity, agitation Unpredictable responses Trembling, poor motor coordination
Perception and attention changes	Feelings of increased arousal and alertness Uses learning to adapt	Narrowed focus of attention Able to focus but selectively inattentive Learning slightly impaired	Inability to focus or concentrate Easily distracted Learning severely impaired	Perception distorted or exaggerated Unable to learn or function
Respiratory and circulatory changes	None	Slightly increased respiratory and heart rates	Tachycardia, hyperventilation	Dyspnea, palpitations, choking, chest pain or pressure
Other changes	None	Mild gastric symptoms, e.g., "butterflies in the stomach"	Headache, dizziness, nausea	Feeling of impending doom Paresthesia, sweating

Source: Data from Carpenito, L. J. (2002). Nursing diagnosis: Application to clinical practice (9th ed.). Philadelphia: Lippincott Williams & Wilkins; and Fontaine (2003) Essentials of mental health nursing (5th ed.) Upper Saddle River, NJ. Prentice Hall.

verbal manner, it is considered a positive emotion. Anger can be a sign of emotional maturity when growth and positive interactions result from it.

A verbal expression of anger is a signal of internal psychological discomfort and a call for assistance to deal with perceived stress. Anger, hostility, violence, and aggression differ:

- *Hostility* is usually marked by antagonism and harmful or destructive behavior.
- *Aggression* is an unprovoked attack or a hostile, injurious, or destructive action or outlook.
- *Violence* is the exertion of physical force to injure or abuse. Verbally expressed anger is not the same as hostility, aggression, or violence. However, if anger persists unabated, it can lead to destructiveness and violence.

When an angry person tells another person about the anger and carefully identifies the source, this is constructive. Clear communication gets the anger out into the open so it can be dealt with appropriately. The angry person "gets it off the chest" and an emotional buildup is prevented.

DEPRESSION. Depression is a common reaction to overwhelming or negative events. The signs and symptoms of depression vary with the client. Emotional symptoms can include feelings of tiredness, sadness, emptiness, or numbness. Behavioral signs of depression include irritability, inability to concentrate, difficulty making decisions, loss of sexual desire, crying, sleep disturbance, and social withdrawal. Physical signs of depression may include loss of appetite, weight loss, constipation, headache, and dizziness. Most people experience short periods of depression in response to overwhelming stressful events, such as the death of a loved one or loss of a job. When depression is prolonged, it is a cause for concern and may require treatment.

◆ Coping

Coping means dealing with problems and situations successfully. A **coping strategy** (coping mechanism) is an inborn or learned way of responding to a changing environment, specific problem, or situation. Two types of coping strategies are problem-focused and emotion-focused coping. *Problem-focused coping* involves taking action to improve a situation. *Emotion-focused coping* involves using thoughts and actions to relieve emotional distress. Emotion-focused coping does not improve the situation but may help alleviate anxiety.

Coping can also be adaptive or maladaptive:

- *Adaptive coping* helps the person to deal effectively with stressful events and minimizes distress associated with them.
- *Maladaptive coping* can result in unnecessary distress for the person. Effective coping results in adaptation; ineffective coping results in maladaptation. When clients exhibit inappropriate behavior, nurses should remember that clients are attempting to cope through such behavior.

MediaLink ◆ Adequacy and Security Needs

BOX 30-2 FACTORS INFLUENCING THE EFFECTIVENESS OF COPING

- The number, duration, and intensity of the stressors
- Past experiences of the individual
- Support systems available to the individual
- Personal qualities of the person

How well a person copes is influenced by a number of factors, which are listed in Box 30-2 ◆. When a person is under stress beyond the ability to cope, he or she will become exhausted and be at risk for developing health problems. Family members who undertake the care of a person in the home for a long period develop long-term stress called *caregiver burden.* Responses such as chronic fatigue, sleeping difficulties, and high blood pressure are common in caregivers. When coping strategies or defense mechanisms become ineffective, the individual may experience interpersonal problems, work difficulties, and inability to meet basic human needs. Sometimes, prolonged stress can result in mental illness. Examples of effects of stress on basic human needs are shown in Table 30-3 ◆.

DEFENSE MECHANISMS

Adaptive mechanisms may be conscious or unconscious. Unconscious ego **defense mechanisms** are psychologic adaptive mechanisms. Sigmund Freud (1946) described them as mental mechanisms that develop as the personality attempts to defend itself, establish compromises among con-

TABLE 30-3	EXAMPLES OF THE EFFECTS OF STRESS ON BASIC HUMAN NEEDS	
NEEDS	**EXAMPLE**
Physiologic	Altered elimination pattern Change in appetite Altered sleep pattern
Safety and security	Expresses nervousness and feelings of being threatened Focuses on stressors and inattention to safety measures
Love and belonging	Isolated and withdrawn Becomes overly dependent Blames others for own problems
Self-esteem	Fails to socialize with others Becomes a workaholic Draws attention to self
Self-actualization	Preoccupied with own problems Shows lack of control Unable to accept reality

flicting impulses, and allay inner tensions. Defense mechanisms are the unconscious mind working to protect the person from anxiety. They can be considered precursors to conscious cognitive coping mechanisms that will ultimately solve the problem. Like some verbal and motor responses, defense mechanisms release tension. Table 30-4 ◆ describes these mechanisms and lists examples of their adaptive and maladaptive use.

NURSING CARE

 ## ASSESSING

When assessing a client's stress and coping patterns, the nurse examines the client for indicators of stress (e.g., nail biting, nervousness, weight changes) or stress-related health problems (e.g., hypertension, dyspnea). When obtaining the nursing history of any client, the nurse asks about stressful incidents in the client's life. The nurse also discusses signs and symptoms of stress and coping strategies used in the past. During the physical examination the nurse observes for verbal, motor, cognitive, or other physical manifestations of stress.

The nurse should be aware of expected developmental transitions (see Table 30-1 ◆). This knowledge helps the nurse identify additional stressors that may be present and the client's response to them. Questions about the client's stress and coping patterns are shown in Box 30-3 ◆.

 ## DIAGNOSING, PLANNING, and IMPLEMENTING

The North American Nursing Diagnosis Association (NANDA) includes several diagnostic labels related to stress, adaptation, and coping. Examples of these are Anxiety, Ineffective Coping, and Fear.

Examples of desired outcomes would be:

◆ Describes causes of anxiety as appropriate
◆ Identifies personal strengths
◆ Describes usual coping patterns

Clients with varying levels of anxiety are found in the acute hospital setting. Acute and chronic physical illness are stress producing. Illness, coupled with necessary adjustments to an unfamiliar environment, can manifest itself in behaviors such as anger, agitation, fear, withdrawal, or inappropriate behavior (see Box 30-5). The nurse can help the client adjust in several ways:

◆ Provide compassionate, consistent care.
◆ Do not take the client's reactions personally.
◆ Keep the client informed.

BOX 30-3 ASSESSING CLIENTS: STRESS AND COPING PATTERNS

◆ On a scale of 1 to 10, how would you rate the stress you are experiencing in the following areas?
  Home
  Work or school
  Finance
  Recent illness or loss of loved one
  Your health
  Family responsibilities
  Ethnic or cultural group
  Religion
  Relationships with friends
  Relationship with parents or children
  Relationship with partner
  Recent hospitalization
  Other (specify)
◆ How long have you been dealing with these stressor(s)?
◆ How do you usually handle stressful situations?
  Cry
  Get angry
  Become verbally abusive
  Talk to someone (Who?)
  Withdraw from the situation
  Structure and control others or situation
  Go for a walk or physical exercise
  Try to arrive at a solution
  Pray for wisdom and courage
  Laugh, joke, or use some other expression of humor
  Meditate or use some other relaxation technique such as yoga or guided imagery
◆ How well does your usual coping strategy work?

Encouraging Health-Promotion Strategies

Health care professionals at all levels should be role models for health promotion strategies. Physical exercise, optimal nutrition, adequate rest and sleep, and time management are all ways to promote health and reduce stress.

Exercise. Regular exercise promotes both physical and emotional health. Physiologic benefits include improved muscle tone, increased cardiopulmonary function, and weight control. Psychological benefits include relief of tension, a feeling of well-being, and relaxation. In general, health guidelines recommend exercise at least three times a week for 30 to 45 minutes.

Nutrition. Optimal nutrition is essential for health and in increasing the body's resistance to stress. To minimize the effects of a stress response (e.g., irritability, hyperactivity, anxiety), people need to avoid excessive caffeine, salt, sugar, and fat and deficiencies in vitamins and minerals. Guidelines for a well-balanced, healthy diet are detailed in Chapter 17. ⌘

TABLE 30-4 DEFENSE MECHANISMS

DEFENSE MECHANISM	EXAMPLE(S)	USE/PURPOSE
Compensation Covering up weaknesses by emphasizing a more desirable trait or by overachievement in a more comfortable area.	A high school student too small to play football becomes the star long-distance runner for the track team.	Allows a person to overcome weakness and achieve success.
Denial An attempt to screen or ignore unacceptable realities by refusing to acknowledge them.	A woman, though told her father has metastatic cancer, continues to plan a family reunion 18 months in advance.	Temporarily isolates a person from the full impact of a traumatic situation. See also Box 29-7. ↪
Displacement The transferring or discharging of emotional reactions from one object or person to another object or person.	A husband and wife are fighting, and the husband becomes so angry he hits a door instead of his wife. A student gets a C on a paper she worked hard on and goes home and yells at her family.	Allows for feelings to be expressed through or to less dangerous objects or people.
Identification An attempt to manage anxiety by imitating the behavior of someone feared or respected.	A student nurse imitating the nurturing behavior she observes one of her instructors using with clients.	Helps a person avoid self-devaluation.
Intellectualization A mechanism by which an emotional response that normally would accompany an uncomfortable or painful incident is evaded by the use of rational explanations that remove from the incident any personal significance and feelings.	The pain over a parent's sudden death is reduced by saying, "He wouldn't have wanted to live disabled."	Protects a person from pain and traumatic events.
Introjection A form of identification that allows for the acceptance of others' norms and values into oneself, even when contrary to one's previous assumptions.	A 7-year-old tells his little sister, "Don't talk to strangers." He has introjected this value from the instructions of parents and teachers.	Helps a person avoid social retaliation and punishment; particularly important for the child's development of superego.
Minimization Not acknowledging the significance of one's behavior.	A person says, "Don't believe everything my wife tells you. I wasn't so drunk I couldn't drive."	Allows a person to decrease responsibility for own behavior.
Projection A process in which blame is attached to others or the environment for unacceptable desires, thoughts, shortcomings, and mistakes.	A mother is told her child must repeat a grade in school, and she blames this on the teacher's poor instruction. A husband forgets to pay a bill and blames his wife for not giving it to him earlier.	Allows a person to deny the existence of shortcomings and mistakes; protects self-image.
Rationalization Justification of certain behaviors by faulty logic and ascription of motives that are socially acceptable but did not in fact inspire the behavior.	A mother spanks her toddler too hard and says it was all right because he couldn't feel it through the diapers anyway.	Helps a person cope with the inability to meet goals or certain standards.
Reaction formation A mechanism that causes people to act exactly opposite to the way they feel.	An executive resents his bosses for calling in a consulting firm to make recommendations for change in his department, but verbalizes complete support of the idea and is exceedingly polite and cooperative.	Aids in reinforcing repression by allowing feelings to be acted out in a more acceptable way.

(continues)

DEFENSE MECHANISM	EXAMPLE(S)	USE/PURPOSE
Regression Resorting to an earlier, more comfortable level of functioning that is characteristically less demanding and responsible.	An adult throws a temper tantrum when he does not get his own way. A critically ill client allows the nurse to bathe and feed him.	Allows a person to return to a point in development when nurturing and dependency were needed and accepted with comfort.
Repression An unconscious mechanism by which threatening thoughts, feelings, and desires are kept from becoming conscious; the repressed material is denied entry into consciousness.	A teenager, seeing his best friend killed in a car accident, becomes amnesic about the circumstances surrounding the accident.	Protects a person from a traumatic experience until he or she has the resources to cope.
Sublimation Displacement of energy associated with more primitive sexual or aggressive drives into socially acceptable activities.	A person with excessive, primitive sexual drives invests psychic energy into a well-defined religious value system.	Protects a person from behaving in irrational, impulsive ways.
Substitution The replacement of a highly valued, unacceptable, or unavailable object by a less valuable, acceptable, or available object.	A woman wants to marry a man exactly like her dead father and settles for someone who looks a little bit like him.	Helps a person achieve goals and minimizes frustration and disappointment.
Undoing An action or words designed to cancel some disapproved thoughts, impulses, or acts in which the person relieves guilt by making reparation.	A father spanks his child and the next evening brings home a present for him. A teacher writes an exam that is far too easy, then constructs a grading curve that makes it difficult to earn a high grade.	Allows a person to appease guilty feelings and atone for mistakes.

Source: Fontaine, K. L. (2003). Essentials of mental health nursing (5th ed.). Upper Saddle River, NJ: Prentice Hall. pp. 11–12. Reprinted with permission.

Rest and Sleep. Rest and sleep restore the body's energy levels and are an essential aspect of stress management. To ensure adequate rest and sleep, clients may need comfort measures such as pain management. Nurses may need to teach techniques that promote peace of mind and relaxation.

Several relaxation techniques can be used to quiet the mind, release tension, and counteract the fight-or-flight responses of GAS discussed earlier in this chapter. Nurses can teach these techniques to clients and encourage their use during and after hospitalization. Relaxation tapes can be purchased if desired. Some clients make their own recordings. Specific relaxation techniques that may be used are summarized in Box 30-4 ◆. (Rest and sleep are discussed further in Chapter 20. ⃝)

Time Management. People who manage their time effectively usually experience less stress because they feel more in control of their circumstances. Feeling overwhelmed may indicate the need to prioritize tasks and make modifications in role demands. Responding appropriately to the demands of others is also an important aspect of effective time management. Since all requests made by others cannot always be met, individuals must decide which requests they can honor without undue stress, which ones can be negotiated, and which ones need to be declined. Another way to manage time effectively is to schedule daily or weekly times to do specific tasks. When people feel overwhelmed, they need to reexamine the "should, ought, and must" approach to their actions and develop more realistic self-expectations.

BOX 30-4 COMPLEMENTARY THERAPY: RELAXATION TECHNIQUES

- Breathing exercises
- Massage
- Progressive relaxation
- Imagery
- Biofeedback
- Yoga
- Meditation
- Therapeutic touch
- Music therapy
- Humor and laughter

See Chapter 20 for details about these techniques.

Minimizing Anxiety

Nurses have always carried out measures to minimize clients' anxiety and stress. For example, nurses encourage clients to take deep breaths before an injection; explain procedures before they are implemented, including sensations likely to be experienced during the procedure; administer a back or neck rub to help the client relax; and offer support to clients and families during times of illness.

Mediating Anger

Often, nurses find clients' anger difficult to handle. Caring for the client who is angry is difficult for two reasons:

1. Clients rarely state, "I feel angry or frustrated," and rarely indicate the reason for their anger. Instead, they may refuse treatment, become verbally abusive or demanding, threaten violence, or become overly critical. Their complaints rarely reflect the cause of their anger.
2. Anger from clients can elicit fear and anger in the nurse, who may respond in a manner that intensifies the client's anger, even to the point of violence. The majority of nurses respond in a way that reduces their own stress rather than the client's stress. Box 30-5 ◆ provides strategies for dealing with client's anger (Fontaine, 2003).

Crisis Intervention

A **crisis** is an acute, time-limited state of emotional inbalance resulting from sources of stress. It can be defined as a turning point in a person's life—a point at which usual resources and coping skills are no longer effective. A person in crisis is temporarily unable to cope with or adapt to the stressor by using previous methods of problem solving. People in crisis generally see a stressor as overwhelming. They often do not have adequate situational support, and do not have adequate coping mechanisms. Common characteristics of crises are shown in Box 30-6 ◆.

Because a state of emotional imbalance is so uncomfortable, a crisis is self-limiting. However, a person experiencing a crisis alone has more difficulty handling the situation than a person working through a crisis with help.

Nurses in acute care or short-term care settings may not see the long-term effects of their crisis interventions. Typically, nurses in these settings assess the crisis and begin implementing a crisis intervention plan.

◆ EVALUATING

The desired outcomes developed during the planning stage will be evaluated by collecting data about the clients current status. In order to determine if the outcome has been achieved, the nurse will ask questions such as:

◆ How does the client perceive the problem?
◆ Is there an underlying problem that has not been identified?
◆ How does the client perceive the effectiveness of the new coping strategies?
◆ Have family members and significant others provided effective support?

Although stress is part of daily life, it is also highly individual. One person may be stressed by a situation that would not concern another person. Some methods for reducing stress will be effective for one person; other methods will be appropriate for a different person. Nurses need to be sensitive to clients' needs and reactions, and choose methods of intervention that will be most effective for each individual. Possible interventions for such clients include encouraging health promotion, minimizing anxiety, mediating anger, teaching relaxation techniques, and intervening in crisis situations.

BOX 30-5
NURSING CARE CHECKLIST

STRATEGIES FOR DEALING WITH ANGER

Fontaine (2003) recommends the following strategies for dealing with clients' anger:

☑ Know and understand your own response to the feelings and expressions of anger.

☑ Accept the client's right to be angry; feelings are real and cannot be discounted or ignored.

☑ Ask the client in what way you may have contributed to the anger.

☑ Help the client "own" the anger—do not assume responsibility for her or his feelings.

BOX 30-6
COMMON CHARACTERISTICS OF CRISES

◆ All crises are experienced as sudden. The person is usually not aware of a warning signal, even if others could "see it coming." The individual or family may feel that they have little or no preparation for the event or trauma.

◆ The crisis is often experienced as ultimately life threatening, whether this perception is realistic or not.

◆ Communication with significant others is often decreased or cut off.

◆ There may be perceived or real displacement from familiar surroundings or loved ones.

◆ All crises have an aspect of loss, whether actual or perceived. The losses can include an object, a person, a hope, a dream, or any significant factor for that individual.

DISCHARGE CONSIDERATIONS

Clients who are experiencing stress may require ongoing nursing support or referral to community agencies after discharge. The determination of how much and what type of planning and home care follow-up is based in great part on the nurse's knowledge of how the client and family have coped with previous stressors and the nature of the present stressor. Box 30-7 ◆ describes data to be gathered for discharge to home care or follow-up.

Nursing Process Case Study: CLIENT WITH STRESS

Ms. Levitt is a 37-year-old divorced mother of three, ages 8, 11, and 14. In addition to her full-time job, she transports her children to numerous extracurricular activities, is active in her synagogue, and is attending school part time in order to obtain a better-paying job. Ms. Levitt's ex-husband left the state years ago and does not assist her financially with the care of the children. Ms. Levitt is brought to the employee clinic by a coworker for evaluation to rule out a heart attack.

Assessment

◆ VS: T 98.6°F (37°C), P 102, R 30, BP 134/78
◆ Pale, diaphoretic
◆ Complains of chest pain rated as 5/10; holding chest and rubbing arm
◆ Weight 189 (admits to a 20-lb. weight gain over last year)
◆ Began smoking again 6 months ago after 7 years of non-smoking
◆ Complains of frequent feelings of nausea, her heart "pounding," headaches, and unusual fatigue of 3 weeks duration.
◆ ECG normal
◆ Client states "I thought I was having a heart attack, but I am too young."

Evaluation by nurse practitioner does not reveal a CVS disorder. It is determined that Mrs. Levitt is experiencing a panic attack.

Diagnosis The following nursing diagnoses are identified for Ms. Levitt:

◆ Anxiety related to situational crisis
◆ Ineffective Coping related personal vulnerability
◆ Risk for Powerlessness related to ineffective coping skills
◆ Compromised Family Coping related to lack of available support for client

Expected Outcomes The expected outcomes of the plan of care specify that Ms. Levitt will:

◆ Have vital signs that reflect baseline or decreased sympathetic stimulation
◆ Verbalize ability to cope and ask for help when needed

BOX 30-7 ASSESSING FOR DISCHARGE: STRESS AND COPING

Client

◆ **Knowledge:** Client's understanding of the nature of the stressors
◆ **Current coping strategies:** Effectiveness of current coping strategies and willingness to learn new stress management techniques
◆ **Self-care abilities:** Physical, emotional, social, and financial ability to minimize associated stressors
◆ **Role expectations:** Client's perception of the need to return to prior roles and possible stressors associated with these roles

Family

◆ **Knowledge:** Family members' and significant others' understanding of the nature of the client's stressors and their own relationship with client stressors
◆ **Family coping strategies:** Effectiveness of family members' and significant others' coping strategies and willingness to learn new stress management techniques
◆ **Role expectations:** Family members' and significant others' perception of the need for the client to return to family and work roles
◆ **Support people's availability and skills:** Family and significant others' sensitivity to the client's emotional and physical needs and ability to provide a supportive environment

Community

◆ **Resources:** Availability of and familiarity with possible sources of assistance for stress management such as massage therapists, religious or spiritual centers, physical care providers, support groups, and so on.
◆ Let clients talk about their anger.
◆ After the interaction is completed, take time to process your feelings and your responses to the client with your colleagues.

◆ Identify factors that are uncontrollable
◆ Verbalize internal resources to help deal with family situation

Planning and Implementation The following interventions are planned and implemented:

◆ Assess client's level of anxiety and physical reaction to anxiety (e.g., tachycardia, tachypnea, nonverbal expression of anxiety).
◆ Explore coping skills previously used by the client to relieve anxiety; reinforce these skills and explore other outlets.
◆ Encourage use of appropriate community resources.

◆ Provide client and family members with information to help distinguish between a panic attack and serious physical illness.

◆ Teach client and family to problem solve.

◆ Teach relaxation techniques.

◆ Encourage moderate aerobic exercise.

◆ Observe for causes of ineffective coping such as poor self-concept, lack of problem-solving skills, lack of support, or changes in life situation.

◆ Teach stress reduction, relaxation, and imagery.

◆ Teach cognitive activities, such as self-talk.

◆ Help client practice assertive communication technique.

◆ Refer to support group, pastoral care, or social services.

◆ Observe for causative and contributing factors.

◆ Note other stressors (e.g., financial, job-related).

Evaluation Ms. Levitt returns to the clinic in 1 week. Vital signs are within normal limits. She reports that she had one additional episode during the last week. She has been practicing stress-relieving relaxation and worked out at the company gym twice during the week.

Critical Thinking in the Nursing Process

1. Speculate about the stressors that Ms. Levitt is experiencing.

2. From the data provided, how do you think Ms. Levitt is responding to the stressors you identified?

3. Explore anger as a possible cause of Ms. Levitt's symptoms.

4. What cues would alert you that Ms. Levitt is adapting to the stressors in her life in a positive and healthy manner?

 Stress Management for Nurses

Nurses, like clients, are susceptible to experiencing anxiety and stress. Nursing practice involves many stressors related to both clients and the work environment, for example, understaffing and increasing client care assignments and adjusting to various work shifts. Although most nurses cope effectively with the physical and emotional demands of nursing, in some situations nurses become overwhelmed and develop burnout, a complex syndrome of behaviors that can be likened to the exhaustion stage of the general adaptation syndrome. The nurse with burnout has little physical and emotional energy, has a negative attitude and self-concept, and experiences feelings of helplessness and hopelessness.

Nurses can prevent burnout by using the stress-management techniques discussed earlier. Nurses must first recognize their stress. They must recognize feelings of being overwhelmed; fatigue; angry outbursts; physical illness; and increases in coffee drinking, smoking, or other substance abuse as responses to overwhelming stress. Nurses then need to identify which situations cause the strongest responses so that steps may be taken to reduce these stressors. Suggestions for reducing stress that can lead to burnout include:

◆ Plan a daily relaxation program with meaningful quiet times to reduce tension (e.g., read a novel, listen to music, soak in a hot tub, or meditate).

◆ Establish a regular exercise program to direct energy outward (e.g., jog, play badminton, or join an aerobics dance class).

◆ Develop assertiveness techniques to overcome feelings of powerlessness in relationships with others. Learn to say no.

◆ Learn to accept failures—your own and others'—and make it a constructive learning experience. Recognize that most people do the best they can. Learn to ask for help, to show your feelings with colleagues, and to support your colleagues in times of need.

◆ Accept what cannot be changed. There are certain limitations in every situation. Get involved in constructive change efforts if organizational policies and procedures cause stress.

◆ Develop support groups to deal with feelings and anxieties generated in the work setting.

Note: Bibliography listings for this and all chapters have been compiled at the back of the book.

Chapter Review

Key Terms by Topics

Use the audio glossary feature of either the CD-ROM or the Companion Website to hear the correct pronunciation of the following key terms.

Introduction
stress

Concepts of stress
stressor, fight or flight, anxiety, fear, anger, depression

Coping
coping, coping strategy, defense mechanism

Nursing care
crisis

Key Points

* Stress is a state of physiological and psychological tension that affects the whole person—physically, emotionally, intellectually, socially, and spiritually.

* Physiologic responses to stress are described by the General Adaptation Syndrome (GAS).

* There are physiologic, psychological, and cognitive indicators of stress.

* Common psychological indicators are anxiety, fear, anger, and depression. Anxiety, the most common response, has four levels: mild, moderate, severe, and panic. Unconscious ego defense mechanisms such as denial, rationalization, compensation, and sublimation protect individuals from anxiety.

* Prolonged stress and ineffective coping interfere with the meeting of basic needs and can affect physical and mental health.

* Nursing interventions for clients who are stressed are aimed at encouraging health-promotion strategies (exercise, balanced diet, adequate rest, and time management), minimizing anxiety, mediating anger, teaching abut specific relaxation techniques, and implementing crisis interventions as needed.

* Because nursing practice involves many stressors related to both clients and the work environment, nurses are susceptible to anxiety and in some cases burnout. Like clients, they need to implement stress-reduction measures.

EXPLORE MediaLink

Additional interactive resources for this chapter can be found on the Companion Website at www.prenhall.com/ramont. Click on Chapter 30 and "Begin" to select the activities for this chapter.

For chapter-related NCLEX-style questions and an audio glossary, access the accompanying CD-ROM in this book.

Animation:
* Diazepam
* Fluoxetine

∞ For Further Study

For additional information about nutrition and a healthy diet, see Chapter 17.

For more information about nursing interventions to promote rest and sleep, see Chapter 20.

For ways to handle sexually inappropriate responses, see Box 29-7.

Critical Thinking Care Map

Caring for a Client with Myocardial Infarction

NCLEX-PN Focus Area: Psychosocial Integrity Coping and Adaptation

Case Study: Darryl Johnson, a 47-year-old accountant, was admitted to the emergency department with a heart attack. He says, "I'm scared about this. My dad died of a heart attack when he was 48 years old." He appears restless, questions everything that is going on, and is hyperventilating.

Nursing Diagnosis: Anxiety

COLLECT DATA

Subjective	Objective
_____	_____
_____	_____
_____	_____
_____	_____
_____	_____
_____	_____
_____	_____

Would you report this data? Yes/No

If yes, to: _____

Nursing Care

_____
_____
_____
_____
_____
_____
_____
_____
_____
_____
_____
_____
_____

How would you document this? _____
_____
_____
_____
_____

Data Collected
(use those that apply)

- Alert and oriented to time, place, and person
- VS: T 99.6°F (37.5°C), P 88, R 28, BP 140/82
- Peripheral pulse strong and equal
- Cap refill less than 3 seconds
- Lungs clear
- Pale; skin cool and diaphoretic
- Nail bed pink
- ECG normal sinus rythmn
- Severe chest pain

Nursing Interventions
(use those that apply)

- Assess client's level of anxiety and physical reaction to anxiety.
- Avoid confrontation.
- Assess for subtle signs of denial.
- Validate observations by asking client, "Are you feeling anxious now?"
- Assess source of fear with client.
- Allow and reinforce client's personal reaction to or expression of pain, discomfort, or threat to well-being.
- Explain all activities, procedures, and issues that involve the client; use nonmedical terms and calm, slow speech. Do this is advance of procedures when possible, and validate client's understanding.
- Encourage realistic and achievable goal setting.
- Explore coping skills previously used by the client to relieve anxiety; reinforce these skills and explore other outlets.
- Provide back rub to decrease anxiety.

NCLEX-PN Exam Preparation

1. Mentally healthy individuals:
   a. Can cope with all crises
   b. Demonstrate difficulty in solving complex problems
   c. Frequently experience work-related difficulty
   d. Work, form relationships, and cope simultaneously

2. The nurse is caring for a client who had a myocardial infarction 2 days ago. The client has been on bed rest, being allowed up in the chair for meals. When you enter the room the client is sitting on the floor doing sit-ups. This is an example of the defense mechanism known as:
   a. Repression
   b. Sublimation
   c. Identification
   d. Denial

3. A client who was driving when involved in a motor vehicle accident has just learned that the passenger in the vehicle has died. The police are attempting to obtain information from the survivor, but the client is unable to recall even being in the car. The nurse on duty realizes that this is an example of:
   a. Dissociation
   b. Denial
   c. Regression
   d. Transference

4. Anxiety can manifest itself on four levels. Of the following, which one produces a slight arousal state that enhances perception, learning, and productive abilities?
   a. Mild
   b. Moderate
   c. Severe
   d. Panic

5. A client on your medical unit is experiencing dyspnea. You also sense that the client is anxious. As the nurse caring for this client, you:
   a. Ignore the anxiety, since it will probably go away when the client is breathing better.
   b. Notify the doctor immediately.
   c. Reassure the client that this is only temporary.
   d. Remain with the client and be supportive.

6. In order for nurses to prevent burnout, they must first:
   a. Identify which situations cause the strongest responses.
   b. Recognize their stress.
   c. Decrease use of substances such as coffee, alcohol, and tobacco.
   d. Take steps to reduce stress.

7. Physiologic responses to stress are described by:
   a. Coping responses
   b. Local adaptation syndrome
   c. General adaptation syndrome
   d. Stimulus-based stress model

8. Stress manifests itself differently at different developmental ages. Of the following stages, which one is associated with accepting changing physique and developing relationships involving sexual attraction?
   a. Adolescent
   b. Young adult
   c. Middle adult
   d. Older adult

9. The autonomic nervous system reacts to a perceived threat with release of adrenaline. This is known as:
   a. A crisis
   b. Stress
   c. Fight or flight
   d. Anxiety

10. A male college student who is overweight and unable to participate in competitive sports becomes the life of the party and drives a new sporty car. He is displaying:
    a. Compensation
    b. Reaction formation
    c. Transference
    d. Identification

Chapter 31

Loss, Grieving, and Death

SHARING experiences

Seeing someone sick and dying can make a big impact on your life, especially being a nurse. You know you are the last one they may see and you are there to make sure they are as comfortable as possible. Touching someone's life is why I want to be a nurse. Nursing is more than an occupation. It is an opportunity to make a difference in the world and in someone's life.

Lana Knapp, LPN student, Idaho State University, Pocatello, ID.

LEARNING outcomes

After completing this chapter, you will be able to:
- Discuss the relationship between loss and grief.
- Discuss and identify stages and clinical symptoms of grieving, and factors that affect a grief response.
- Identify measures that facilitate the grieving process.
- List clinical signs of impending and actual death.
- Describe essential aspects of the Patient Self-Determination Act.
- Identify the nurse's legal responsibilities regarding client death and issues such as advance directives, certification of death, labeling of the deceased, autopsy, organ donation, inquest, euthanasia, and do-not-resuscitate (DNR) orders.
- Describe nursing measures for care of the body after death.
- Describe the role of the nurse in working with families or caregivers of dying clients.

MediaLink

www.prenhall.com/ramont

Use the address above to access the free, interactive Companion Website created for this textbook. Get hints, instant feedback, and textbook references to chapter-related NCLEX-style questions. Link to other interesting sites.

Audio Glossary:
Use the Companion Website, or the CD-ROM disk enclosed with your textbook, to hear the pronunciation of key terms in the chapter.

Loss, grieving, and death are experienced by everyone at some time during life. People may suffer the loss of valued relationships through life changes, such as moving from one city to another, separation, divorce, or the death of a parent, spouse, or friend. People may grieve changing life roles as they watch grown children leave home or they retire from their lifelong work. The loss of valued material objects through theft or natural disaster can evoke feelings of grief and loss. When people's lives are affected by civil or national strife, they may grieve the loss of valued ideals such as safety, freedom, or democracy.

Nurses may interact with dying clients and their families or caregivers in a variety of settings, from a fetal demise to the adolescent victim of an accident, to the elderly client who finally succumbs to a chronic illness. Nurses must recognize the various influences on the dying process—legal, ethical, religious and spiritual, biologic, personal—and be prepared to provide sensitive, skilled, and supportive care to all those affected.

 Loss and Grief

Loss is an actual or potential situation in which something that is valued is changed, no longer available, or gone. People can experience the loss of body image, a significant other, a sense of well-being, a job, personal possessions, beliefs, or a sense of self. Illness and hospitalization often produce losses.

 Grief, Bereavement, and Mourning

Grief is the total response to the emotional experience related to loss. Grief is manifested in thoughts, feelings, and behaviors associated with overwhelming distress or sorrow. **Bereavement** is the subjective response experienced by the surviving loved ones after the death of a person with whom they have shared a significant relationship. **Mourning** is the behavioral process through which grief is eventually resolved or altered. It is often influenced by culture, spiritual beliefs, and customs. Grief and mourning are experienced not only by the person who faces the death of a loved one but also by the person who suffers other kinds of loses. Grieving is essential for good mental and physical health. It permits the individual to cope with the loss gradually and to accept it as part of reality. Grief is a social process; it is best shared and carried out with the assistance of others.

Working through one's grief is important, because bereavement has been shown to have potentially devastating effects on health. Among the symptoms that can accompany grief are anxiety, depression, weight loss, difficulties in swallowing, vomiting, fatigue, headaches, dizziness, fainting, blurred vision, skin rashes, excessive sweating, menstrual disturbances, palpitations, chest pain, dyspnea, and infection.

The bereaved may also experience alterations in libido, concentration, and patterns of eating, sleeping, activity, and communication.

STAGES OF GRIEVING

Many authors have described stages or phases of grieving. Perhaps the most famous of them was Kübler-Ross, who has described five stages: denial, anger, bargaining, depression, and acceptance (Kübler-Ross, 1969). Table 31-1 ◆ provides a description of these stages.

MANIFESTATIONS OF GRIEF

After a loss, the nurse assesses the grieving client or family members to determine the stage of grieving. Physiologically, the body responds to a current or anticipated loss with a stress reaction. The nurse can assess the clinical signs of this response. See Chapter 30 for a discussion of stress and the stress reaction. 🔗

Manifestations of grief that would be considered normal include:

◆ Speaking about the loss
◆ Crying
◆ Sleep disturbance
◆ Loss of appetite
◆ Difficulty concentrating

Dysfunctional grieving may be characterized by extended time of denial, depression, severe physiologic symptoms, or suicidal thoughts.

FACTORS INFLUENCING LOSS AND GRIEF RESPONSES

A number of factors affect a person's response to a loss or death. These factors include age, significance of the loss, culture, spiritual beliefs, gender, socioeconomic status, support systems, and the cause of the loss or death. Nurses learn general concepts about the influence of these factors of the grieving experience, but it is important to remember that these factors and their significance vary from individual to individual.

Age

Age affects a person's understanding of and reaction to loss. With experience, people usually increase their understanding and acceptance of life, loss, and death.

CHILDHOOD. Children differ from adults not only in their understanding of loss and death but also in how they are affected by the loss of others. The child's patterns progress rapidly; adult patterns of growth and development are generally stable. The loss of a parent or other significant person can threaten the child's ability to develop, and regression sometimes results. Assisting the child with the grief experience includes helping the child regain the normal continuity and pace of emotional development.

In situations of crisis and loss, children are sometimes pushed aside or protected from the pain. They can feel afraid,

TABLE 31-1	CLIENT RESPONSES AND NURSING IMPLICATIONS IN KÜBLER-ROSS'S STAGES OF GRIEVING	
STAGE	BEHAVIORAL RESPONSES	NURSING IMPLICATIONS
Denial	Refuses to believe that loss is happening Is unready to deal with practical problems, such as prosthesis after loss of leg May assume artificial cheerfulness to prolong denial	Verbally support client but do not reinforce denial. Examine your own behavior to ensure that you do not share in client's denial.
Anger	Client or family may direct anger at nurse or staff about matters that normally would not bother them	Help client understand that anger is a normal response to feelings of loss and powerlessness. Avoid withdrawal or retaliation; do not take anger personally. Deal with needs underlying any angry reaction. Provide structure and continuity to promote feelings of security. Allow clients as much control as possible over their lives.
Bargaining	Seeks to bargain to avoid loss May express feelings of guilt or fear of punishment for past sins, real or imagined	Listen attentively, and encourage client to talk to relieve guilt and irrational fear. If appropriate, offer spiritual support.
Depression	Grieves over what has happened and what cannot be May talk freely (e.g., reviewing past losses such as money or job), or may withdraw	Allow client to express sadness. Communicate nonverbally by sitting quietly without expecting conversation. Convey caring by touch.
Acceptance	Comes to terms with loss May have decreased interest in surroundings and support people May wish to begin making plans (e.g., will, prosthesis, altered living arrangements)	Help family and friends understand client's decreased need to socialize. Encourage client to participate as much as possible in the treatment program.

abandoned, and lonely. Careful work with bereaved children is especially necessary because experiencing a loss in childhood can have serious effects later in life.

EARLY AND MIDDLE ADULTHOOD. As people grow, they come to experience loss as part of normal development. By middle age, for example, the loss of a parent through death seems a normal occurrence compared to the death of a younger person. Coping with the death of an aged parent has even been viewed as a necessary developmental task of the middle-aged adult.

The middle-aged adult can experience losses other than death. For example, losses resulting from impaired health or body function and losses of various role functions can be difficult for the middle-aged adult. How the middle-aged adult responds to such losses is influenced by previous experiences with loss, the person's sense of self-esteem, and the strength and availability of support.

LATE ADULTHOOD. Losses experienced by older adults include loss of health, loss of mobility, loss of independence, and loss of work role (see Chapter 24). ⊙⊙ Limited income and the need to change one's living accommodations can also lead to feelings of loss and grieving.

For older adults, the loss through death of a longtime mate is profound (Figure 31-1 ◆). Although individuals differ in their ability to deal with such a loss, research suggests that health problems for widows and widowers increase during the first year following the death of the spouse (Richter, 1984). Because the majority of deaths occur among elderly people,

Figure 31-1. ◆ Losing friends and loved ones is one difficult aspect of growing older.

and because the number of elderly people is increasing in North America, nurses will need to be especially alert to the potential problems of older grieving adults.

Culture

Culture influences an individual's reaction to loss. How grief is expressed is often determined by the customs of the culture. In the United States and Canada, unless an extended family structure exists, grief is usually handled by the nuclear family. The death of a family member in a typical nuclear European-American family leaves a great void, because the same few individuals fill most of the roles. In cultures in which several generations and extended family members either live in the same household or are physically close, the impact of a family member's death may be softened, because the roles of the deceased are quickly filled by other relatives (Figure 31-2 ◆).

Many Americans appear to have adopted the belief that grief is a private matter to be endured internally. Therefore, feelings tend to be repressed and may remain unidentified. People who have been socialized to "be strong" and "make the best of the situation" may not express deep feelings or personal concerns when they experience a serious loss.

Some cultural groups value social support and the expression of loss (see also Chapter 26). ⊂⊃ In some groups, the expression of grief through wailing, crying, physical prostration, and other outward demonstrations are acceptable and encouraged. Other groups may frown on this demonstration as a loss of control, favoring a more quiet and stoic expression of grief. In cultural groups in which strong kinship ties are maintained, physical and emotional support and assistance are provided by family members.

Spiritual Beliefs

Spiritual beliefs and practices greatly influence both a person's reaction to loss and subsequent behavior. Most religious groups have practices related to dying, and these are often important to the client and support people. To provide support at a time of death, nurses need to understand the client's particular beliefs and practices.

Gender

The gender roles into which many people are socialized in the United States and Canada affect their reactions at times of loss. Men are frequently expected to "be strong" and show very little emotion during grief, whereas it is acceptable for women to show grief by crying. Often, when a wife dies, the husband, who is the chief mourner, is expected to repress his own emotions and to comfort sons and daughters in their grieving.

Socioeconomic Status

The socioeconomic status of an individual often affects the support system available at the time of a loss. A pension plan or insurance, for example, can offer a widowed or disabled person a choice of ways to deal with a loss: A person who loses a hand and can no longer carry out work-related tasks may be able to pursue vocational reeducation. A wealthy person whose spouse has died may decide to take a cruise or visit relatives in Europe. On the other hand, a person who is confronted with both severe loss and economic hardship may not be able to cope with either.

Support Systems

The people closest to the grieving individual are often the first to recognize and provide needed emotional, physical, and functional assistance. However, because many people are uncomfortable or inexperienced in dealing with losses, the usual support people may instead withdraw from the grieving individual. Also, support may be available when the loss is first recognized, but as the support people return to their usual activities, the need for ongoing support may be unmet. Sometimes, the grieving individual is unable or unready to accept support when it is offered.

Cause of Loss or Death

Individual and societal views on the cause of a loss or death may significantly influence the grief response. Some diseases, such as cardiovascular disorders, are considered "clean." They engender compassion, whereas others may be viewed as repulsive and less unfortunate. A loss or death that is beyond the control of those involved may be more acceptable than one that is preventable, such as a drunk driving accident. Injuries or deaths occurring during respected activities, such as a firefighter who dies "in the line of duty," are considered honorable. Deaths that occur during illicit activities may be considered the individual's just rewards.

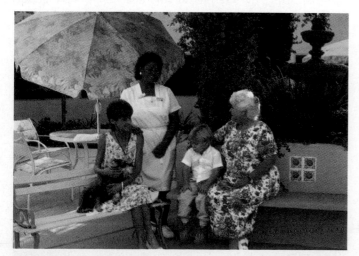

Figure 31-2. ◆ When there is close contact among several generations, families sometimes can cope better with loss and death.

NURSING CARE

 ASSESSING

Nursing assessment of the client experiencing a loss includes the nursing history, an assessment of personal coping resources, and the physical assessment. During the routine health assessment of every client, the nurse poses questions about previous and current losses. The nature of the loss and the meaning of such losses to the client must be explored.

If there is a current or recent loss, greater detail is needed in the assessment. Because clients do not always associate physical ailments with emotional responses such as grief, the nurse may need to probe to identify possible loss-related stresses. If the client reports significant losses, it is important to examine how the client usually copes with loss and what resources are available to assist the client in coping. This information is needed in order to determine a plan of care. Box 31-1 ◆ details assessment questions for interviews about loss and grief.

In assessing the client's response to a current loss, the nurse may identify dysfunctional grief. This is best treated by a health care professional who is expert in assisting such clients. If the nursing assessment reveals severe physical or psychologic signs and symptoms, the client should be referred to an appropriate care provider.

 ## DIAGNOSING, PLANNING, and IMPLEMENTING

Nursing diagnoses relating specifically to grieving include the following:

- Grieving
- Anticipatory Grieving
- Dysfunctional Grieving

The overall goals for clients who are grieving the loss of body function or a body part are to adjust to the changed ability and to redirect both physical and emotional energy into rehabilitation. The goals for clients who are grieving the loss of a loved one are to remember that person without feeling intense pain, to redirect emotional energy into one's own life, and to adjust to the actual or impending loss.

Specific desired outcomes might include:

- Shares loss with significant others
- Reports increased involvement in usual activities
- Reports adequate sleep and nutritional intake
- Participates in decision making about daily activities
- Identifies support people and resources available to assist during difficult episodes
- Verbalizes positive expectations for the future

In supporting the grieving client, it is often helpful to teach about common aspects of the grieving process that are typically experienced. For example, inform the client of the stages that he or she can expect to experience over time. Particular emphasis should be placed on the significance of holidays and other important dates that may evoke memories. Also, prepare clients for feelings of guilt that may arise as they recover from the initial impact of a loss.

Additional teaching should include providing the client with resources that can be used in the future. For some people,

BOX 31-1 ASSESSING CLIENTS: INTERVIEW FOR LOSS AND GRIEVING

Previous Losses

- Have you ever lost someone or something very important to you?
- Have you or your family ever moved to a new home?
- What was it like for you when you first started school? Moved away from home? Got a job? Retired?
- Are you physically able to do all the things you like to do? Used to do?
- Has anyone important or close to you died?
- Do you think there will be any losses in your life in the near future?

Previous Grieving

- Tell me about (the loss). What was losing _____ like for you?
- Did you have trouble sleeping? Eating? Concentrating?
- What kinds of things did you do to make yourself feel better when something like that happened?
- Are there spiritual or cultural practices you observed when you had a loss like that?
- Who was a person you could turn to if you were very upset about (the loss)?

events long after a loss will renew painful feelings associated with the loss. These feelings are often alarming to someone who thought they had "gotten over it." Preparation for such an occurrence and information about support groups and counseling are important aspects of teaching.

The skills most relevant to situations of loss and grief are attentive listening, silence, open and closed questioning, paraphrasing, clarifying and reflecting feelings, and summarizing. It is less helpful to clients to respond by giving advice and evaluating, by interpreting and analyzing, or by giving unwarranted reassurance. To ensure effective communication, the nurse must make an accurate assessment of what is appropriate for the client.

Communication with grieving clients needs to be relevant to their stage of grief. Whether the client is angry or depressed affects how he or she hears messages and how the nurse interprets the client's statements. Implications for nurse–client communication are related to Kübler-Ross's five stages (see Table 31-1).

EVALUATING

Evaluating the effectiveness of nursing care of the grieving client is difficult because of the long-term nature of the life transition. Criteria for evaluation must be based on goals set by the client and family.

Client goals and related desired outcomes for a grieving client depend on the characteristics of the loss and the client. For example, the nurse might ask about a client's participation in rehabilitation therapy sessions, or about whether the client is now sleeping through the night. Weight gain is an observable outcome in someone who has had no appetite during the first months of grief.

If outcomes are not achieved, the nurse needs to explore why the plan was unsuccessful. Such exploration begins with reassessing the client to determine whether nursing diagnoses are appropriate.

Nursing Process Case Study: CLIENT WITH METASTATIC CARCINOMA OF THE BOWEL

John Yee, age 63, was diagnosed with metastatic carcinoma of the bowel 4½ months ago. A colostomy was done at that time to relieve a bowel obstruction. No further treatment was available and Mr. Yee was discharged home on hospice care.

Assessment Roger Hadrick, Mr. Yee's hospice nurse, has noted that Mr. Yee has become profoundly weak over the past week and is no longer able to walk to the bathroom. His abdomen is greatly distended, firm, and tender, and he complains of feeling bloated and nauseated. Bowel sounds are sluggish. Although he complains of having no appetite, his wife has been encouraging him to eat several times a day. Over the past 2 months he has become increasingly jaundiced. Mr. Yee describes his pain as 8 out of 10, even though he is taking a long-acting morphine preparation twice a day. On this visit, he tells his nurse, "I know I haven't long to live. Why can't they just give me a big dose of morphine and get it over with?"

Diagnosis The current nursing diagnoses for Mr. Yee are as follows:

◆ Hopelessness related to deteriorating physiologic condition
◆ Powerlessness related to terminal illness
◆ Pain related to increased tumor growth

Expected Outcomes The expected outcomes specify that Mr. Yee will:

◆ Participate in self-care activities in accordance with health status.
◆ Make choices related to care and treatment.
◆ Maintain physiologic comfort.
◆ Share values and personal meaning of life.

Planning and Implementation The following nursing interventions are planned and implemented:

◆ Encourage client and family to maintain pain diary.
◆ Monitor use of breakthrough pain medication.

◆ Evaluate efficacy of pain regimen.
◆ Administer antiemetics and antianxiety medications as ordered.
◆ Teach client and family about the dying process.
◆ Instruct family regarding decreasing nutritional needs of a dying person.
◆ Allow client to verbalize feelings.
◆ Identify support systems available to client and family.

Evaluation After 3 days of monitoring and adjusting Mr. Yee's medications, his symptoms are under control. His long-acting morphine has been increased and his wife administers the short acting morphine at the onset of breakthrough pain, when Mr. Yee requests. Also, his wife has told him to ask for food if he is hungry, rather than offering food and encouraging him to eat. Although he is spending more time sleeping, his waking moments often include short conversations with his wife and children. He no longer expresses a desire to hasten his death.

Critical Thinking in the Nursing Process

1. Why is Mr. Yee's appetite decreased?
2. What is the rationale for giving both long-acting and short-acting preparations of morphine?

Dying and Death

The concept of death develops over time, as people grow, experience loss, and think about concrete and abstract concepts. Table 31-2 ◆ describes some of the specific beliefs common to different age groups. Knowledge of these developmental stages helps in understanding a client's responses to a life-threatening situation.

RESPONSES TO DYING AND DEATH

The reaction of any person to another person's impending or real death, or to the potential reality of one's own death, depends on all the factors discussed earlier in this chapter. Yet, responses do tend to cluster in the phases described by Kübler-Ross and other theorists (see Table 31-1).

Both the dying client and the family members grieve as they recognize the loss. Clients and their families may experience denial, guilt, anger, despair, feelings of worthlessness, crying, and inability to concentrate. These reactions may extend to thoughts of suicide, delusions, and hallucinations. Fear, the feeling of disruption that is related to an identifiable source (in this case someone's death), may also be present. Many of the characteristics seen in a fearful person are similar to those of grieving (crying, immobility, increased pulse and respirations, dry mouth, anorexia, difficulty sleeping, and

MediaLink ♦ Stages of Dying

TABLE 31-2	DEVELOPMENT OF THE CONCEPT OF DEATH
AGE	**BELIEFS/ATTITUDES**
Infancy–5 years	Does not understand concept of death Infant's sense of separation forms basis for later understanding of loss and death Believes death is reversible, a temporary departure, or sleep Emphasizes immobility and inactivity as attributes of death
5–9 years	Understands that death is final Believes own death can be avoided Associates death with aggression or violence Believes wishes or unrelated actions can be responsible for death
9–12 years	Understands death as the inevitable end of life Begins to understand own mortality, expressed as interest in afterlife or as fear of death
12–18 years	Fears a lingering death May fantasize that death can be defied, acting out defiance through reckless behaviors (e.g., dangerous driving, substance abuse) Seldom thinks about death, but views it in religious and philosophic terms May seem to reach "adult" perception of death but be emotionally unable to accept it May still hold concepts from previous developmental stages
18–45 years	Has attitude toward death influenced by religious and cultural beliefs
45–65 years	Accepts own mortality Encounters death of parents and some peers Experiences peaks of death anxiety Death anxiety diminishes with emotional well-being
65+ years	Fears prolonged illness Encounters death of family members and peers Sees death as having multiple meanings, (e.g., freedom from pain, reunion with already deceased family members)

nightmares). **Hopelessness** occurs when the person perceives no solutions to a problem—when the death becomes inevitable and the person is unable to see how to move beyond the death. A hopeless person may make statements such as, "I'm never going to get over this." The nurse may observe apa-

thy, pessimism, and inability to make decisions. A person who does perceive a solution to the problem but does not believe that it is possible to implement the solution may be said to experience **powerlessness.** This loss of control may be manifested by anger, violence, acting out, or depression and passive behavior.

Nurse's Responses to Dying and Death

Caring for the dying and the bereaved is one of the nurse's most complex and challenging responsibilities, bringing into play all the skills needed for holistic physiologic and psychosocial care. To be effective, nurses must come to grips with their own attitudes toward loss, death, and dying, because these attitudes directly affect their ability to provide care.

DEFINITIONS AND SIGNS OF DEATH

The traditional clinical signs of **death** were cessation of the apical pulse, respirations, and blood pressure, also referred to as heart-lung death. However, since the advent of artificial means to maintain respirations and blood circulation, identifying death is more difficult. If a person is connected to an artificial means of life support, death is determined by an absence of brain wave activity (measured by electroencephalogram) for at least 24 hours. Some would also include cerebral death (irreversible damage to the cerebral cortex) within the definition of death, even though a person might still be able to breathe. In this case, an irreversible state of unconscious **(vegetative state)** becomes a defining factor. Box 31-2 ◆ lists indications of death.

LEGALITIES RELATED TO DEATH

The nurse's role in legal issues related to death are prescribed by the laws of the region and the policies of the health care institution. For example, in some states a nasogastric feeding tube cannot be removed from a person in a persistent vegetative state without a prior directive from the client. In other states, the removal is allowed at the family's request or a physician's order. Many of these legal issues stimulate strong ethical concerns. The nurse needs support from other team

---

BOX 31-2
INDICATIONS OF DEATH

- ◆ Total lack of response to external stimuli
- ◆ No muscular movement, especially breathing
- ◆ No reflexes
- ◆ Flat encephalogram
- ◆ For people on artificial support, absence of electric currents from the brain (measured by an electroencephalogram) for at least 24 hours
- ◆ Irreversible destruction of the cerebral cortex (cerebral death or higher brain death); the client may still be able to breathe but is irreversibly unconscious.

members in understanding and providing appropriate care to clients facing death (see Chapter 2). ⊂⊃

Advance Directives

The Patient Self-Determination Act, implemented in 1991, requires all health care facilities receiving Medicare and Medicaid reimbursement to do the following:

◆ Recognize advance directives.
◆ Ask clients whether they have advance directives.
◆ Provide educational materials advising clients of their rights to declare their personal wishes regarding treatment decisions, including the right to refuse medical treatment.

There are two types of advance medical directives: the living will and the health care proxy or surrogate. The **living will** provides specific instructions about what medical treatment the client chooses to omit or refuse (e.g., cardiopulmonary resuscitation [CPR], intubation, ventilatory support) in the event that the client is unable to make those decisions.

The health care proxy, also referred to as durable **power of attorney for health care,** is a written statement appointing someone else (e.g., a relative or trusted friend) to manage health care treatment decisions when the client is unable to do so. For example, it is often used for specific clients who are in a coma, are having life-sustaining procedures, or are receiving artificial nutrition or hydration.

Nurses should learn the law regarding client self-determination for the state in which they practice. They are also responsible to know the policy and procedures for implementation in the institution where they work. The legally binding nature and specific requirements of advance medical directives are determined by individual state legislation (Springhouse, 1996, pp. 156–177).

In most states, advance directives must be witnessed by two people but do not require review by an attorney or notarization. Some states do not permit relatives, heirs, or physicians to witness advance directives.

Certification of Death

The formal determination, or *pronouncement*, of death must be performed by a physician, a coroner, or a nurse. In some areas, police officers or paramedics are also permitted to pronounce death. Again, the granting of the authority to nurses to pronounce death is regulated by the state or province. It may be limited to nurses in long-term care, home health, and hospice agencies, or to advanced practice nurses. By law, a death certificate must be made out when a person dies. It is usually signed by the attending physician and filed with a local health or other government office. The family is usually given a copy to use for legal matters, such as insurance claims.

Labeling of the Deceased

Nurses have a duty to handle the deceased with dignity and to label the corpse appropriately. Mishandling can cause emotional distress to survivors. Mislabeling can create legal prob-

lems if the body is inappropriately identified and prepared incorrectly for burial or a funeral. In the hospital, the deceased's wrist identification tag is left on, and another tag is tied to the client's ankle, in case one of the tags becomes detached. A third tag is attached to the shroud. All identification tags should include the client's name, hospital number, and physician's name.

Autopsy

An **autopsy** or postmortem examination is an examination of the body after death. It is performed only in certain cases. The law describes under what circumstances an autopsy must be performed, such as when death is sudden or occurs within 48 hours of admission to a hospital. The organs and tissues of the body are examined to establish the exact cause of death, to learn more about a disease, or to assist in the accumulation of statistical data.

It is the responsibility of the physician or, in some instances, of a designated person in the hospital to obtain consent for autopsy. Consent must be given by the individual in a legal document before death or by the next of kin. Laws in many states and provinces prioritize the family members who can provide consent as follows: surviving spouse, adult children, parents, siblings. After autopsy, hospitals cannot retain any tissues or organs without the permission of the person who consented to the autopsy.

Organ Donation

Under the Uniform Anatomical Gift Act and the National Organ Transplant Act in the United States or the Human Tissue Act in Canada, people who are 18 years or older and of sound mind may become **organ donors.** That is, they make a gift of all or any part of their own body for the following purposes: for medical or dental education, research, advancement of medical or dental science, therapy, or transplantation. The donation can be made by a provision in a will or by signing a card-like form. This card is usually carried at all times by the person who signed it. In most states and provinces, the gift can be revoked, either by destroying the card or by revoking the gift orally in the presence of two witnesses. Nurses may serve as witnesses for people consenting to donate organs. In 28 states, health care workers are required to ask survivors for consent to donate the deceased's organs.

Inquest

An **inquest** is a legal inquiry into the cause or manner of a death. When a death is the result of an accident, for example, an inquest is held into the circumstances of the accident to determine any blame. The inquest is conducted under the jurisdiction of a coroner or medical examiner. A *coroner* is a public official, not necessarily a physician, appointed or elected to inquire into the causes of death, when appropriate. A *medical examiner* is a physician and usually has advanced education in pathology or forensic medicine. Agency policy dictates who is responsible for reporting deaths to the coroner or medical examiner.

Euthanasia

Euthanasia is the act of painlessly putting to death persons suffering from incurable or distressing disease. It is sometimes referred to as "mercy killing." Regardless of compassion and good intentions or moral convictions, euthanasia is illegal in both Canada and the United States. It can lead to criminal charges of homicide or to a civil lawsuit for withholding treatment or providing an unacceptable standard of care.

Voluntary euthanasia, or **assisted suicide,** refers to situations in which the dying individual desires some control over the time and manner of death. All forms of euthanasia are illegal, except in Oregon where a physician-assisted suicide statute was passed in 1994. That statute permits physicians to prescribe lethal doses of medications to clients who request them and meet certain criteria. After several legal challenges, the law took effect late in 1997. Since Oregon's action, several other states have proposed similar laws and legal challenges continue.

Do-Not-Resuscitate Orders

Physicians may order "no code" or **do not resuscitate (DNR)** for clients who are in a stage of terminal, irreversible illness or expected death. A DNR order is generally written when the client or surrogate has expressed the wish for no resuscitation in the event of a respiratory or cardiac arrest. Many physicians are reluctant to write such an order if there is any conflict between the client and family members or among family members. A comfort measures only order is written to indicate that the goal of treatment is a comfortable, dignified death and that further life-sustaining measures are not indicated. Many states permit clients living at home to arrange special orders so that emergency technicians called to the home in the event of a cardiopulmonary arrest will respect the client's wish not to be resuscitated. Nurses should be familiar with the federal and state or provincial laws and the policies of their agency concerning withholding life-sustaining measures.

DEATH-RELATED RELIGIOUS AND CULTURAL PRACTICES

Various cultural and religious traditions and practices associated with death, dying, and the grieving process help people cope with these experiences. Nurses are often present through the dying process and at the moment of death. Knowledge of the client's religious and cultural heritage helps nurses provide individualized care to clients and their families, even though they may not participate in the rituals associated with death.

Beliefs and attitudes about death, its cause, and the soul vary among cultures. Unnatural deaths, or "bad deaths," are sometimes distinguished from "good deaths." Also, the death of a person who has behaved well in life may be considered less threatening based on the belief that the person will be reincarnated into a good life.

Beliefs about preparation of the body, autopsy, organ donation, cremation, and prolonging life are closely allied to the person's religion. Autopsy, for example, may be prohibited, opposed, or discouraged by Eastern Orthodox religions,

Muslims, Jehovah's Witnesses, and Orthodox Jews. Some religions prohibit the removal of body parts and dictate that all body parts be given appropriate burial. Organ donation is prohibited by Jehovah's Witnesses and Muslims, whereas Buddhists in America consider it an act of mercy and encourage it. Cremation is discouraged, opposed, or prohibited by the Mormon, Eastern Orthodox, Islamic, and Jewish faiths. Hindus, in contrast, prefer cremation and cast the ashes in a holy river. Prolongation of life is generally encouraged; however, some religions, such as Christian Science, are unlikely to use medical means to prolong life, and the Jewish faith generally opposes prolonging life after irreversible brain damage. In hopeless illness, Buddhists may permit euthanasia.

Nurses also need to be knowledgeable about the client's death-related rituals, such as last rites and administration of Holy Communion, chanting at the bedside, and other rituals, such as special procedures for washing, dressing, positioning, and shrouding the dead. For example, certain immigrants may wish to retain their native customs, in which family members of the same sex wash and prepare the body for burial and cremation. Muslims also customarily turn the body toward Mecca. Nurses need to ask family members about their preference and verify who will carry out these activities. Burial clothes and other cultural or religious items are often important symbols for the funeral. For example, faithful Mormons are often dressed in their "temple clothes." Some Native Americans may be dressed in elaborate apparel and jewelry and wrapped in new blankets with money. The nurse must ensure that any ritual items present in the health care agency be given to the family or to the funeral home.

HOSPICE AND HOME CARE

Hospice care, palliative care, and home care focus on support and care of the dying person and family, with the goal of facilitating a peaceful and dignified death. **Hospice care** is based on holistic concepts that emphasize care to improve the quality of life rather than to cure (Figure 31-3 ◆). The hospice movement was founded by the physician Cecily Saunders in London, England, in 1967 and was later extended to the United States. The number of hospice programs in the United States grew rapidly after the enactment of the Medicare Hospice Benefit in 1983.

The principles of hospice care can be carried out in a variety of settings, the most common being the client's or family's home or in extended care facilities. Autonomous hospice and hospital-based palliative care units are also sometimes available. Palliative care is special care that is challenging and requires skillful interpersonal relationships and compassion. Services range from comprehensive to a focus on selected areas, such as symptom control and pain management, in some palliative care units. Home care services for the dying client maintain the client in the natural home environment until that is no longer possible or until death. Hospice care is always provided by a team of both health professionals and nonprofessionals to ensure a full range of care services.

Figure 31-3. ◆ The touch of your hand may be the dying person's last memory.

NURSING CARE

◆ ASSESSING

To gather a complete database that allows accurate analysis and identification of appropriate nursing diagnoses for dying clients and their families, the nurse first needs to recognize the state of awareness the client and family manifest. Three types of awareness that have been described:

♦ In *closed awareness*, the client and family are unaware of impending death. They may not completely understand why the client is ill, and they believe the client will recover.
♦ With *mutual pretense*, the client, family, and health personnel know that the prognosis is terminal but do not talk about it and make an effort not to raise the subject.
♦ With open awareness, however, the client and people around know about the impending death and feel comfortable discussing it, even though it is difficult. The type of awareness exhibited by the client and family must be considered in planning care and communicated to all caregivers.

Nursing care and support for the dying client and family include making an accurate assessment of the physiologic signs of approaching death. In addition to signs related to the client's specific disease, certain other physical signs are indicative of impending death. The four main characteristic changes are loss of muscle tone, slowing of the circulation, changes in respirations, and sensory impairment (see Box 31-2).

Various consciousness levels occur just before death. Some clients are alert, whereas others are drowsy, stuporous, or comatose. Hearing is thought to be the last sense lost.

◆ DIAGNOSING, PLANNING, and IMPLEMENTING

Nursing diagnoses address both physiologic and psychosocial needs. Those that can be applied to the dying client and their caregivers include the following:

♦ Fear
♦ Hopelessness
♦ Powerlessness
♦ Risk for Caregiver Role Strain
♦ Interrupted Family Processes

Major goals of dying clients are (a) maintaining physiologic and psychologic comfort and (b) achieving a dignified and peaceful death, which includes maintaining personal control and accepting declining health status. When planning care with these clients, the Dying Person's Bill of Rights can be a useful guide (Figure 31-4 ◆).

The major nursing responsibility for clients who are dying is to assist the client to a peaceful death. More specific responsibilities include the following:

♦ To provide relief from loneliness, fear, and depression
♦ To maintain the client's sense of security, self-confidence, dignity, and self-worth
♦ To maintain hope
♦ To help the client accept losses
♦ To provide physical comfort

Meeting Physiologic Needs of the Dying Client

The physiologic needs of people who are dying are related to a slowing of body processes and to homeostatic imbalances. Interventions include providing personal hygiene measures; controlling pain (see Chapter 15 ⊘); relieving respiratory difficulties; assisting with movement, nutrition, hydration, and elimination; and providing measures related to sensory changes. Table 31-3 ◆ describes nursing interventions to meet the needs of a dying person.

Providing Spiritual Support

Spiritual support is of great importance in dealing with death. Although not all clients identify with a specific religious faith or belief, the majority have a need for meaning in their lives, particularly as they experience a terminal illness.

The nurse has a responsibility to ensure that the client's spiritual needs are attended to, either through direct intervention or by arranging access to individuals who can provide spiritual care. It is important for nurses to establish an effective interdisciplinary relationship with spiritual support specialists. Death-related beliefs and practices of selected groups are discussed earlier in this chapter.

Supporting the Family

The most important aspect of providing support to the family members of a dying client involves using therapeutic communication to facilitate their expression of feelings. When no interventions can reverse the inevitable dying process, the nurse can provide an empathetic and caring presence. The nurse also serves as a teacher, explaining what is happening and what the family can expect. Due to the effects of the stress of moving through the grieving process, family members may not absorb what they are told and need to have information

The Dying Person's Bill of Rights

As we face death, what are our rights as human beings? This bill of rights was created at a workshop on "The Terminally III Patient and the Helping Person," sponsored by the Southwestern Michigan Insurance Education Council and conducted by Amelia J. Barbus.

- I have the right to be treated as a living human being until I die.
- I have the right to maintain a sense of hopefulness, however changing its focus may be.
- I have the right to be cared for by those who can maintain a sense of hopefulness, however changing this might be.
- I have the right to express my feelings and emotions about my approaching death in my own way.
- I have the right to participate in decisions concerning my care.
- I have the right to expect continuing medical and nursing attention even though "cure" goals must be changed to "comfort" goals.
- I have the right not to die alone.
- I have the right to be free from pain.
- I have the right to have my questions answered honestly.
- I have the right not to be deceived.
- I have the right to have help from and for my family in accepting my death.
- I have the right to die in peace and dignity.
- I have the right to retain my individuality and not be judged for my decisions which may be contrary to beliefs of others.
- I have the right to discuss and enlarge my religious and/or spiritual experiences, whatever these may mean to others.
- I have the right to expect that the sanctity of the human body will be respected after death.
- I have the right to be cared for by caring, sensitive, knowledgeable people who will attempt to understand my needs and will be able to gain some satisfaction in helping me face my death.

Figure 31-4. ◆ The dying person's bill of rights.

provided repeatedly. The nurse must present a calm and patient demeanor.

Family members should be encouraged to participate in the physical care of the dying person as much as they wish to and are able. The nurse can suggest they assist with bathing, speak or read to the client, and hold hands. The nurse must not, however, have specific expectations for family members' participation. Those who feel unable to be with the dying person also require support from the nurse and from other family members. They should be shown an appropriate waiting area if they wish to remain nearby.

Providing Postmortem Care

After death, some characteristic physical changes occur. **Rigor mortis** is the stiffening of the body that occurs about 2 to 4 hours after death. It results from a lack of adenosine triphosphate (ATP), which is not synthesized because of a lack of glycogen in the body. ATP is necessary for muscle fiber relaxation. Its lack causes the muscles to contract, which in turn immobilizes the joints. Rigor mortis starts in the involuntary muscles (heart, bladder, etc.), then progresses to the head, neck, and trunk, and finally reaches the extremities. Rigor mortis usually leaves the body about 96 hours after death.

Algor mortis is the gradual decrease of the body's temperature after death. When blood circulation terminates and the hypothalamus ceases to function, body temperature falls about 1° C (1.8° F) per hour until it reaches room temperature. Simultaneously, the skin loses its elasticity and can easily be broken when removing dressings and adhesive tape.

After blood circulation has ceased, the red blood cells break down, releasing hemoglobin, which discolors the surrounding tissues. This discoloration, referred to as **livor mortis,** appears in the lowermost or dependent areas of the body.

Tissues after death become soft and eventually liquefied by bacterial fermentation. The hotter the temperature, the more rapid the change. Therefore, bodies are often stored in cool places to delay this process. Embalming prevents the process through injection of chemicals into the body to destroy the bacteria.

Nursing personnel may be responsible for care of a body after death. Postmortem care should be carried out according to the policy of the hospital or agency. Because care of the body may be influenced by religious law, the nurse should check the client's religion and make every attempt to comply. If the deceased's family or friends wish to view the body, it is important to make the environment as clean and pleasant as possible and to make the body appear natural and comfortable. All equipment, soiled linen, and supplies should be removed from the bedside. Some agencies require that all tubes in the body remain in place; in other agencies, tubes may be cut to within 2.5 cm (1 in) of the skin and taped in place; in others, all tubes may be removed.

TABLE 31-3	PHYSIOLOGIC NEEDS OF DYING PERSONS
PROBLEM	**NURSING INTERVENTIONS**
Ineffective Airway Clearance	Fowler's position: conscious clients Throat suctioning: conscious clients Lateral position: unconscious clients
Self-Care Deficit: Bathing/Hygiene	Frequent baths and linen changes if diaphoretic Mouth care as needed for dry mouth
Impaired Physical Mobility	Assist client out of bed periodically, if client is able Regularly change bedridden client's position Support client's position with pillows, blanket rolls, or towels as needed Elevate client's legs when sitting up, to prevent pooling of blood
Imbalanced Nutrition: Less Than Body Requirements	Antiemetics or small amount of alcoholic beverage to stimulate appetite Encourage liquid foods as tolerated
Constipation	Dietary fiber as tolerated Laxatives as needed to prevent constipation
Impaired Urinary Elimination	Skin care in response to incontinence of urine or feces Bedpan, urinal, or commode chair within easy reach Call light within reach for assistance onto bedpan or commode Absorbent pads placed under incontinent client; linen changed as often as needed Catheterization, if necessary Keep room as clean and odor free as possible
Sensory/Perceptual Alterations: Visual, Tactile	Clients prefer a light room Hearing is not diminished; speak clearly and do not whisper Touch is diminished, but client will feel pressure of touch

Normally the body is placed in a supine position with the arms either at the sides, palms down, or across the abdomen. One or two pillows are placed under the head and shoulders, or the head of the bed is elevated 30 degrees, to prevent blood from discoloring the face by settling in it. The eyelids are closed and held in place for a few seconds. Often, the eyes and mouth do not remain closed and require a mortician's intervention.

Soiled areas of the body are washed. However, a complete bath is not necessary, because the body will be washed by the *mortician* (also referred to as an undertaker), a person trained in care of the dead. Absorbent pads are placed under the buttocks to take up any feces and urine released because of relaxation of the sphincter muscles. A clean gown is placed on the client, and the hair is brushed and combed. All jewelry is removed, except a wedding band in some instances, which is taped to the finger. The top bed linens are adjusted neatly to cover the client to the shoulders. Soft lighting and chairs are provided for the family.

In the hospital, after the body has been viewed by the family, additional identification tags are applied. The body is wrapped in a *shroud*, a large piece of plastic or cotton material used to enclose a body after death. Identification is then applied to the outside of the shroud. The body is taken to the morgue if arrangements have not been make to have a mortician pick it up from the client's room.

 ## Evaluating

To evaluate the achievement of client goals, the nurse might do the following:

◆ Listen to the client's reports of feeling in control of the environment surrounding death, such as control over pain relief, visitation of family and support people, or treatment plans
◆ Observe the client's relationship with significant others
◆ Listen to the client's thoughts and feelings related to hopelessness or powerlessness

Note: The bibliography listings for this and all chapters have been compiled at the back of the book.

Chapter Review

Key Terms by Topics

Use the audio glossary feature of either the CD-ROM or the Companion Website to hear the correct pronunciation of the following key terms.

Loss and grief
loss, grief, bereavement, mourning, dysfunctional grieving

Dying and death
hopelessness, powerlessness, death, vegetative state, living will, power of attorney for health care, autopsy, organ donor, inquest, euthanasia, assisted suicide, do not resuscitate (DNR), hospice care

Nursing care
rigor mortis, algor mortis, livor mortis

Key Points

* Nurses help clients deal with all kinds of losses, including loss of body image, loss of a loved one, loss of a sense of well-being, and loss of a job.

* Grieving is a normal, subjective emotional response to loss; it is essential for mental and physical health. Grieving allows the bereaved person to cope with loss gradually and to accept it as part of reality.

* Knowledge of different stages or phases of grieving and factors that influence the loss reaction can help the nurse understand the responses and needs of clients.

* How an individual deals with loss is closely related to the individual's stage of development, personal resources, and social support system.

* Caring for the dying and the bereaved is one of the nurse's most complex and challenging responsibilities. Nurses themselves must be allowed to resolve their grief at the loss of a client.

* Nurses must consider the entire family as requiring care in situations involving loss, especially death.

* Nurses must be knowledgeable about their responsibilities in regard to legal issues surrounding death: advance directives, certification of death, labeling of the deceased, autopsy, organ donation, inquest, euthanasia, and do-not-resuscitate orders.

* Dying clients require open communication, physical help, and emotional and spiritual support to ensure a peaceful and dignified death. They need to maintain a sense of control in managing the events preceding death.

EXPLORE MediaLink

Additional interactive resources for this chapter can be found on the Companion Website at www.prenhall.com/ramont. Click on Chapter 31 and "Begin" to select the activities for this chapter.

For chapter-related NCLEX-style questions and an audio glossary, access the accompanying CD-ROM in this book.

Animations:
* Diazepam
* Fluoxetine

For Further Study

For further study about legal and ethical issues related to nursing care, see Chapter 2.

For more information about assisting clients with chronic pain, see Chapter 15.

For more information about age-related factors, see Chapter 24.

For information about practices of religious groups related to dying, see Chapter 26.

See Chapter 30 for causes and indicators of stress.

Critical Thinking Care Map

Caring for a Client with Anticipatory Grieving

NCLEX-PN Focus Area: Coping and Adaptation

Teresa Jimenez's son Ramon, age 15, has advanced cystic fibrosis. Mother and son are waiting for an appropriate donor for a heart–lung transplant. She says, "We've been called to the transplant unit twice, but things didn't work out. Ramon gets his hopes all geared up, and then he's deflated. I can't eat or sleep for worrying. I don't know what I'll do if he doesn't get that transplant. He's all I've got since my husband left us 6 years ago."

Nursing Diagnosis: Anticipatory Grieving

COLLECT DATA

Subjective	Objective
_____	_____
_____	_____
_____	_____
_____	_____
_____	_____
_____	_____

Would you report this data? Yes/No

If yes, to: _____

Nursing Care

_____
_____
_____
_____
_____
_____
_____
_____
_____
_____
_____
_____
_____

How would you document this? _____
_____
_____
_____
_____

Data Collected
(use those that apply)

- Easily fatigued
- Reports poor appetite
- Recent weight gain
- BP is 128/80
- Neglects personal hygiene
- Attends church regularly
- Crying episodes
- Labile affect
- Sleeps 7 to 8 hours/night
- Difficulty concentrating
- Complains of frequent headaches
- Nausea and vomiting

Nursing Interventions
(use those that apply)

- Note emotional responses such as anger, crying.
- Instruct client to begin exercise program.
- Encourage high carbohydrate, low fat diet.
- Provide information about grief reactions.
- Provide a list of local support groups for parents of gravely ill children.
- Review experiences with loss and coping.
- Use therapeutic communication skills of active listening, silence, and acknowledgment.
- Determine parent's perception of anticipated loss.
- Discuss and assist in planning for funeral.
- Provide assurance that everything will be all right.

NCLEX-PN Exam Preparation

1. Both a client in end-stage renal failure and her family are aware of the signs of approaching death, but they do not talk about it. They are manifesting which state of awareness?
   a. Closed awareness
   b. Mutual pretense
   c. Open awareness
   d. Undisclosed pretense

2. A client diagnosed with inoperable lung cancer states, "Please get my discharge papers ready. We had vacation plans before I got this cold, and I feel well enough to go." The client is experiencing which stage of the grief process?
   a. Denial
   b. Anger
   c. Bargaining
   d. Acceptance

3. An unmarried adult is admitted following a motor vehicle accident. He is unresponsive and has been placed on life support. His mother and his domestic partner arrive. His mother states, "I can't bear to take him off life support. I know he would want everything to be done." The domestic partner produces a notarized Durable Power of Attorney for Health Care that states no life support is to be used and that gives control to the partner. The physician must consider:
   a. The mother's wishes
   b. The domestic partner's wishes
   c. The instructions outlined in the document
   d. The ER physician's assessment

4. Following the death of a client, the nursing assistant leaves the room quickly and is found sobbing in the utility room. Which action would be the most supportive?
   a. Sending the nursing assistant home for the rest of the shift
   b. Reassigning the nursing assistant to an area where it is unlikely that a client may die
   c. Sitting with her and allowing her to express how she feels
   d. Insisting that she perform postmortem care for the client

5. A terminally ill client is alert but death seems imminent. He does not want any measures to prolong his life. What is your most important nursing action at this time?
   a. Sit quietly and hold the dying client's hand.
   b. Move the client to the hall so he can be observed.
   c. Place him in a single room near the nursing station.
   d. Tell him to put on his call light if he needs anything.

6. The parents of a stillborn infant wish to see the baby. The nurse should:
   a. Show them the baby but not allow them to touch the baby.
   b. Wash and clean the baby and wrap it in a soft baby blanket prior to allowing the parents to see and hold the baby.
   c. Request that only the mother see the baby.
   d. Not allow the mother to remove the blanket from the baby.

7. A client has terminal cancer and the physician has recommended hospice care to the family. The most appropriate explanation of hospice is:
   a. "Hospice nurses give better care than the hospital nurses."
   b. "Hospice care is cheaper than hospital care."
   c. "Hospice allows terminal clients to be cared for at home."
   d. "Hospice uses specialized equipment not available in the hospital."

8. Which of the following criteria must be met in order for the physician to pronounce the client on life support dead?
   a. The family must agree to discontinuance of life support.
   b. Absence of brain activity for at least 24 hours.
   c. The client may still be able to breathe but is irreversibly unconscious.
   d. A court order to discontinue life support.

9. A widower reports headache, loss of appetite, and inability to sleep following his wife's death. He relates that his symptoms increased on his wife's birthday. He states he would just like to die and be with her. The most appropriate nursing diagnosis is:
   a. Anticipatory Grief
   b. Ineffective Family Coping
   c. Ineffective Individual Coping
   d. Dysfunctional Grieving

10. An 11-year-old child's grandfather has just died. Of the following statements, which is most developmentally appropriate?
    a. "Grampa will get better and come home soon."
    b. "I got mad because my grandfather would not buy me a video game. That is why he got sick."
    c. " What happens after someone dies? Will Grampa's body go to heaven or just his heart?"
    d. "When people die they go to live with God. I'm sad but Grampa isn't sick anymore, so that is good."

Answers for Review Questions, as well as discussion of Case Study and Critical Thinking Care Map questions, appear in Appendix IV.

Thinking Strategically About...

You have been assigned your first case as an LPN working for a community hospice agency. The client is a 68-year-old Hispanic woman whose breast cancer has metastasized to her spine. The RN completed the intake interview with the family yesterday at the hospital. The client has been discharged to her home. You have reviewed her discharge plan and see that no additional treatment has been recommended because of her rapidly advancing disease.

When you arrive at home, the client's daughter meets you in the driveway and asks you to remove your name badge, which indicates you are from the hospice organization. She states, "Mother doesn't know how sick she is. We want her last days to be happy. We don't want her to think about dying." The daughter asks you to say that the doctor sent you to help with her bath and to see if all the equipment arrived.

You observe that the family relationship is very close and loving, but that there seems to be an underlying strain. You adhere to the daughter's request during that visit, but when you return to the agency you ask to have a conference with the RN and the social worker.

CULTURAL COMPETENCY

- Do you think that keeping the terminal diagnosis from the client has any relationship to culture?
- How can a nurse who adheres to values of honesty and individualism maintain integrity while honoring this client's culture?

CRITICAL THINKING

- What legal and ethical issues occur when a client's "right to know" is not addressed?
- What are the implications of this for health care institutions and workers?

COMPASSIONATE CARING

- How can you help the client to obtain a sense of closure if the family refuses to talk about the impending death?
- What tools are available that do not violate the family's specific request?

COMMUNITY CARE STRATEGIES

Arrange a visit to a family support group for people in hospice. Observe how the facilitator works with families to draw them out. List communication strategies used in these settings to allow people to face the death of a loved one and to cope with their grief.

UNIT V

Becoming a Licensed Nurse

Chapter 32 ▸ Introduction to Leadership

Chapter 33 ▸ Preparing to Take the Licensure Exam

Chapter 34 ▸ Finding that First Job

Chapter 32

Introduction to Leadership

SHARING experiences

After struggling with a long string of low-paying jobs, I decided to go back to school and further my education. I chose the LPN program because it meant I would always be employed. Upon entering my clinicals, I realized that nursing was my passion, so much so that I decided to continue my education to become an RN. Having my LPN license allowed me to obtain a good paying job. The job expanded my knowledge and strengthened the foundation for my RN studies.

Susan Palmer, RN, ADN, Parkmoor View Medical Center, Colorado Springs, CO.

LEARNING outcomes

After completing this chapter, you will be able to:
- Discuss factors that govern licensure, standards of care, and nurse practice acts.
- Identify the purpose and ways of implementing HIPPA.
- Identify important attributes of effective leaders.
- Describe the purpose of the nurse practice act.
- Describe the advantages of professional networks.
- Define conflict.
- Describe the advantages of each method of nursing care delivery.

MediaLink

www.prenhall.com/ramont

Use the address above to access the free, interactive Companion Website created for this textbook. Get hints, instant feedback, and textbook references to chapter-related NCLEX-style questions. Link to other interesting sites.

Audio Glossary:
Use the Companion Website, or the CD-ROM disk enclosed with your textbook, to hear the pronunciation of key terms in the chapter.

A graduate of a practical/vocational nursing program cannot use the title of Licensed Practical/Vocational Nurse until the licensing exam has been taken and passed, and the *license* (legal written permit) has been issued.

◆ Licensure

Licensure is a process by which a government agency gives permission for an individual to engage in an occupation or profession. It certifies that the individual has attained the minimum requirements necessary to protect the public safety and welfare. These requirements for a nursing license are outlined in the nurse practice act in each state.

The requirements for obtaining a license vary from state to state. In general, the requirements are as follows:

1. The applicant must have completed a minimum of 2 years of high school or its equivalent. (Many states now require a high school diploma.)
2. The applicant must have completed an approved course in practical/vocational nursing.
3. The applicant must be a citizen of the United States or have a current visa.

If these requirements have been met, the applicant will be eligible to take the examination. Following the exam the state board of nursing will review the application and issue the license.

All the work you have done up to this point was in preparation to take the licensing exam. The exam is designed to measure your knowledge in a number of areas. Passing of the exam certifies that you have enough knowledge to practice safely and competently as an entry-level licensed practical/vocational nurse (LPN/LVN).

At one time, each state had its own licensing exam. Today, there is a national exam developed by the National Council of State Boards of Nursing. The exam is the NCLEX-PN (National Council Licensure Examination for Practical Nurses—see Chapter 33). ⌘ The examination is administered by testing agencies throughout the community. The agencies provide the state board of nursing with the names of the individuals who have passed the examination. The Board is responsible for issuing the license. Licenses may not be issued to persons convicted of certain crimes, people who are mentally ill or people who are addicted to alcohol or other drugs. In Texas and California, the license is for vocational nursing. In all other states, nurses are known as licensed practical nurses.

Licenses are issued for a specific period of time, determined by the board that issued the license. It is the responsibility of the licensee to keep his or her license current and to meet any continuing education requirements. It is a violation of the nurse practice acts to function as an LPN/LVN without a current license.

SUSPENSION OR REVOCATION

The state board of nursing has a responsibility to protect the public. The board has the authority, under the nurse practice act, to suspend or revoke a nursing license if the licensee is found guilty of an offense. See Box 32-1 ◆ for some causes of license suspension or revocation.

When action is taken against a licensee, the nurse must be notified of the charges and given a hearing before the board. The individual (either in person or through an attorney) has the right to enter a defense.

In addition to suspending or revoking a license, the board can, for just cause, place a licensee on probation, refuse to issue or renew a license, or issue a letter of reprimand.

Actions taken against a licensed nurse are a matter of public record. In many states, the information can be obtained by any community member by telephone or from the board's Web site. Individual state boards can be linked from www.ncsbn.org/public/regulation/boards_of_nursing_board.htm.

STANDARDS OF CARE

Standards of care are used to determine what a nurse should or should not do. They can be used to determine if appropriate action was taken. All health care professionals must adhere to certain standards. A physician's standards of care are different from those of a registered nurse. Similarly, an LPN/LVN's standards differ from those of the RN. Each nurse must be aware of these standards of care to which they will be held accountable. Standards of care come from various sources: state licensing laws, nurse practice acts, nursing organizations, journal articles, and policies or procedures of individual facilities.

NURSE PRACTICE ACTS

Nurse practice acts, in general, provide a definition of who is a nurse, establish a board of nursing, outline the requirements for licensure, and define the circumstances for suspending and

---

BOX 32-1 CAUSES OF LICENSE SUSPENSION OR REVOCATION

◆ Conviction for
  ◆ Felony
  ◆ Moral turpitude or gross immorality
◆ Found guilty of
  ◆ Fraud or deceit in obtaining a license
  ◆ Willful neglect of a client
◆ Mental incompetence
◆ Chemical dependence or abuse, including alcohol
◆ Suspension or revocation of license in another jurisdiction
◆ Unfit by reason of neglect

MediaLink Code of Ethics

revoking licenses. These acts are specific for each state or territory. They facilitate recognition of possible conflicts between the scope of practice and the tasks being performed by the LPN/LVN. Although the acts differ from state to state, some standardized terminology is used. Understanding these terms will be helpful as you assume the role of a licensed nurse within your state. See Table 32-1 ◆ for terms and their explanation.

The National Association of Practical Nurse Education and Service (NAPNES) issued the following statement of the responsibilities of practice of the practical/vocational nurse, in its 1998 Code of Ethics for Licensed Practical/Vocational Nurses (NAPNES, 1998). Statements from professional organizations are not state law and so they merely serve as guidelines for practice. See Box 32-2 ◆ for statement.

HEALTH INSURANCE PORTABILITY AND ACCOUNTABILITY ACT (HIPPA)

HIPPA, the Health Insurance Portability and Accountability Act, was passed to control the use and disclosure of client-identifiable information. Its purposes are:

* To guarantee that persons leaving their jobs would not lose certain health care coverage
* To standardize how health information is collected and transmitted for claim submission
* To decrease fraud and abuse
* To guarantee security and privacy of health information

Compliance with HIPPA Privacy Standards was required by all health care agencies and providers by April 14, 2003. According to these standards, client information is controlled by the client and is protected by law. Clients alone can autho-

BOX 32-2 CODE OF ETHICS FOR THE LICENSED PRACTICAL/VOCATIONAL NURSE

The Licensed Practical and Licensed Vocational Nurse shall:

* Consider as a basic obligation the conservation of life and the prevention of disease.
* Promote and protect the physical, mental, emotional, and spiritual health of the client and his/her family.
* Fulfill all duties faithfully and efficiently.
* Function within established legal guidelines.
* Accept personal responsibility for his/her acts, and seek to merit the respect and confidence of all members of the health team.
* Hold in confidence all matters coming to his/her knowledge, in the practice of his/her profession, and in no way at no time violate this confidence.
* Give conscientious service and charge just remuneration.
* Learn and respect the religious and cultural beliefs of his/her client and of all people.
* Meet the obligation to the client by keeping abreast of current trends in health care through reading and continuing education.
* As a citizen of the United States of America, uphold the laws of the land and seek to promote legislation that will meet the health needs of its people.

Source: Reprinted by permission of the National Association of Practical Nurse Education and Service.

TABLE 32-1 COMMON TERMS USED IN NURSE PRACTICE ACTS

TERMS	EXPLANATION
Basic Nursing Care	Nursing care that is predictable and does not require modification, based on the knowledge and skills obtained during an educational program and those which can be safely performed by an LPN/LVN.
Basic Client Situation	Situations in which the client's condition is predictable and clinical condition requires only basic nursing care. Medical and nursing orders are continuously changing and do not contain complex modifications. The situation is determined by the RN.
Complex Nursing Situation	Client's clinical condition is not predictable and requires frequent changes in medical or nursing orders or complex modifications. Nursing care expectations are beyond that learned by the LPN/LVN during the educational program.
Delegated Medical Act	Doctor's orders given to the RN or LPN/LVN.
Delegated Nursing Act	Nursing orders given to an RN or LPN/LVN by an RN.
Direct Supervision	Supervisor is continuously present to coordinate, inspect, or direct nursing care.
General Supervision	Supervisor regularly coordinates, inspects, or directs nursing care. The supervisor is available within the building or by telephone.

rize release of their information, and it can be released only to individuals who have a business need to know. Some ways for health care providers to protect client information are listed in Box 32-3.

Compliance with HIPPA regulations is mandatory. Noncompliance can bring civil penalties of up to $25,000 per calender year for multiple violations of a single standard. There can also be heavy criminal penalties:

- Up to $50,000 and/or imprisonment for up to 1 year
- For false pretenses, $100,000 and/or imprisonment for up to 5 years
- For noncompliance for your commercial advantage, personal gain, or malicious harm, $250,000 and/or imprisonment for up to 10 years

BOX 32-3 PROTECTING THE PRIVACY OF CLIENT INFORMATION

Paper

- Do not leave paper unattended in an area where others can see it.
- Don't leave papers, specimens, labels, or forms with client information lying on counters, on carts in hallways, or on doors.
- Dispose of paper, addressograph plates, and labels by approved methods.
- Don't leave paper on printers, fax machines, copiers, or in trash bins in common areas or walkways.
- Always use a fax cover sheet with a confidentiality statement over the document.

Conversation

- Be sure you know to whom you are speaking before you release client information.
- Disclose information only to individuals with a business need to know and provide only the minimum necessary to accomplish the job.
- Keep your voice down and speak in a tone that others will not overhear.
- Don't leave information in clients' rooms.
- Knock before entering a client's room.
- When possible, close the client's doors or draw privacy curtains.
- Do not speak about client information in hallways, cafeterias, elevators, or any other public areas.

Computers

- Use privacy screens for monitors.
- Don't share your ID and password with anyone.
- Log out of programs when you finish using them.
- Use computers for business purposes only.
- Be sure monitors are not facing out to public view.

It is part of your job responsibility to report instances of suspected privacy policy violations. These would be reported to the supervisor or Privacy Officer. An anonymous Confidential Compliance Hotline is also available. Further information about HIPPA guidelines can be obtained through health care facilities and at the web site http://aspe.hhs.gov /admnsimp/.

 # Leadership

The transition from graduate to licensed nurse happens quickly. You will need to begin to think differently about yourself. **Leadership** is a process used to move a group toward setting and achieving goals. This definition is compatible with nursing leadership. The process can be used by anyone; therefore, anyone can, in theory, be a leader. As you begin your career, you will have the opportunity to observe nursing leaders. While watching and learning, you will begin to develop your own leadership style.

There are several leadership styles. Each one has good and not so good characteristics. There are situations in which one style may be more effective than another. Experienced leaders adapt their style in order to maximize their leadership effectiveness.

TYPES OF LEADERS

The Autocrat

The **autocratic** (authoritarian) leader makes unilateral decisions while dominating the team members. This approach can result in passive resistance from the team. This style requires constant control from the leader in order to have objectives met. The authoritarian approach generally is not successful in getting the best performance from a team. There are, however, some instances when the autocratic style may be more appropriate. For example, when there is a need for immediate action, this style may be the most effective.

Most people are familiar with the autocratic style and have little trouble adopting it. In some situations subordinates may actually prefer being directed by an autocrat.

The Laissez-Faire Manager

The **laissez-faire** manager (French for "let it be") exercises little control over the group. The manager leaves them alone to tackle their work, sort out their roles, and solve problems. This approach often leaves the team floundering, with little motivation or direction.

There are situations in which the laissez-faire approach is effective. It can be appropriate with highly motivated and skilled team members who have produced excellent work in the past. Once the leader has established the team as competent, confident, and motivated, it may be appropriate to back off and allow the team to function. By handing over ownership of the project, the leader empowers the team. Self-motivated

MediaLink **★LINK** Together Everyone Accomplishes More

teams can take ownership and will most likely achieve their goals.

The Democrat

The **democratic** leader makes decisions after consulting with team members. Although the team enters into the decision-making process, the leader still maintains control. The team is allowed to decide how the task will be accomplished and who will be responsible for each task. Being a democratic leader can be viewed positively or negatively.

The good democratic leader delegates wisely and encourages participation, but the leader never loses sight of the fact that the ultimate responsibility belongs to him or her. The leader values group discussion and input. The leader draws from the team members' strengths and knowledge in order to obtain the best performance from the team.

Poor democratic leaders can be seen as being unsure of themselves and their relationships with their subordinates, especially if it appears that everything is a matter of group decision. This type of leader is seen as not leading at all.

TEAM LEADING

The first leadership role you might experience as an LPN/LVN may be that of a **team leader.** In this role you will be responsible for guiding and directing care for a group of clients. You will also be responsible for supervising the members of the team, including nursing assistants.

The duties of the team leader include:

◆ Making assignments
◆ Taking report
◆ Making rounds and assessing clients
◆ Giving report to team members on assigned clients
◆ Assisting in administration of medications and treatments
◆ Facilitating team conferences
◆ Collaborating with an RN supervisor or clinical nurse specialist (CNS)

DELEGATION

The sign of a good leader is to know how and when to delegate. The leader will understand the scope of all team members so that delegation of tasks will be appropriate.

The first step in the **delegation** process is to prioritize activities and available resources. The purpose of delegation is efficiency. No one person can do all the work; therefore, some work must be passed on. It is important to remember that even though a task has been delegated, the ultimate responsibility for the task belongs to the nurse-leader.

Some leaders have difficulty in delegating. This presents several problems. First, the leader who does not delegate becomes overworked, tired, and ineffective. When delegation is not utilized, some team members become lazy or bored. Team members who are never given responsibility through delegation may feel that the leader is unappreciative of their contribution and think they are incapable; this leads to a breakdown of the team.

Many facilities have *unlicensed assistive personnel (UAP)*, people who work alongside the LVN/LPN. You may be called on to supervise their performance and delegate tasks to them. It is important that you provide good instruction and feedback so that they are able to complete the tasks appropriately. Many LPN/LVNs have found unlicensed help to be very valuable. UAP should be treated with respect and encouraged to use their skills as a career ladder to licensed nursing.

clinical ALERT

UAP are tremendously valuable and can be your extra pair of hands. Remember, though, that if you do not treat them as valuable members of the team, they may not work as part of the team when you most need them.

Groups with a leader who makes use of delegation benefit in the following ways:

◆ Their sense of responsibility increases.
◆ Their job satisfaction is heightened.
◆ Their knowledge is increased.

The reason why leaders may delegate poorly or not at all may be that they simply do not know how. Delegation skills can be learned and perfected. Delegation works best when assignments are specific. Team members may be afraid to accept the assignment for fear of failure. They need to have the opportunity to ask questions and seek clarification before being expected to take on the task. They need to know they can trust the leader to support them in their efforts. The leader should be ready to reward the group for successful completion of delegated activities. Group members whose contributions are appreciated will be motivated to accept further responsibility. A simple word of thanks can go along way.

Ultimately, delegation promotes happiness within the group; morale will improve, as will productivity. In other words, it will help the team function at its peak.

 ## Reporting Techniques

In nursing giving report is very much related to delegation. Reporting to other nurses at the change of shifts is both delegation of responsibility and an accounting of what has been done.

SHIFT REPORT

Shift report is the most effective way to pass information from one shift to another. The report can take on many forms. It may be oral face-to-face with the staff arriving for the next shift. It may be done in a room or as a part of walking rounds. The report may be taped by the nurse going off duty to be listened to by the on-coming nurse. It may be written. There are advantages and disadvantages of each type of reporting. No matter which form a facility uses, some important issues must be addressed. Each form of report is discussed below, with its advantages and disadvantages.

Taped Report

Taped report has been adopted by many facilities in an effort to save time and provide floor coverage during report. The nurses going off duty can tape the report on their clients one at a time, leaving the other staff to provide coverage for all the clients. Nurses coming on shift can listen to the tape while the previous shift continues to cover the clients. There are a few disadvantages of taped reports. Sometimes they are difficult to hear or understand. Also, questions must be saved until the end, when they must be addressed to the nurse who may be anxious to go off duty. Box 32-4 ◆ provides guidelines for giving and taking a taped report.

Oral Report

Oral report is very much like a taped report. It can be delivered in a report room or while the nurses are making client rounds. Advantages of an oral report are that questions can be addressed immediately. If it is done during rounds, clients can be checked at the same time. Disadvantages are that the report can't start until all staff has arrived. If clients are in semiprivate rooms, confidentiality may be breached when report is given in the presence of other clients or visitors.

WRITTEN REPORT

Written report is frequently used in long-term care facilities. Each nurse's station has a report or communication book. Because residents have a *lower acuity* (less immediately threatening conditions), there is less to report. The nurses are well acquainted with the residents, since they been under their care for a long time. Written report should be concise. State the resident's name, the problem, what has been done, and what if anything needs to be done by the on-coming shift. Before the entry, list time and date. If more details are needed, the on-coming nurse can be referred to the chart.

BOX 32-4
NURSING CARE CHECKLIST

TAPED REPORTS

Giving Report on Tape

- ☑ Give your name/shift/date
- ☑ Room number
- ☑ Client's full name
- ☑ Age of client
- ☑ Diagnosis/Admission date/Surgical date
- ☑ Primary or admitting physician
- ☑ Proceed with information. Remember that the nurse coming on may not know the client as well as you do. Be complete. Don't drag. Give pertinent information. Most nurses follow the Kardex and then add changes. For example:
  Complains of gas pains/What did you do?
  BP was elevated/What was it?/What did you do?
  No Code
  Specimens needed
  Accucheck AC/HS/What were the blood sugars, and was insulin coverage given?
  Drainage from NGT/JP/Hemovac/How much teaching?/Did client demonstrate/understand dressing change?
  Pet Peeve: Don't belittle the client on tape. If you don't like a client, keep it to yourself. Personal comments about clients make the nurse look unprofessional.
- ☑ Remember not to mumble or yawn too much. You can always stop the tape if you forgot something. Put the tape on pause, gather information, and restart the recorder.
- ☑ If you have had a particularly hard shift and haven't finished something like a dressing which was not a priority, make sure to let the next shift know. Don't let them just find it. You need to be honest. Don't let it become a habit to leave things undone.
- ☑ *Insight:* Clients sometimes like to play nurse against nurse, shift against shift. Don't play into it. Remember nursing is continuity of care and it is a team effort even if it happens on someone else's shift. If infighting occurs, it is the client who suffers or gains.
- ☑ End on a good note—have a good day!

Receiving Shift Information from a Taped Report

- ☑ Taped messages can be difficult to hear at first. Tune out other noises and concentrate. It may be necessary to let the staff know you can't hear, especially if they are socializing. Ask others for help if you can't make out words. Nurses usually know their clients and have a trained ear.

Receiving Change of Shift information from a Taped Report

- ☑ Taped report can be difficult to hear at first. It may be necessary to let the staff know you can't hear, especially if they are socializing.
- ☑ Listen for pertinent data and changes:
  Age/diagnosis
  Temperature elevation, BP changes
  Altered mental status
  Dressing changes
  Unusual problems
  Pain/whether medication is controlling it
- ☑ Information such as diet/VS/I&O can be obtained from the Kardex©, so don't be too worried if you don't get all the details.

Paperwork Reponsibilities

You may have heard seasoned nurses complain about the increasing amount of paperwork. Over the years, changes have been made to control the amount of writing a nurse must do. Narrative notes have been replaced with flow sheets and other forms of abbreviated charting. However, increased regulations, licensing requirements, and government restrictions have created additional need for documentation. See Chapters 8 and 9 for more information about types of documentation. ∞

PHYSICIAN'S ORDERS

Physician's orders are a part of the client's medical record. As a nurse, you need to have an order for all areas of client care. The client cannot even be admitted to the hospital without an order from a physician. Table 32-2 ◆ provides clinical guidelines for use when calling the physician.

Physician's orders take different forms:

◆ Handwritten by the physician during hospital rounds
◆ Verbal orders
◆ Preprinted or standing orders to cover admissions for certain conditions or surgeries (e.g., postpartum care follow-ing an uncomplicated delivery or total knee replacement surgery)
◆ Telephone orders (see Chapter 9 for additional information on taking phone orders, and Chapter 21 for orders specific to medications) ∞

Transcription of Orders

Some facilities employee a clerical person, whose job it is to transcribe physician's orders. This individual may have the title of ward or unit secretary or ward clerk. If no unit secretaries are employed on evening and night shift or in long-term care facilities, the LPN/LVN may be expected to transcribe physicians' orders for their clients.

Handwritten orders may be difficult to read. With practice, though, you will learn the commonalities of a physician's handwriting and will be able to read what has been written.

clinical ALERT

Seek a second opinion if you are having trouble deciphering an order—never guess. When in doubt, seek clarification from the physician. Never carry out an unclear order until it has been clarified.

TABLE 32-2	CONFLICT RESOLUTION STRATEGIES	
STRATEGIES	**DESCRIPTION**	**USES**
Competition	Winner takes all; results in a win–lose situation	During an emergency when there is no time for discussion **Situation:** During a code blue situation; someone must direct the code team without discussion.
Accommodation	One person in the group is willing to yield to the other	When preserving relationships; or encouraging others to express themselves and learn by actions **Situation:** Used by two team leaders when deciding who will get the extra float nurse.
Avoidance	Lose–lose, one side denied that the problem exists or withdraws so that there is no active resolution. Nurses use avoidance as primary strategy for resolution of conflicts	When others may resolve the conflict more effectively; both sides see issue as minor or the negative impact is too costly to meet issue head on **Situation:** After a heated discussion with a physician, a nurse asks another to make rounds until he has time to calm down.
Compromise	Negotiation, trade-offs; each person gets something and gives up something; win–lose/win–lose for both sides	When there is a need to reach an agreement between equally empowered sides. Conflicts resolved by finding a common ground **Situation:** A nurse volunteers to stay over to cover a shift if another colleague agrees to come early.
Collaboration	Both parties meet problem on an even playing field. Each has equal concern for the issues, allows everyone to win by identifying areas of agreement and differences. Alternatives are evaluated and solutions are selected. There is full support and commitment from both sides.	Can be used to solve a previously irreconcilable and long-standing problem **Situation:** A manager assigns two feuding nurses to work together to solve chronic unit problems.

Note: Nurses use avoidance as a primary strategy for resolution of conflicts.

Medication orders can present a particular problem. When the spelling of a medication is in question, refer to the PDR (*Physician's Desk Reference*) or a list of commonly prescribed medications. With the number of new drugs being developed and the use of both generic and trade names, it is impossible to know all drugs by sight. Use available resources to protect your clients from receiving an incorrect medication.

Verbal and telephone orders are taken by a licensed nurse and recorded on the physician order sheet. Policies regarding verbal and phone orders differ from facility to facility.

It is important for the LPN/LVN to know the state board policy on verbal and phone orders. These policies vary from state to state. Federal Hospital Certification regulation 42 CFR 482.223 I(2)(i) states that when telephone or oral orders must be used, they must be: "Accepted only by personnel that are authorized to do so by the medical staff, and policies and procedures, such rulings must be consistent with Federal and State laws."

Orders given by telephone or verbally have an increased opportunity for error. Clarify the order by repeating it back to the physician. This gives the nurse and the physician the opportunity to hear the order and make corrections if necessary. Verbal or telephone orders should be written immediately. Verbal and phone orders must be signed by the physician. Each facility will have a policy as to when the orders must be signed; policies may vary between one facility and the next.

INCIDENT REPORTS

Incident report (or occurrence report) is completed when client care was not consistent with expected standards of care. Issues involve omitted medications or treatments, or medications administration that violated one of the "five rights." Any unusual occurrence, one that did cause or may have caused harm, needs to be documented on an incident report. Injury to a client, employee, or visitor also requires a report.

Incident reports do not become a part of the client medical record. They are usually filed with the risk management department.

When completing an incident report, be sure to include all pertinent details. List time, date, and an objective observation of the incident. Guilt should not be admitted. Other staff members who witnessed the incident or were involved should also be listed. The completed report should be turned over to the supervisor or individual designated by the facility to investigate.

The purpose of the incident report is to help the facility prevent future problems through correction and education. When the incident is reported in the medical chart, the completion of the incident report is usually not documented. See Figure 32-1 ◆ for an example of an incident report.

◆ Conflict Resolution

Conflict can be defined as disagreement or antagonism between groups, individuals, or ideas. The presence of conflict is not necessarily a negative situation. Well-managed conflicts can stimulate healthy competition, can bring new ideas to the table and can identify legitimate differences and problems within the organization.

Most of us were taught as children to manage conflicts passively. We were sent to the corner or "time-out" when we couldn't get along. In nursing, conflicts cannot be ignored. Instead, they must be dealt with and managed no matter how difficult that might be.

Managing conflicts is not an automatic skill for most people, but it can be learned. The ability to manage conflicts is a critical skill which a nurse must develop. Use of these skills can help the nurse to be more productive.

There are several common approaches to conflict resolution. It is important to select a strategy that is appropriate to the situation. Frequently, nurses select strategies with which they are comfortable, rather than those that may be more effective. The conflict resolution strategy most frequently used by staff nurses is avoidance. Table 32-3 lists approaches to conflict resolution and situations in which they are used.

STAGES OF CONFLICT

On-the-job conflicts produce reactions within the person, much like any other psychosocial problem. There are six stages of conflict:

1. *Disbelief* is an initial emotional reaction. This frequently happens when values that are held in high regard are disagreed with or discounted.
2. *Disconnectedness*. This stage follows the shock of the first stage. The individual feels confused and taken back.
3. *Obsession*. The individual becomes obsessed with the situation, and soon it is all the person can think about. Many times, this results in inability to sleep; wakeful nights are spent thinking about what to do.
4. *Frenzied activity* follows. Many people find this a way of reducing the bitterness, pain, and frustration they feel. The conflicted person may acquire boundless energy, working endlessly to seek information that will help him or her understand the problem. Colleagues are consulted one after another, trying to redefine the situation. The individual aggressively takes on new tasks, or may be involved in numerous activities simultaneously.
5. *Balance or burnout*. As the frenzied search for clues subsides, the individual either begins to reestablish balance or succumbs to symptoms of burnout—withdrawal, depression, and apathy. In intense conflicts, the individual may turn the negative feelings inward. When this occurs, purposeful alienation follows: the individual places emotional and perhaps even physical space between self and colleagues. This is a self-preservation move.
6. *Caution*. A caution is adopted as the individual controls verbalization and self-preservation. This move provides a rest or refuge for all involved parties. Once the conflict is

CONFIDENTIAL REPORT OF UNUSUAL OCCURRENCE
NOT a part of the Medical Record - Please forward to RISK MANAGEMENT

I. (COMPLETE IF ADDRESSOGRAPH UNAVAILABLE)

PATIENT/VISITOR_____ PHYSICIAN _____

MEDICAL RECORD #_____ DATE OF BIRTH _____

ADDRESSOGRAPH

II. DATE OF OCCURRENCE _____ TIME OF OCCURRENCE _____ LOCATION (ROOM OR FLOOR) _____

NAME OF M.D. NOTIFIED_____PATIENT AWARE OF OCCURRENCE: YES___NO___FAMILY AWARE OF OCCURRENCE: YES___NO___

REPORT COMPLETED BY_____OTHERS FAMILIAR WITH OCCURRENCE _____

III. ADMITTING DIAGNOSIS _____

PATIENT CONDITION PRIOR TO OCCURRENCE: ALERT_____ ASLEEP_____ ANESTHETIZED_____ DISORIENTED_____ OTHER_____

IF SEDATIVE/NARCOTICS/DIURETICS GIVEN IN LAST 12 HOURS (WHERE APPLICABLE) PLEASE COMPLETE: (MED, DOSE, TIME)

IV. EVENT

FALLS
- 100 Unobserved Fall
- 101 Assisted to Floor
- 102 Fell from Bed
- 103 Fell from Table/Equipment
- 104 Fell in Bathroom
- 105 Walking/Standing/Slip & Fall
- 106 Sitting Commode/Wheelchair
- 107 Restrained Prior to Fall
- 108 Restrained After Fall
- 109 Bed Rails Up (1 2 3 4)
- 110 Bed Rails Down (1 2 3 4)
- 112 Visitor Fall
- 113 Outpatient Fall
- 119 Other_____

BURNS
- 120 Electrical/Chemical Burn
- 121 Spill
- 122 Fire
- 129 Other_____

ALTERCATION/COMPLAINTS
- 130 Pt/Family/Employee/Visitor
- 131 Complaint-Waiting Time
- 132 Complaint-Billing Services
- 133 Complaint-Food Services
- 134 Complaint-Housekeeping/Ancillary
- 135 Complaint-Nursing
- 136 Complaint-Medical Staff
- 137 Complaint-Security
- 139 Other_____

MISCELLANEOUS
- 140 Suicide/Attempt
- 141 Left AMA/Elopement
- 142 Equipment-Struck/Failure
- 143 Property Loss/Damage
- 144 Unexpected Death
- 145 Non-Compliant Smoking
- 148 Development of Pressure Ulcer
- 149 Other_____

MEDICATIONS Drug_____
- 150 Order (Computer Entry)
- 151 Wrong Time
- 152 Wrong Dosage
- 153 Wrong Route
- 154 Wrong Drug
- 155 Wrong Patient
- 156 Omission
- 157 Adverse Drug Reaction
- 158 Prescribing Error
- 159 Other_____

INTRAVENOUS Sol._____
- 160 Infiltration
- 161 Wrong Rate
- 162 Wrong Solution
- 163 Wrong Time
- 164 Order (Computer Entry)
- 165 Infected Site/Phlebitis
- 169 Other_____

BLOOD TRANSFUSION
- 170 Allergic/Adverse Reaction
- 171 Delay in Administration
- 172 Incorrect Flow Rate
- 173 Infiltration
- 174 Omitted/Patient Refusal
- 175 Wrong Amount
- 176 Wrong/Omitted Filter
- 177 Wrong Component
- 178 Biological Product Deviation
- 179 Other_____

PATHOLOGY
- 180 Reference Laboratory Error
- 181 Lost/Mishandled Specimen
- 182 Specimen Collection Error
- 183 Cytology/Biopsy Discrepancy
- 184 Biopsy/Resection Discrepancy
- 185 Autopsy Suggests Serious Clinical Discrepancy
- 186 Frozen Section/Pathological Discrepancy
- 187 Error Performing Test/Error Reporting Results
- 188 Delayed Draw
- 189 Hematoma Following Draw
- 190 Other_____

OR/PACU/OPS/WOR
- 200 Removal Foreign Body
- 210 Incorrect Count-Sponge/Needle/Instr
- 202 X-rays Taken/Deferred
- 203 Arrest
- 204 Wrong Pt/Side/Site/Procedure
- 205 OPS Pt Admitted Post-Op
- 206 Unplanned Organ Repair/Removal
- 207 Lac/Tear/Puncture-Organ/Body Part
- 208 Canceled Surg-Prep/Equipment Problem
- 209 Unplanned Return to OR
- 210 Surgery Delayed
- 211 Consent Incorrect/Incomplete/Not Done
- 212 Reddened Area
- 213 Unsterile Situation
- 214 Specimen Problem
- 215 Eye Irritation/Injury
- 216 Post Arterial Hematoma
- 217 Improper Discharge
- 219 Other_____

ANESTHESIA
- 220 Unexpected Arrest
- 221 Canceled Surgery After Induction
- 222 Injury/Death Post Induction
- 223 Tooth/Face/Lip/Mandible Damage
- 224 CNS Injury/Brain Damage
- 225 Unplanned Transfer to Special Care Unit
- 226 Aspiration
- 229 Other_____

EMERGENCY DEPARTMENT
- 230 Arrives DOA After Discharge/Seen in ED within Past 7 Days
- 231 Seen for Complication Post Treatment/Procedure from Prev. Hospitalization
- 232 Left AMA
- 239 Other_____

OB/GYN/INFANT CARE
- 240 Delivery Occurred Outside L&D Area
- 241 Mother Transferred to ICU
- 241 Unplanned Return to Surgery
- 243 Stirrup Related Injury
- 244 Delivery Unattended by any Physician
- 245 Blood Loss > 1500 cc
- 246 Cord Blood Gas pH <7.0
- 247 Cardiac/Respiratory Arrest
- 248 Infant Seizures in Delivery Room
- 249 Apgar Score 5 or Less at 5 Minutes
- 250 Unusual Condition - Child
- 251 Infant Injury-skull fx/paralysis/palsy
- 252 Transfer From NB Nursery to ISC/NICU
- 253 Instrumented Delivery-Injury
- 259 Other_____

ADULT/PEDIATRIC CARE
- 260 Unexpected Tx – Higher Care Level
- 261 Significant Neurosensory/Functional Deficit/Intractable Pain not Present upon Admit
- 262 Acute MI/CVA within 48 hours of Surgery/Procedure
- 263 Death within 48 hours of Surgery/Procedure
- 264 Nosocomial Infection Prolonging Stay or Complicating Pt's Condition > 5 days
- 265 Patient Found Unresponsive
- 266 Self Extubation
- 267 Arrest – Code Team Activation
- 268 Soft Tissue Injury
- 269 Other_____

TESTS/TREATMENTS
- 270 Wrong Patient
- 271 Wrong Test/Treatment
- 272 Treatment Delayed
- 273 MD Ordered-Not Done
- 274 Complication Resulting in Injury
- 275 Computer Entry
- 276 Infection Control issue
- 279 Other_____

RADIOLOGY/RAD ONC/IMAGING
- 280 Complication Requiring Surgical Correction
- 281 New Onset Nerve Deficit
- 282 Reaction to Contrast Agent
- 283 Overexposure to Radiation
- 284 Cardiac/Respiratory Arrest
- 285 Treatment Delayed Worsening Condition
- 286 Unplanned Repeat Diagnostic Procedure
- 287 Monitored Inadequately
- 288 X-ray Inaccurately Read
- 289 Equipment Failure
- 290 Lack of Prep-Cancel Procedure
- 291 Wrong Pt/Side/Site/Prodedure
- 299 Other_____

V. OUTCOME

SEVERITY OF OUTCOME
- 350 No Injury/Unaffected
- *351 Minor Injury
- *352 Major Injury/Consequential

*_SPECIFY INJURY BELOW –

GENERAL
- 300 Delay in Therapy
- 301 Embolism
- 302 Reaction/Toxic Effect
- 303 Death
- 304 Prolonged Hospital Stay
- 305 Neurological Sensory
- 306 Decubitus
- 307 Arrest/CPR
- 309 Other_____

OBSTETRICAL
- 310 Unusually Low Apgar
- 311 Fetal Injury
- 312 Fetal Death
- 313 Maternal Injury
- 314 Maternal Death
- 319 Other_____

SKELETAL
- 320 Fracture
- 321 Dislocation
- 322 Teeth
- 323 Sprain
- 329 Other_____

TISSUE
- 330 Hematoma/Contusion
- 331 Necrosis
- 332 Laceration
- 333 Fistula
- 334 Dehiscence
- 335 Abrasion/Blister
- 336 Swelling
- 337 Reddened Area/Ecchymosis
- 338 Skin Tear
- 339 Other_____

VI. BRIEF COMMENTS IF NECESSARY _____

1004952 (9/01)

Figure 32-1. ◆ Example of an incident report.

TABLE 32-3	GUIDELINES WHEN CALLING A PHYSICIAN	
TIMING	**CRITICAL THINKING AND PREPARATION**	

Prior to calling	1. Why am I calling the physician? What do I want from the physician?
	2. Have I seen and assessed this client myself before I call?
	3. Are there standing orders?
	4. Do I have at hand:
	  a. The chart
	  b. List of current meds, IV fluids, and labs
	  c. Most recent vital signs
	  d. If reporting lab work, date and time this test was done and results of previous tests for comparison
	  e. Code status
	5. Have I read the most recent MD progress notes and notes from the nurse who worked the previous shift?
	6. Have I discussed the call with my charge nurse? Are there any other nurses in the unit who also need to talk to this same physician?	

During the call	7. When making the call:
	  a. Introduce yourself, unit, client, and room number.
	  b. State admitting diagnosis, which physician is the attending, and date of admission.
	  c. Briefly state the problem, what it is, when it happened or started and how severe it is, and how it was treated if it previously occurred in the hospitalization.
	8. Read back all telephone orders received from the MD prior to documentation in the medical record for clarification.
	9. Document the name of the physician (e.g., Dr. H. Smith) you spoke with, the date and time of call, and a brief summary of the conversation.
	10. Thank the physician. Ask if there is anything else.
	  a. If there are other nurses who also need to talk to the same physician, let the physician know and hand the phone over to the next nurse.
	  b. If there are no other nurses who also need to talk to the same physician, end the call.	

resolved positively, the individual may gain personal insight into how to handle future conflicts.

Nurses will have to be prepared to deal with conflicts in all areas of nursing practice. Knowing how and when to use appropriate strategies will promote successful conflict resolution.

Nursing Trends

Throughout the years the delivery of nursing services has continued to change. It is important that nursing professionals understand these trends and be proactive in making personal changes to meet the needs of their careers.

NURSING CARE DELIVERY METHODS

The oldest delivery method of nursing services is the *case method,* in which a nurse is responsible for care provided for clients during one shift. Intensive care units frequently operate under the case method. Private-duty nurses and home care nurses can also be described as nursing by the case method.

In the **functional nursing** system, each team member is assigned specific tasks or functions. Although functional nursing is efficient, it can create fragmented delivery of client care. Functional nursing also makes it somewhat more difficult to establish a therapeutic relationship between nurse and

client, because of the large number of team care professionals interacting with the client.

In *primary nursing,* a professional nurse has total responsibility for a group of clients. This is a more recent development in delivery methods. Primary nursing in the purest sense gives responsibility to the nurse 24 hours a day 7 days a week, from admission through discharge. The purpose of this method is to provide continuity and coordination of care. If the RN is not physically in attendance, the care may be delegated to an associate (another RN or an LPN/LVN). Many hospitals ascribe to primary nursing, but in a way that resembles the case method. While the nurse is at work, the responsibility for the assigned client is his or hers.

Team nursing has been used since the early 1950s. It was replaced with primary nursing in the 1970s. The purpose of this concept was to reduce the fragmentation that was present in the functional method. Team nursing is again becoming popular given the nursing shortage and low ratio of nurses to clients. The nursing team in the acute hospital is usually directed by an RN. The remainder of the team is made up of LPN/LVNs and UAP (e.g., nursing assistants, client care technicians). A nursing unit may have two or more nursing teams caring for 10 or more clients. Team members work together to use their diverse skills and education to best care for the assigned clients. Care planning is done in team meetings in which all members have input.

MEN IN NURSING

Throughout history, men have made significant contributions to the nursing profession. Current trends show that increased numbers of men are entering the nursing profession. At one time, men sought positions in specialty areas such as psychiatry, emergency and trauma nursing, correctional institutions and rehabilitation, as well as medical–surgical nursing. They sought administrative positions. More recently, there has been increased interest by men in hospice work, pediatrics, neonatology, and teaching in schools of nursing. More men entering the profession have brought a different perspective and an increase in salary and benefits.

No matter whether a nurse is male or female, or what the work setting (acute hospital, ambulatory care, specialty, or long-term care), it is important to be aware of current trends. Being well informed will help you to be a more effective nurse and a valuable member of the health care community, as you carry out the roles and responsibilities of an LPN/LVN. Box 32-5 ◆ describes these roles and responsibilities.

 ## Community Service

Your community has provided you with many opportunities. If you received your training in a public institution, your community has supported you in reaching your goal to become a nurse. It is now time that you do the same for others.

BOX 32-5 ROLES AND RESPONSIBILITIES OF LPN/LVN

- ◆ Recognize the LPN/LVN's role in the health care delivery system and articulate that role with those of other health care team members.
- ◆ Maintain accountability for one's own nursing practice within the ethical and legal framework.
- ◆ Serve as a client advocate.
- ◆ Accept the role in maintaining and developing standards of practice in providing health care.
- ◆ Seek further growth through educational opportunities.

Community service is one very important way to fulfill this challenge. There are many opportunities for nurses to contribute to the community. You can volunteer to use your skills at schools, community activities, senior centers, or churches. You can provide community health care education, or you can become involved with activities such as Race for the Cure, Relay for Life, or a Memory Walk. These give you the opportunity to raise money for the sponsoring agencies, educate your sponsors, and provide you with an opportunity to exercise. Giving back to the community will benefit you and others and strengthen you emotionally and professionally.

Note: The bibliography listings for this and all chapters have been compiled at the back of the book.

Chapter Review

Key Terms by Topics

Use the audio glossary feature of either the CD-ROM or the Companion Website to hear the correct pronunciation of the following key terms.

Licensure
licensure

Leadership
leadership, autocratic, laissez-faire, democratic, team leader, delegation

Reporting techniques
shift report, taped report, oral report, written report

Paperwork responsibilities
incident report

Conflict resolution
conflict

Nursing trends
functional nursing

Key Points

* Licensure certifies that the individual has attained the minimum requirements necessary to protect the public safety and welfare.
* Licenses may not be issued to persons convicted of certain crimes, to people who are mentally ill, or to people who are addicted to alcohol or other drugs.
* The State Board of Nursing has a responsibility to protect the public.
* The Board has the authority, under the nurse practice act, to suspend or revoke a nursing license, if the licensee is found guilty of an offense.
* Nurse practice acts provide a definition for nurse, establish a board of nursing, outline the requirements for licensure, and provide the circumstances for suspension and revocation of the license.
* The sign of a good leader is to know how and when to delegate.
* The leader must understand the scope of practice of all team members so that delegation of tasks will be appropriate.
* Incident report is completed when client care was not consistent with standards for expected care.

EXPLORE MediaLink

Additional interactive resources for this chapter can be found on the Companion Website at www.prenhall.com/ramont. Click on Chapter 32 and "Begin" to select the activities for this chapter.

For chapter-related NCLEX-style questions and an audio glossary, access the accompanying CD-ROM in this book.

For Further Study

For admission, transfer, and discharge documents, see Chapter 8.
For more information about documentation, see Chapter 9.
For orders specific to medications and transcription of orders, see Chapter 21.
For more about the NCLEX-PN examination, see Chapter 33.

NCLEX-PN Exam Preparation

TEST-TAKING TIP

Always focus on the client's feelings first. If an answer reflects the client's feelings, select that answer.

1. The most frequent conflict resolution strategy used by staff nurses is:
   a. Collaboration
   b. Accommodation
   c. Avoidance
   d. Competition

2. A new LPN is assigned to your unit. She appears to have a great need to be liked. Which of the following conflict resolution strategies will this individual likely use?
   a. Collaboration
   b. Accommodation
   c. Avoidance
   d. Competition

3. Your hospital has begun to hire unlicensed assistive personnel to alleviate some of the workload of the licensed nurses. You will be delegating some activities to the UAP. The most frequent reason delegated activities are not completed as expected is:
   a. The need to avoid conflict
   b. Inappropriate supervision
   c. Poor UAP attitudes
   d. Inadequate communication

4. Which of the following job titles requires a license to practice?
   a. Care partner
   b. Nursing assistant
   c. LPN or LVN
   d. Orderly

5. You have been studying accountability in nursing as it relates to delegation of tasks. One of your classmates asks you to define the term. Which of the following definitions most accurately describes *accountability*?
   a. The provision of guidance, direction, evaluation, and follow-up by a licensed nurse
   b. Being responsible and answerable for actions of self and others in the context of delegation
   c. Delegating nursing activities to be performed by an individual consistent with his or her licensed scope of practice
   d. Transferring to a competent individual the authority to perform a selected nursing task in a selected situation

6. You are working as a certified nursing assistant on weekends while enrolled in your vocational nursing program. Your supervisor knows that you are a student and asks you to pass medications that she had prepared. Of the following, which is the best response to her request?
   a. "I can't do that because I am not licensed yet. I would think you would know better than to ask me."

   b. "I have been trained to pass medications in my program. I can pass them, but you will have to sign the MAR."
   c. "I have my own work to do—I don't have time."
   d. "I'm sorry, medications are not within the scope of practice for a nursing assistant. Perhaps I could assist you by giving your clients their baths or making their beds."

7. You have been discussing leadership styles in class. Your instructor describes a manager who leaves the unit staff alone to tackle their work, sort out their roles, and solve problems, leaving the team floundering with little motivation or direction. You know that this is a description of which style of management?
   a. Autocratic
   b. Laissez-faire
   c. Authoritative
   d. Democratic

8. The nursing system in which establishing a therapeutic relationship between nurse and client is somewhat more difficult because of the large number of team care professionals interacting with the client is known as:
   a. Team nursing
   b. Primary nursing
   c. Functional nursing
   d. Case method

9. Under the nurse practice act, who has the responsibility to suspend or revoke a nursing license?
   a. The National Council for Licensure Examination for Practical Nurses (NCLEX-PN)
   b. The attorney general of the state in which the license was issued
   c. The State Board of Nursing in the state in which the license was issued
   d. The superior court judge if the nurse is convicted of a felony

10. You are assigned to a nursing team that consists of an RN, two unlicensed assistive personnel (UAP), and you (the LPN). You observe that both assistants have left the floor for their lunch break at the same time. What is your most appropriate action to remedy the situation?
    a. Have them paged on the overhead pager to return to the floor, and tell them never to do that again.
    b. When they return, inquire as to why they both left at the same time, and discuss with them the floor policy and the safety issues that may have occurred.
    c. When they return, tell them that you will have to report them to the RN.
    d. Report their behavior to the RN, mentioning how irresponsible they are being.

Answers for Review Questions appear in Appendix IV.

Preparing to Take the Licensure Exam

Chapter 33

SHARING experiences

Practicing healthy coping skills and positive thinking has helped me to reduce the stress and anxiety that surfaces before a test. I know that studying the NCLEX-PN workbook now will equip me with the advantage of being familiar with the different types of questions. In addition, it will give me the confidence that comes from preparation.

Shawna Thurman, LVN student, Austin Community College, Austin, TX.

MediaLink

www.prenhall.com/ramont

Use the address above to access the free, interactive Companion Website created for this textbook. Get hints, instant feedback, and textbook references to chapter-related NCLEX-style questions. Link to other interesting sites.

Audio Glossary:

Use the Companion Website, or the CD-ROM disk enclosed with your textbook, to hear the pronunciation of key terms in the chapter.

LEARNING outcomes

After completing this chapter, you will be able to:

- Identify the time to begin studying for the NCLEX-PN Examination.
- Describe the purpose of the examination.
- Explain how the National Council of State Boards of Nursing develops the test plan and the test.
- Identify how to get a copy of the current NCLEX-PN test plan.
- Explain the concept of a multistate compact.
- Describe the four categories of client needs and their subcategories.
- Describe selected aspects of the test itself.
- Develop an individualized plan for reviewing for the NCLEX-PN.
- Assess personal readiness for the examination.
- Explain how to apply to take the examination.
- Describe how to overcome test anxiety.
- Describe what to do the day before, day of, and during the examination to increase the chances of success on the examination.

From the minute you enter nursing school until you graduate, you must be aware that, in order to practice as a licensed practical/vocational nurse (LPN/LVN):

1. You need to acquire a certain body of nursing knowledge and nursing skills.
2. You must pass the National Council Licensure Examination for Practical/Vocational Nurses (NCLEX-PN).

The purpose of this examination is to protect the public by ensuring that all licensed entry-level nurses have the competencies they need to practice safely and effectively.

◆ Development of the NCLEX-PN

The National Council of State Boards of Nursing, Inc. (NCSBN) develops the NCLEX-PN based on a test plan. In developing the test plan and then the test, the NCSBN considers the legal scope of practical/vocational nursing practice as governed by each state's laws and regulations, including the various nurse practice acts. The NCSBN also conducts a vocational nursing job analysis study every three years (e.g., 2000, 2003). This analysis is also used to develop the framework for the current NCLEX-PN. Test questions on the NCLEX-PN focus on the job tasks identified as those normally carried out by entry-level PNs in their first year of nursing employment. The test plan is available on the National Council from the National State Boards of Nursing Web site: www.ncsbn.org or by writing the National Council of State Boards of Nursing, 676 St. Clair Street, Suite 550, Chicago, Illinois 60611-2921.

AVAILABILITY OF THE NCLEX-PN

The NCLEX-PN is available in every state in the United States and in the various territories of the United States, including the District of Columbia, American Samoa, Guam, the Northern Mariana Islands, Puerto Rico, and the U.S. Virgin Islands. As of 2002, The Board of Nursing in Puerto Rico had its own unique examination in Spanish. However, students could elect to take the NCLEX-PN, which is in English. The fact that these states and territories use the NCLEX-PN to assist them in making licensure decisions makes it possible for you to get licensure by endorsement from a state board of nursing in a state other than the one in which you took the examination, should you decide to work in another state.

Multistate Compact

In addition to endorsement, the concept of a **multistate compact** became reality when, in 2000, Utah became the first state to enact multistate licensure legislation. Arkansas, Maryland, North Carolina, Texas, Iowa, Nebraska, South Dakota, Wisconsin, Mississippi, Maine, Delaware, and Idaho quickly joined Utah. If the state where you pass your NCLEX-

PN is part of this multistate compact, you can practice in another state that is part of the compact, as long as you follow the nurse practice act and the rules and regulations pertaining to the act. See also Chapter 2. ⚭

◆ Understanding the NCLEX-PN Plan

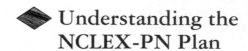

COGNITIVE LEVELS OF QUESTIONS

The NCLEX-PN questions are developed at the cognitive levels of knowledge, comprehension, application, and analysis. Table 33-1 ◆ describes the cognitive levels of testing and provides some examples. Your nursing instructors will give you tests and examinations at these cognitive levels throughout your nursing courses. These will help prepare you for the examination and be more comfortable with each level of question.

TEST PLAN FRAMEWORK

"Client Needs" was chosen as the framework of the test plan. Client needs is a universal concept that is applicable to a variety of clients in a wide spectrum of health care settings.

Client Needs

The test plan is organized around four categories of client needs across the life span in a variety of settings:

1. Safe, effective care environment
2. Health promotion and maintenance
3. Psychosocial integrity
4. Physiologic integrity

Box 33-1 ◆ lists the categories and subcategories of the test, and the percentage of questions given for each category.

A number of concepts and processes that students learn well before graduation are integrated throughout the categories of client needs. They include: Nursing Process (see Chapter 4 ⚭), Caring, Communication, Documentation, Cultural Awareness, Self-care, and Teaching/Learning.

Percentages of questions from each of the 10 subcategories are set by the National State Boards of Nursing, Inc. These percentages can be obtained by visiting the Web site cited above or by writing to the NSBN for a test plan. (See the 2002–2003 plan percentages in Box 33-1.) Percentages can change from one test plan revision to the next.

NCLEX-PN QUESTIONS BY CLIENT NEEDS. The questions in Box 33-2 ◆ will give you some idea of the format of the NCLEX-PN questions. Provided in the discussion of the answer is the category of client needs as well as the subcategory (see Box 33-1). Students do not need to know how to identify these categories and subcategories to test well. You will not be asked to identify them. This information is provided for those students who want an example of the various categories and subcategories of client needs on the test plan.

TABLE 33-1	COGNITIVE LEVELS OF TESTING (BLOOM'S TAXONOMY)
COGNITIVE LEVEL	**DESCRIPTION AND EXAMPLE**
Knowledge	Questions at a knowledge level test a person's memory of a fact or recall of a given piece of information *Example:* Which of the following numbers of questions is the maximum number of questions a test taker can receive when taking the NCLEX-PN? (*Answer:* 205. This tests simple memory of this fact.)
Comprehension	Comprehension questions test a person's understanding of concepts or principles. It is an understanding of what something means or how something is related to something else. It can involve reorganizing or restating learned information to demonstrate understanding. *Example:* After completing the teaching of insulin injection to a diabetic client, the nurse will have the most confidence in the client's understanding of the teaching if the client does which of the following things? (*Answer:* Demonstrates self-injection principle: Most people learn better by doing rather than seeing or hearing.)
Application	Application questions test a person's ability to use information such as concepts, theories, principles, and formulas in new situations, or to come up with a solution to a problem.
Analysis	Analysis questions provide information that needs to be separated, sorted, and examined looking at the various parts and a conclusion drawn to clarify meaning or show how something is structured. *Example:* From a list of behaviors of a client with a diagnosis of schizophrenia, determine which are normal growth and development and which one behavior is associated with the diagnosis of schizophrenia.

COMPUTERIZED ADAPTIVE TESTING (CAT)

Prior to April 1994, the examination for licensure as a licensed practical/vocational nurse was a paper-and-pencil test administered by each state board of nursing. Large numbers of candidates for licensure took the exam in a room monitored by proctors. Examinations were usually given only twice a year. Test security was a major concern, with large numbers of people taking the same examination at the same time and with versions of the test being administered again from time to time.

In April 1994, candidates for licensure began to take the licensure examination on the computer. The computer uses a method called **Computerized Adaptive Testing (CAT)** to provide each student a unique examination, selecting the test questions as the student takes the examination. In April 2001, those taking the exam could use a computer mouse for the first time, and a drop-down calculator became available.

The test questions for the NCLEX-PN exams are stored in an extremely large test bank. Questions are categorized according to their fit into various categories of the test plan

---

BOX 33-1 FRAMEWORK OF NCLEX-PN EXAM

Client Needs Categories and Percentage of Questions

1. Safe, effective care environment:
   a. Coordinated care (6–12%)
   b. Safety and infection control (7–13%)
2. Health promotion and maintenance:
   a. Growth and development through the life span (4–10%)
   b. Prevention and early detection of disease (4–10%)
3. Psychosocial integrity:
   a. Coping and adaptation (6–12%)
   b. Psychosocial adaptation (4–10%)
4. Physiological integrity:
   a. Basic care and comfort (10–16%)
   b. Pharmacological therapies (5–11%)
   c. Reduction of risk potential (11–17%)
   d. Physiological adaptation (13–19%)

Additional Concepts and Processes

◆ Nursing process
◆ Caring
◆ Communication
◆ Documentation
◆ Cultural awareness
◆ Self-care
◆ Teaching/learning

Test Plan Contact Information

Information on the current test plan can be found on the web pages of NCSBN at: www.ncsbn.org or you can write to National Council of State Boards of Nursing, 676 St. Clair Street, Suite 550, Chicago, Illinois 60611-2921.

BOX 33-2 SAMPLE NCLEX-PN TYPE QUESTIONS BY CLIENT NEEDS CATEGORY

1. Your assigned client asks you for something for pain. The physician has ordered meperidine (Demerol) 125 mg and promethazine hydrochloride (Phenergan) 25 mg every 4 hours prn. In addition to checking for allergies and when the last dose of the medication was given, it would be most important to do which of the following?
   a. Check the client's respiration rate before giving the injection.
   b. Put the side rails up after the injection.
   c. Teach client not to wait until pain is bad to ask for medication.
   d. Identify the location and intensity of the pain.
   Answer: A. Since Demerol is likely to depress respirations, the nurse must check the respiratory rate to ensure that it is 12 breaths per minute or above before giving the pain medication. *This question is at the client need category of physiological integrity and subcategory of reduction of risk potential.*

2. When working with a client who has been admitted with a diagnosis of alcohol dependency, the nurse asks the client to describe the problems that caused him to be admitted. The client says that he does not have any problems and it is his spouse who has the problems. The nurse realizes that the client is using which of the following defense mechanisms?

   a. Denial
   b. Suppression
   c. Rationalization
   d. Identification
   Answer: A. The client is using denial. Persons with alcohol or other drug abuse or dependency most often use the defense mechanism of denial. They frequently deny that they have a problem to avoid getting treatment. *This question is at the level of evaluation in nursing process. It is in the client needs category of psychosocial integrity and the subcategory of coping and adaptation.*

3. The nurse is doing some teaching on recognizing the early warning signs of diabetes. Which of the following warning signs will the nurse include as an early warning sign of diabetes?
   a. Pain on urination
   b. Lack of appetite
   c. Increased thirst
   d. Scant voidings
   Answer: C. The early warning signs of diabetes include increased urination, increased hunger, and increased thirst. *This question is in the health promotion and maintenance category of client needs and the subcategory of prevention and early detection of disease.*

structure. In addition, questions are categorized according to the level of difficulty. Each candidate is given a unique examination to test her or his knowledge and abilities while meeting the test plan requirements.

When you take this exam and answer a question correctly, the computer will scan the test bank and give you a more difficult question. On the other hand, if you select an incorrect answer, the computer will scan the test bank and give you an easier question.

In addition to the "real" questions that will determine if you are a safe practitioner or not, you will be given an additional 25 questions that will not count for or against you. These 25 additional questions are often referred to as "tryout" questions. These questions are being field-tested or "pilot tested." In other words, they are being tested or tried out on real exam takers to see if they are appropriate questions for future NCLEX examinations. These questions do not count for or against you.

The maximum testing period is 5 hours. If you are still testing at the end of 5 hours, you will receive no more questions. The maximum number of questions you can receive is 205, which consists of 180 real questions and 25 tryout questions. If you are testing and finish the 205th question, you will get no more questions. That is the end of your testing. The minimum number of questions you can receive is 85, which consists of 60 real questions and 25 tryout questions. The

National Council of State Boards of Nursing believes that 60 carefully chosen questions is the minimum number of questions that can determine whether you are a safe practitioner.

You will test until (1) the computer's program determines that you have clearly met the test plan requirements, or (2) you have failed, or (3) you have run out of time. You can pass or fail with either the minimum number or the maximum number or any number between 85 and 205.

To understand how you can pass or fail with the same number of questions, it is helpful to realize that if you answer a question correctly, you will be given a harder question. If you answer a question incorrectly, you will be given an easier question. The computer ends your examination when it calculates with a 95% degree of confidence that you have tested in a way that indicates you are a safe/competent practitioner or you are not.

Alternate Format Questions

Beginning April 2003, alternate item formats will have been introduced into the examination. The alternate items are based on the current test plan and do not have an effect on the length of the test. Initially, less than 2% of the items in the question pool will be of the alternate type. This means that a candidate taking the minimum length examination may have one item in the alternate format. Questions would give the candidate the opportunity to demonstrate entry-level nursing competence in ways that are different from the standard multiple-choice items. Some of the alternate format question types ask the candidates to perform calculations without the benefit of selecting the answer from four answer options. Another form is a fill-in-the-blank which requires the candidate to type in an answer to the question. Some of the new items present four or more response options, and they may require the candidate to select more than one option. The final question type can be used to evaluate the candidate's skill. This type is referred to as "Hot Spot." This item includes an anatomical drawing and requests the candidate to identify the appropriate spot for obtaining assessment information.

Specific example questions can be viewed at www.ncsbn.org or in the NCLEX examination candidate bulletin.

◆ Preparing and Reviewing for the Exam

PREPARING FOR THE EXAM

Have you ever been in a class where some of the students asked the instructor to cover only what would be on the exam, suggesting that if it is not on the exam, it is not important? This is not the way to prepare yourself for the licensure exam or to prepare yourself to provide good nursing care. Preparation begins the day you start your first nursing class and includes but is not limited to the following:

- Reading assignments for class
- Completing practice quizzes at the end of assigned chapters
- Using the computerized test banks that come with the texts to practice taking tests of key concepts
- Participating in class
- Learning **mnemonics** (techniques for developing memory)

Mnemonics can help you remember key concepts that you need to recall for the NCLEX-PN, as well as important information for giving safe care to your clients. An example of a mnemonic for blood pressure readings is using the words "sit down." "Sit" stands for systolic as the first/top number; "down" stands for diastolic or the bottom/last number in a blood pressure reading. When you say "sit down", you think, "sit" is for systolic (the first number and the one on top); down is for diastolic (the bottom and last number in the blood pressure reading). Mnemonics are useful for any key things that you must remember quickly and retain forever, not just for a quiz, midterm, or final exam.

REVIEWING FOR THE EXAM

Review for the NCLEX-PN examination needs to begin early. Plan to devote some time each day or a certain number of hours per week to such activities as working in an NCLEX-

PN review book or studying with a study group. Closer to the time of the examination, you can consider taking a professional review course for the NCLEX-PN and taking a mock NCLEX examination. Some schools of nursing require students to take a mock NCLEX examination.

NCLEX-PN Review Books

There are a variety of NCLEX-PN review books published by major nursing publishing companies. These books do not contain the questions from the NCLEX-PN itself. (The questions in that bank are confidential.) However, these review books do contain similar questions and cover the key concepts as well as the areas and categories that are tested in the licensing exam. While the review books may vary in their presentation, most are divided into units of specialized content, each with a review of key concepts, a practice exam on the content, and a section of answers with rationales for the correct answer.

To maximize your readiness to take the exam, you need to begin using a review book long before you take the licensing exam (Figure 33-1 ◆). You could start at least 6 months before the exam and try to review a set number of pages each day or each week so you will have sufficient time to firm the key concepts in your mind. You would benefit from reviewing more than one NCLEX-PN book. You and a fellow student might each buy different review books and trade books at some point.

Study Groups

In addition to using NCLEX-PN review books, many students find they benefit from a study group. The study group can be used not only for course tests but also to review and discuss the rationales for answers to questions in the review books. Setting aside time to work with a study group each week will benefit most students.

Figure 33-1. ◆ Taking regular times to prepare for the NCLEX-PN will help you study better and remember more.

Some students claim that a study group only confuses them. Why is this? Occasionally, one or two students in a group monopolize the group's time or say things that are incorrect or not needed by the others in the group. Several alternative solutions to this problem come to mind. One solution is for other members of the group to insist on members taking turns in the group or speaking up when the topic has been sufficiently covered. Another solution is to join a different group, and a third solution is to study with just one strong student. If a group study simply won't work for you, try setting aside time to study in the library or a quiet place alone.

Professional Review Courses

There are professional review courses that are usually 1 to 2 days in length, requiring advanced registration and payment of a course fee. Your instructor, director of your program, or your State Board of Nursing will usually be able to advise you of dates and costs of these review courses.

Mock NCLEX Examination

Some programs of practical/vocational nursing require, or offer a chance for, students to take a mock NCLEX-PN examination just prior to graduation. While these examinations are not free, they do provide a student with a percentile score for each category of client needs found on the examination. The student receives information on questions they got wrong and a list of the correct answers, along with an explanation and the rationales for the correct answers and for the distracters for each question. If you can take a mock NCLEX-PN exam, the information you receive on completion will help you to identify the areas where you need to focus your study time.

◆ Evaluating Your Readiness to Take the Examination

You have finished your formal nursing program and received your diploma. Are you ready to take the NCLEX-PN, or do you suppose putting off taking the exam would improve your chances of passing? Usually, people completing practical nursing programs are anxious to take the NCLEX-PN soon after completing the program for several reasons. Taking the exam soon means you are taking it while you are accustomed to testing and while much of what you have learned is fresh in your mind. From a practical and economic standpoint, you may also want to get your license so you can make more money. You probably want to get to work as a licensed practical/vocational nurse and sign your name with LPN (LVN if in Texas or California). If you did well on the Mock NCLEX-PN and/or if you have done well in answering most or all of the questions from all the various sections of your NCLEX-PN review book or books, you will probably decide that you are ready to take the examination. You have many indicators that you have a great chance of passing the examination.

If you have indicators that you may not do well on the NCLEX-PN exam, you should consider taking a review class. There are two types of classes. The first format reviews course work; the other is designed to prepare you to take the test. It provides test-taking tips and assistance in dealing with different types of questions. Time is also devoted to working through some of the psychological aspects of testing, such as test anxiety.

Delaying the exam does not necessarily improve your chances of passing the examination. In fact, there is some evidence that the probability of failure increases the longer a graduate waits.

It is important to remember that the NCLEX-PN exam is testing your ability to be a safe entry-level practitioner. Don't let your fears prevent you from being successful.

◆ Applying to Take the NCLEX-PN

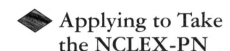

The National Council of State Boards of Nursing Web site has information on scheduling your NCLEX-PN examination. You can also get this information by writing to NCSBN for a copy of the test plan. In general, you will do the following:

1. Fill out an application for a license to the board of nursing of your state. The director of your nursing program or the faculty will probably provide you with this application, instructing you on the fees and size and type of pictures that must be submitted with the application.
2. After processing your application as satisfactory, the board of nursing of your state will advise the testing service selected by NCSBN to administer the examination, of your eligibility to test. The testing service selected most recently is National Computer Systems, Inc., which is part of Pearson Education.
3. Receive an NCLEX Examination Candidate Bulletin from the board of nursing.
4. Receive from the testing service an authorization to test and a booklet, which will tell you about the test centers and how to schedule your examination.
5. Register with, and schedule an appointment with, the testing service, which has been selected by NCSBN to administer the examination. Beginning October 1, 2002, candidates schedule with Pearson Professional Testing to take the licensing examination.

◆ Coping with Test Anxiety

Test anxiety seems to occur among students, as if on a continuum from low to high: from a normal mild level of uneasiness, which can be controlled easily and used as energy to do well on the exam, to a level of uneasiness and fear that immobilizes the test taker. Some students have a great deal of test anxiety before and/or during every quiz, midterm, and final exam and find themselves having difficulty focusing on the quiz or exam. Grades may suffer because of test anxiety. Other students seem to enjoy exams, concentrate fully, and look at them as a challenge.

WAYS TO OVERCOME TEST ANXIETY

If you are one of the students who are very nervous before or during tests, you need to start now to reduce your nervousness and anxiety around test taking. (See also Chapter 30. ⊂⊃) You would probably benefit from working with a counselor on these issues. If your test anxiety is not overwhelming, some simple strategies may reduce it. Sit down in a quiet place and write down 10 things you think would help you to reduce your test anxiety. You are the expert on you and may be able to come up with exactly what you need. Perhaps you will have on your list some of the following suggestions:

1. Learn some relaxation techniques, such as closing your eyes and tensing then relaxing each part of your body beginning at the head and neck and working downward. Check with your library to see if they have a relaxation tape and some books on relaxation that you can check out.
2. Try picturing yourself taking the exam, being in control, and doing well with the answers to the questions.
3. Imagine your mind as a blackboard and erase any negative thoughts that lead to believing you might not do well. Write on your imaginary board, "I will do well on the test/exam."
4. Refuse to think about anything that you can't see, smell, feel, or touch. You can't see, feel, smell, or touch a worry about not doing well.
5. Desensitize yourself about your fear of failing a test. Take some short tests until you are doing well and seeing your success. Build up to bigger tests. You could enlist the help of an instructor.
6. Count from 10 to 1 when you begin to feel nervous.

◆ Taking the Examination

Preparation on the day before and the day of the examination can help you arrive at the test prepared and relaxed. Try following these suggestions:

1. Do not cram the night before the examination. Relax your body and your mind. This could mean a pleasant movie or light reading. Some people relax by doing relaxation exercises or yoga or relaxing in warm water.
2. It is usually best to avoid using stimulants or depressants the evening before the examination. This includes caffeine drinks, alcohol, and other forms of stimulants and depressants.
3. Select some comfortable clothing for the next day. Perhaps something "layered" so you can take something off or put something on in case it is too warm or too cool for your comfort in the testing room.

4. Lay out anything you will have to take to the examination with you. This includes your instructions, required forms of identification, and your vehicle keys. You don't want to be searching for your vehicle keys when it is time to leave for the examination. You may want to take a power snack and a bottle of water to the examination with you to consume on your 10-minute break during the examination.
5. Get sufficient sleep the night before taking the test. Go to bed at the usual time and arise at the usual time. If crises are apt to occur at your home, make plans to sleep in a more restful environment. Getting into an argument with your roommate, significant other, or spouse the night before the exam will almost always not help you do well on the exam.

The day of the examination:

1. Eat moderately and finish your meal at least 1 to 2 hours before the exam. Avoid sugared foods, and include some protein in your meal. This will mean that you will have a more stable blood sugar than you would from just eating sugared foods. Do not rush your meal or overeat before the examination. If you overeat, blood will leave your brain to aid in digestion. This is blood you need to keep your brain working.
2. Be certain you have the required identification with you as you leave home to go to the examination.
3. Wear a watch. When taking the NCLEX-PN computer examination, you can take as long as you wish to review a question (also referred to as an item) and select an answer. Consider two things in deciding how long to take in reviewing a question and trying to determine the answer: (a) Once you have recorded your answer, the question will disappear and you cannot get it back. You will have to answer the question on the screen before you can get another question. Even if you need to guess, you must answer each question; (b) You will have 5 hours for the exam, so while you don't have to rush, you cannot afford to take a half hour or more per question. Taking an extremely long time to answer a question will not increase your chances of getting the right answer and will probably increase your anxiety.
4. Push negative thoughts out of your mind. Replace negative thoughts with positive ones.
5. You will receive instructions and practice questions before the actual exam begins. You will not need prior computer experience to take the examination because you will only be using the cursor, the space bar, and the enter key and there are no other functional keys. The use of the computer has been made very simple.
6. Don't waste time looking for a pattern to the answers or making your educated guesses based on a pattern. All answers are random.
7. There will be very few if any questions that ask you to determine the answer that is "not correct" or the action

that is "inappropriate." However, you need to read your questions very carefully to determine exactly what the question is asking. Answer what is being asked. The choices may include a correct statement that does not answer the question. Reading the question carefully will help you avoid selecting the statement that is correct but is not the right answer.

8. When answering questions, discipline yourself to answer based on the idea that the vast majority of the time your selected answer is true or best. Some test takers miss questions because they are searching for the one instance they know of, or have heard of, in which this answer might not be true or best.

9. If you find yourself not liking the question or wishing it were reworded, put your feelings aside and just do your best to answer the question as it is.

10. Concentrate fully on the exam. If you find yourself being distracted, tell yourself to focus and concentrate deeper.

◆ Waiting for Your Results

Stay calm while waiting for your results. Your state board of nursing will mail your results in about a month. Some states provide a 900 telephone number that the candidate can call for a fee. If your state participates, you will be given the information on when and how to obtain results by phone.

During the waiting period you may find that you are recalling and worrying about some questions you feel certain that you missed on the examination. While looking up the answers so you will have this knowledge, you want to try to avoid worrying as some of the questions you missed are likely to be the pilot questions that do not count against you and almost everyone will miss some of the "real" questions.

The best news that you can receive is that you have passed the examination. In this event, you are now a licensed practical nurse (or, if you are testing in Texas or California, you are a licensed vocational nurse). Congratulations! You now have all the benefits and responsibilities of being an LVN/LPN. Your lifelong learning continues.

The only other news you could receive is that you have failed the examination. Failing the exam means two things: one is that you need to identify any factors that you could change to increase your chances of passing. The other is that you need to develop a plan to prepare yourself better to take the examination.

A **diagnostic profile** is provided to candidates who fail the examination. The diagnostic profile is mailed to these candidates by their respective boards of nursing, along with the results of the examination. The profile aids the candidate in determining their areas of relative strength and weakness based on the test plan and in designing their study accordingly, prior to retaking the exam.

Stop any worrying that you are doing and begin to prepare. Do not say anything negative to or about yourself. This only wastes energy you need in preparing to take and pass the examination. You might make and hang some posters saying "SUCCESS" or "I WILL BE SUCCESSFUL" in your study area. If that isn't possible, then put sticky notes with that message in your study book.

There is a minimum number of days set by the NCSBN that you must wait before retaking the NCLEX-PN. Your state board of nursing can set a longer period of time, but not a shorter period. This time period is of course designed to allow you time to prepare yourself for success.

If you failed the examination, you will benefit from doing some or all of the following:

◆ Talking with the director of your nursing program
◆ Working on a plan to be prepared when you retake the examination
◆ Getting a tutor
◆ Taking a review course
◆ Obtaining another NCLEX review book
◆ Spending more time reviewing
◆ Getting professional help for test anxiety

Note: The bibliography listings for this and all chapters have been compiled at the back of the book.

Chapter Review

Key Terms by Topics

Use the audio glossary feature of either the CD-ROM or the Companion Website to hear the correct pronunciation of the following key terms.

Development of the NCLEX-PN
multistate compact

Understanding the NCLEX-PN plan
Computerized Adaptive Testing (CAT)

Preparing and reviewing for the exam
mnemonics

Coping with test anxiety
test anxiety

Waiting for your results
diagnostic profile

Key Points

* Preparation for the NCLEX-PN examination needs to begin when a student first enters the school of nursing.

* Students must pass the NCLEX-PN test in order to practice. The plan takes into consideration the legal scope of practical/vocational nursing of each state and a practical/vocational nursing job analysis.

* The purpose of the NCLEX-PN examination is to protect the public by ensuring that all who pass and receive a license to practice the entry level competencies needed to practice safely and effectively.

* Test questions on the NCLEX-PN are at the cognitive levels of knowledge, comprehension, application, and analysis.

* The test plan is organized around four categories of client needs across the life span in a variety of settings. The categories of human needs are: safe, effective care environment, health promotion and maintenance, psychosocial integrity, and physiologic integrity.

* The maximum testing period is 5 hours with the maximum number of questions being 205 and the minimum 85. A student can pass or fail with the minimum or maximum number of questions or any number in between.

* Mnemonics are a way to help a person recall key concepts.

* It is a good idea to get an NCLEX review book and begin using this book at least 6 months before taking the NCLEX-PN examination. Study groups and review groups also help most students do better on the NCLEX-PN.

* Readiness for the NCLEX-PN can be judged by looking at one's performance on tests and examinations in the nursing program, performance on mock NCLEX examinations, and results of practice tests in an NCLEX-PN review book.

* Learning techniques for reducing test anxiety can greatly improve your NCLEX-PN results.

* Prepare before the examination by avoiding stimulants or depressants the night before the test, determining the route to the examination, laying out everything needed for the examination ahead of time, relaxing, and getting enough sleep.

* Pace yourself during the exam so you can finish within five hours. Don't waste time looking for patterns to answers. Select the best answer, and concentrate fully on the examination.

EXPLORE MediaLink

Additional interactive resources for this chapter can be found on the Companion Website at www.prenhall.com/ramont. Click on Chapter 33 and "Begin" to select the activities for this chapter.

For chapter-related NCLEX-style questions and an audio glossary, access the accompanying CD-ROM in this book.

For Further Study

For further study about legal and ethical issues, see Chapter 2.
For in-depth discussion about the nursing process, see Chapter 4.
For more information about stress and coping, see Chapter 30.

NCLEX-PN Exam Preparation

1. When is the best time for a student who is enrolled in a practical nursing program to begin preparing for the NCLEX-PN?
   a. On the first day of the nursing program
   b. After the completion of the first nursing course
   c. Six months before completion of the program
   d. As soon as the nursing program is completed

2. You have been asked to answer this question: When is the best time for a student who is enrolled in a practical nursing program to begin preparing for the NCLEX-PN? This question is an example of testing at which of the following levels of comprehension?
   a. Knowledge
   b. Comprehension
   c. Application
   d. Analysis

3. The NCLEX-PN examination is revised periodically with the time period for review based on:
   a. An annual analysis of how secure the test questions in the test bank are
   b. Completion of a new job analysis of the tasks of licensed vocational nurses
   c. A vote of the member states of the National Council of State Boards of Nursing
   d. When substantial changes in the nurse practice acts of the states have occurred

4. In order to prepare for the NCLEX-PN, a nursing student needs what degree of computer expertise?
   a. Extensive
   b. Above average
   c. Average
   d. None

5. A student finds that he is worrying before, during, and after tests in his nursing courses because the tests are so difficult. Which of the following actions would be best on this student's part?
   a. Use the grievance procedure and complain about the test difficulty.
   b. Seek help in designing effective methods of studying and relaxing.
   c. Talk with peers about how much you are worried and how you worry.
   d. Wait and see if it gets easier in another course with another teacher.

6. The night before the examination, it is usually best to go to bed at which of the following times?
   a. About 8 to 10 hours before time to awaken
   b. No later than midnight
   c. The usual time you normally go to bed
   d. Whenever you feel tired

7. In taking the tests in nursing courses and answering questions in the NCLEX-PN review books, you find that even though you memorize a lot of things, the questions don't seem to test these facts. The best explanation for this is:
   a. You are not studying the facts needed for these questions.
   b. You are having difficulty memorizing enough.
   c. The teacher is not very good at writing tests on what was taught.
   d. The level of the testing is at comprehension, analysis, or synthesis.

8. You must not forget to take which of the following things to the NCLEX-PN testing location with you?
   a. Watch
   b. Calculator
   c. Identification
   d. Scratch paper

9. The maximum testing period during which you can answer questions on the NCLEX-PN is which of the following?
   a. 1 hour
   b. 3 hours
   c. 4 hours
   d. 5 hours

10. The minimum number of questions you could be given on the NCLEX-PN is:
    a. 50
    b. 85
    c. 125
    d. 300

Answers for Review Questions appear in Appendix IV.

Finding That First Job

SHARING experiences

I have always loved helping people, and when I am done with this program, I will get to do it and get paid for it! What a treat! Nursing has such a large impact on people's lives, more so than any other health care profession, in my opinion.

Holly Zamora, LPN student, Idaho State University, Pocatello, ID.

LEARNING outcomes

After completing this chapter, you will be able to:
- Describe the components of a portfolio
- Develop a cover letter for an entry level job
- Prepare a résumé
- Define professional behavior
- Describe a career ladder for the nursing profession

MediaLink

www.prenhall.com/ramont

Use the address above to access the free, interactive Companion Website created for this textbook. Get hints, instant feedback, and textbook references to chapter-related NCLEX-style questions. Link to other interesting sites.

Audio Glossary:
Use the Companion Website, or the CD-ROM disk enclosed with your textbook, to hear the pronunciation of key terms in the chapter.

There are many differences between student and graduate nurses. For example, as a student you have an instructor on hand to observe you as you carry out your duties. As a graduate you will be expected to make decisions independently. Once you are out of school, reality hits.

Most new graduates feel unprepared, overwhelmed, and scared. The good news is that no employer, whether a hospital or other agency, expects you to know everything. You will continue to learn as you begin your first job. You may even come to think of that first position as being another phase of your education.

You may be realizing a lifelong dream to be a nurse, embarking on a new career, or returning to the workforce. No matter what it was that brought you to this place, you are now a new member of a profession, and you have much to contribute. This chapter will provide you with a survival plan as you transition from student to licensed practical or vocational nurse.

Making the transition from student to licensed nurse is in many ways like planning a trip to a foreign country. You need to make preparations. You need to:

◆ Decide where you want to go.
◆ Be sure you have all your documents.
◆ Prepare the appropriate wardrobe.
◆ Have your timeline and contact persons well in mind.

Thinking about all of these ahead of time will keep you from feeling lost as you begin the job search process.

You may have a particular facility in mind where you would like to work. It may be one you were assigned to as a student, one where you have worked as an unlicensed health care worker, or one that was recruiting at a job fair. Learn as much as you can about each facility and its parent company before making an application.

Portfolio

Your next step is to review your **portfolio.** A portfolio is an itemized visual account of your skills and best practices that are related to the position you are seeking. You compile a portfolio so that when you leave school you can walk into an interview with all the information you need to emphasize your strengths, education, and experience, and to present yourself as a professional practical/vocational nurse. You do not compile your portfolio overnight. Ideally, you begin developing it halfway into your nursing program.

A leather type three-ring binder is an appropriate way to display your personal portfolio. A complete portfolio includes:

◆ Title page
◆ Table of contents
◆ Cover letter/Introduction letter
◆ Application
◆ Résumé
◆ Work Samples (two), for example:

◆ Nursing care plans
◆ Narrative charting samples
◆ Lesson plan for client teaching
◆ Writing samples (one of the following):
  ◆ Case studies
  ◆ Research projects
  ◆ Observation studies
◆ Student reflection (e.g., journal entry)
◆ Community service
◆ Clinical evaluations
◆ Awards/Achievements
◆ Recommendation letters
◆ Sample thank you letter
◆ Sample resignation letter

WORK SAMPLES

Work samples are items you have used in the workplace. Individualized nursing care plans are an excellent way to display your critical thinking and understanding of rationales. Charting is an important way to present your writing skills related to the workplace. It demonstrates your flexibility with different methods and strategies of documentation. Lesson plans for client teaching under the direction of the RN can provide further evidence of your abilities in problem solving and intervention implementation. As mentioned earlier, you can compile this information as you progress through your program, to underscore your strengths in the nursing field.

WRITING SAMPLES

Effective writing that is organized, clear, correctly spelled, and uses correct grammar is a meaningful workplace skill. Use a sample of your work that is researched and includes a bibliography. This item stresses your ability to write in a logical order using correct format and shows your attention to detail. A journal entry or a student reflection piece would serve as an additional writing sample.

COMMUNITY SERVICE

Document ways you give back to the community by doing community service. Society looks to the nursing profession for leadership and guidance. Health professionals' involvement in community service demonstrates commitment and dedication to organizations that contribute to the well being of the community. Employers consider participation in community service a positive attribute.

CLINICAL EVALUATION

Provide a copy of your best evaluation signed by your clinical instructor. This instructor may also be on your reference list.

SAMPLE THANK YOU LETTER

A brief thank you letter to the interviewers can remind them of you and your abilities. Be positive about the interview process, and thank them for their time and consideration. Again, use correct grammar and spelling. Having a sample letter in your portfolio will make this a simple task when needed.

SAMPLE LETTER OF RESIGNATION

It is customary to write a letter of resignation for your position when you are leaving. A 2-week notice is appropriate. Be positive about your work environment and position. Thank your employers for the experience and professional growth you have gained. The first person you notify about your resignation should be your boss. It is not wise to have him or her hear it through the grapevine before you deliver the letter of resignation. Appropriate reasons for leaving are new challenges, increase in pay, relocation, family matters, or career advancements.

The portfolio is an ideal place to store copies of your license, CPR card, or other certifications you receive (e.g., intravenous therapy or blood withdrawal). You also may wish to include a list of references with their contact information and a sample completed application. These will be helpful to you when you are asked to fill out an application on site.

From the beginning of your student program, have a file set aside to collect documents for your portfolio. You can keep a note card of classes you especially enjoyed, positive comments from teachers, and dates of meetings you attended. All these will remind you of the steps you have taken throughout your program, and they will be useful when the time comes to build an attractive portfolio.

◆ Job Search

There are many ways to look for potential practical/vocational nurse positions. Many companies advertise on the Internet. You can check newspaper ads, job boards, nursing magazines, and the place where you currently work. There are job fairs just for nursing positions.

Make a list of questions before making application to an organization. Decide what priorities you have in searching for a position. Examples include:

◆ What information does the advertisement give you about the organization?
◆ What experience is required?
◆ Is there a hiring-on benefit?
◆ Are the shifts 8 or 12 hours?
◆ What is the starting pay?
◆ Is there advancement for an LPN/LVN?
◆ Is there a plan for school reimbursement?
◆ Does the organization provide continuing education classes, and is there a fee for employees?
◆ What benefits are available?
◆ Who is the contact person?

On the Internet, you can find the average salaries for LPNs and LVNs. This will help you determine where the organization stands in comparison to the average for the county, state, and nation in which you are applying.

Internet sites that are easily accessed are:

◆ *Monster.com*
◆ *State.bls.gov*
◆ *Classifieds.yahoo.com*

THE COVER LETTER

Once you have found a job or jobs to which you wish to make application, you will need to prepare a **cover letter.** A cover letter is what your potential employer uses to determine whether he or she wants to find out more about your qualifications. It must be brief and to the point, but it also should highlight your best professional and educational attributes. This concise, one-page letter must reflect correct grammar, good spelling, and appropriate format.

Address the letter appropriately. Think about what you do with mail that is addressed "To Occupant." If you do not want your cover letter and résumé to be tossed in the "circular file," do your homework. Get the name of the person you are addressing, and make a point to spell it correctly. Establish his or her title or position. This is all part of making a favorable first impression.

The introductory paragraph should immediately explain the letter's purpose. Begin your paragraph by introducing yourself. Explain your intent to apply for the position of licensed practical/vocational nurse. Give the details of your response to an ad, job listing, Web site, or other source that disclosed this job offering. If you are a new graduate, include your school and date of graduation.

The body or second paragraph contains your highlighted qualifications. This is where you address your enthusiasm for this particular job. State how you have been prepared by your education. Describe briefly the skills and strengths that you will contribute to the position. Write about what sets you apart from the other applicants. Include a statement about the facility to which you are applying and why you want to be part of a "recognized staff and organization." This is the time to write about your experience and competencies. If you have limited clinical experience, mention your diverse clinical rotations. Include major accomplishments and awards. Since this is your first position in this capacity, avoid using words like *best, expert*, and *excellent* to describe yourself. Evade flowery words or phrases that do not sound professional. Write out any industry-specific abbreviations you may be using.

The closing paragraph restates your interest and conveys your anticipation in obtaining an interview. Indicate when and how you will follow up your letter. Refer to your enclosed résumé.

Your cover letter must include your name, address, and telephone number. Printed letterhead is acceptable. Use the same, top-quality bond paper for both your cover letter and résumé. Cream, beige, or light gray paper is suggested. Review your letter for errors and have someone else read it also. If your letter is computer generated, use spell and grammar check, but never rely on them alone. (They will not catch errors like "I come *form* (not *from*) the Midwest.") Refer to Box 34-1 ◆ for a sample cover letter.

RÉSUMÉ

The **résumé** is a concise, systematic summary of your professional experience and educational background. This is a marketing tool to give your potential employer a snapshot glimpse into your nursing background and experience. A one-page document is preferred, with two pages being the maximum.

Remember, if you become too wordy or if the employer has to search to find information, your résumé may end up in the trash. Your résumé needs to be well planned, informative, and organized. Take the time necessary to be neat and accurate.

There are three types of résumé formats: chronological, functional, and combination format.

◆ The chronological format highlights your employment in a *reverse chronological order* (i.e., from your current or most recent job to your least recent job). This type is the most traditional.
◆ The functional résumé emphasizes your skills.
◆ The combination résumé combines your previous jobs and your list of skills.

The next step is to assemble data that illustrates your professional qualifications. It is important for a new graduate to list accomplishments that would give the employer an insight into your work ethic and commitment. Include such areas as community service, serving as a class officer, competi-

---

BOX 34-1 SAMPLE COVER LETTER

Mary J. Fuller LPN
4123 W. Green Street
Martinsville, Iowa 92222
999 555-1212
e-mail mjf24@aol.com

January 24, 2003

Roseanne Blake, RN
Director of Nurses
St. Catherine's Hospital
1002 Main Street
Marysville, Iowa 92223

Dear Ms. Blake:

It is with great interest that I apply for the licensed practical nurse position advertised in the Marysville Times on Sunday. I am a recently licensed practical nurse, having completed the nursing program at the Waterloo Vocational and Technical School.

I have more than 7 years' experience as a certified nursing assistant in the acute care setting. My background as a nursing assistant, as well as the clinical experience obtained during my practical nursing program, have built a firm foundation for my first nursing position.

I graduated first in my class and received the faculty award for clinical excellence. I received a Silver Medal in practical nursing skills at the Health Occupation Students of America National Leadership Conference in June. I will consider any clinical area, depending on your needs. I am enthusiastic and dependable, and I am committed to quality client care.

I have enclosed my résumé for your consideration. If you need additional information, please feel free to contact me at my home number listed above. Thank you for your time and consideration. I will call your office next week to discuss further the possibilities of employment.

Sincerely,

Mary S. Fuller, LPN

Mary J. Fuller, LPN

Enclosure

tive event awards from Health Occupations Students of America, scholarships, or other honors. Use action words to describe your qualifications. See Box 34-2 ◆ for a list of action words.

Your educational history lists years of education completed, dates of school attendance, year of graduation, school name and location, certification, and diploma information. Again, this is usually presented in a reverse chronological order in which the first entry is the most current.

Employment experience would include dates, positions, and employing agencies. Note on your résumé that references are available upon request. (See "References" on page 748.)

Most résumés are computer-generated today. However, at the very least, your résumé must be typed on quality paper (usually the same light-colored paper that you used for your cover letter). Many computer résumé programs are available. You may want to start there, but be sure that you individualize it. Make a résumé that is unique to you.

Many students have learned to use graphics from computer files. Remember to keep your résumé professional; no hearts or stethoscopes should detract from the purpose and content. Have an experienced professional nurse review your résumé for spelling, grammatical errors, and appearance. This is not a document to be taken lightly, and it will take more than one draft to complete. Use a consistent format and follow it throughout the document.

Everything surrounding your résumé should be professional. If your e-mail address is not professional, you might want to create a separate address for work-related business.

Also remember that when you have sent a résumé, you may receive a phone call. Make sure your message machine is working properly and that there is a professional message left for callers.

Résumé Components

Résumé components should be provided in the following order:

1. *Résumé heading*. This includes your name, complete address, phone number, and an e-mail address (if available).
2. *Job objective*. Not everyone agrees that you need an objective on your résumé today. However, in your objective you are stating your professional career goal. You can be general in your goal or more specific. This will help the Human Resource Department determine whether you may be qualified for the position they are looking to fill. Your job objective should be one sentence.
3. *Summary of qualifications*. This summary is used to assist a new nurse to stress strong points. Be sure to include why you are qualified to meet your objective. You can bullet the summary for easier reading.
4. *Educational history*. In this section, start with your most recent education. Include the name of the school, and then enter city and state. List your certification, license, degree or focus of education, and graduation date. Follow through with other educational background.
5. *Experience*. Again, start with your current or most recent work experience. Include full-time and part-time employment. State the position clearly and succinctly. Describe the duties, responsibilities assigned, and dates employed. Your work history is important to employers, and they look for gaps in time. Use the same format as you did with your education.
6. *Achievements*. This section highlights your value to the employer. Your accomplishments as a student are important. Use them to your advantage. Perfect attendance, faculty awards for clinical excellence, academic excellence, and Health Occupations Students of America competitive awards all demonstrate value. Include any community service you have done; it displays personal commitment and involvement. Completion of Intravenous Therapy and Blood Withdrawal and Telemetry classes are additional tickets that may increase your marketability.

When your résumé is complete, Human Resources can keep it on file for positions that become available. If you have access to a computer, you can send your résumé electronically (and *e-résumé*) to prospective employers. This is a quick and efficient way to cover a lot of ground. Keep your cover e-mail short and concise. Identify the position for which you are applying. Let your prospective employer know if you are willing to relocate. Don't forget to attach your résumé to your e-mail. See Figure 34-1 ◆ for a sample résumé.

BOX 34-2
ACTION WORDS

Accomplished	Observed
Achieved	Organized
Analyzed	Planned
Built	Presented
Chaired	Prevented
Collaborated	Provided
Communicated	Reduced
Created	Reorganized
Delegated	Served
Designed	Simplified
Developed	Standardized
Devoted	Studied
Dispensed	Taught
Ensured	Transformed
Evaluated	Unified
Expanded	Validated
Focused	Worked
Formulated	Wrote
Implemented	

Luz Marina Balderas
555 Main Street
Any Town, CA 99999
(555) 555-1234

OBJECTIVES:

To obtain a challenging position in the Nursing QI/QM field where I can utilize my clinical knowledge and quality management experience in an environment that will promote career and educational opportunities.

SKILLS:

Project
Management:
- Time management and project deadline compliance
- Critical thinking and conflict resolution
- Data collection and statistical data analysis
- Delegation and team work management

Business:
- Accurately type and data enter 120 words per minute.
- Computer proficiency in Word, Excel, Access, PowerPoint, E-Z Cap, SPSS, MedCore
- Strong Customer Relations background
- Public speaking and project presentation experience
- Employee training and compliance assurance
- Policy and procedure development and implementation

EXPERIENCE:

Position: Market Research Analyst
Company: MedPartners, Inc.
Location: Long Beach, California
Employment: September 1997 through July 2000

Position: IPA Quality Improvement Coordinator
Company: MedPartners, Inc.
Location: Long Beach, California
Employment: June 1993 through September 1997

Position: QI Nursing Representative
Company: MedPartners, Inc.
Location: Long Beach, California
Employment: May 1991 through June 1993

Position: Specialty Clinic – Back Office Medical Assistant
Company: MedPartners, Inc.
Location: Long Beach, California
Employment: July 1988 through May 1991

Figure 34-1. ◆ Sample résumé.

Luz Marina Balderas
555 Main Street
Any Town, CA 99999
(555) 555-1234

Page 2

EDUCATION:

North Orange County ROP:	Licensed Vocational Nursing Program	Aug. 2000 - July 2002
Cypress Community College:	Limited X-Ray Technician Program	Sept. 1984 - Sept. 1986
Cerritos Community College:	Medical Assisting Program	Sept. 1982 - Sept. 1984
Downey Adult Ed. Program:	Nurses' Assistant Program	July 1982 - Dec. 1983
University of Calif., Irvine:	Bachelor's in Science - Psychology	Sept. 1978 - June 1982

AWARDS & ACHIEVEMENTS:

Kaiser Permanente Health Care Issues State Scholarship: 1st Place, March 2002
HOSA State Leadership Conference: Gold Medallist - Pathophysiology, March 2002
HOSA State Leadership Conference: Bronze Medallist - Bio Medical Debate, March 2002
Kaiser Permanente Health Care Issues National Scholarship: 1st Place, June 2002
HOSA National Leadership Conference: Gold Medallist - Pathophysiology, June 2002
HOSA National Leadership Conference: 1st Place - Health Education Pilot Event, June 2002
Class Valedictorian: NOCROP – LVN Program, Graduating Nursing Class A, July 2002

PRESENTATIONS:

"Cushing's Syndrome"   NOCROP – LVN Program, Pharmacology Module, October 2001
"Traumatic Head Injuries"   NOCROP – LVN Program, Neurology Module, May 2002

CERTIFICATIONS & LICENSES:

Basic Cardiac Life Support Certification
Phlebotomy Certified
Medical Assistant Certification
Limited X-Ray License: Expired
Nursing Assistant Certification: Expired

REFERENCES:

Available upon request

Figure 34-1. ◆ Sample résumé. *(continued)*

REFERENCES

References are people who agree to provide a written or verbal assessment of you to a potential employer. Two of these people should be professionals connected to the type of job you are seeking. The others can be personal references. Three to four references are adequate.

You should never assume that you can use a teacher, employer, or personal acquaintance as a reference. Be sure to contact each person you would like as a reference and obtain permission to use his or her names, addresses, phone numbers, and e-mail addresses (if available).

A list of your references (names, regular address and e-mail address, and phone numbers) should be made on a single typed or computer-generated sheet of paper. A copy of your references should always be available in your portfolio in case of a request.

APPLICATION

An application may seem like an easy task. However, the more attention you pay to detail, the better you represent yourself to your employer. Many employers will have you fill out the application on site. Have all the information required at your fingertips. Being prepared gives you an advantage. The following guidelines may be useful to you:

◆ Practice completing applications. If you plan to apply to a facility you have worked at as a student, ask for an application and practice completing it ahead of time. Some employers have their applications online; you can download a copy and fill it out before you actually apply.

◆ Never leave lines blank. If some question on the form is not applicable to you, write "N/A" (not applicable) in the space provided.

◆ Type the application if you can. If you are completing it in the office by hand, be neat, legible, avoid abbreviations, and use ink.

INTERVIEWS

Getting an interview means that the employer is interested in what you have said in your cover letter and résumé. This is where you sell yourself to the employer. A face-to-face meeting gives you the chance to make a good first impression. Whether or not the interview results in employment, the experience will provide you with insight into your ability to speak logically and think critically. Did you get your message across? Did your nervousness get the best of you, or did practice pay off? One-on-one interviews are less nerve wracking, but today you may be faced with two or three interviewers firing questions at you. If you are well prepared, you can have a successful interview. See Chapters 25 and 33. 🔗

In order to be prepared for an interview, you must practice and rehearse a variety of questions. Mock interviews will help you gain poise and allow you to think about what you need to modify before you are in the midst of an actual interview. See Box 34-3 ◆ for Examples of Interview questions.

BOX 34-3
EXAMPLES OF INTERVIEW QUESTIONS

◆ Describe your education and experience as it relates to the position.
◆ What is one quality you like about yourself?
◆ How would you handle an irritated family member?
◆ What can you bring or contribute to this company or facility?
◆ What interested you in applying for this facility?
◆ Where do you see yourself in 5 years?
◆ How would you handle a combative client?
◆ How do you view yourself as a worker?
◆ What skill, personal or professional, do you feel you need improvement on to make you a better employee?
◆ How do you rate yourself in the area of problem solving on a scale of 1 to 5, with 5 being the highest?
◆ Describe the process used and give an example. (Remember to use Nursing Process!)
◆ What are your strengths/weaknesses? Elaborate on each.
◆ What do you like most about your job?
◆ What are some things you have learned from clients?
◆ What would you do if you believed a doctor was causing harm to the client?
◆ If you were asked to do something out of your scope of practice, what would be your course of action?
◆ If you could change one thing in nursing, what would it be and why?
◆ As a new graduate, why would I hire you over someone with 2 years' experience?
◆ What is the biggest issue facing nursing today?
◆ How do you feel about floating to an area unfamiliar to you?

Physical Appearance

Dress professionally. Professional dress means different things to different people. What does it mean to you? For a male, it is a conservative suit, dress shirt and tie, and clean-shaven face. If you wear a beard, it must be trimmed and neat. For the female, the most suitable professional dress is a medium length skirt with a blouse and jacket. (If you are tugging at your skirt when you sit, it is too short. If you have to ask "Is this appropriate?," you should find something else to wear.) A pantsuit is permissible.

Clothes should be neatly pressed. Closed-toed shoes with nylons are proper dress. Avoid plunging necklines and skirts with thigh-high slits. It is permissible to wear your uniform, although business attire is preferred. However, remember you are trying to make an impression.

Adopt a clean, moderate, controlled hairstyle and appearance. Styles that mean so much today may seem silly next year; style always needs to be tempered with conservatism. One set

Chapter 34 Finding That First Job ◆ 749

of stud earrings is always acceptable. Neutral moderate makeup and nails are essential. Hygiene is understood.

Timing and Attitude

Arrive at the interview at least 15 minutes early. Identify yourself with the front desk or secretary, and say who you are there to meet.

Take charge of your attitude. Be positive, polite, and confident. Your enthusiasm for the position will come across, and even if you are not the most qualified and experienced, that refreshing attitude can have an effect on your rating. Convince the interviewer about your commitment and motivation. Be aware of your verbal and nonverbal communication. Avoid phrases like "you guys," "like, you know," and be aware of how many "ums" you might say. If your hands tend to shake, put them on your lap. Also avoid touching and playing with your hair.

Be prepared to wait if the previous interview extends into your assigned time. Be patient and use the time to review what you know about the facility and staff where you are applying.

Introductions

When you enter the interview offices, use a firm handshake with each panel member. Smile (it breaks the ice) and once again state your name clearly. Address the panel members by Miss, Mrs., or Mr. Remain standing until you are asked to take a seat.

Body of Interview

Avoid fidgeting, sit upright and a little forward in the chair, and be attentive. Do not chew gum during an interview; it leaves a negative impact. Do make eye contact; it conveys confidence and credibility in your answers. Answer questions succinctly but completely; use examples if appropriate. (Roughly six to ten questions will be presented.) Be interesting and avoid rambling. The usual time period for an interview is 15 to 20 minutes. Discuss your qualifications and experiences related to the position. As a new graduate you can use your clinical rotation and any associated work experiences. Offer your portfolio for their review; point out highlights that you feel would be of particular interest.

If the opportunity arises, articulate why you have chosen this facility for application. For example, it might be the compassionate care that you observed firsthand as a student. It may be their renowned staff and cutting-edge cancer research, or may be the physician–nurse respect and interdisciplinary approach used in client care. If you don't know firsthand about the facility, look into the facility on its Web site or speak with staff members.

Follow-up Questions

When the interview is finished, the interviewer will ask you for any questions that you may have. Have at least two questions ready to pose. Suitable questions to be considered include:

- What is the normal staff-to-client ratio?
- What types of continuing education or classes are offered, and are there is a fee to enroll?
- Does this organization offer tuition reimbursement for higher education?
- How long is the new graduate orientation, and what is the process?
- What are full-time benefits?
- Are there job advancement opportunities or level changes?
- When and how will you be notified about their decision concerning the position?
- What is the involvement of the nursing staff in community service?

There are differing points of view on asking questions about salary. One is that it isn't discussed until the job is offered. However, if you have a condition about salary, and entry-level pay is unacceptable, it is better to clarify this early in the process.

At the end of the interview, express your appreciation for the interviewers' time and for the opportunity to interview for this position. Shake hands with the panel and exit promptly. Write a short thank you note following the interview. It reminds the interviewer of your interest. To be effective, the note should be received within a week of the interview. Refer to Box 34-4 ◆ for a rubric on interview skills. Reviewing this will assist you to self-evaluate your abilities in this area.

Illegal Questions

There are questions that interviewers cannot legally ask. The Civil Rights Act and state laws protect citizens against these questions. You are not required to answer these questions. However, should a question be asked, be prepared to decline tactfully or to veer the discussion to another topic. Examples of illegal questions include:

- Are you married?
- What are your child care arrangements?
- What is your religion?
- How old are you? What is your birth date?
- Where were you born?
- What is your race (or any race-related question)?

Avoid putting the panel on the defensive. If you point out an illegal question, the interview and your chance for a position may be terminated early. There are ways to answer questions that will not alienate the interviewer. Answer in a controlled manner. Do not offer more personal information than is necessary. Maintain a positive attitude, and keep your voice conversational and upbeat. If an interviewer consistently asks personal questions, think twice about taking that job.

Suggested responses to this type of questioning are:

- "I'm not sure how that question pertains to this position."
- "Child care arrangements are not an issue; please do not be concerned."
- "If you mean am I over 18, yes I am."

BOX 34-4 INTERVIEW RUBRIC

Interview Skills

A successful interviewee. . .

◆ Exhibits professional dress and demeanor.
◆ Arrives early for the interview, with all necessary documents.
◆ Speaks clearly and confidently about skills and qualifications.
◆ Uses effective verbal and nonverbal communication skills.
◆ Understands the importance of following up the interview.

Advanced	Student arrives early for the interview, with all necessary documents, and exhibits professionalism in both appearance and demeanor. The student can list important documents that may be requested at the interview, including the following: resume; letters of reference; work samples; and photocopies of diplomas, awards, certificates, driver's license, Social Security card, and any military papers. Student demonstrates appropriate verbal and nonverbal communication before, during, and after the interview, shaking hands and making eye contact with all interviewers. He/she demonstrates a high degree of knowledge of the company and/or position and demonstrates interest by asking a minimum of two appropriate questions. All interview questions are answered in an organized, professional manner, using supporting details and/or examples. Language is appropriate to the available position, and student's demeanor and voice tone are pleasant. The student demonstrates interview follow-up by writing a thank you letter to the interviewer and/or calling the company to inquire about the company's hiring decision in a sophisticated, professional manner.
Proficient	Student arrives early for the interview, with all necessary documents, and exhibits professionalism in both appearance and demeanor. The student can explain the purpose of a job interview. Questions are answered clearly and confidently, using language appropriate to the available position. Supporting details and/or examples may be missing. Oral delivery is clear but needs improvement in one to two of the following areas: tone of voice, pace, energy, and/or nonverbal communication. The student demonstrates interview follow-up, including writing a thank you letter to the interviewer and/or calling the company to inquire about the company's hiring decision. Demonstrates some interest in asking a question about the position or company.
Basic	The student does not demonstrate a basic understanding of the job interview, as indicated by any of the following behaviors: • He/she does not arrive early and/or is missing necessary documents. • Dress and demeanor are not professional. • Questions are not answered completely; supporting details and/or examples are weak or absent. • Oral delivery demonstrates deficiencies in three or more of the following areas: tone of voice, pace, energy, and/or nonverbal communication. Has no questions of the interviewer. • There is no interview follow-up.

Source: Courtesy of Lynne Porter, RN, North Orange County ROP, Anaheim, CA.

AWAITING A RESPONSE

Once you have completed the interview process, you need to wait patiently for the panel to make their decision and check your references. If during the interview they told you when they would be making their decision, it is permissible to call the human resource or nursing office after that time to check on the status of the position. Making this call can be difficult, but it will let you know if you are still being considered or if you should pursue other options.

◆ The Hiring Process

When you receive the offer of employment, you will be very excited. Contain yourself long enough to get all the details as well as time and dates of your orientation. If you have received more than one job offer and need time to make a decision, thank the caller for the offer and state that you will get back to them at a specific time with your answer.

ORIENTATION

Orientation is a program or time period provided for newly hired individuals to prepare them to take on the responsibilities of the position for which they were hired.

Most facilities have new employees complete all the paperwork during the first day of orientation. You may be required to complete a physical, drug test, or finger printing prior to that date. It is a good idea to ask about proper dress for the first orientation day (e.g., business attire or nursing uniform). Be sure you know where to park and the exact time and place to report. Plan to spend the full day. You may be finished early, but do not count on it.

Most facilities provide several weeks of orientation. Some may offer a longer new graduate program. The first week is normally on the day shift, with additional time provided on the shift to which you are assigned.

It is a good idea to arrive for orientation with a notebook. You will be given a lot of information, and it is wise to write it down to refer to later.

You have now made that transition from student to licensed nurse. Congratulations! All your hard work and dedication has paid off. You are now a member of a worthy profession.

PROFESSION/PROFESSIONALISM

A **profession** is defined as an occupation that requires extensive education or a calling that requires special knowledge, skill, and preparation. Licensed practical/vocational nursing is an integral part of the nursing profession. As a LPN/LVN working in a hospital or other health care agency, you will be expected to demonstrate certain characteristics and behaviors that demonstrate **professionalism,** as described in Box 34-5 ◆. By emulating these behaviors, you will be well on your way to being a successful licensed nurse.

Long-term success in nursing requires more than a license and an orientation. You will learn many life lessons in your first year as an LPN/LVN. See Box 34-6 ◆ for tips to thrive (not just survive) in your first year as an LPN/LVN.

PROBATIONARY PERIOD AND PERFORMANCE EVALUATION

Each health care facility has a **probationary period** for newly hired employees. During this time, your immediate supervisor will be evaluating your performance. At the end of this time, you will be given a **performance evaluation** and mostly likely a small increase in salary. Your attendance and promptness will be an important consideration, as will your ability to work as a team member, complete your assignments in a timely manner, and perfect your skills.

BOX 34-5 PROFESSIONAL CHARACTERISTICS AND BEHAVIORS

A practicing nurse (LPN/LVN) should possess professional qualifies of warmth and empathy. These characteristics include but are not limited to:

◆ Ability to develop relationships that exhibit a caring philosophy
◆ An ethic of caring (reflected by appropriate emotional responses, communication, punctuality, hygiene, and attire) that seeks to preserve the wholeness and dignity of self and others.
◆ Adherence to confidentiality of clients and others
◆ Behavior that reflects responsibility and accountability for safety of clients, self, and others
◆ Demonstration of knowledge regarding scope of practice of the LPN/LVN
◆ Demonstration of interpersonal skills needed to function as an effective team member
◆ Demonstration of problem-solving skills applying the concepts of the nursing process within the scope of the practical/vocational nurse
◆ An awareness of available resources for continued personal and professional growth

BOX 34-6 THRIVING DURING THE FIRST YEAR ON THE JOB

◆ **Be patient.** It takes time to gain experience. Some say it takes up to 2 years to be able to handle most situations.
◆ **Be positive.** Every day write down something good you did or learned, and review your list often. Focus on the positive; it will become your reality.
◆ **Be a seeker.** Don't wait for someone to tell you to do a procedure. Seek out opportunities to do new things. If you don't know how, request the opportunity to observe a more experienced colleague. Show your willingness to learn.
◆ **Be a helper.** It is never too soon to lend a hand to a co-worker. Be sure to be available to students; remember, you were there once.
◆ **Be a buddy.** Buddy up with a co-worker after whom you would like to model yourself. You can learn from people, no matter what their title.
◆ **Be a team player.** Introduce yourself to co-workers on all shifts, to physicians, and to other hospital personnel. Have lunch with someone you don't know. Become a part of the team.
◆ **Be a lifelong learner.** Use references and policy and procedure manuals, ask questions, and do your homework at the end of each day by looking up things that are new to you.
◆ **Be a joiner.** Become a member of a professional organization; develop close ties with colleagues on a state and national level. Organizations provide cutting-edge information.
◆ **Be a tracker.** Track your progress. Don't lose track of the progress you have already made. Review this often; see how far you have come.
◆ **Be a stress buster.** Stress should be managed, not just tolerated (see Chapter 30). ◉ Make time for yourself for socializing, for leisure activities, for hobbies. Take care of yourself so you can give care to others.
◆ **Be focused.** Keep moving forward. You can do it!

After the initial evaluation, most facilities evaluate employees on an annual basis. Annual evaluations may include skills testing and renewal of CPR or other certifications. You are expected to keep track of these requirements yourself, since expired certifications may prevent you from working.

◆ Pursuing Your Career

CONTINUING EDUCATION

All state boards of nursing have continuing education requirements for licensed nurses. The number of hours varies with the individual board. It is your responsibility to know the requirements for your state. Requirements can be met with on-site classes, professional conferences, home study courses, or courses on the Internet. It is important that classes be completed prior to the renewal date of your license. Once continuing education classes are completed, keep the certificates on file. Your portfolio is an excellent storage location for a copy, since state nursing boards conduct random audits of license holders. Continuing education is designed to help keep you current in the field, but they also can introduce you to new skills or even a new specialty. The possibilities are limited only by time and interest.

CAREER LADDER

A **career ladder** can be described as progression from one level in a profession to another through educational pursuits and professional experience. Figure 34-2 ◆ is a sketch of a career ladder.

Career ladder programs offer a variety of options. An individual who already has a practical or vocational nursing license can enter an associate nursing degree (ADN or AS) program by taking a transition course. Some training programs have direct *articulation* with schools of registered nursing. Direct articulation can be described as when LPN/LVNs receive advanced placement, courses are waived because of an agreement between the schools.

Another option is to enroll in a 2-year ADN program and exit after the first year, after completing the practical nurse option. These options better meet the individual's needs for employment and continuing education.

Many LPN/LVNs have a desire to progress beyond the ADN level of registered nursing. The availability for lifelong learning and advanced practice opportunities are many.

Some new graduates are ready to dive right into additional schooling. Others need to seek full-time employment to support themselves or family. Still others may need a well-deserved break from school. With nursing, the option of further education is always there, either now or in the future.

Your career goal may be fulfilled when you become an LPN/LVN, or you may wish to continue up the ladder. Whatever your professional goal, it is important never to stop learning and always to strive to be a competent and compassionate nurse.

MediaLink ◆ Career Ladder

PROFESSIONAL ORGANIZATIONS

The first **professional nursing organization** was established in 1893. Nurses found that if they united to achieve common goals and missions, they could have a greater impact on their chosen profession.

The National League of Nursing (NLN) was established under the name of the American Society of Superintendents of Training Schools for Nurses in the United States and Canada. In 1912, the name was changed to the NLN. Their purpose was to standardize and improve nursing education. There are two levels of membership in the NLN: individual and agency. Schools of nursing and other agencies that provide nursing care are eligible for agency membership. In 1943, lay members were permitted to join the organization, which had previously been open only to nurses. The NLN is the accrediting organization for nursing programs. A graduate of an NLN-accredited program will be recognized nationally and credits will be recognized by other NLN-approved program when the nurse chooses to continue his or her education.

The American Nurses Association (ANA) is a professional organization for limited to registered nurses. The National Federation of Licensed Practical Nurses (NFLPN) and The National Association for Practical Nurse Education and Services (NAPNES) are professional organizations for the LPN/LVN. Membership in a professional organization provides the licensed nurse with many services. These organizations are your representative on a national level, providing continuing education opportunities and opportunities for networking. There are specialty organizations for nurses working in pediatrics, geriatrics, or obstetrics, to name a few. Participation in a local or national organization is a worthwhile activity for a graduate nurse.

NETWORKING AND COLLABORATION

Nursing is not a career that one can pursue in a vacuum. **Networking** is described as the deliberate effort to make connections among people for a variety of interests, including employment opportunities. Networking may be casual or formal (Kurzen, 2001). Formal networking is done in the context of a professional organization or in a work situation while casual networking is done in social settings. (e.g., your cousin introduces you to a friend who is the clinical nurse educator in a hospital where you wish to apply.)

Collaborative nursing practice or interdependent nursing practice is working jointly with other health care professionals, including physicians, in the performance of nursing roles within the scope of practice. Learning to network and collaborate with other nurses and health care providers is extremely important. You can begin to learn these skills by participating in staff or unit minutes. In the beginning, you may feel you have little to contribute, but as you listen to your colleagues and progress in your nursing practice you will see ways to improve client care and unit operations. Once you are comfortable in a small group, volunteer for a hospital or sys-

Nursing Instructor
Professor
D.NS, PhD, EdD

Nurse Practitioner
Certified Nurse Midwife

Clinical Nurse
Specialist
MSN

Registered Nurse
Associate Degree
BSN

Licensed Practical
Licensed Vocational
Nurse

Certified Nursing
Assistant
Home Health Aide

Allied Health
Medical Assistant
EMT

Figure 34-2. ◆ LPNs and LVNs have much room for advancement up the career ladder.

tem-wide committee. As a member of a professional organization, your networking and collaborative opportunities will increase as your circle of professional associates increases.

Note: The bibliography listings for this and all chapters have been compiled at the back of the book.

Chapter Review

Key Terms by Topics

Use the audio glossary feature of either the CD-ROM or the Companion Website to hear the correct pronunciation of the following key terms.

Portfolio
portfolio, work samples

Job search
cover letter, résumé, references

The hiring process
orientation, profession, professionalism, probationary period, performance evaluation

Pursuing your career
career ladder, professional nursing organization, networking

Key Points

* You will continue to learn as you begin your first job. You may even come to think of that first position as being another phase of your education.

* Learn as much as you can about the facility and its parent company before making application.

* A portfolio is an itemized visual account of your skills and best practices related to the position you are seeking.

* Most résumés are computer generated today, but at the very least, your résumé must be typed on quality paper and should be printed on the same light-colored paper that you used for your cover letter.

* A face-to-face meeting gives a first impression. Whether it results in employment or not, it is an experience that can give you insight into your ability to speak logically and think critically.

* Continuing education is required by all state boards of nursing. The licensed nurse needs to be aware of the specific requirements of the state in which he or she is licensed.

* Professional organizations represent the members' interests nationally; they also provide educational and networking opportunities.

EXPLORE MediaLink

Additional interactive resources for this chapter can be found on the Companion Website at www.prenhall.com/ramont. Click on Chapter 34 and "Begin" to select the activities for this chapter.

For chapter-related NCLEX-style questions and an audio glossary, access the accompanying CD-ROM in this book.

For Further Study

For more information about ways to communicate well, see Chapter 25.

For further discussion of stress and coping skills, see Chapter 30.

For review of ways to prepare for examinations, see Chapter 33.

NCLEX-PN Exam Preparation

1. A cover letter should contain three paragraphs. The first paragraph is where you would:
   a. Highlight your particular qualifications.
   b. Identify yourself and the job that is being sought.
   c. Convey your anticipation in obtaining an interview.
   d. Express your enthusiasm for this particular job.

2. You have a significant gap in your work history following a lay-off from a previous job. Which of the following is the best way to address the gap on an employment application?
   a. Skip that time period. Prospective employers are not interested in times when you were not employed.
   b. Leave the area on the application blank where it asks why you left that job.
   c. Identify the time period and highlight educational or volunteer activities during that time.
   d. Write an explanation of why you were laid off, so they know it was not your fault.

3. If subjected to a question concerning your religion during the hiring process, which of the following would be the best response?
   a. "Civil rights laws prohibit you from asking me personal questions."
   b. "I would really rather not answer that question."
   c. "I will need time off on religious holidays to fulfill my personal obligations. I hope that will not be a problem."
   d. "My religious beliefs will not interfere with my ability to carry out the responsibilities of this position."

4. One of your fellow students has applied to several health care facilities, but has not received one call back. You notice that her cover letter and résumé are addressed "To Whom It May Concern." What is the most likely reason for the lack of response?
   a. The facilities do not like to hire new graduates.
   b. Her cover letter and résumé did not demonstrate an effort on her part to find out pertinent information about the facility and staff.
   c. The facility knew she was applying to others and did not want to waste their time if she really wasn't interested.
   d. Because the letter was not addressed to a person, it did not reach the person doing the hiring.

5. A profession can be described in many ways. The definition that best describes nursing as a profession is:
   a. An occupation to which one devotes oneself and in which one has specialized expertise
   b. A job that requires post-baccalaureate education
   c. A lifelong career that provides upward mobility
   d. An occupation that has a continuing education requirement

6. You are scheduled for an interview at a hospital where you were employed as a nursing assistant throughout your nursing program. The interview is scheduled at 9 A.M. after you come off night shift. Which is the most appropriate view about attire for the interview?
   a. "I will wear my uniform; that way I will not be rushed and can relax before the meeting."
   b. "Since the director of nursing and human resource director already know me, it won't matter how I am dressed."
   c. "I will go home, shower, and dress in business attire. This will show respect for the interview team and the position for which I am applying."
   d. "I will tell my supervisor I need to leave early because this interview is really important."

7. Which of the following would be considered to be casual networking for a job?
   a. Attending a presentation with classmates on a new facility that is recruiting LPNs
   b. Attending a job fair at a local college
   c. Hearing about the advantages of a new job while having coffee with a friend
   d. Discussing job opportunities on a hospital internet website

8. There are several types of résumé formats. Which of the following formats emphasizes skills?
   a. Chronological
   b. Functional
   c. Combination
   d. E-résumé

9. It is important to include writing samples in your portfolio because they demonstrate:
   a. Your ability to write in a logical order using correct format and your attention to detail
   b. That academic skills were a part of your nursing program
   c. Your ability to chart effectively
   d. Your level of computer skills

10. The first professional nursing organization, American Society of Superintendents of Training Schools for Nurses in the United States and Canada later changed its name to:
    a. The American Nurses Association
    b. The National Association for Practical Nursing
    c. The North American Nursing Diagnosis Association
    d. The National League of Nursing

Answers for Review Questions appear in Appendix IV.

Thinking Strategically About...

You are a recent graduate from a vocational nursing program. You successfully passed your licensure exam and have been hired as night shift charge nurse for a skilled nursing facility. Your orientation went well, and now this is your first night alone on the unit.

A client from the assisted living unit was sent to the ED of the local hospital for IVs to treat dehydration resulting from several days of nausea and vomiting. The IV line has been placed. He will be discharged from the ED and will be coming to your unit. You are not yet IV certified but are planning to take the class after receiving your first paycheck.

You attempt to reach the Director of Nursing (DON) by phone and find that she is out of town. You call the Assistant DON and inform her that no nurse in the building is IV certified. You request that the client be kept at the hospital until morning. You explain your lack of certification to the ADON. She hesitates, then asks what care will be needed during the night. There is no medication to be given IV, but fluids will needed to be added to the IV at about 5 A.M. You have watched the procedure many times and realize that although you are not legally qualified, it is a relatively easy procedure.

COMMUNICATION AND TEAM BUILDING

Using your knowledge of communication and team building, what solutions could you suggest to the ADON? List several possibilities.

CRITICAL THINKING

The ADON says, "Well, you've watched these things being done a dozen times. It's not that big a deal. Can't you just do it?" When you hesitate, she lashes out and states, "I knew there would be a problem hiring you new grads. If you can't solve your problems, maybe we need to rethink your charge nurse position." What responses would be appropriate in this situation?

CONFLICT RESOLUTION

After this conflict, you are concerned about your relationship with the ADON. You want to try to resolve the tension over the IV issue. How might you approach the ADON to change the situation? If you are concerned that the ADON might tried to get you fired, what steps should you take to protect your position?

Appendix I   2003–2004 NANDA-Approved Nursing Diagnoses

Activity Intolerance
Activity Intolerance, Risk for
Adaptive Capacity: Intracranial, Decreased
Adjustment, Impaired
Airway Clearance, Ineffective
Anxiety
Anxiety, Death
Aspiration, Risk for
Attachment, Parent/Infant/Child, Risk for Impaired
Body Image, Disturbed
Body Temperature: Imbalanced, Risk for
Bowel Incontinence
Breastfeeding, Effective
Breastfeeding, Ineffective
Breastfeeding, Interrupted
Breathing Pattern, Ineffective
Cardiac Output, Decreased
Caregiver Role Strain
Caregiver Role Strain, Risk for
Communication, Readiness for Enhanced
Communication: Verbal, Impaired
Confusion, Acute
Confusion, Chronic
Constipation
Constipation, Perceived
Constipation, Risk for
Coping: Community, Ineffective
Coping: Community, Readiness for Enhanced
Coping, Defensive
Coping: Family, Compromised
Coping: Family, Disabled
Coping: Family, Readiness for Enhanced
Coping (Individual), Readiness for Enhanced
Coping, Ineffective
Decisional Conflict (Specify)
Denial, Ineffective
Dentition, Impaired
Development: Delayed, Risk for
Diarrhea
Disuse Syndrome, Risk for
Diversional Activity, Deficient

Dysreflexia, Autonomic
Dysreflexia, Autonomic, Risk for
Energy Field, Disturbed
Environmental Interpretation Syndrome, Impaired
Failure to Thrive, Adult
Falls, Risk for
Family Processes, Dysfunctional: Alcoholism
Family Processes, Interrupted
Family Processes, Readiness for Enhanced
Fatigue
Fear
Fluid Balance, Readiness for Enhanced
Fluid Volume, Deficient
Fluid Volume, Deficient, Risk for
Fluid Volume, Excess
Fluid Volume, Imbalanced, Risk for
Gas Exchange, Impaired
Grieving, Anticipatory
Grieving, Dysfunctional
Growth, Disproportionate, Risk for
Growth and Development, Delayed
Health Maintenance, Ineffective
Health Seeking Behaviors (Specify)
Home Maintenance, Impaired
Hopelessness
Hyperthermia
Hypothermia
Identity: Personal, Disturbed
Infant Behavior, Disorganized
Infant Behavior: Disorganized, Risk for
Infant Behavior: Organized, Readiness for Enhanced
Infant Feeding Pattern, Ineffective
Infection, Risk for
Injury, Risk for
Knowledge, Deficient (Specify)
Knowledge (specify), Readiness for Enhanced
Latex Allergy Response
Latex Allergy Response, Risk for
Loneliness, Risk for
Memory, Impaired
Mobility: Bed, Impaired

Mobility: Physical, Impaired
Mobility: Wheelchair, Impaired
Nausea
Neurovascular Dysfunction: Peripheral, Risk for
Noncompliance (Specify)
Nutrition, Imbalanced: Less than Body Requirements
Nutrition, Imbalanced: More than Body Requirements
Nutrition, Imbalanced: More than Body Requirements,
  Risk for
Nutrition, Readiness for Enhanced
Oral Mucous Membrane, Impaired
Pain, Acute
Pain, Chronic
Parenting, Impaired
Parenting, Readiness for Enhanced
Parenting, Risk for Impaired
Perioperative Positioning Injury, Risk for
Poisoning, Risk for
Post-Trauma Syndrome
Post-Trauma Syndrome, Risk for
Powerlessness
Powerlessness, Risk for
Protection, Ineffective
Rape-Trauma Syndrome
Rape-Trauma Syndrome: Compound Reaction
Rape-Trauma Syndrome: Silent Reaction
Relocation Stress Syndrome
Relocation Stress Syndrome, Risk for
Role Conflict, Parental
Role Performance, Ineffective
Self-Care Deficit: Bathing/Hygiene
Self-Care Deficit: Dressing/Grooming
Self-Care Deficit: Feeding
Self-Care Deficit: Toileting
Self-Concept, Readiness for Enhanced
Self-Esteem, Chronic Low
Self-Esteem, Situational Low
Self-Esteem, Risk for Situational Low
Self-Mutilation
Self-Mutilation, Risk for
Sensory Perception, Disturbed (Specify: Visual, Auditory,
  Kinesthetic, Gustatory, Tactile, Olfactory)
Sexual Dysfunction
Sexuality Patterns, Ineffective
Skin Integrity, Impaired
Skin Integrity, Risk for Impaired

Sleep Deprivation
Sleep Pattern, Disturbed
Sleep, Readiness for Enhanced
Social Interaction, Impaired
Social Isolation
Sorrow, Chronic
Spiritual Distress
Spiritual Distress, Risk for
Spiritual Well-Being, Readiness for Enhanced
Spontaneous Ventilation, Impaired
Sudden Infant Death Syndrome, Risk for
Suffocation, Risk for
Suicide, Risk for
Surgical Recovery, Delayed
Swallowing, Impaired
Therapeutic Regimen Management: Community,
  Ineffective
Therapeutic Regimen Management, Effective
Therapeutic Regimen Management: Family, Ineffective
Therapeutic Regimen Management, Ineffective
Therapeutic Regimen Management, Readiness for
  Enhanced
Thermoregulation, Ineffective
Thought Processes, Disturbed
Tissue Integrity, Impaired
Tissue Perfusion, Ineffective (Specify type: renal, cerebral,
  cardiopulmonary, gastrointestinal, peripheral)
Tissue Perfusion, Ineffective (Peripheral)
Transfer Ability, Impaired
Trauma, Risk for
Unilateral Neglect
Urinary Elimination, Impaired
Urinary Elimination, Readiness for Enhanced
Urinary Incontinence, Functional
Urinary Incontinence, Reflex
Urinary Incontinence, Stress
Urinary Incontinence, Total
Urinary Incontinence, Urge
Urinary Incontinence, Risk for Urge
Urinary Retention
Ventilatory Weaning Response, Dysfunctional
Violence: Other-Directed, Risk for
Violence: Self-Directed, Risk for
Walking, Impaired
Wandering

Source: NANDA nursing diagnoses: Definitions and classification, 2003–2004. Philadelphia, PA: North American Nursing Diagnosis Association. Used with permission.

Appendix II *Sample Critical Pathway for Client Following Total Mastectomy*

◆ Assessment Data

NURSING ASSESSMENT FOR HELEN MORTON

Mrs. Helen Morton, 36 years old, was admitted for a right mastectomy. She had a positive biopsy for breast cancer two weeks prior to admission. On admission to ambulatory surgery, Mrs. Morton asked the nurse, "Will I ever look normal again?" She also told the nurse, "I don't want any visitors after surgery; I don't want anyone to see how I look." The day following surgery, Mrs. Morton states, "I don't want to look at it," when the physician starts the dressing change.

Physical Examination
Height: 167.6 cm (5'6")
Weight: 65 kg (143 lb)
Temperature: 37C (98.6F)
Pulse rate: 76 bpm
Respirations: 20/minute

Blood pressure: 120/80 mm Hg
Skin warm, dry, pink, and pale
Mastectomy incision clean, dry, and well approximated

Diagnostic Data
RBC: 4.2 million/μL
Hgb: 10.2 g/dL
Hct: 39%
Urine: negative
Expected length of stay: 3 to 4 days
Daily outcomes
Tests and treatments
Knowledge deficit
Diet
Activity
Medications
Body image
Psychosocial
Transfer/discharge plans

EXPECTED LENGTH OF STAY: 3 TO 4 DAYS			
	DATE _____ **FIRST 24 HOURS POSTOPERATIVE**	**DATE** _____ **48 HOURS POSTOPERATIVE**	**DATE** _____ **3–4 DAYS POSTOPERATIVE**
Daily outcomes	Client will ◆ Be afebrile. ◆ Have clean, dry dressing. ◆ Recover from anesthesia as evidenced by vital signs return to baseline; being awake, alert, and oriented. ◆ Verbalize understanding and demonstrate cooperation with turning, coughing, deep breathing, and splinting. ◆ Tolerate ordered diet without nausea and vomiting. ◆ Verbalize control of incisional pain. ◆ Verbalize ability to cope.	Client will ◆ Be afebrile. ◆ Have clean, dry wound with edges well approximated, healing by first intention. ◆ Demonstrate cooperation with turning, coughing, deep breathing, and splinting. ◆ Tolerate ordered diet without nausea and vomiting. ◆ Ambulate 4 times per day in hallway. ◆ Verbalize control of incisional pain. ◆ Verbalize beginning ability to cope with changes in body image. ◆ Verbalize ability to cope. ◆ Verbalize beginning understanding of home care instructions.	Client will ◆ Be afebrile. ◆ Have clean, dry wound with edges well approximated, healing by first intention. ◆ Manages pain with oral medications and/or nonpharmacologic measures. ◆ Be independent in self-care. ◆ Be fully ambulatory. ◆ Have resumed preadmission urine and bowel elimination pattern. ◆ Verbalize home care instructions. ◆ Tolerate usual diet. ◆ Verbalize ability to cope with changes in body image and ongoing stressors.

(continues)

	DATE _____ FIRST 24 HOURS POSTOPERATIVE	DATE _____ 48 HOURS POSTOPERATIVE	DATE _____ 3–4 DAYS POSTOPERATIVE
Daily outcomes			◆ Demonstrate progressive upper extremity exercises that include external rotation and abduction of the affected shoulder when the stitches are removed 7 to 10 days after surgery.
Tests and treatments	Vital signs and O$_2$ saturation, neurovascular assessment, dressing and wound drainage assessment q15min × 4; q30min × 4; q1h × 4 and then q4h if stable. NO BLOOD PRESSURES OR VENIPUNCTURE ON AFFECTED ARM. Assess respiratory status q4h and prn. Incentive spirometer q2h. Intake and output q shift. Assess voiding—if unable to void, try suggestive voiding techniques or catheterize q8h or prn.	Vital signs and dressing and wound drainage assessment q4h. NO BLOOD PRESSURES OR VENIPUNCTURE ON AFFECTED ARM. Assess respiratory status q4h. Incentive spirometer q2h until fully ambulatory. Intake and output q shift. Assess voiding pattern q shift. Dressing change by surgeon.	Vital signs and dressing and wound drainage assessment q4h–8h. NO BLOOD PRESSURES OR VENIPUNCTURE ON AFFECTED ARM. Assess respiratory status q4h–8h. Assess wound and apply dry sterile dressing q day and prn.
Knowledge deficit	Orient to room and surroundings. Provide simple, brief instructions. Review preoperative preparation, including hospital and specific postoperative care: turning, coughing, deep breathing, incentive spirometer, mobilization, intravenous infusions, pain management.	Review plan of care and importance of early mobilization. Begin discharge teaching regarding wound care/dressing change, diet, and activity. Review written discharge instructions with client and support person.	Complete discharge teaching to include wound care, diet, follow-up care, signs and symptoms to report, activity, and medication: frequency, dose, route, and side effects. Provide client with written discharge instructions including upper arm and shoulder exercises for affected arm.
Diet	Clear to full liquids as tolerated.	Full liquids to usual diet to tolerance.	Usual diet to tolerance.
Activity	Provide safety precautions. Ambulate 4 times in room. Encourage finger, wrist, and elbow movement and use of affected arm for ADLs and personal hygiene.	Fully ambulatory in room. Walk in hall 4 to 6 times per day. Encourage finger, wrist, and elbow movement and use of affected arm for ADLs and personal hygiene. Instruct client in progressive upper arm exercises.	Fully ambulatory. Encourage finger, wrist, and elbow movement and use of affected arm for ADLs and personal hygiene. Reinforce instructions regarding progressive exercises.
Medications	IM or IV/PCA analgesics. IV antibiotics. IV fluids.	PO, IM, or IV/PCA analgesics. IV antibiotics. Intermittent IV device.	PO analgesics. Discontinue IV device.
Body image	Establish a trusting relationship with client. Encourage client and significant others to verbalize their feelings about the mastectomy. Listen to client and significant others and show interest and concern rather than giving advice. Allow the client to respond to loss of body part and changed body image with denial, shock, anger, depression, and other grieving behaviors. Support the client's strengths and assist her to look at herself in totality.	Maintain trusting relationship with client. Encourage client and significant others to verbalize their feelings about the mastectomy. Listen to client and significant others and show interest and concern rather than giving advice. Allow the client to respond to loss of body part and changed body image with denial, shock, anger, depression, and other grieving behaviors. Support the client's strengths and assist her to look at herself in totality.	Provide opportunities to verbalize ongoing concerns regarding changes in body image and self-concept. Encourage and provide opportunities for self-care of wound and dressing. Provide opportunity for client to meet with volunteer from Reach to Recovery. Assist client to obtain temporary breast prosthesis. Answer questions and provide information on breast reconstruction.

	DATE _____ FIRST 24 HOURS POSTOPERATIVE	DATE _____ 48 HOURS POSTOPERATIVE	DATE _____ 3–4 DAYS POSTOPERATIVE
Psychosocial	Assess coping status. Use active listening. Provide a nonthreatening environment. Determine support people and resources available to the client. Assess responses of support people. Allow for client's input regarding sequence of care. Be supportive of client's effective coping behaviors.	Assess coping status. Use active listening. Provide a nonthreatening environment. Assist client to identify and develop support system and resources. Assess responses of support people. Allow for client's input regarding sequence of care. Be supportive of client's effective coping behaviors.	Assess coping status. Use active listening. Provide a nonthreatening environment. Determine support people and resources available to the client. Assess responses of support people. Allow for client's input regarding sequence of care. Be supportive of client's effective coping behaviors.
Transfer/ discharge plans	Determine discharge needs with client and support people. Begin home care instructions.	Review progress toward discharge goals. Finalize discharge plans. Refer to Reach to Recovery.	Complete discharge instructions.

Appendix III Glossary

(Note: Glossary terms may appear in several chapters. The number(s) in parentheses in boldface after the glossary term show the primary chapter in which the term is defined. Other words or terms that may require definitions are italicized in the text and are defined there.)

Ablative: removal by surgery (as a diseased body part) (22)

Absorption: process by which the drug passes into the blood stream (21)

Accommodation: alternating change in pupil size (constrict when looking at the near object, dilate when looking at the distant one) (11)

Active listening: listening for key themes in communication with clients; use of attentive behaviors (25)

Active range of motion: full normal movement of the extremities and joints by the client through a systematic series of motions (11)

Acute pain: pain that lasts only through the expected recovery period (15)

Adenosine triphosphate (ATP): energy compound of cells (10)

Admission: hospital admission is entry into the hospital (8)

Adventitious breath sounds: Abnormal breath sounds (11)

Adverse effect: More severe side effects, or drug reactions (21)

Advocate: one who expresses and defends the cause of another (2)

Afebrile: without fever (14)

Affective domain: aspects of learning that includes feelings, emotions, interests, attitudes, and appreciations (23)

Afternoon care: care of client that often includes providing a bedpan or urinal, washing the hands and face, and assisting with oral care (13)

Against Medical Advice: situation of a client leaving the hospital or health care facility without the written permission of a physician (8)

Algor mortis: gradual decrease of the body's temperature after death (31)

Alopecia: hair loss (13)

Ambulation: act of walking (20)

Amino acids: end products of protein digestion (17)

Ampule: clear glass container with a distinctive shape usually designed to hold a single dose of a drug (21)

Anabolism: process of building tissue (17)

Analysis: interpretation of a variety of data and recognition of the commonalities, differences, and interrelationships among ideas (1)

Anatomic position: normal standing positions; body is upright, facing front, arms at the sides with the palms facing forward, and feet parallel (10)

Anatomy: study of body structure (10)

Anemia: condition of too few red blood cells that contain too little or abnormal hemoglobin (16)

Anesthesia: alteration in the level of sensation and consciousness; classified as *general* (comprehensive) or *regional* (specific) (22)

Anger: emotional state that includes feelings of animosity or strong displeasure (30)

Angina pectoris: chest pain, usually caused by lack of oxygen to the coronary vessels (16)

Ankylosed: permanently immobile (20)

Anticipatory Grieving: The state in which an individual or group experiences reactions in response to an expected significant loss (31)

Antiemboli stockings: firm elastic hose that compress the veins of the legs and facilitate the return of venous blood to the heart (22)

Antigens: markers that identify the type of cell and help the immune system determine whether the cell is foreign to the organism (7)

Antiseptics: agents that inhibit the growth of some microorganisms

Anuria: lack of urine production, with no effective urinary output (18)

Anxiety: state of mental uneasiness, apprehension, dread;

feeling of helplessness related to an unidentified threat to self or significant relationships (30)

Apical: at the apex of the heart (14)

Apnea: periods of no breathing (16)

Apothecaries' system: system of measurements that predates the metric system (21)

Application: utilizing knowledge and understanding in a particular case (1)

Asepsis: absence of disease-causing microorganisms (7)

Aseptic technique: method used to prevent the transmission of microorganisms from one place or person to another (7)

As-needed (prn) care: care provided as required by the client (13)

Assault: an attempt or threat to touch another person unjustifiably (2)

Assessment: systematic collection, organization, *validation* (proving or supporting), and documentation of *data* (information) (4)

Assisted suicide: also called voluntary euthanasia; situations in which the dying individual has some control over the time and manner of death (31)

Atelectasis: collapse of the alveoli, of a lobe, or of an entire lung (20)

Atherosclerosis: narrowing and obstruction of circulatory vessels; most common cause of ischemia (16)

Atherosclerotic plaque: fat deposits within the blood vessels (16)

Atrophy: unused muscles atrophy (decrease in size), losing most of their normal strength and function (20)

Attitudes: mental positions or feelings toward a person, object, or idea (2)

Auscultation: process of listening to sounds produced within the body (11)

Autocratic: making unilateral decisions while dominating team-members (32)

Autonomy: the right to make one's own decisions (2)

Autopsy: postmortem examination; examination of the body after death (31)

Bacteria: most common microorganisms causing disease in humans (7)

Bactericidal agent: agent that destroys bacteria (7)

Bacteriostatic agent: agent that prevents growth and reproduction of only some bacteria (7)

Bagging: means of enclosing dirty, contaminated, or hazardous materials in plastic bags for safe removal and disposal (6)

Basal metabolic rate (BMR): rate at which the body metabolizes (burns) food to maintain energy (14)

Battery: the willful and unjustifiable touching of a person or personal items; it may or may not cause harm (2)

Bed cradle: (Anderson frame) a device designed to keep the top bedclothes off the feet, legs, and even abdomen of a client (13)

Behavior modification: system of positive reinforcement in which desirable behavior is regarded and undesirable behavior is ignored (23)

Behaviorism: belief that environment influences behavior, which is the essential factor determining human action (23)

Beliefs: interpretations or conclusions which people accept as being true; they do not necessarily involve values (2)

Bereavement: subjective response experienced by the surviving loved ones after the death of a person with whom they have shared a significant relationship (31)

Bevel: part of the needle which is the slanted part of the tip (21)

Bioethics: ethics as applied to life (2)

Blood pressure: measure of the pressure exerted by the blood as it flows through the arteries (14)

Body image: how a person perceives the size, appearance, and functioning of the body and its parts (28)

Body mechanics: term used to describe safe, efficient use of the body to move objects and carry out activities of daily living (6)

Bradypnea: abnormally slow respiratory rate (16)

Buccal: pertaining to the cheek; in medication administration, it means next to the mucous membranes of the cheek (21)

Buffers: chemicals that help maintain acid-base balance by neutralizing excess acids or bases (17)

Calculi: stones (18)

Calories: units of heat energy (17)

Cannula: shaft part of the needle which is attached to the hub (21)

Capillary refill: return of blood to tissue (such as the nail bed) after being pressed; return of normal color to tissue (11)

Cardiac output: amount of blood pumped by the heart in one minute (14)

Cardiopulmonary resuscitation (CPR): combination of oral resuscitation (mouth-to-mouth breathing) and external cardiac massage (chest compression); procedure is intended to provide oxygen to the lungs and reestablish cardiac function and blood circulation (16)

Care plan: written guide that organizes information about the client's care (4)

Career ladder: progression from one level in a profession to another through educational pursuits and professional experience (34)

Carrier: person or animal, which has a pathogenic microorganism living inside of them (7)

Case management: range of models for integrating health care services for individuals or groups (5)

Case method: system in which one nurse is responsible for the comprehensive care of a group of clients during an 8- or 12-hour shift (5)

Catabolism: process of breaking down tissue (17)

Cathartic: medication that stimulates bowel activity and assists fecal elimination (19)

Catheterization: introduction of a catheter through the urethra into the urinary bladder (18)

Cell membrane: "skin" of a cell; plasma membrane (10)

Cell: basic unit of all life (10)

Center of gravity: point at which all of the body's mass is centered and the base of support of the foundation on which the body achieves balance (20)

Cerumen: earwax (13)

Change-of-shift report: a report given to all nurses on the incoming shift (9)

Channels: openings that permit the passage of certain materials into or out of the cell (10)

Charting: recording; documenting; process of making an entry on a client's record (9)

Chronic pain: pain that lasts beyond the typical healing period (15)

Chyme: waste products that leave the stomach through the small intestine and then pass through the ileocecal valve (19)

Cilia: hairlike projections on the surface of some cells (10)

Circumcision: removal of the foreskin of the penis (29)

Cleaning baths: baths given chiefly for hygiene purposes (13)

Client: (in this text) recipient of nursing care; includes individuals, families, and communities (1)

Client education: integrated and multifaceted teaching–learning process in which the nurse and client work together to change unhealthy client behaviors (23)

Client-focused care: delivery model that brings all services and care providers to the clients (5)

Clinical pathway: method for tracking the client's progress, planning care, and providing client teaching and discharge planning (5)

Clinical record: chart, client record; formal, legal document that provides evidence of a client's care (9)

Closed wound drainage system: a drain connected directly from the wound or from an incision near the wound to a suction device; it promotes healing by allowing excess serosanguineous fluid and purulent material to drain (22)

Closed-ended questions: questions that generally require only "yes" or "no" or short factual answers (25)

Code of ethics: formal statement of a group's ideals and values (2)

Cognitive: related to awareness; perceiving; thinking (24)

Cognitive domain: area of learning that includes knowing, comprehending, and applying (23)

Cognitivism: definition of learning as largely a complex thinking process; emphasizes individual perception and motivation, as well as the teacher–learner relationship and environment (23)

Coitus: copulation; heterosexual genital intercourse (29)

Collaborate: to cooperate, to work together with someone in a different position or specialty (4)

Collaborative actions: nursing activities that reflect the overlapping responsibilities between health personnel (4)

Colostomy: an opening into the *colon* (large bowel) (19)

Communicable disease: disease spread or transmitted by direct or indirect contact (7)

Communication: exchange of information or thoughts between two or more people through language, the arts, or body actions (25)

Compliance: extent to which a person's behavior coincides with medical or health advice (23)

Comprehension: knowledge and understanding of information (1)

Computerized Adaptive Testing (CAT): method of testing in which the computer selects a unique set of test questions for each test taker from a large test bank of questions. It provides a set percentage of questions from predetermined categories (33)

Confer: to consult another person for advice, information, ideas, or instructions (9)

Conflict: competitive or antagonistic state; mental state resulting from opposing needs, wishes, or demands (32)

Connective tissue: supporting fabric of the body (10)

Conscious sedation: a minimal form of anesthesia in which a client is conscious and has an increased pain threshold during surgery (22)

Consensual response: constriction of one eye when a bright light is shown into the opposite pupil, removed, and shown a second time (11)

Constipation: fewer than three bowel movements per week (19)

Consumer: individual, group of people, or community that uses a service or commodity (1)

Continuous feedings: feedings generally administered over a 24-hour period using an infusion pump that guarantees a constant flow (17)

COPD: chronic obstructive pulmonary disease; persistent obstruction of bronchial air flow (16)

Coping behavior: behavior people perform in times of crisis or stress, in an attempt to deal with their feelings (8)

Coping: dealing with problems and situations successfully (30)

Coping strategy (coping mechanism): inborn or learned way of responding to a changing environment, specific problem, or situation (30)

Cover letter: concise, one-page letter that highlights professional and educational attributes for a potential employer (34)

Crime: act committed in violation of public (criminal) law and punishable by a fine or imprisonment (2)

Crisis: stage in fever marked by excessive sweating and hot, flushed skin due to sudden vasodilatation; acute, time-limited state of emotional imbalance resulting from sources of stress (14, 30)

Critical thinking: process of examining one's own thinking and assumptions to arrive at a broader viewpoint (3)

Cultural competence: the knowledge, skill, and ability to provide safe and effective health care regardless of population or setting (26)

Culture: learned, shared, and transmitted values, beliefs, norms, and life way practices of a particular group that guide thinking, decisions, and actions in patterned ways (26)

Culture-specifics: values, beliefs, and patterns of behavior that tend to be unique to a designated culture rather than shared with members of other cultures (26)

Culture-universals: commonalities of values, norms of behavior, and life patterns among different cultures (26)

Cumulative effect: buildup of the drug in the blood because of impaired metabolism or excretion (21)

Cutaneous pain: pain that originates in the skin or subcutaneous tissue (15)

Cyanosis: bluish tinge of skin that usually indicates poor oxygenation (11)

Cytoplasm: main substance filling the inside of the cell; a colloidal (jellylike) suspension (10)

Dandruff: diffuse scaling of the scalp (13)

DAR: diagnosis (**D**), action (**A**), and response (**R**); means of organizing progress notes into data (9)

Database: baseline data; information about a client gathered from many sources; a reference point to assess changes in the client's condition (4)

Data collection: process of gathering information (4)

Date rape: situation in which one person manipulates a social interaction in order to have nonconsensual intercourse with another (29)

Death: cessation of the apical pulse, respirations, and blood pressure, also referred to as heart–lung death (31)

Debridement: removal of necrotic material (12)

Deductive reasoning: reasoning from the general to the specific (3)

Defamation: communication that is false, or made with a careless disregard for the truth, and that results in injury to the reputation of a person (2)

Defecation: bowel movement; expulsion of feces from the anus and rectum (19)

Defense mechanisms: psychologic adaptive mechanisms that develop as the personality attempts to defend itself, establish compromises among conflicting impulses, and allay inner tensions (30)

Dehiscence: partial or total rupturing of a sutured wound (12)

Dehumanization: process in which unique human qualities are ignored (as in hospitalized clients having to surrender their belongings, privacy, and independence) (8)

Delegation: distribution of tasks in a way that prioritizes activities and available resources (32)

Democratic: making decisions that reflect input from team members (32)

Depression: common reaction to overwhelming or negative events (30)

Desired outcome: goal; a description, in terms of observable client responses, of what the nurse hopes the client will achieve by implementing the nursing orders (4)

Development: an increase in the complexity of function and skill progression and in adaptation to the environment (24)

Diagnostic: used to confirm or establish a diagnosis (22)

Diagnostic profile: information provided to students who fail the NCLEX-PN, giving them data on performance in the various categories of the test (33)

Diagnostic related groups (DRGs): Classification of clinical conditions used for reimbursement by Medicare to health care provider or facility (1)

Diarrhea: passage of liquid feces and increased frequency of defecation (19)

Diastole: period in which the ventricles of the heart relax (11)

Diastolic pressure: pressure when the ventricles are at rest; the lower pressure that is present at all times within the arteries (14)

Diffusion: the movement of gases or other particles from an area of greater pressure or concentration to an area of lower pressure or concentration (16)

Direct response: constriction or tightening of a pupil when a bright light is shown into it (11)

Discharge: official procedure by which the client leaves the health care facility and returns home or to another setting (8)

Discrimination: differential treatment of individuals or groups based on categories such as race, ethnicity, gender, social class, or exceptionality (26)

Disease: process with distinctive signs and symptoms of infection (7)

Disinfectants: agents that destroy pathogens other than spores (7)

Diuresis: production and excretion of large amounts of urine (18)

Diuretics: chemicals that increase urine formation by preventing the reabsorption of water and electrolytes from the tubules of the kidney into the bloodstream (18)

Diversity: the fact or state of being different (26)

Do not resuscitate (DNR): order given for clients who are in a stage of terminal, irreversible illness or expected death (31)

Documenting: process of making an entry on a client record (9)

Drug allergy: immunologic reaction to a drug (21)

Drug interaction: problem that occurs when the administration of one drug alters the effect of another drug (21)

Drug tolerance: occurs when a person requires increases in dosage to maintain the therapeutic effect (21)

Drug toxicity: deleterious effects of a drug on an organism or tissue resulting from overdosage or from ingestion of a drug intended for external use (21)

Dysfunctional grieving: grieving characterized by extended time of denial, depression, severe physiologic symptoms, or suicidal thoughts (31)

Dysmenorrhea: painful menstruation (29)

Dyspareunia: pain during sexual activity and intercourse (29)

Dyspnea: difficult or labored breathing (16)

Dysrhythmias: abnormalities of the heart rate and rhythm (16)

Early morning care: care provided to clients as they awaken in the morning (13)

Edema: presence of excess interstitial fluid in tissue; causes a puffy appearance (11)

Effleurage: technique used in massage to promote relaxation and rest; light massage (20)

Effluent: fecal material (19)

Elective surgery: surgery performed when a condition is not immediately life threatening or to improve the client's life (22)

Electrocardiography: graphic recording of the heart's electrical activity (16)

Electrolytes: charged ions that can conduct electricity; present in all body fluids and fluid compartments (17)

Emboli: clots moved from their place of origin, causing circulatory obstruction elsewhere; may lodge in vessels supplying vital organs (20)

Embolus: thrombus that has broken loose (16)

Emergency surgery: surgery performed immediately to preserve function or the life of the client (22)

Endocrine glands: glands that do not have ducts; secretions (hormones) are transported away from the gland by blood flowing through the gland (10)

Endogenous opioids: naturally occurring opioids (enkephalins, dynorphins, and beta endorphins) that bind to opiate receptor sites in the central and peripheral nervous system, decreasing or blocking any pain impulse (15)

Endoplasmic reticulum: network of membrane-bound tubules that extend from the cell membrane to the nuclear membrane (10)

Enema: solution introduced into the rectum and large intestine to distend the intestines and sometimes to irritate the intestinal mucosa to promote peristalsis and remove feces and flatus (19)

Enteral nutrition: EN, also called total enteral nutrition (TEN); nutrients provided when the client is unable to ingest or absorb foods (17)

Environment: internal and external surroundings that affect the client (3)

Enzymes: proteins that speed up chemical reactions that occur at the cell membrane (10)

Epiglottis: inlet to the larynx that closes during swallowing, routing food to the esophagus (16)

Epithelium: tissue that forms a covering or lining (10)

Equilibrium: sense of balance (20)

Erectile dysfunction: (see *Impotence*) (29)

Eructation: belching or burping (19)

Erythema: redness associated with a variety of rashes (11)

Erythrocytes: red blood cells (16)

Eschar: scar tissue (12)

Ethics: method of inquiry that helps people to understand the morality of human behavior; the practices or beliefs of a certain group; the expected standards of moral behavior of a particular group (2)

Ethnicity: consciousness of belonging to a group that is differentiated from others by symbolic markers (culture, biology, territory) (26)

Ethnocentrism: the view that the beliefs and values of one's own culture are superior to those of other cultures (26)

Etiology: identification of factors contributing to, or probable causes of, a health problem (4)

Eupnea: normal respiration; it is quiet, rhythmic, and effortless (16)

Euthanasia: act of painlessly putting to death persons suffering from incurable or distressing disease (31)

Evaluation: review of interventions to determine their effectiveness (4)

Evisceration: protrusion of internal viscera and tissue through an incision (12)

Exacerbations: flare-ups of a chronic disease (16)

Examination: physical assessment; a systematic method of collecting physical data about a client (4)

Exogenous opioid: analgesics (e.g., morphine) that bind to receptor sites to provide pain relief (15)

Expiration: exhalation; air moving out of the lungs as part of ventilation (16)

External disasters: events outside the hospital that produce a large number of victims (e.g., fires, plane or train accidents, earthquakes or violent civil disturbances) (6)

External respiration: refers to the interchange of oxygen and carbon dioxide between the alveoli of the lungs and the pulmonary blood (14)

Extracellular fluid (ECF): fluid found outside the cells; accounts for about one third of total body fluid (17)

Exudate: material that has escaped from blood vessels during the inflammatory process and is deposited in tissue or on tissue surfaces (12)

False imprisonment: unlawful restraint or detention of another person against his or her wishes (2)

Fear: emotion or feeling of apprehension aroused by impending danger, pain, or other perceived threat (30)

Feces: or *stool* excreted waste products (19)

Feedback: shared information that relates a person's performance to the desired goal (23)

Fiber: high-residue food that stimulates peristalsis to maintain regularity (19)

Fight or flight: a generalized body response to an emergency situation (30)

Fistula: abnormal passage between a hollow organ and the skin or between two hollow organs (12)

Flagellum: long whiplike extension from a cell that is used to move the cell itself (10)

Flatulence: presence of excessive *flatus* (gas) in the intestines (19)

Flatus: air and by-products of the digestion of carbohydrates within the bowel; gas (19)

Flowsheets: abbreviated progress notes that enable nurses to record nursing data quickly and concisely and provide an easy-to-read record of the client's condition over time (9)

Folk medicine: health beliefs and practices that derive from cultural traditions rather than from modern medicine's scientific base (26)

Fontanelles: gaps in the bone structure of an infant's skull that close gradually (24)

Friction: force acting parallel to the skin surface (12)

Fulcrum: fixed point about which a lever moves (6)

Functional method: delivery model that focuses on the jobs to be completed, using personnel with less preparation than the professional nurse to perform less complex care requirements (5)

Functional nursing: system in which each team member is assigned specific tasks or functions (32)

Fungi: microorganisms classified as either yeasts or molds (7)

Gamete: sperm or egg cell (10)

Gastrostomy: surgical creation of an artificial opening into the stomach (17)

Gate control theory: theory stating that peripheral nerve fibers carrying pain to the spinal cord can have their message modified at the spinal cord level (the "gate") before transmission to the brain (15)

Generic: family name of a drug (21)

Gland: tissue that produces some form of secretion (10)

Glycogen: stored form of glucose (17)

Goal: (see *Desired outcome*) (4)

Golgi apparatus: site where materials are synthesized and sorted for secretion from the cell (10)

Granulation tissue: translucent red tissue that grows in a wound (12)

Grief: total response to the emotional experience related to loss (31)

Grieving: process of reacting to loss; natural human response involving psychosocial and physiologic reactions to an actual or perceived loss (24)

Group: two or more people who have shared needs and goals, who take each other into account in their actions, and who thus are held together and set apart from others because of their interactions (25)

Growth: physical change and increase in size, including height, weight, bone size, and dentition (24)

Gustatory: dealing with the sense of taste (27)

Half-life: time interval required for the body's elimination processes to reduce the concentration of the drug in the body by one half (21)

Health: degree of wellness or well-being that the client experiences (3)

Health behaviors: actions people take to understand their health state, maintain an optimal state of health, prevent illness and injury, and reach their maximum physical and mental potential (26)

Health beliefs: concepts about health that an individual believes true; may or may not be founded on fact (26)

Health care system: totality of services offered by all health disciplines (5)

Health Maintenance Organizations (HMO): group health care agency that provides basic and supplemental health maintenance and treatment services to voluntary enrollees; fee is set without regard to the amount or kind of services provided (5)

Health status: state of health of an individual at a given time (26)

Hearing aid: battery-powered, sound-amplifying device used by hearing-impaired persons (13)

Hematocrit: measurement of the percentage of erythrocytes in the blood (16)

Hemoglobin: oxygen-carrying red pigment in the red blood cells (16)

Hemoptysis: blood in the sputum (16)

Hemostasis: the arrest of bleeding (12)

Hemothorax: blood in the pleural space (16)

Hermaphroditism: presence of both testicular and ovarian tissue in an infant at birth (29)

Hirsutism: growth of excessive body hair (13)

Holistic: approach that takes into account the client as a physical, mental, emotional, and spiritual being (3)

Homeostasis: state of balance, when all the components of a system are working properly; normal ranges of fluids and electrolytes and of acids and bases (10)

Hopelessness: reaction that occurs when the person perceives no solutions to a problem (31)

Hormones: secretions of (ductless) endocrine glands (10)

Hospice care: care of dying people based on holistic concepts that emphasize quality of life rather than cure (31)

Hour of sleep (HS): care provided to clients before they retire for the night (13)

Household system: measures commonly used in the home, including drops, teaspoons, tablespoons, cups, and glasses (21)

Hub: part of the needle which fits onto the syringe (21)

Humanism: humanistic learning theory; focuses on both cognitive and affective qualities of the learner (23)

Hygiene: science of health and its maintenance (13)

Hypercapnia: accumulation of excessive carbon dioxide in the blood; hypercarbia (16)

Hypercarbia: See *Hypercapnia* (16)

Hypersomnia: excessive daytime sleep (20)

Hyperthermia: body temperature above the usual range; fever (14)

Hypertonic: having a greater concentration of solutes than plasma (17)

Hyperventilation: increased rate and depth of respirations (16)

Hypervolemia: excess blood volume such as might result from fluid retention or kidney failure (16)

Hypothermia: core body temperature below the lower limit of normal (14)

Hypotonic: having a lesser concentration of solutes (17)

Hypovolemia: inadequate blood volume such as might result from hemorrhage or severe dehydration (16)

Hypoxia: condition of insufficient oxygen anywhere in the body (16)

Iatrogenic disease: disease caused unintentionally by medical therapy (21)

Iatrogenic infection: infection directly caused by any diagnostic or therapeutic source (7)

Idiosyncratic effect: unexpected unique bodily response that causes unpredictable abnormal symptoms in clients (21)

Ileostomy: an opening into the *ileum* (small bowel) (19)

Illness: highly individualized response to disease (1)

Immunity: resistance of the body to infection (7)

Impaction: mass or collection of hardened, puttylike feces in the folds of the rectum (19)

Impaired nurse: a nurse whose practice has been negatively affected by chemical abuse, specifically the use of alcohol and drugs (2)

Implementation: fourth step of nursing process, in which selected nursing interventions (actions) are performed (4)

Impotence: erectile dysfunction; the inability to achieve or maintain an erection sufficient for sexual satisfaction for oneself or one's partner (29)

Incident: any unexpected event (9)

Incident report: occurrence report; form completed when client care was not consistent with standards for expected care (32)

Incontinence: inability to control excretion (18)

Independent Practice Associations (IPA): similar to HMOs and PPOs except that clients pay a fixed prospective payment to the IPA, and the IPA pays the provider (5)

Indigenous: related to traditional folkways (26)

Inductive reasoning: forming generalizations from a set of facts or observations (3)

Infarction: death of tissue (20)

Infection: invasion and growth of microorganisms in a body tissue (7)

Infertility: inability to conceive a child (29)

Infibulation: excision of the clitoris, the labia minora, and the labia majora, or closure of the vagina (29)

Inflammatory response: local nonspecific defense reaction of tissues when they are exposed to infection or injury (7)

Inquest: a legal inquiry into the cause or manner of a death (31)

Insomnia: inability to obtain an adequate amount or quality of sleep, is the most common sleep disorder (20)

Inspection: visual examination; assessing by using the sense of sight (11)

Inspiration: inhalation; air flowing into the lungs as part of ventilation (16)

Intake and output (I & O): measurement and recording of all fluid taken in and excreted during a 24-hour period (17)

Integrated delivery system: incorporates acute care services, home health care, extended and skilled care facilities, and outpatient services to provide care throughout the life span (5)

Integumentary system: skin and its associated structures (hair, nails, oil and sweat glands, blood vessels, nerves, and sensory organs) (10)

Intercourse: the sexual union of two persons (29)

Intermittent feeding: administration of 300–500 mL of enteral formula several times per day (17)

Internal disasters: events within the hospital that interrupt services and produce victims (e.g., utility interruption or chemical spill) (6)

Internal respiration: interchange of oxygen and carbon dioxide between the circulating blood and the cells of the body tissues (14)

Interstitial fluid: fluid between cells; transports wastes from cells via lymph system, as well as directly into blood plasma through capillaries (17)

Interventions: (see also Nursing interventions) actions performed by a nurse. 1. *Independent interventions:* activities nurses are licensed to initiate on the basis of their knowledge and skills. 2. *Dependent interventions:* activities carried out under the physician's orders or supervision, or according to specified routines (4)

Interview: planned communication; conversation with a purpose (4)

Intracellular fluid (ICF): fluid within the cells of the body; about two thirds of the total body fluid in adults (17)

Intractable pain: Chronic pain that persists despite therapeutic interventions (15)

Intradermal: ID; injection into the dermis or skin (21)

Intramuscular: IM; injection into the muscle (21)

Intravenous: IV; injection into the vein (21)

Invasion of privacy: direct wrong of a personal nature that injures the feelings of the person and does not take into account the effect of revealed information on the standing of the person in the community (2)

Irrigation: flushing or washing out with a specified solution; *lavage* (18)

Ischemia: lack of blood supply to tissues and organs due to obstructed circulation (12)

Isotonic: having the same concentration of solutes as blood plasma (17)

Jejunostomy: surgical creation of a permanent opening through the abdominal wall into the jejunum (17)

Kardex®: a widely used, concise method of organizing and recording data about a client (9)

Keloid: hypertrophic (progressively enlarging) scar (12)

Kinesthetic: awareness of the position and movement of body parts (27)

Knowledge: recall of information (1)

Kussmaul's breathing: hyperventilation that accompanies metabolic acidosis; rapid, deep breaths that attempt to rid the body of excess body acids by blowing off the carbon dioxide (16)

Labyrinth: inner ear or consists of the cochlea, vestibule, and semicircular canals (20)

Laissez-faire: exercising little control or guidance of the group (32)

Lanugo: fine hair on the body of the fetus; down or woolly hair (13)

Law: "rules made by humans which regulate social conduct in a formally prescribed and legally binding manner" (Bernzweig, 1996, p. 3) (2)

Laxative: medication that stimulates bowel activity and assist fecal elimination; less potent than a cathartic (19)

Leadership: process used to move a group toward setting and achieving goals (32)

Learning: life-long process of acquiring knowledge or skills that cannot be solely accounted for by human growth; it is demonstrated by changes in behavior (23)

Lesion: alteration in normal skin appearance (11)

Level of consciousness: state of alertness; LOC can range from alert and oriented to coma (11)

Liability: being legally responsible for one's acts and omissions (2)

Libel: defamation by means of print, writing, or pictures (2)

Licensure: process by which a government agency gives permission for an individual to engage in an occupation or profession (32)

Line of gravity: imaginary vertical line drawn through the body's center of gravity (20)

Lipids: organic substances that are greasy and insoluble in water but soluble in alcohol or ether (17)

Living will: a type of advanced medical directive that provides specific instructions about what medical treatment the client chooses to omit or refuse (e.g., CPR, intubation, ventilatory support) in the event that the client is unable to make those decisions (31)

Livor mortis: discoloration of tissues after blood circulation has ceased (31)

Local infection: illness caused by microorganisms that are only in a specific part of the body (7)

Loss: an actual or potential situation in which someone or something that is valued is changed, no longer available, or gone (31)

Maceration: softening of tissue by prolonged wetting (12)

Magico-religious: belief that health and illness are controlled by supernatural forces (26)

Malpractice: negligence that occurs while a person is performing as a professional (2)

Managed care: health care system established to provide cost-effective, quality care for groups of clients (5)

Manifestations: combination of subjective and objective data (4)

Matrix: network of nonliving, intracellular material (10)

Meatus: opening of the urethra on the external body (18)

Medicaid: federal public assistance program paid out of general taxes to people who require financial assistance (5)

Medical asepsis: all practices used to confine a specific microorganism to a specific area (7)

Medicare: amendment to the Social Security Act that provided a national and state health insurance program for older adults (5)

Medication: substance administered for the diagnosis, cure, treatment, relief, or prevention of disease; *drug* (21)

Meiosis: type of cell division responsible for the formation of sex cells (10)

Menstruation: monthly uterine bleeding (29)

Metabolic acidosis: condition that occurs when bicarbonate is lost or acid is increased within the plasma (17)

Metabolic alkalosis: condition that occurs when the plasma loses hydrogen ions (acid) and gains bicarbonate (17)

Metric system: decimal system based on units of ten (21)

Micturition: process of emptying the urinary bladder (18)

Midstream: term for a clean-catch urine specimen collected after voiding a small amount of urine to clear the urethra (18)

Mitochondria: large organelles where adenosine triphosphate (ATP) is produced (10)

Mitosis: division of a single parent cell into two genetically identical daughter cells (10)

Mnemonics: techniques for developing memory (33)

Moral: having to do with judgments of right or wrong (24)

Morning care: care provided after clients have breakfast (13)

Motivation: desire (23)

Motor development: the development of abilities to move and to control the body (24)

Mourning: behavioral process through which grief is eventually resolved or altered (31)

Multistate compact: an agreement among several state boards of nursing that a nurse licensed in one of these states can work in any other state that has signed the agreement without having to obtain a separate license (33)

Myocardial infarction: MI or heart attack (16)

Narcolepsy: poorly understood disorder, possibly genetic or autoimmune; sufferers experience regular REM onset sleep attacks lasting from a few seconds to several hours (20)

NCLEX-PN: National Council Licensure Examination for Practical/Vocational Nurses; a test given to ensure that graduates of practical/vocational nursing schools meet the minimum standards to practice safely as LPNs/LVNs (1)

Negligence: misconduct or practice that is below the standard expected of an ordinary, reasonable, and prudent practitioner, which places another person at risk for harm (2)

Nerve block: chemical interruption of a nerve pathway, effected by injecting a local anesthetic into the nerve (15)

Networking: deliberately making connections among people for interests and employment opportunities (34)

Neuropathic pain: pain felt as the result of a disturbance of the nerve pathways either from past or continuing tissue damage (15)

Nitrogen balance: measure of intake and loss of nitrogen (17)

Nociceptors: receptors that transmit pain sensation (15)

Nomogram: Body surface area determined by using a child's height and weight; considered to be the most accurate method of calculating a child's dose (21)

Nonspecific defenses: defenses that protect the body against all microorganisms (7)

Nosocomial infections: infections that occur as a result of health care delivery in a health care setting (7)

NPO: nothing by mouth (21)

NREM sleep: non–rapid eye movement sleep; a deep, restful sleep with some decreased physiologic function (20)

Nucleus: most prominent organelle; control center that contains the cell's genetic material (DNA) (10)

Nurse practice acts: acts that legally define and describe the scope of nursing practice and that protect the public; legal acts that regulate the practice of nursing in the United States and Canada (1)

Nursing: attributes, characteristics, and actions of the nurse providing care on behalf of, or in conjunction with, the client; the diagnosis and treatment of human responses to actual and potential health problems (1)

Nursing care conference: meeting of a group of nurses to discuss possible solutions to client problems (9)

Nursing diagnosis: clinical judgment about individual, family, or community responses to actual and potential health problems or life processes (4)

Nursing interventions: actions initiated by the nurse to achieve client goals (4)

Nursing process: systematic, logical method of providing individualized nursing care; it includes assessment, diagnosis, planning, implementation, and evaluation (4)

Nursing rounds: procedures in which a group of nurses visit selected clients at each client's bedside (9)

Nutrients: organic, inorganic, and energy-producing substances found in food (17)

Nutrition: result of the interaction between nutrients and the human body (17)

Obesity: body weight that exceeds ideal by more than 20 percent (17)

Objective data: signs that are detectable by an observer or can be tested against an accepted standard (3)

Observation: process of gathering data by using the senses (4)

Occult blood: hidden blood, as in stool (19)

Olfactory: having to do with the sense of smell (27)

Oliguria: low urine output (18)

Omnibus Budget Reconciliation Act (OBRA): legislation to bring a measure of quality improvement to the nursing home and extended-care facility industry (5)

Open-ended questions: questions that invite a person to explore their thoughts or feelings (25)

Ophthalmics: preparations for the eye (21)

Oral report: taped report delivered in a report room or while nurses are making client rounds (32)

Orchiectomy: removal of the testicles (29)

Organ donors: a gift of all or any part of one's own body for medical or dental education, research, advancement of medical or dental science, therapy, or transplantation (31)

Organ system: organs that function together for the same general purpose (10)

Orgasmic dysfunction: the inability of a woman to achieve orgasm (29)

Orientation: introduction of clients to the people and facility in which they are admitted; awareness of place and time and family members; program or time period provided for newly hired individuals to prepare them for their position (8, 11, 34)

Orthostatic hypotension: sudden decrease in central blood pressure with position changes (14)

Osteoporosis: demineralization process, continues during immobility; bones become spongy and deformed, and they fracture easily (20)

Ostomy: an opening in the abdominal wall for the elimination of feces or urine (19)

Otics: ear preparations (21)

Pain: sensation that is highly subjective and individual; one of the body's defense mechanisms indicating that there is a problem (15)

Pain reaction: pain responses including the autonomic nervous system and behavioral responses (15)

Pain threshold: amount of pain stimulation a person requires in order to feel pain (15)

Pain tolerance: maximum amount and duration of pain that an individual is willing to endure (15)

Palliative: for relief or reduction of symptoms of a disease; does not produce a cure (22)

Pallor: pale appearance caused by lack of circulating blood or hemoglobin, which results in reduced amounts of oxygen being carried to body tissues (11)

Palpation: examination of the body using the sense of touch (11)

Paralytic ileus: temporary cessation of intestinal movement (19)

Parasites: microorganisms that live on other living organisms (7)

Parasomnia: behavior that may interfere with sleep, such as sleepwalking (20)

Parenteral: injectable medications (21)

Parenteral nutrition: nutrients provided, usually intravenously, when the client is unable to ingest or absorb foods (17)

Passive range of motion: movement of the client's extremities and joints by a caregiver (11)

Pathogens: microorganisms that cause disease (7)

Patient: person who is waiting for or undergoing medical treatment and care (1)

Pediculosis: infestation with lice (13)

Percussion: act of striking a part with short, sharp blows (1) to help gather data about internal organs; (2) to assist in massage; (3) to help a client to clear the respiratory tract (11)

Performance: relates what a person does in a particular role to the behaviors expected of that role (28)

Performance evaluation: a review (usually annual) of on-the-job activity (including attendance and promptness, skills, work as a team member, and ability to complete assignments in a timely manner) (34)

Perfusion: blood supply to an area (11)

Perioperative period: time surrounding a surgery, consisting of *preoperative phase* (prior to surgery); *intraoperative phase* (during surgery); and *postoperative phase* (following surgery) (22)

Peripheral pulse: pulse located in the periphery of the body (foot, hand, or neck) (14)

Peripheral vascular system: all the blood vessels that carry oxygenated blood to body tissues and organs, and that return deoxygenated blood to the heart and lungs (11)

Peristalsis: wavelike motion that propels intestinal contents forward (19)

PERRLA: pupils equally round and react to light and accommodation (11)

Personal identity: conscious sense of individuality and uniqueness that continually evolves throughout life (28)

Petrissage: technique used in massage to stimulate muscles; deep massage (20)

Phagocytosis: engulfing of microorganisms and cellular debris by white blood cells known as phagocytes (12)

Phantom pain: a painful sensation perceived in a body part that is missing (15)

Physical assessment: one of three types of examination of the body: (a) complete assessment, (b) focused assessment by body systems, (c) focused assessment of a body part (11)

Physiologic: having to do with physical processes in the human body (24)

Physiology: study of how the body functions (10)

Plane: imaginary flat surface that divides a structure into two portions; *frontal plane:* separates into front and back; *sagittal plane:* separates into left and right; *midsagittal:* indicates equal left and right; *transverse:* cuts horizontally, creating a superior and inferior portion (10)

Planning: third step of nursing process; decision making, prioritizing, and problem solving to achieve desired client outcomes (4)

Pleural effusion: fluid in the pleural space (16)

Pneumothorax: air in the pleural space (16)

Polyuria: production of abnormally large amounts of urine by the kidneys (18)

Portfolio: itemized visual account of skills and best practices related to the position one is seeking (34)

Postural tonus: sustained muscle contraction required to maintain the upright position (20)

Power of attorney for health care: a written statement appointing someone else (e.g., a relative or trusted friend) to manage health care treatment decisions when the client is unable to do so (31)

Powerlessness: state in which a person perceives a solution to a problem but does not believe that it is possible to implement the solution (31)

Preemptive analgesia: administration of analgesics prior to an invasive or operative procedure; also includes around-the-clock (ATC) analgesia (15)

Preferred Provider Arrangements (PPA): similar to PPOs but can be contracted with individual health care providers, rather than an organization of health care providers (5)

Preferred Provider Organizations: group of physicians and perhaps a health care agency (often hospitals) that provide an insurance company or employer with health services at a discounted rate (5)

Prejudice: a strongly held positive or negative opinion about some topic or group of people; it may be based on experience, fear, or misinformation (26)

Prescription: written direction for the preparation and administration of a drug (21)

Pressure ulcers: decubitus ulcers, pressure sores, or bedsores; lesions caused by unrelieved pressure that results in damage to underlying tissue (12)

Primary nursing: system in which one nurse is responsible for total care of a number of clients 24 hours a day, 7 days a week (5)

Priority setting: process of identifying most important to least important (4)

PRN order: "as needed order," permits the nurse to give a medication when the client requires it (21)

Probationary period: time during which an immediate supervisor evaluates a new employee's performance (34)

Problem-oriented medical record (POMR): or problem-oriented record (POR); arrangement of data according to individual problems the client has rather than by the source of the information (9)

Procedures: technical, *psychomotor* (hands-on) skills that involve nursing actions such as manipulating equipment, giving injections, or repositioning clients (4)

Profession: occupation to which one devotes oneself and in which one has specialized expertise (34)

Professional: highly structured and maintained by individuals who have completed formal studies (26)

Professional nursing organization: organization established to help nurses achieve common goals and missions (34)

Professionalism: a courteous, conscientious, and generally businesslike manner in the workplace (34)

Prospective Payment System: legislation that limits the amount paid to hospitals that are reimbursed by Medicare (5)

Prosthesis: artificial limb or part (22)

Protein-calorie malnutrition: significant problem of clients with cancer and chronic disease; characterized by weight loss, and visible muscle and fat wasting (17)

Psychomotor domain: area of learning that includes motor skills (such as giving an injection) (23)

Psychosocial: having to do with relationships with oneself and others (24)

Puberty: period in which sexual organs mature and secondary sexual characteristics develop (29)

Pulmonary function tests: testing done to measure lung volume and capacity (16)

Pulse: heartbeat (11)

Pulse deficit: differences between the apical and radial pulse rates (14)

Pyrexia: hyperthermia, fever, body temperature above the usual range (14)

Race: classification of people according to shared biologic characteristics, genetic markers, or features such as skin color (26)

Radiating pain: pain perceived at the source of the pain that extends to nearby tissues (15)

Range of motion (ROM): maximum movement possible for that joint (20)

Rape: sexual intercourse in which one person is an unwilling or unconsenting party (29)

Rationale: scientific principle given as the reason for selecting a particular nursing intervention (4)

Reactive hyperemia: Reaction in which skin takes on a bright red flush when pressure is relieved (12)

Readiness: motivation to learn at a specific time (23)

Receptors: points of attachment for materials on the surface of the cell membrane; nerve cells that receive a stimulus and convert it to a nerve impulse (10, 27)

Reconstructive: performed to restore function or appearance that has been lost or reduced (22)

Record: a written or computer-based collection of data (9)

References: people who agree to provide a written or verbal assessment to a potential employer (34)

Referred pain: pain felt in a part of the body that is considerably removed from the tissues causing the pain (15)

Reflecting: directing ideas, feelings, questions, or content back to clients to enable them to explore their own ideas and feelings about a situation (25)

Reflexes: unconscious, involuntary responses that are neither learned nor consciously carried out; nervous system responses to stimuli (24)

Relevance: importance or applicability (23)

REM sleep: rapid eye movement sleep; part of sleep in which dreams occur (20)

Report: a means of conveying information about changes in a client's condition promptly (9)

Reservoir: place where a microorganism naturally lives (7)

Resident flora: microorganisms that are normal in a particular body area (7)

Residual urine: urine remaining in the bladder following voiding (18)

Respiration: the act of breathing (14)

Respiratory acidosis: a state of excessive carbon dioxide in the body; hypercapnia (17)

Respiratory alkalosis: a state of excessive loss of carbon dioxide in the body (17)

Résumé: concise systematic summary of professional experience and educational background (34)

Retention: holding, keeping; in the case of learning, active remembering (23)

Rigor mortis: stiffening of the body that occurs about 2 to 4 hours after death (31)

Role: set of expectations about how the person occupying one position behaves toward a person occupying another position (28)

Sanguineous: hemorrhagic; consisting of large amounts of red blood cells (12)

Scabies: contagious skin infestation by the itch mite (13)

Scope of practice: document developed by the board of nursing which governs practice within each state (2)

Sebum: oily skin secretion that softens and lubricates the hair and skin (13)

Secondary sex characteristics: traits associated with gender but not directly necessary for reproduction (10)

Self-concept: a complex idea that includes all aspects of how one perceives oneself (28)

Self-esteem: one's judgment of one's own worth (28)

Sensory deficit: impaired reception, perception, or both, of one or more of the senses (27)

Sensory deprivation: decrease in or lack of meaningful stimuli (27)

Sensory overload: excessive stimulation; generally occurs when a person is unable to process or manage the amount or intensity of sensory stimuli (27)

Sensory perception: the conscious organization and translation of data or stimuli into meaningful information (27)

Sensory reception: process of receiving stimuli or data (27)

Sepsis: presence of infection (7)

Septicemia: condition that exists when bacteria enters the bloodstream and spreads though all of the body's systems (7)

Sequential compression device (SCD): device such as elastic stockings that promotes venous return from the legs (22)

Serosanguineous: blood-tinged (12)

Sex: term most commonly used to denote biologic male or female status; also, sexual intercourse (29)

Sexual abuse: any involvement of a child in an act designed to provide sexual gratification to an adult (29)

Sexual dysfunction: undesired, altered sexual function (29)

Sexual harassment: "unwelcome sexual advances, requests for sexual favors, and other verbal or physical conduct of a sexual nature" (EEOC) (2)

Sexual orientation: preference of a person for one sex or the other (29)

Sexuality: dimension of personality, broader than one's capacity for erotic response alone (29)

Sexually transmitted diseases (STDs): diseases spread by sexual activity (29)

Shearing force: combination of friction and pressure (12)

Shift report: report to other nurses at the change of shifts to delegate responsibility and describe what has been done (32)

Shortness of breath (SOB): feeling of being unable to get enough air (16)

Side effect: unintended drug action (21)

Sigmoidoscopy: diagnostic procedures for visualizing the sigmoid colon (19)

Signs: (see *Objective data*) (4)

Single order: "one-time order"; medication is given once at a specified time (21)

Sitz bath: therapeutic bath for soaking a client's pelvic area (12)

Slander: defamation by the spoken word, stating information or false words, which can cause damage to a person's reputation (2)

Sleep apnea: periodic cessation of breathing during sleep (20)

Somatic pain: diffuse pain that arises from ligaments, tendons, bones, blood vessels, and nerves (15)

Source-oriented record: a record in which information about a particular problem is documented under different sources (9)

Specific defenses: immune defenses; antibody-mediated and cell-mediated defenses against identified foreign proteins such as bacteria, fungi, viruses, and other infectious agents (7)

Specific gravity: a measure of concentration, or the amount of solutes present in the solution (e.g., urine) (18)

Spiritual: having to do with relationship with God or a higher power (24)

Sputum: mucous secretion from the lungs, bronchi, and trachea (16)

Standard Precautions: precautions used with all clients to prevent spread of microorganisms; applied to all body fluids, blood, secretions, excretions (except sweat), mucus membranes, and nonintact skin (7)

Standing order: may or may not have a termination date; medication can be given indefinitely (21)

Stat order: medication to be given immediately and only once (21)

Statute of limitations: limit to the amount of time that can pass between recognition of harm and the bringing of a suit (2)

Stereognosis: ability to recognize objects by touching or manipulating them (27)

Stereotyping: assumption that all members of a culture or ethnic group are alike (26)

Sterile field: microorganism-free area (7)

Stimulus: agent or act that stimulates a nerve receptor (27)

Stooping: acute flexion of the back with hips and knees straight (6)

Stress: universal phenomenon described as tension between two opposing forces (30)

Stressors: sources of stress that are classified as either internal or external (30)

Stridor: harsh, high-pitched sound (16)

Subculture: smaller group sharing specific cultural characteristics (26)

Subcutaneous: (SC or SQ) below the skin (21)

Subjective data: symptoms; facts, perceptions, or sensations apparent only to the person affected (3)

Sublingual: administration of drug under the tongue (21)

Suctioning: aspirating secretions through a catheter connected to a suction machine or wall suction outlet (16)

Suffocation: asphyxiation; lack of oxygen due to interrupted breathing (6)

Supplemental Security Income (SSI): special benefits for disabled or blind persons and people not eligible for Social Security; payments are not restricted to health care costs (5)

Suppuration: process of pus formation (12)

Surgery: a unique experience of a planned physical alteration (22)

Surgical asepsis: sterile technique; practice that keeps an object or an area completely free of microorganisms and spores (7)

Susceptible host: individual who has difficulty combating microorganisms and is at risk for developing an infection (7)

Sutures: threads used to sew body tissues together (22)

Symptoms: (see *Subjective data*) (4)

Syringes: equipment used to administer parenteral medications (21)

Systemic infection: illness caused by microorganisms that spread to and damage other body areas (7)

Systole: period in which the ventricles of the heart contract (11)

Systolic pressure: pressure of the blood as a result of contraction of the ventricles; the pressure of the height of the blood wave (14)

Tachypnea: rapid breathing rate (16)

Taped report: report spoken into a tape recorder by nurses going off duty (32)

Tarry: red or black stool (19)

Teaching: system of activities intended to produce specific learning (23)

Team leader: person who guides and directs the care of a group of clients and supervises the members of the team (32)

Team nursing: delivery of individualized nursing care to clients by a nursing team led by a professional nurse; members use diverse skills and education to deliver client care (5)

Test anxiety: range of feelings from uneasiness about an upcoming test or uneasiness during a test, to extreme and excessive worry about failing (33)

Theories: ways of looking at a discipline—such as nursing— in clear, explicit terms that can be communicated to others (3)

Therapeutic baths: baths given for physical effects, such as to soothe irritated skin or to treat an area (13)

Therapeutic communication: client-centered, goal-directed and time-limited communication (25)

Therapeutic effect: desired effect; reason the drug is prescribed (21)

Thrombophlebitis: one or more clots loosely attached to an inflamed vessel wall (20)

Thrombus: blood clot (16)

Ticks: small, gray-brown parasites that bite into tissue and suck blood (13)

Tissue: cells with similar structures and functions (10)

Tissue perfusion: passage of oxygen-carrying blood through the vessels to tissues (22)

Tort: civil wrong committed against a person or a person's property (2)

Tracheostomy: surgical incision in the trachea just below the larynx through which a tracheostomy tube is inserted (16)

Transfer: move to another unit or to a different facility as a result of a client or physician request (8)

Transmission: manner in which the microorganism gets to the host; *direct:* infected person has direct contact with another person through touch, droplets, kissing, or sexual intercourse; *indirect:* requires a vector or vehicle to carry the microorganism to the host; *airborne:* droplet nuclei (remains of droplets coming from an infected person) are spread to another person (7)

Transmission Based Precautions: used in addition to Standard Precautions for any client with known or suspected infections that are spread by airborne or droplet transmission, or by physical contact (7)

Transplant: surgical replacement of a malfunctioning structure (22)

Transporters: proteins that actively move materials through the cell membrane in both directions (10)

Triage: means of assessing a large number of emergency victims quickly. Victims are prioritized according to their care needs, from most severe to least (6)

Triglycerides: fatty acids (17)

Turgor: elasticity (fullness) of the skin (11)

Twisting: rotation of the thoracolumbar spine (6)

Undernutrition: nutrient intake insufficient to meet daily energy requirements (17)

Urinary diversion: surgical rerouting of urine from the kidneys to a site other than the bladder (18)

Urinary retention: accumulation of urine in the bladder and inability of the bladder to empty itself (18)

Urinary stasis: stagnation of urine flow (20)

Validation: form of feedback that provides confirmation that both parties have the same basic understanding of the message and the feedback (25)

Valsalva maneuver: straining associated with constipation; often accompanied by holding the breath (19)

Values: freely chosen, enduring beliefs or attitudes about the worth of a person, object, idea, or action (2)

Vector: object or animal by which organisms are transmitted (an insect, or a used drinking glass, for instance) (7)

Vegetative state: an irreversible state of unconsciousness (31)

Ventilation: (breathing) movement of air between the atmosphere and the alveoli of the lungs (16)

Vertigo: strong sensation of spinning around in space, which impairs balance (20)

Vial: small glass bottle with a sealed rubber cap, contains medication (21)

Virulence: microorganism's ability to produce disease (7)

Viruses: microorganisms made primarily of a substance called nucleic acid; they must enter living cells in order to reproduce (7)

Visceral: having to do with any large interior organ (27)

Visceral pain: pain that results from stimulation of pain receptors in the abdominal cavity, cranium, and thorax (15)

Viscosity: physical property that results from friction of molecules in a fluid (14)

Vital capacity: maximum volume of air that can be exhaled after maximum inhalation (20)

Vital signs: measurements of temperature, pulse, respirations, and blood pressure; assessment of pain is sometimes called the fifth vital sign (11)

Vitamin: organic compound that cannot be manufactured by the body and is needed in small quantities to *catalyze* (or trigger) metabolic processes (17)

Voiding: urination; the process of emptying the urinary bladder (18)

Voluntary euthanasia: assisted suicide; situations in which the dying individual exerts control over the time and manner of death (31)

Wellness: state of well-being (1)

Work samples: résumé items used in the workplace, such as individualized nursing care plans, lesson plans for client teaching, etc. (34)

Written report: report, frequently used in long-term care facilities, that is written in a communication or report book (32)

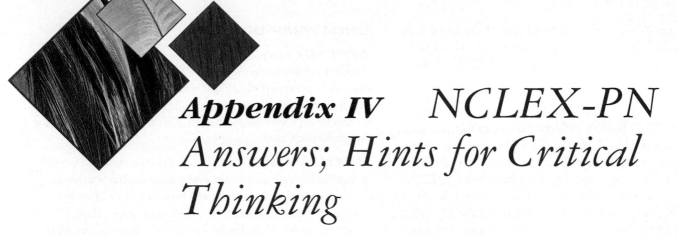

Appendix IV NCLEX-PN Answers; Hints for Critical Thinking

CHAPTER 1

NCLEX-PN ANSWERS **1. B.** Florence Nightingale received her nurse's training at the hospital founded by the Order of Deaconesses in Kaiserwerth, Germany. The other choices have a connection to her life. She lived in Italy as a child. She cared for soldiers during the Crimean War in Turkey, and she founded a training school in London. **2. C.** American Poet Walt Whitman served as a nurse in the Civil War. Charles Dickens was an English writer. Robert Frost wrote many volumes about Abraham Lincoln, but never served in the war as a nurse. Gore Vidal was a twentieth-century writer. **3. B.** Clara Barton. Lavinia Dock was instrumental in women's voting rights. Mary Breckinridge founded the Frontier Nursing Service. Lillian Wald is considered to be the founder of public health nursing. **4. C.** Application. Questions of knowledge simply test facts. Comprehension questions require you to understand the meaning of a word (such as cathartic) and use the knowledge to arrive at an answer. Application involves knowledge and comprehension, plus use of that information in a fresh situation. Analysis questions are more complex than application questions. **5. B.** 1897. **6. C.** Provided federal funding for practical nurse education. **7. C.** Operating under the umbrella of a professional organization distinguishes a profession from an occupation. **8. C.** National Federation of Licensed Practical Nurses. Lillian Wald founded the Henry Street Settlement. **9. C.** The NCLEX-PN is a computer adaptive test that is mostly multiple-choice questions. The questions are used to determine whether a person can function safely and effectively as an entry-level LPN/LVN. **10. B.** Each state has its own nurse practice act, which provides the scope of nursing for its jurisdiction. Nurses are responsible for knowing the limits of practice wherever they work.

CHAPTER 2

NCLEX-PN ANSWERS **1. A.** The client may be anxious and have some family issues. However, the real concern here is that the client has agreed to treatment without enough information to make an independent decision. The nurse should be concerned whether the consent was informed. **2. B.** Restraint without an order, or failing to follow facility poli-

cies on restraints, constitutes false imprisonment. Negligence and ethical considerations may enter into the discussion, but they are not the best answer in this situation. Defamation has to do with false communication, not restraints. **3. C.** Negligence is practice that is below the accepted standard expected by an ordinary, reasonable, prudent practitioner. A prudent nurse will always recheck a physician's order if the client has questions about medication or treatment. **4. B.** Slander is defamation by the spoken word. Libel is defamation in the form of a printed or written word or picture. Invasion of privacy and breach of confidence have to do with confidentiality. When a nurse discredits another staff member, he or she is guilty of defamation. **5. B.** Failure to observe and take appropriate action is malpractice related to failure to report a client's complaint or concern. **6. C.** The National League of Nursing is a private agency responsible for the accreditation of basic nursing programs. The individual state boards of nursing are responsible for the other tasks. **7. C.** Completion of an incident report is the duty of the nurse who discovers the incident. This may be the nurse involved in the incident, but does not have to be. The supervisor and the risk management department will review the report. **8. B.** The ADA prohibits discrimination on the basis of disability in employment, public service, and public accommodations. This act is enforced by the federal government. **9. B.** The concept of autonomy involves people's right to make their own decisions. **10. B.** Computerized medical records present specific security concerns. The best thing staff members can do is protect their personal security codes and follow the facility's policies for use.

CHAPTER 3

NCLEX-PN ANSWERS **1. C.** Environment (according to Nightingale) is related to internal and external factors such as light and excessive noise. A represents health; B represents person/client; D represents nursing. **2. B.** Newman's theory focuses on reaction to stress in the environment; Roy focuses on the adaptation to the changes in the environment; Orem's theory focuses on self-care; and Leininger focuses on cultural care. **3. B.** The art of thinking about thinking represents critical thinking; A—although the word critical can mean fault finding, in this context critical means discerning; C and D are characteristics of natural rather than critical thinking. 4. **A.** During the assessment/data collection phase, the nurse must consider personal assumptions or biases that may affect judgment. 5. **A.** Environmental Theory—Nightingale; Adaptation Model—Roy; Systems Model—Newman; Cultural Care Diversity—Leininger. 6. **A.** A nurse who is using critical thinking skills will evaluate the client's cognitive ability or limitations prior to beginning health-related teaching. 7. **C.** Client C's pulse is somewhat elevated; capillary refill time is slow; and blood pressure is low. Through the use of critical thinking and by comparing these results against normal, a nurse will determine the need to report observations about client C. 8. **A.** With inductive reasoning, certain bits of information suggest a particular interpretation when viewed together. 9. **D.** Leininger's theory is based on universal human caring, although ways of caring vary across cultures. 10. **B.** This statement infers that aspirin is the cause of Reye's syndrome, so any child receiving it would have a risk of developing Reye's syndrome. A is a statement of fact; C is judgment; and D is an opinion.

CHAPTER 4

NCLEX-PN ANSWERS 1. **C.** Assessment involves data collection related to the client's current health status, while evaluation is concerned with accomplishment of the goals. 2. **C.** The second phase of the nursing process is diagnosing. During this phase collected data are analyzed and problems are identified. 3. **B.** Goals must have a subject (client), verb (walk), condition or modifier (the length of hall), criteria for desired outcome (with assistance of two staff members, two times per day), and timeline (in two days). The other choices are missing one or more required components. 4. **A.** Rationales are the reason why a particular intervention was tried. They identify the scientific basis for the intervention. 5. **D.** The care plan is the culmination of the planning phase. Choosing interventions occurs before the care plan, and evaluation of effectiveness of interventions is part of the evaluation phase. Delegating interventions is part of implementation. 6. **C.** Explain why an intervention of vital sign and pulse oximeter readings should be included. A is an intervention; B and D are statements of evidence for evaluation. 7. **B.** Although the care plan is written in the planning stage, it is put into action in the implementation stage. 8. **C.** Once the care plan has been implemented, the licensed nurse will decide what tasks can be carried out by other nursing personnel and also how much supervision they will need to complete them. 9. **A.** Evaluations must include a conclusion (goal met, not met, or partially met) and data that provide evidence for the stated conclusion. 10. **C.** Although the other choices contribute to the nursing process, C provides a clear definition of Nursing Process as an organized framework for professional nursing practice.

UNIT I WRAP-UP

COMMUNITY Long-term care is "home" for many of the residents. A nurse who seems abusive may be creating an environment that affects all the people who live there. He or she may make them all more anxious about how they might be treated. In this sense, a staff member who is abusive is equivalent to a "neighborhood bully."

CRITICAL THINKING

◆ Whistleblowers are people who expose negligence, abuse, or dangers (such as professional misconduct or incompetence) in the organization in which they work. They become whistle-blowers because normal quality control is neglected by those in charge.

◆ This situation has both ethical and legal implications. Carlos was motivated by his concern for the client and the nursing code of ethics. Depending on the jurisdiction in which Carlos works, there may be legal ramifications if he does not report his observations. It may be necessary to report the abuse outside of the organization. In many jurisdictions, legislation requires that child abuse or abuse of vulnerable adults be reported.

◆ It would probably be difficult for Carlos to prove that he was being ostracized by the staff. If other staff members would testify to the racial slurs, he may have some recourse, although legal action would not improve his work situation.

COMMUNICATION Role-playing these scenes negatively and discussing the feelings that they raise can be useful. However, it is even more important to role-play positive alternatives to these scenarios, because these are what nurses will need. Making a long list of possible alternatives is also a valuable class activity.

CONFLICT RESOLUTION Carlos could have done several things differently. He could have gathered facts about the situation and ascertained the risks, then spoken privately to other staff members and to the resident to determine whether abuse had occurred. He could have sought relevant information directly from the nurse whose behavior or practice raised concerns. ("Is this client giving you problems?") The nurse may not have realized that her behavior was viewed by others as abusive. He could have modeled good nursing behavior in relation to the client. As charge nurse, he could have called a team conference to discuss aspects of this client's care. He could have requested in-service training for all nurses to help in dealing with client behavior issues.

CHAPTER 5

NCLEX-PN ANSWERS 1. **B.** Included in this bill are the right of clients to considerate and respectful care; privacy for the clients, confidentiality of records and communications regarding their care; and the right to make decisions about their care, including right to refuse treatment. 2. **A.** OBRA instituted requirements for nurse's aide training. Specifically, they include a minimum of 75 hours of training and competence evaluation of aides. **3. C.** All of these may be an issue with a homeless client. However, the living environment and the exposure to disease, poor nutrition, and the elements would be the major concern. **4. D.** Team nursing is a collaborative effort of direct client care, with health care workers from two or more levels. Care is allocated according to the scope of practice of the individual team members. **5. D.** The 1965 Medicare amendments (Title 18) to the Social Security Act provided for national and state health insurance for older adults. Medicaid and Medi-cal are health insurance for individuals needing federal and/or state assistance. Medicare is a federal program; Medi-cal is one of numerous state programs. **6. C.** In 1983 the U.S. Congress passed legislation putting the prospective payment system into effect. Reimbursement is made according to a classification system called diagnostic-related groups (DRGs). **7. D.** Paramedical is defined as having some training to do with medicine. A spiritual support person attends to the client's spiritual needs but is not required to have health care training. Occupational therapists, physiotherapists, and dietitians are interdisciplinary team members specially trained to meet specific health needs. **8. A.** Although managed care may mean that the number of hospital days may be reduced and allocation of services may be more efficient, the purpose of managed care is to provide the client with the most effective treatment. Managed care can be used with any nursing model. **9. B.** Health maintenance organizations provide capitated care. In other words, a monthly fee is paid for each member, whether or not they received treatment during that time period. **10. A.** Primary care includes preventive care, health education, environmental protection, as well as early detection and treatment. Secondary care includes acute care and diagnosis and treatment. Tertiary care includes rehabilitation and care of the terminally ill.

CHAPTER 6

NCLEX-PN ANSWERS **1. C.** Children are curious and have not developed the judgment needed to understand danger. Bad behavior and parental neglect can cause injury, but unfounded accusation should not be made. New walkers frequently fall, but a child-safe environment can protect from injury. **2. A.** Restraining a client without physician's orders constitutes false imprisonment. Facility policy and family permission are not sufficient to allow restraints. Restraining for a short period until physician's orders are received can only be done in an emergency when the client is uncontrolled by other means. **3. D.** A vest restraint is the safest choice. Mitten and elbow restraints would impair hand and arm use but would not keep the child in bed. The belt would limit movement to a sitting position; belts frequently become displaced on small children, causing a choking hazard. The wrist restraint with one arm secured to the bed would not be used; a child could be seriously injured trying to climb out of bed. **4. C.** The walker will

need to be used at all times until he is fully recovered. The other choices show good understanding of his discharge needs. **5. B.** Body mechanics is a safe and efficient way to move the body. Physical therapy is treatment of large muscle groups; occupational therapy deals with small muscle groups. Nursing interventions are nursing actions to help clients meet goals. **6. B.** OSHA, the Occupational Safety and Health Administration, is the government agency responsible for safe work environments. The CDC is the Centers for Disease Control and Prevention. The Department of Labor is concerned with all work-related issues, not specifically safety. JCAHO is not a government agency; it is responsible for accreditation of health care organizations. **7. C.** The CDC recommends that isolation linens be removed promptly from the room by bagging them. Linens are not disposable, so they should not be placed in a refuse container. **8. C.** Triage is defined as the prioritization of victims according to their treatment needs. **9. C.** The inability to change position independently proves the greatest risk to clients with paralysis. Clients with paralysis do not necessarily take more pain medication than other clients. Although clients with paralysis frequently have problems with incontinence and muscle atrophy, these problems are not inevitable. They can be prevented, as can associated injury. **10. A.** Stress can reduce the person's ability to concentrate. Reduced sensory perception awareness will affect ability to perceive environmental stimuli. Inability to communicate can present safety hazards because of an inability to receive and convey information. Stress can affect cognitive awareness and the person's ability to respond appropriately through thought and action.

CASE STUDY HINTS

1. Restraints should be used only as a last resort. Studies have not shown that restraining a client prevents falls or injury. Restraints lessen the client's movement and independence, which infringes on their rights. The restraints can cause injury (e.g., pressure ulcers, skin tears, or death from strangulation). Restraints can interfere with treatment. Restraints can increase health problems such as poor circulation. They can be embarrassing to both the client and family members.

2. Several factors could affect Mr. Moore's safety. These include, but are not limited to: age greater than 65; history of falls, recent hip surgery to repair fracture may impair his mobility; and possibility that he is weaker now than before surgery. He may resume normal activities before he is strong enough. Mr. Moore may not be able to meet his nutritional needs as he will be preparing all meals but one each day. He is a greater risk for injury while preparing his own food. He may not understand the precautions necessary to protect his own safety.

3. He has been physically and socially active and independent; he has a strong family support system (his son will visit daily); he has access to community resources; his

rooms are on one level and his home is small; he has pets to decrease his loneliness; he has no other chronic illnesses that would interfere with his healing process.

CRITICAL THINKING CARE MAP

Subjective Data Mrs. Whitman expressed concerns about his upcoming discharge; lives alone in a two-story house; does yard work; socializes with the neighbors; daughter and three grandchildren live 75 miles away; Mrs. Whitman and the daughter feel they should move to a retirement apartment; Mr. Whitman expressed, "Selling the house would be a sign that I am just giving up."

Objective Data Rigidity due to the Parkinson's; difficulty in swallowing; large bruise on his left leg and right forearm; VS: BP 140/88, P/76, R 20, T 98.2°F (36.7°C); H&H 13.2, 40.4; PT 13.5 sec; PTT 90 sec.

Report Yes, bruising on left leg and right arm. Would report to MD. Client is on anticoagulation therapy.

Interventions Take temperature, pulse, and blood pressure q4h. Observe nutritional status. Work with dietitian to increase nutritional status. Monitor risk for bleeding. Teach client and family signs of bleeding, precautions to take to prevent bleeding.

Documentation Areas of bruising on left thigh and right forearm. Client resting in bed. H&H 13.2, 40.4; PT 13.5 sec; PTT 90 sec. 9 A.M. heparin held, physician notified. K. Smartt LPN

CHAPTER 7

NCLEX-PN ANSWERS 1. **D.** The wound and the dressing are contaminating the environment, and because the dressing is wet it may be transmitting other organisms to the wound itself. The physician would not ordinarily order medications for a temperature below 101°F (38.3°C). Elevation of the leg and placing the client in isolation may be done later. 2. **B.** The tuberculosis organism is transmitted through the air in droplets. Tier 2 or transmission-based precautions are specific for this condition. Tier 1 or Standard Precautions and the use of clean gowns do not address airborne organisms. The nurse would use the mask to prevent inhalation of the tuberculosis organism. 3. **C.** Metal and glass items are autoclaved. Plastic and rubber items are gas sterilized to prevent melting. The items must be put into separate, properly labeled bags. The bags must be impervious to drainage and are usually colored (red). None of the items can be disposed of in an ordinary fashion because they would contaminate the environment. 4. **A.** The items are contaminated, so they must be cleaned. However, throwing toys and clothes away is costly and unnecessary. Exposing them to air will not kill any of the organisms. Washing the items in hot water will clean them before they

are used again and destroy most bacteria. 5. **A.** Covering the client will not prevent the spread of airborne organisms, nor will the wearing of gloves. The client, not the transporter, should wear the mask to prevent the spread of organisms when he or she coughs or sneezes. Informing the radiology department that the client is still infectious will allow them to take appropriate precautions. 6. **D.** Using sterile forceps is appropriate, but not reaching across the field, since organisms could fall on it and contaminate it. Only sterile gloves are worn while handling the contents of the tray so as to not contaminate them. All sterile trays and materials should be covered with sterile towels immediately if they are not in use. 7. **C.** The gloves are contaminated and must be removed first in sequence before the ties of the mask or gown are touched. Otherwise, the person's head, neck, and back can become contaminated. Only the ties of the mask are handled, and they are undone next. Finally, the ties of the gown are loosened and the gown is removed. 8. **B.** A compromised host is someone who is already at high risk for getting infections for one or more reasons. The client is elderly and has a history of emphysema, two other predisposing problems. A susceptible host is just at risk for developing an infection. 9. **C.** The CDC continues to recommend soap and water washing for hands that are visibly soiled with blood and body fluids. Otherwise, research has shown that the alcohol-based cleaner is very effective in destroying pathogens on hands. It is not recommended that gloves be worn for all client contact. Hands should be cleaned after gloves are removed. It is recommended that the alcohol-based cleaner be placed in the palm of one hand and rubbed against the other hand covering all surfaces until it dries. 10. **C.** Itching is not considered part of the inflammatory process but a possible result. The hallmark signs of inflammation are swelling or edema, and redness as well as heat due to increased circulation in the area. Bruising generally does not occur with inflammation, and the wound does not need to be weeping to be inflamed.

CASE STUDY HINTS

1. Because Mrs. Chase is elderly and has a history of emphysema, she is at risk for respiratory infection. In addition she smokes, which decreases ciliary function and makes infection more likely. By caring for her grandchild who was ill with a strep infection, she was exposed to bacteria that her immune system was unable to fight off.

2. Microorganisms from Mrs. Chase's respiratory tract are transmitted to the tissues through mucus and saliva. Because the tissues have touched the bed linens, the linens are now also contaminated. The nurse who removes the tissues must wear gloves to avoid further transmission of microorganisms.

3. Mrs. Chase has an elevated temperature, is coughing up yellow-green tinged sputum, and has an elevated white count. Her abnormal chest x-ray indicates pneumonia.

...s less than 60 or above ...P would be a reason to ...espiratory rate is a con- ...analgesic. Apical–radial ...quacy of peripheral circu- ...s, low-pitched, coarse, gur- ...moaning or snoring quality, ...e heard on both inspiration ...by coughing. Crackles (rales) ...ling sounds; alveolar rales are ...spiration. May not be cleared ...superficial grating or creaking ...on and expiration, unrelieved by ...tinuous, high-pitched, squeaky ...on expiration, not usually altered ...ht upper quadrant (RUQ) contains ...odenum, head of pancreas, right ...e of right kidney, hepatic flexure of ...ng colon, and a section of transverse ...quadrant (RLQ) contains the lower ...cecum, appendix, section of ascending ...ght fallopian tube, right ureter, right ...part of uterus. The left upper quadrant ...left lobe of the liver, stomach, spleen, ...eft kidney, pancreas, left adrenal gland, ...colon, a section of transverse colon, and a ...ling colon. The left lower quadrant (LLQ) ...r lobe of the left kidney, sigmoid colon, sec- ...ng colon, left ovary, left fallopian tube, left ...matic cord, and part of the uterus. 9. D. Skin ...pinched shape and returns to normal slowly is ...enting, seen in dehydration. Normal skin is soft ...d returns to shape quickly. Loose skin has lost it ...om aging or significant weight loss. Tight skin ...n edema. 10. B. Moods, affect, judgment, abilities, ...le are part of a psychosocial assessment. A history ...cal are a record of previous and present health issues. ...assessment concentrates on body systems. Family ...istory records pertinent family health problems which ...bearing on the client.

Franklin's blood pressure was low and her pulse ele- ...due to blood loss. As her blood pressure dropped, ...ulse increased to compensate and force more blood to ...tal organs.

...Ms. Franklin's blood pressure was low, the blood was ...ng her head slowly, resulting in dizziness.

...or Delayed Bonding with Baby is appropriate ...e it is possible that breast-feeding would be inter- ...due to Ms. Franklin's intolerance to activity and a ...o be off the postpartum floor for a procedure to con- ...e bleeding.

CRITICAL THINKING CARE MAP

Subjective Data Family not present, uninvolved in care of client. Client unmotivated to get better. Complains of dizziness on standing. Complains of loss of appetite over the past week.

Objective Data BP 128/80, 110/72, 90/50: lying/sitting/ standing. Pitcher of water is on the left side of the bed and is full. Saline lock in place and patent. Crackles noted in lower lobes of lungs, bilaterally. Nonproductive cough. P 89, T 99.0°F (37.2°C), R 18 and shallow at rest, 26 and shallow on exertion. Skin is pale and client is diaphoretic.

Report Yes, report the change in blood pressure, complaint of dizziness, and crackles noted in lower lobes of lungs bilaterally, to team leader.

Interventions Place water pitcher on client's right side, within reach. Instruct client to sit up in bed for a few minutes before standing. Put a bed alarm in place according to agency policy. Check physician's orders for IV fluid administration and discuss with RN. Encourage client to increase clear fluid intake. Instruct client to call for assistance before ambulating. Use a walking belt when ambulating client. When mobilizing client, monitor for orthostatic hypotension accompanied by dizziness or fainting. Encourage client to change positions slowly. Slow pace of care, allowing client extra time to carry out activities.

Documentation 9/1/04, 11:30 AM Complains of dizziness on standing, BP 129/80, 110/72, 90/50: lying/sitting/standing; skin dry and flaky, oral mucosa dry. Crackles noted in lower lobes of lungs bilaterally. O₂ sat. 98%, nonproductive cough noted. Encouraged increased fluid intake. Bed alarm placed on bed. Instructed client to call for assistance before ambulating. K. Hirota, LVN

CHAPTER 12

NCLEX-PN ANSWERS 1. B. The first intervention would be to change position as a preventive measure. Q2h is the standard recommendation for repositioning an immobile client. Airflow mattress and protective pads are preventive measures but not the nurse's immediate response. 2. D. When the dry dressing is removed, it eliminates necrotic debris, which has been softened by the dressing solution. Cooling is an effect of a wet dressing. The purpose of this type of dressing is to debride. Antipruritic medication stops itching. A nevus is a mole. 3. A. The open wound becomes a portal for microorganisms to enter the body. An open wound is susceptible to infection and can become contaminated at the time of injury or as healing progresses. Vitamin D synthesis, lubrication, and excretion are functions of the integumentary system. 4. D. Stage IV includes full-thickness skin loss with necrosis and/or damage to muscle, bone, or other supporting structures. Sinus tracts can also be associated with the Stage IV ulcer and are

CRITICAL THINKING CARE MAP

Subjective Data Complains of burning pain in area of wound, says his foot is cold, says he hasn't washed right leg in several days, states he left wound open because "air is good for it."

Objective Data Yellow-green secretions, foul odor from wound and secretions, poor pedal pulses, feet appear slightly cyanotic.

Report Yes, to RN, charge nurse, and physician.

Interventions Administer analgesics as ordered by physician. Report poor pedal pulses and edema. Cleanse wound and apply wound dressings as ordered. Keep feet warm. Put feet in a dependent position. Teach client about airborne contamination. Consult with dietitian regarding diet.

Documentation 10-27-2005, 0800. On admission ulcerated area noted on lower, inner aspect of right leg. No apparent dressing. Moderate amount of thick yellow-green drainage observed. Foul odor noted. Area 15 cm long, 6 cm wide, 1.5 cm deep. Pedal pulses present but weak, foot slightly cyanotic with +2 edema. Wound edges red, surrounding skin hot. States wound has "stinging pain." Charge nurse notified. Wound cleansed with sterile normal saline, wet-to-dry dressing applied. Foot placed in dependent position, with blanket for warmth. Acetaminophen 500 mg given PO per physician's order. Started on high-protein diet. Teaching about wound contamination done. M. Penn, LVN

CHAPTER 8

NCLEX-PN ANSWERS 1. D. The nurse refers to the client properly by her last name, does not relay health information, and does not refer to the client as a diagnosis. A is incorrect because the nurse refers to the client as a diagnosis; this can result in a loss of self-identity. In B the nurse refers to the client by his first name, which some people find offensive. C is incorrect because the client is referred to by room number and not by last name. 2. D. During the initial interview, language skills and understanding should be assessed and arrangements made for an interpreter. A is wrong because Indian was an incorrect name for native people that was adopted early in our country's history. B is incorrect because in some cultures, the informal use of a client's first name is offensive. C is incorrect; it is important to speak clearly and use simple words without slang, but nurses need not speak above their normal tone. 3. A. Individualized client care during admission, transfer, and discharge reduces anxiety; it also promotes safety and improved health status. B is incorrect because discharge planning does not require a physician order and should begin on admission. C and D are incorrect; the client's coping skills and knowledge deficit should be incorporated into the individualized plan for care. 4. D. Lack of oxygen is life threatening, so breathing is always a priority consideration. The nurse should anticipate that the client's oxygen need will increase with

activity and anxiety. Oxygen delivery can be maintained during transfer by securing a portable oxygen tank. A and C are good but not the priority. B: The LPN/LVN may answer questions related to the transfer and would call the RN if the client or significant other has unanswered questions. 5. C. The Joint Commission on Accreditation of Healthcare Organizations (JCAHO) requires that a registered nurse perform the admission assessment. A and D are incorrect because formulation of nursing diagnoses and development of the treatment plan are RN responsibilities. B is incorrect. The LPN/LVN may collect data related to the confused client but should report findings to the charge nurse, not apply a restrictive device. 6. B. The first choice should be to send any valuables home with a significant other. If this is not possible, the valuables may be stored in the hospital safe. A is incorrect: Only the personal items that a client needs (such as glasses, dentures, and hearing aid) should stay by the client's bedside. They should be recorded on the inventory list. C and D are not the best solution. 7. C. The nurse can anticipate that a client who needs to learn self-monitoring administration of insulin will need additional planning and coordination. The LPN/LVN will need to collaborate with the RN to clarify teaching and discharge goals for this client. A, B, and D are incorrect because the LPN/LVN would be able to clarify goals and discharge planning needs independently for these clients. 8. A. Client safety should be the nurse's first concern. The nurse should check the identification band before performing any procedure or giving any medication. With B, C, or D, a medical error might occur. 9. A. Children may experience separation anxiety if the parent is not allowed to stay through the admission process. B is incorrect. Since the nurse is a stranger, trying to hold the child may increase the child's anxiety. C is correct but it is not the best answer because the priority goal is to reduce the client's anxiety related to the admission process. D is incorrect because the nurse–client relationship is harmed when the nurse does not tell the truth. 10. C. Nursing actions during transfer should be directed toward managing the transfer process in an efficient and calm manner. When the nurse shares information, anxiety is decreased and compliance increased. A is wrong; placing the client on the side may not be possible. Nurses should introduce the client using first and last name. D is incorrect because the client may not understand the information presented and may become more anxious.

CASE STUDY HINTS

1. The reason for Mr. Reynolds's admission (potential myocardial infarction) led Janet to address nursing care issues related to his physical status. Specifically, she observed his color and level of pain, monitored his vital signs, and completed the required systems assessment. She also observed and listened to his reaction to his medical situation. Mr. Reynolds gave evidence of having emotional as well as physical nursing care issues. Janet routinely informs the nursing team leader that a new client's admis-

sion has been completed, and reports particular problems requiring the team leader's attention. Regarding Mr. Reynolds, Janet reported that he was experiencing a high degree of anxiety. There were several considerations in making her report. Janet understood that fear and anxiety could exacerbate his symptoms. The physician may have ordered anxiety-reducing medication that would be administered by the nursing team leader (RN). Janet did not have meds certification. She would also discuss with the nursing team leader the nature of Mr. Reynolds's concerns because the anxiety they produced represented a nursing care issue that would be noted in the nursing care plan and require team response.

2. There were several verbal and nonverbal indications that Mr. Reynolds was experiencing fear and anxiety. Certainly what Mr. Reynolds said and how he said it would indicate that he thought he was having a heart attack, that he might die, and he might never see his wife again. His sentences were short and clear. His behavior could also be interpreted as anxious. Mr. Reynolds seemed to be taking his carotid pulse. His face was grimaced. Janet observed Mr. Reynolds's nonverbal behavior and listened to what he said in order to anticipate and recognize clues related to anxiety and fear. Janet empathically understood that anyone in Mr. Reynolds's situation would most likely experience some degree of fear and anxiety.

3. Arranging a room might seem insignificant, but Janet realized that chaos tends to increase anxiety. She understood that establishing order does not in itself reduce fear and anxiety. However, giving Mr. Reynolds choices and listening to his preferences could enable him to feel more control over his situation. It could help him settle in physically and emotionally, and prepare him to face his health issues.

CRITICAL THINKING CARE MAP

Subjective Data "My cats need me, and I can make do." Chart indicates noncompliance with discharge plan to assisted living facility; daughter says client very independent.

Objective Data Unsafe environment at home (outdoor entry and metal stairs).

Report Yes, to charge nurse.

Interventions Maintain a calm, quiet manner; Demonstrate firmness in seeking cooperation; assess level of understanding regarding discharge and transfer; explain purpose of transfer to assisted living; encourage statement of concerns; Allow time to answer questions about the assisted living facility; Inquire about family members who live in the area.

Documentation 1/30/05, 1430. Discharge interview for transfer to rehab attempted. Daughter did not arrive as scheduled. Client resistant to discussion of rehab, even as temporary. Stated "I'm not going there! I'm going home," turned

chair to window. Told client would talk after dinner. Reported to charge nurse. R. Perry, LPN

CHAPTER 9

NCLEX-PN ANSWERS 1. C. This answer is most accurate and reflects the need to inform the doctor of the client's emotional status. 2. D. There is no reason to discuss a client's condition with someone not directly involved with care. C would respect client confidentiality as you are explaining to a visitor what the contact isolation means, not what is wrong with the client. 3. B. You would initial the original medication administration record, not the copy. The other statements are reasonable requests to ensure confidentiality of information. 4. A. This is the correct procedure for most agencies. While the chart does belong to the facility, the client generally has a right to a copy after making a request. There may be a copy fee. 5. C. It is not necessary to cross out an entry or entries so that your notes are in chronological order. A late entry made with the event's time and labeled as a late entry is appropriate. 6. C. Requesting assistance from your charge nurse is appropriate as he/she may be more familiar with the physician's handwriting. If you and your charge nurse are unable to read the orders, you would then call the doctor for clarification. 7. D. Every facility defines the duties of its LPN/LVNs in a job description, which may or may not be similar to job descriptions at other facilities. 8. A. You should always indicate the time the event happened when making your entry. 9. B. Faxing information to a physician's office is appropriate (if permitted by your agency), but should be followed up with a call to the office to ensure that they received the fax. Include the name of the person you spoke with in your nurse's notes. 10. B. When client information is discussed on "walking rounds," care must be taken to ensure that your comments are appropriate and are not overheard by people in the hall. Caution must also be taken when speaking in front of the client, because terminology may be misunderstood or misinterpreted.

CASE STUDY HINTS

1. Maintain aseptic/neutropenic environment. Maintain freedom from infection.
2. Wearing a mask reduces Amy's risk of contracting a disease since her immune system is compromised.
3. Notify the physician. These are signs and symptoms of infection.
4. The steroids suppress the immune system and permit the chemotherapeutics to work more effectively.

CRITICAL THINKING CARE MAP

Subjective Data States "I don't know how to cook for one person"; decreased social activity; crying; talks as if spouse alive.

Objective Data Weight loss since admission; not wearing make-up, hair not combed; decreased interest in surroundings.

Report Yes, to attending physician and care coordinator

INTERVENTIONS

Obtain referrals to grief counselor, appropria[te] group; arrange dietitian consult for mea[l] charge; suggest to family that the client's [?] ularly; schedule time during the shift wh[en] 1:1 time with client; encourage client to talk

Documentation Date 11/25/05. Time 1230. Client ate 25% of supper, declined supplemen[t] hungry. S. Randall LVN. Date 11/27/05. Time 1[?] Notes. Family here to visit reports changes in cli[ent] habits with weight loss over last 2 years. Also repo[rts] cries frequently over death of husband 2 years ago. Fam[ily] reports that client's current lack of interest in chur[ch] grooming was not present prior to death of spouse. S. Ran[dall] LVN. Date 11/27/05. Time 1600. Nurses Notes. Dr. Jone[s] here to see client. Notified of weight loss and family reports (see note above). New orders noted for grief counselor referral and Dietitian Consult. S. Randall LVN. Date 11/27/05. Time 1630. Nurses Notes. Dietary notified of consult order. Client and family notified of orders and of presence of two grief counselors in their area. Son states will choose one and call back in A.M. with choice. S. Randall LVN.

UNIT II WRAP-UP

CRITICAL THINKING

Remember ABC priority when seeing clients in an emergency situation. Mr. Suarez's breathing is compromised; this will be the priority nursing concern. Based upon information gained from the intake inquiry, he may have a communicable disease. Mr. and Mrs. Suarez should be escorted to a private holding area in the emergency department, where Mr. Suarez can rest and his vital signs can be taken. Until Mr. Suarez is removed to an isolated area, he will need to wear a mask. Anyone attending to Mr. Suarez would utilize strict respiratory and contact isolation precautions.

COLLABORATIVE CARE

The triage nurse would be called immediately. A radiology technician and lab technician would be required. The IV team or assigned RN should be notified to start a peripheral line. An infectious control consult would be called. The infectious control manager of the hospital should be alerted. It might also be necessary to contact the county Public Health Department.

CULTURAL COMPETENCY

A translator should be summoned stat to speak to Mr. Suarez and to obtain further information from Mrs. Suarez. The nurse should be sensitive to the fact that Mr. Suarez gave all information, in spite of difficulty breathing. His role may be threatened if caregivers refer questions and decisions to his wife.

COMPASSIONATE CARING

Nursing care for clients with significant respiratory complications focus on maintaining airway clearance, ease of breathing,

...tion and compare it to a baseline. Resu[lt] 100 could be signs of toxicity. Low [?] hold hypertensive medication. Low [?] cern when administering narcotic [?] pulses are assessed to determine [?] lation. 7. B. Gurgles are continuou[s] gling, harsh, louder sounds with a[?] best heard on expiration but can [?] and expiration. May be altered [?] are fine, short, interrupted crac[kles] high-pitched. Best heard on [?] by coughing. Friction rub i[s] sounds heard during inspira[tion] coughing. Wheezes are co[?] musical sounds best heard [?] by coughing. 8. A. The ri[ght?] the liver, gallbladder, d[?] adrenal gland, upper lob[e?] colon, section of ascend[ing?] colon. The right lowe[r?] lobe of right kidney, r[?] colon, right ovary, [?] spermatic cord, and [?] (LUQ) contains the [?] upper lobe of the [?] splenic flexure of [?] section of descen[ding?] contains the low[er?] tion of descend[ing?] ureter, left sp[?] that retains th[?] described as [?] and elastic a[?] elasticity fr[?] results from [?] and lifesty[le?] and phys[ical?] Focused [?] health [?] have [?]

r. [?]
cor[?]
same [?]
cells a[?]
describe [?]
ducts, an[d?]
ported awa[y?]
gland. 10. C. [?]
sis, are often fo[und?]
lum.

CHAPTER 11

NCLEX-PN ANSWERS 1. [?] sidered to be a focused a[ssessment?] plete assessment, and histo[ry?] assessments. 2. B. All assessm[ent?] client's complaints. Nursing [?] response to problems identifie[d?] Physician and nursing orders are c[?] mentation stage of the nursing proce[ss?] for tactile discrimination. Auscultatio[n?] aid of a stethoscope. Inspection uses se[?] tion. 4. A. Eye, motor, and verbal respo[nse?] the Glasgow Coma Scale. Heart rate, respira[tion?] tone, and reflex response are measured wit[h?] Circulation, movement, and sensation (CMS) a[re?] musculoskeletal and nervous system conditions. [?] sion, rigidity, and guarding are related to a pain [?] 5. C. Perfusion, capillary refill, vital signs, and [?] assessed when a cast application has been comple[ted?] vein thrombosis is assessed with Homan's sign. Hip [?] traction and TKR with CPM is assessed with c[?] movement, and sensation. 6. C. Digoxin is a cardio[?] It is important to assess the apical pulse prior to a[?]

not always easily identified. **5. A.** Maceration is a softening of the skin, which can lead to further skin breakdown. Frequent dressing changes occur with wet dressings. Debridement is the desired outcome of a wet-to-dry dressing. Ischemia is decreased blood flow to the area. **6. A.** The second phase of healing includes granulation tissue. Capillaries grow across the wound bringing oxygen and nutrients. The tissue is a translucent red color and easily bleeds. Phagocytosis is a process to ingest and digest bacteria and cellular debris. Necrosis is blackened dead tissue. Exudate is drainage of fluid and cells from a wound. **7. D.** Shearing force is caused by skin that is not moving in relationship to the downward sliding body movement in bed. Evisceration describes the protrusion of the internal viscera through an incision. Hematoma is a localized collection of blood underneath the skin that appears as a reddish-blue swelling. Reactive hyperemia occurs once pressure has been relieved; the area is flooded with extra blood to compensate for the blood flow that was impeded. **8. C.** Handwashing is health care personnel's primary defense against nosocomial infections. Incisions open to air promote healing. Surgical and clean techniques are utilized in dressing changes. Incisions are cleaned from clean to contaminated areas. **9. A.** Diabetes is a systemic disease and affects organs and blood vessels of the body. Peripheral vascular disease decreases the blood flow and contributes to the formation of ulcers. **10. B.** Alcohol has a drying effect on the skin and evaporates rapidly. Maceration softens the skin. Suppuration is a pus formation.

CASE STUDY HINTS

1. It is important to reinforce diabetes teaching to encourage regimen compliance. Diabetes is a systemic disease and is difficult to control under normal conditions. When the body is compromised with an open wound, the blood sugars rise, causing vascular changes and slowing healing. Diabetes hastens hardening and closing of blood vessels and decreases blood flow. It is important to have Mrs. Lee keep a record of her glucose levels, to become an active participant in her care, and to record her blood sugar progress. Remind her of the healing process and the role that blood flow plays in healing.

3. Stage III involves a full-thickness skin loss involving damage or necrosis of subcutaneous tissue that may extend down to, but not through, underlying fascia. The ulcer presents as a deep crater with or without undermining of adjacent tissue. Stage IV is also full-thickness skin loss with extensive destruction, tissue necrosis or damage to muscle, bone, or supporting structures. Undermining and sinus tracts are associated with this stage. Treatment for necrosis can involve enzymatic medications to break down the dead tissue for easier removal. Necrosis needs to be removed because it contains bacteria and must be eliminated to allow healing to take place. Wet-to-dry dressing with a cleansing solution allows for mechanical debride-

ment. Wound packing strategies vary. With a Stage III, the whole wound is visible. In a Stage IV, the wound may have sinus tracts, which, if allowed to heal over, can develop pockets of infection and prolong the healing process. Grafting can be another method of treatment. Nutritional needs increase protein, vitamin C, multivitamins to assist in healing.

CRITICAL THINKING CARE MAP

Subjective Data Difficulty ambulating; client states "I'm not hungry most of the time"; general malaise; decreased sensation to his entire right side.

Objective Data Height 6 ft; weight 135; incontinent of urine; deeply reddened coccyx, right hip, and peritoneal area; right-sided weakness.

Report Yes, report the reddened coccyx, right hip, and peritoneal area to both the charge nurse and physician.

Nursing Interventions Turn client q2h. Steadily increase ambulation. Monitor reddened area. Offer urinal frequently.

Documentation 2/9/05 1430. Client has reddened coccyx (2" × 2"), right hip (2" × 3") and peritoneal area, no open areas noted, physician notified. Client turned q2h and ambulated six feet to the restroom. Urinal offered at frequent intervals, incontinent ×1 this shift. Will continue to monitor reddened areas and offer urinal. D. Stormer, LVN

CHAPTER 13

NCLEX-PN ANSWERS 1. C. Early AM care includes washing the face and hands and giving oral care or assisting the client in doing hygiene tasks. It also includes offering the urinal or bedpan if the client is on bed rest. **2. A.** It is best to follow the client's preferences as long as they are compatible with client's health and equipment. This action on the part of the nurse provides the client with a sense of participation and control, helps the client's self-esteem, and provides a familiar, comforting routine. **3. A.** Loose bed linen and wrinkles can cause irritation and possible skin breakdown. Massaging with alcohol will dry the skin further. It is not recommended that feet be rubbed briskly. Top sheet should be tucked in loosely or with toe pleat in order to keep feet in proper alignment and to prevent pressure in feet. **4. C.** The nursing staff and others caring for elderly clients need to offer water throughout the day because well-hydrated skin is less prone to injury and breakdown. **5. B.** Position the unconscious client in a side-lying position, with the head of the bed lowered. In this position, the saliva automatically runs out by gravity rather than being aspirated into the lungs. This position is the one of choice for the unconscious client receiving mouth care. If the client's head cannot be lowered, turn it to one side. The fluid will readily run out of the mouth or pool in the side of the mouth, where it can be suctioned. **6. D.** Sebum is an oily substance secreted by the skin. It not only lubricates the skin, but also prevents heat loss, kills bacteria, and produces and absorbs vitamin D. **7. C.** When the client is not going to be using the hearing aid for several days, the batteries need to be removed. **8. B.** Students with tinea pedis can spread it by going barefoot in the shower room. Students can get it by going barefoot in the shower room where others with the fungus have walked barefoot. **9. B.** The nurse needs to use a different cotton ball for each wipe. Use normal saline, not tap water, and wipe from inner to outer canthus. The eye shield is used if the corneal reflex is absent and the doctor gives an order for it. **10. C.** It is important to hold dirty linens away from your uniform and not to shake the linens, because that could spread harmful microorganisms.

CASE STUDY HINTS

1. Mr. Bucholz stated that no one "ever told me I shouldn't cut my nails." He was probably told this when he was first diagnosed with diabetes, but he may have been overwhelmed with all the information that came with the diagnosis. Giving a client an easy to follow pamphlet regarding important subjects such as foot care may help reinforce the instructions given.
2. Getting into the habit of having a podiatrist cut his nails may help deter Mr. Bucholz from attempting to cut them at home.

CRITICAL THINKING CARE MAP

Subjective Data States, "I can't remember when I last saw a dentist."

Objective Data VS: T 99.2°F (37.3°C), P 78, R 20 BP 134/82. Pulse ox 98% on room air. Teeth stained from heavy smoking. One large cavity evident in second lower left molar. Tartar buildup along gum margins. Pronounced halitosis. Gums are reddened in some areas and bleed when flossed.

Report Yes, to admitting physician.

Interventions Inspect oral cavity at least once daily and note any discoloration, lesions, edema, bleeding, exudate, or dryness. Determine client's usual method of oral care and address any concerns related to oral care. Use tap water or normal saline to provide oral care; do not use commercial mouthwash containing alcohol or hydrogen peroxide. Identify reasons client has not seen a dentist. Use foam sticks to moisten the oral mucous membrane, clean out debris, and swab while client is NPO. Keep lips well lubricated using petroleum jelly or a similar product.

Documentation 11/23/05. 0930. Focus: Oral mucosa. **D:** Teeth stained. Gums are reddened in some areas and bleed when flossed. One large cavity evident in second lower left molar. Tartar buildup along gum margins. Pronounced halitosis. **A:** Oral care provided with foam stick. Rinsed, cautioned not to swallow due to NPO status. Flossed. Petroleum jelly

applied to lips. **R:** No evidence of bleeding from flossing. Mucosa dry, no exudates. Daren Stiefle, LPN

CHAPTER 14

NCLEX-PN ANSWERS **1. C.** A temperature of 101.8°F (38.7°C) (A) is considered to be one degree lower than an oral temp. A temperature of 102.8°F (39.3°C) would warrant immediate reporting. BP above 140 should be compared to the client's last reading. A pulse of 100 or above should be reassessed after client has rested. **2. B.** Blood pressure should not be taken on the arm on the side of a mastectomy. It also should not be taken on an arm that has sustained an injury. It is best to obtain a larger cuff and take the pressure on the thigh. **3. A.** A cuff with a bladder that is too narrow will result in a falsely high blood pressure reading. **4. B.** Phase 5 of the Korotkoff's sounds is considered to be the adult diastolic pressure, which is followed by a period of silence. **5. D.** When converting Celsius temperature to Fahrenheit, 38.6 converts to 101.48, and is rounded to 101.5. **6. D.** Pulse for children under 3 years of age is more frequently assessed apically. **7. A.** Normal systolic blood pressure for a child is 80 + 2 × the child's age. **8. A.** Orthostatic hypotension will be evident when blood pressure drops with position changes. **9. C.** Prior to administration of digoxin, the apical pulse must be assessed. The medication is held if the apical pulse is less than 60 or more than 100. **10. C.** Morphine sulfate depresses respirations; the client needs to be assessed for 30 seconds following administration.

CASE STUDY HINTS

1. It is important to perform activities of daily living as independently as possible. Perform activities at a comfortable pace, take a rest break as soon as you get tired. Plan to walk twice daily at a comfortable pace. Increase distance weekly until you are able to walk 1 to 2 miles without shortness of breath. You should be able to do 2 miles in 40 minutes, within 6 weeks. After distance is reached, decrease time to 30 minutes, with no dyspnea.
2. Caution Mrs. Munson to discuss the herbal medicine with her physician. "Mrs. Munson, even though the herbs you are taking are natural, they can interact with food and other medication. Notify your physician if any side effects occur. You should have your blood pressure monitored once a week. Report any abnormal readings to your physician. (An abnormal BP would be 30 mm above or below your baseline.) Continue to adhere to diet and report any headaches or visual disturbance to the physician immediately."

CRITICAL THINKING CARE MAP

Subjective Data Chest pain radiating to back and down arm 9/10. Pain 5/10 following medication. "I probably won't live to an old age. I have bad genes for heart attack and stroke." Mother had stroke at 60. Father died at 56 of heart attack. "I normally eat fast food for lunch; my wife makes healthy dinners." Lives with wife. One son. Employed as history teacher at community college. Head injury 1 week ago MVA.

Objective Data African American male. VS: T 99.8°F (37.6°C), P 100, R 24, BP 158/90. Ht. 5'10" Wt. 295 lbs. Sinus tachycardia with occasional PVC.

Report Yes, report head injury 1 week ago MVA to physician.

Interventions Assess client's feelings, values, and reasons for not following prescribed plan of care. Discuss client's beliefs about health and his ability to maintain health. Identify barriers and benefits to being healthy. Determine client's height and weight. Compare results with standards for age and heights. Encourage client to eat a diet that contains fresh foods and is low in saturated fat and no added salt. Assess for the influences of cultural beliefs, norms, and values on the client's beliefs about health.

Documentation Focus. Health-seeking behavior. 1120. **D:** Family hx of CVA and MI, being treated for hypertension, Verapamil 180 mg bid. VS 99.8/100/24 158/90. Client describes diet as fast food regularly for lunch, healthy dinners. **A:** Provided information on cardiac diet to enhance treatment of hypertension. Discuss food likes and dislikes. **R:** Client able to explain benefits of appropriate diet and choose daily menu which meets the prescribed criteria. K. Turner LVN. **D** = Data; **A** = Action; **R** = Results.

CHAPTER 15

NCLEX-PN ANSWERS **1. C.** The client is the best source of information about the pain being experienced; A and B place the responsibility for control on the health care professional; participation in the plan by the client will result in a more satisfying experience; D discounts the client's input and understanding. **2. B.** Using a numerical pain rating scale is the most effective way of assessing the severity of the pain. A is a closed-ended question, which rarely provides good data for the assessment. C and D are vague and subjective. **3. D.** Acute pain lasts only through the expected recovery period, whether its onset is sudden or slow and regardless of the intensity. Chronic pain lasts beyond the typical healing time period. Chronic pain that persists despite therapeutic interventions is classified as intractable. Referred pain is pain felt in a part of the body that is considerably removed from the tissues causing the pain. **4. A.** Constipation is a side effect and occurs frequently with opioids. Rashes and anaphylaxis are symptoms of an allergic reaction. Respiratory depression can occur with opioids; respiratory distress can be life-threatening reaction. **5. C.** Many clients have had good response to anticonvulsants when dealing with nerve pain. NSAIDs work well for muscle pain and inflammation. Nonopioids are effective for mild pain; opioids are more appropriate for severe pain (7 to 10 on a rating scale). **6. B.** Time of onset, duration, and recurrence or intervals without pain are referring to the pain pattern. Intensity and

severity are rated with a pain scale; duration refers to how long the pain episode lasts. **7. C.** Duragesic, an opioid analgesic, comes in the form of a patch that is placed on the skin (transdermal). Patient-controlled analgesia (PCA) is IV pain control that it accessed by a push button available to the client. It has a lockout mechanism to prevent overdose. Intravenous analgesia is usually given IV push by the RN. Intraspinal analgesia is delivered via catheter into the subarachnoid or epidural space. **8. D.** Level 4 of sedation is characterized by minimal or no response to stimuli; level 1 is easily arousable; level 2 is awake and alert; level 3 is frequently drowsy, arousable, and drifts off to sleep during conversation. **9. B.** Tissue ischemia is a chemical type of pain stimuli. Tumors and trauma to body tissues (e.g., surgery) and blockage of a body duct are mechanical stimuli. **10. B.** Nerve block requires an injection, which is invasive. Transcutaneous electrical nerve stimulation (TENS) is noninvasive; it is accomplished through electrodes placed on the skin. Distraction and guided imagery are pain therapy that depend on the mind–body connection to control pain.

CASE STUDY HINTS

1. There are subjective data (rating pain as 5) and objective data (vital signs, position, holding abdomen, rigid position) to support that Mrs. Lundahl is experiencing pain. However, no conclusions can be drawn about the intensity, location, quality, or pattern of her pain.
2. It would be incorrect to assume that Mrs. Lundahl needs no interventions for her pain with a self-assessment of 5. People rate their pain differently based on their past pain experiences, their pain tolerance, their ethnic/cultural values. Mrs. Lundahl should be asked if she needs pain intervention.
3. Mrs. Lundahl is most likely experiencing acute pain from her surgery. Depending on the amount of manipulation of bowel, blood vessels, and so on, within her abdomen, she may also be experiencing visceral pain.
4. In addition to pain medication, interventions such as changing position, back massage, use of cutaneous stimulator, and distraction may be helpful.
5. The most reliable method of determining that Mrs. Lundahl's pain has been relieved is for her to tell you so. Objective data may include decreased blood pressure and respirations when compared to preintervention values; Mrs. Lundahl resting quietly or asleep; pink color, absence of perspiration; relaxed facial expression and so on.

CRITICAL THINKING CARE MAP

Subjective Data Client complains of pain (7 on a scale of 1 to 10). "I am cold and tired, I wish I could sleep." Complains of being thirsty. Complains of nausea but no vomiting.

Objective Data Height: 188 cm (6'3"). Weight: 90.0 kg (200 lbs). T 37°C (98.6°F). Lying in dorsal recumbent position with legs drawn up. P 90, R 24, BP 158/82. Skin pale and moist, pupils dilated. NPO, intravenous infusion of D_5H NS at 125 cc/hr left arm, nasogastric tube to low intermittent suction. Restless. Midline abdominal incision, sutures dry and intact. Chest x-ray and urinalysis negative, WBC 12,000.

Report No.

Interventions Medicate before an activity to increase participation. Evaluate the effectiveness of the pain control measures used through ongoing assessment. Assess wound drainage at each dressing change. Determine analgesic selections (narcotic, nonnarcotic, or NSAID) based on type and severity of pain. Institute safety precautions as appropriate if receiving narcotic analgesics. Instruct client to request prn pain medication before the pain is severe. Create a quiet, nondisruptive environment with dim lights and comfortable temperature when possible.

Documentation 06/04/05, 1640. Client restless; lying in bed with legs drawn up. C/o pain 7/10 in abdomen. Abdomen distended, NG to low intermittent suction. c/o thirst and nausea. NG irrigated with 30 cc NSS. Reconnected to low suction, 300 cc of brown fluid drained. Demerol 75 mg IM given. G. Nugent LVN. 1715. Abdomen soft, reports pain decreased to 2/10; no c/o of nausea. NG draining. Resting comfortably. Asked "Please turn off the TV and pull the curtain, I think I can take a nap now." G. Nugent LVN.

CHAPTER 16

NCLEX-PN ANSWERS 1. **D.** High-Fowler's position (~90 degrees) allows gravity to aid in lowering the diaphragm, allowing greater chest expansion. Trendelenberg is a head-down, feet-up position. Abdominal contents would be pushed up on the diaphragm resulting in *less* chest expansion. In low-Fowler's position, the head of the bed is elevated only ~30 degrees. The gravitational pull is significantly less than high-Fowler's. Sims' position is a side-lying position and as a result, restricts the movement of the chest on the dependent side. 2. **C.** Cheyne–Stokes is the pattern described in this question. Kussmaul's respirations are seen in clients who are hyperventilating. There is an increase in both rate and depth; no periods of apnea. Tachypnea refers solely to respiratory rate; specifically a faster than normal rate. Eupnea is normal breathing: regular, quiet, effortless. 3. **D.** All three of these assessments are essential elements of a respiratory assessment. Restlessness can be an early sign of hypoxia (lack of oxygen to the brain). None of the data is a priority, with the possible exception of pain. Pupil size is more a neurologic concern; sneezing is not a priority complaint. BP and sweating would be more significant for a client with a cardiac diagnosis. Capillary refill is more directly related to perfusion. Trembling is irrelevant. The amount of sputum is important, but not the *most* important. 4. **B.** An open airway with adequate gas exchange takes the highest priority (airway and breathing always take priority; then circulation). Reducing anxiety is a desired goal but

should not receive the highest priority. Talking about feelings is an important goal, but is superceded by the need for a patent airway. Maintaining fluid balance is important, but not the most essential element to sustain life. 5. **D.** Orthopnea is a respiratory condition in which the client complains of difficulty breathing in any position except sitting or standing. It is seen in heart failure, pulmonary edema, and severe emphysema. The question asked for a definition of orthopnea. A, B, and C are not definitions of orthopnea. 6. **C.** A tracheostomy tube is inserted into the trachea to create an artificial airway. A tracheostomy tube cannot be used for nutrition; it is inserted in the airway, not the esophagus. A tube to remove flatus would be inserted in the rectum. A tracheostomy tube decreases dead space. 7. **A.** The ABCs (*a*irway, *b*reathing, *c*irculation) are always the first priority. Rapid, irregular respirations of 32/min require immediate intervention. B, C, and D do not take priority over increased respirations. 8. **D.** Dyspnea means difficult breathing or difficulty breathing (taken from the Latin *dys* for "difficult" and *pnea* for "breath"). Shallow respirations do not necessarily mean that the client's gas exchange is compromised. Rapid breathing is called tachypnea and could be a physiologic compensatory mechanism. C is a definition of orthopnea. 9. **B.** Oxygen is a highly combustible gas that can easily ignite on contact with a spark. Posting "No Smoking" signs promotes client safety. All rooms should be well ventilated, regardless of oxygen use. One liter difference in flow rate does not increase combustibility of oxygen. Skin lotions do not interfere with oxygen, nor do they pose a danger. 10. **B.** Hypoxia is a diminished oxygen supply to the cells of the body resulting in the symptoms listed. The respiratory control center is located in the brain; therefore, judgment can also be impaired. A and C are *late* signs of hypoxia. D Crowing respirations are characteristic of an obstructed airway.

CASE STUDY HINTS

1. Mr. Markert is at risk for respiratory complications related to his chest trauma. The pulse can detect changes in oxygen status, such as hyperemia, before clinical manifestations develop. If complications are noted early in their development, actions can be taken to stop progression of the problem.

2. Important nursing care involves frequent monitoring of Mr. Markert's respiratory and cardiac status and his oxygen saturations; monitoring the patency of his drainage system; maintaining the integrity of his water-seal drainage; never raising the drainage system above his chest; implementing emergency measures should an air leak develop; and providing Mr. Markert with information and reassurance.

3. Mr. Markert would benefit from sitting or lying in a position that enhances respiration, engaging in deep breathing exercises, ambulating or exercising, and maintaining adequate fluid intake.

CRITICAL THINKING CARE MAP

Subjective Data Fatigue; "bad cold for several weeks that just wouldn't go away"; dieting for several weeks and skipping meals; works full time and is attending college; smoked one pack of cigarettes per day since 18 years of age.

Objective Data Weight 120 lbs; VS: T 103°F (39.4°C), P 82, R 24, BP 118/70; skin pale; cheeks flushed; chills; nasal flaring; use of accessory muscles; inspiratory crackles with diminished breath sounds right base; thick, yellow sputum; chest x-ray: right lobar infiltration WBC 14,000; pH 7.48; $PaCO_2$ 33 mm Hg; HCO_3 20 mEq/L; $PaCo_2$ 80 mm Hg.

Report Yes, to physician.

Interventions Encourage her to take a deep breath, hold for two seconds, and cough two or three times in succession; encourage use of incentive spirometry, as appropriate; monitor rate, rhythm, depth, and effort of respirations; auscultate breath sounds, noting area of decreased or absent ventilations and presence of adventitious sounds; monitor respiratory secretions; monitor increased restlessness, anxiety, and air hunger.

Documentation 1/23/06, 0900. Focus area: Cough. **D:** Yellow, thick sputum, expectorated following C/DB and respiratory treatment. Complains of discomfort right chest, pale, lips cyanotic, diaphoretic. **A:** Breath sounds assessed; assisted to high-Fowler's position; cough preparation administered per physician's order. **R:** Color improved, lips pink, sitting up in bed. States "my chest doesn't hurt as much now." W. Poole LPN.

CHAPTER 17

NCLEX-PN ANSWERS 1. A. The protein in a diet provides amino acids, the structural material for building body tissues. Although protein intake is related to fat intake, this answer does not satisfy the question being asked. Calories are primarily gained from consumption of carbohydrates, not proteins. Calcium may be present in protein, but supplements are often given to those at risk for decreased bone density. 2. C. When clients believe that they can make a difference in the outcome of their health, they are more likely to succeed at making dietary changes. Relying on others, looking for approval, or lacking belief that dietary changes can influence health outcome all suggest less likelihood of success. 3. B. To calculate the answer, you add the urine output and the amount of emesis to gain an accurate result. 4. B. Cream sauces tend to be high in fat, which would increase LDL cholesterol. It is not necessary to shop in specialty stores. The substitutes in answer D contain salt and may promote hypertension. 5. C. A person who is 20% over IBW is obese and remains at risk even though he or she may be physically active. 6. B. No feeding is to be started until placement is clearly and positively identified. There is no prioritized need to weigh the client before restarting tube feeding. Do not give the client trials of eating food without evidence of safety in swallowing, including swallow studies and physician orders. This could lead to aspiration. 7. A. Insulation is a function of fats. Protein provides building blocks for body repair. Although carbohydrates may supply fiber, their primary function is to provide energy for the body. 8. B. The milkshake, apricot nectar, and creamed soups are not transparent. 9. C. The smaller blue port (A) is for air exchange. Giving medications through may cause inadequate function of the tube. B would be unsafe and unacceptable nursing practice; do not give the client medications orally unless physician's order precisely directs you to do this. Medications must continue to be given even in the presence of a NG tube. 10. A. The primary function of potassium is smooth muscle conduction. Calcium regulates muscle contraction and relaxation. The primary function of magnesium is aiding in ATP production.

CASE STUDY HINTS

1. The nurse would attempt to encourage the client to consume a greater part of the diet provided. If the nurse can establish a trusting relationship, it may be possible to identify some foods that would be preferred, and to discuss the client's self-perception of being overweight. Although other means would be attempted first, it may be necessary to provide parenteral nutrition to the client to maintain or restore electrolyte balance.
2. Anorexia is a psychological disorder. A trained psychologist might be able to help the client understand what caused the feelings of being overweight to occur, and what other feelings might be standing in the way of a healthier self-image.
3. Disturbed Body Image is appropriate because the client feels huge, ugly, and overweight when she is in fact in danger of starving to death. At this point, she is not capable of seeing her real image clearly.

CRITICAL THINKING CARE MAP

Subjective Data Mood: irritable, anxious; states she is very thirsty.

Objective Data Weight: 145; BP 98/62; P 110, regular; R 16; oxygen saturation: 93% on room air; Nausea and vomiting present; mucous membranes dry; skin turgor poor; urine dark amber, 50 mL in last voiding.

Report Yes, to physician and/or charge nurse

Interventions Monitor and report abnormal lab results; monitor and document intake and output; encourage fluid intake; teach client to stand slowly; monitor color, amount, and frequency of fluid loss; assess for vertigo and hypotension; daily weights; give and monitor effectiveness of antinausea medication as ordered; give and monitor effectiveness of antidiarrheal medications as ordered. Monitor orthostatic blood pressure q4h; Administer IV therapy as ordered; provide frequent oral care.

Documentation Client states thirsty, mucous membranes dry. Instructed on intake/output. Safety precautions instructed, rise slowly. Oral care for comfort. IV fluids initiated per orders. Orthostatic BP, pulse as ordered. I. Sharpsaddle, LPN

CHAPTER 18

NCLEX-PN ANSWERS **1. B.** Women are prone to urinary tract infections because of their short urethra and the proximity of the urinary meatus to the vagina and anus. **2. D.** Diuresis is the production and excretion of large amounts of urine. Oliguria is low urine output; anuria refers to a lack of urine production, without effective urinary output. Polydipsia is excessive thirst. **3. C.** The kidneys produce urine at a rate of approximately 60 mL per hour or about 1,500 mL per day. **4. A.** Urine culture is ordered to identify microorganisms that are causing urinary tract infection. **5. B.** At the start of the collection period, have the client void and discard this first urine. **6. C.** Clamp the catheter for 30 minutes. This allows fresh urine to collect in the catheter. **7. B.** The specific gravity of water is 1.000; the specific gravity of urine is 1.010 to 1.025 and is a measure of its concentration. **8. C.** Increasing fluid for a client with kidney disease may be contraindicated related to the functional ability of the kidneys. Renal calculi and UTI would require increasing fluid intake. **9. D.** Increase the acidity of urine by the use of vitamin C or drinking cranberry juices. This inhibits bacterial formation. Increased fluids, showering rather than bathing, and use of cotton underclothes are preventive measures. **10. D.** The suprapubic catheter is inserted through the abdominal wall above the symphysis pubis and into the urinary bladder.

CASE STUDY HINTS

1. Wash hands prior to any procedure; this is the single most effective practice to inhibit contamination. Use disposable gloves and cleanse the area where the needle will be inserted with a disinfectant. This will remove microorganisms on the surface of the catheter. Be careful not to puncture the tube, compromising the closed system. When transferring the urine to the specimen container, do not allow the needle to touch the side of the container; this would contaminate the sterile container.
2. Measures to prevent the development of a urinary tract infection are to increase fluid intake and wipe the perineal area from front to back following urination or defecation. Catheter care will prevent organisms from traveling up the catheter into the bladder. Encourage fluids that increase the acidity of urine through intake of vitamin C and cranberry juices, which inhibit bacterial growth. Early removal of the catheter per physicians order will decrease the risk for infection.

CRITICAL THINKING CARE MAP

Subjective Data Diabetes out of control; weakened; tired; thirst; diabetic care compliance.

Objective Data Incontinent; foul-smelling, cloudy urine; mucous threads; diminished pedal pulses; glucose 440; T 99°F (37.2°C); catheter to gravity drainage.

Report Yes, notify the physician of: glucose 440; client's complaint of thirst; cloudy, foul-smelling urine with mucous threads; T 99°F; diminished pedal pulses.

Interventions Monitor lab tests; observe urine for output; assess urine for abnormal constituents; maintain catheter asepsis; VS q4h.

Documentation 1600. Client's urine is cloudy, foul smelling with mucous threads. 18″ urinary catheter placed, per order. Output spontaneous 300 mL. Client tolerated procedure well. T 99°F. Glucose 440, physician notified, medicated client with 10 U of regular insulin. Lab results pending. D. Haus LVN

CHAPTER 19 ANSWERS

NCLEX-PN ANSWERS **1. D.** Surgery that involves direct handling of the intestines can cause the intestinal movement to cease temporarily. It usually lasts 24 to 48 hours. Constipation is defined as fewer than three bowel movements per week. The stool becomes dry and hardened. Volvulus is a twisting of the bowel. Ulcerative colitis is an inflammatory disease of the colon that results in severe diarrhea. **2. C.** Rectal stimulation is contraindicated for those with cardiac disease because it may result in cardiac arrythmias. **3. D.** Wavelike motion that propels intestinal contents forward and occurs with both circular and longitudinal muscle contraction is known as peristalsis. **4. C.** Oil retention enema lubricates and softens the stool prior to manual removal. **5. A.** Digestive enzymes break down large molecules to simple chemicals; therefore, if these enzymes come in contact with the skin, they cause breakdown and irritation. **6. C.** Guaiac test is used to determine blood in the stool, as is testing for occult (hidden) blood. **7. B.** Fluid and electrolytes (potassium) are not being reabsorbed, they are being eliminated from the body. **8. B.** Codeine decreases gastrointestinal motility. Colace is a stool softener; catapres and clonidine are antihypertensives. **9. C.** Ambulation increases peristalsis and therefore can facilitate gas movement. Use of a straw may increase gulping air, adding to the problem. Lomotil is an antidiarrheal medication. **10. C.** When the skin is irritated the site should be treated and assessed q 24 to 48 hours. Five days would be the length of time that the appliance remains intact.

CASE STUDY HINTS

1. The expulsion of feces from the anus and rectum is known as defecation. The frequency is individual and can vary from daily to every third day or more. Peristalsis moves feces into the sigmoid colon and rectum; the sensory nerves in the rectum are stimulated; and the individual becomes aware of the need to defecate. Expulsion of feces

is assisted by contraction of the abdominal muscles and the diaphragm. This causes intra-abdominal pressure, which moves the feces through the anal canal.

2. Diet is important in providing bulk, which stimulates peristalsis to move the feces along the canal. Activity and exercise increase peristalsis. Fluid intake is a factor that affects the consistency of the stool; 2,000 to 3,000 mL per day promote normal soft stool. Individuals who eat at the same times every day usually have a regularly timed physiologic response to the food intake and regular pattern of peristaltic activity in the colon.

CRITICAL THINKING CARE MAP

Subjective Data Client c/o pain; anxious; fearful.

Objective Data Ileostomy right abdomen; stoma brick red; effluent watery, dark brown, new flecks of blood; peristomal area reddened; weight 110; hemoglobin 10; WBC 12,000; T 99.4°F (37.4°C); skin turgor slow; client not looking at stoma.

Report Yes, report to physician: low-grade temp, WBC 12,000, hemoglobin 10, flecks of blood, reddened peristomal area, slow skin turgor, client's denial regarding ostomy. Inform the enterostomal nurse regarding the peristomal area.

Interventions Monitor intake and output; assess skin turgor; daily weights; VS q4h; increase fluid intake; assess stoma; peristomal inspection; include family in teaching; referrals to Ostomy Association; monitor WBC, hemoglobin lab values; assess coping mechanisms.

Documentation 1400. Client is having difficulty accepting ileostomy, evidenced by covering head when staff empties bag, encouraged verbalization. Enterostomal nurse changed appliance at 1330. Included family members when reinforcing ostomy care. Client assisting minimally with ostomy. Temp. 99.4, skin turgor slow, encouraged fluids. Monitoring daily wts. Stoma brick red color, peristomal area reddened, no breakdown. Effluent dark brown with flecks of blood. Fecal output at 500 mL. Physician notified. D. Haus LVN

CHAPTER 20

NCLEX-PN ANSWERS 1. B. Center of gravity is where the body's mass and base of support are centered and balance is achieved. Line of gravity is an imaginary vertical line through the center of gravity. Postural tonus is muscle contraction needed to maintain an upright position. 2. C. Osteoporosis is a demineralization process of the bones, which occurs without the stress of weight-bearing activity. Contractures are permanent shorting of the muscles which cause permanent fixation of joints. Orthostatic hypotension is a drop in blood pressure following a rapid change in position. Disuse atrophy is loss of normal strength and function and size of unused muscles. 3. D. Bed rest decreased the production of surfactant which

enables the alveoli to remain open. This, along with mucus plugged bronchiole, can cause a lung to collapse. 4. A. Crutches must be adjusted so that weight is on the forearm, not the axilla, since pressure on the underarm can damage the brachial plexus. Understanding the need for nonslip shoes and rubber tips on the crutches and removal of hazards in the home demonstrates successful learning. 5. C. The orthopneic position is modified Fowler's, which aids in air exchange in respiratory and heart clients. 6. C. Stage III occurs when heart and respiratory rates and other body processes slow and are dominated by the parasympathetic nervous system. The sleeper becomes more difficult to arouse. Stages I and II are light sleep; stage IV is deep sleep. 7. C. Hypothyroidism decreases stage IV sleep. Hyperthyroidism lengthens presleep time, making it difficult to fall asleep. 8. B. Treatment of insomnia routinely includes behavior modification in which the client learns new habits to foster sleep. Long-term sleep-inducing medication is not recommended since it does not treat the cause and can result in dependency. Antidepressants and beta blockers can cause nightmares and daytime drowsiness. 9. A. *Somnambulism* is a term meaning sleepwalking; bedwetting is enuresis, and teeth grinding is bruxism. 10. A. Even mild conditioning can strengthen the legs and increase circulation, which will help relieve postural hypotension.

CASE STUDY HINTS

1. Check traction for proper alignment and ensure that weights are hanging free. Traction will maintain the position of the fracture and help relieve muscle spasms. Encourage Kevin to do active ROM to unaffected extremities. Encourage position changes with aid of trapeze.
2. Once Kevin's bowel sounds have returned, he should be permitted a regular diet. Request the physician to write an order that food can be brought in from home. Have dietitian talk with Kevin about food likes and dislikes, provide nutritious snacks, fresh fruit, dairy products, and protein. Discuss the need for calcium and protein to promote healing. Allow Kevin to make informed choices.
3. Distractions might include handheld video games, DVD movies, music, Internet access (if possible) to help him keep up with school work, and interactions with family and peers. Roommate selection is very important if long-term hospitalization is necessary. It is important for Kevin to have contact with his peers at his developmental level.

CRITICAL THINKING CARE MAP

Subjective States she has a problem falling asleep since her mastectomy 2 months ago; says fears of prognosis become prominent when she is not active and busy; has tried reading or watching TV but neither make her sleepy or relaxed.

Objective Weight 126, a 10-pound weight loss since surgery; R 16; skin pale; dark circles around eyes; radiation site irritated and red; appears agitated and restless.

Interventions Assess client's sleep patterns and usual bedtime rituals and incorporate these into the plan of care; assess for signs of new onset of depression; depressed mood state, statement of hopelessness, poor appetite; observe client's diet and medication and caffeine intake. Look for hidden sources of caffeine; advise client to avoid use of alcohol or hypnotics to induce sleep.

Documentation 10/14/05. 1300. Focus: Insomnia. **D:** Anxious and agitated, states she has not been sleeping well since surgery, admitted to dwelling on prognosis. **A:** Discussed bedtime rituals and caffeine intake. Suggested keeping a sleep diary until next visit. **R:** Agreed to keep diary and replace bedtime tea with decaffeinated or herbal tea. M.Tunny LPN.

CHAPTER 21

NCLEX-PN ANSWERS 1. C. When a portion of a unit dose of a controlled substance is not used, it must be disposed of in the presence of another licensed person. Both must acknowledge the wasting in writing. Never dispose of a controlled substance in the tubex in the sharps container, because it could be retrieved and used illicitly. Allowing a client to remain without medication could be considered neglect. 2. A. The nurse is responsible for his or her actions. Although the error could have been discovered by any of the other parties, the responsibility belongs to the nurse. 3. C. The reason a drug is prescribed is the therapeutic effect; the other answers are adverse effects of the drug. 4. B. The idiosyncratic effect is an unexpected individualized reaction. Drug tolerance occurs when more drug is required to cause the same effect. Drug interaction is what occurs when two or more drugs affect each other. Iatrogenic disease is a disease caused unintentionally by medical therapy. 5. B. A "stat" order is one that is to be given immediately and only once. A prn order is given as needed. An order that has no d/c date is known as a standing order. The times a drug is given may be determined by facility policy (e.g., qid could be at 0900, 1300, 1700, and 2100 or at 0600, 1100, 1800, 2400), but the order must be written by the physician. 6. B. 1/60 grain = 1 mg; on hand you have 1 mg/mL, so you would give 0.2 mL to the client. All the others would be too much: 1 mL would equal 5 times the ordered dose; 2 mg would be 10 times the dose; 1/3 mL would be approximately .33 mL, which would be about 1½ the ordered dose. 7. D. Using a medicine cup is the most accurate way for the mother to measure the medication. A household teaspoon can overmeasure by almost a half more. Mixing medication with essential food can alter the taste, and the child may be reluctant to eat it in the future. The medication is ordered q6h, which means it needs to be given around the clock. Giving it with meals and at bedtime would not be appropriate. 8. B. A tuberculin syringe can be used for medication when less than 1 cc is to be given SQ; 4,000 U would equal 0.8 cc. The attached needle is of the appropriate length and gauge for an SQ injection. Insulin syringes are used only for insulin; insulin units and heparin units are not equal. In 2- and 3-cc syringes it is difficult to measure less than 1 cc exactly, and the needle gauge or length is not appropriate for an SQ injection. 9. A. The primary reason for wearing gloves is to prevent the spread of microorganisms from the skin. Some topical medications can cause an effect in the nurse (e.g., nitro patches can cause headaches if the nurse comes in contact with the medication). The typical medication will not be passed on to another client if the nurse follows Standard Precautions and washes hands between clients. Unless there are open wounds (like burns), topical application of medication is not usually done as a sterile procedure. 10. B. The gluteal muscles are developed by walking. They should not be used until the child has been walking for at least 1 year. All muscles absorb medication at the same rate. Bruising results from technique and type of medication rather than location. A child must be held securely to prevent injury, no matter what site you use.

CASE STUDY HINTS

1. Side effects are not related to allergic reaction and do not produce the same symptoms as allergies do. Allergic reactions have a distinct pattern of reaction (e.g., skin rash, pruritus, rhinitis, tearing, nausea, vomiting, wheezing, dyspnea, or diarrhea).
2. The appropriate injection site depends on factors such as client's body weight, the healthiness of the muscle tissue, access to the site, the frequency with which the site has been used for previous injections, the condition of the skin over the site, and the client's preference. The ventrogluteal site is generally preferred because the area contains no large nerves or blood vesssels and has less fat than the buttock area.
3. Some drugs are better absorbed when given on an empty stomach; others cause gastrointestinal irritation and should be given with meals or after meals.

CRITICAL THINKING CARE MAP

Subjective Data "It will be hard to follow the diet at home, I don't eat on a regular schedule on my school nights and my roommates are big snackers." States " I have been so tired, but it is probably because I am working and going to school." Complains of excessive thirst and frequent urination; client hesitant to perform monitoring and injections herself.

Objective Data Weight 156 lbs; fasting blood sugar 164 mg/mL; urine shows presence of ketones; VS: T 99°F (37.2°C), P 132, R 28, BP 100/54. Started on insulin injection and BGM; 1,800-cal ADA diet.

Report Yes, to the diabetes educator and the physician.

Interventions Provide information about the therapeutic regimen in various formats (video, brochures, written instructions). Deliberate with the client on changes that are possible to meet therapeutic goals. Demonstrate and allow client to perform monitoring and self-injection under supervision.

Documentation 05/30/02, 0730. Has completed diabetic education program. BGM performed by client. Able to complete all steps accurately. Prepared insulin injection per sliding scale and routine NPH order under supervision. Client still hesitant to inject self. Discussed reluctance. Expressed concern with associated pain. Stated "I am just a chicken." Injection given by nurse in abdomen. Client admitted to very little discomfort, and stated she will try to do it herself next time. V. Dawson LPN.

CHAPTER 22

NCLEX-PN ANSWERS 1. B. Although the length of the hospital stay may not be shortened, good preoperative teaching aids recovery. Pain will still be present, but client will be better equipped to deal with the pain and may need less medication. Teaching decreases anxiety. **2. D.** A client may retain his or her wedding ring as long as it is secured with tape, unless he or she is having arm or hand surgery or a surgical procedure that may produce arm or hand swelling. A modified radical mastectomy involves removal of the lymph nodes, which can result in swelling. **3. B.** Once vital signs are stabilized, they are taken every hour ×4 and then q4h for 2 days. A client 3 hours post op would continue to have hourly vital signs taken even if stable. A and D would have q4h vital signs, and C would still need q15 min vital signs because they have not stabilized. **4. C.** It is recommended that the client remain flat following spinal anesthesia for at least 8 hours. Unconscious clients are positioned on their sides until fully awake. Semi-Fowler's and reverse Trendelenburg are not used postoperatively. **5. A.** The client should be in Fowler's or semi-Fowler's position during coughing and deep breathing. **6. D.** Pain severity is best described by the client; teaching the client to use the 0–10 pain scale is the most accurate. **7. C.** Early ambulation is key in promoting postoperative recovery. Explaining this to the client is empowering and encourages compliance. **8. C.** It is the physician's responsibility to explain the procedure to the client (informed consent). If the client is unsure of the procedure, the physician needs to see the client prior to his or her being transported to the OR. Although it is important that the physician be informed of vital signs and allergies, they can be noted on the chart. Frequently, a physician will allow necessary medication with small sips of water; notify the OR and note on the chart. **9. B.** Gastric contents follow the path of least resistance, so vent tube must be kept higher than the stomach to prevent reflux. **10. C.** Evisceration is the protrusion of a body organ from a wound dehiscence. Dehiscence is a separation in layers of the incisional wound. Secondary intention refers to the healing when the wound is large, gaping, and irregular. Granulation is new tissue filling in the wound.

CASE STUDY HINTS

1. Factors that may increase Mr. Teng's risk may include: Mr. Teng is 77 years old, placing him at a greater risk than younger adults; his respiratory status is compromised and he runs a greater risk for developing postoperative atelectasis or lung infection; he may be taking medications that will slow healing such as corticosteroids.
2. A major disadvantage of general anesthesia is that it depresses the respiratory and the circulatory systems, so regional anesthesia was probably chosen so as not to further compromise his respiratory status.
3. Specific precautions may include: promoting adequate hydration to replace fluids lost during surgery or fluid limitations prior to surgery; early movement and ambulation to foster maximum lung expansion, and prevent lung infection; deep breathing exercises to remove mucus and prevent stasis of lung secretions; pain control so that he can ambulate and cough more effectively; and leg exercises to prevent thrombophlebitis.

CRITICAL THINKING CARE MAP

Subjective Data Complains of pain; "I wish I had died in the accident; life will never be the same."

Objective Data Vital signs stable; refuses to respond to nurse's questions about pain level; will not look at limb during dressing change; dressing dry and intact; wound healing without signs of infection.

Report Yes, to social worker.

Interventions Contact physician for social worker or psychologist referral; acknowledge denial, anger, or depression as normal; encourage client to make own decisions, participate in plan of care and accept both inadequacies and strengths; allow client gradual exposure to body change; help client to accept help from others; teach family appropriate care of surgical site.

Documentation Client turned toward wall during dressing change. Refused to look at limb. Stated "I wish I had died in the accident, life will never be the same." Complaining of pain, unable to describe the level. H. Mobley LVN.

CHAPTER 23

NCLEX-PN ANSWERS 1. B. Modeling focuses on imitation, the process by which individuals copy and reproduce what they have observed. Lecture, handouts, and written testing are used in cognitive theory. Rewards are positive reinforcement and are part of behaviorism theory. **2. C.** Restoration involves information about what is being done as well as self-care skills and resources. **3. D.** Pain is a barrier to learning because it decreases concentration. Pain needs to be dealt with prior to initiating teaching. **4. B.** It is important to use words that the client understands, for example, that bathing and shower, as well as washing the incision with soap and water, could interfere with the healing process. **5. A.** The client apparently has the physical capabilities to prepare her insulin injections, because earlier there was no evidence of sensory or cognitive deficits. She is likely overwhelmed by the process of caring for herself without support when she gets home and is feeling a lack of control of the situation. **6. C.** Many cultural groups, especially from east Asia, are reluctant to maintain eye contact with professionals, feeling that it is a lack of respect. It does not mean that they are confused or that they are not interested. The client probably would not make eye contact with the physician if he or she was giving the instructions. **7. C.** Young school-age children relate to and learn better from imaginary figures. They tend to give life to inanimate objects (*animism*). Stories, puppets, and colorful items are the best reinforcement of learning in this age group. Lecture and handouts are used better with individuals who can read and who have a longer attention span. Food that can be manipulated and placed on the pyramid can be used with school-age children as a return demonstration. Cooking class works well for older school-age children as they enter the stage of industry. **8. C.** Understanding that it is not safe to leave the client alone for extended periods each day is important to home safety. When a client suffers from dementia, he may forget that he should not use the stove, or forget to turn it off after use. Posting a number is a good idea, but in an emergency the client with dementia will not be able to process quickly who should be called. Although it is hard for the family to see their loved one like this, this statement does not address the safety issues. **9. A.** Negative feedback will cause the client to avoid the nurse; it is never appropriate and should not be used in a teaching situation. **10. B.** It is better to wait until the client and all caregivers are available so that clear, complete instructions can be given. Since the client and the husband both have sensory deficits, waiting for the daughter is imperative.

CASE STUDY HINTS

1. Early detection of the signs and symptoms of infection may decrease the need for very aggressive treatment of the infection. If the infection is not discovered until it is severe, the client may need to be readmitted to the hospital and aggressive action would be taken.
2. In order for the nurse to be sure the client is able to clean and dress his wound correctly, he or she must see the client perform these actions. If a client is familiar with the equipment needed for wound care, he will be less likely to have difficulty performing his wound care once he is at home.

CRITICAL THINKING CARE MAP

Subjective Data Complains of shortness of breath upon mild exertion; complains of occasional mild chest pain; states she rests a lot after work so she doesn't overwork her heart; states she has smoked 1 pack of cigarettes a day for 25 years.

Objective Data Weight 180 lbs; height 5'1"; BP 140/100; P 80; T 98.5°F (36.9°C); blood oxygen level 98%; lung sounds clear bilaterally.

Report Yes, report blood pressure, any present complaint of chest pain to RN.

Interventions Encourage client to make dietary changes. Stress importance of cutting back on fat, especially saturated fats, which may help reduce cholesterol. Encourage client to eat a well-balanced diet with at least five servings of fruits and vegetables a day. Obtain a physician's order for the client to meet with the hospital dietitian. Explain to client that physical activity can reduce her risk of heart attack. However, her doctor will prescribe how much activity she may do based on the severity of her coronary artery disease. Explain to client that smoking is a major risk factor and that by quitting she can significantly cut her risk of a heart attack.

Documentation 3/9/06. Complains of shortness of breath upon exertion and occasional, mild chest pains. BP 140/100, P 80, T 98.5, blood oxygen level 98%. Lungs clear bilaterally. Weight 180 lbs, height 5'1". T Abundali, LPN

UNIT III WRAP-UP

TIME MANAGEMENT

After report, the nurse should first visit each client's room to introduce himself or herself and make a quick assessment of each client. The LPN can assess vital signs and surgical sites at this time (or delegate vital signs to UAP). It is important to check the MAR, Kardex, or chart for any new orders. Since Mr. Drew and Mr. Melezack are quiet at the moment, it will be a priority to deal with Mr. Ramos's agitation. Check to see if he can be medicated for anxiety. Make sure his catheter irrigation is running, and determine if the irrigation needs to be increased to flush out clots, which may be causing him discomfort. Bring in someone to sit with Mr. Ramos until he is calm again, and administer medication. Then inform his doctor of the agitation; discuss the need for physical restraints if he cannot be controlled by other means. At this point, if you are informed of Mr. Melezack's nausea and vomiting and pain, this will become your priority. While documenting, review lab work. When you find that Mr. Drew has not had an MI, you will need to schedule time to begin his discharge teaching. This is of lower priority, and may be accomplished at the end of visiting hours while you are providing HS care.

CRITICAL THINKING

Teach Mr. Drew some of the things that can be done to decrease recurrent angina: avoid overexertion; decrease anxiety and stress (causes blood vessels to constrict); avoid overeating (increases workload of the heart); avoid cold weather (constricts blood vessels to conserve heat); avoid hot, humid conditions (increase workload of the heart); avoid walking uphill and/or against the wind (increases workload of the heart). Also teach ways to control risk factors: stop smoking; decrease intake of fat content foods/cholesterol; decrease weight; increase exercise (gradually if not used to exercise); decrease hypertension by above activities; decrease stressors (some stress is normal), especially if they precipitate chest discomfort; take medication as prescribed by physician.

COMPASSIONATE CARING

Although the first concern is for the physiologic status of Mr. Ramos, the nurse must also be concerned with the stress the roommate is experiencing because of his behavior. While you are assessing your client, the nurse assigned to the roommate should (if possible) remove him from the area. He could be taken to the solarium in a wheelchair, if necessary, while arrangements are made to move him to a different room. It will be necessary to obtain an interpreter in order to assess Mr. Ramos's pain and anxiety level properly. It will be important to take the client's vitals signs and observe the catheter bags for the condition of the drainage. It will be necessary to have a Spanish-speaking sitter stay with the client until he can be calmed down, since climbing out of bed could result in a fall and injury, and he could dislodge his IV or catheter if he climbs out of bed. Client safety is a priority—it will be necessary to medicate or temporarily restrain the client to prevent injury.

COMMUNICATION AND TEAM BUILDING

Date: 8/31/04; Time: 1630. Focus: NG tube. **D:** NGT clamped since 12 noon, clear liquid lunch; 50% consumed and tolerated. C/o stabbing abdominal pain 8/10. Vomited 500 cc dark brown emesis. **A:** NGT unclamped; irrigated with 100 cc of NSS, connected to low intermittent wall suction. Medicated for pain Meperidine 75mg with Vistaril 25mg IM. Dr. Sample notified, order to continue suction. **R:** Client resting comfortably; pain 2/10. No c/o of nausea. NGT drain moderate amt. of dark brown emesis. L. Fellows LPN.

Report client's condition to the charge nurse or RN team leader. Since NG tube cannot be removed, MD should be notified. Discuss client's needs with the care assistant and give instructions to provide mouth care, ice chips, partial bath, and gown and bed change as necessary.

CHAPTER 24

NCLEX-PN ANSWERS 1. B. The best response is to explain how development occurs cephalocaudally, and that it is very individualized. False reassurance such as in choice A or generalized statements as in C and D will not relieve the mother's concerns. 2. C. Your client's developmental needs are not being met and thus despair is being expressed. A coincides with the toddler year, B occurs during middle adult years, and D is related to the young adult period. 3. B. A child between the ages of 6 and 11 is in Erikson's stage of industry versus inferiority. Children at this age want to be productive and need to feel that they can do a task well. 4. C. An infant's weight at 5 months will be approximately double the birth weight. D would be the approximate weight at 1 year. 5. C.

Although growth has slowed somewhat by the preschool period, the extremities tend to grow a bit faster than the trunk. 6. C. Right behavior is obeying the law and following the rules. At this stage, the circumstances are not taken into account. 7. D. The individual becomes less dogmatic at this stage and is aware of truth from a variety of viewpoints. 8. D. Is one of the six developmental tasks described by Havighurst during the age period of later maturity. 9. D. During maturity, an individual whose developmental needs have been met will be able to accept the uniqueness of one's own life and death. If needs are not met, the individual will experience a sense of loss and despair. 10. C. In older adults, changes in cognitive abilities are more often a difference in speed than in ability. Confusion and senility are not the norm. Older adults need fewer but higher-quality calories in order to maintain ultimate weight and nutritional status.

CASE STUDY HINTS

1. Sandra's burns could be an attempt to get attention from her family. Her behaviors have been alienating her children, but because they love her and are concerned, they will respond to the injuries. Self-inflicted injuries can also be a way of releasing tension or anxiety. Depression can result in a lack of concentration, so her injuries may be a result of not concentrating on a task when she is in the kitchen. It is also possible that the injuries are a result of some physiologic problem. She should have a complete medical workup, including hormone levels.

2. Now that Sandra's children are raised and she has less responsibility, she will need to become involved in activities that will give her a feeling of self-worth. Social or civic responsibilities can be a source of self-worth. Leisure activities will help her to establish new friendships and help to relieve tension. Sandra and her husband need to relate to each other as individuals. Now that their parenting roles and responsibilities have changed, their relationship may have changed also.

3. Avoiding contact with Sandra will only increase her critical attitude toward her family. Sandra and her children should begin to make changes in their relationship. Interacting with each other as adults is difficult but very necessary if they are to have a harmonious relationship. Sandra needs to bring herself to look at her children as adults with families of their own. It is very important that parents, especially mothers, work at these adult interactions prior to the arrival of grandchildren.

CRITICAL THINKING CARE MAP

Subjective Data Lives with parents; half-sister, child of father's previous marriage visits alternate weekends; both parents work outside the home. Todd is cared for by maternal grandmother during the week. Diet: appetite fair; grandmother has trouble getting him to sit down for meals, usually resorts to finger food, takes a bottle at night. Mother states

"Opened medicine bottles from home medicine cabinet"; "able to open patio door near backyard jacuzzi." Mother states she is "worn out from chasing Todd."

Objective Data Two-year-old male child; T 98.8°F (37.1°C) (tympanic), P 80, R 18; weight 29 lbs; height 34 inches. Climbing on furniture, opening cupboard, pulling paper from exam table. Mother chasing child around room.

Report Yes, report mother's concerns about home safety and her own physical state and stress level to the physician.

Interventions Teach caregiver the need for close supervision of young children. Provide poison control number to mother. Instruct parent to keep syrup of ipecac in home first aid kit. Assist parents in devising a plan to childproof home. Inform parents of available CPR and first aid training in the community. Suggest group activities would channel some of his energy.

Documentation Two-year-old active, well-developed child to see physician for follow-up for antibiotic therapy (amoxicillin 500 mg tid × 10 days). Course completed 2 days ago. Mother expressed concerns for child safety related to ability to open medicine bottles from cabinet and patio door leading to jacuzzi area. Mother asked if degree of activity is normal for a two-year-old. Marge Smith LPN.

CHAPTER 25

NCLEX-PN ANSWERS 1. **B.** Personal space is the distance people prefer in interaction with others; sitting on the bed invades that space. 2. **C.** Closed-ended questions frequently can be answered with a yes, no, or a single word (e.g., "How old are you?"). 3. **A.** The opening sets the tone for the whole interview. The closing states appreciation for what has been accomplished. The body is the time for the client to communicate what she or he thinks, feels, knows, or perceives. The orientation gives the nurse the opportunity to state the purpose of the interview. 4. **B.** Interpreting nonverbal behavior is done by a systematic assessment of physical appearance, posture, gait, facial expression, and gestures. Interpreting nonverbal behaviors does not contradict the client's verbal communication, although it may identify some incongruencies. The client, not the nurse, is communicating nonverbally. The nurse's observations are designed to interpret the client's action, not to make judgments. 5. **A.** Telling the client that you are available and how much time you have will help to establish a therapeutic relationship. 6. **B.** Giving personal opinions, false reassurance, and changing the subject to talk about your own experiences will set up barriers to a therapeutic relationship. 7. **B.** Active listening demonstrates an interest in what the client is saying with eye contact, posture, and gestures. Interrupting, making notes, and looking at your watch do not demonstrate interest. 8. **C.** A leading question is one in which the questioner inadvertently gives the answer with the question. 9. **D.** The body of the interview is the time for the client to communicate what

she or he thinks, feels, knows, or perceives in response to the nurse's question. 10. **B.** Expressing enjoyment for the time together and appreciation for what was accomplished is an excellent way to allow the client to know the interview is coming to an end. Abruptly cutting off conversation or changing position will not allow the client to express additional needs or wants. Telling the client you have other people you must see may make him or her feel unimportant and place a barrier for future communication.

CASE STUDY HINTS

1. The nurse sat with client, asked questions and expressed compassion.
2. The nurse did not validate Mrs. Levowitz's feelings when she said, "The news can't be that bad." She used false reassurance when she said, "Everything will be OK for you. It will turn out just fine." In this situation, the nurse did not think before she spoke; she did not sit quietly and listen attentively.
3. Pulling up a chair conveyed that she was not in a hurry, but saying that she had other clients to attend to made her words and nonverbal communication *incongruent* (contradictory).

CRITICAL THINKING CARE MAP

Subjective Data Feels she is fat; lost 15 pounds in 2 months; LMP 3 months ago; regularly exercises more than 2 hours per day; mother's relationship with client appears very controlling; mother seems to be in denial about eating disorder; "eats lunch at school"; mother thinks client may be pregnant; takes laxatives for constipation.

Objective Data Height 5'9"; weight 98 lbs; VS: T 96.8°F (36°C) BP 90/66.

Report Yes, report to physician for possible referral to counselor: significant weight loss and amenorrea for 2 months; mother's lack of recognition of eating disorder; possibility that client's life is planned and controlled by mother.

Interventions Review with family members the congruence and incongruence of family behaviors and health related goals. Collaborate with other consultants regarding strategies for working with families. Facilitate modeling and role-playing for family regarding healthy ways to communicate and interact. Establish open and trusting relationship within the family. Provide sufficient knowledge to support family decisions regarding therapeutic regimens. Review symptoms of specific disorder and work with family toward developing a greater awareness of symptoms.

Documentation An 18-year-old female with anorexia nervosa; appointed for college physical. Mother reluctant to allow daughter to be seen without her being present. Mother questioned if client could be pregnant, amenorrhea ×2 months. Client and mother unaware of seriousness and symptoms of disorder. Fifteen lb. weight loss; complains of constipation; taking laxative. Suggested that client see physician alone while mother and nurse discuss proper diet for active teenager. R. Dunheim LVN.

CHAPTER 26

NCLEX-PN ANSWERS 1. **D.** Even though a nurse may understand the client's culture, health care professionals are part of the "medical" subculture, which affects their beliefs about health. 2. **B.** Race is the classification of people according to shared biological characteristics, genetic markers, and features such as skin color, bone structure, facial features, hair texture, and blood type. Different ethnic groups can belong to the same race. 3. **A.** The indigenous health care system refers to traditional folk methods of health care. 4. **C.** In health care, ethnocentrism can include the view that the only valid health care beliefs and practices are those held by health care professionals. 5. **A.** Classifying clients' responses to care and treatment by ethnicity is considered to be stereotyping. 6. **D.** The magico-religious view suggests that health and wellness are based on supernatural forces, independent of medical treatment. 7. **B.** In some families the man is considered to be the provider and the decision maker. The woman may need to consult her husband prior to making decisions about medical treatment for her child. 8. **C.** Always consider the client's culture before assuming that people do not understand or are being resistant. Modesty is a real issue with hospitalized clients of many cultures. 9. **D.** Many religious groups have specific dietary laws which they must follow. These needs can be met while hospitalized by consulting with the dietitian. 10. **B.** The nurse should avoid using family members to interpret to limit biased responses. Interpreters who are the same sex as the client are preferred to provide translation.

CASE STUDY HINTS

1. Cultural values often determine interactions between roles of family members. Identify who will have the "authority" to make decisions on the client's behalf. Without clear guidelines about which cultural practices Rachel follows, it may be difficult to provide culturally sensitive care during this important period of Rachel's life.
2. Rachel's culture will dictate whether or not she dies with family present, whether any rites or rituals are performed, and whether she dies at home or in the hospital. Religion is more likely to influence the care of her body following her death than is her culture. It will provide guidelines for postmortem care and burial.

CRITICAL THINKING CARE MAP

Subjective Data Father reports, "Her grandmother, who lives with us, performs Giac on her. In our culture, in order to draw out a bad force within the child, we place small, heated glasses on the skin, which form suction. This leaves a red circular mark." URI of 3 days' duration.

Objective Data One-year-old Vietnamese female child; snuffy nose, cough, wheezing; T 102.2°F (39°C), R 28 and shallow; nasal flaring and retraction; bright red circular dermabrasions covering back, legs, and arms. Chest x-ray nonspecific inflammation. Viral culture of nasal swab revealed RSV (respiratory syncytial virus).

Report Yes, to the hospital social worker.

Interventions Negotiate with family regarding aspects of health behavior that will need to be modified. Assess for the influences of cultural beliefs, norms, values, and expectations on the family experience of caregiving. Negotiate with client regarding the aspects of caregiving that can be modified and still honor cultural beliefs. Encourage family support groups or other service providers. Acknowledge racial/ethnic differences at the onset of care.

Documentation One-year-old Vietnamese female accompanied by father for treatment of URI of 3 days' duration. Dx. of RSV. Covered with red marks on back, arms, and legs. Father reports that they are a result of Giac, folk remedy to relieve "bad forces" which are causing illness. Admitted to isolation room. Social worker notified, is to meet with staff to assist in delivery of culturally sensitive care. P. Farmer LVN

CHAPTER 27

NCLEX-PN ANSWERS 1. **B.** Stimulus; A is the receptor; C is impulse; D describes perception. 2. **C.** The client who is not oriented to time, place, and person is disoriented. The client with reduced awareness and who is easily bewildered is confused. A semicomatose individual can be aroused by extreme or repeated stimuli. 3. **D.** Conversing in a foreign language may cause sensory deprivation for the clients. This should be explained to the staff, since they may not be aware of it. 4. **C.** Placing a clock and an activity list in type large enough for the resident to read easily will allow the individual to be independent. Referring him to the activity board may cause confusion, and it is not readily available for him to check. Sending someone for him would not promote independence. Overhead paging can cause sensory overload for these residents as well as others. It should be avoided in residential care facilities. 5. **B.** Hearing many times is still intact even when a client is unconscious, so talking to the client and explaining what you are doing can help relieve anxiety. 6. **A.** Always give your arm to a visually impaired client, allowing him or her to choose your dominant or nondominant one. Walking about one foot ahead allows you to evaluate hazards and promote safe ambulation. 7. **B.** Sudden loss of a loved one is one of the primary causes of confusion in the elderly who are cared for in their own home. 8. **A.** Safety and prevention of sensory deprivation are the priority. The other things have little bearing if a safe, stimulating environment is not maintained. 9. **A.** All adults over 40 should have a visual exam every 3 to 5 years. If there is a family history of glaucoma, they should be examined more frequently. Waiting until symptoms occur may result in irreversible deficits. 10. C. Reorient the client, offer to stay with her until she falls asleep, and offer to make contact with husband in the morning. Threatening the client with restraints or medication is never an acceptable solution. The nurse should never tell a client that a family member has been contacted and that eveything is fine, unless it has actually been done.

CASE STUDY HINTS

1. She is being bombarded by the noise of her monitors and ventilator, which may be distorted and meaningless due to the sedation she is receiving. Her pain and inability to communicate also contribute to her sensory overload as they increase her feelings of being overwhelmed and out of control.

2. Interventions include, but are not limited to: reducing lights; decreasing noise to the degree possible (close curtains or doors); orienting the client to person, place, and time; speaking in a soft unhurried manner; and limiting visitors.

3. Client cared for at home may experience either sensory deprivation or overload depending on the environment. If it is a busy, active environment with several family members, they may experience overload. If clients live alone, have few supportive family members, or are seldom contacted, they are more likely to experience social isolation. They may become withdrawn or uncommunicative, or lose interest in their usual activities. Interventions for home care or ICU clients are similar and adapted to the specific needs of the client, regardless of setting.

CRITICAL THINKING CARE MAP

Subjective Data She states, "I'm afraid of all of these strange creatures in this orphanage." Cared for herself independently for 15 years in her own home. Her children were concerned about her physical safety, lack of socialization.

Objective Data Height: 63″, weight 122 lbs; VS: T 98.6°F (37°C), P 72, R 18, BP 128/74: Underwent surgery for the removal of cataracts; Rinne test: negative, experienced more difficulty with hearing; chest x-ray, CBC, and urinalysis all negative. Somewhat confused and disoriented to person, place, and time. Appears restless, withdrawn. Syntax is sometimes inappropriate.

Report Yes, to physician.

Interventions Provide a consistent physical environment and a daily routine. Provide caregiver who is familiar to Mrs. Hagstrom. Provide low-stimulation environment for Mrs. Hagstrom because disorientation may be increased by overstimulation. Provide for adequate rest, sleep, and daytime naps. Facilitate use of hearing aids, as appropriate. Obtain Mrs. Hagstrom's attention through touch.

Documentation 11/05/06, 0730. Eighty-year-old female admitted 3 days ago to extended care facility, disoriented to person, place, and time. States, "I am afraid of all these strange creatures in this orphanage." Bilateral cataract removal status post × 2 weeks. Complains of of increased difficulty with hearing. Reoriented to person, time, and place. Is able to identify primary nurse by name and expresses a desire to go home for Thanksgiving in 3 weeks. Asked that batteries be checked in her hearing aid. M. Smythe LPN

CHAPTER 28

NCLEX-PN ANSWERS 1. B. Self-concept has four dimensions: (1) self-knowledge: the knowledge that one has about oneself, including insights into one's abilities, nature, and limitations; (2) self-expectation: what one expects of oneself, may be realistic or unrealistic expectation; (3) social self: how a person is perceived by others and society; (4) social evaluation: the appraisal of oneself in relationship to others, events, or situations. 2. C. Psychosocial development theory was developed by Erikson; Sigmund Freud's theory was psychosexual development; Kohlberg was concerned with the theory of moral development; Aaron Beck was concerned with cognitive theory. 3. D. Self-concept is established when the inborn tendencies of the individual connect with reality and is brought into compliance with the demand of society. 4. B. Although any of these diagnoses could be used for this medical diagnosis, Disturbed Body Image is evident when the individual does not recognize serious weight loss when viewing own body. 5. D. Making eye contact and a gentle touch can convey caring and let the client know you are available to him or her. Lack of eye contact and a reluctance to touch a client may give the client the feeling of being unworthy. 6. B. "I can't" statements reinforce negative self-concept. Worry or concerns of health or status changes are normal and demonstrate the client's efforts to cope with the change. 7. C. Validating the client's feelings and offering to be there for the client are the best ways to show empathy. The other choices discount feelings and offer false reassurance. 8. A. Self-esteem can be assessed in terms of the goals a client can set for him/herself. 9. B. Therapeutic relationships should be client centered and aimed at assisting clients to evaluate their own behavior and initiate change. 10. C. Asking open-ended questions, those that require more than a yes or no answer, will give the nurse most access to information. The other choices can be answered with a yes or no.

CASE STUDY HINTS

1. Brian needs to feel that what is said will be kept confidential, and that the nurse will respond nonjudgmentally. Provide a private area for Brian to talk. Listen attentively, without interrupting. Be careful not to offer approval or disapproval. This subject may be uncomfortable for you, and it is all right to let him know that you are somewhat uncomfortable, but express your desire to learn more about his feelings. If you are unable to get past your own feelings, help him to make contact with someone who is

better suited to establishing this relationship. Validate his feelings, state implied feelings and thoughts. This will let him know you are paying attention, that you care, and that you are willing to help.

2. Brian is an adult, but apparently his family and their response to his feelings are very important to him. Explain to the father that you cannot discuss Brian's treatment plan with him, but that Brian wishes his family to be involved in decisions that he needs to make. Suggest that he take the opportunity to speak with the counselor by attending the session with Brian, let him know that he can make arrangements with the counselor to be seen privately if the need arises. Reassure him that the session is an opportunity to talk about concerns that both he and Brian may have in a nonthreatening atmosphere. Thank him for his concern and encourage him to be supportive of his son.

3. Decisions such as the ones Brian is considering are life altering. He needs to be provided with correct reliable information. Encourage him to seek additional opinions and to discuss his feelings with the counselor and other trusted professionals. The nurse needs to be supportive of whatever decision the client makes and let him know that no matter the outcome, he is still a very important worthy individual and that you want the best for him. Be sure to provide him with crisis intervention resources, since decisions such as this can cause severe anxiety and even thoughts of suicide. Make sure he knows that life is always the best option.

CRITICAL THINKING CARE MAP

Subjective Data Mother very supportive; father is grief stricken and having difficulty dealing with Craig's condition because Craig is captain of his college basketball team and had aspirations of becoming a professional basketball player. Client usually an outgoing individual.

Objective Data Twenty-year-old male student; automobile accident 3 days ago; mother at bedside; traumatic amputation; condition is stable; rehabilitation program to begin immediately; to be fitted for a prosthesis; somber and nontalkative; does not look at his limb when dressings are being changed; refuses to discuss rehabilitation.

Interventions Actively listen to, demonstrate respect for, and accept the client; have client list strengths; accept client's own pace in working through grief and crisis situation; assess for unhealthly coping mechanisms such as substance abuse; provide information about support groups; assess client's support system.

Report Yes, to the primary physician or a mental health professional: usually outgoing but now somber, quiet; does not look at his limb when dressings are being changed; refuses to discuss his rehabilitation program.

Documentation Focus: body image. D: Somber, nontalkative, unwilling to look at surgical site or discuss rehab program. A: Dressing changed; approach in nonthreatening manner. Procedure explained. Encouraged to ask questions. R: Was able to look at residual limb after redressed. Asked if swelling and pain is normal. S. Garcia LVN.

CHAPTER 29

NCLEX-PN ANSWERS 1. D. Alcohol is a relaxant and central nervous system depressant. Chronic alcoholism is associated with impotence. While alcohol may lower inhibitions and impair judgment, it is not a sexual stimulant. 2. A. The position that offers the most pleasure and is acceptable to both partners is the correct one. 3. B. During early adolescence primary and secondary sex characteristics develop and for boys this involves an increase in the size of the testes and scrotum and the darkening of the skin over the scrotum. 4. C. All states have child abuse laws that require professionals, including nurses to report suspected child abuse. 5. C. In 1996 the U.S. Congress passed legislation making the practice of any form of female genital mutilation on girls under 18 a federal criminal offense. 6. A. Females are more at risk of cervical cancer if they have human papillomavirus or multiple sexual partners. 7. B. Coitus interruptus should be taught as far less effective than the other methods listed. 8. D. Gender determination can be made by 11 to 14 weeks of gestation. 9. C. Most cases of orgasmic dysfunction have psychological causes. 10. B. The nurse will teach the client who has had heart surgery or been hospitalized for alterations in heart function to avoid sexual intercourse after large meals and/or consumption of alcoholic beverages.

CASE STUDY HINTS

1. Mr. Stevens was engaged in sexual intercourse when he experienced a myocardial infarction. This would have a likely effect of making him concerned about sexual activity. He may be making inappropriate sexual suggestions as a way of denying to himself that his sexual activity must change because of his condition. However, he also directly expresses that he is concerned he won't be able to continue his sexual relationship with his wife as it was. Mr. Stevens' remarks may be a way of asking for help.

2. It would have been helpful to know Mr. Stevens' activities prior to his MI (e.g., hours and activity at work) and prior to other episodes of chest pain. Family history of heart disease is also important.

3. Mrs. Stevens should be involved in all discussions about Mr. Stevens' health and condition. This is important both because of the way the condition affects his sexual activity and because the experience may be overwhelming for him. Having a second person there to listen will be useful. Contact with others who have recovered from MIs and with a counselor will also be beneficial.

CRITICAL THINKING CARE MAP

Subjective Data States she will never be the same. States husband deserves more.

Objective Data Looking down when speaking. Holds robe tightly around chest. Ate 10% of breakfast and lunch. Stayed in bed with face covered all morning. Refused to ambulate in the hall. Looked through mail brought to room by volunteer.

Report Yes, to the nurse in charge of the unit and physician.

Interventions Encourage client to express feelings about the way she feels about sexuality related to loss of the breast. Discuss the usual feelings of clients who are postoperative mastectomy and ways to cope. Discuss with client importance of Reach for Recovery. Instruct in the importance of communication with husband to work through feelings toward acceptance. Discuss available support groups in the community and obtain necessary contacts for follow-up (American Cancer Society). Encourage client to discuss sexuality issues with the primary health care provider.

Documentation 5/5/05, 1300. States, "I'll never be the same" and "My husband deserves more." Discussed with client why she stated, "I'll never be the same." Client expressed concern over her appearance and working in the office. Questioned about Reach for Recovery Program contact, and client states she does not need their assistance. Reported to charge nurse and physician. Discussed the purpose of Reach for Recovery and assistance provided. Agreed to call and schedule follow-up. Janie Miller, LVN.

CHAPTER 30

NCLEX-PN ANSWERS 1. **D.** A mentally healthy individual is able to cope with life while working and forming relationships, not just cope with crises. The other responses are symptoms of an individual who is experiencing a mental illness or emotional imbalance. 2. **D.** Denial is an unconscious refusal to accept situations as they are. 3. **A.** The client has temporarily separated from the painful situation and put it out of his consciousness. 4. **A.** Mild anxiety heightens the person's response. Higher levels of anxiety decrease the person's ability to respond and cope. 5. **D.** A client experiencing physical symptoms related to anxiety needs to have support from the nurse. Ignoring the anxiety or discounting it will not validate the importance of the client's feelings. The episode should be documented, but it is not necessary to notify the physician immediately. 6. **B.** The nurse, in order to prevent burnout, must first recognize his or her stress. The other interventions can follow. 7. **C.** Regardless of the cause, circumstances, or psychological interpretation of a demanding situation, the response is a pattern of physiologic responses known as the general adaptation syndrome. 8. **A.** Adolescents have rapid physical and sexual development. This plus identity and role confusion issues are major stressors during this period. 9. **C.** Fight or flight is a physiologic response to the release of adrenaline, when an individual is feeling personal danger. 10. **A.** Compensation is a defense mechanism which allows an individual to make up for inadequacies in one area of life by substituting attributes or behaviors in another area.

CASE STUDY HINTS

1. Ms. Levitt's stressors may include: the sole responsibility of three children; lack of financial assistance from her husband; the demands being placed on her by her job, school, and community activities; the lack of emotional support systems; possible financial problems; weight gain; and not having adequate time for rest and leisure.
2. Mrs. Levitt seems to have predominantly physiologic manifestations to stress, because she has physical problems with no apparent cause.
3. No data support that Ms. Levitt is angry. However, she has anger that she is not expressing. Any of her stressors could provoke anger on her behalf, and suppression of that anger could result in physical signs and symptoms.
4. Some of the changes that would serve as cues to positive adaptation may include: decreased or absent symptoms produced by stress; lifestyle changes such as decreased activities; change in diet; balancing leisure with work, or taking time for herself.

CRITICAL THINKING CARE MAP

Subjective Data He says, "I'm scared about this. My dad died of a heart attack when he was 48 years old." Severe chest pain.

Objective Data Lungs clear; pale; skin cool and diaphoretic; nail bed pink; ECG normal sinus rhythm; alert and oriented to time, place, and person; VS: T 99.6°F (37.5°C), P 88, R 28, BP 140/82; peripheral pulses strong and equal; cap refill less than 3 seconds; appears restless; questions everything that is going on; hyperventilating.

Report Yes, to the physician.

Interventions Assess client's level of anxiety and physical reaction to anxiety. Validate observations by asking client, "Are you feeling anxious now?" Allow and reinforce client's personal reaction to or expression of pain, discomfort, or threat to well-being. Explain all activities, procedures, and issues that involve the client. Use nonmedical terms in calm, slow speech. Do this in advance of procedures when possible, and validate client's understanding. Explore coping skills previously used by the client to relieve anxiety; reinforce these skills and explore other outlets. Provide back rub to decrease anxiety.

Documentation Client presented at the ER complaining of chest pain, nitro sublinguial given ×1, hyperventilating, other VS within normal limits. ECG normal sinus rhythm. Stated, "My father died of a heart attack, and having chest pain really scares me." Demonstrated relaxation techniques. Explained the importance of stress control. E. Keene, LPN

CHAPTER 31

NCLEX-PN ANSWERS **1. B.** In mutual pretense the family and health personnel know the prognosis but no one talks about it. With closed awareness, the client and the family are unaware of the impending death. In open awareness, the client and the people around know about the impending death and feel comfortable discussing it, even though it is difficult. **2. A.** When the client is in the denial stage there is a refusal to believe that the loss is happening. The client may be artificially cheerful to prolong denial. **3. C.** A notarized document that outlines the client's wishes should be followed. In some states the wishes of a domestic partner cannot overrule the wishes of the family. The ER physician's assessment determines the status of the client; once this has been determined, the notarized durable power of attorney will be the basis for the decisions. **4. C.** Expressing feelings to an understanding listener helps to facilitate the grieving process. Communication helps people deal openly with their emotions and feelings, which is healthier than suppressing them. Being sent home or changing assignment would not help promote grieving. Asking the CNA to perform postmortem care in the emotional state would show disregard for the trauma the individual may be experiencing. **5. A.** Dying clients tend to become isolated and deserted by the staff. The primary objective in this case should be to provide a physical presence to listen and support the client as death draws near. All other choices involve leaving the client alone to die. **6. D.** When the parents wish to see their stillborn baby, the baby can be cleaned and wrapped in a baby blanket. The mother and father of the baby should be allowed to see, touch, and hold their baby. Although some parents may not wish to view the baby, doing so allows them to close the cycle of birth and death and accept the fact that their baby is dead. **7. C.** Hospice, which usually takes place in the home or a specialized facility, is dedicated to the care of terminally ill clients. It is designed to provide quality of life when quantity is not possible. It is not done as a cost-saving measure or because of special equipment. Although hospice nurses have special training, they do not have more or less skill than hospital nurses. **8. B.** A client on life support must have an absence of electric currents from the brain (measured by an electroencephalogram) for at least 24 hours. Clients continue to have respirations as long as the respirator is functioning. A court order is not necessary unless the client has left no instructions or there is a disagreement between family members. **9. D.** Dysfunctional grieving is characterized by physical and psychological reactions, and thoughts of suicide. **10. C.** Children from 9 to 12 years express an interest in the afterlife; 5-year-olds look at death as reversible or temporary; 5- to 9-year-olds believe that unrelated events can be responsible for death; 12- to 18-year-olds view it in religious or philosophic terms.

CASE STUDY HINTS

1. Decreased appetite occurs for many reasons. First, he has tumor growth in his abdomen, giving a feeling of fullness. Second, toxins from liver involvement (which gives rise to his jaundice) and tumor growth may cause nausea and decreased appetite. Third, during the dying process, body systems are failing, activity is decreasing, and nutritional needs are greatly diminished.
2. The long-acting morphine is designed to decrease pain over a long period of time, eliminating the need for frequent doses of pain medication. Because there are sometimes episodes of acute pain, known as breakthrough pain, short-acting morphine is often made available. Ideally, breakthrough pain medication should be required only two to three times a day.

CRITICAL THINKING CARE MAP

Subjective Data Easily fatigued; reports poor appetite; difficulty concentrating; complains of frequent headaches.

Objective Data Neglects personal hygiene; nausea, vomiting; crying episodes; labile affect.

Report Yes, report all data to charge nurse.

Interventions Note emotional responses such as anger, crying; provide information about grief reactions; provide a list of local support groups for parents of gravely ill children; review experiences with loss and coping; use therapeutic communication skills of active listening, silence, acknowledgment; determine parent's perception of anticipated loss.

Documentation 12-2-03, 0930. Client expressing concerns that transplant may be unavailable. States "I don't know what I'll do . . . He's all I've got." Reported to charge nurse. Roger Hadrick, LVN.

UNIT IV WRAP-UP

CULTURAL COMPETENCY

* In many cultures it is common for the family to keep the diagnosis from a client with a serious diagnosis, such as cancer. It is thought that knowing the diagnosis may create a sense of hopelessness and hasten the death.
* Often, the dying client knows the truth but is reluctant to discuss it with the family. A sensitive nurse can be open to providing a therapeutic environment for the client so he or she can discuss concerns when the family is not around. The nurse can also make time to listen to family members' concerns out of earshot of the client.

CRITICAL THINKING

With the current federal laws under the Health Insurance Portability and Accountability Act (HIPPA), information cannot be given to anyone other than the client without prior permission. The scenario described here would occur only if the client had signed a document saying that a designated family member would be the primary decision maker, or if the physician or other caregivers ignored HIPPA. Ethically, it is difficult not to give a dying person the opportunity to bring closure to his or her life. Most people value the chance to say goodbye and resolve unfinished business. Health care institutions and workers must develop a means for handling such situations in a legal and ethical manner.

COMPASSIONATE CARING

If you suspect that the client is aware of the diagnosis, you can encourage him or her to make a journal or to record messages for the family on tape. You can listen while clients talk about their life, and encourage them to express to family any wishes they want carried out when death comes. If sufficient time is available, the nurse may be able to support the client so that he or she will be able to raise the subject with family and say goodbyes in person.

COMMUNITY CARE STRATEGIES

Remember, the "experts" in caregiving learn every day from their clients. You don't need to have all the answers when you begin to practice. Good listening skills and a caring attitude will help you learn ways to give excellent nursing care.

CHAPTER 32

NCLEX-PN ANSWERS 1. C. Although it is not the best way to resolve conflicts, avoidance is the most frequently used. Many staff nurses feel if it is ignored it will resolve itself. Both sides see issue as minor or fear that the negative impact is too costly to meet issue head on. 2. B. Accommodation is used when one person or group is willing to yield to the other and when preserving relationships is the most important task. A staff member who is trying to get others to like him or her would use this strategy, either consciously or unconsciously. 3. D. Lack of communication, especially incomplete instructions, are the most frequent reason why delegated tasks are not completed as expected. A UAP cannot be expected to perform unless he or she has been adequately prepared to complete the task. Avoidance of conflict, poor attitudes, and lack of supervision can have an effect but they are not the primary reasons. 4. C. Care partners, nursing assistants, and orderlies are unlicensed assistive personnel. The LPN/LVN's is the only job title listed that requires a license. 5. B. Accountability is related to responsibility (being responsible for one's own actions and the actions of those to whom you have delegated work). The other choices have to do with supervision and delegation. 6. D. Politely decline to carry out tasks which are outside of the job for which you were hired. Offering to assist with appropriate tasks within your job description will relieve the nurse, so she can complete work you cannot do for her. A and C are rude responses and should not be made from a subordinate to a supervisor. B should never be considered. Skills learned as a student can only be done under the supervision of an instructor and when in the capacity of a student. Performing these duties while working as a UAP could jeopardize your future

license and the facility. 7. B. A management style that is unstructured and leaves the decisions up to the group is known as laissez-faire. The autocratic leader makes unilateral decisions while dominating the team members. The democratic leader makes decisions after consulting with team members. *Authoritarian* is another term for autocratic. 8. C. Although functional nursing is efficient, it can create fragmented delivery of client care. In primary nursing, a professional nurse has total responsibility for a group of clients. Case method is when a nurse is responsible for care provided for clients during one shift. The purpose of team nursing was to reduce fragmentation that was present in the functional method. 9. C. The state boards of nursing have a duty to protect the public when a licensed nurse violates the provisions of the license. The state board has jurisdiction of that license. NCLEX is responsible for the licensing exam. If a crime has been committed the Attorney General and the courts will become involved, but the decision regarding the license is up to the state board. 10. B. Dealing with the supervision of UAP can be difficult. It is best to discuss the issue, determine why the incident happened, and provide information about facility policies and the importance of adequate staffing for the safety of the clients. Although the RN may need to be informed, reporting should not be used as a threat. Reporting them before talking to them and overhead paging may adversely affect your working relationship with them.

CHAPTER 33

NCLEX-PN ANSWERS 1. A. Reviewing and studying as you move through the program will help you retain the knowledge and information you are learning. It also will prevent "cramming" just before you take the examination. 2. A. You are being asked to recall a fact or statement presented to you. 3. B. Although ongoing review and analysis do occur, the revision is based on completion of a new job analysis of the tasks of licensed vocational nurses. Changes in the nurse practice acts of the states may occur at any time and are not linked to test revision. 4. D. The test is set up so that any student can follow the computer instructions and take the test. 5. B. Taking a proactive approach is most helpful. There are useful techniques that can improve both your study methods and your ability to relax. 6. C. A sudden change in sleep time can disturb your biorhythms and cause you to feel more tired and less alert. 7. D. Questions of comprehension, analysis, or synthesis require you to do more than memorize facts. They require you to put information together and think more in depth. 8. C. Identification is essential in order to sit for the exam. The computer program for the test contains a pull-down calculator. Most likely, there will be a clock in the exam room. 9. D. Depending on your answers, you may complete the test in much less time than 5 hours. However, if 5 hours pass and you have not completed enough questions to pass, the exam will end. 10. B. You will receive 25 pilot questions, along with a minimum of 60 test question. Sixty questions were determined to be the minimum a person had to answer correctly in order to prove competence and awareness of safety.

CHAPTER 34

NCLEX-PN ANSWERS **1. B.** Use the first paragraph to identify yourself and the job you are interested in. This will help you get your letter to the correct person. The other choices are found in your second and third paragraphs. **2. C.** Employers will be concerned with time gaps on applications. By highlighting your activities during the gap, it will demonstrate your interest to improve your skills or contribute to the community. It is never appropriate to leave blanks on an application or ignore large time gaps on an application. Writing an explanation is not necessary and looks like an excuse. **3. D.** Although you are not required to answer personal questions, an answer that could alleviate concerns of the interviewer without revealing personal information is the best solution. Quoting the law, stating that you won't answer the question, or using it to make stipulations on the job may put the interviewer on the defensive and prevent you from being considered. **4. B.** Although all of these reasons are possible, nonspecific résumés and letters not addressed to a name and title show lack of research into the position for which the applicant is applying. **5. A.** A profession is characterized by devotion and expertise. Most nurses consider themselves to be part of the profession even after retirement. Although continuing education is necessary, it is not what defines a profession. **6. C.** The best response is to shower and dress professionally. Wearing your uniform is acceptable unless it is soiled, which is a possibility after working all night. Even though the interviewers know you, you want them to look at you as a professional nurse. Dressing appropriately will help them see you in that way. **7. C.** Having coffee with a friend can provide valuable job search information in a casual setting. The other choices are planned activities and they are considered to be formal networking. **8. B.** The functional résumé focuses on the skills an individual possesses, while a chronological résumé presents education and skills in reverse chronological order. An e-résumé highlights key words; employers file e-résumés by these key words. **9. A.** The main reason for including a writing sample is to highlight your ability to write in a logical order using correct format and showing your attention to detail. **10. D.** The NLN was the name given to the American Society of Superintendents of Training Schools for Nurses in the United States and Canada in 1912.

UNIT V WRAP-UP

COMMUNICATION AND TEAM BUILDING

You can tell her you looked at the schedule and an IV-certified nurse will be coming in at 6 A.M. You could call him, asking him to come in 1 hour early, and offer to relieve him an hour early the next day. You could ask the ADON to come in to do the IV. You could repeat your suggestion to have the client stay at the hospital another day. You could ask her to approve having a registry nurse or a home health nurse come in to do the IV.

CRITICAL THINKING

No matter what the result, do not jeopardize your hard-earned license. The ADON is not demonstrating good managerial or leadership skills by asking you to do a procedure that is outside your scope of practice. Let her know that you are unwilling to break the law and that if a solution is not reached prior to the time the solution must be added, you will be forced to call the administrator. If no one has arrived to add the IV fluids at the prescribed time, call the administrator and leave the matter in his or her hands.

CONFLICT RESOLUTION

You could tell the ADON that you intend to take the IV certification class as soon as you get paid. (Most facilities do not provide training but may front the cost for newly graduated employees.) Tell her that you want to be fully prepared for your job.

For your own records, document the interaction as exactly as possible and keep it in your home file, along with any further related exchanges. Do your job well and document carefully. Chances are, the situation will be forgotten. If, however, the ADON wants you fired, you need to have your own documentation of consequences, including changed assignments, imbalanced scheduling, denials of requests for time off, constant criticisms without balancing encouragement, and so on.

Bibliography

CHAPTER 1

Baer, E. D., D'Antonio, P., Rinker, S., & Lynaugh, J. E. (Eds.) (2000). *Enduring issues in American nursing*. Philadelphia, PA: Springhouse.

Barber, M. F. (1992). In R. Smolan, P. Moffitt (Contributor), & M. Naythims (Contributor), *The power to heal: Ancient arts & modern medicine*. Upper Saddle River, NJ: Prentice Hall.

Creighton, J. (1998, December 28). Nurse on cap hunt. *The Toronto Sun*. A-28.

Dolan, J. A., Fitzpatrick, M. L., & Herrmann, E. K. (1983). *Nursing in society: A historical perspective*. (15th ed.) Philadelphia, PA: Saunders.

Edmonds, S. E., & Leonard, E. D. (1999). *Memoirs of a soldier, nurse and spy: A woman's adventures in the Union Army*. DeKalb, IL: Northern Illinois University Press.

Ellis, J. R., & Hartley, C. L. (2001). *Nursing in today's world: Challenges, issues & trends* (7th ed.). Philadelphia, PA: Lippincott Williams & Wilkins.

Hamilton, P. M. (1999). *Realities of contemporary nursing* (2nd ed.). Menlo Park, CA: Addison-Wesley.

Kelly, L. Y., & Joel, L. A. (1999). *Dimensions of professional nursing* (8th ed.). New York: McGraw-Hill.

Kowalski, K., Burton, L., & Rehwaldt, M. (1997, September/October). Revisioning, re-educating, regenerating, and recommitting nursing for the twenty-first century. *Nursing Outlook, 45*, 220-223.

Lang-Otsuka, P. A. (Ed.). (2002). *Pathophysiology made incredibly easy*. Philadelphia, PA: Springhouse–Lippincott William & Wilkins.

Nelson, S. (2002). The fork in the road: Nursing history vs. the history of nursing. *Nursing History Review*, Vol. 10. Lanoka, NJ: American Association for the History of Nursing Inc.

Nightingale, F. (1860). *Notes on nursing: What it is, and what it is not* (Commemorative Edition). Philadelphia, PA: Lippincott.

Norman, E. (2000). *We band of angels*. New York: Pocket Books.

Porter, Lynne. Notes on how to read a textbook. North Orange County Regional Occupational Program. Anaheim, CA. Unpublished.

Ramsom, C. B. (2003). *Clara Barton History Maker Bios*. Berkeley, CA: Lerner Publication Company.

Sandelowski, M. (2000). *Devices & desires: Gender, technology and American nursing*. Chapel Hill, NC: University of North Carolina Press.

Schuyler, C. B. (1992). Florence Nightingale. In F. Nightingale, *Notes on nursing: What it is, and what it is not* (Commemorative Edition) (pp. 3-17). Philadelphia, PA: Lippincott.

Schorr, T. M. with Kennedy, M. S. (1999). *100 years of American nursing*. Philadelphia, PA: Lippincott.

Sorel, N. C. (2000). *The women who wrote the war*. New York: Harper Perennial.

Wake, R. (1998). *The Nightingale Training School 1860-1996*. London: Haggerstown Press.

Wood, W. (Ed.). Century in review. (1999, December 13). *Nurseweek, 12*(25), 1.

Zerwekh, J., & Claborn, J. C. (2002). *Nursing today: Transition and trends* (3rd ed.). Philadelphia, PA: Saunders.

CHAPTER 2

American Nurses Association. (1998). *Standards of clinical nursing practice* (2nd ed.). Washington, DC: Author.

Anderson, M. A. (2001). *Nursing leadership, management, and professional practice for the LPN LVN* (2nd ed.). Philadelphia, PA: Davis.

Burke, L., Weill, B. (2000). *Information technology for health care professionals*. Upper Saddle River, NJ: Prentice Hall.

Brent, N. J. (1997). *Nurses and the law*. Philadelphia, PA: Saunders.

Equal Employment Opportunity Commission. (1980). Sex discrimination guidelines. In *EEOC Rules and Regulation*. Chicago: Commerce Clearing House.

Norman, J. C. (2000). HIV/AIDS: Epidemic update. *CME Resources, 67*(7), 12-36.

Smith, K. V. (1996). Ethical decision-making by staff nurses. *Nursing Ethics: An International Journal for Health Care Professionals, 3*(1), 17-25.

Taylor, P., & Ferszt, G. (1998, August). The nurse as patient advocate. *Nursing 98, 28*(8), 70-71.

United States Department of Health, CDC. (2001). *Guidelines for HIV Counseling, Testing and Referral*. Atlanta, GA: Author.

Wood, L. C., & DelPapa, L. A. (1996). Nurses' attitudes, ethical reasons, and knowledge of the law concerning advance directives. *Image: Journal of Nursing Scholarship, 28*(4), 371.

CHAPTER 3

Andrews, M. M., & Boyle, V. S. (1999). *Transcultural concepts in nursing care* (3rd ed.). Philadelphia, PA: Lippincott.

Fawcett, J. (2000). *Analysis and evaluation of contemporary nursing knowledge: Nursing models and theories*. Philadelphia, PA: Davis.

Kurzen, C. (2001). *Contemporary practical/vocational nursing* (4th ed.). Philadelphia, PA: Lippincott.

LeMone, P., & Burke, K. (2000). *Medical surgical nursing: Critical thinking in client care* (2nd ed.). Upper Saddle River, NJ: Prentice Hall Health.

Paul, R. W., & Elder, L. (2001). *Critical thinking*. Upper Saddle River, NJ: Pearson Education.

CHAPTER 4

Ackley, B. J., & Ladwig, G. B. (2002). *Nursing diagnosis handbook: A guide to planning care* (5th ed.). St. Louis, MO: Mosby.

Alfaro-LeFevre, R. (2002). Applying the nursing process: Promoting *collaborative care* (5th ed.). Philadelphia/New York: Lippincott Williams & Wilkins.

American Nurses Association. (1998). *Standards of clinical nursing practice* (2nd ed.). Kansas City, MO: Author.

Anderson, M. A. (2000). *Nursing leadership, management and professional practice for the LPN/LVN* (2nd ed.). Philadelphia, PA: Davis.

Boucher, M. A. (1998, February). Delegation alert. *American Journal of Nursing, 98*(2), 26–32.

Carpenito, L. J. (2002). *Handbook of nursing diagnosis* (9th ed.). Philadelphia, PA: Lippincott Williams & Wilkins.

Carpenito, L. J. (2002). *Nursing diagnosis: Application to clinical practice* (9th ed.). Philadelphia: Lippincott Williams & Wilkins.

Doenges, M. E., Moorhouse, M. F., & Burley, J. T. (2000). *Application of nursing process and nursing diagnosis: An interactive text for diagnostic reasoning* (3rd ed.). Philadelphia, PA: Davis.

Joint Commission on Accreditation of Healthcare Organizations. (2000). *Accreditation manual for hospitals*. Chicago: Author.

McCloskey, J. C., & Bulechek, G. M. (Eds.). (2000). *Nursing intervention classifications* (NIC) (3rd ed.). St. Louis, MO: Mosby.

North American Nursing Diagnosis Association. (2001). *Nursing diagnoses: Definitions & classification, 2001–2002*. Philadelphia, PA: Author.

CHAPTER 5

Abrams, W., Beers, M., & Berkow, R. (Eds.) (2000). *The Merck manual of geriatrics* (3rd ed.). Whitehouse Station, NJ: Merck.

American Academy of Nursing Panel on Women's Health. (1997). Women's health and women's health care: Recommendations of the 1996 AAN expert panel on women's health. *Nursing Outlook, 45*(1), 7–15.

American Hospital Association. (1992). *A patient's bill of rights*. Chicago: Author.

Hansten, R., & Washburn, M. J. (1998, March). Professional practice: Facts and impact. *American Journal of Nursing, 98*(3), 42–45.

Ignani, K. (1995). Navigating the health care marketplace. *Health affairs, 14*(1), 221–225.

Lairson, D., Schulmeier, G., Begley, C., Aday, L., Coyle, Y., & Slater, C. (1997). Managed care and community-oriented care: Conflict or complement? *Journal of Health Care for the Poor and Underserved, 8*(1), 36–55.

U.S. Department of Health and Human Services. (2000). *Healthy people 2010: Understanding and improving health* (2nd ed.). Washington, DC: U.S. Government Printing Office.

U.S. Department of Labor, Bureau of Labor Statistics (1999 and various years). *Employee benefit survey*. Washington, DC: U.S. Government Printing Office.

CHAPTER 6

Arias, K. M. (Ed.). (2000). *Quick reference to outbreak investigation and control in health care facilities*. New York: Aspen.

Bonder, B., & Wagner, M. B. (2001). *Functional performance in older adults*. Philadelphia, PA: Davis.

Brenner, Z. R. (1998, December). Toward restraint-free care. *American Journal of Nursing, 98*(12), 16F–16I.

Carpenito, L. J. (2002). Nursing diagnosis: Applications to clinical practice (9th ed.). Philadelphia, PA: Lippincott.

Charney, W. (Ed.). (1999). *Handbook of modern hospital safety*. Boca Raton, FL: Lewis Publishing.

Doenges, M. E., & Moorhouse, M. F. (2003). *Application of nursing process and nursing diagnoses: An interactive text for diagnostic reasoning* (4th ed.). Philadelphia: Davis.

Edelman, C. L., & Mandle, C. L. (2002). *Health promotion throughout the lifespan* (5th ed.). St. Louis, MO: Mosby.

Hutton, J. T., Elias, W., Shroyer, J. A., Curry, Z. (2000). *Preventing falls: A defensive approach*. Amherst, NY: Prometheus Books.

Kobs, A. (1998, January). Questions and answers from the JCAHO. Restraints revisited. *Nursing Management, 29*(1), 17–18.

Springhouse Corporation (1998). *Healthcare professionals guide: Safety and infection control*. Springhouse, PA: Author.

Tai, E. (2000). OSHA Compliance Management: A Guide for Long-Term Health Care Facilities (2000). Boca Raton, FL: Lewis Publishing.

Tideiksaar, R. (2002). *Falls in older persons*. Baltimore, MD: Health Professions Press.

Wagner, K. D., Rounds, C. D., Spurgin, R., & Biello, L. (1998). Philadelphia, PA: Saunders.

CHAPTER 7

Bonten, M. J. M., Weinstein, R. A. (1996, March). The role of colonization in the pathogenesis of nosocomial infections. *Infection Control and Hospital Epidemiology, 17*, 193–200.

Carpenito, L. J. (1997). *Handbook of nursing diagnosis* (7th ed.). Philadelphia, PA: Lippincott.

Centers for Disease Control and Prevention. (1994). Guidelines for preventing the transmission of tuberculosis in health care facilities. *Federal Register, Vol. 59* no. 22 (208).

Centers for Disease Control and Prevention. (1996a). Guidelines for isolation precautions in hospitals, Part 1: Evolution of isolation practices. *American Journal of Infection Control, 24*(1), 24–31.

Harkness, G. A., & Dincher, J. K. (1999). *Medical–surgical nursing: Total patient care* (10th ed.). St. Louis, MO: Mosby.

LeMone, P., Burke, K. M. (2000). *Medical surgical nursing: Critical thinking in client care* (2nd ed.). Upper Saddle River, NJ: Prentice Hall.

North American Nursing Diagnosis Association. (1999). *Nursing diagnoses: Definitions and classification 1999–2000*. Philadelphia, PA: Author.

Smith, S. F., Duell, D. J., & Martin, B. C. (2000). *Clinical nursing skills: Basic to advanced* (5th ed.) Upper Saddle River, NJ: Prentice Hall.

Springhouse Corporation. (1998). *Healthcare professional guides: Safety and infection control*. Springhouse, PA: Author.

Nettina, S. M. (Ed.) (2000). *The Lippincott manual of nursing practice* (7th ed.). Philadelphia, PA: Lippincott Williams & Wilkins.

Timby, B. K., Scherer, J. C., & Smith, N. E. (1999). *Introductory medical-surgical nursing* (7th ed.). Philadelphia, PA: Lippincott.

U.S. Department of Health and Human Services, Centers for Disease Control and Prevention (1997, September 8). Draft guidelines for infection control in health care personnel, 1997. *Federal Register, 62*(173).

CHAPTER 8

Grubbs, P., & Blasband, B. (2000). *The long-term care nursing assistant* (2nd ed.). Upper Saddle River, NJ: Prentice Hall.

Kellter, P. G., Sucher, K. P. (1990, November). Diet counseling in a multicultural society. *Diabetes Education, 39* (127-134).

Meils, C., & England, T. (1999). *From nursing assistant to clinical care associate*. Upper Saddle River, NJ: Prentice Hall.

Pulliam, J. (2002). *The nursing assistant: Acute, subacute and long-term care* (3rd ed.). Upper Saddle River, NJ: Prentice Hall.

CHAPTER 9

American Nurses Association. (1985). *Code for nurses*. Kansas City, MO: Author.

Barbera, M. L. (1994). Giving report: How to sidestep common pitfalls. *Nursing, 24*(9), 41.

Chase, S. K. (1997). Charting critical thinking: Nursing judgments and patient outcomes, *Dimensions of Critical Care Nursing, 16*(2), 102-111.

Cirone, N. (1998, August). Taking orders by phone? *Nursing98, 28*(8), 56-57.

Coty, E., Davis, J., & Angell, L. (2002). *Documentation: The language of nursing*. Upper Saddle River, NJ: Prentice Hall.

Cox, S. S. (1994). Taping report: Tips to record by. *Nursing, 24*(3), 64.

Eggland, E. T., & Heinemann, D. S. (1994). *Nursing documentation: Charting, recording, and reporting*. Philadelphia, PA: Lippincott.

Iyer, P. W. (1991a, June). Thirteen charting rules. *Nursing91, 21*, 40-44.

Iyer, P. W. (1991b, July). Six more charting rules to keep you legally safe. *Nursing91, 21*, 34-39.

Iyer, P. W., & Camp, N. H. (1995). *Nursing documentation: A nursing process approach* (2nd ed.). St. Louis, MO: Mosby.

Iyer, P. W., & Camp, N. H. (1999). *Nursing documentation handbook* (3rd ed.). St. Louis, MO: Elsevier.

Joint Commission on Accreditation of Healthcare Organizations. (2000). *2000 accreditation manual for hospitals*. Chicago: Author.

Joint Commission on Accreditation of Healthcare Organizations. (2002). *Management of information update 3/14/02*. Chicago: Author.

Mandell, M. (1994). Not documented, not done. *Nursing, 24*(8), 62-63.

Marrelli, T. M. (2000). *Nursing documentation handbook*. St. Louis, MO: Elsevier.

Mosher, C., & Bontomasi, R. (1996). How to improve your shift report. *American Journal of Nursing, 96*(8), 32-34.

Murphy, J., & Burke, L. J. (1990, May). Charting by exception: A more efficient way to document. *Nursing90, 20*, 65, 68-69.

Rasmussen, N. (1994). Clinical pathways of care: The route to better communication. *Nursing, 24*(2), 47-49.

Simpson, R. L. (1994). Ensuring patient data privacy, confidentiality, and security. *Nursing Management, 25*(7), 18-20.

Springhouse. (1995). *Mastering documentation*. Springhouse, PA: Author.

CHAPTER 10

Cohen, B. J., et al. (2000). *Memmler's the human body in health and disease* (9th ed.). Philadelphia: Lippincott Williams & Wilkins.

Marieb, E. N. (2001). *Human anatomy & physiology* (5th ed.). Upper Saddle River, NJ: Pearson Education, Inc. (publishing as Benjamin Cummings).

Scanlon, V. C., & Sanders, T. (2003). *Essentials of anatomy and physiology* (4th ed.). Philadelphia: Davis.

Seeley, R. R., et al. (1995). *Anatomy & physiology* (3rd ed.). St. Louis, MO: Mosby-Year Book.

Spence, A. P., et al. (1992). *Human anatomy & physiology* (4th ed.). West Publishing Company.

Van De Graff, K. M., Fox, S. I. (1999). *Concepts of human anatomy & physiology* (5th ed.). New York: WCB/McGraw Hill.

CHAPTER 11

Barkauskas, V., Baumann, L. C., Stoltenberg-Allen, K., & Darling-Fisher, C. (1998). *Barkauskas' health and physical assessment* (2nd ed.). St. Louis, MO: Mosby.

Berman, A., Snyder, S., Kozier, B., & Erb, G. (2002). *Kozier and Erb's techniques in clinical nursing*. Upper Saddle River, NJ: Prentice Hall.

Leifer, G. (1999). *Thompson's introduction to maternity and pediatric nursing* (3rd ed.). Philadelphia, PA: Saunders.

Memmler, R. L., Cohen, B. J., & Wood, D. L. (2000). *Structure and function of the human body* (7th ed.). Philadelphia, PA: Lippincott-Raven.

O'Hanlon-Nichols, T. (1998, April). Basic assessment series: Gastrointestinal system. *American Journal of Nursing, 98*(4), 48-53.

O'Hanlon-Nichols, T. (1998, June). Basic assessment series. A review of the adult musculoskeletal system: A guide to a key aspect of client care. *American Journal of Nursing, 98*(6), 48-52.

Owen, A. (1998, April). Respiratory assessment revisited: Refresh your technique for spotting pulmonary problems. *Nursing98, 28*(4), 48-49.

CHAPTER 12

Capobianco, M. L., & McDonald, D. D. (1996, November/December). Factors affecting the predictive validity of the Braden Scale. *Advances in Wound Care: The Journal for Prevention and Healing, 9*, 32-36.

Carpenito, L. J. (1999). *Handbook of nursing diagnosis* (8th ed.). Philadelphia: Lippincott.

Hahn, J. F., Olsen, C. L., Tomaselli, N., & Goldberg, M., (2000, revised 2002). *Wounds: Nursing care and product selection—Part I*. (Electronic Version). Nursing Spectrum.

Hess, C. T. (2002, January). *Clinical guide to wound care* (4th ed.). Philadelphia: Lippincott Williams & Wilkins.

International Committee on Wound Management. (1996). ICWM World Council consensus statement on cost effective wound care. Evaluating your supply use to prepare for managed care. *Ostomy/Wound Management, 42*(2), 72, 74-76.

Maklebust J., & Sieggreen, M. (2000). *Pressure ulcers: Guidelines for prevention and nursing management* (2nd ed.). Springhouse, PA: Springhouse.

McConnell, E. A. (1997, May). Clinical do's and don'ts: Using dry heat to promote healing. *Nursing, 27*(5), 22.

North American Nursing Diagnosis Association. (1999). *Nursing diagnoses: Definitions and classification 1999-2000.* Philadelphia, PA: Author.

Pieper, B., Sugrue, M., Weiland, M., Sprague, K., & Heiman, C. (1998, January). Risk factors, prevention methods, and wound care for patients with pressure ulcers. *Clinical Nurse Specialist, 12*(1), 7-14.

Sisk, B. (2002). *Pressure sore update* (Electronic Version). Nurse Scribe.

Sterling, C. (1996, November). Methods of wound assessment documentation: A study. *Nursing Standard, 11*(10), 38-41.

Stotts, N. A. (1990, February). Seeing red, yellow, and black: The three-color concept of wound care. *Nursing90, 20,* 59-61.

Van Rijswijk, L. (1996, August). The fundamentals of wound assessment. *Ostomy/Wound Management, 42*(7), 40-42, 44, 46, 48-50.

Web Sites:

National Pressure Ulcer Advisory Panel (NPUAP). www.npuap.org/ Default.htm. Current research, newsletter, conferences, and information about pressure ulcers.

The National Decubitus Foundation. www.decubitus.org. Describes wound care.

Wound Care Information Network. www.medialedu.com/default. htm. Site maintained by two MDs: A. Freedline and T. Fishman; information based on National Guidelines.

CHAPTER 13

Berman, A., Snyder, S., Kozier, B., and Erb, G. (2002). *Kozier and Erb's techniques in clinical nursing.* Upper Saddle River, NJ: Prentice Hall.

Beuscher, T. L. (1998, January). Community outreach: Foot care for the elderly: A winning proposition. *Home Healthcare Nurse, 16*(1), 37-44.

Calianno, C. (2002, June). Patient hygiene part 2—Skin care: Keeping the outside healthy. *Nursing2002, 32*(6). Page supplement.

Carpenito, L. J. (2002). *Handbook of nursing diagnosis* (9th ed.). Philadelphia, PA: Lippincott.

Claphan, L. (1997, September). Preventing foot problems in patients with diabetes. *Professional Nurse, 12*(12), 851-853.

Dugan, M. B. (2003). *Living with hearing loss.* Washington, DC: Gallaudet University Press.

Eshleman, J., & Davidhizar, R. (2002, December). When your patient complains of hair loss. *Home Health Care Nurse, 20*(12), 778-782.

Kydd, A. (2002, August). Focusing nursing care on the older person. *Nursing Times, 98*(33), 13.

Lassieur, A. (2000). *Head lice (my health).* New York: Frank Watts, Inc.

Little, J. W. (Ed.). (2002). *Dental management of medically compromised patient.* St. Louis, MO: Mosby.

Marieb, E. N. (2001). *Human anatomy and physiology* (5th ed.). Menlo Park, CA: Pearson/Benjamin Cummings.

Mauizio, S. J., & Rogers, J. L. (1997, March). Prevention update: Oral hygiene to the home care patient. *Caring, 16*(3), 54-55.

North American Nursing Diagnosis Association. (2001). *Nursing diagnoses: Definitions and classification 2001-2002.* Philadelphia, PA: Author

Reed, S. (2002, June). Implementing best practices in pressure ulcer prevention. *Nursing Times, 97*(24), 69.

Wilkinson, J. (1999). *Nursing diagnosis handbook with NIC interventions and NOC outcomes* (7th ed.). Upper Saddle River, NJ: Prentice Hall.

Wilkinson, J. (2001, May). Patient hygiene part I, Oral Care: The inside story. *Nursing, 31*(5), 1.

CHAPTER 14

Ackley, B. J., & Ladwig, G. B. (2002). *Nursing diagnosis handbook—A guide to planning care* (5th ed.) St. Louis, MO: Mosby.

American Heart Association. (1993). Recommendations for human blood pressure determination by sphygmomanometers (6th ed.). Product no. 88:2460-2467. Dallas, TX: Author.

American Heart Association. (1997, January). Consult stat. Guidelines for monitoring BP at home. *RN, 60,* 57.

Bickley, L., & Szilagyi, P. C. (2002). *Bates' guide to physical examination and history taking* (7th ed.). Philadelphia, PA: Lippincott Williams & Wilkins.

Erickson, R. S., Meyer, L. T., & Woo, T. M. (1996, Spring). Accuracy of chemical dot thermometers in critically ill adults and young children. *Image, 14,* 23-28.

Guyton, A. C., & Hall, J. (2000). *Textbook of medical physiology* (10th ed.). Philadelphia, PA: Saunders.

Jones, D., Engelke, M. K., & Brown, S. T., et al. (1996, April). A comparison of two noninvasive methods of blood pressure measurement in the triage area. *Journal of Emergency Nursing, 22*(2), 111-115.

Ladewig, P. W., London, M. L., Moberly, S. M., & Olds, S. B. (2002). *Maternal-newborn nursing care: The nurse, the family, and the community* (5th ed.). Upper Saddle River, NJ: Prentice Hall.

Marieb, E. N. (2001). *Human anatomy and physiology* (5th ed.). Menlo Park, CA: Pearson/Benjamin Cummings.

Roper, M. (1996, August). Back to basics: Assessing orthostatic vital signs. *American Journal of Nursing, 96,* 43-46.

Thomas, D. O. (1996, April). Assessing children—It's different. *RN, 59,* 38-45, 53.

CHAPTER 15

Ackley, B. J., & Ladwig, G. B. (2002). *Nursing diagnosis handbook* (5th ed.). St. Louis, MO: Mosby.

American Academy of Pain Medicine. (2002). The use of opioids for the treatment of chronic pain (Joint consensus statement from the American Academy of Pain Medicine and the American Pain Society). www.productpub/statements.painmed.org/.

Blanchard, R. (2002). Why study pain? A qualitative analysis of medical and nursing faculty and students' knowledge of and attitudes to cancer pain management. *Journal of Palliative Medicine, 5*(1), 57.

Briggs, E. (2002). The nursing management of pain in older people. *Nursing Older People, 14*(7), 23-29.

Bucknall, T., Manias, E., Botti, M. (2001). Acute pain management: Implications of scientific evidence for nursing practice in the postoperative context. *International Journal of Nursing Practice, 7*(4), 266.

Edwards, H. E., Nash, R. E., Najman, J. M., Yates, P. M., Fentiman, B. J., Dewar, A., Walsh, A. M., McDowell, J. K., & Skerman, H. M. (2001). Determinants of nurses' intention to administer opioids for pain relief. *Nursing & Health Sciences, 3*(3), 149.

Guyton, A., & Hall, J. E. (2000). *Textbook of medical physiology* (10th ed.). Philadelphia, PA: Saunders.

Houldin, A. D. (2002). *Patients with cancer: Understanding the psychological pain.* Philadelphia: Lippincott Williams & Wilkins.

Slaughter, A., Pasero, C., & Manworren, R. (2002, May). Unacceptable pain levels approaches to prompt pain relief. *American Journal of Nursing, 102*(5), 75.

Kanner, R. (2001). *Pain management secrets.* Philadelphia, PA: Lippincott Williams & Wilkins.

McCaffery, M. (1979). *Nursing management of the patient with pain* (2nd ed.). Philadelphia, PA: Lippincott. (Classic.)

McCaffery, M. (2002). *Pain management revised—The nurse's active role in opioid administration* (CD-ROM). Philadelphia, PA: Lippincott Williams & Wilkins.

McCaffery, M., & Beebe, A. (1989). *Pain: Clinical manual for nursing practice.* St. Louis, MO: Mosby.

McCaffery, M., & Pasero, C. L. (1998, March). Pain control. Talking with patients and families about addiction. *American Journal of Nursing, 98*(3), 18–21.

North American Nursing Diagnosis Association. (2001). *Nursing diagnoses: Definitions and classification 2001-2002.* Philadelphia, PA: Author.

Pinnell, N. *Nursing Pharmacology.* (1996). Philadelphia, PA: W. B. Saunders.

Schechter, N. L., Berde, C. B., & Yaster, M. (2002). *Pain in infants, children and adolescents.* Philadelphia, PA: Lippincott Williams & Wilkins.

Slaughter, A., Padero, C., & Manworren, R. Unacceptable pain levels. (2002, May). *American Journal of Nursing, 102*(5), 75–77.

Unacceptable pain levels. (2002, May). *American Journal of Nursing, 102,* 75–77.

Vega-Stromberg, T., Holmes, S., Gorski, L., & Johnson, B. P. (2002). Road to excellence in pain management: Research, outcomes and direction (ROAD). *Journal of Nursing Care Quality, 17*(1), 15.

Wong, D. L. (2001). *Whaley and Wong's essentials of pediatric nursing* (6th ed.). St. Louis, MO: Mosby.

CHAPTER 16

Brown, P. (2000, April). DVT: What every nurse should know. *RN, 63*(4), 58–62.

Burke, K. M., LeMone, P., & Mohn-Brown, E. L. (2003). *Medical surgical nursing care.* Upper Saddle River, NJ: Prentice Hall.

Carroll, P. (2001, May). How to intervene before asthma turns deadly. *RN, 64*(5), 52–58.

Davies, P. (2002, March). Guarding your patient against ARDS. *Nursing2002, 32*(3), 36–41.

Fort, C. W. (2002, September). Get pumped to prevent DVT. *Nursing2002, 32*(9), 50–52.

Lazzara, D. (2002, June). Eliminate the air of mystery from chest tubes. *Nursing2002, 32*(6), 36–43.

McConnell, E. A. (2002, April). Applying antiembolism stockings. *Nursing2002, 32*(4), 17.

Perkins, L. A., & Shortall, S. P. (2000, January). Ventilation without intubation. *RN, 63*(1), 34–38.

Pope, B. B. (2002, May). Asthma: Patient education series. *Nursing2002, 32*(5), 44.

Siomko, A. J. (2000, January). Demystifying cardiac markers. *American Journal of Nursing, 100*(1), 36–40.

West, J. B. (2001, January 15). *Pulmonary physiology and pathophysiology: An integrated, case-based approach.* Philadelphia, PA: Lippincott Williams & Wilkins.

CHAPTER 17

Como, D. (Ed.). (2002). *Mosby's medical, nursing, and allied health dictionary.* St. Louis, MO: Mosby.

Lane, K. (Ed.). (1999). *The Merck manual.* West Point, PA: Merck.

McPhee, A. T. (1997). *Fluids and electrolytes made incredibly easy.* Springhouse, PA: Springhouse.

Nettina, S. M. (Ed.). (2001). *The Lippincott manual of nursing practice.* Philadelphia, PA: Lippincott-Raven.

Pagana, K. D., & Pagana, T. J. (2003). *Mosby's diagnostic and laboratory test reference.* St. Louis, MO: Mosby.

Phillips, L. (2001). *Manual of I.V. therapeutics.* Philadelphia, PA: Davis.

Venes, D. (Ed.). (2001). *Taber's cyclopedic medical dictionary.* Philadelphia, PA: Davis.

Whitney, E. N., Cataldo, C. B., & Rolfes, S. R. (2002). *Understanding normal and clinical nutrition.* Belmount, CA: Wadsworth/ Thomson Learning.

Wilkinson, J. M. (2000). Nursing diagnosis handbook. Upper Saddle River, NJ: Prentice Hall Health.

CHAPTER 18

Ackley, B. J., & Ladwig, G. B. (1997). Nursing diagnosis handbook: A guide to planning care (3rd ed.). St. Louis, MO: Mosby.

Bradley, M., & Pupiales, M. (1997, July). Essential elements of ostomy care. *American Journal of Nursing, 97*(7), 38–46.

Nettina, S. M. (2001). *Lippincott manual of nursing practice* (7th ed.). Philadelphia: Lippincott Williams & Wilkins.

Newman, D. K. (2002). *Managing and treating urinary incontinence* (1st ed.). Baltimore, MD: Health Professions Press.

Carpenito, L. J. (1999). *Handbook of nursing diagnosis* (8th ed.). Philadelphia, PA: Lippincott.

Colley, W. (1997, March). Know how: Male catheterization. *Nursing Times, 93*(11), 32–33.

Mahony, C. (1997, December). The impact of incontinence problems on self-esteem. *Nursing Times, 93*(52), 58, 60.

Marchiondo, K. (1998, March). A new look at urinary tract infection. *American Journal of Nursing, 98*(3), 34–39.

Polick, T. (2001). *Slaying the myths concerning women and urinary incontinence* (Electronic Version). Nursing Spectrum.

Schakenbach, L. (1997, July). Consult stat. The proper way to manage a distended bladder. *RN, 60*(7), 63.

Web Sites

National Association for Continence. www.nafc.org.

Simon Foundation for Continence. www.simonfoundation.org.

CHAPTER 19

Bryant, D., Fleischer, I. (2000, November). Changing an ostomy appliance (Electronic Version). *Nursing, 30*(11), 51.

Butler, M. (1998, January). Laxatives and rectal preparations. *Nursing Times, 94*(3), 56-58.

Carpenito, L. J. (1999). *Handbook of nursing diagnosis* (8th ed.). Philadelphia, PA: Lippincott.

Guyton, A. C., & Hall, J. E. (2000). *Textbook of medical physiology* (10th ed.). Philadelphia, PA: Saunders.

Jensen, L. L. (1997, September). Fecal incontinence: Evaluation and treatment. *Journal of Wound, Ostomy and Continence Nursing, 24*(5), 277-282.

Nettina, S. M. (2001). *Lippincott manual of nursing practice* (7th ed.). Lippincott Williams & Wilkins.

North American Nursing Diagnosis Association. (1999). *Nursing diagnoses: Definitions and classification 1999-2000*. Philadelphia, PA: Author.

Petticrew, M. (1997, November). Treatment of constipation in older people. *Nursing Times, 93*(48), 55-56.

Vickery, G. (1997, July/August). Basics of constipation. *Gastroenterology Nursing, 20*(4), 125-128.

Web Sites

National Institute of Diabetes & Digestive & Kidney Diseases. (See listing for Constipation, Diarrhea, Ileostomy, Colostomy, and Ileoanal Reservoir Surgery and Digestive Disease Statistics.) www.niddk.nih.gov/health/digest/nddic.htm.

National Association for Continence (NAFC). www.nafc.org.

The Simon Foundation for Continence. http://simonfoundation.org.

CHAPTER 20

Ackley, B. J., & Ladwig, G. B. (2002). *Nursing diagnosis handbook: A guide to planning care*. St. Louis, MO: Mosby.

Ancoli-Israel, S. (1997, January). Sleep problems in older adults: Putting myths to bed. *Geriatrics, 52*(1), 20-22, 25-26, 28.

Beck-Little, R., & Weinrich, S. P. (1998, April). Assessment and management of sleep disorders in the elderly. *Journal of Gerontological Nursing, 24*(4), 21-29.

Carpenito, L. J. (2002). *Handbook of nursing diagnosis* (9th ed.). Philadelphia, PA: Lippincott.

Graves, G. (1998, March). The 9 habits of highly successful sleepers. *Good Housekeeping*, 82, 84, 88.

Guyton, A. C., & Hall, J. E. (1996). *Textbook of medical physiology* (9th ed.). Philadelphia, PA: Saunders.

Haigh, C., & Peacok, L. (1998, February). Dilemmas in moving and handling patients. *Community Nurse, 4*(1), 26-28.

Melillo, K. D., Williamson, E., Futrell, M., & Chamberlain, C. (1997, June). A self-assessment tool to measure older adults' perceptions regarding physical fitness and exercise activity. *Journal of Advanced Nursing, 25*(6), 1220-1226.

Schuldenfrei, P. (1998, September). No heavy lifting. *American Journal of Nursing, 98*(9), 46-48.

Sobezak, J. (1998, February). Exercising for better health and mobility. *Community Nurse, 4*(1), 20-22.

Krahn, L., Black, J., & Silber, M. (2001). Subspecialty clinics: sleep disorders: narcolepsy—new understanding of irresistible sleep. *Mayo Clinic Proceedings, 76*, 185-194.

Thomason, M., Huggins, M., Beier, S., & Watkins, T. (2002). *The autoimmune hypothesis in narcolepsy* (electronically published manuscript). Retrieved from the World Wide Web July 16, 2002. Available at: www.tonto.stanford.edu/^john/205/watkins.pdf.

CHAPTER 21

Ackley, B. J., & Ladwig, G. B. (2002). *Nursing diagnosis handbook* (5th ed.). St. Louis, MO: Mosby.

Beyea, S., & Nicoll, L. (1996, January). Back to basics: Administering IM injections the right way. *American Journal of Nursing, 96*(1), 34-35.

Cohen, M. R. (2002). *Medication errors*. Huntingdon Valley, PA: American Pharmaceutical Association.

edruginfo.com. (2002). *Clinical pearls*. Philadelphia, PA: Lippincott Williams & Wilkins.

Glazer, G. (2002, February 28). NursingWorld OJIN: Legislative Column: "Medication administration interventions that must be performed by a registered nurse." Online Journal of Issues in Nursing. Available at www.nursingworld.org/ojin/tpclg/leg_ 12.htm.

Highleyman, L. (2002, September). Preventing HCV Transmission in Personal Care Settings. San Francisco: Hepatitis Support Project.

McCloskey, J. C., & Bulechek, G. M. (2000). *Nursing interventions classification (NIC)* (3rd ed.). St. Louis, MO: Mosby-Year Book.

Miller, D. (2000). *Nurse's clinical guide: Medication administration*. Philadelphia, PA: Springhouse-Lippincott Williams & Wilkins.

Moses, S. (2000). Cation-exchange resin. Family Practice Notebook. (online publication). Retrieved January 29, 2003. Available at www.fpnotebook.com/REN101.htm.

National Institute for Occupational Safety and Health (1999, November). *Alert—Preventing needlestick injuries in health care settings*. Cincinnati, OH: DHHS (NIOSH) Publication No. 2000-108.

National League for Nursing (2001, April 18). *Basic proficiency in medication administration* (4th Version). New York: Author.

Sifton, D. W. (Ed.) *Physician's desk reference* (56th ed.). Montvale, NJ: Medical Economics.

Smith, S. F., Duell, D. J., & Martin, B. C. (2000). *Clinical Nursing Skills: Basic to advanced skills*. Upper Saddle River, NJ: Prentice Hall.

Wilson, B. A., Shannon, M. T., & Stang, C. L. (2003). *Nurse's drug guide*. Upper Saddle River, NJ: Prentice Hall.

Wolfe, S. (Ed.). (2001, October). Safer needle devices, part 1. *RN, 62*(10), 59.

Worthington, K. A. (2002, May). Hazardous drugs: Handling medications can pose danger to nurses. *American Journal of Nursing, 102*(5), 120.

CHAPTER 22

Ackley, B. J., & Ladwig, G. B. (2002). *Nursing diagnosis handbook* (5th ed.). St. Louis, MO: Mosby.

Benko, T., Cooke, E. A., McNally, M. A., & Mollan, R. (2000). Graduated compression stockings—knee length or thigh length. *Clinical Orthopaedics and Related Research, 383*, 197-203.

Brown, B. (2001, November). Promoting patient safety through preoperative patient verification. *AORN Journal, 74*(11), 690.

Busen, N. (2001, February). Perioperative preparation of the adolescent surgical patient. (AORN) *Journal of Association Perioperative RN* 73(2), 464.

Carroll, P. (1993). Deep venous thrombosis: Implications for orthopaedic nursing. *Orthopaedic Nursing, 12*(3), 33-43.

Church, V. (2000). Staying on guard for DVT & PE. *Nursing2000, 30*(2), 34.

Dealey, C. (2000). *The care of wounds: A guide for nurses* (2nd ed.). Boston: Blackwell Science.

Garbee, G. (2001, September). Creating a positive surgical experience for patients. *AORN Journal, 74*(9), 333.

Munden, J. (2002). *Pathophysiology made incredibly easy* (2nd ed.). Springhouse, PA: Lippincott Williams & Wilkins.

North American Nursing Diagnosis Association. (2001). *Nursing Diagnosis: Definitions and classification 2001-2002.* Philadelphia, PA: Author.

Tappen, C. (2001, February). Perioperative assessment and discharge planning for older adults undergoing ambulatory surgery. *AORN Journal, 73*(2), 464.

Walton, J. (2001, March). Helping high-risk surgical patients beat the odds. *Nursing2001, 31*(3), 54.

Winslow, E. H., & Crenshaw, J.T. (2002, May). Preoperative fasting: Old habits die hard. *American Journal of Nursing, 102*(5), 36-44.

CHAPTER 23

Bandura, A. (1971). Analysis of modeling processes. In A. Bandura (Ed.), *Psychological modeling*. Chicago: Aldine.

Byrnes, James P. (2001). *Cognitive development and learning in instructional context.* Boston: Allyn & Bacon.

Carpenito, L. J. (1997). *Nursing diagnosis: Application to clinical practice* (7th ed.). Philadelphia, PA: Lippincott.

Doak, C. C., Doak, L. G., & Root, J. H. (1996). *Teaching patients with low literacy skills* (2nd ed.). Philadelphia, PA: Lippincott.

Messner, R. I. (1997, August). Patient teaching tips from the horse's mouth. *RN, 60*(8), 29-31.

Rankin, S. H., & Stallings, K. D. (1996). *Patient education: Issues, principles, practices* (3rd ed.). Philadelphia, PA: Lippincott.

Redman, B. K. (1993). *The process of patient education* (7th ed.). St. Louis, MO: Mosby.

Robinson, A., & Miller, M. (1996). Making information accessible: Developing plain English discharge instructions. *Journal of Advanced Nursing, 24*(3), 528-535.

Rutledge, D. N., & Donaldson, N. E. (1998, June). Improving readability of print materials in patient care and health services. *Online Journal of Clinical Innovations, 1*(3), 1-27.

Stephens, S. T. (1992, January/February). Patient educational materials: Are they readable? *Oncology Nursing Forum, 19*(1), 84.

CHAPTER 24

Barkauskas, V., Bauman, L. C., & Stoltenberg-Allen, K., & Darling-Fisher, C. (1998). *Barkauskas health and physical assessment* (2nd ed.). St. Louis, MO: Mosby.

Cicchetti, D. (2000). The promotion of wellness in children and adolescents: Issues in children's and families' lives. Stamford, CT: Appleton & Lange.

Edelman, C., & Mandle, C. L. (2002). Health promotion throughout the life span (5th ed.). St. Louis, MO: Mosby.

Eliopoulos, C. (2001). *Gerontological nursing* (5th ed.). Philadelphia, PA: Lippincott.

Erikson, E. H. (1963). *Childhood and society* (2nd ed.). New York: Norton. (Classic.)

Erikson, E. H. (1982). The life cycle completed: A review. New York: Norton. (Classic.)

Erikson, E. H., and Joan, M. (1997). *The life cycle completed.* New York: Norton.

Fontaine, K. L. (2003). *Mental health nursing* (5th ed.). Upper Saddle River, NJ: Prentice Hall.

Piaget, J. (1966). *Origins of intelligence in children.* New York: Norton. (Classic.)

Population. U.S. Bureau of the Census: (2000). Washington, DC: U.S. Government Printing Office.

Wold, G. (1999). *Basic geriatric nursing* (2nd ed.). St. Louis, MO: Mosby-Year Book.

Zator-Estes, M. E. (2001). *Health assessment & physical examination* (2nd ed.). Clifton Park, NY: Delmar Publishing.

CHAPTER 25

Ackley, B. J., & Ladwig G. B. (2002) Nursing diagnosis handbook (5th ed.). St. Louis, MO: Mosby.

Anderson, M.A. (2001). Nursing leadership: Management and professional practice for the LPN/LVN (2nd ed.). Philadelphia, PA: Davis.

Anderson, M.A. (2000). To be a nurse: Personal/Vocational relations for LPN/LVN. Philadelphia: Davis.

Arnold, E., and Boggs, K.U. (1999). *Interpersonal relationships: Professional communication skills for nurses* (3rd ed.). Philadelphia, PA: Saunders.

Bateson, G. (1979). *Mind and nature.* New York: Dutton.

Carpenito, L. J. (1997). *Nursing diagnosis: Application to clinical practice* (7th ed.). Philadelphia: Lippincott.

Deering, C. G. (1999, January). To speak or not to speak? Self-disclosure with patients. *American Journal of Nursing, 99*(1), 34-39.

Egan, G. (1998). *The skilled helper: A problem-management approach to helping* (6th ed.). Pacific Grove, CA: Brooks/Cole.

Fontaine, K. L. (2003). *Mental health nursing* (5th ed.). Upper Saddle River, NJ: Prentice Hall.

Hersey, P., Blanchard, K. H., & Johnson, D. E. (2001). Effective Communication. In *Management of organizational behavior: Leading human resources* (8th ed.). Upper Saddle River, NJ: Prentice Hall.

Miller, K. L. (1995, November). Keeping the care in nursing care. Our biggest challenge. *Journal of Nursing Administration, 25*(11), 29-32.

Milstead, J. A. (1996, January/February). Basic tools for the orthopaedic staff nurse: Assertiveness. *Orthopaedic Nursing, 15*, 23-29.

Morse, J. (1996, Fourth Quarter). The science of comforting. *Reflections, 22*(4), 6-7.

Morse, J. M., Bottorff, J., Anderson, G., O'Brien, B., & Solberg, S. (1992, July). Beyond empathy: Expanding expressions of caring. *Journal of Advanced Nursing, 17*(7), 809-821.

Purnell, L. D., & Paulanka, B. J. (1998). *Transcultural health care—A culturally competent approach.* Philadelphia, PA: Davis.

Sieh, A., & Brentin, L. K. (1997). *The nurse communicates.* Philadelphia, PA: Saunders.

Smith, M. K., & Sullivan, J. M. (1997, March/April). Nurses' and patients' perceptions of most important caring behaviors in a long-term care setting. *Geriatric Nursing, 18*(2), 70-73.

Tannen, D. (1991). *You just don't understand: Women and men in conversation.* New York: Ballantine.

CHAPTER 26

Andrews, M. M., & Boyle, J. S. (1999). *Transcultural concepts in nursing care* (3rd ed.). Philadelphia, PA: Lippincott.

Doswell, W. M., & Erlen, J. A. (1998, June). Multicultural issues and ethical concerns in the delivery of nursing care interventions. *Nursing Clinics of North America, 33*, 353-361.

Glanti, G. A. (1997). *Caring for patients from different cultures* (2nd ed.). Philadelphia, PA: University of Pennsylvania Press.

Leininger, M. M. (1988, November). Leininger's theory of nursing: Cultural care diversity and universality. *Nursing Science Quarterly, 14*, 152-160.

Lipson, J. G., Dibble, S. L., & Minarik, P. A. (1996). *Culture and nursing care: A pocket guide.* San Francisico: UCSF Nursing Press.

Purnell, L. D., & Paulanka, B. J. (1998). *Transcultural health care—A culturally competent approach.* Philadelphia, PA: Davis.

Spector, R. E. (2000a). *Cultural diversity in health and illness* (5th ed.). Upper Saddle River, NJ: Prentice Hall.

Spector, R. E. (2000b). *Cultural care guides to heritage assessment and health traditions* (2nd ed.). Upper Saddle River, NJ: Prentice Hall.

CHAPTER 27

Bernstein, D. K., & Tiegerman-Farber, E. (2001). *Language and communication disorders in children* (5th ed.). Boston: Allyn & Bacon.

Centers for Disease Control, National Center for Birth Defects and Developmental Disabilities, Early Hearing Detection and Intervention Program. What is EHDI? Retrieved from the world wide web October 15, 2001. Available at: www.cdc.gov/ncbddd/ ehdi/ehdi.htm.

Ebersole, P., & Hess, P. (2001). *Geriatric nursing & healthy aging.* St. Louis, MO: Mosby.

Hasselkus, A., Tenenholtz, E., & Brown, J. (2002, June). Speech-language pathologists add value to home care. *Home Healthcare Nurse, 20*(6), 393-398.

Jarvis, C. (2000). *Pocket companion for physical examination and health assessment.* Philadelphia, PA: Saunders.

McConnell, E. A. (1996, May). Caring for a patient who has a vision impairment. *Nursing96, 26*(5), 28.

McConnell, E. A. (2002, August). Clinical do's and don'ts: Talking with a hearing-impaired patient. *Nursing2002, 32*(8), 20.

North American Nursing Diagnosis Association. (2001). *Nursing Diagnoses: Definitions and Classification 2001-2002.* Philadelphia, PA: Author.

Papalia, D. E., Olds, S. W., & Feldman, R. D. (2001). *Human development* (8th ed.). Columbus, OH: McGraw-Hill.

Trummer, K. H., Foster, B. B., Hartman, L., Lewis-Vais, C., & Sullivan, H. (1996, July). Protecting confused patients from falls. *American Journal of Nursing, 96*(7), 16R-16X.

CHAPTER 28

Arnold, E., & Boggs, K.U. (1999) *Interpersonal Relationships—Professional communication skills for nurses* (3rd ed.). Philadelphia, PA: Saunders.

Carpenito, L. J. (2001). *Nursing diagnosis: Application to clinical practice* (8th ed.). Philadelphia, PA: Lippincott.

Edelman, C. L., & Mandle, C. L. (1998). *Health promotion throughout the life span* (4th ed.). St. Louis, MO: Mosby.

Erikson, E. H. (1963). *Childhood and society* (2nd ed.). New York: Norton. (Classic.)

Erikson, E. H., & Erikson, J. M. (1997). *The life cycle completed.* New York: Norton.

Neeb, K. (2001). *Fundamentals of mental health nursing* (2nd ed.). Philadelphia: Davis.

North American Nursing Diagnosis Association. (1999). *Nursing Diagnoses: Definitions and Classification 1999-2000.* Philadelphia, PA: Author.

CHAPTER 29

American Cancer Society. (2001). *Cancer facts and figures—2001.* Atlanta, GA: Author.

Anderson, K. N. (Ed.) *Mosby's medical, nursing, and allied health dictionary (2002)* (6th ed.). St. Louis, MO: Mosby, 808.

Ball, J., & Bindler, R. (1999). *Pediatric nursing: Caring for children.* Upper Saddle River, NJ: Prentice Hall.

Brady, M. (1998, September). Female genital mutilation. *Nursing98, 28*(9), 50-51.

Carpenito, L. J. (2002). *Handbook of nursing diagnosis* (9th ed.). Philadelphia, PA: Lippincott Williams & Wilkins.

Clark, M. J. (2003). *Community health nursing: Caring for the population* (4th ed.). Upper Saddle River, NJ: Pearson Education.

Clayton, B. D., & Stock, Y. (2001). *Basic pharmacology for nurses* (12th ed.). St. Louis, MO: Mosby.

Hofland, S. L., & Powers, L. (1996). Sexual dysfunction in the menopausal woman: Hormonal causes and management issues. *Geriatric Nursing, 17*(4), 161-165.

Leifer, G. (1999). *Thompson's introduction to maternity and pediatric nursing* (3rd ed.) (p. 252). Philadephia, PA: Saunders.

Masters, W. H., & Johnson, V. E. (1966). *Human sexual response.* Boston: Little, Brown.

Masters, W. H., Johnson, V. E., & Kolodny, R. C. (1995). *Human sexuality* (5th ed.). New York: HarperCollins College.

Napoli, M. (1999, December 31). Expanding the Viagra market to include women. *HealthFacts, 24*(12), 1-2.

Nettina, S. (2001). *The Lippincott manual of nursing practice* (7th ed.) (p. 1115). Philadelphia, PA: Lippincott Williams & Wilkins.

Novak, J. C., & Broom, B. L. (1999). *Ingalls and Salerno's maternal and child health nursing* (9th ed.) (pp 295, 863). St. Louis, MO: Mosby.

Olds, S., London, M., & Ladewig, P. (1996). *Maternal-newborn nursing* (5th ed.). Menlo Park, CA: Addison-Wesley Nursing.

Porth, C. M. *Pathophysiology: Concepts in altered health states.* (2003). Philadelphia, PA: Lippincott Williams & Wilkins.

Sherwen, L. N., Scoloven, M.A., & Weingarten, C.T. (1999). *Maternity nursing: Care of the childbearing family.* (pp. 83, 87). Stamford, CT: Appleton & Lange.

CHAPTER 30

Carpenito, L. J. (2002). *Nursing diagnosis: Application to clinical practice* (9th ed.). Philadelphia, PA: Lippincott.

Fontaine, K. L. (2003). *Mental health nursing* (5th ed.). Upper Saddle River, NJ: Prentice Hall.

Freud, S. (1946). *The ego and the mechanisms of defense.* New York: International Universities Press. (Classic.)

Holmes, T. H., & Rahe, R. H. (1967, August). The social re-adjustment rating scale. *Journal of Psychomatic Research, 11,* 213–218. (Classic.)

Kurzen, C. R. (2001). *Contemporary practical/vocational nursing* (4th ed.). Philadelphia, PA: Lippincott.

Lazarus, R. S. (1998a). *The life and work of an eminent psychologist.* New York: Springer.

Lazarus, R. S. (1998b). *Fifty years of research and theory of R. S. Lazarus: An analysis of historical perennial issues.* New York: Lawrence Erlbaum.

LeMone, P., & Burke, K. M. (2000). *Medical–surgical nursing: Critical thinking in client care.* Upper Saddle River, NJ: Prentice Hall.

Monat, A., & Lazarus, R. S. (Eds.). (1991). *Stress and coping* (3rd ed.). New York: Columbia University Press.

Neeb, K. (2001). *Fundamentals of mental health nursing* (2nd ed.). Philadelphia, PA: Davis.

Selye, H. (1976). *The stress of life* (revised ed.). New York: McGraw-Hill. (Classic.)

Thomas, C. L. (Ed.). (2001). *Taber's cyclopedic medical dictionary* (19th ed.). Philadelphia, PA: Davis.

CHAPTER 31

Anweiler, N. (2000, November). Another dying patient. *Nursing2000, 30,* 11, 32.

Benton, R. E. (1978). *Death and dying: Principles and practices in patient care.* New York: Van Nostrand.

Carpenito, L. J. (1997). *Handbook of nursing diagnosis* (7th ed.). Philadelphia, PA: Lippincott.

Engel, G. L. (1964, September). Grief and grieving. *American Journal of Nursing, 64,* 93–98. (Classic.)

Furman, J. (2002, February). What you should know about chronic grief. *Nursing2002, 32,* 56.

Hospice and Palliative Nurses Association. (1999). *Hospice and palliative nursing practice review* (3rd ed.). Dubuque IA: Kendall/Hunt.

Kübler-Ross, E. (1969). *On death and dying.* New York: Macmillan. (Classic.)

Kübler-Ross, E. (1974). *Questions and answers on death and dying.* New York: Macmillan. (Classic.)

Kübler-Ross, E. (1975). *Death: The final stage of growth.* Englewood Cliffs, NJ: Prentice Hall. (Classic.)

Kübler-Ross, E. (1978). *To live until we say good-bye.* Englewood Cliffs, NJ: Prentice Hall. (Classic.)

North American Nursing Diagnosis Association. (1999). *Nursing diagnoses: Definitions and classification 1999–2000.* Philadelphia, PA: Author.

Ross, H. (2001, April). Islamic tradition at the end of life. *Medsurg Nursing, 10*(2), p. 83.

Springhouse. (1996). *Nurse's legal handbook* (3rd ed.). Springhouse, PA: Author.

Ufema, J. (Monthly column). Insights on death and dying. *Nursing2002,* February, April, June, October, November 2001: January, March 2002.

Wrede-Seaman, L. (1999). *Symptom management algorithms: A handbook for palliative care* (2nd ed.). Washington, DC: Intellicard, Inc.

CHAPTER 32

Anderson, M. A. (2000). *Nursing leadership, management, and professional practice for LPN/LVN* (2nd ed.). Philadelphia, PA: Davis.

Hansten, R. I., & Washburn, M. J. (1998). *Clinical delegation skills—A handbook for professional practice* (2nd ed.). Gaitherburg, MD: Aspen Publishing.

Kurzen, C. R. (2001). *Contemporary practical/vocational nursing* (4th ed.). Philadelphia, PA: Lippincott.

National Association of Practical Nurse Education and Service. (1998). *Code of ethics for licensed practical/vocational nurses.* Silver Springs, MD: Author.

Walczak, M. B., & Absolon, P. L. (2001). Essentials for effective communication in oncology nursing: Assertiveness, conflict management, delegation and motivation. *Journal of Nurses Staff Developments, 17*(3), 159–162.

CHAPTER 33

Gronlund, N. (2000). *How to write and use instructional objectives.* Upper Saddle River, NJ: Prentice Hall.

Hill, S., & Howlett, H. (2001). *Success in practical/vocational nursing: From student to leader.* Philadelphia, PA: Saunders.

National Council of State Boards of Nursing, Inc. (2002). *NCLEX-PN examination effective date: April 2002.* Chicago: Author.

Smith, S. (1997). *Review questions for the NCLEX-PN CAT* (3rd ed.). Upper Saddle River, NJ: Prentice Hall.

Wilson, B., Shannon, S., & Strang, C. (2002). *Nurse's drug guide 2002.* Upper Saddle River, NJ: Prentice Hall.

CHAPTER 34

Anderson, M. (2001). *Nursing leadership, management, and professional practice for the LPN/LVN* (2nd ed.). Philadelphia, PA: Davis.

Anderson, M. (2000). *To be a nurse—Personal/vocational relationships for the LPN/LVN.* Philadelphia, PA: Davis.

Bozell, J. (1999). *Anatomy of a job search.* Philadelphia, PA: Springhouse.

Harrington, N., Smith, N. E. & Spratt, W. E. (1996). LPN to RN transition. Philadelphia, PA: Lippincott.

Hill, S. S., Howlett, H. S., & Howlett, H. A. (2001). *Success in practical/vocational nursing from student to leader.* St. Louis, MO: Mosby.

Kurzen, C. (2001). *Contemporary practical/vocational nursing* (4th ed.). Philadelphia, PA: Lippincott.

Makely, S. (2000). *The Health Care Worker's Primer on Professionalism.* Upper Saddle River, NJ: Brady/Prentice Hall.

Porter, L. (2000). *Rubrics.* Anaheim, CA: North Orange County Regional Occupational Program. Unpublished.

Index

Pages followed by *f* indicate figure; those followed by *t* indicate table.

A

Abbreviations, 157*t*
Abdomen
  assessment of, 207–8, 208*f*, 209*f*, 216*f*
  injury to, 420–21
Abdominal breathing, 356
Abdominal cavity, 193, 194, 194*f*
Abdominopelvic cavity, 193–94
Abduction, 460*t*
Ablative surgery, 543. *See also* Surgery
Abortion, 32
Abrasions, 223*t*, 255*t*
Absorption, of medications, 503
Academic skills
  reading and, 13
  test taking and, 13–15
  time management and, 15–16
Accessory reproductive organs, 191
Accidental hypothermia, 294
Accidents. *See also* Falls; Safety
  incident report for, 27, 28
  malpractice actions due to, 21
  preventing equipment-related, 92
Accommodation, pupil, 204
Accreditation, 23
Acetone, 410*t*, 413
Acid-base balance
  discharge considerations and, 391
  explanation of, 386–87
  intravenous therapy and, 390
  nursing care and, 388, 390–91
  problems with, 387–88
Acidosis, 387–88
Acne, 255*t*
Acquired immune deficiency syndrome
    (AIDs). *See* HIV/AIDS
Action words, 62, 745
Active-assistive ROM exercises, 469
Active immunity, 116, 117*t*
Active involvement, 569, 569*f*
Active listening, 620, 623*f*
Active or second-generation low air loss bed,
    232*t*
Active range of motion, 209
Active ROM exercises, 469
Activities of daily living (ADLs), 170, 337
Activity. *See also* Body movement; Exercise;
    Immobility
  assessment tolerance for, 466
  growth and development and, 460
  mental health and, 460

normal movement and, 459–60, 460*t*
  nursing care and, 464–72
  nutrition and, 460
  physical health and, 460
Acupressure, 332
Acupuncture, 331
Acupuncturists, 79
Acute infection, 113
Acute pain, 325, 338. *See also* Pain; Pain
    management
Adduction, 460*t*
A-delta fibers, 327
Adenosine triphosphate (ATP), 182,
    710
Adjuvant analgesics, 331
Admission
  of client from emergency care, 143–44
  common responses to, 138
  cultural considerations regarding, 138
  diagnosing, planning, and implementing,
    141–43
  evaluation of, 143
  explanation of, 138
  nursing care and, 141–43
  procedures for, 138, 139*f*–140*f*, 141
Adolescents. *See also* Children
  cognitive development in, 600
  concept of death and, 706
  growth and development in, 588*t*
  health assessment and promotion in, 599*t*,
    601
  moral development in, 600
  pain management for, 338*t*
  physical development in, 599–600
  psychosocial development in, 600, 658*t*
  safety measures for, 88–89
  sexual abuse of, 671
  sexual development in, 668, 669*t*
  stress and, 687
  vital signs in, 292*t*
Adults. *See* Middle-aged adults; Older
    adults; Young adults
Advance directives, 707
Adventitious breath sounds, 206, 207*t*
Adverse effects of medications, 501
Advocacy, 33–34
Aerosol sprays, 500*t*
Afebrile, 293
Affective domain, 568, 578–79
Affective responses, 337
Afghanistan, 4
African Americans
  blood pressure and, 305
  hair care for, 261, 261*f*, 278
Afternoon care, 253

Age
  blood pressure and, 305
  body temperature and, 293
  defecation and, 438
  infection and, 115
  learning and, 570*t*
  pressure ulcers and, 237
  pulse rate and, 298
  reaction to loss and, 701–3
  safety and, 87
  wound healing and, 225
Agencies, nurses employed by, 24
Agency fires, 89
Agents, infectious, 114
Aggression, 690
AIDS. *See* HIV/AIDS
Airborne transmission
  explanation of, 114–15
  precautions for, 119
Air-fluidized beds, 232*t*
Airway obstruction, 348
Albumin, 377
Alcohol consumption
  fluid output and, 407
  sleep and, 475
Alcoholics Anonymous, 77, 616
Alcott, Louisa May, 4
Aldosterone, 405
Alexian brothers, 8
Algor mortis, 710
Alkaline, 386
Alkalosis, 387, 388
Allergies, 502, 502*t*
Altered nutrition, 383–84
Altered protection, 173
Alternating pressure mattresses, 232*t*
Alternative care providers, 79
Altitude, 302*t*
Alveolar ducts, 345, 346
Alveolar gas exchange, 346
Alveoli, 345, 346*f*
Ambulation
  assisting clients with, 469, 472, 492–94,
    492*f*, 493*f*
  explanation of, 469
  postoperative, 551
Ambulatory care centers, 74
American Academy of Nursing (AAN), 79
American Civil War. *See* Civil War
American Committee for Devastated France,
    6
American Heart Association, 94, 359
American Hospital Association (AHA), 77,
    567
American Medical Association (AMA), 7

American Nurses Association (ANA)
  assisted suicide and, 33
  Center for Ethics and Human Rights, 32
  function of, 752
  nursing definition of, 3
  practical/vocational nursing position of, 9
American Red Cross, 6, 359
American Society of Superintendents of
    Training Schools for Nurses of the
    United States and Canada, 6
Americans with Disabilities Act (ADA),
    27–28
Amino acids, 377
Ammonia dermatitis, 255t
Amphetamines, 476
Ampules
  explanation of, 514, 514f
  preparing medications from, 527–28,
    527f
Amputation, 564
Anabolism, 377
Anal canal, 437–38
Analgesics
  adjuvant, 331
  effects of, 551
  patient-controlled, 331, 333f, 334t–335t,
    550
  preemptive, 331
Analysis questions, 14t
Anaphase, 182
Anatomical terms, 192
Anatomic positions, 192–93, 192f, 193f
Anatomy, 181
Andrews, Margaret, 631
Anemia, 350
Anesthesia
  defecation and, 439
  effects of, 551
  types of, 546
Angel of Mercy image, 3, 5
Anger
  explanation of, 689–70
  oxygenation and, 351
  strategies for dealing with, 694
Angina, 461
Angina pectoris, 349
Angioedema, 502t
Angiography, 353
Anions, 385
Ankylosed joints, 461
Anorexia, 462
Anoscopy, 442
Anterior, 192
Antibiotics
  negative aspects of, 116
  overuse of, 113
  proper use of, 113, 114
  wound healing and, 226
Antibody-mediated defense, 116

Anticholinergics, 545
Antidepressants, 476
Antidiuretic hormone (ADH), 405, 407
Antiemboli stockings
  explanation of, 358, 546
  procedure for applying, 557–58, 557f
Antiflatulent medication, 446
Antigens, 181
Antihistamines, 545
Antihypertensive medication, 678
Anti-inflammatory medication, 225
Antiseptics, 117
Antispasmodic medication, 513
Anuria, 408
Anus, 437
Anxiety. See also Stress
  due to hospital admission, 138
  explanation of, 688–89
  indicators of levels of, 689t
  minimizing, 694
  pain experience and, 329, 331
Aorta, 349
Apgar scoring, 591, 594t
Apical pulse
  assessment of, 301, 315–16
  explanation of, 298, 300, 301
Apical-radial pulse, 301, 316–17
Apical site, 299, 299f, 299t
APIE charting, 162, 163f
Apnea, 304, 348
Apocrine glands, 600
Apothecaries' system, 508, 508t
Appearance. See Hygienic care; Personal ap-
    pearance
Appendectomy, 521–23
Application questions, 14t
Aquamatic pads, 230
Aquathermia pads, 230, 235
Aqueous solutions, 500t
Aqueous suspensions, 500t
Arbitration, 24
Around-the-clock (ATC), 331
Arousal mechanism, 493
Arrhythmia, 300
Arterial blood gas (ABG) test, 387–88, 390
Arteries, 298
Artificial airways, 354
Artificial eyes, 267, 267f
Artificial immunity, 117t
Ascending colostomy, 441
Asepsis, 117. See also Infection control
Aseptic technique, 117
As-needed (prn) care, 253
Asphyxiation, 90
Aspiration pneumonia, 548t
Aspirin, 439, 543
Assault, 22
Assessment. See also Physical health assess-
    ment

  of accident or injury risk, 98–99
  data organization and, 52–53
  for discharge, 146, 149
  explanation of, 52, 52t
  function of, 52t
  of infection risk, 120–21
  of newly admitted clients, 141, 169
  nursing care and, 200–201, 204–10
  steps involved in, 52–54, 54t
Assisted-living centers, 76
Assisted suicide, 33, 708. See also Euthanasia
Asymptomatic infections, 112
Atelectasis, 462, 548t
Atherosclerosis, 350, 351
Atherosclerotic plaque, 349
Atria, 349
Atrophy, 461
Atropine, 545
Attitude, 30, 749
Audits, 155
Ausculatory gap, 309
Auscultation
  assessment by, 206–7, 216
  explanation of, 201
  pulse rate and, 300
Autoclaves, 117
Autocratic leaders, 721
Autonomic nervous system response, 326
Autonomy, 30
Autopsies
  explanation of, 707
  religious views of, 635, 708
Awareness
  states of, 643
  types of, 709
Axons, 185

B

Babinski reflex, 590
Back injury, 102–3, 103f
Back massage, 494–95, 494f
Bacteremia, 113
Bacteria, 112
Bacterial endocarditis, 350
Bactericidal, 253
Bactericidal agents, 117
Bacteriostatic agents, 117
Bag baths, 253–54
Bagging, 93, 120
Bag shampoos, 261
Ballard School, 8, 9t
Bandages, 229, 234, 234f
Bandura, Albert, 568
Barber, Margaret Fairless, 3
Barium, 440
Barium enema, 442
Barrack Hospital (Turkey), 4
Barton, Clara, 4–6, 6f
Basal metabolic rate (BMR), 292–93, 478

Medications. *See also specific medications*
  actions on body of, 502–3
  antidiarrheal, 445
  antiflatulent, 446
  blood pressure and, 305
  cathartic and laxative, 446–47, 446t
  culture and, 503, 645
  defecation and, 439, 440
  derived from pork, 635
  dry mouth from, 262
  effects of, 501–3, 502t
  to enhance sleep, 478
  explanation of, 500
  forms of, 500, 500t
  infection and, 115–16
  interactions between, 502
  names for, 500
  oxygenation and, 351
  for pain management, 328, 330–31, 334t–335t
  preoperative, 545
  preparation of, 527–30, 527f, 528f
  pulse rate and, 298
  respiratory rate and, 302–3, 302t
  sexual function and, 677, 678
  sleep and, 475
  standards for, 500–501
  urinary retention and, 407
  wound healing and, 225–26
Meditation, 331
Meiosis, 183, 183f
Mena, Juan de, 8
Menopause, 351
Menstruation, 668, 686f
Mental status impairment
  informed consent and, 26
  learning and, 570t
  pressure ulcers and, 237
  sexuality and, 679
  thermal tolerance and, 230
Meperidine hydrochloride (Demerol), 475, 545
Mercury-in-glass thermometers, 296
Metabolic acidosis, 387–88
Metabolic system
  immobility and, 462–63
  stress and, 686
Metabolism, 478
Metaphase, 182
Metered-dose inhaler (MDI), 520, 521
Methicillin-resistant *Staphylococcus aureus* (MRSA), 113, 114
Method of transmission, 114–15
Methylphenidate (Ritalin), 476
Metric system
  converting weights within, 508–9
  explanation of, 507–8
  volume equivalents in, 508t
Microminerals, 378

Micronutrients, 377–78
Microorganisms
  chain of infection and, 114
  common infectious, 115t
  control of environmental, 116–17
  explanation of, 112
  harmful actions of, 112–13
  helpful actions of, 112
  types of, 112
Micturition, 406. *See also* Urinary elimination
Middle-aged adults
  cognitive, moral, and spiritual development in, 603
  concept of death and, 706
  explanation of, 588t, 601
  health promotion in, 602t–603t, 603
  physical development in, 603
  psychosocial development in, 603, 659t
  reaction to loss by, 701–2
  sexuality and, 670t
  stress and, 687
Midsagittal, 193
Midstream voided specimen, 411
Milia, 202
Mineral oil, 265
Minerals, 378
Minimization, 692t
Minimum Data Set (MDS), 170
Minors, 26
Minor surgery, 543. *See also* Surgery
Misdemeanor, 23
Mitering, 270, 271f
Mitochondria, 182
Mitosis, 182–83, 182f
Mitotic event, 182
Mitral valve, 349
Mobility. *See also* Immobility
  discharge and, 465, 472
  joint, 459, 460t
  nursing care and, 464–69, 470t–471t, 472, 472f
  physical health and, 460
  safety and, 87
Mobility devices
  canes, 463, 464f
  crutches, 463–64, 464f
  walkers, 463, 464f
Monilia infection, 679
Monosaccharides, 376
Montgomery straps, 228, 228f
Moral concepts, 30–31
Moral development
  in adolescents, 600
  in children, 598
  explanation of, 587
  in infants, 591
  Kohlberg's stages of, 596t
  in middle-aged adults, 603

in older
in pres
in tod
in you
Morality.
Moral pr
Mormor
Morning
Moro re
Morphi
Motivat
  expla
  for l
  sleep
Motor
Mourr
Mouth
  asse
  nu
Mout
Mout
Mucc
Mult
Mul
Mul
Mus

Cimetidine (Taga
Circadian rhythm
Circular turns, 2
Circulating imm
Circulation impa
Circulatory syste
Circumcision, 67
Circumduction, 4
Civil law
  criminal law vs
  explanation of,
  false communic
  intentional tort
  loss of client pr
  unintentional tc
Civil War, 4, 5, 6,
Clean-catch specin
Cleaning baths, 25
Cleansing enemas,
Clean voided speci
Clear liquid diet, 3
Clean wounds, 223
Clear liquid diet
Client advocacy, 33
Client education. S
  for ambulation d
  areas for, 567
  for client with la
  cultural consider
    577, 578
  factors that inhib
  guidelines for, 57
  implementation c
  learning theories
  motivation and, 5
  nursing care and,
  overview of, 567
  process for, 571
Client-focused care,
Client records. *See al*
  ports
  confidentiality of,
  data on, 52, 53, 54
  diagnosing, planni
    and, 169–70,
  documentation me
  evaluation and, 17
  guidelines for recor
    158–59, 158f
  health history and,
  of nursing care, 169
  problem-oriented,
  purposes of, 155
  source-oriented, 16
Clients
  cultural assessment
  dying, 10
  explanation of, 9
  incorrectly identifyi

Basic life support (BLS). *See* Cardiopul-
    monary resuscitation (CPR)
Bataan March, 4
Baths
  cleaning, 253–54
  equipment for, 272
  function of, 254
  of infants and newborns, 256
  perineal-genital care and, 257, 274–75
  procedures for, 272–74
  therapeutic, 253
Battery, 22
Beard care, 261
Bed baths, 272–74
Bedboards, 467
Bedclothes, 547
Bed cradles, 270
Bed exit monitoring devices, 90, 91f, 106–7
Bedpans
  discomfort in use of, 463
  placing and removing, 445, 446f
  types of, 444, 445f
Beds
  changing occupied, 270, 271f, 286–87, 286f
  changing unoccupied, 284–86, 284f, 285f
  for clients with pressure ulcers, 232t
  explanation of, 268–70
  moving and turning clients in, 469, 484–88, 484f, 485f, 486f, 487f, 488f
  positions of, 269, 269t, 468, 470t–471t
  transferring clients from, 469, 488–91, 489f, 490f, 491f
Bedsores. *See* Pressure ulcers
Behavioral response, 326, 337–38
Behaviorism, 568, 579
Behavior modification, 577
Behaviors
  assessment of, 211
  associated with psychosocial development stages, 658t
Beliefs, 30
Beneficence, 30
Benzodiazepines, 478
Bereavement, 701
Beta blockers, 475
Bevel, of needles, 510, 511
Bicarbonate, 386–87, 386t
Bicuspid valve, 349
Biekerdyke, Mother, 4
Binders, 229, 234–35
Bioethics, 30
Biofeedback, 331
Bisexuals, 675
Bladder
  function of, 405–6, 406f
  palpitation of, 209, 209f, 217
  removal of, 418

Bladder irrigations
  explanation of, 418, 418f
  procedure for, 431–32
Bladder training programs, 414, 415
Blood
  alterations of, 350
  in feces, 443, 444
  functions of, 350
  handling of, 118f
  infections in, 115t
  nosocomial infections in, 113t
  in urine, 410t, 413
  viscosity of, 305
Bloodborne Pathogens Standards, 92
Blood chemistries, 352
Blood clots, 224, 350, 356
Blood coagulation studies, 231
Blood glucose, 381, 392
Blood pressure
  assessment sites for, 308
  determinants of, 304–5
  equipment for measuring, 306–8
  errors in assessing, 309, 310t
  explanation of, 304
  factors affecting, 305
  hypertension and, 305, 351
  hypotension and, 305–6
  methods for measuring, 308, 309f, 318–20
  nursing care and, 309–10
  nursing diagnosis for, 309
Blood pressure cuffs, 306, 306f, 307, 307f, 308f
Blood pressure equipment, 120
Blood tests, 352
Blood urea nitrogen (BUN), 408
Blood vessels, 349–50
Blood volume, 305, 350
Bloom, B., 568
Bloom's taxonomy, 733t
B lymphocytes, 116
Body alignment
  assessment of, 464–65, 464f
  explanation of, 459, 459f
  factors affecting, 460
  positioning client in good, 467
Body cavities, 193–94, 193f, 194f
Body fluids
  composition of, 384–85
  discharge considerations and, 391
  explanation of, 384, 385f
  nursing care and, 388–91
  regulation of, 385–86
Body image
  assessment of, 660
  assisting clients with disturbed, 662
  self-concept and, 657–58
  sexuality and, 673
Body language. *See* Nonverbal communica-
    tion

Body mass index (BMI), 379–80
Body mechanics
  back injury prevention and, 102–3, 102f
  explanation of, 101–2
  guidelines and principles related to, 104t
  lifting and, 103, 105
  for pivoting, 105
  for pushing or pulling, 105
Body movement, 459. *See also* Activity
  elements of normal, 459–60, 460t
  factors affecting, 460
Body odor, 205
Body planes, 193, 193f
Body pressure areas, 241f
Body surface area, 509
Body temperature. *See also* Thermometers
  alterations in, 293–95, 294f
  discharge considerations and, 298
  explanation of, 292–93, 292f, 293f
  factors affecting, 293
  measurement of, 295–98, 311–13
  nursing care and, 297–98
  pressure ulcers and, 237
  regulation of, 293
  scales for, 297
  sites for measuring, 295t
  sleep and, 475
Body weight, 379–80
Bones, 218
Bounding pulse, 300
Bowel diversion ostomies. *See* Fecal diversion
    ostomies
Bowel incontinence. *See* Fecal incontinence
Bowel movements. *See* Feces; Gastrointesti-
    nal elimination
Bowel training programs, 448
Bowleg, 202
Bowman's capsule, 405, 405f
Boyle, Joyceen, 631
Brachial site, 299, 299f, 299t
Braden Scale for Predicting Pressure Sore
    Risk, 237–38, 239f
Bradley, Ruby, 4
Bradycardia, 300
Bradypnea, 304, 348
Brand names for medications, 500. *See also*
    Medications; *specific medications*
Breast cancer screening, 672–73, 672f, 673f
Breast self-examination (BSE), 672–73,
    672f, 674
Breathing. *See* Respiration
Breathing exercises, 356, 356f, 551, 556
Breckinridge, Mary, 6–7, 7f
Brewster, Mary, 6
British Pharmacopoeia, 501
Bromhidrosis, 205
Bronchi, 345
Bronchial tree, 345
Bronchodilators, 520

Bubbling, 304
Buccal medicatio...
512, 512f
Buddhists, 635
Buffers, 386–87
Bulbourethral gla...
Burns, 21, 89

C

Caffeine, 407
Calcium, 386t
Calcium balance,...
Calculation questi...
Calculi, 462
Calculus, 407–8
Canada
aid at accident s...
categories of ass...
credentialing in,...
criminal categor...
nursing diagnosi...
Canada Food and D...
Canadian Narcotic...
Cancer screening, 6...
Candida, 671
Candidiasis, 672t
Canes
explanation of, 4...
teaching client to...
Cannula, 510
Caplets, 500t
Capsules, 500t
Carbohydrates, 376–
Carbon dioxide, 346
Cardiac arrest, 359
Cardiac monitoring,...
Cardiac muscle, 185
Cardiac output
explanation of, 30...
heart structure and...
Cardiac reserve, 461
Cardiopulmonary res...
94–95, 95f, 3...
Cardiovascular diseas...
gender and, 351
heartbeat and puls...
as surgical risk fact...
Cardiovascular system...
alterations in funct...
assessment of, 206,...
blood and, 350
blood vessels and, 3...
explanation of, 348...
heart and, 348–49
immobility and, 46...
nursing care and, 3...
Career building
continuing educatio...

Legal issues (continued)
related to death/dying, 706–7
restraints and, 95, 96
sexual harassment and, 29
student nurses and, 25
Leg exercises, 551, 555, 555f
Leininger, Madeleine, 46t–47t, 631
Leininger's Culture Care, Diversity, and Universality Theory, 46t–47t
Lesions, 205
Leukocytes, 115, 231
Level of consciousness (LOC)
assessment of, 211–12
explanation of, 204, 204t
postoperative, 547
Liability insurance, 25
Libel, 22
Libido, 671, 673. See also Sexuality
Licensed practical nurses (LPNs), 8. See also LPN/LVNs (Licensed practical nurses/licensed vocational nurses)
Licensed vocational nurses (LVNs), 8. See also LPN/LVNs (Licensed practical nurses/licensed vocational nurses)
Licensure
explanation of, 8, 23, 719
Health Insurance Portability and Accountability Act and, 720–21
nurse practice acts and, 719–20, 720t
standards of care and, 719
suspension or revocation of, 719
Lifestyle
safety and, 87
sleep and, 475
stimuli and, 645
Lifting, 103, 103f, 105
Light diet, 381
Linen handling, 118f, 120
Line of gravity, 459, 459f
Liniments, 500t
Lipid profiles, 377
Lipids, 377
Lipoproteins, 377
Liquid connective tissue, 184
Listening, active, 620, 623f
Liver disease, 543
Living will, 707
Local anesthesia, 546
Local infection, 113
Loeb Center for Nursing and Rehabilitation, 82
Long-term care documentation, 170, 172
Long-term care facilities
beds in, 269
environment in, 268–69
explanation of, 75–76
Long-term care plans, 63
Long-term goals, 60

Lordosis, 202, 464
Loss. See also Grief/grieving
cause of, 703
explanation of, 701
factors affecting response to, 701–3
nursing care for clients suffering from, 175, 703–5
Lotions, 500t
Lozenges, 500t
LPN/LVNs (Licensed practical nurses/licensed vocational nurses). See also Nurses; Nursing practice
credentialing of, 23
delegating and supervising opportunities for, 64, 65
nursing process role of, 51, 52 (See also Nursing process)
opportunities for, 11, 13
practice settings for, 11
practice standards for, 12
professional associations for, 11
responsibilities of, 43, 728
student organizations for, 11
Lungs
assessment of, 202, 203, 206
function of, 345–47
immobility and, 462
Lung scans, 353
Luteinizing hormone (LH), 191
Lymphatic system, 189, 189f
Lymphocytes, 116, 119
Lysosomes, 182

Maceration, 236, 414
Machismo, 632
Macrominerals, 378
Macronutrients, 376–77
Macrophages, 224
Magico-religious health beliefs, 631
Magnesium, 385, 386t
Major surgery, 543. See also Surgery
Male nurses, 7–8, 728
Malnutrition, 543
Malpractice
explanation of, 20, 21
protections against, 24, 25
Malpractice insurance, 25
Managed care, 80, 82
Marcella, 3
Marion Laboratories, 238
Martin Chuzzlewit (Dickens), 5
Masks, 118f, 120
Maslow, Abraham, 568
Maslow's hierarchy of needs
explanation of, 43, 62f
hospital admission and, 138

nursing...
teaching...
Massage, ...
Material S...
Mattresses...
explana...
types o...
Maturatio...
Meals, 3...
Measure...
Meatus,...
Medial,...
Medicai...
Medical...
Medica...
Medica...
Medica...
Medic...

Urinary diversions, 418–19, 419f
Urinary drainage devices, 414–15
Urinary elimination
assessment of, 217
bladder and, 405–6
client with abdominal injury and, 420–21
explanation of, 405, 406
factors affecting, 406–7, 407t
kidneys and, 405
maintaining normal, 413
measurement of, 409–11
nursing care and, 408–21
pathologic conditions affecting, 407–8, 409t
postoperative, 551–52
through life span, 407t
ureters and, 405
urethra and, 406
Urinary incontinence
explanation of, 409t
management of, 413–14
pressure ulcers and, 236
Urinary irrigations
explanation of, 418, 418f
procedure for, 431–32
Urinary pH, 412
Urinary retention
immobility and, 462–63
management of, 415
postoperative, 549t
Urinary stasis, 462
Urinary stones, 407–8
Urinary tract
discharge considerations and, 420
explanation of, 191, 191f, 405f, 406f
immobility and, 462–63
nursing care and, 408–20
structure and function of, 405–6
Urinary tract infections (UTIs)
catheter-associated, 415, 416
explanation of, 113t, 115t, 406, 413
postoperative, 549t
prevention of, 413, 420
Urine
altered production of, 408
characteristics of, 408, 410t, 412–13
color of, 407, 410t
explanation of, 385
residual, 411
retention of, 407
Urine ketone tests, 413
Urine output, 409–11
Urine specimens
clean-catch, 422–23
to evaluation oxygenation, 353
explanation of, 411–12, 411f, 412f
Urine tests, 412–13
Urinometer, 412, 412f, 413

Uterine tubes, 191
Uterus, 191

V

Vagina, 112, 191
Vaginal medications, 504t, 519, 537–38, 538f
Valium, 262
Valsalva maneuver, 440, 461
Values, 29–30
Van-comycin-resistant Enterococci (VRE), 113
Variance documentation, 166, 166t
Vascular response, 116
Vasocongestion, 675
Vasoconstriction, 229, 230
Vasodilation
explanation of, 236
from heat application, 229, 230
Vastus lateralis site, 517–18, 518f
Vegetarianism, 635
Veins, 350
Venous stasis, 358–59
Venous vasodilation, 461, 461f
Ventilation
explanation of, 269, 302, 345–46
immobility and, 462
Ventral, 192
Ventral cavity, 193
Ventricles, 349
Ventrogluteal site, 517, 517f
Venturi mask, 353
Veracity, 30–31
Verbal communication, 616, 618, 621, 633. See also Communication
Verbal response, 212
Vernix caseosa, 202, 589
Vertigo, 460
Veterans Administration (VA), 74
Vials
explanation of, 514, 514f
preparing medications from, 528–29, 528f
Vibration, 357
Vietnam War, 4, 5f
Violence, 690
Virulence, 112
Viruses, 112
Visceral pain, 325. See also Pain; Pain management
Visceral stimuli, 643
Visualization procedures
to evaluate urinary function, 408
to evaluation oxygenation, 353
for gastrointestinal tract, 442
Visually impaired clients, 650
Vital capacity, 462

Vital signs. See also specific vital signs
age variations in, 292t
assessment of, 204–5
blood pressure, 304–10, 318–20
body temperature, 292–98, 311–13
explanation of, 292, 309–10
postoperative, 547
preoperative monitoring of, 546
pulse, 298–301, 313–17
respirations, 302–4, 317–18
sample nurse's notes containing, 310
time to assess, 297
Vitamins, 377–78
Voiding, 406. See also Urinary elimination
Volume expanders, 390
Voluntary muscle, 185
Vomiting, 502t, 549t
Voting rights, 6
Voyeurism, 677
Vulva, 191

Wald, Lillian, 6, 6f
Walkers
explanation of, 463, 464f
teaching client to use, 465
Walking reflex, 590
War, 4, 5, 8
Waste, 92–93, 93
Water, 376
Water beds, 232t
Water-soluble vitamins, 378
Wedges, 232t
Weed, Lawrence, 160
Weight, 205
Wellness, 10
Wellness models, 41
Wet-to-damp technique, 226, 228t, 240
Wet-to-dry technique, 228t
Wet-to-wet technique, 228t
Wheeze, 206, 304
Wheezing, 502t
Whistle-blowing, 27
Whitman, Walt, 4
Women's health, 79
Women's movement, 6, 6f, 11, 79
Wong/Baker Faces Rating Scale, 336, 336f
Work samples, 742
World Health Organization (WHO), 328, 671
World War II, 4, 81
Wound dressings
application of gauze, 228t
explanation of, 226
hydrocolloid, 227–28, 227t, 245

postoperative assessment of, 547, 552

securing methods for, 228, 233, 234*f*

transparent, 226–27, 227*t,* 228*f,* 244–45

types of, 226*f,* 227*t*

Wounds. *See also* Pressure ulcers

bandages and binders for, 229, 234–35

cleaning, 226

cleaning sutured, 561–62

discharge considerations and, 236

drainage of, 224–25, 246–47

healing of, 223–24, 231–33

heat and cold applications for, 229–31, 229*t,* 230*f,* 235–36

irrigation and packing, 226, 233, 247–48

mechanical devices to reducing pressure on, 232*t*

nursing care and, 231–36

postoperative care of, 552–53, 561–62

postoperative problems with, 550*t*

specimens of, 231, 246–47

supporting and immobilizing, 228–29, 237, 238*f*

treated, 232

types of, 223, 223*t*

untreated, 231

Writing samples, 742

Written reports, 723

X-rays, 353, 442

Yeast infections, 671

Yom Kippur, 635

Young adults

cognitive, moral, and spiritual development in, 601

growth and development in, 588*t*

health promotion in, 601, 602*t*–603*t*

physical development in, 601

psychosocial development in, 601, 658*t*

reaction to loss by, 702

sexuality and, 669*t*

stress and, 687

Young Women's Christian Association (YWCA), 8

Zantac, 545

Z-track technique, 518

Zygote, 191

SINGLE PC LICENSE AGREEMENT AND LIMITED WARRANTY

READ THIS LICENSE CAREFULLY BEFORE OPENING THIS PACKAGE. BY OPENING THIS PACKAGE, YOU ARE AGREEING TO THE TERMS AND CONDITIONS OF THIS LICENSE. IF YOU DO NOT AGREE, DO NOT OPEN THE PACKAGE. PROMPTLY RETURN THE UNOPENED PACKAGE AND ALL ACCOMPANYING ITEMS TO THE PLACE YOU OBTAINED THEM. *THESE TERMS APPLY TO ALL LICENSED SOFTWARE ON THE DISK EXCEPT THAT THE TERMS FOR USE OF ANY SHAREWARE OR FREEWARE ON THE DISKETTES ARE AS SET FORTH IN THE ELECTRONIC LICENSE LOCATED ON THE DISK:*

1. GRANT OF LICENSE and OWNERSHIP: The enclosed computer programs and data ("Software") are licensed, not sold, to you by Pearson Education, Inc. ("We" or the "Company") and in consideration of your purchase or adoption of the accompanying Company textbooks and/or other materials, and your agreement to these terms. We reserve any rights not granted to you. You own only the disk(s) but we and/or our licensors own the Software itself. This license allows you to use and display your copy of the Software on a single computer (i.e., with a single CPU) at a single location for <u>academic</u> use only, so long as you comply with the terms of this Agreement. You may make one copy for back up, or transfer your copy to another CPU, provided that the Software is usable on only one computer

2. RESTRICTIONS: You may <u>not</u> transfer or distribute the Software or documentation to anyone else. Except for backup, you may <u>not</u> copy the documentation or the Software. You may <u>not</u> network the Software or otherwise use it on more than one computer or computer terminal at the same time. You may <u>not</u> reverse engineer, disassemble, decompile, modify, adapt, translate, or create derivative works based on the Software or the Documentation. You may be held legally responsible for any copying or copyright infringement which is caused by your
failure to abide by the terms of these restrictions.

3. TERMINATION: This license is effective until terminated. This license will terminate automatically without notice from the Company if you fail to comply with any provisions or limitations of this license. Upon termination, you shall destroy the Documentation and all copies of the Software. All provisions of this Agreement as to limitation and disclaimer of warranties, limitation of liability, remedies or damages, and our ownership
rights shall survive termination.

4. LIMITED WARRANTY AND DISCLAIMER OF WARRANTY: Company warrants that for a period of 60 days from the date you purchase this SOFTWARE (or purchase or adopt the accompanying textbook), the Software, when properly installed and used in accordance with the Documentation, will operate in substantial conformity with the description of the Software set forth in the Documentation, and that for a period of 30 days the disk(s) on which the Software is delivered shall be free from defects in materials and workmanship under normal use. The Company does not warrant that the Software will meet your requirements or that the operation of the Software will be uninterrupted or error-free. Your only remedy and the Company's only obligation under these limited warranties is, at the Company's option, return of the disk for a refund of any amounts paid for it by you or replacement of the disk. THIS LIMITED WARRANTY IS THE ONLY WARRANTY PROVIDED BY THE COMPANY AND ITS LICENSORS, AND THE COMPANY AND ITS LICENSORS DISCLAIM ALL OTHER WARRANTIES, EXPRESS OR IMPLIED, INCLUDING WITHOUT LIMITATION, THE IMPLIED WARRANTIES OF MERCHANTABILITY AND FITNESS FOR A PARTICULAR PURPOSE. THE COMPANY DOES NOT WARRANT, GUARANTEE OR MAKE ANY REPRESENTATION REGARDING THE ACCURACY, RELIABILITY, CURRENTNESS, USE, OR RESULTS OF USE, OF THE
SOFTWARE.

5. LIMITATION OF REMEDIES AND DAMAGES: IN NO EVENT, SHALL THE COMPANY OR ITS EMPLOYEES, AGENTS, LICENSORS, OR CONTRACTORS BE LIABLE FOR ANY INCIDENTAL, INDIRECT, SPECIAL, OR CONSEQUENTIAL DAMAGES ARISING OUT OF OR IN CONNECTION WITH THIS LICENSE OR THE SOFTWARE, INCLUDING FOR LOSS OF USE, LOSS OF DATA, LOSS OF INCOME OR PROFIT, OR OTHER LOSSES, SUSTAINED AS A RESULT OF INJURY TO ANY PERSON, OR LOSS OF OR DAMAGE TO PROPERTY, OR CLAIMS OF THIRD PARTIES, EVEN IF THE COMPANY OR AN AUTHORIZED REPRESENTATIVE OF THE COMPANY HAS BEEN ADVISED OF THE POSSIBILITY OF SUCH DAMAGES. IN NO EVENT SHALL THE LIABILITY OF THE COMPANY FOR DAMAGES WITH RESPECT TO THE SOFTWARE EXCEED THE AMOUNTS ACTUALLY PAID BY YOU, IF ANY, FOR THE SOFTWARE OR THE ACCOMPANYING TEXTBOOK. BECAUSE SOME JURISDICTIONS DO NOT ALLOW THE LIMITATION OF LIABILITY IN CERTAIN CIRCUMSTANCES, THE ABOVE LIMITATIONS MAY NOT
ALWAYS APPLY TO YOU.

6. GENERAL: THIS AGREEMENT SHALL BE CONSTRUED IN ACCORDANCE WITH THE LAWS OF THE UNITED STATES OF AMERICA AND THE STATE OF NEW YORK, APPLICABLE TO CONTRACTS MADE IN NEW YORK, AND SHALL BENEFIT THE COMPANY, ITS AFFILIATES AND ASSIGNEES. HIS AGREEMENT IS THE COMPLETE AND EXCLUSIVE STATEMENT OF THE AGREEMENT BETWEEN YOU AND THE COMPANY AND SUPERSEDES ALL PROPOSALS OR PRIOR AGREEMENTS, ORAL, OR WRITTEN, AND ANY OTHER COMMUNICATIONS BETWEEN YOU AND THE COMPANY OR ANY REPRESENTATIVE OF THE COMPANY RELATING TO THE SUBJECT MATTER OF THIS AGREEMENT. If you are a U.S. Government user, this Software is licensed with "restricted rights" as set forth in subparagraphs (a)-(d) of the Commercial Computer-Restricted Rights clause at FAR 52.227-19 or in subparagraphs (c)(1)(ii) of the Rights in Technical Data and Computer Software clause at DFARS 252.227-7013, and similar clauses, as applicable.

Should you have any questions concerning this agreement or if you wish to contact the Company for any reason, please contact in writing: Prentice-Hall, New Media Department, One Lake Street, Upper Saddle River, NJ 07458.